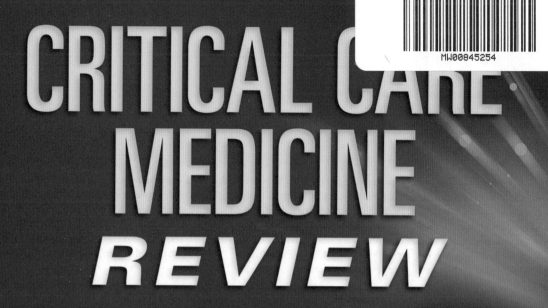

# CRITICAL CARE MEDICINE *REVIEW*

## 1000 QUESTIONS AND ANSWERS

**Abraham Sonny, MD, FASE**

Assistant Professor
Department of Anesthesia, Critical Care and Pain Medicine
Massachusetts General Hospital
Harvard Medical School, Boston, Massachusetts

**Edward A. Bittner, MD, PhD, MS.Ed, FCCM**

Associate Professor
Program Director, Critical Care Anesthesiology Fellowship
Department of Anesthesia, Critical Care and Pain Medicine
Massachusetts General Hospital
Harvard Medical School, Boston, Massachusetts

**Ryan J. Horvath, MD, PhD**

Instructor in Anesthesia
Department of Anesthesia, Critical Care and Pain Medicine
Massachusetts General Hospital
Harvard Medical School, Boston, Massachusetts

**Sheri M. Berg, MD**

Instructor in Anesthesia
Medical Director, Post Anesthesia Care Units
Department of Anesthesia, Critical Care and Pain Medicine
Massachusetts General Hospital
Harvard Medical School, Boston, Massachusetts

### ASSOCIATE EDITOR

**Hassan Farhan, MD**

Anesthesia Resident
Department of Anesthesia, Critical Care and Pain medicine
Massachusetts General Hospital
Harvard Medical School, Boston, Massachusetts.

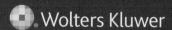

. Wolters Kluwer

Philadelphia • Baltimore • New York • London
Buenos Aires • Hong Kong • Sydney • Tokyo

*Acquisitions Editor:* Keith Donnellan
*Development Editor:* Ashley Fischer
*Editorial Coordinator:* Tim Rinehart
*Production Project Manager:* Kim Cox
*Design Coordinator:* Stephen Druding
*Manufacturing Coordinator:* Beth Welsh
*Prepress Vendor:* TNQ Technologies

9  8  7  6  5  4  3  2  1

Printed in China

**Library of Congress Cataloging-in-Publication Data**

ISBN-13: 978-1-975102-90-6

Cataloging in Publication data available on request from publisher.

shop.lww.com

# CRITICAL CARE MEDICINE
## REVIEW

# 1000
## QUESTIONS AND ANSWERS

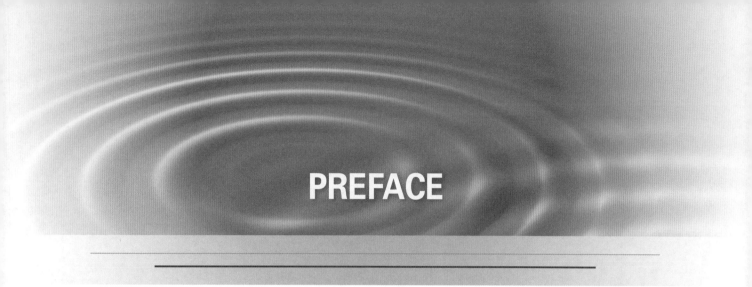

# PREFACE

This book was conceived as a result of feedback from our critical care fellows on the absence of a comprehensive question and answer book to learn from, during fellowship training. Subsequently, we compiled this book, over a span of one year, to bridge this gap in educational resource.

Our goal was to create a resource equipped to help all trainees in critical care, irrespective of their primary discipline. The content of this book was developed from keywords in critical care published by various boards, specifically American board of Anesthesiology, Internal Medicine, Neurology, and Surgery. The chapters were contributed by critical care fellows and junior faculty from various reputed institutions across the United States, working in conjunction with senior authors who are recognized experts in their discipline.

This book covers all topics pertinent to the practice of critical care in a question and answer format, divided into twelve section and 123 chapters. A large majority of the questions are clinically oriented with case scenarios, making it pertinent to your clinical practice. After each question, the readers are directed toward relevant references and resources, for additional reading on a certain topic. Furthermore, this book also provides a "grab bag" chapter which contains a random collection of questions from various common topics in critical care.

We hope this book can improve your knowledge in critical care medicine especially during fellowship training and also serve as reference guide in future.

Abraham Sonny, MD, FASE
Edward A. Bittner, MD, PhD, MS.Ed, FCCM
Ryan J. Horvath, MD, PhD
Sheri M. Berg, MD
Boston, Massachusetts

# CONTRIBUTORS

**Noor Abdalla, MD**
Resident
Lahey Hospital
Burlington, Massachusetts

**Fatima I. Adhi, MD**
Fellow Physician, Critical Care Medicine
Respiratory Institute
Cleveland Clinic
Cleveland, Ohio

**Avneep Aggarwal, MD**
Staff physician
Anesthesiology Institute
Center for Critical Care Medicine
Cleveland Clinic
Cleveland, Ohio

**Abdulaziz S. Almehlisi, MBBS**
Assistant Professor
Department of Emergency Medicine
King Saud University
Riyadh, Saudi Arabia

**Reem Almuqati, MD**
Critical care fellow
Department of Anesthesiology
Cleveland clinic foundation
Cleveland, Ohio

**John Andre, MD**
Chief of Skills and Simulation
Department of General Surgery
Loyola University Medical Center
Maywood, Illinois

**Daniel Austin, MD**
Resident
Department of Anesthesia & Perioperative Care
University of California
San Francisco, California

**Ji Sun Christina Baek, MD**
Department of Anesthesiology
University of California,
San Diego, California

**Theresa Barnes, MD, MPH**
Associate Professor
Department of Anesthesiology
Emory University
Atlanta, Georgia

**Sean M. Baskin, DO, MA**
Resident
Department of Anesthesiology and Perioperative
    Medicine
Penn State Milton S. Hershey Medical Center
Hershey, Pennsylvania

**DaMarcus Baymon, MD**
Resident
Department of Emergency Medicine
Massachusetts General Hospital - Harvard
Boston, Massachusetts

**Lisa M. Bebell, MD**
Instructor, Harvard Medical School
Assistant in Medicine, Massachusetts General
    Hospital
Infectious Diseases Unit
Boston, Massachusetts

**William J. Benedetto, MD**
Assistant Professor
Department of Anesthesia, Critical Care and Pain
    Medicine
Massachusetts General Hospital
Boston, Massachusetts

**Sheri M. Berg, MD**
Instructor in Anesthesia
Medical Director, Post Anesthesia Care Units
Department of Anesthesia, Critical Care and
    Pain Medicine
Massachusetts General Hospital
Harvard Medical School
Boston, Massachusetts

**Lorenzo Berra, MD**
Reginald Jenney Associate Professor of Anaesthesia
Harvard Medical School
Massachusetts General Hospital
Boston, Massachusetts

**Leah N. Bess, MD**
Resident
Department of Anesthesiology and Perioperative
    Medicine
Penn State University Milton S. Hershey Medical
    Center
Hershey, Pennsylvania

**Annie van Beuningen, MD**
Fellow in Cardiovascular Medicine
Department of Medicine
Massachusetts General Hospital
Boston, Massachusetts

**Somnath Bose, MD**
Instructor of Anesthesiology, Harvard Medical
    School
Department of Anesthesiology, Critical Care and
    Pain Medicine
Beth Israel Deaconess Medical Center
Boston, Massachusetts

**Jason K. Bowman, MD**
Chief Resident
Departments of Emergency Medicine
Massachusetts General Hospital
Brigham and Women's Hospital
Boston, Massachusetts

**Joanna Brenneman, MD**
Staff Anesthesiology & Critical Care Medicine
Cleveland Clinic Akron General
Akron, Ohio

**Edward A. Bittner, MD, PhD, MS.Ed, FCCM**
Associate Professor
Program Director, Critical Care Anesthesiology
    Fellowship
Department of Anesthesia, Critical Care and
    Pain Medicine
Massachusetts General Hospital
Harvard Medical School
Boston, Massachusetts

**Erika Lore Brinson, MD**
Assistant Clinical Professor of Anesthesia
Department of Anesthesia and Perioperative Care
University of California, San Francisco
San Francisco, California

**Lundy Campbell, MD**
Professor, Department of Anesthesiology
Chief, Division of Cardiothoracic Anesthesiology
University of California
San Francisco, California

**Marvin G. Chang, MD**
Faculty
Department of Anesthesia
Massachusetts General Hospital
Boston, Massachusetts

**Anoop Chhina, MD**
Anesthesiologist and Intensivist
Department of Anesthesiology
Henry Ford Hospital
Detroit, Michigan

**Christine Choi, MD**
Assistant Professor
Department of Anesthesiology
University of California, San Diego
San Diego, California

**Margaret R. Connolly, MD**
Resident
Department of Surgery
Massachusetts General Hospital
Boston, Massachusetts

**Jennifer Cottral, MD**
Clinical Fellow in Anaesthesia
Department of Anesthesia, Critical Care, and Pain
    Medicine
Massachusetts General Hospital
Boston, Massachusetts

**Phat Tan Dang, MD**
Anesthesiology Critical Care Fellow
Department of Anesthesiology
University of California, San Diego
La Jolla, California

**Christopher Dinh, MD**
Critical Care Fellow
Department of Anesthesiology
University of California, San Diego
San Diego, California

**David M. Dudzinski, MD, JD**
Director, Cardiac Intensive Care Unit
Massachusetts General Hospital
Assistant Professor
Harvard Medical School
Boston, Massachusetts

**Brett Elo, DO**
Department of Anesthesia and Critical Care
Cleveland Clinic
Cleveland, Ohio

**Faith Natalie Factora, MD**
Medical Director
Surgical Intensive Care Unit
Cleveland Clinic
Cleveland, Ohio

**Peter Fagenholz, MD**
Assistant Professor of Surgery
Harvard Medical School
Attending Surgeon
Division of Trauma, Emergency Surgery, and
    Critical Care
Department of Surgery
Massachusetts General Hospital
Boston, Massachusetts

**Hassan Farhan, MD**
Anesthesia Resident
Department of Anesthesia, Critical Care and
    Pain medicine
Massachusetts General Hospital
Harvard Medical School
Boston, Massachusetts

**Raffaele Di Fenza, MD**
Resident
School of Anesthesia, Critical Care and
    Pain Medicine
University of Milan-Bicocca
Milan, Italy

**Rachel C. Frank, MD**
Cardiovascular Medicine Fellow
Division of Cardiology
Massachusetts General Hospital
Boston, Massachusetts

**Kevin E. Galicia, MD, MA**
Resident
Department of General Surgery
Loyola University Medical Center
Maywood, Illinois

**Mariya Geube, MD, FASE**
Assistant Professor
Cleveland Clinic Lerner College of Medicine
Department of Cardiothoracic Anesthesiology
Cleveland Clinic Foundation
Cleveland, Ohio

**Jeffrey Gotts, MD, PhD**
Assistant Professor
Department of Medicine
University of California San Francisco
San Francisco, California

**Ngoc-Tram Ha, MD**
Pulmonary and Critical Care Fellow
Department of Pulmonary and Critical Care
    Medicine
Geisinger Medical Center
Danville, Pennsylvania

**Dusan Hanidziar, MD, PhD**
Instructor in Anesthesia
Department of Anesthesia
Critical Care and Pain Medicine
Massachusetts General Hospital
Boston, Massachusetts

**Charles Corey Hardin, MD, PhD**
Assistant Professor of Medicine
Division of Pulmonary and Critical Care
Massachusetts General Hospital
Boston, Massachusetts

**Qasim AlHassan, MBBS**
Anesthesiology Critical Care Fellow
Department of Anesthesiology
Cleveland Clinic Foundation
Cleveland, Ohio

**Kathryn A. Hibbert, MD**
Instructor in Medicine
Director, Medical ICU
Massachusetts General Hospital
Harvard Medical School
Boston, Massachusetts

**Kristen Holler, DO**
Anesthesiology Institute
The Cleveland Clinic Foundation
Cleveland, Ohio

**Ryan J. Horvath, MD, PhD**
Instructor in Anesthesia
Department of Anesthesia, Critical Care and
    Pain Medicine
Massachusetts General Hospital
Harvard Medical School
Boston, Massachusetts

**Steven Hur, MD**
Fellow
Department of Anesthesia & Perioperative Care
University of California, San Francisco
San Francisco, California

**John O. Hwabejire, MD, MPH**
Clinical Fellow in Trauma, Acute Care Surgery, and
   Surgical Critical Care
Massachusetts General Hospital and Harvard
   Medical School
Boston, Massachusetts

**Saef Izzy, MD**
Neurocritical Care faculty
Divisions of Stroke, Cerebrovascular, and
   Critical Care Neurology
Assistant Professor in Neurology
Department of Neurology
Brigham and Women's hospital
Harvard Medical School
Boston, Massachusetts

**Ceena N. Jacob, MD**
Internal Medicine
Cleveland Clinic Foundation
Cleveland, Ohio

**Todd A. Jaffe, MD**
Emergency Medicine Resident
Harvard Affiliated Emergency Medicine Residency
Brigham and Women's/Massachusetts General
   Hospital
Boston, Massachusetts

**Paul S. Jansson, MD, MS**
Critical Care Medicine Fellow
Brigham and Women's Hospital
Harvard Medical School
Boston, Massachusetts

**Teny M. John, MD**
Assistant Professor
Department of Infectious Disease, Infection Control
   & Employee Health
The University of Texas MD Anderson Cancer
   Center
Houston, Texas

**Sonia John, MD**
Critical Care Fellow
Department of Anesthesiology
Massachusetts General Hospital
Boston, Massachusetts

**Sneha Kannan, MD**
Resident, Department of Medicine
Massachusetts General Hospital
Boston, Massachusetts

**Kunal Karamchandani, MD, FCCP**
Associate Professor
Department of Anesthesiology and Perioperative
   Medicine
Penn State Health Milton S. Hershey Medical Center
Hershey, Pennsylvania

**Riaz M. Karukappadath, MD**
Assistant Professor
Department of Anesthesiology and Critical Care
University of Alabama at Birmingham
Birmingham, Alabama

**Sandeep Khanna, MD**
Assistant Professor
Cleveland Clinic Lerner College of Medicine
Staff, Department of General Anesthesiology,
   Department of Outcomes Research
Cleveland Clinic Foundation, Ohio

**Mina Khorashadi, MD**
Department of Anesthesia and Perioperative Care
University of California San Francisco
San Francisco, California

**Thomas J. Krall, MD**
Assistant Professor
Department of Anesthesia and Perioperative Care
University of California - San Francisco
San Francisco, California

**Nitin Das Kunnathu Puthanveedu, MD**
Fellow Infectious Disease
Cleveland clinic
Cleveland, Ohio

**Jean Kwo, MD**
Assistant Professor
Department of Anesthesia, Critical Care, and
   Pain Medicine
Massachusetts General Hospital
Boston, Massachusetts

**Yvonne Lai, MD**
Clinical Instructor
Associate Residency Program Director
Department of Anesthesia, Critical Care, and Pain
Management Massachusetts General Hospital
Boston, Massachusetts

**Jarone Lee, MD, MPH, FCCM**
Associate Professor
Harvard Medical School
Boston, Massachusetts

**Nathan M. Lee, MD**
Assistant Professor
Department of Anesthesia and Critical Care
University of Chicago Medical Center
Chicago, Illinois

**Brian P. Lemkuil, MD**
Associate Professor
Department of Anesthesiology
University of California
San Diego, California

**David P. Lerner, MD**
Assistant Professor
Department of Neurology
Lahey Hospital and Medical Center
Burlington, Massachusetts

**Casey McBride Luckhurst, MD**
Surgical Critical Care Fellow
Massachusetts General Hospital
Boston, Massachusetts

**Jason H. Maley, MD**
Fellow
Pulmonary and Critical Care Medicine
Massachusetts General Hospital
Boston, Massachusetts

**Francisco Jesús Marco Canosa, MD**
Fellow
Infectious Disease Department
Cleveland Clinic Foundation
Cleveland, Ohio

**Maram Marouki, MD**
Critical Care Anesthesia Fellow
Anesthesia Institute
Cleveland Clinic Foundation
Cleveland, Ohio

**Lydia R. Maurer, MD**
General Surgery Resident
Department of Surgery
Massachusetts General Hospital
Boston, Massachusetts

**Zeb McMillan, MD**
Associate Professor
Department of Anesthesiology
Division of Critical Care
University of California San Diego
San Diego, California

**Jenna McNeill, MD**
Pulmonary and Critical Care Fellow
Department of Pulmonary and Critical Care
Massachusetts General Hospital
Boston, Massachusetts

**April E. Mendoza, MD, MPH**
Instructor
Department of Surgery
Massachusetts General Hospital
Boston, Massachusetts

**Nino Mihatov, MD**
Fellow in Cardiovascular Medicine
Chief Medical Resident
Massachusetts General Hospital
Boston, Massachusetts

**Yuk Ming Liu, MD, MPH**
Assistant Professor
Department of Surgery
Loyola University Medical Center
Maywood, Illinois

**Anushirvan Minokadeh, MD**
Professor
Department of Anesthesiology
UC San Diego Health
San Diego, California

**Ilan Mizrahi, MD**
Instructor of Anesthesia
Department of Anesthesia, Critical Care, and
    Pain Medicine
Massachusetts General Hospital
Boston, Massachusetts

**Christoph G. S. Nabzdyk, MD, MEd**
Cardiothoracic and Critical Care Anesthesia Fellow
Department of Anesthesia, Critical Care and Pain
    Medicine
Massachusetts General Hospital
Boston, Massachusetts

**Revati Nafday, MD**
Adult Cardiothoracic Anesthesiology Fellow
Department of Anesthesia and Perioperative Care
University of California, San Francisco
San Francisco, California

**Alexander Nagrebetsky, MD, MSc**
Assistant Professor
Department of Anesthesia, Critical Care and
    Pain Medicine
Massachusetts General Hospital, Harvard Medical
    School
Boston, Massachusetts

**Alan S. Nova, DO**
Neurocritical Care Fellow
Department of Neurosciences
University of California San Diego
La Jolla, California

**Nandini C. Palaniappa, MD**
Assistant Professor
Department of Anesthesia and Perioperative Care
University of California, San Francisco
San Francisco, California

**Riccardo Pinciroli, MD**
Assistant Professor of Anesthesia
University of Milan-Bicocca, School of Medicine and
    Surgery
Anesthesiologist and Intensivist
Department of Anesthesia and Critical Care
Niguarda Hospital
Milan, Italy

**Alexandra Plichta, MD**
Critical Care Fellow
Department of Anesthesia, Critical Care, and
    Pain Medicine
Massachusetts General Hospital
Boston, Massachusetts

**Kenneth Potter, MD**
Assistant Professor
Department of Anesthesiology
Virginia Commonwealth University Health System
Richmond, Virginia

**Irfan Qureshi, MD, MS**
Clinical instructor Trauma Surgery
Department of Surgery
Colorado Plains Medical Center
Morgan, Colorado

**Jeremy T. Rainey, DO**
Fellow
Center for Critical Care Medicine Anesthesiology
    Institute
Cleveland Clinic
Cleveland, Ohio

**Phillip Ramirez, MD**
Anesthesia Institute
Cleveland Clinic Foundation
Cleveland, Ohio

**Kimberly S. Robbins, MD**
Associate Clinical Professor
Department of Anesthesiology and Critical Care
UC San Diego Medical Center
La Jolla, California

**Martin G. Rosenthal, MD**
Instructor in Surgery
Department of Trauma, Emergency Surgery, Surgical
    Critical Care
Massachusetts General Hospital
Boston, Massachusetts

**Galen Royce-Nagel, MD**
Department of Anesthesia, Critical Care, and
    Pain Medicine
Massachusetts General Hospital
Boston, Massachusetts

**Ofer Sadan, MD, PhD**
Department of Neurology and Neurosugery
Division of Neurocritical Care
Emory University Hospital
Atlanta, Georgia

**Debdoot Saha, MD**
Fellow
Critical Care Medicine
Geisinger Medical Center
Danville, Pennsylvania

**Ulrich Schmidt, MD, PhD, MBA**
Vice Chair Critical Care Medicine
Clinical Professor of Anesthesiology
University of California San Diego
San Diego, California

**Milad Sharifpour, MD, MS**
Assistant Professor
Department of Anesthesiology and Critical Care
    Medicine
Emory University Hospital
Atlanta, Georgia

**Archit Sharma, MD, MBA**
Fellowship Director, Critical Care Fellowship
Department of Anesthesiology
University of Iowa Carver College of Medicine
Iowa City, Iowa

**Hasan Khalid Siddiqi, MD**
Fellow
Division of Cardiovascular Medicine
Brigham and Women's Hospital
Boston, Massachusetts

**Wendy Smith, MD**
Assistant Clinical Professor
Department of Anesthesia & Perioperative Care
University of California at San Francisco
San Francisco, California

**Abraham Sonny, MD, FASE**
Assistant Professor
Department of Anesthesia, Critical Care and
    Pain Medicine
Massachusetts General Hospital
Harvard Medical School
Boston, Massachusetts

**Jamie Sparling, MD**
Associate in Anesthesia
Department of Anesthesia, Critical Care and
    Pain Medicine
Boston, Massachusetts

**Roshni Sreedharan, MD**
Program Director, Anesthesiology Critical Care
    Medicine Fellowship
Assistant Professor of Anesthesiology, CCLCM
Faculty, Center for Excellence in Healthcare
    Communication
Department of General Anesthesiology
Anesthesiology Institute/Center for Critical Care
    Medicine
Cleveland Clinic
Cleveland, Ohio
Chair, In-training section of the SCCM

**Rachel Steinhorn, MD**
Resident physician
Massachusetts General Hospital
Boston, Massachusetts

**Alex T. Suginaka, DO**
Fellow in Critical Care Medicine
Department of Anesthesiology
University of Iowa Hospitals & Clinics
Iowa City, Iowa

**Jaya Prakash Sugunaraj, MD**
Assistant Professor
Department of Pulmonary & Critical Care
Geisinger
Danville, Pennsylvania

**Kristina Sullivan, MD**
Professor
Department of Anesthesia and Perioperative Care
University of California, San Francisco
San Francisco, California

**Madiha Syed, MD**
Clinical Assistant Professor
Anesthesiology Institute and Center for Critical Care
Cleveland Clinic Foundation
Cleveland, Ohio

**Maryam Bita Tabrizi, MD, FACS**
Clinical Instructor Harvard University
Department of Surgery
Massachusetts General Hospital
Boston, Massachusetts

**Kevin C. Thornton, MD**
Clinical Professor
Department of Anesthesia and Perioperative Care
University of California San Francisco
San Francisco, California

**Minh Hai Tran, MBBS**
Assistant Clinical Professor
Department of Anesthesiology
University of California San Diego
San Diego, California

**William J. Trudo, MD**
Resident Physician
Department of Anesthesiology
Emory School of Medicine
Atlanta, Georgia

**Aaron C. Tyagi, MD**
Emergency Medicine Critical Care Fellow
Department of Anesthesia
University of Iowa Hospitals and Clinics

**Bharathram Vasudevan, MBBS, MD**
Critical care fellow
Department of Anesthesiology
University of Iowa Hospitals and Clinics
Iowa City, Iowa

**Anand Venkatraman, MD**
Resident
Department of Neurology
Massachussets General Hospital/Brigham and
    Women's Hospital/Harvard Medical School
Boston, Massachusetts

**Brett J. Wakefield, MD**
Critical Care Medicine Fellow
Department of Anesthesiology
Washington University - Barnes Jewish Hospital
St Louis, Missouri

**Anureet K. Walia, MD**
Clinical Assistant Professor
Department of Anesthesiology
Department of Psychiatry
University of Iowa Carver College of Medicine
Iowa city, Iowa

**Daniel P. Walsh, MD**
Instructor in Anesthesia
Beth Israel Deaconess Medical Center
Harvard Medical School
Boston, Massachusetts

**Sarah Welch, PharmD, BCCCP**
Surgical Intensive Care Pharmacy Specialist
Department of Pharmacy
Cleveland Clinic
Cleveland, Ohio

**Jeanine P. Wiener-Kronish, MD**
Henry Isaiah Dorr Professor of Research and
    Teaching in Anaesthetics and Anaesthesia
Department of Anesthesia, Critical Care and Pain
    Medicine
Harvard Medical School
Anesthetist-in-Chief
Massachusetts General Hospital
Boston, Massachusetts

**Dario Winterton, MD**
School of Anesthesia Critical Care and Pain
    Medicine
University of Milan-Bicocca
Milano, Italy

**Amanda S. Xi, MD, MSE**
Anesthesia Critical Care Fellow
Department of Anesthesia, Critical Care and Pain
    Medicine
Massachusetts General Hospital
Boston, Massachusetts

**Howard Zee, MD**
Resident
Department of Anesthesia, Critical Care and Pain
    Medicine
Massachusetts General Hospital
Boston, Massachusetts

# TABLE OF CONTENTS

# NEUROLOGIC
# DISORDERS

# 1

# BRAIN DEATH AND DEGENERATIVE DISEASES

David P. Lerner, Anand Venkatraman, and Saef Izzy

1. An 84-year-old man with coronary artery disease and atrial fibrillation had a ST-segment elevation myocardial infarction that was complicated by a ventricular fibrillation cardiac arrest with 45 minutes of pulselessness. His initial management included evaluation in the cardiac catheterization lab with placement of a bare metal stent into the right coronary artery. He underwent 24 hours of cooling post cardiac arrest, but following this he has had limited neurologic recovery. Post arrest day 6, neurology is consulted. Which of the following is MOST correct?

   A. The most accurate prognostic test for poor neurologic outcome is electroencephalography.
   B. If there are no corneal responses 6 days post cardiac arrest, there is no anticipated neurologic recovery.
   C. Neuron-specific enolase is not affected by cooling and can be used for prognosis at 6 days post cardiac arrest.
   D. A magnetic resonance imaging (MRI) can assist with prognosis, and the most commonly affected area of the brain is the cortical region.

2. A 54-year-old woman is admitted to the intensive care unit (ICU) with a subarachnoid hemorrhage due to a left middle cerebral artery aneurysm rupture. Early external ventricular drain was placed because of a poor neurological examination. Over the course of 7 days, there have been ongoing issues with refractory elevated intracranial pressure and poor neurologic examination, progressing to no cranial nerve responses. Her examination is as follows: pupils 5 mm and nonreactive, absent oculocephalic reflexes, absent corneal reflexes, absence of facial grimace, absent gag, and absent cough. The only evoked motor response is minimal triple flexion in the bilateral legs. An apnea test was completed and there were no spontaneous respirations with an increase in $pCO_2$ 20 mm Hg more than baseline. Which of the following is MOST true?

   A. Because of the motor response present, the patient does not meet criteria for brain death.
   B. An ancillary test (EEG, cerebral angiogram, nuclear scan) should be completed to diagnose brain death.
   C. We need to repeat the apnea test.
   D. The current examination is consistent with brain death.

3. A 28-year-old previously healthy male is admitted to the ICU with altered mental status and hypoxic respiratory failure following a traumatic brain injury. There is limited history of his actual injury, but the night before his admission, he was intoxicated with friends when he got in an altercation and was hit on left side of his head and did have a brief loss of consciousness. His friends took him home, and at that time he was confused, complaining of a headache but was still talking and walking. He went to bed and he was checked on 10 hours later and was unresponsive. Emergency medical services (EMS) was called, and on arrival he was unresponsive with fixed, dilated pupils and no movements to painful stimulation and was intubated without sedation or paralytic. A head computed tomography (CT) was completed on arrival to the emergency department and demonstrated a 1.4 cm left-sided holocephalic subdural with 1.2 cm of left-to-right midline shift including uncal herniation and midbrain compression. His examination demonstrates lack of brain stem responses, no spontaneous breathing, and no movement to painful stimulation. An apnea test was attempted to evaluate for brain death but was unable to be completed because of hemodynamic instability. A whole brain positron emission tomography (PET) scan was completed and showed no activity in the brain stem and cortex. What is the MOST correct statement regarding the patient?

   A. The patient does not meet brain death criteria because the ancillary study does not support the diagnosis of brain death.
   B. The patient does not meet brain death criteria because he was unable to complete an apnea test.
   C. The patient does meet brain death criteria because his clinical examination is consistent with this and did not need an ancillary study.
   D. The patient does meet brain death criteria because his clinical examination is consistent with this and the ancillary study supports this diagnosis.

4. A 58-year-old woman with amyotrophic lateral sclerosis (ALS) presents to the emergency department complaining of increased weakness and difficulty with feeding herself. Her daughter inquires if there are any interventions which have been proven to increase life expectancy in ALS patients. Which of these is the MOST appropriate answer?

   A. Amantadine
   B. Noninvasive ventilation
   C. Colostomy
   D. Prophylactic antibiotics
   E. Indwelling nasogastric tube

5. A 74-year-old man with hypertension, coronary artery disease, and Parkinson disease is admitted to the ICU for management of pneumonia. He is intubated and started on broad-spectrum antibiotics. Six days after admission, he is found to have worsening fever, rigidity, and is no longer following commands. What is the MOST likely etiology for his condition?

   A. Status epilepticus
   B. Meningitis
   C. Serotonin syndrome
   D. Neuroleptic malignant syndrome (NMS)
   E. Infective endocarditis

# Chapter 1 ▪ Answers

1. Correct Answer: D

**Rationale:**
The extent of brain injury is the key factor for prognostication after cardiac arrest. Clinical examination has been the staple of prognosis—absent pupillary reflexes, absent corneal reflexes, motor response of extensor posturing, or no movement. These findings have come into question in the era of therapeutic cooling. Most importantly, absence of corneal reflexes does not necessarily portent a poor prognosis. Although electroencephalography is for the detection of seizures, the prognostication value has not been validated. Somatosensory evoked potentials (SSEPs) have been studied and the largest study evaluated 407 patients with cardiac arrest, and of the patients with bilaterally absent cortical sensory responses, all had poor neurologic outcome. Pertinent biomarkers include neuron-specific enolase, which was studied in the same SSEP study and levels higher than 33 µg/L predicting a poor outcome, but this study was performed before cooling. Hypothermia can attenuate release of neuron-specific enolase, and there are reports

of good outcome with levels greater than 100 µg/L. Although there are limitations to imaging, many use MRI with most useful imaging coming 3 to 5 days post arrest. Common findings are diffuse cortical diffusion restriction and changes in the basal ganglia.

Consideration of Evaluation for Prognosis after Cardiac Arrest

| 0-24 HOURS | 24-48 HOURS | 48-72 HOURS (POSTARREST OR POST REWARMING) | 3-5 DAYS (POSTARREST OR POST REWARMING) |
|---|---|---|---|
| • Clinical examination | • Clinical examination | • Clinical examination | • Clinical examination |
| • Continuous EEG | • Continuous EEG | • SSEP | • EEG (if indicated) |
| | • Consider NSE | • CT | • MRI |
| | | • EEG (if indicated) | |
| | | • Consider NSE | |

*CT, computed tomography; EEG, electroencephalography; MRI, magnetic resonance imaging; NSE, neuro-specific enolase; SSEP, somatosensory evoked potential.*
*Adopted from Greer DM. Cardiac arrest and postanoxic encephalopathy. Continuum. 2015;21:1384-1396.*

References

1. Wijdicks EF, Hijdra A, Young GB, et al. Practice parameter: prediction of outcome in comatose survivors after cardiopulmonary resuscitation (an evidence-based review): report of the Quality Standards Subcommittee of the American Academy of Neurology. *Neurology*. 2006;67:203-210.
2. Booth CM, Boone RH, Tomlinson G, et el. Is this patient dead, vegetative, or severely neurologically impaired? Assessing outcome for comatose survivors of cardiac arrest. *JAMA*. 2004;291:870-879.
3. Sandroni C, Cavallaro F, Callaway CW, et al. Predictors of poor neurological outcome in adult comatose survivors of cardiac arrest: a systematic review and meta-analysis. Part 1: patients not treated with therapeutic hypothermia. *Resuscitation*. 2013;84:1310-1323.

**2.** Correct Answer: D

**Rationale:**
The clinical findings necessary to confirm irreversible cessation of all functions of the entire brain, including the brain stem: coma, absence of brain stem reflexes, and apnea. The above patient does demonstrate all three of these criteria consistent with brain death. There are multiple reported reflexive movements that can be seen in patients with the diagnosis of brain death. Patient's apnea test is consistent with brain death criteria, which is based on increase $pCO_2$ >60 mm Hg or 20 mm Hg more than baseline. Single apnea test is required. No ancillary tests are required if the full clinical examination is consistent with brain death. In some institutions, two assessments of brain stem reflexes are required before declaring brain death.

References

1. Wijdicks EF, Varelas PN, Gronseth GS, et al. Evidence-based guideline update: determining brain death in adults. *Neurology*. 2010;74:1911-1918.
2. Han SG, Kim GM, Lee KH, et al. Reflex movements in patients with brain death: a prospecitve study in a tertiary medical center. *J Korean Med Sci*. 2006;21:588-590.

**3.** Correct Answer: D

**Rationale:**
The diagnosis of brain death is primarily clinical. However, ancillary tests are performed when the clinical criteria cannot be applied reliably. Irreversible coma that is explained by neuroimaging, lack of other etiology that could explain brain death (CNS-depressant drugs, paralytics, electrolyte abnormalities, profound hypothermia, hypotension), and clinical examination are all criteria required to make the diagnosis. The diagnosis of brain death can be challenging in cases when there is unreliable clinical examination or it is not possible to perform apnea test, for which ancillary tests should be performed. In this patient's case, apnea test was not completed because of hemodynamic instability for which ancillary test is required. There are several ancillary tests including EEG, cerebral angiography, nuclear scan, transcranial Dopplers, CT angiography, and magnetic resonance angiography (MRA). The ideal ancillary test is one with no confounding effects from sedatives or metabolic disturbances and preferable with no false positives. Evaluating cerebral perfusion with four-vessel cerebral angiography and nuclear scan of blood flow is commonly utilized. However, CT angiography and MRA may soon be found to be equally suitable.

### References

1. Wijdisks EF, Varelas PN, Gronseth GS, et al. Evidence-based guideline update: determining brain death in adults. *Neurology*. 2010;74:1911-1918.
2. Karantanas AH, Hadjigeorgiou GM, Paterakis K, et al. Contribution of MRI and MR angiography in early diagnosis of brain death. *Eur Radiol*. 2002;12:2710-2716.
3. Saposnik G, Maurino J, Bueri J. Movements in brain death. *Eur J Neurol*. 2001;8:209-213.
4. Mandel S, Arenas A, Scasta D. Spinal automatism in cerebral death. *N Engl J Med*. 1982;307:501.

---

**4.** Correct Answer: B

**Rationale:**

Patients with ALS have progressive degeneration of both upper and lower motor neurons causing weakness, difficulty swallowing, and respiratory insufficiency. Although many different approaches have been tried to manage these patients, there are only a few which have shown benefits in increasing life expectancy. Noninvasive ventilation, specifically with optimized bilevel positive airway pressure (BiPAP) protocols, helps to avoid hypercarbia, secondary to diaphragm and respiratory muscle weakness. Other interventions include riluzole, a medication that is thought to work on the neuronal level and shown to increase survival by few months and delay the onset of tracheostomy and ventilator dependence in selected ALS patients. Amantadine is used to promote alertness in patients with neurological injury; however, it has not been shown to be of benefit in ALS. Although patients with ALS often get gastrostomy tubes for safer feeding, colostomy and indwelling nasogastric tubes have not been shown to increase life expectancy. Prophylactic antibiotics are not recommended for ALS as there is no immune suppression.

### References

1. *Amyotrophic Lateral Sclerosis (ALS) Fact Sheet*. 2019. Available at https://www.ninds.nih.gov/Disorders/Patient-Caregiver-Education/Fact-Sheets/Amyotrophic-Lateral-Sclerosis-ALS-Fact-Sheet. Retrieved January 24, 2019.
2. Karam CY, Paganoni S, Joyce N, et al. Palliative care issues in amyotrophic lateral sclerosis: an evidenced-based review. *Am J Hosp Palliat Care*. 2016;33(1):84-92.
3. Hardiman O, Al-Chalabi A, Chio A, et al. Amyotrophic lateral sclerosis. *Nat Rev Dis Primers*. 2017;3:17071.

---

**5.** Correct Answer: D

**Rationale:**

NMS is an uncommon but often life-threatening illness characterized by fever, rigidity, obtundation, and autonomic instability. Elevated serum creatine kinase levels can also be seen. Though the pathogenesis is not well understood, it is thought to be related to a sudden decrease in dopaminergic signaling, which may be caused by stopping dopaminergic drugs such as levodopa as well as the use of neuroleptics. It is commonly confused with serotonin syndrome, which is a much more rapidly developing condition caused by excess serotonin signaling. This patient is unlikely to have status epilepticus or stroke, as that is unlikely to cause worsening fevers with rigidity. Infective endocarditis would present with fevers and potentially with neurological deficits if it leads to septic emboli to the brain; however, rigidity, obtundation, and autonomic instability are not typical for infective endocarditis.

### References

1. Hashimoto T, Tokuda T, Hanyu N, et al. Withdrawal of levodopa and other risk factors for malignant syndrome in Parkinson's disease. *Parkinsonism Relat Disord*. 2003;9:25-30.
2. Guzé BH, Baxter LR. Neuroleptic malignant syndrome. *N Engl J Med*. 1985;313(3):163-166.

# 2

# CEREBROVASCULAR DISEASES

David P. Lerner and Saef Izzy

**1.** A 49-year-old man with no past medical history is admitted to the medicine service for 2 weeks of intermittent night sweats, myalgia, and progressive headache. Other than febrile, his vital signs are normal at the time of admission. His neurologic examination at the time of admission is normal, and basic laboratory workup is unrevealing. A lumbar puncture is performed with a normal opening pressure, pleocytosis with 41 white blood cells/microL (94% polymorphonuclear cells), 5 red blood cells/microL, glucose 58 mg/dL, and protein 53 mg/dL. There was concern for potential infectious meningitis, so vancomycin, ceftriaxone, and acyclovir were started. One day following the lumbar puncture, the patient had acute onset of marked expressive aphasia and right facial weakness. A head computed tomography (CT) was completed and demonstrated in the figure that follows.

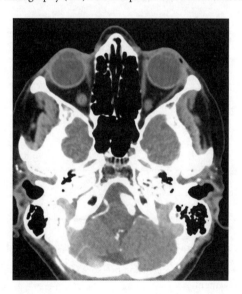

Additional workup was completed to determine the etiology of his stroke, and he was found to have a mobile target on the anterior leaflet of the mitral valve, concerning for endocarditis (shown in the figure that follows), and the mitral valve has severe mitral valve regurgitation.

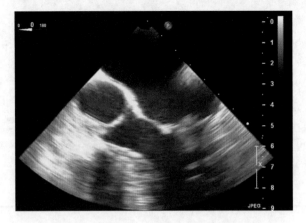

What is the next best step in management of the patient's possible endocarditis?

**A.** The patient should undergo urgent (within 5 days) mitral valve replacement.
**B.** The patient should undergo urgent (within 5 days) mitral valve repair.
**C.** The patient should undergo delayed (~4 weeks) mitral valve replacement.
**D.** The patient should undergo delayed (~4 weeks) mitral vale repair.
**E.** Only antibiotics therapy is needed, and current antibiotics should remain the same.

2. A 53-year-old woman is postbleed day 8 from a subarachnoid hemorrhage (SAH) from a, now secured, right middle cerebral artery (MCA) aneurysm. Since admission, the patient has been closely watched and the data from her external ventricular drain (EVD), brain tissue oxygenation monitor, and microdialysis catheter are all monitored. Recordings from the previous day shows $PbtO_2$ (partial pressure of brain tissue $O_2$) to be consistently greater than 25 and lactate/pyruvate (L/P) ratio less than 35, while her most recent readings from this morning are noted in the table that follows.

|  | 7 AM | 8 AM | 9 AM | 10 AM | 11 AM |
| --- | --- | --- | --- | --- | --- |
| $PbtO_2$ | 22 | 15 | 15 | 28 | 29 |
| Brain temp | 37.9 | 38.2 | 38.2 | 38.2 | 37.6 |
| Cerebral perfusion pressure (CPP) | 86 | 74 | 78 | 101 | 109 |
| Lactate (L) | 6.3 | 7.9 | 8.1 | 8.2 | 7 |
| Pyruvate (P) | 150 | 172 | 180 | 221 | 199 |
| L/P ratio | 42.1 | 46 | 45 | 36.9 | 35.1 |

What is the best next step in management to reduce the patient's risk of delayed cerebral ischemia?

**A.** Continue to maintain increased cerebral perfusion pressure (CPP)
**B.** Targeted temperature management
**C.** Transfuse one unit of packed red blood cells
**D.** Start continuous electroencephalogram (cEEG) monitoring

3. A 47-year-old male with untreated hypertension was brought to the emergency department for loss of consciousness while at home and an episode of emesis. A head CT demonstrated a diffuse SAH with intraventricular extension and early signs of hydrocephalus. A CT angiogram demonstrated a 6 mm fusiform aneurysm from the distal right posterior inferior cerebellar artery (PICA). He was admitted to the intensive care unit for ongoing management. Over the course of the evening, there was progressive somnolence and an EVD was placed with an elevated opening pressure. Once placed, the EVD remained clamped. Given the need to delay definitive management of the aneurysm, transexamic acid (TXA) was started. Within 8 hours of admission, there was acute worsening of the examination and an acute increase in the intracranial pressure (ICP), and on opening the EVD, blood actively drained. What of the following is MOST true of aneurysmal rerupture?

A. Aneurysm rerupture does not change functional outcome of those who survive.

B. Posterior circulation aneurysms are more common to have rerupture than anterior circulation aneurysms.

C. The use of TXA decreases the risk of rebleeding and improves clinical outcomes.

D. Placement of an EVD increases the risk of rebleeding.

E. Rerupture more commonly occurs within the first 3 to 5 days, following the initial aneurysm rupture.

---

4. A 67-year-old female has had progressive tinnitus over the last 4 years. Initial laboratory workup has been unrevealing, so additional workup with brain imaging was completed. The CT angiogram is shown in the figure that follows.

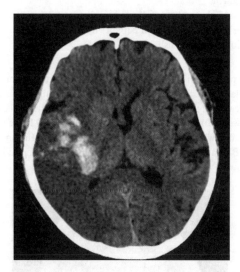

Which of the following is MOST true regarding incidentally discovered aneurysms?

A. Saccular aneurysms are most amenable to treatment with intra-arterial coiling.

B. Incidentally discovered aneurysms without any symptoms do not warrant further evaluation or intervention.

C. Aneurysms located in the posterior circulation have a higher risk of rupture than the anterior circulation.

D. The average annual rupture rate of all incidentally discovered aneurysm is around 10%.

---

5. A 69-year-old male, who has not seen a doctor in at least 10 years, presents to the emergency department for left-sided numbness and weakness. He initially had symptoms 1 day before presentation that lasted for 30 minutes with complete recovery. A head CT did not demonstrate any ischemic changes. A magnetic resonance imaging (MRI) did not demonstrate any infarction. A magnetic resonance angiogram (MRA) of the intracranial and neck vessels demonstrated severe stenosis of the right MCA. What is the next best step management?

A. Consultation to endovascular service for angioplasty and placement of a stent across the right MCA stenosis

B. Start intravenous (IV) heparin infusion with bolus of heparin

C. Start dual antiplatelet therapy with aspirin and clopidogrel

D. Start single antiplatelet therapy with aspirin following a loading dose

---

6. A 73-year-old woman, with prior parietal intraparenchymal hemorrhage approximately 6 months prior and ischemic stroke approximately 2 years prior, presents to the emergency department after being found slumped in a chair at home and unresponsive. She was intubated for airway protection, and a head CT demonstrated a large left frontal intracerebral hemorrhage with intraventricular extension and SAH as well as 5 mm of left-to-right midline shift. Her pertinent medications at home are metoprolol 25 mg daily and aspirin 81 mg daily. Her vital signs in the emergency department are heart rate (HR) 86, blood pressure (BP) 124/68, and $SpO_2$ 98% on 40% $FiO_2$. Her basic metabolic panel and complete blood count are normal. Her only medication at the time of evaluation is propofol for sedation. What medications/treatments should be added to the patient's current regimen?

A. Platelet transfusion

B. Platelet transfusion and levetiracetam

C. Platelet transfusion, levetiracetam, and labetalol infusion

D. Levetiracetam and labetalol infusion

E. No additional medications are needed

7. A 64-year-old man with hypertension is brought to the emergency department for acute-onset (within the last 60 minutes) left face, arm, and leg weakness. A noncontrast head CT is completed and does not demonstrate a hemorrhage or early ischemic changes. His vitals are BP 174/120, HR 76, and SpO$_2$ 99% on room air. A finger-stick blood glucose was obtained and was 127, but other labs are pending. What is the next BEST step in management for the patient?

   A. Administration of tissue plasminogen activator (tPA) at 0.9 mg/kg with initial bolus of 10% total dose and 90% via infusion.
   B. Await coagulation profile (international normalized ratio [INR] and partial thromboplastin time [PTT]) and platelet count before treatment.
   C. Place a nasogastric tube and Foley catheter followed by administration of tPA.
   D. Administration of 182 mg rectal aspirin, given patient's dysarthria.
   E. Administration of labetolol 10 mg IV push.

8. A 69-year-old female with hypertension presents to the emergency department from home following acute onset of slurred speech and left facial droop. She was with her family watching television when her daughter noted the symptoms. Emergency medical services (EMS) was called and noted left facial droop, left arm weakness, and dysarthria. Her initial vitals were unremarkable other than a BP of 212/92. She was treated with IV labetolol with BP improvement and was treated with IV tPA. Thirty minutes into the infusion she complained of a headache and became less responsive. Her BP was 190/86, and the tPA was stopped. A repeat head CT was completed and is shown in the figure that follows.

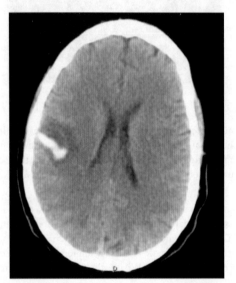

Axial noncontrast head CT. There is a large right MCA acute ischemic stroke with edema and effacement of the sulci. There is hemorrhage present within the area of ischemia centered in the right basal ganglia and insula.

Other than BP management, what is the next best step in management of her current neurologic issue?

   A. Administration of 10 mg IV vitamin K followed by 5 mg IV daily for 3 days
   B. Administration of at least 2500 units of prothombin complex concentrate
   C. Administration of aminocaproic acid (Amicar) 10 g IV in 250 mL NS IV over 1 hour or TXA with load of 1 g over 10 minutes and 1 g over the following 8 hours
   D. Administration of cryoprecipitate
   E. Administration of fresh frozen plasma

9. A 54-year-old man with no past medical history was brought into the emergency department by his wife for altered mental status. On arrival to the emergency department, the only pertinent history and findings were an ongoing holocephalic headache and some confusion. A noncontrast head CT demonstrated a right frontoparietal intraparenchymal hemorrhage. The patient was stabilized and taken for a diagnostic angiogram, which is shown in the figure that follows. The figure is a right internal carotid injection projected as an anterior-posterior view. He was diagnosed with an arteriovenous malformation (AVM).

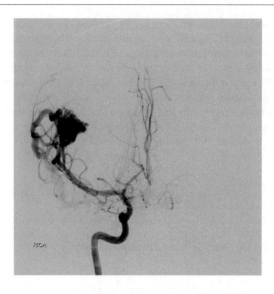

Which of the following statements is true regarding this patient and his AVM?

**A.** This AVM is not concerning, given that it does not arise directly from the internal carotid artery.
**B.** Because the AMV has already bled, there is a lower risk of rehemorrhage in the future.
**C.** AVMs are typically congenital and increase the lifetime risk of seizure and intracerebral hemorrhage.
**D.** An AVM is a direct connection between arteries and veins with normal brain tissue surrounding the abnormal vessels.

# Chapter 2 ▪ Answers

**1.** Correct Answer: D

**Rationale:**
The patient meets Duke criteria for possible endocarditis, given he has one major criteria (transthoracic echocardiography [TTE] with new regurgitation and mobile target) and two minor criteria (fever and emboli). The patient has a severe mitral regurgitation, which will require surgical repair. There are mixed criteria for early intervention, but the American Heart Association recommends early intervention if any of the following is observed:
- Valve dysfunction causing symptoms or signs of heart failure
- Paravalvular extension of infection with development of annular or aortic abscess
- Destructive or penetrating lesion causing heart block
- Infection from a difficult-to-treat pathogen such as fungal or highly resistant organism
- Persistent infection after the start of appropriate antibiotics

This patient does not meet the criteria above, and there is no need to repair his mitral valve urgently. In addition, given his intraparenchymal hemorrhage, undergoing anticoagulation is not an option at this acute time of his presentation. Overall, endocarditis patients with intracerebral hemorrhage are at high risk for clinical worsening during the first month after symptom onset and have a higher mortality than those without (75% vs. 40%).

## References
1. Durack DT, Lukes AS, Bright DK. New criteria for diagnosis of infective endocarditis: utilization of specific echocardiographic findings. Duke Endocarditis Service. *Am J Med.* 1994;96:200-209.
2. Baddour LM, Wilson WR, Bayer AS, et al. Infective endocarditis in adults: diagnosis, antimicrobial therapy, and management of complications: a scientific statement for healthcare professional from the American Heart Association. *Circulation.* 2015;132:1435-1486.

**2.** Correct Answer: A

**Rationale:**
All SAH patients are at risk for delayed cerebral ischemia and cerebral infarction during the acute and subacute stages of their disease. Some centers use multimodality monitoring for evaluation of delayed cerebral ischemia as well as evaluation of interventions attempting to prevent or treat this disease. This particular patient has a brain tissue sensor which measures the partial pressure of oxygen in the brain interstitial cortical tissue. $PbtO_2$ is a balance between oxygen delivery and oxygen consumption in brain cells. It can be affected by a number of parameters, such as

cerebral metabolism, cerebral blood flow, sedation, low inspired oxygen, ICP and CPP changes, and other traumatic changes in the cellular environment. The microdialysis catheter is a semipermeable membrane that allows diffusion of water and solutes down the concentration gradient, and is used to measure the concentrations of these solutes. This particular example has both glucose, lactate, and pyruvate as markers of cerebral metabolism. During times of oligemia, glucose level will drop and lactate levels will rise, marking a shift to anaerobic metabolism.

In this scenario, $PbtO_2$ and lactate-pyruvate ratio (LPR) were within goal the day before and changed significantly this morning to show low brain oxygenation and increased LPR as shown in the table. The goal with $PbtO_2$ monitoring is to assess which change will have the greatest effect on $PbtO_2$ trends. In this case, increasing CPPs (as shown in the table) reversed the changes in $PbtO_2$ and LPR (this morning) and improved brain oxygenation ($PbtO_2$) and metabolism.

### References

1. Helbok R, Olson DM, Le Roux PD, Vespa P. Intracranial pressure and cerebral perfusion pressure monitoring in non-TBI patients: special considerations. *Neurocrit Care*. 2014;21(suppl 2):S85-S94.
2. Ngwenya LB, Burke JF, Manley GT. Brain tissue oxygen monitoring and the intersection of brain and lung: a comprehensive review. *Resp Care*. 2016;69:1232-1244.
3. de Lima Oliveira M, Kairalla AN, Fonoff ET, et al. Cerebral microdialysis in traumatic brain injury and subarachnoid hemorrhage: state of the art. *Neurocrit Care*. 2014;21:152-162.

### 3. Correct Answer: E

**Rationale:**

This SAH patient has suffered a rerupture of his PICA aneurysm. Rebleeding is a major complication of SAH and a major cause of mortality, which can occur at any time during the course. Early rebleeding has been commonly reported to take place between 3 and 5 days, yet the exact period of great risk is still debated. The correlation between risk of rebleeding and predictors such as poor clinical SAH grades, loss of consciousness, external ventricular drainage, and size of aneurysm has been debated. Posterior circulation aneurysms are more likely to rupture, yet overall they are not associated with an increased risk of rerupture.

In an attempt to decrease the risk of rebleeding, TXA has been evaluated in SAH patients and has shown to decrease the rate of early rebreeding; however, it did not associate with improvement in clinical outcome.

### References

1. Naidech AM, Janjua N, Kreiter KT, et al. Predictors and impact of aneurysmal rebleeding after subarachnoid hemorrhage. *Arch Neurol*. 2005;62:410-416.
2. Starke RM, Connolly ES Jr; Participants in the International Multi-Disciplinary Consensus Conference on the Critical Care Management of Subarachnoid Hemorrhage. Rebleeding after aneurysmal subarachnoid hemorrhage. *Neurocrit Care*. 2011;15:24106.

### 4. Correct Answer: C

**Rationale:**

The tinnitus is likely an unrelated symptom, but there is CT angiogram evidence of an incidentally discovered broad-based unruptured aneurysm arising from the left vertebral artery. The overall annual incidence of aneurysm rupture is 1.1% to 1.4%. Patient factors that increase the risk of aneurysmal rupture include smoking, female sex, and posterior circulation, and patient age inversely (younger patients at higher risk) increased the risk of rupture. Aneurysm factors that increase the risk of rupture include larger size in anterior circulation >7 and >6 mm in posterior circulation, multilobulated aneurysm, posterior circulation, and aneurysm growth in serial imaging are associated with increased risk of rupture. The different approaches to management of unruptured, and ruptured, aneurysm are open surgery with ligation or wrapping of the aneurysm and endovascular therapy with coiling of the aneurysm with or without stent assistance.

### References

1. Juvela S, Poussa K, Lehto H, et al. Natural history of unruptured intracranial aneurysms: a long-term follow-up study. *Stroke*. 2013;44:2414-2421.
2. Wermer MJH, van der Schaff IC, Algra A, et al. Risk of rupture of unruptured intracranial aneurysms in relation to patient and aneurysm characteristics. *Stroke*. 2007;38:1404-1410.

### 5. Correct Answer: C

**Rationale:**

This patient presents with a crescendo transient ischemic attack (TIA), defined as recurrent episodes of TIAs over hours to as long as 1 week. The potential mechanism may be embolic or hemodynamic. There are prior studies that examine patients with stroke or TIA attributed to stenosis of 70% to 99% diameter of a major intracranial artery—SAMPRIS trial. In this trial, patients were randomized to percutaneous transluminal angioplasty and stenting with aggressive medical management versus aggressive medical management alone (aspirin and clopidogrel, management of primary and secondary risk factors including lifestyle modification). In those undergoing stenting there was increased risk of stroke and death at 30 days and 1 year compared to medical therapy alone.

A second trial (POINT) evaluated the use of dual antiplatelet therapy versus single antiplatelet agent in patients with small ischemic stroke or TIAs due to intracranial atherosclerotic disease in China. Dual antiplatelet therapy is associated with a reduction in stroke recurrence from 11.7% to 8.2%. Although some advocate for anticoagulation in crescendo TIA, there is limited evidence of efficacy, but there are data that heparinization is safe.

## References

1. Johnston DCC, Hill MD. The patient with transient cerebral ischemia: a golden opportunity for stroke prevention. *CMAJ*. 2004;107:1134-1137.
2. Chimowitz MI, Lynn MJ, Derdeyn CP, et al. Stenting versus aggressive medical therapy for intracranial arterial stenosis. *N Engl J Med*. 2011;365:993-1003.
3. Wang Y, Wang Y, Zhao X. Clopidogrel with aspiring in acute minor stroke or ischemic attack. *N Engl J Med*. 2013;369:11-19.

**6.** Correct Answer: E

**Rationale:**

There are no additional medications that are needed at this time. Given her intracerebral hemorrhage, she should have aggressive BP management to maintain a systolic BP goal of <140 for at least the first 24 hours. The patient's BP is currently below the goal target of 140 mm Hg, so no additional intervention is needed. Intracerebral hemorrhage can result in early clinical seizure, but these early seizures do not change clinical outcomes and the use of prophylactic antiepileptics is not recommended as they might worsen patient's outcome. Lastly, the use of antiplatelet agents before an intracerebral hemorrhage can be a confounding factor. Based on the results of the PATCH study, platelet transfusions are not recommended for use in the setting of intracerebral hemorrhage while taking antiplatelet medication as they appear to increase risk of death or dependence.

## References

1. Anderson CS, Heeley E, Huang Y, et al. Rapid blood-pressure lowering in patients with acute intracerebral hemorrhage. *N Engl J Med*. 2013;368:2355-2365.
2. Beg E, D'Alessandro R, Beretta S, et al. Incidence and predictors of acute symptomatic seizures after stroke. *Neurology*. 2011;77:1785-1793.
3. Hemphill JC, Greenberg SM, Anderson CS, et al. Guidelines for the management of spontaneous intracerebral hemorrhage: a guideline for healthcare professionals from the American Heart Association/American Stroke Association. *Stroke*. 2015;46:1-29.

**7.** Correct Answer: E

**Rationale:**

Ischemic stroke is a common neurologic emergency that can result in permanent disability and death. Intravenous tPA has been studied in multiple trials and been found to be effective in acute stroke treatment. The American Heart Association, American Academy of Neurology, and the American Stroke Association have recommendations on the use of tPA in the treatment of ischemic stroke. There are exclusion criteria for treatment with tPA. The initial American tPA study was the NINDS trial, which demonstrated safety (same mortality at 90 days) and efficacy (improved neurologic outcome at 90 days) with use of tPA within 3 hours of neurologic symptoms. ECASS-II and ECASS-III extended the time window from last known well to 4.5 hours. These data demonstrate improved neurologic outcome with treatment in the 3 to 4.5 hour window but further extended to 6 hours with no difference in mortality or outcome. The feared complication of intracerebral hemorrhage can occur with IV tPA treatment. In the case above, the patient has an absolute contraindication to tPA administration, which is BP >185/>110. Treatment of the BP to below this level can then allow for tPA administration, so option E is the right choice.

| ABSOLUTE CONTRAINDICATION | RELATIVE CONTRAINDICATION |
| --- | --- |
| Acute intracranial hemorrhage | Early ischemic changes on head CT |
| History of intracranial hemorrhage | Advanced age (>75 y old) |
| Severe uncontrolled hypertension | Mild or improving symptoms |
| Serious head trauma or stroke within 3 mo | Severe stroke and coma |
| Thrombocytopenia or coagulopathyIncluding use of direct thrombin inhibitor, factor Xa inhibitor, and heparinoids unless able to demonstrate lack of drug | Recent major surgery |
| Severe hypo/hyperglycemia | Arterial puncture of noncompressible vessel |
| | Recent gastrointestinal or genitourinary hemorrhage |

| ABSOLUTE CONTRAINDICATION | RELATIVE CONTRAINDICATION |
| --- | --- |
| | Seizure at onset |
| | Recent myocardial infarction |
| | Central nervous system lesionNeoplasm, AVM, or aneurysm |
| | Dementia |

### References

1. Jauch EC, Saver JL, Adams HP Jr, et al. AHA/ASA guideline: guidelines for the early management of patients with acute ischemic stroke. *Stroke*. 2013;44:870-947.
2. Fugate JE, Rabinstein AA. Absolute and relative contraindications to IV rt-PA for acute ischemic stroke. *Neurohospitalist*. 2015;5:110-121.

**8.** Correct Answer: D

**Rationale:**

For every 100 patients treated with tPA, 1 patient will experience a severely disabled or fatal outcome as a result of tPA-related hemorrhage. The treatment of symptomatic hemorrhage following tPA administration has not been studied in a randomized fashion. In patients with hypofibrinoemia (level <150 mg/dL) post tPA, cryoprecipitate is recommended to increase this level as those with low fibrinogen had hematoma expansion and worse outcomes. Although fresh frozen plasma contains the same clotting factors as cryoprecipitate, they are not as concentrated and would require a larger volume and would not correct the low fibrinogen level as quickly. TXA and aminocaproic acid can be used for uncontrolled and life-threatening hemorrhage following tPA administration, but these should not be considered first-line therapy, given the complications of prothrombic state that can occur. The dose noted for TXA listed above was studied in trauma patients and demonstrated decreased risk of death. Lastly, use of prothrombin complex concentrate and vitamin K can be used for vitamin K antagonist hemorrhage but play little role in treatment of tPA hemorrhage.

### References

1. The NINDS t-PA Stroke study Group. Intracerebral hemorrhage after intravenous t-PA therapy for ischemic stroke. *Stroke*. 1997;28:2109-2118.
2. Morgenstern LB, Hemphill JC III, Anderson C, et al. Guidelines for the management of spontaneous intracerebal hemorrhage: a guideline for healthcare professionals for the American Heart Association/American Stroke Association. *Stroke*. 2010;41:2108-2129.

**9.** Correct Answer: C

**Rationale:**

AVMs are abnormal, direct connections between arteries and veins without intervening capillary beds and no normal brain tissue among the blood vessels. AVMs are typically congenital but can grow with time. Typical presenting symptoms of AVMs are seizures and intraparenchymal hemorrhage as these may not be isolated to the brain. The risks of AVM surgical mortality and morbidity are characterized based on the AVM size, location, and type of venous drainage. With increased use of intracranial imaging, asymptomatic AVMs are increasingly documented, which should be closely followed.

### References

1. Kucharaczyk W, Lemme-Pleghos L, Usake A, et al. Intracranial vascular malformations: MR and CT imaging. *Radiology*. 1985;56:383-389.
2. da Costa L, Wallace C, tre Brugge KG, et al. The natural history and predictive features of hemorrhage from brain arteriovenous malformations. *Stroke*. 2009;40:100-105.

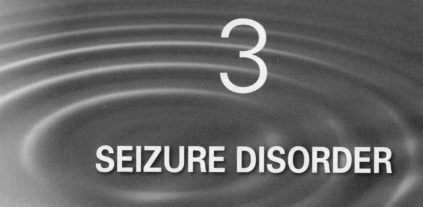

# 3

# SEIZURE DISORDER

David P. Lerner, Anand Venkatraman, and Saef Izzy

1. A 19-year-old male with known generalized epilepsy was brought to the emergency department for convulsive status epileptics. He has had nausea, emesis, and a low grade fever for the last 5 days and has been unable to take his home antiepileptic drug. He is having ongoing low amplitude, rhythmic clonic movements of his bilateral arms and legs. His vitals are as follows: heart rate 86, blood pressure 106/68, SpO$_2$ 100% on 2 L nasal canula, temperature 100.2°C. EMS administered 2 mg of lorazepam and had cessation of clonic movements but still altered and not back to baseline mental state. What is the next best medication treatment for this patient?

   A. Intubate the patient and start propofol
   B. Monitor the patients for few hours and order EEG
   C. Additional lorazepam to dose of 0.1 mg/kg followed by fosphenytoin with loading dose of 15 mg/kg IV
   D. Obtain CT head to further evaluate the etiology and rule out structural abnormalities

2. A 74-year-old man presents to the hospital after falling down a flight of stairs. EMS found him on the ground moaning with left-sided weakness but able to answer questions. On arrival to the emergency department he remained neurologically stable. A head CT demonstrated a 5 mm right holohemispheric subdural hemorrhage. Neurosurgery was consulted and recommended initiation of an antiepileptic drug (AED). Valproic acid was started. Which of the following are concerns related to the use of valproic acid?

   A. It has the same early seizure prevention as phenytoin but it associates with improved mortality rate
   B. It is an inducer of the CYP system with multiple drug interactions
   C. It can result in acute renal injury and possible renal failure
   D. It can result in a coagulopathy which potentially could increase the size of the patient's subdural hemorrhage

3. A 56-year-old female is admitted to the intensive care unit for management of a complete right middle cerebral artery ischemic stroke. During her stay within the intensive care unit, she has progressive somnolence over the course of 96 hours with only minor changes on her CT scan and no midline shift. Given her profound stupor, an EEG was ordered and a portion of the recording is shown in the figure that follows. Her current neurologic examination showed symmetric and reactive pupils at 3 mm, right gaze preference but crosses midline, profound upper motor neuron facial droop on the left, left arm and leg weakness. Patient did not follow commands or open eyes, but she continues to localize with the right arm.

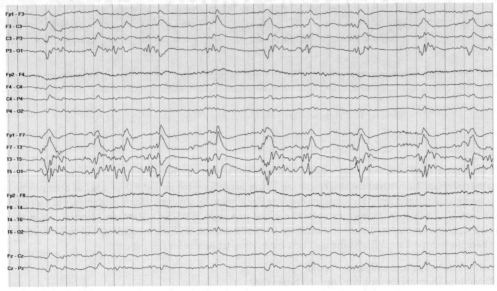

Standard 10 to 20 electrode placement with representation as "double banana" with left over right representation. There is diffuse slowing.

What is the next best step in management for this patient?

A. Continue with supportive care and no change to medications
B. Initiation of antiepileptic medication—levetiracetam 500 mg twice a day
C. Benzodiazepine trial—lorazepam 1 mg IV once
D. Neurosurgery consultation for craniectomy

4. A 48-year-old man with subacute progressive headache and confusion was brought in to the emergency department via EMS for convulsive status epileptics. He received a total of 8 mg of IV lorazepam by EMS and was intubated in the field due to respiratory depression. He has continued to have rhythmic clonic movements of his limbs following intubation. He has now had ongoing seizure activity for 30 minutes. He is then treated with IV phenytoin at a dose of 20 mg/kg at a rate of 50 mg/min. During the infusion he has hypotension requiring vasoactive medications to maintain a mean arterial pressure of 65 mm Hg. What is the underlying cause of hypotension associated with intravenous phenytoin?

A. Loss of vascular sympathetic tone due to voltage-gated sodium channel blockade
B. CNS suppression via voltage-gated sodium channel blockade results in loss of sympathetic tone
C. Ongoing seizure activity has resulted in hypoxia and hemodynamic instability
D. Ongoing seizure activity has resulted in lactic acidosis and hemodynamic instability

5. A 43-year-old woman is brought to the emergency department for ongoing convulsive activity. She has a history of traumatic brain injury 5 years ago with residual encephalomalacia in the left parietal lobe, which has resulted in cognitive impairment and partial epilepsy with secondary generalization. She is maintained on levetiracetam, carbamazepine, and clobazam at home. She is admitted to the ICU, and exam reveals an obese female with tachycardia, BP 134/82, and oxygen saturation of 96%. Her labs show a serum sodium of 128. Which of the following MOST likely is the cause of hyponatremia in this patient?

A. Poor oral intake of solute
B. Medication side effect
C. Cerebral salt wasting secondary to brain trauma
D. Hypothalamic involvement during epileptiform activity
E. Hepatic impairment

6. A 70-year-old man with a history of coronary artery disease, Alzheimer dementia, epilepsy, and chronic kidney disease is admitted to the ICU after presenting with respiratory failure. He started spiking high fevers on the third day and grew *Staphylococcus aureus* in his sputum. On the fourth day of admission, he starts to have rhythmic jerking of his left upper extremity with gaze deviation. With lorazepam treatment the episode resolves. An MRI of the brain after the event shows atrophy, prominent in the right temporoparietal regions, with some ex vacuo ventricular dilation. Which of the following is the MOST likely explanation for this event?

   A. Staphylococcal meningitis in the setting of advanced age
   B. Mycotic aneurysms in the cerebral vasculature as a result of hematogenous spread
   C. Lowered seizure threshold in the setting of critical illness
   D. Amyloid spells in advanced Alzheimer disease, in the setting of critical illness
   E. Late manifestation of hypoxic injury in a patient with baseline brain atrophy

7. A 69-year-old woman with excessive alcohol intake (2 bottles of wine a day) suffers an out-of-hospital cardiac arrest. She receives several rounds of cardiopulmonary resuscitation, achieves return of spontaneous circulation, and is brought to the hospital. She undergoes 24 hours of therapeutic hypothermia. Her urine drug screen is positive for benzodiazepines. After rewarming, she is found to have rapid twitching movements of her face and extremities. An EEG is attached and it shows abnormal rhythmic activity. Which of the following is MOST true about this condition?

   A. Presence of EEG activity is an indicator of high chance of recovery at 6 months.
   B. Postanoxic myoclonic status epilepticus is an indicator of poor prognosis
   C. Oxcarbazepine and topiramate are the only agents with proven efficacy in controlling these movements
   D. Diagnostic lumbar puncture is essential to rule out meningitis in these cases
   E. This is likely a manifestation of brain irritability secondary to benzodiazepine withdrawal

# Chapter 3 ▪ Answers

1. Correct Answer: C

**Rationale:**
The patient has history of generalized epilepsy and presented with likely breakthrough seizures which in this case meets the diagnosis of convulsive status epilepticus. Benzodiazepine is the first-line therapy. Lorazepam, diazepam, or midazolam are appropriate choices of benzodiazepine. In this case, patient already received an initial dose of an appropriate first-line agent (lorazepam) but not at an appropriate total dose. Lorazepam dose is 0.1 mg/kg with max dose of 4 mg/dose and may be repeated once if seizures persisted. At this point, readministration of a benzodiazepine is appropriate. There is no evidence-based preferred second-line agent for management of status epilepticus. The recommended agents for control of status epileptics are IV fosphenytoin/phenytoin and sodium valproate. The use of levetiracetam in treating status epilepticus is controversial, although it has been used in many institutions as a second-line agent. If none of these agents are available, IV phenobarbital can be considered. If patient continues to seize despite first- and second-line therapies, redosing second-line agent, securing airway, and anesthetic doses of either midazolam, propofol, or less likely phenobarbital should be considered. Further seizure evaluation is needed including comprehensive metabolic and infectious panel, given history of fevers, as well as imaging of the head, especially if he has any neurological exam abnormalities, once his underlying status epilepticus is under control.

References
1. Brophy GM, Bell R, Claassen J, et al. Guidelines for the evaluation and management of status epilepticus. *Neurocrit Care.* 2012;17:3-23.
2. Eue S, Grumbt M, Muller M, et al. Two years of experience in the treatment of status epilepticus with intervenous levetiracetam. *Epilepsy Behav.* 2009;15:467-469.

2. Correct Answer: D

**Rationale:**
Valproic acid is a highly protein-bound organic acid that has antiepileptic properties via blockage of the voltage-dependent Na$^+$ channels, gamma-aminobutyric acid (GABA) potentiation, and glutamate/NMDA inhibition. Valproic acid is degraded in the liver via the CYP system into glucuronidation and then 50% renally cleared from the body. There are no risks of renal injury with the medication, but there are risks of liver injury and pancreatitis. Valproate is an inhibitor of mainly CYP2C9 but other CYP enzymes as well. On evaluation of phenytoin and valproic acid, the

two drugs have similar early seizure prevention, no change in late seizure prevention, but there was a trend toward higher mortality with those treated with valproic acid. Lastly, there are coagulation effects of valproic acid. The mechanism of VPA-induced coagulopathy is not well-identified and may include multiple mechanisms. VPA can decrease platelet count and has an inhibitory effect of platelets similar to that of aspirin, and it can also decrease procoagulant factors including factor VII and VIII which could theoretically increase the risk of bleeding from surgery. Paying special attention to the changes in blood coagulation studies in the preoperative assessment may be of clinical importance in VPA-treated patients.

### References

1. Loscher W. Basic pharmacology of valproate: a review after 35 years of clinical use for the treatment of epilepsy. *CNS Drugs*. 2002;16:669-694.
2. Wen X, Wang JS, Kivisto KT, et al. In vitro evaluation of valproic acid as an inhibitor of human cytochrome P450 isoforms: preferential inhibition of cytochrome P450 2C9 (CYP2C9). *Br J Clin Pharmacol*. 2001;52:547-553.
3. Temkin NR, Dikmen SS, Anders GD, et al. Valproate therapy for prevention of posttraumatic seizures: a randomized trial. *J Neurosurg*. 1999;91:593-600.

---

**3.** Correct Answer: A

### Rationale:

Patient's neurological examination is consistent with her right middle cerebral artery stroke. There is no clear clinical signs of seizures noted. The EEG was done to further her mental status which demonstrates spikes or sharp waves occurring at an approximately regular interval which is called periodic lateralized epileptiform discharges (PLEDs). There are no electrographic signs of seizures. The PLD nomenclature was adopted in 2012 to simplify the discussion of EEG findings within the ICU which are meant to be more descriptive while removing ambiguity from prior naming schema. PLEDs are commonly seen in patients with multiple CNS diseases such as acute ischemic stroke, tumor, infection, hemorrhage, and metabolic. In this case presentation acute stroke is the likely etiology. Given stable CT head with no signs of midline shift, there is no indication of decompressive craniectomy at this point. There are no signs of clinical or electrographic seizures, so option B and C are not indicated at this point. Continue supportive care is the right choice for now.

### References

1. Hirsch LJ, LaRoche SM, Gaspard N, et al. American Clinical Neurophysiology Society's Standardized Crticial Care EEG Terminology: 2012 version. *J Clin Neurophysiol*. 2013;30:1-27.
2. Chu NS. Periodic lateralized epileptiform discharges with preexisting focal brain lesions. *Arch Neurol*. 1980;37:551-554.

---

**4.** Correct Answer: A

### Rationale:

Intravenous phenytoin is a well-established treatment of status epilepticus and is considered a second-line agent in treatment following administration of benzodiazepine medications. The mechanism of action within the CNS is blockade of the sodium channels within the central nervous system which prevents sustained repetitive firing of neurons. In addition, phenytoin also blocks the sodium channels outside the central nervous system including both the cardiac and peripheral vasculature which could result in hypotension in the setting of ventricular fibrillation and negative ionotropic effects and peripheral vasodilation.

### References

1. Brophy GM, Bell R, Claassen J, et al. Guidelines for the evaluation and management of status epilepticus. *Neurocrit Care*. 2012;17:3-23.
2. Treiman DM, Meyers PD, Walton NY, et al. A comparison of four treatment for generalized nonconvulsive status epilepticus. Veterans affairs status epilepticus cooperative study group. *N Engl J Med*. 1998;339:792-798.

---

**5.** Correct Answer: B

### Rationale:

This patient has been on chronic carbamazepine for seizure control. Hyponatremia is one of the most common side effects associated with carbamazepine use and should be monitored for. The mechanism is thought to be excessive production of antidiuretic hormone. While cerebral salt wasting and the syndrome of inappropriate antidiuretic hormone secretion (SIADH) can be seen in brain trauma, it is rare for them to manifest 5 years after the insult. There is no evidence from the history of any hepatic impairment, though hyponatremia can certainly be seen in patients with impaired liver function.

### References

1. Maan JS, Saadabadi A. Carbamazepine. Treasure Island (FL): StatPearls Publishing; 2019.
2. Van Amelsvoort T, Bakshi R, Devaux C, et al. Hyponatremia associated with carbamazepine and oxcarbazepine therapy: a review. *Epilepsia*. 1994;35(1):181-188.

**6.** Correct Answer: C

**Rationale:**

Critical illness is commonly known to lower the threshold for seizures, especially in a patient with prior history of epilepsy. Even in those without a history of epilepsy, infections are a common trigger for seizures. Elderly patients and those with underlying structural brain disease are commonly affected. The common seizure triggers associated with critical illness are metabolic and electrolyte abnormalities, infections, and medication. Meningitis is a possibility in the setting of a known infection but would be less likely than breakthrough seizure in the setting of infection. Mycotic aneurysms may occur in patients with bacteremia, but there is no evidence of that in this patient. Amyloid spells are spectrum of transient focal neurological episodes reported to occur in cerebral amyloid angiopathy patients. Overall, they are not common and less likely seen in intubated, critically ill patients. Hypoxic injury is a possibility in this patient who has had respiratory failure, but with an MRI that does not demonstrate any early cortical ischemic changes and a presentation consistent with seizures, this option will be lower on the differential.

References

1. Mirski MA, Varelas PN. Seizures and status epilepticus in the critically ill. *Crit Care Clin.* 2008;24(1):115-147.
2. Delanty N, Vaughan CJ, French JA. Medical causes of seizures. *Lancet.* 1998;352(9125):383-390.

**7.** Correct Answer: B

**Rationale:**

Postanoxic myoclonic status epilepticus can be seen after hypoxic-ischemic brain injury following cardiac arrest. Its presence generally portends a poor prognosis. In some cases, they may be noticed only after rewarming from therapeutic hypothermia. Levetiracetam and valproic acid have shown some benefit in controlling these phenomena Although presence of EEG activity is a better sign than having no EEG activity at all after a cardiac arrest, postanoxic myoclonic status epilepticus has poor prognostics values. Given urine drug screen is positive for benzodiazepines, patient is at risk of benzodiazepine withdrawal which could rarely present as seizures only, yet, given patient's alcohol history, it should be on the differential diagnosis. Given there is no report of fever or other evidence for ongoing infection, there is no acute indication for a lumbar puncture.

References

1. Wijdicks EF, Parisi JE, Sharbrough FW. Prognostic value of myoclonus status in comatose survivors of cardiac arrest. *Ann Neurol.* 1994;35(2):239-243.
2. Beretta S, Coppo A, Bianchi E, et al. Neurologic outcome of postanoxic refractory status epilepticus after aggressive treatment. *Neurology.* 2018;91(23):e2153-e2162.

# 4

# NEUROMUSCULAR DISORDERS

David P. Lerner and Saef Izzy

1. A 51-year-old woman with antibody-positive myasthenia gravis, on immunosuppressive therapy with azathioprine, is admitted to the intensive care unit for increased work of breathing. Two weeks prior she had an upper respiratory tract infection, and when it did not improve, she was prescribed a course of levofloxacin, which she started 3 days ago. Since that time she has had a progressive dyspnea and was unable to walk up a flight of stairs. Her initial vital signs in the emergency department (ED) were normal and her oxygen saturation was 98% on room air with a respiratory rate of 24. She appeared comfortable, and although tachypneic she did not have accessory muscle use. She underwent bedside spirometry testing and was found to have a negative inspiratory force of −40 mm Hg and forced vital capacity of 0.75 L (weight 79.6 kg). An arterial blood gas was obtained in the intensive care unit and was pH 7.32, $pCO_2$ 32, and $pO_2$ 171. Should this patient be intubated?

   A. Yes, given her tachypnea, low-forced vital capacity, and respiratory alkalosis, she should be intubated. Intubation should be completed using a depolarizing neuromuscular blocker.
   B. Yes, given her tachypnea, low-forced vital capacity, and respiratory alkalosis, she should be intubated. Intubation should be completed using a nondepolarizing neuromuscular blocker.
   C. No, given her comfortable appearance, appropriate negative inspiratory force, and respiratory alkalosis, she should not be intubated and continue with close neurologic and respiratory monitoring.
   D. No, given her comfortable appearance, appropriate negative inspiratory force, and respiratory alkalosis, she should not be intubated, however, bilevel positive airway pressure support (BiPAP) should be initiated.

2. A 14-year-old woman with medically intractable epilepsy presents to ED in status epilepticus. Three weeks prior, she had a "virallike illness" and had never fully returned to normal. She was having increased seizure frequency during that time. While in the ED, she was intubated for airway protection. Her workup reveals pyelonephritis, and she is treated with an appropriate course of antibiotics with improvement in her vitals and laboratory results. She had limited improvement in her mental status initially, and long-term electroencephalogram (EEG) monitoring revealed subclinical status epilepticus. Following 24 hours of burst suppression with propofol and midazolam, she had improvement in her EEG. Over the course of the next 72 hours, she had improvement in her mental status but was unable to be weaned from the ventilator because of poor tidal volumes during spontaneous breathing trials. On examination, she has marked proximal weakness in all four extremities. Electodiagnostic testing is completed, which demonstrates prolonged compound muscle action potential (CMAP) on nerve conduction studies and positive sharp waves and decreased recruitment on electromyography. What is the MOST likely cause of her weakness?

   A. Critical illness neuropathy
   B. Critical illness myopathy
   C. Acute demyelinating encephalomyelitis (ADEM)
   D. Guillain-Barré syndrome (GBS)
   E. Inflammatory myopathy (eg polymyositis)

3. A 56-year-old man with essential thrombocytosis (baseline approximately 800 000) and prior renal cell carcinoma status post left nephrectomy 5 years before presentation presents with progressive bilateral lower extremity weakness and ascending paresthesia over the course of 7 days. He has mild proximal weakness in his bilateral legs, but is able to ambulate, and decreased sensation in his bilateral legs to mid-shin. No reflexes noted on examination. Additional testing including a lumbar puncture, demonstrating elevated protein with no white blood cells, and nerve conduction study, demonstrating dispersion of motor and sensory nerve responses with conduction block, confirms the diagnosis of GBS. What is the most appropriate treatment?

   A. Intravenous immunoglobulin (IVIg) at 2 g/kg in divided doses of 0.4 g/kg/d for 5 days
   B. Plasmapheresis (PLEX) exchange volume 250 mL/kg for five sessions on alternating days
   C. Intravenous methylprednisolone at 1 g/day for 5 days
   D. PLEX exchange volume 250 mL/kg for five sessions on alternating days followed by IVIg at 2 g/kg in divided doses of 0.4 g/kg/d for 5 days

4. A previously healthy 36-year-old male was admitted to the medical intensive care unit following a cardiac arrest. On the day of admission to the hospital, he was getting ready for work, but felt quite fatigued and short of breath. He was talking with his wife, and she noted that he looked "blue" and then fell to the floor. He did not have a pulse, and she started emergency medical services (CPR) and contacted emergency medical services (EMS). On arrival, he did not have a pulse and received one dose of epinephrine and was intubated in the field with return of spontaneous circulation. On arrival to the ED, he was hemodynamically stable with normal vital signs, localizing with his arms and opening his eyes to noxious stimulation. He remained intubated and his mental status recovered, but he was unsuccessfully extubated because of hypercarbic respiratory failure over the course of several hours. A full cardiac and pulmonary workup was completed without underlying etiology for his respiratory failure. The neurology serviced was consulted for evaluation of failure to wean. Further history noted progressive dyspnea and fatigue over the last 6 months, but he attributed this to his stress at work. Also, he noted more difficulty with lifting his young children. His neurologic examination was pertinent for mild symmetric deltoid weakness and moderate symmetric hip flexion weakness. The remainder of the neurologic examination was normal. Electrodiagnostic tests were completed with normal nerve conduction studies, but abnormal electromyography with positive sharp waves and fibrillation potentials demonstrated in the deltoid, supraspinatus, iliopsoas, and thoracic paraspinal musculature. The paraspinal musculature also demonstrated complex repetitive discharges and myotonic discharges. What is the MOST likely underlying cause of the patient's presentation?

   A. Acid maltase deficiency
   B. C9orf72 genetic mutation
   C. Glucose-6-phosphatase deficiency
   D. Laminin A/C gene mutation
   E. Zinc finger 9 genetic mutation

# Chapter 4 ■ Answers

1. Correct Answer: D

   **Rationale:**
   This patient is presenting with myasthenic crisis, which can occur for a number of reasons, most importantly for this patient likely secondary to infection and use of a fluoroquinolone antibiotic. Other common medications that can worsen myasthenia include macrolides, aminoglycosides, beta-blockers, magnesium-containing medications, and steroids. Early initiation of noninvasive ventilatory support with BiPAP may avert the need for endotracheal intubation. Although there are no strict guidelines on admission criteria into the intensive care unit, close respiratory monitoring is needed as these patients can quickly develop hypercarbic respiratory failure and require endotracheal intubation. The assessment of respiratory function included the bulbar muscular function as those with bulbar weakness may have overt aspiration. Signs of respiratory weakness including hypophonia, pausing while talking to breathe, rapid/shallow breathing, and paradoxical abdominal breathing. The two commonly used bedside tests are the vital capacity and negative inspiratory force. Consideration for intubation should occur if the vital capacity falls below 15 to 20 mL/kg (ideal body weight) or the negative inspiratory force is less than −25 to −30 mm Hg. These values should not be taken in isolation the clinical context, which needs to be evaluated as well. This patient does not require intubation at this time, but if progression

of her weakness were to occur intubation with either a nondepolarizing agent (eg rocuronium) or depolarizing agent (eg succinylcholine) can be used, but nonstandard dosing needs to be considered. Given there is decreased functional acetylcholine receptors, there is a need for a higher dose of depolarizing agents and decreased dosage of nondepolarizing agents. Given the sensitivity and unpredictable response to nondepolarizing agents, depolarizing agents are typically used.

### References

1. Wendell LC, Levine JM. "Myasthenic crisis." *Neurohospitalist.* 2011;1:16-22.
2. Myasthenia Gravis Foundation in America. "Drugs to Avoid". Online at: myasthenia.org. Accessed May 2016.
3. Senevirante J, Mandrekar J, Wijdicks EF, Rabinstein AA. "Noninvasive ventilation in myasthenia crisis." *Arch Neurol.* 2008;65: 54-58.
4. Godoy DA, Vaz de Mello LJ, Masotti L, et al. "The myasthenic patient in crisis: an update of the management in Neurointensive Care Unit." *Arq Neuropsiquiatr.* 2013;71:627-639.
5. Martyn JA, hite DA, Gronert GA, et al. "Up-and-down regulation of skeletal muscle acetylcholine receptors. Effects on neuromuscular blockers." *Anesthesiology.* 1992;76:822-830.

## 2. Correct Answer: B

**Rationale:**

The patient has quadriparesis including respiratory weakness with electrodiagnostic testing consistent with a myopathic disease process. Given her recent intubation, sedation, sepsis, and limited mobility due to burst suppression, these point to critical illness myopathy as the underlying disease process. Risk factors for critical illness myopathy include sepsis, high-dose glucocorticoids, prolonged neuromuscular blockade, hyperglycemia, immobility, vasopressor use, renal replacement therapy, and trauma. In critical illness neuropathy, the common findings are decreased amplitude of both sensory and motor nerve responses with normal spontaneous activity on EMG. Although not required to make the diagnosis, muscle biopsy in critical illness myopathy will typically demonstrate loss of myosin. There are no specific treatments for critical illness myopathy although strict glucose control can decrease the risk and early mobility may improve function. Although the patient had a "virallike illness" before her presentation, the nerve conduction findings are not consistent with a demyelinating disease process such as GBS. Although ADEM can present with quadriparesis due to high cervical cord involvement, the nerve conduction findings are not consistent with this diagnosis. Although an inflammatory myopathy is unlikely the cause, given her other ongoing critical illness.

### References

1. Latronico N, Bolton CF. "Critical illness polyneuropathy and myopathy: a major cause of muscle weakness and paralysis." *Lancet Neurol.* 2011;10:931-941.
2. Bolton CF, Gilbert JJ, Hahn AF, Sibbald WJ. "Polyneuropathy in critically ill patients." *J Neurol Neurosurg Psychiatry.* 1984;47:1223-1231.

## 3. Correct Answer: B

**Rationale:**

There are several types of GBS, classified by the part of the peripheral nerve involved in this disease. Acute inflammatory demyelinating polyradiculoneuropathy (AIDP) is the most common etiology, but there is also an axonal type, which typically results in worse recovery. This patient presents with the stereotypical presentation of GBS: ascending paresthesias, progressive ascending weakness, and loss of deep tendon reflexes. Confirmatory testing includes lumbar puncture, which demonstrates a cytoalbuminologic gap and nerve conduction study suggestive of demyelinating features. Although not presented in the case, there are a number of disease-related complications including labile blood pressure, arrhythmias, gastroparesis, urinary retention, and syndrome of inappropriate antidiuretic hormone (SIADH). Treatment of GBS has two treatments: IVIg and PLEX. The American Academy of Neurology recommendations for treatment of GBS in ambulatory patients within 2 weeks of neuropathic symptoms advocates for PLEX. Another reason for use of PLEX over IVIg in this patient is the complications of treatment. IVIg can results in thrombosis because of hyperviscosity. Given his underlying thrombocytosis, IVIg could place him at even higher risk worsening thrombocytosis and in turn increase the risk of bleeding especially with platelet counts over 1 000 000. Studies showed that sequential treatment with PLEX followed by IVIg does not have a greater benefit than either treatment given alone. In addition, AAN guideline does not recommend steroids for the treatment of GBS patients (Level A, Class 1).

### References

1. Yuki N, Hartung HP. "Guillain-Barre syndrome." *N Engl J Med.* 2012;366:2294-2304.
2. Plasma Exchange/Sandoglobulin Guillain-Barré Syndrome Trial Group. Randomised trial of plasma exchange, intravenous immunoglobulin, and combined treatments in Guillain-Barré syndrome. *Lancet.* 1997;349:225-230.

**4.** Correct Answer: A

**Rationale:**

The neurologic etiologies of failure to wean from the ventilator are quite broad and can be divided into central (bi-hemispheric, bithalamic, brain stem, and cervical cord), peripheral nerve, neuromuscular junction, and muscle. The pattern of weakness can help determine the underlying etiology, and electrodiagnostic tests can further determine the underlying cause. In this case, examination demonstrates myopathic pattern of weakness and this is confirmed with the electrodiagnostic testing. The patient has a limb-girdle pattern of weakness with the striking finding of abnormal electromyography within the paraspinal muscles. The clinical history and EMG findings are most consistent with late onset Pompe disease, which is a deficiency in acid maltase. Although muscle biopsy can confirm the diagnosis, there are now blood tests: leukocyte isolates from whole blood for GAA activity and blood spot assay for acid alpha-glucosidase activity. Making this diagnosis is crucial as there is enzyme replacement therapy which can improve survival. C9orf72 genetic mutation is associated with ALS-FTD spectrum disorders. Glucose-6-phosphatase deficiency is associated with von Gierke disease, which presents in infancy with hepatosplenomegaly, hypoglycemia during fasting, epilepsy, and lactic acidosis. Laminin A/C is associated with limb-girdle muscle dystrophy, which can present similar but will not have the respiratory and paraspinal muscle findings as Pompe. Zinc finger 9 is associated with myotonic dystrophy type 2 that has a very characteristic "hatchet face" appearance and myotonia on examination.

## References

1. Boles JM, Bion J, Connors A, et al. Weaning from mechanical ventilation. *Eur Respir J*. 2007;29:1033-1056.
2. Muller-Feller W, Horvath R, Gempei K, et al. Late onset Pompe disease: clinical and neurophysiological spectrum of 38 patients including long-term followup in 18 patients." *Neuromuscl Disord*. 2007;17:698-706.

# 5

# INCREASED INTRACRANIAL PRESSURE

David P. Lerner and Saef Izzy

1. A 79-year-old female with history of hypertension and right-sided subdural hemorrhage status-post right hemicraniectomy and cranioplasty presented to the emergency department with progressive head and focal right arm twitching concerning for a focal seizure. A head CT was obtained and is shown in the figure that follows.

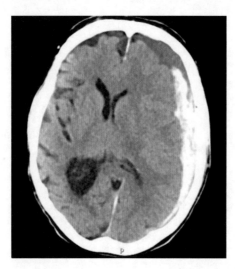

What type of herniation is demonstrated on the head CT and what are the anticipated neurologic findings on examination?

A. Fungating herniation—contralateral > ipsilateral weakness
B. Subfalcine herniation—contralateral > ipsilateral leg weakness
C. Transtentorial (uncal) herniation—contralateral weakness and anisocoria
D. Tonsillar herniation—marked depressed level of consciousness and bulbar dysfunction

2. A 22-year-old male has an external ventricular drain placed for intracranial pressure monitoring following a traumatic brain injury. The patient continues to have a poor neurologic examination. There are episodes of time when he has an elevation in his intracranial pressure to 20 mm Hg that will last for 10 to 20 minutes at a time. During this time there are no changes to other vital signs. A tracing of the external ventricular drain (EVD) is shown below. What is the phenomenon depicted?

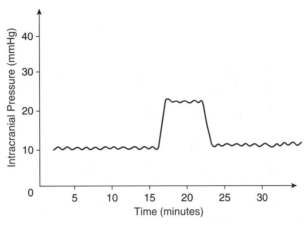

   A. Lundberg A wave
   B. Lundberg B wave
   C. Lundberg C wave
   D. Autonomic storming

3. An 18-year-old male is brought in to the emergency department after a motor vehicle crash. He was on a motorcycle and was found 30 feet away from his vehicle in unconscious state without a helmet. He has noted trauma to his left forearm, active bleeding from the left posterior portion of his scalp. He was intubated in the field with EMS. On arrival he is tachycardic (heart rate 120s), blood pressure 110/62. He was recently paralyzed for intubation and does not have twitches present on train of four testing. A head CT is completed which demonstrates a large left-sided subdural hematoma with 6 mm midline shift. In the interval, as neurosurgery team is taking the patient to the OR, hyperventilation is started to decrease cerebral edema. How does hyperventilation decrease intracranial pressure?

   A. Change in CSF pH results in constriction of vascular smooth muscle
   B. Change in intracranial blood pH results in constriction of vascular smooth muscle
   C. Change in CSF pH results in electrical quiescence of neurons, decreased metabolic demand, and decreased cerebral blood flow
   D. Change in $pCO_2$ sensed by carotid body chemoreceptors results in vasoconstriction
   E. A drop in $pCO_2$ leads to a large osmotic gradient and worsening interstitial edema

4. A 32-year-old female with chronic alcoholism and cirrhosis was brought to the emergency department following a night of binge drinking. She was found unresponsive at home and EMS was called. On arrival to the emergency department she was intubated for airway protection. She did not require sedation for intubation and is not currently on any sedation. A head CT was completed and demonstrated diffuse cerebral edema with effacement of the sulci and ventricular system. Her lab results were remarkable for an elevation in AST and ALT (2000, 1000 units/L respectively), total bilirubin 5.6 mg/dL, and ammonia 3642 μm/L. Her examination remains poor, with only extensor posturing to motor stimulation. Her pupils are 5 mm and sluggishly reactive to light. Given the findings on head CT what is the next best step in management?

   A. Hyperventilate the patient with goal $pCO_2$ 20 mm Hg
   B. Start sedation with a midazolam infusion at 1 mg/h
   C. Placement of an intraparenchymal monitor for intracranial pressure monitoring and guidance of therapy
   D. Infusion of mannitol at 1 g/kg and if needed repeat every 6 hours
   E. Emergent liver transplantation

**5.** A 62-year-old male was admitted with diffuse subarachnoid hemorrhage, intraventicular extension of the hemorrhage, and early signs of hydrocephalus. An EVD was placed without complication. The EVD has functioned well and following placement the patient's examination improved. The figure that follows is the waveform produced. What occurs during the P3 peak?

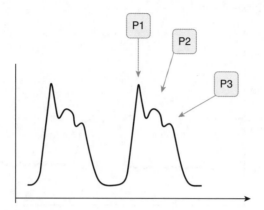

**A.** P3 represents the arterial pulse
**B.** P3 represents the cerebral compliance
**C.** P3 represents the respiratory ICP wave
**D.** P3 represents the dicrotic notch

**6.** A 59-year-old female with no past medical history is admitted to the neurointensive care unit following a large right middle cerebral artery ischemic stroke. She was not a candidate for intravenous tPA nor intra-arterial therapy. She has had progressive somnolence and anisocoria with a right larger than left pupil that was not responsive to direct or consensual light testing. She was started on hyperosmolar therapy followed by a decompressive hemicraniectomy. She is now poststroke day 5 and continues to have malignant cerebral edema. Prior to her next dose of mannitol her lab values are as follows:

Na 150, K 3.4, Cl 116, HCO 24, BUN 10, Cr 0.32, Glucose 187, Calcium 7.3, Osmolality 314

What is her osmolar gap?

**A.** 0
**B.** 6
**C.** 14
**D.** 53

**7.** A 53-year-old, right-handed, previously independent male with no past medical history was found down at home. He was brought to the emergency department where he was found to have a large, well-established L MCA ischemic stroke on CT with a proximal L M1 thrombus on CT angiogram. He was not a candidate for IV tPA or intra-arterial therapy given the well established infarction and his last known well-being over 12 hours prior to presentation. He was admitted to the intensive care unit for ongoing management. Over the course of the next 24 hours he has progressive decline in his mental status and required intubation. A repeat head CT shows evolution of the ischemic stroke with left-to-right midline shift. What is the best description of the anticipated outcome following a hemicraniectomy for malignant ischemic stroke?

**A.** A hemicraniectomy can potentially be a life-saving intervention and will improve neurologic recovery
**B.** A hemicraniectomy can potentially be a life-saving intervention but will not improve neurologic recovery
**C.** Because the ischemic stroke is on the dominate hemisphere, hemicraniectomy should be completed as there is a higher chance of recovery
**D.** Hemicraniectomy without durotomy is preferred as there is a lower risk of infection as compared to hemicraniectomy with durotomy

# Chapter 5 ▪ Answers

**1.** Correct Answer: B

**Rationale:**

The head CT above demonstrates an acute on subacute left-sided subdural hemorrhage with left-to-right midline shift and compression of the left lateral ventricle and potential trapping of the right lateral ventricle. The timing of the subdural hemorrhage is based on the density of the blood product. Acute blood appears hyperdense to brain parenchyma. After approximately 3 days the blood product begins to break down and will reach an isodense characteristic compared to brain parenchyma, typically around 10 to 14 days. After 21 days, the blood product becomes hypodense to brain tissue and is similar to cerebrospinal fluid. The herniation demonstrated on this image is subfalcine with left frontal lobe shift under the falx into the right hemisphere. Subfalcine herniation results with cingulate gyrus herniation across the falx and compression of the pericallosal arteries resulting in contralateral (and commonly bilateral) leg weakness. Transtentorial or uncal herniation occurs with the medial temporal lobe and uncus compresses the ipsilateral cerebral peduncle resulting in compression of the ipsilateral third cranial nerve resulting in an enlarged and fixed or sluggishly reactive pupil and contralateral weakness. Tonsillar herniation occurs when there is a pressure within the cerebellum resulting in herniation of the cerebellar tonsil into the foramen magnum and compression of the fourth ventricle resulting in noncommunicating hydrocephalus and obtundation. Fungating herniation occurs when there is a skull defect and herniation of brain tissue outside the cranial vault. All herniation occurs due to a pressure gradient from one compartment (left-right hemisphere, or supra-infratentorial compartment).

References

1. Brant WE, Helms CA. *Fundamentals of Diagnostic Radiology*. Lippincott Williams & Wilkins; 2007.
2. Blumenfeld H. *Neuroanatomy Through Clinical Cases*. 2nd ed. Sinauer Associates; 2010.

**2.** Correct Answer: A

**Rationale:**

The intracranial pressure (ICP) waveform shown is the Lundberg A, which are a sustained elevation in ICP with amplitude of 50 to 100 mm Hg (higher than Lundberg B and C waves). They typically last for 5 to 20 minutes and they are always pathological as they represent reduced cerebral compliance and increase intracranial pressure. Lundberg B waves are short elevation of ICP with amplitude of 5 to 20 mm Hg at a frequency of 0.5 to 2 waves/min, which last for 1 to 5 minutes. They are thought to be normal waves with probably some association with unstable ICP and vasospasm. Lundberg C waves are rapid oscillations of 4 to 8 waves/min with low amplitude of <20 mm Hg. They are normal waves with changes related to cardiac and respiratory cycles. Without changes in other physiologic parameters, it is unlikely the ICP change is due to autonomic storming. Common features include increase in blood pressure, respiratory rate, heart rate, worsening level of consciousness, muscle rigidity, and hyperhidrosis.

References

1. Beaumont A. Intracranial pressure and cerebral blood flow monitoring. neuromonitoring. In: Torbey M, ed. *Neurocritical Care Book*. Cambridge press; 2009:109-114.
2. Fernandez-Ortega JF, Prietro-Palomino MA, Garcia-Caballero M, et al. Paroxysmal sympathetic hyperactivity after traumatic brain injury: clinical and prognostic implications. *J Neurotrauma*. 2012;29:1364-1370.

**3.** Correct Answer: D

**Rationale:**

The intracranial pressure is influenced by $pCO_2$. A rise in $pCO_2$ will result in brain blood vessel dilatation and then increase in the cerebral blood volume. In contrast, when the $pCO_2$ drops, the blood vessel diameter decreases and results in decreased cerebral blood volume. Although hypocarbic strategy promotes transient decrease in ICP and considered one of the effective intracranial hypertension temporizing measures, hyperventilation carries a serious risk of significant reduction in cerebral blood flow (CBF) and cerebral ischemia. In addition, studies showed prolonged hypocapnia can lead to rebound ICP. For this reason the Brain Trauma Foundation changed recently their 2017 guidelines about hyperventilation and stated that "prolonged prophylactic hyperventilation with partial pressure of carbon dioxide in arterial blood ($PaCO_2$) of 25 mm Hg or less is not recommended" (Level IIB).

The change in cerebral blood flow is independent of the pH as there is no change with metabolic acidosis and alkalosis. There is rapid $CO_2$ equilibration between the arterial blood and CSF, and the change in pH of the CSF acts directly in the vasculature resulting in relaxation or contraction.

## References

1. Souter MJ, Lam AM. Neurocritical Care. In: Miller RD, Erickssno LI, Fleisher L, Wiener-Kroonish JP, et al. eds. *Miller's Anesthesia*. 7th ed. Philadephia PA: Churchill Livingstone;2009:2899-2921.
2. Sato M, Pawlik G, Heiss WD. Comparative studies of regional CNS blood flow autogregulation and responses to $CO_2$ in the cat. Effexts of altering aterial blood pressure and $PaCO_2$ on rCBF of cerebrum, cerebellum and spinal cord. *Stroke*. 1984;15:91-97.
3. Schieve JF, Wilson WP. The changes in cerebral vascular resistance of man in experimental alkalosis and acidosis. *J Clin Invest*. 1953;32:33.
4. Muizelaar JP, Marmarou A, Ward JD, et al. Adverse effects of prolonged hyperventilation in patients with severe head injury: a randompized clinical trial. *J Neurosurg*. 1991;75:731-739.
5. Kinoshita K. Traumatic brain injury: pathophysiology for neurocritical care. *J Intensive Care*. 2016;v4;29.
6. Yoon SH, Zuccarello M, Rapoport RM. $pCO_2$ and pH regulation of cerebral blood flow. *Front Physiol*. 2012;3:265.
7. Carney N, Totten AM, O'Reilly C, et al. Guidelines for the management of severe traumatic brain injury, fourth edition. *Neurosurgery*. 2017;80:6-15.

## 4. Correct Answer: D

### Rationale:

Fulminant liver failure is frequently associated with worsening cerebral edema and elevation in ICP. The detoxification of high ammonia levels to glutamine in astrocytes results in increased intracellular osmolality and cerebral edema. Given the extremely high mortality rate associated with the development of cerebral edema, it is prudent to aggressively manage this pathology. There is a step-wise approach in the management of intracranial hypertension which starts with head of bed elevation, and securing airways should always take priority and starting the patient on sedation could help controlling ICP. In liver failure patients, midazolam, which through multiple CYP pathways, will accumulate and cause complications. Propofol might be a safer option; however, it is thoroughly studied in this cohort of patients.

The use of hyperosmolar therapy (mannitol and hypertonic saline) for increased ICP in acute liver failure is extrapolated from its use in head trauma. Smaller studies showed that hypertonic saline helps reducing ICP when was used in patients with grade III and IV hepatic encephalopathy and mannitol helps reducing cerebral edema and improves survival in patients with fulminant hepatic failure.

Overall, the common practice is to place an intracranial monitor to best manage these patients. However, given the possibly underlying coagulopathy in these patients, hemorrhages related to ICP monitor placement can be catastrophic and may add to the overall mortality. Smaller studies showed that epidural catheters have lower hemorrhage rates and precision relative to subdural bolts and intraparenchymal catheters.

Regarding other ICP management options, hyperventilation is a temporizing measure which can result in lowered ICP but prolonged hyperventilation carries a serious risk of significant reduction in cerebral blood flow (CBF) and cerebral ischemia.

Although transplantation can be potentially considered, treating intracranial hypertension at this point takes priority.

## References

1. Cordoba J, Blei AT. Cerebral edema and intracranial pressure monitoring. *Liver Transplant Surg*. 1995;1:187-194.
2. Conn HO. Hyperammonemia and intracranial hypertension: lying in wait for patients with hepatic disorders. *Am J Gasteroenterol*. 2000;95:814-816.
3. Rossi S, Buzzi F, Paparella A, et al. Complications and safety associated with ICP monitoring: a study of 542 patients. *Acta Neurochir Suppl*. 1998;71:91-93.
4. Karvellas CJ, Fix OK, Battenhouse H, et al. Outcomes and complications of intracranial pressure monitoring in acute liver failure: a retrospective cohort study. *Crit Care Med*. 2014;42:1157-1167.
5. Amarapurkar DN. Prescribing medications in patients with decompensated liver cirrhosis. *Int J of Hepatology*. 2011;2011:5.

## 5. Correct Answer: D

### Rationale:

An external ventricular drain is a soft catheter than can be placed within the ventricular system of the brain for management of elevated intracranial pressure and both communicating and noncommunicating hydrocephalus by means of allowing for diversion of cerebrospinal fluid and potentially clearing the obstructive fluid like blood and pus. The above wave is a normal waveform that is produced during a normal cardiac cycle. The first peak found in the wave is P1 or percussion wave; it correlates with the arterial pulse transmitted through the choroid plexus into the CSF. The second peak is P2, or tidal wave, which represents cerebral compliance as it correlates with arterial pulse bouncing off the brain parenchyma. The third peak is P3, or dicrotic wave; it correlates with the closure of the aortic valve. In normal ICP, P1 > P2 > P3. If P2 > P1, it is indicated that ICP is likely elevated and the intracranial compliance is likely decreased. The respiratory ICP waveform correlates with the respiratory cycle.

References

1. Cardoso ER, Rowan JO, Galbraith S. Analysis of the cerebrospinal fluid pulse wave in intracranial pressure. *J Neurosurg.* 1983;59:817-821.
2. Doyle DJ, Mark PW. Analysis of intracranial pressure. *J Clin Monit.* 1992;8:81-90.
3. Oshio K, Onodera J, Uchida M, et al. Assessment of brain compliance using ICP waveform analysis in water intoxication rat model. *Acta Neurochir Suppl.* 2013;118:219-221.
4. Kirkness CJ, Mitchell PH, Curr RL, et al. Intracranial pressure waveform analysis: clinical and research implications. *J Neurosci Nurs.* 2000;32:271-277.

**6.** Correct Answer: A

**Rationale:**

The osmolar gap estimates the unknown osmotic agent in the blood, which in this patient's case is mannitol. To calculate the osmolar gap we need to calculate the calculated osms.

$$\text{Calculated osm} = (2 \times \text{Na}) + (\text{BUN}/2.8) + (\text{Glu}/10)$$

$$\text{Osm Gap} = \text{Measured Osm} - \text{Calculated Osm}$$

Mannitol is a hypertonic solution of sugar that is used to treat cerebral edema. The medication works as an osmotic diuretic which causes large volume urinary output due to high concentrated urine within the distal collecting duct and allows for extraction of extracellular fluid into the bloodstream due to the osmotic gradient between the intravascular and extravascular, extracellular compartment. There are a number of complications that can occur with mannitol therapy including volume depletion, electrolytes imbalance such as hyponatremia, and metabolic acidosis. Acute kidney injury can also occur secondary to dehydration and mannitol accumulation. Therefore, mannitol should only be given within specific parameters including osmolar gap <12 (the gap value varies between institution). In our patient's case her osmolar gap is 0 and therefore, she should receive mannitol 0.25 to 1 g/kg every 6 to 8 hours.

References

1. Gipstein RM, Boyle JD. Hypernatremia colicationting prolonged mannitol diuresis. *N Engl J Med.* 1965;272:1116.
2. Aviram A, Pfau A, Czaczkes JW, et al. Hyperosmolality with hyponatremia caused by inappropriate administation of mannitol. *Am J Med.* 1967;42:648.
3. Dorman HR, Sondheimer JH, Cadnapaphornchai P. Mannitol-induced acute renal failure. *Medicine.* 1990;69:153.
4. Brain Trauma Foundation; American Association of Neurological Surgeons; Congress of Neurological Surgeons. Guidelines for the management of severe traumatic brain injury. *J Neurotrauma.* 2007;24(suppl 1):1-106.

**7.** Correct Answer: B

**Rationale:**

There have been a number of trials that have evaluated hemicraniectomy with durotomy for malignant MCA ischemic strokes: DESTINY, DECIMAL, DECIMAL 2, and HAMLET. The trials involved a total of 314 patients and demonstrated a decrease in mortality from 71% to 30% (odds ratio 0.19) with number needed to treat 2.4. With the pooled data there was increase in patients with slight disability and increase in moderate to severe disability which outweighed the slight disability improvement.

Treatment choice should not depend on hemispheric involvement. Mortality, functional outcome, and quality of life do not seem to depend on the dominate hemisphere involved. Rather, neuropscholoigcal defects seen in patients with infarcts in the nondominant hemisphere may be as disabling as language deficits. The surgical procedure involves removal of a generous bone flap and durotomy which has been demonstrated to provide further decrease in intracerebral pressure and is not associated with increased complications.

References

1. Vahedi K, Vicaut E, Mateo J, et al. Sequential-design, multicenter, randomized, controlled trial of early decompressive craniotomy in malignant middle cerebral artery infarction (DECIMAL trial). *Stroke.* 2007;38:2506-2517.
2. Frank JL, Schumm LP, Wroblewski K, et al. Hemicraniectomy and durotomy upon deterioration from infarction-related swelling trial: randomized pilot clinical trial. *Stroke.* 2014;45:781-787.
3. Juttler E, Schwab S, Schmiedek P, et al. Decompressive surgery for the treatment of malignant infarction of the middle cerebral artery (DESTINY): a randomized, controlled trial. *Stroke.* 2007;38:2518-2525.
4. Hofmeijer J, Kappelle LJ, Algra A, et al. Surgical decompression for space-occupying cerebral infarction (the hemicraniectomy after middle cerebral artery infarction with life-threatening edema trial [HAMLET]): a multicenter, open, randomized trial. *Lancet Neurol.* 2009;8:326-333.
5. Juttler E, Bösel J, Amiri H, et al. DESTINY II: DEcompressive Surgery for the Treatment of malignant INfarction in the middle cerebral arterY II. *Int J Stroke.* 2011;6:79-86.
6. Staykov D, Gupta R. Topical revie imaging: hemicraniectomy in malignant middle cerebral artery infarction. *Stroke.* 2011;42:513-516.
7. Hutchinson P, Timofeev I, Kirkpatrick P. Surgery for brain edema. *Neurosurg Focus.* 2007;15:E14.
8. Schneck MJ, Origitano TC. Hemicraniectomy and durotomy for malignant middle cerebral artery infarction. *Neurol Clinics.* 2007;24:715-727.

# 6

# NEUROTRAUMA

David P. Lerner, Anand Venkatraman, and Saef Izzy

1. A 15-year-old boy was struck by a car traveling 35 miles per hour and was thrown 15 feet. He was unresponsive and posturing upon arrival. He was intubated without use of paralytic or anesthetic agents. His examination prior to intubation was Glascow Coma Scale (GCS) 3 with reactive pupils at 4 mm. Following intubation and trauma screen, he was taken to CT scan, which demonstrated diffuse subarachnoid hemorrhage (SAH) and diffuse cerebral edema. He was admitted to the neurocritical care unit for ongoing management. Ten days into his hospital course, he was noted to have events of tachycardia, extensor posturing, and tachypnea in the setting of being bathed. Which of the following is true regarding his likely diagnosis?

   A. Start antiepileptic medications to better control seizure activities.
   B. The most common cause of this disease is traumatic brain injury (TBI).
   C. The pathophysiology of this disease results from basal ganglia or thalamic synchronous neuronal firing.
   D. The patient's age is not associated with this disease process.

2. A 73-year-old female with hypertension, hyperlipedemia, and atrial fibrillation on oral anticoagulation with coumadin sustained a mechanical fall backwards and hit the right posterior aspect of her head. Following the fall, there was no loss of consciousness. On initial arrival to the emergency department (ED), she was interactive, but over the course of 30 minutes, she had neurologic deterioration with loss of spontaneous movement on the left side and multiple episodes of emesis and was intubated for airway protection. A head CT was completed at that time and is shown below. Her labs are remarkable for an elevated international normalized ratio (INR) of 2.1, Cr 1.4. Vitals are remarkable for blood pressure (BP) 126/88 mm Hg, pulse 80 but irregular. What is the age of the hemorrhage that is present on the noncontrast head CT?

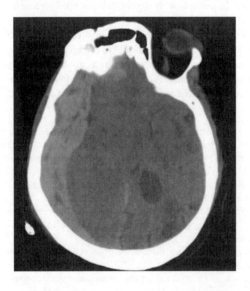

A. There is only acute subdural hemorrhage.
B. There is mixed acute and subacute subdural hemorrhage.
C. There is mixed acute and chronic subdural hemorrhage.
D. There is only chronic subdural hemorrhage.
E. There is only acute epidural hemorrhage.

3. A 45-year-old female was riding her bicycle when she was struck by a car. She suffered a severe TBI requiring intracranial pressure (ICP) monitoring and treatment of elevated ICP with hyperosmolar therapy. Patient's neurological status remained poor despite aggressive medical treatment, and she was eventually discharged to a skilled nursing facility following placement of a tracheostomy and gastrostomy tube. Six weeks following her initial injury, she was able to spontaneously open her eyes, track family, move all her extremities spontaneously, and reach for objects but not following commands. She had no verbal output or attempts at verbalization. Amantadine was considered by the primary team. Which of the below comments is correct?

   A. Amantadine can speed the rate of recovery.
   B. Amantadine can lower the seizure threshold and commonly results in seizures.
   C. Amantadine is the only studied pharmacologic agent in severe TBI that has shown improvement in functional outcomes.
   D. Amantadine can improve multiple behavioral domains, and the most commonly affected is vocalization.
   E. Although not fully elucidated, the mechanism by which amantadine works is through tubuloinfandibular pathway D2 receptor.

4. A 21-year-old male with no past medical history is brought in via emergency medical services (EMS) for evaluation of a gunshot wound to the head. Police and EMS were called, and he was found at the scene awake, interactive but confused. There appeared to be a left frontotemporal entry site without an exit site. His initial vital signs were heart rate 136, BP 95/54, and $SpO_2$ 98% on 2 L nasal cannula (NC). His initial examination demonstrated an uncomfortable young man oriented to person only, following simple commands with antigravity movements throughout his extremities with some decreased movement on the right homebody. A head CT was completed (see figures that follow).

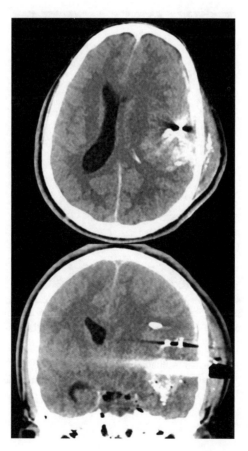

Which of these statements is most correct regarding penetrating head trauma?

**A.** Prognosis is better for penetrating head trauma than blunt head trauma.
**B.** Extensive debridement of the scalp and bony wound should be undertaken, and accessible intraparenchymal bone and bullet fragments should be removed.
**C.** Antibiotic prophylaxis with vancomycin should be started.
**D.** Retained fragments in eloquent cortex increase the risk of epilepsy following penetrating head.
**E.** The SAH demonstrated on the CT commonly leads to vasospasm and worse outcome.

**5.** A 24-year-old male was a nonhelmeted motorcyclist hit by a car. EMS arrived to find him with labored breathing and intubated him. His GCS was 6 prior to intubation: eyes did not open, incomprehensible speech, and withdrawal of all extremities to painful stimulation. On presentation to the ED, he underwent a trauma evaluation and had nondisplaced parietal bone fracture, mastoid fracture, and multiple noncongruent rib fractures. His head CT demonstrated small bifrontal and temporal lobe intraparenchymal hemorrhages, a small amount of bilateral frontal SAH, and a 2 mm right frontal subdural hemorrhage. He was admitted to the neurologic intensive care unit (ICU) where a bolt was placed, which demonstrated a normal ICP. He continued in the same comatose state for 12 hours with a repeat head CT that was stable. What is the next best test?

**A.** MRI of the brain with imaging including gradient echo sequence (GRE)
**B.** Long-term EEG monitoring (LTM)
**C.** Start hyperosmolar therapy to control pericontusional edema
**D.** Transcranial Doppler ultrasound for evaluation of possible vasospasm in the setting patient's underlying SAH

**6.** A 60-year-old male with prior deep vein thrombosis (DVT) and pulmonary embolism (PE) on therapeutic anticoagulation, hypertension, and alcohol abuse is brought to the ED after being found down at the bottom of a flight of stairs. His GCS was 6 (eyes did not open 1, no verbal output 1, withdrawal of all extremities to painful stimulation 4). Given his poor neurologic examination, he was intubated. A head CT was completed and is shown in the image that follows. His initial trauma evaluation did not demonstrate any major injury, and his vital signs are normal. What is the next best step in management of the patient?

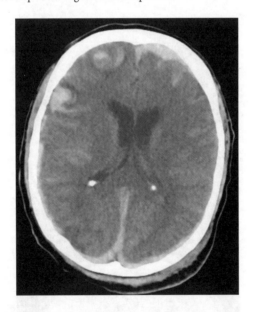

Axial noncontrast head CT. Bilateral acute subdural hemorrhage with parafalcine subdural hemorrhage. There is cortical subarachnoid hemorrhage. Bilateral right more than left frontal contusions with intraparenchymal hemorrhage.

**A.** Obtain an MRI of the brain to further evaluate the extent of TBI
**B.** Obtain a computed tomography angiography (CTA) head and neck for evaluation of potential intracranial aneurysm
**C.** Place a subdural ICP monitor
**D.** Start IV fluids with dextrose source

**7.** A 29-year-old male was riding a motorcycle and was involved in a collision with a truck. He was placed in a cervical collar, and his GCS at the site was 7 for which he was intubated. After 3 days in the ICU, he started to move all extremities to command. An MRI of the brain is obtained, and it showed scattered foci of bleeding, as follows.

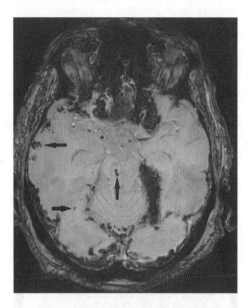

**Axial susceptibility weighted imaging (SWI) on MRI. The arrows point to areas of microhemorrhages within the brain stem and temporal lobes. There is also tentorial subdural hematoma present.**

Based on what is seen on the MRI, which of the following is true?

**A.** Immediate hemicraniectomy will reduce risk of long-term disability.
**B.** He is likely to return back to baseline and have no clinical deficits 30 days from admission.
**C.** He will likely have focal seizures after 6 months from the event.
**D.** He is likely to have cervical spinal cord injury.
**E.** The distribution of the hemorrhagic areas is helpful in determining severity of injury.

**8.** A 47-year-old female with a past medical history of diabetes mellitus and asthma fell down a flight of stairs. When EMS arrives, she is unconscious (GCS 4). She is intubated in the field and brought to the ED. In the ED, she is found to have extensor posturing. CT head is obtained and shown below:

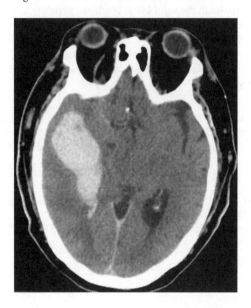

Axial noncontrast head CT. There is a large right temporal intraparenchymal hemorrhage with surrounding edema. There is mass effect with uncal herniation and compression of the midbrain and loss of the quadrageminal and ambient cisterns.

Which of the following is true about decompressive hemicraniectomy?

A. It reduces long-term disability.
B. It reduces mortality rates.
C. Smaller hemicraniectomies are preferable to larger ones.
D. The primary benefit is in reducing the risk of posttraumatic epilepsy.
E. The skull on the opposite side of the contusion must be removed to reduce contrecoup swelling.

9. A 52-year-old female is admitted to the neuro ICU after a fall down five stairs. She did not lose consciousness but was confused for several hours after the fall. She is not intubated. A CT head was obtained and demonstrated SAH overlaying the cerebral cortex.

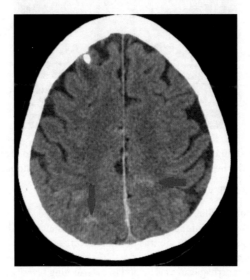

Axial noncontrast head CT. The arrows point out areas of subarachnoid hemorrhage present in the deep sulci of the bilateral frontal lobes.

Which of the following is true about this patient?

A. She is at high risk for vasospasm in the 4 to 14 days postbleed period.
B. A catheter angiogram is to be obtained within the first 48 hours to rule out vascular malformations and repeated in 1 week if the first one was negative.
C. She does not need to be worked up for polycystic kidney disease.
D. She is at high risk of ischemic stroke in the left middle cerebral artery (MCA) territory.
E. She is likely to have a coagulopathy.

10. A 47-year-old male is found to have refractory elevation in ICP following a TBI in the setting of a motor vehicle accident. His neuro examination is poor, with GCS of 5. A head CT was obtained which demonstrated signs of bilateral frontal and temporal contusions. Which of the following methods will help reduce ICP?

A. Loading with topiramate
B. Cooling to 34°C
C. Supination with flat head of the bed
D. Maintaining a serum sodium strictly less than 145 mg/dL
E. Adjusting the ventilator to target $PaCO_2$ of 35 to 40

# Chapter 6 ▪ Answers

**1.** Correct Answer: B

**Rationale:**

Paroxysmal sympathetic hyperactivity (PSH) is a syndrome associated with multiple different brain injuries, including TBI, anoxic brain injury, stroke, and autoimmune encephalitis. The prevalence of PSH has been reported in between 7.5% and 33% of patients admitted to the ICU. Risk factors associated with the development of PSH following TBI are the severity of initial injury, younger age, and male gender. The pathophysiology of PSH nor anatomic etiology is fully understood, but there is a final common pathway of imbalance of adrenergic outflow. An excitatory-inhibitory ratio model which also describes spinal cord modulation via diencephalic centers and loss of these centers into the mesencephlaom results in loss of control of allodynic inhibition. The episodes typically consist of worsening mental status, increased heart rate, BP, respiratory rate, diaphoresis, and posturing, but all do not need to be present to make the diagnosis. There is limited evidence to pharmacologic treatment of PSH, and medications currently are targeted at managing the symptoms associated with PSH and include opiates, nonselective beta-blockers, dopamine agonists, alpha 2-agonists, GABAergic agents, benzodiazepines, and muscle relaxants. There can be delay in diagnosing PSH as this can appear similar to seizures, but given the hemodynamics and posturing part of the presentation, the more likely diagnosis is PSH. There is no clear clinical seizure activity, so there is no need to start seizure treatment at this point.

References

1. Samuel S, Allison TA, Lee K, et al. Pharmacologic management of paroxysmal sympathetic hyperactivity after brain injury. *J Neurosci Nursing.* 2016;48:82-89.
2. Perkes I, Baguley IJ, Nott MT, et al. A review of paroxysmal sympathetic hyperactivity after acquired brain injury. *Ann Neurol.* 2010;68:126-135.
3. Fearnside MR, Cook RJ, McDougall P, et al. The Westmead head injury project outcome in severe head injury. A comparative analysis of pre-hospital, clinial and CT variables. *Brit J Neurosurg.* 1993;7:267-269.
4. Carmel PW. Vegetative dysfunction of the hypothalamus. *Acta Neurochirurgica.* 1985;75:113-121.
5. Choi HA, Jeon SB, Samuel S, et al. Paroxysmal sympathetic hyperactivity after acute brain injury. *Curr Neurol Neurosci Rep.* 2013;13:370
6. Baguley IJ, Nott MT, Slewa-Younan S, et al. Diagnosing dysautonomia after acute traumatic brain injury: evidence for overresponsiveness to afferent stimuli. *Arch Phys Med Rehabil.* 2009;90:580-586.

**2.** Correct Answer: A

**Rationale:**

The head CT demonstrates a large right-sided subdural hemorrhage. This blood collection accumulates in the space between the dura and arachnoid mater. This hemorrhage is not limited by the cranial sutures as is the case with an epidural hemorrhage. Subdural hemorrhages are seen in all ages, most commonly due to trauma. Subdural hemorrhages are typically formed from stretching and tearing of bridging critical veins as they cross the subdural space. In the hyperacute (first hour) phase, the hemorrhage typically will have a swirled appearance due to a mixture of clot, serum, and unclotted blood. An acute subdural hemorrhage is typically a homogenous hyperdense extra-axial collection and can have areas of unclotted blood causing mixed densities within the hemorrhage. A subacute subdural hemorhage (between day 3 and 21) will become isodense to the adjacent cortex. Lastly, a chronic subdural hemorrhage becomes hypodense and appears similar to cerebrospinal fluid (CSF) and can mimic subdural hygromas.

Although not pictured here, MRI imaging can be used to age hemorrhage.

|                      | T1         | T2     |
| -------------------- | ---------- | ------ |
| Hyperacute (4-6 h)   | Isointense | Bright |
| Acute (7-72 h)       | Isointense | Dark   |
| Subacute (4-7 d)     | Bright     | Dark   |
| Subacute 2 (1-4 wk)  | Bright     | Bright |
| Chronic (months)     | Dark       | Dark   |

## References

1. Jallo J, Loftus CM. *Neurotrauma and Critical Care of the Arin*. Thieme Medical Publication; 2009.
2. Brant WE, Helms CA. *Fundamentals of Diagnostic Radiology*. Lippincott Williams & Wilkins; 2007.
3. Atlas SW, Thulborn KR. *Intracranial Hemorrhage. Magnetic Resonance Imaging of the Brain and Spine*. 3rd ed. Philadelphia, PA: Lippincott Williams & Wilkins; 2002:773-832.

**3.** Correct Answer: A

**Rationale:**

Approximately 10% to 15% of patients with severe TBI are discharged from acute care in a vegetative state. Amantadine is a weak antagonist of the N-methyl-D-aspartate (NMDA) glutamate receptor, which increases dopamine release and blocks dopamine reuptake. The largest study of amantadine evaluated its use in the subacute setting (approximately 1-2 months following TBI) and involved 184 patients. All patients were in a minimally conscious state or vegetative state. Of those that received amantadine, the initial dose was 100 mg twice a day and could be increased to 200 mg twice a day. Those that received the medication had a more rapid improvement in the behavioral domains examined and of those the most affected was object recognition with the least affected being verbal output. At the end of the 4-week study, there was a 2 week washout phase all patients had continued improvement, but those in the placebo group had more rapid recovery and improvement to the same functional outcome. There were no differences in the number of adverse events with the medication as compared to placebo, and specifically there were two patients in the treatment and four patients in the placebo group with seizures. Although postulated in the trial, there is an uncertain mechanism of action for amantadine's activation in severe TBI. Studies have demonstrated increase in PET activity in the prefrontal cortex as well as increase in striatal D2 dopamine-receptor availability.

## References

1. Levin HS, Saydjari C, Eisenberg HM, et al. Vegetative state after closed head injury: a traumatic coma data bank report. *Arch Neurol*. 1991;48:580-585.
2. Dunn JP, Henkel JG, Gianutsos G. Pharmacological activity of amantadine: effect on N-alkyl substitution. *J Pharm Pmaracol*. 1986;38:353-356.
3. Giacino JT, Whyte J, Bagiella E, et al. Placebo-controlled trial of amantadine for severe traumatic brain injury. *N Eng J Med*. 2012;366:819-826.
4. Kraus MF, Smith GS, Butters M, et al. Effects of the dopaminergic and NMDA receptor antagonist amantadine on cognitive function, cerebral glucose metabolism and D2 receptor availability in chronic traumatic brain injury: a study using positron emission tomography (PET). *Brain Inj*. 2005;19:471-479.
5. Schnakers C, Hustinx R, Vandewalle G, et al. Measuring the effect of amantadine in chronic anoxic minimally conscious state. *J Neurol Neurosurg Psychiatry*. 2008;79:225-227

**4.** Correct Answer: D

**Rationale:**

Penetrating head trauma has limited data compared to nonpenetrating head trauma with much of the literature and treatment paradigms extrapolated from military interventions. The head CT in this case demonstrates a number of findings: retained bullet fragments in eloquent cortex, intraparenchymal bone fragments, crossing of the midline with involvement of the bilateral hemispheres, and small epidural and SAH. The prognosis from penetrating head trauma is worse than nonpenetrating head trauma. Initial evaluation of penetrating head trauma is similar to other trauma with evaluation of airway, breathing, and circulation (ABC), then a trauma assessment. There is need for careful evaluation of the entry and potential exit wound. Specific evaluation of any CSF leakage, brain parenchymal, and ongoing bleeding at these sites is crucial. A detailed neurologic examination should be completed as well. Following this neuroimaging will assist with determination of surgical planning if needed. Imaging can reveal intracranial fragments, missile tract and relationship to blood vessels, intracranial air, ventricular injury, basal ganglia and brain stem injury, basal cistern effacement, herniation, and mass effect. CT and CTA are the standard imaging modalities for penetrating brain imaging. There are high-risk vascular areas including near the Sylvian fissure, supraclinoid carotid artery, vertebrobasilar vessel, aversions signs, and major dural venous sinuses. Other common findings on imaging are the presence of blood product including within the subarachnoid space. This type of hemorrhage is due to vascular injury and although there is risk of cerebral vasospasm similar to the typical aneurysmal SAH. As is in this case, there are retained fragments, and this places the patient at higher risk for intracranial infection. There are varying treatment paradigms for prophylactic antibiotic use, but it is recommended. The common infections are skin flora including *Staphylococcus aureus*, but also gram-negative organisms can cause infection. Therefore, broad-spectrum antibiotic therapy with a cephalosporin, vancomycin, and aerobic coverage (metronidazole) is considered mainstay therapy, but the duration of therapy is quite variable from 7 to 14 days up to 6 weeks. Lastly, following penetrating head injury, it is common to have epilepsy. About 50% of penetrating TBI patients may develop epilepsy in during the 15 years post injury.

References

1. Guidelinesfor the management of penetrating brain injury. *J Trauma*. 2001;51:S3-S6.
2. Kazim SF, Shamim MS, Tahir MZ, et al. Management of penetrating brain injury. *J Emerg Trauma Shock*. 2011;4:395-402.
3. Offiah C, Twigg S. Imaging assessment of penetrating craniocerebral and spinal trauma. *Clan Radiol*. 2009;64:1146-1157.
4. Kordestani RK, Counelis GJ, McBride DQ, Martin NA. Cerebral arterial spasm after penetrating craniocerebral gunshot wounds: Transcranial Doppler and cerebral blood flow findings. *Neurosurgery*. 1997;41:351-359.
5. Bastion R, de Louvois J, Brown EM, et al. Use of antibiotics in penetrating craniocerebral injuries. Infection in neurosurgery working party of British Society for Antimicrobial Chemotherapy. *Lancet*. 2000;355:1813-1817.
6. Timken NR, Dikmen SS, Winn HR. Post-traumatic seizures. In: Eisenberg HM, Aldrich EF, eds. *Management of Head Injury*. W. B. Saunders: Philadelphia; 1991:425-435.

**5.** Correct Answer: B

**Rationale:**

Nonconvulsive status epilepticus is a common (22%) finding in severe TBI. Those who have prolonged, unexplained depressed level of consciousness within the ICU should undergo prolonged EEG monitoring for evaluation of possible nonconvulsive seizures and status epilepticus. In comatose patients, it frequently takes 24 hours of monitoring to capture the first seizure. Further prolonged EEG monitoring can still capture further electrographic seizures; however, there are no recommendations regarding the length of EEG monitoring. Patient's multicompartment contusions will make him at higher risk of seizures. The other answers may be appropriate in certain clinical settings but are not the best answers. GRE is a specific MRI sequence that evaluates for iron deposition and is related to the extent of diffuse axonal injury, which is overall helpful in guiding our outcome prognostication. Cerebral vasospasm can occur with traumatic SAH, within 48 hours of the initial head injury. The hyperacuity of the patient's current presentation is likely to exclude vasospasm. There is no clear need to start hyperosmolar therapy; patient's bolt shows normal ICPs and his repeat head CT that was stable.

References

1. Vespa PM, Nuwer MR, Nenov V, et al. Increased incidence and impact of no convulsive and convulsive seizures after traumatic brain injury as detected by continuous electroencephalographic monitoring. *J Neurosurg*. 1999;91:750-756.
2. Claassen J, Mayer SA, Kowalski RG, et al. Detection of electrographic seizures with continuous EEG monitoring in critically ill patients. *Neurology*. 2004;62:1743-1748.
3. Claassen J, Taccone FS, Horn P, et al. Recommendations on the use of EEG monitoring in critically ill patients: consensus statement from the neurointensive care section of the ESICM. *Intensive Care Med*. 2013;39:1337-1351.
4. Liu J, Kou Z, Tian Y. Diffuse axonal injury after traumatic cerebral microbleeds: an evaluation of imaging techniques. *Neural Regen Res*. 2014;9:1222-1230.

**6.** Correct Answer: C

**Rationale:**

ICP monitoring should be offered to patients with severe TBI (GCS 3-8) and an abnormal head CT (hematoma, contusion, swelling, herniation, or compressed basal cisterns) or severe TBI with normal head CT and two of the following: over 40 years of age, unilateral or bilateral motor posturing, or systolic BP <90 mm Hg. Although there is initial brain injury at the time of impact, there is significant risk for secondary injury including cerebral hypoperfusion and hypoxia. The goal of ICP monitoring is to limit hypoperfusion. The mainstay of management is appropriate cerebral perfusion pressure (calculated vale: mean arterial pressure – intracranial pressure), with values <50 associated with poor outcomes. ICP monitoring can be the first sign of worsening intracranial pathology. Although MRI can assist with prognosis, it is not necessary in the acute setting for ongoing initial management. MRI can be useful during the course of management to guide our outcome prognostication. Although the CT scan demonstrates SAH, it is caused by the trauma, and a CT angiogram is not needed at this time unless vascular injury (eg, carotid dissection) is suspected. Lastly, administration of dextrose prior to thiamine could precipitate Wernicke encephalopathy. Although extremely rare, and if the patient had hypoglycemia it should be treated prior to thiamine administration, there are reports of worsening neurologic symptoms in the setting of dextrose administration.

References

1. Brain Trauma Foundation. Guidelines for the management of severe traumatic brain injury. 3rd Edition. *J Neurotrauma*. 2017;24(S1):1-106.
2. Chambers IR, Treadwell L, Mendelow AD. The cause and incidence of secondary insults in severely het-injured adults and children. *Br J Neurosurg*. 2000;14:424-431.
3. Servadei F, Antonelli V, Giuliani G, et al. Evolving lesions in traumatic subarachnoid hemorrhage: prospect study of 110 patients with emphasis on the role of ICP monitoring. *Acta Neurochir Suppl*. 2002;81:81-82.
4. Haghbayan H, Boutin A, Laflamme M, et al. The prognostic value of magnetic resonance imaging in moderate and severe traumatic brain injury: a systematic review and meta-analysis protocol. *Cyst Rev*. 2016;19:10-21.
5. Charness ME, Simon RP, Greenberg DA. Ethanol and the nervous system. *N Engl J Med*. 1989;321:442-454.

**7.** Correct Answer: E

**Rationale:**

This patient's MRI brain demonstrates scattered foci of microbleeds following head trauma, which caused alterations in his mental status. This pattern is suggestive of diffuse axonal injury (DAI), which is a form of shear injury caused in the setting of abrupt rotational or torsional trauma to the head. DAI has been graded into three grades of severity, based on the distribution of the microbleeds on imaging. Grade I, if microbleeds are limited to the cortex; grade II, if they involve the corpus callosum as well; and grade III, if involving the brain stem. Overall, the higher grades are associated with more severe injury. However, recent studies suggest that we need to pay more attention to the location and proximity of microbleeds to the arousal nuclei as not all microbleeds in the brain stem carry the same prognostication value. There is no indication for hemicraniectomy in the management of isolated DAI, unless there is other evidence of increased ICP or underlying mass effect. Patients with DAI often have a prolonged ICU, hospital, and rehabilitation course. DAI outcome prognostication is challenging; it is unlikely that our patient will not have any clinical deficits in 30 days from admission. Seizures may happen after traumatic brain injuries, especially in the acute phase, but there is no evidence that DAI patients are more likely to have seizures several months after the injury. Cervical spinal cord injury can be seen in patients with traumatic brain injury, but in this case presentation, there is no clinical red flag to suggest spinal cord injury. Patient was able to move his extremities to commands.

### References

1. Abu Hamdeh S, Marklund N, Lannsjö M, et al. Extended anatomical grading in diffuse axonal injury using MRI: hemorrhagic lesions in the substantia nigra and mesencephalic tegmentum indicate poor long-term outcome. *J Neurotrauma*. 2017;34(2), 341-352.
2. Mesfin FB, Dulebohn SC. *Diffuse Axonal Injury (DAI) StatPearls* [Internet]: StatPearls Publishing; 2018.
3. Adams JH, Doyle D, Ford I, et al. Diffuse axonal injury in head injury: definition, diagnosis and grading. *Histopathology*. 1989;15(1), 49-59.
4. Izzy S, Mazwi NL, Martinez S, et al. Revisiting grade 3 diffuse axonal injury: not all brainstem microbleeds are prognostically equal. *Neurocritical Care*. 2017;27(2), 199-207.
5. Meythaler JM, Peduzzi JD, Eleftheriou E, et al. Current concepts: diffuse axonal injury–associated traumatic brain injury. *Arch Phys Med Rehabil*. 2001;82(10), 1461-1471.

**8.** Correct Answer: B

**Rationale:**

Decompressive hemicraniectomy is a major life-saving surgical procedure that has been shown to reduce mortality in patients with severe TBI. It helps to relieve the pressure on brain structures by removing some portions of the skull, allowing the brain to swell outward. Based on the brain trauma foundation guidelines, large decompressive hemicraniectomies are recommended over smaller ones and are generally done on the side with the large contusions. Though they have been shown to reduce mortality, they achieve this by moving more of these patients into the "disabled" category. Posttraumatic epilepsy is occasionally seen after traumatic brain injuries, but preventing future seizures is not the primary reason for performing decompressive hemicraniectomy in TBI.

### References

1. Cooper DJ, Rosenfeld JV, Murray L, et al. Decompressive craniectomy in diffuse traumatic brain injury. *N Engl J Med*. 2011;364(16), 1493-1502.
2. Hutchinson PJ, Kolias AG, Timofeev IS, et al. Trial of decompressive craniectomy for traumatic intracranial hypertension. *N Engl J Med*. 2016;375(12), 1119-1130.
3. Moon JW, Hyun DK. Decompressive craniectomy in traumatic brain injury: a review article. *Korean J Neurotrauma*. 2017;13(1):1-8.
4. Zhang D, Xue Q, Chen J, et al. Decompressive craniectomy in the management of intracranial hypertension after traumatic brain injury: a systematic review and meta-analysis. *Sci Rep*. 2017;7(1):8800.
5. Carney N, Totten AM, O'reilly C, et al. Guidelines for the management of severe traumatic brain injury. *Neurosurgery*. 2017;80(1), 6-15.

**9.** Correct Answer: C

**Rationale:**

Trauma to the head can be associated with small foci of cortical SAH. Usually these are caused by the rupture of small superficial cortical vessels. Polycystic kidney disease can be associated with berry aneurysms causing aneurysmal subarachnoid bleeds, but not with traumatic hemorrhages. Unlike aneurysmal SAH, the risk of clinically significant vasospasm is low in these superficial traumatic SAHs. While a CT angiogram is a good way to rule out underlying vascular lesions, a catheter angiogram is not usually indicated to investigate traumatic SAH unless there is a high suspicion for vasospasm or an underlying vascular abnormality. Patients with normal coagulation profiles can still have small traumatic subarachnoid bleeds following head trauma, and this in itself is not concerning for a clotting disorder. Mild trauma of this nature is not a risk factor for large territorial strokes.

### References

1. Pirson Y, Chauveau D, Torres V. Management of cerebral aneurysms in autosomal dominant polycystic kidney disease. *J Am Soc Nephrol.* 2002;13(1):269-276.
2. Paiva WS, Muniz R, Paganelli P, et al. The prognosis of the traumatic subarachnoid hemorrhage: a prospective report of 121 patients. *Int Surg.* 2010;95(2):172-176.
3. Izzy S, Muehlschlegel S. Cerebral vasospasm after aneurysmal subarachnoid hemorrhage and traumatic brain injury. *Curr Treat Options Neurol.* 2014;16(1):278.
4. Witiw CD, Byrne JP, Nassiri F, et al. Isolated traumatic subarachnoid hemorrhage: an evaluation of critical care unit admission practices and outcomes from a North American perspective. *Crit Care Med.* 2018;46(3):430-436.
5. Servadei F, Murray GD, Teasdale GM, et al. Traumatic subarachnoid hemorrhage: demographic and clinical study of 750 patients from the European brain injury consortium survey of head injuries. *Neurosurgery.* 2002;50(2):261-269.

**10.** Correct Answer: B

**Rationale:**

Elevated ICP is a common complication of acute severe TBI. There is a stepwise approach in the management of intracranial hypertension which starts with head of bed elevation, and hyperosmolar therapy (mannitol and hypertonic saline). Securing airways should always take priority and starting the patient on sedation like propofol and versed could help controlling ICP. ICP monitors should always be considered to guide treatment and provide CSF drainage if needed. If ICP remains refractory, other measures including barbiturates, to provide more sedation and reduce brain metabolism, and neuromuscular paralysis, to control shivering, should be also considered. Therapeutic hypothermia is one of the effective treatments to reduce ICP if less invasive approaches were ineffective. The effect of therapeutic hypothermia on clinical outcomes in TBI with refractory ICPs remains debated. While hyperventilation ($PaCO_2$ of 25-30) is a good way to acutely lower ICP, it should not be used for more than 30 minutes due to the risk of rebound elevation in ICP when the $PaCO_2$ is normalized. Elevated serum sodium is likely to benefit patients with elevated ICP, and therefore there is no reason to strictly maintain sodium below 145. Controlling seizures is helpful in keeping ICP low, but topiramate is rarely the agent used to control active seizure presentation. For intracranial hypertension refractory to initial medical management, CSF drainage, hypothermia, and barbiturate coma, decompressive craniectomy should be considered.

### References

1. Flynn LM, Rhodes J, Andrews PJ. Therapeutic hypothermia reduces intracranial pressure and partial brain oxygen tension in patients with severe traumatic brain injury: preliminary data from the Eurotherm3235 trial. *Ther Hypothermia Temp Manag.* 2015;5(3):143-151.
2. Andrews PJ, Sinclair HL, Rodriguez A, et al. Hypothermia for intracranial hypertension after traumatic brain injury. *N Engl J Med.* 2015;373(25):2403-2412.
3. Polderman KH, Tjong Tjin Joe R, Peerdeman SM, et al. Effects of therapeutic hypothermia on intracranial pressure and outcome in patients with severe head injury. *Intensive Care Med.* 2002;28(11):1563-1573.
4. Rangel-Castillo L, Gopinath S, Robertson CS. Management of intracranial hypertension. *Neurol Clin.* 2008;26(2):521-541.

# 7

# SPINAL CORD INJURY

Leah N. Bess and Kunal Karamchandani

1. A 27-year-old male was brought to the ICU following a motorcycle crash resulting in bilateral open femur fractures, grade IV splenic laceration, and traumatic spinal cord transection at T3. Which of the following is NOT an expected disease-related physiological change?

   A. Decreased systemic vascular resistance
   B. Hypothermia
   C. Increased vital capacity (VC)
   D. Bradycardia

2. A 17-year-old football player presents to the ED with acute onset paraplegia after colliding head-on with another player during a training session. He is awake, alert, and oriented; has stable hemodynamics; and is in no respiratory distress with an oxygen saturation of 100% on room air. Neurological examination reveals lack of sensation below T8 and muscle weakness involving all flexors and extensors. CT scan and MRI examination of the spinal cord is negative for any acute pathology. Over the course of next few hours, his motor strength starts improving. What would be the next course of treatment?

   A. Steroids
   B. EMG
   C. Operative intervention
   D. Close observation

3. Which of the following injuries is LEAST likely to result in spine instability?

   A. A 78-year-old male brought to the ED after a 70-pound box of books fell on his head at the library
   B. A 34-year-old NASCAR driver flown in as a level 1 trauma after a being involved in a head on collision at 120 miles per hour
   C. A 57-year-old female who jumped out of a 7th story window after her curling iron caught on fire and is transferred from outside hospital with bilateral calcaneus fractures
   D. A 18-year-old male involved in a car theft found to have multiple gunshot wounds to his lower back with exit wounds in close proximity to lumbar spine

4. A 88-year-old female presents to the ED after tripping over her cat and landing on her back. She sustains injury to her cervical spinal cord, which is immobilized with a cervical collar, and she is admitted to the ICU. Which of the following interventions are more likely to improve her neurological outcome?

   A. Maintaining systolic blood pressure (SBP) >120 mm Hg
   B. Administering intravenous methylprednisolone
   C. Maintaining mean arterial pressure (MAP) >85 mm Hg
   D. Maintaining her central venous pressure (CVP) > 20 cm $H_2O$
   E. None of the above

**5.** A 40-year-old male is admitted to the ICU after being stabbed in the back during a bar fight. Neurological examination reveals loss of all sensation at the T8 level, loss of proprioception and vibration below T8 on one side, and loss of pain and temperature sensation below T8 on the other side. Motor strength is impaired on the same side as loss of proprioception and vibration. Which of the following syndrome best describes the findings on neurological examination in this patient?

    **A.** Brown-Sequard syndrome (BSS)
    **B.** Central cord syndrome
    **C.** Anterior cord syndrome
    **D.** Complete spinal cord injury (SCI)

# Chapter 7 ▪ Answers

**1.** Correct Answer: C

**Rationale:**

SCI can lead to neurogenic shock, which consists of bradycardia and severe arterial hypotension. It is due to autonomic nervous system malfunction and is caused by the lack of sympathetic activity, through loss of supraspinal control and unopposed parasympathetic tone via intact vagus nerve. Lesions between T1-T4 interrupt the cardiac accelerator fibers resulting in significant bradycardia along with hypotension, decreased vascular tone, and venous pooling.

Lesions at or above T7 cause impaired functioning of intercostal muscles, which causes reduction in VC and expiratory reserve volume, leading to hypoventilation and hypoxia. Disruption of the sympathetic nervous system due to SCI also results in impaired thermoregulatory function secondary to interruption of signal transmission to the hypothalamic temperature regulating center. This leads to hypothermia, which is characteristic of neurogenic shock.

**References**

1. Krassioukov AV, Claydon VE. The clinical problems in cardiovascular control following spinal cord injury: an overview. *Prog Brain Res.* 2007;152:223-229.
2. Grigorean VT, Sandu AM, Popescu M, et al. Cardiac dysfunctions following spinal cord injury. *J Med Life.* 2009;2(2):133-145.
3. Miller RD, Miller ED, Reves JG, et al. *Anesthesia.* Vols. 297–298. 7th ed. New York, NY: Churchill Livingstone; 2009:2299.

**2.** Correct Answer: D

**Rationale:**

This patient has most likely suffered spinal cord concussion (SCC), which is a variant of mild SCI, clinically designated as transient paraplegia or neurapraxia, and characterized by variable degrees of sensory impairment and motor weakness that typically resolve within 24 to 72 hours without permanent deficits. Many patients show signs of recovery with the first few hours after injury and completely recover within 24 hours. Spinal cord injuries are classified as concussions if they met three criteria: (1) spinal trauma immediately preceded the onset of neurological deficits; (2) neurological deficits were consistent with spinal cord involvement at the level of injury; and (3) complete neurological recovery occurred within 72 hours after injury.

SCC is predominantly a sport-related injury occurring in a wide variety of contact sports in adult and pediatric athletes including wrestling, hockey, gymnastics, and diving, but most commonly in American football. Because the injury is self-resolving, no further treatment is needed. There is, however, controversy over whether players who suffer SCC have a higher likelihood of sustaining SCI in future and whether they should be cleared for return-to-play.

**References**

1. Fischer I, Haas C, Raghupathi R, Jin Y. Spinal cord concussion: studying the potential risks of repetitive injury. *Neural Regen Res.* 2016;11(1):58-60.
2. Zwimpfer TJ, Bernstein M. Spinal cord concussion. *J Neurosurg.* 1990;72(6):894-900.

**3.** Correct Answer: D

**Rationale:**

Spinal cord instability results when at least two of the three spinal columns (anterior, middle, and posterior) are disrupted. The most common mechanism of injury is blunt force involving acceleration-deceleration; these patients should be approached with a high degree of suspicion until injuries have been ruled out radiographically. Injuries to the thoracolumbar region are common in the setting of flexion forces and typically involve T11-L3. Bilateral calcaneus fractures typically result from high impact forces and are also associated with an increased incidence of spinal fractures and require a thorough thoracolumbar evaluation. In contrast to blunt spinal cord trauma, penetrating injuries are less likely to result in spinal instability and may not require placement of c-collars and immobilization. Damage caused by penetrating injuries occur at the time of the initial trauma making the risk of subsequent exacerbation less likely than with blunt spinal cord trauma.

### Reference

1. Stuke LE, Pons PT, Guy JS, Chapleau WP, Butler FK, McSwain NE. Prehospital spine immobilization for penetrating trauma–review and recommendations from the prehospital Trauma Life Support Executive Committee. *J Trauma*. 2011;71(3):763-769; discussion 769-770.

### 4. Correct Answer: C

**Rationale:**

SCI results in significant morbidity and mortality. Improving neurological recovery by reducing secondary injury is a major principle in the management of SCI. To minimize secondary injury, maintaining adequate spinal cord perfusion using blood pressure (BP) augmentation has been advocated. Spinal cord perfusion pressure (SCPP) is the difference between the diastolic blood pressure (DBP) and Intraspinal pressure (ISP) or intracranial pressure (ICP). [SCPP = DBP–ISP/ICP]. Increasing the DBP, potentially increases the SCPP, thus improving perfusion to the injured spinal cord. Current recommendations according to the guidelines of the American Association of Neurological Surgeons/Congress of Neurological Surgeons (AANS/CNS) Joint Section on Spine and Peripheral Nerves advise correcting hypotension and maintaining a MAP goal of 85 to 90 mm Hg for 7 days postinjury.

The use of methylprednisolone after acute SCI is debatable, and there is unclear evidence about the efficacy and clinical impact of methylprednisolone in recovery from SCI. Consensus statements consider methylprednisolone as a treatment option for acute SCI, but not a standard of care based on available evidence. SBP or CVP has limited impact on improving spinal cord perfusion.

### References

1. Breslin K, Agrawal D. The use of methylprednisolone in acute spinal cord injury: a review of the evidence, controversies, and recommendations. *Pediatr Emerg Care*. 2012;28(11):1238-1245.
2. Walters BC, Hadley MN, Hurlbert RJ, et al. Guidelines for the management of acute cervical spine and spinal cord injuries: 2013 update. *Neurosurgery*. 2013;60(suppl 1):82-91.
3. Saadeh YS, Smith BW, Joseph JR, et al. The impact of blood pressure management after spinal cord injury: a systematic review of the literature. *Neurosurg Focus*. 2017;43(5):E20.

### 5. Correct Answer: A

**Rationale:**

Incomplete SCI is defined as partial injury to the cord that results in varying degrees of residual sensory and motor function. The site of the injury dictates the findings on neurological examination.

BSS or lateral hemi-section syndrome represents a spinal cord hemi-section in its pure form. It involves injury to the dorsal column, corticospinal tract, and spinothalamic tract unilaterally, which results in weakness, loss of vibration, and proprioception ipsilateral to, and loss of and temperature sensation contralateral to the injury. Sensory loss of all modalities at the level of the lesion is often seen. BSS is usually secondary to penetrating SCI but can be rarely seen from transverse myelitis after influenza vaccination or a ruptured pheochromocytoma. Management is conservative with aggressive early rehabilitation. Surgical intervention is indicated in the presence of cerebrospinal fluid leak, persistent spinal cord/root compression, or progressive deterioration. BSS demonstrates a favorable prognosis compared with other types of incomplete spinal cord injuries.

Central cord syndrome is the most common of the clinical syndromes, often seen in individuals with underlying cervical spondylosis who sustain a hyperextension injury (most commonly from a fall) and may occur with or without fracture and dislocations. This clinically presents as an incomplete injury with greater weakness in the upper limbs than in the lower limbs.

The anterior cord syndrome is a relatively rare syndrome that historically has been related to a decreased or absent blood supply to the anterior two-thirds of the spinal cord. The dorsal columns are spared, but the corticospinal and spinothalamic tracts are compromised. The clinical symptoms include a loss of motor function, pain sensation, and temperature sensation at and below the injury level with preservation of light touch and joint position sense.

Complete SCI would lead to complete paralysis and absence of sensation below the level of the injury.

### References

1. Moskowitz E, Schroeppel T. Brown-Sequard syndrome. *Trauma Surg Acute Care Open*. 2018;3:e000169.
2. Kirshblum SC, Burns SP, Biering-Sorensen F, et al. International standards for neurological classification of spinal cord injury (revised 2011). *J Spinal Cord Med*. 2011;34:535-546.

# ENCEPHALOPATHY AND DELIRIUM

Alexander Nagrebetsky and Jeanine P. Wiener-Kronish

1. A 34-year-old previously healthy female was admitted to the hospital in labor. She was hypertensive on admission and complained of right upper quadrant pain. Fifteen minutes after delivery she developed a generalized onset motor seizure and was intubated and admitted to the ICU. Her seizure is MOST likely:

   A. A late initial manifestation of a preexisting epilepsy
   B. A complication of delivery before normalization of blood pressure
   C. Associated with subcortical vasogenic cerebral edema on imaging
   D. A complication of high dermatomal level of epidural analgesia/anesthesia
   E. Associated with thrombocytosis and cerebral vascular occlusion

2. A 63-year-old man with a history of hypertension controlled with three agents and type 2 diabetes treated with metformin presents with new-onset confusion, nausea, and vomiting. His daughter states that he had self-discontinued his antihypertensive medications. He is normoglycemic but hypertensive with systolic blood pressure consistently above 200 mm Hg. Brain imaging did not show evidence of acute hemorrhage or ischemic changes; chest imaging was unremarkable. Assuming that the patient's symptoms are due to hypertension, the recommended goal for blood pressure reduction during the first hour is:

   A. <140 mm Hg
   B. <160 mm Hg
   C. ≤15%
   D. ≤25%
   E. ≤40%

3. A 67-year-old man with chronic liver disease was admitted to the ICU with confusion and agitation. Laboratory studies are remarkable for hyperammonemia, serum K of 2.9 mEq/L, elevated urine leukocyte esterase, and large quantities of bacteria in urine. Which of the following interventions is LEAST likely to result in improvement of this patient's status?

   A. Diuresis with furosemide
   B. Antibiotics for urinary tract infection
   C. Late-night carbohydrate-rich meal when able to tolerate
   D. Lactulose
   E. Polyethylene glycol

4. A 69-year-old woman with type 2 diabetes has been diagnosed with diabetic nephropathy. If her disease continues to progress to end-stage kidney disease, which of the following neurologic findings is most likely to lead to initiation of renal replacement therapy in this patient.

  A. Acute-onset right hemiplegia
  B. Glove-pattern paresthesia of upper extremities
  C. Overt uremic encephalopathy presenting with seizures
  D. Memory impairment and diminished ability to concentrate
  E. Stupor progressing to coma

5. A 72-year-old man has survived a witnessed cardiac arrest with return of spontaneous circulation after 32 minutes of cardiopulmonary resuscitation. There was a delay with securing advanced airway—an emergency tracheostomy was performed 15 minutes after onset of chest compressions. He is now in the ICU 72 hours after the arrest, intubated, showing no signs of discomfort off of sedative or analgesic medications. Which of the following is MOST likely to predict an adverse clinical outcome in this patient?

  A. Plasma lactate 7 mmol/L
  B. K 6.0 mEq/L
  C. Segmental pulmonary embolus on computed tomography
  D. Urine output 0.1 mL/kg/hr
  E. Extensor response to pain

6. A 17-year-old female patient is admitted to the ICU with acute-onset right-sided hemiparesis and hemianopia. Brain imaging demonstrated parietal cortical and subcortical lesions that do not follow vascular distribution. Her laboratory workup was significant for lactic acidosis. Patient has had similar episodes in the past, occasionally associated with seizures. She has residual motor deficit at baseline and impaired cognitive function. Patient's mother states that her other daughter is suffering from a similar condition. Which of the following is MOST likely to be found during further workup?

  A. Ragged-red muscle fibers
  B. High-grade bilateral stenosis of internal carotid arteries
  C. CSF with moderately elevated protein and moderate pleocytosis
  D. Adrenal hemorrhage on computed tomography
  E. Antimitochondrial antibodies

7. Drug and alcohol withdrawal: A 72-year-old man was admitted to the ICU after surgical control of abdominal sepsis. The patient's shock has resolved, but he remains mechanically ventilated and could not be extubated because of agitation. After morning rounds a medical student approaches you and expresses concern that this patient is at high risk for ICU delirium which, in turn, increases mortality. She asks if there are any pharmacological options to address ICU delirium. Which of the following is currently recommended for prevention or treatment of ICU delirium in this patient?

  A. Haloperidol for prevention
  B. Haloperidol for treatment
  C. Risperidone for prevention
  D. Dexmedetomidine for treatment
  E. Rosuvastatin for prevention

# Chapter 8 ▪ Answers

1. Correct Answer: C

**Rationale:**
Brain imaging obtained in this patient is likely to demonstrate posterior reversible encephalopathy syndrome (PRES), which is found in most (over 90%) patients with eclampsia. Typical features of PRES on brain imaging include sub-cortical vasogenic cerebral edema, most commonly in parietal and occipital regions.

  This patient has developed severe preeclampsia antepartum. Although her blood pressure is not specified, right upper quadrant pain is a severe feature of preeclampsia. Such pain is thought to result from distension of liver capsule and may coexist with HELLP syndrome—Hemolysis, Elevated Liver enzymes, Low Platelets. A combination of hypertension and right upper quadrant pain in a parturient should prompt laboratory testing for HELLP syndrome and consideration of expedient delivery. Rapid delivery of the fetus is the definitive treatment in preeclampsia, eclampsia, and HELLP syndrome and is prioritized over blood pressure control (Answer B).

New-onset generalized motor seizure in a patient with preeclampsia suggests eclampsia. Although the majority of cases of eclampsia occur ante- or intrapartum, eclampsia may also occur postpartum. Given the clinical presentation consistent with eclampsia, it is less likely that seizures in this patient are a manifestation of epilepsy (answer A). High dermatomal level of epidural anesthesia typically presents with upper extremity weakness, respiratory failure, and circulatory shock; seizures due to cerebral hypoxia in the setting of shock and hypoventilation are possible but less likely due to absence of other indications of high level of epidural anesthesia (answer D). Thrombocytopenia, not thrombocytosis, is a component of HELLP syndrome.

### References

1. Brewer J, Owens MY, Wallace K, et al. Posterior reversible encephalopathy syndrome in 46 of 47 patients with eclampsia. *Am J Obstet Gynecol.* 2013;208:468.e1-468.e6.
2. Aagaard-Tillery KM, Belfort MA. Eclampsia: Morbidity, mortality, and management. *Clin Obstet Gynecol.* 2005;48:12-23.
3. McDermott M, Miller EC, Rundek T, et al. Preeclampsia: association with posterior reversible encephalopathy syndrome and stroke. *Stroke.* 2018;49:524-530.

---

**2.** Correct Answer: D

**Rationale:**

This patient presents with a hypertensive emergency defined as acute target organ damage in the setting of significantly elevated blood pressure: systolic blood pressure >180 mm Hg and/or diastolic blood pressure >120 mm Hg. Confusion, nausea, and vomiting suggest hypertensive encephalopathy as the most likely diagnosis.

The current American College of Cardiology/American Heart Association (ACC/AHA) guidelines from 2017 for management of hypertension in adults recommend reducing blood pressure by a maximum of 25% over the first hour. The blood pressure goal for the following 2 to 6 hours is 160/100 to 110 mm Hg. Blood pressure should be normalized over the following 24 to 48 hours. Blood pressure goals for the first hour are different in patients with severe preeclampsia or pheochromocytoma crisis (<140 mm Hg) and aortic dissection (<120 mm Hg). Of note, for patients with markedly elevated blood pressure without evidence of new, progressive, or worsening target organ damage, the JACC/AHA guidelines recommend reinstitution or intensification of oral antihypertensive drug therapy and outpatient follow-up.

### References

1. Whelton PK, Carey RM, Aronow WS, et al. 2017 ACC/AHA/AAPA/ABC/ACPM/AGS/APhA/ASH/ASPC/NMA/PCNA guideline for the prevention, detection, evaluation, and management of high blood pressure in adults: a report of the American College of Cardiology/American Heart Association Task Force on Clinical Practice Guidelines. *J Am Coll Cardiol.* 2018;71:e127-e248.
2. Johnson W, Nguyen ML, Patel R. Hypertension crisis in the emergency department. *Cardiol Clin.* 2012;30:533-543.
3. Ipek E, Oktay AA, Krim SR. Hypertensive crisis: an update on clinical approach and management. *Curr Opin Cardiol.* 2017;32:397-406.

---

**3.** Correct Answer: A

**Rationale:**

In this patient with baseline hypokalemia, diuresis with furosemide is likely to worsen encephalopathy by further decreasing serum potassium level. Hypokalemia increases production of ammonia in the kidneys and may lead to exacerbation of encephalopathy.

The 2014 Practice Guideline by the American Association for the Study of Liver Diseases and the European Association for the Study of the Liver suggests a four-pronged approach to management of patients with overt hepatic encephalopathy:

1. Initiation of care for patients with altered consciousness
2. Identification and treatment of alternative causes of altered mental status
3. Identification of precipitating factors and their correction
4. Commencement of empirical HE treatment

In this patient with altered mental status, elevated urine leukocyte esterase and large quantities of bacteria in urine, treatment of the possible urinary tract infection (Answer B) addresses both the alternative cause of altered mental status (urosepsis) and a potential precipitating factor for hepatic encephalopathy.

Nutritional management of hepatic encephalopathy in patients with cirrhosis is outlined in the 2013 Consensus of the International Society for Hepatic Encephalopathy and Nitrogen Metabolism. When patients with overt hepatic encephalopathy can tolerate oral diet, they should be encouraged to eat small meals throughout the day and a late dinner rich in complex carbohydrates (Answer C) to avoid fasting, which leads to production of glucose from amino acids and accumulation of ammonia.

Lactulose (Answer D) is a component of empirical treatment of hepatic encephalopathy. Transformation of lactulose by colonic flora lowers colonic pH which favors transformation of absorbable ammonia to nonabsorbable ammonium and decreases plasma levels of ammonia. Polyethylene glycol (Answer E) may be utilized for treatment of hepatic encephalopathy. The proposed mechanism of effect is excretion of ammonia in stool. One study (Rahimi et al. 2014) suggested that polyethylene glycol may be superior to lactulose in treatment of hepatic encephalopathy.

### References

1. Vilstrup H, Amodio P, Bajaj J, et al. Hepatic encephalopathy in chronic liver disease: 2014 practice guideline by the american association for the study of liver diseases and the european association for the study of the liver. *Hepatology*. 2014;60:715-735.
2. Amodio P, Bemeur C, Butterworth R, et al. The nutritional management of hepatic encephalopathy in patients with cirrhosis: International society for hepatic encephalopathy and nitrogen metabolism consensus. *Hepatology*. 2013;58:325-336.
3. Rahimi RS, Singal AG, Cuthbert JA, et al. Lactulose vs polyethylene glycol 3350–electrolyte solution for treatment of overt hepatic encephalopathy: the HELP randomized clinical trial. *JAMA Intern Med*. 2014;174:1727-1733.

## 4. Correct Answer: D

**Rationale:**

In a patient with chronic kidney disease, progressive slow cognitive decline is more likely to lead to initiation of renal replacement therapy than overt uremic encephalopathy. There is a trend toward early initiation of renal replacement therapy at higher levels of kidney function, even though results of a large trial (IDEAL) did not support such an approach. Thus, chronic kidney disease patients are likely to start renal replacement therapy long before they develop life-threatening symptoms such as overt encephalopathy.

Overt uremic encephalopathy typically develops in patients with estimated glomerular filtration rate of <5 mL/min/1.73 m$^2$ and presents with severe cognitive impairment such as confusion, stupor, coma, or seizures (Answers C and E). The proposed mechanism for development of uremic seizures is activation of excitatory (NMDA) and inhibition of inhibitory (GABA) receptors.

The severity of uremic encephalopathy likely depends on the rate of renal function loss—encephalopathy may be more severe in acute kidney injury compared to chronic kidney disease. However, in patients with acute kidney injury, renal replacement therapy is likely to be initiated before development of overt encephalopathy for other clinical indications such as severe acidosis (pH < 7.1), diuresis-refractory volume overload, or hyperkalemia. Of note, a meta-analysis of studies comparing early versus late initiation of renal replacement therapy did not find the early initiation to be beneficial, although most of the included studies were described as low quality.

Answers A and B are not consistent with typical presentation of uremic encephalopathy and should not lead to initiation of renal replacement therapy.

### References

1. Stevens PE, Levin A; Kidney disease: improving global outcomes chronic kidney disease guideline development work group members. Evaluation and management of chronic kidney disease. Synopsis of the kidney disease: Improving global outcomes 2012 clinical practice guideline. *Ann Intern Med*. 2013;158:825-830.
2. Seifter JL, Samuels MA. Uremic encephalopathy and other brain disorders associated with renal failure. *Semin Neurol*. 2011;31:139-143.
3. Cooper BA, Branley P, Bulfone L, et al. A randomized, controlled trial of early versus late initiation of dialysis. *N Engl J Med*. 2010;363:609-619.

## 5. Correct Answer: E

**Rationale:**

This patient has likely suffered hypoxic-ischemic brain injury in the setting of cardiac arrest with significant duration of cerebral hypoperfusion. Despite clinical and laboratory evidence of multiorgan failure, his neurologic injury due to global cerebral ischemia is a critical predictor of severe long-term disability. The Quality Standards Subcommittee of the American Academy of Neurology has reported the following level A markers of poor prognosis when assessed 3 days after cardiopulmonary resuscitation:

- absent pupillary light response or corneal reflexes
- extensor or no motor response to pain

The duration of cardiopulmonary resuscitation >30 minutes and anoxia >10 minutes (due to delay with advanced airway) are other risk factors for unfavorable prognosis in this patient.

This patient is suffering from severe tissue hypoxia (Answer A), has signs of organ failure (Answer D) with metabolic abnormalities (Answer B). Both shock and acute renal failure decrease the accuracy of clinical examination-based prognostication in hypoxic-ischemic encephalopathy. Segmental pulmonary embolus is a less reliable predictor of adverse clinical outcome than extensor response to pain, a sign of likely severe neurologic disability.

### References

1. Wijdicks EF, Hijdra A, Young GB, et al. Practice parameter: Prediction of outcome in comatose survivors after cardiopulmonary resuscitation (an evidence-based review): report of the quality standards subcommittee of the American Academy of Neurology. *Neurology*. 2006;67:203-210.

2. Booth CM, Boone RH, Tomlinson G, et al. Is this patient dead, vegetative, or severely neurologically impaired? assessing outcome for comatose survivors of cardiac arrest. *JAMA*. 2004;291:870-879.
3. Golan E, Barrett K, Alali AS, et al. Predicting neurologic outcome after targeted temperature management for cardiac arrest: Systematic review and meta-analysis. *Crit Care Med*. 2014;42:1919-1930.
4. Berek K, Jeschow M, Aichner F. The prognostication of cerebral hypoxia after out-of-hospital cardiac arrest in adults. *Eur Neurol*. 1997;37:135-145.

## 6. Correct Answer: A

**Rationale:**

This patient is most likely suffering from the syndrome of mitochondrial encephalopathy, lactic acidosis, and stroke-like episodes (MELAS). MELAS is caused by mutations of mitochondrial DNA and is characterized by maternal pattern of inheritance and multisystem manifestations. Muscle biopsies demonstrate presence of ragged-red fibers (RRF) in areas of mitochondrial proliferation. The proposed diagnostic criteria for this relatively rare condition were based on an analysis of 69 cases and include:

"Invariant" criteria:
1. Strokelike episode before age of 40
2. Encephalopathy characterized by seizures, dementia, or both
3. Lactic acidosis, RRF, or both

Two of the following factors "secure" the diagnosis, per authors of the proposed diagnostic criteria:
1. Normal early development
2. Recurrent headache
3. Recurrent vomiting

Patients with MELAS typically develop symptoms in childhood. The neurologic component of the presentation includes strokelike episodes with hemiparesis, hemianopia, or cortical blindness. Brain imaging in MELAS patients commonly demonstrates parieto-occipital lesions in the cortex and subcortical areas that may not follow vascular pattern of distribution. The symptoms may partially resolve, but often the neurologic disability progresses with age. Seizures (generalized or focal), dementia, recurrent headaches, vomiting, and hearing loss are also common. Short stature and muscle weakness are frequently observed on physical examination.

High-grade bilateral stenosis of internal carotid arteries (Answer B) would be an unlikely explanation of the neurologic syndrome in this 17-year-old patient without known risk factors for vascular disease. Moderately elevated CSF protein with moderate pleocytosis (Answer C) and normal glucose are typical CSF findings in patients with acute viral encephalitis. This patient, however, does not have other evidence of an ongoing infectious process and has a history of chronic neurologic problems, making the diagnosis of acute encephalitis less likely. Adrenal hemorrhage (Answer D) with acute adrenal gland failure is known as Waterhouse–Friderichsen syndrome. It is typically caused by Neisseria meningitidis infection and is associated with prominent hemorrhagic rash. The patient described above does not have a rash and has no evidence of adrenal gland failure. Antimitochondrial antibodies (Answer E) are a diagnostic finding in primary biliary cirrhosis.

### References
1. Pavlakis SG, Phillips PC, DiMauro S, et al. Mitochondrial myopathy, encephalopathy, lactic acidosis, and strokelike episodes: a distinctive clinical syndrome. *Ann Neurol*. 1984;16:481-488.
2. Dashe JF, Boyer PJ. Case records of the Massachusetts General Hospital. Weekly clinicopathological exercises. Case 39-1998. A 13-year-old girl with a relapsing-remitting neurologic disorder. *N Engl J Med*. 1998;339:1914-1923.
3. Hirano M, Ricci E, Koenigsberger MR, et al. Melas: an original case and clinical criteria for diagnosis. *Neuromuscul Disord*. 1992;2:125-135.

## 7. Correct Answer: D

**Rationale:**

The only current recommendation for pharmacological treatment in delirium is for the use of dexmedetomidine in mechanically ventilated patients who cannot be extubated due to agitation. The recommendation, however, is based on a single small (n = 71) trial that demonstrated an increase in ventilator-free hours in the dexmedetomidine group compared to placebo group.

The 2018 Clinical Practice Guidelines for the Prevention and Management of Pain, Agitation/Sedation, Delirium, Immobility, and Sleep Disruption in Adult Patients in the ICU (PADIS) address pharmacologic interventions in patients with ICU delirium. All of the recommendations regarding pharmacological therapy are deemed conditional by the authors and are based on low-quality evidence.

Haloperidol (Answer A), Haloperidol (Answer A), risperidone (Answer C), and dexmedetomidine have demonstrated effectiveness in preventing delirium in low-quality clinical trials. However, PADIS guideline authors recommended against using these agents in all critically ill patients due to the lack of robust evidence of improved outcomes and potential for side effects. A study of rosuvastatin (Answer E) showed that it did not reduce delirium or cognitive impairment at 12 months. There are some studies to suggest dexmedetomidine helps in the treatment of delirium by decreasing the use of drugs that might be causing delirium, including sedatives and analgesics.

Neither haloperidol (Answer B) nor atypical antipsychotic agents are recommended as treatment for ICU delirium. Currently available evidence suggests that these agents do not reduce mortality, duration of delirium, mechanical ventilation, or ICU length of stay.

The PADIS guidelines recommend using a multicomponent nonpharmacologic intervention aimed at reducing modifiable risk factors for delirium. Existing evidence suggests that improved compliance with the ABCDEF bundle may reduce mortality.

The ABCDEF bundle includes:

- **A**wakening and **B**reathing Coordination
- **C**hoice of drugs
- **D**elirium monitoring and management
- **E**arly mobility
- **F**amily engagement

### References

1. Devlin JW, Skrobik Y, Gelinas C, et al. Clinical practice guidelines for the prevention and management of pain, Agitation/Sedation, delirium, immobility, and sleep disruption in adult patients in the ICU. *Crit Care Med*. 2018;46:e825-e873.
2. Reade MC, Eastwood GM, Bellomo R, et al. Effect of dexmedetomidine added to standard care on ventilator-free time in patients with agitated delirium: a randomized clinical trial. *JAMA*. 2016;315:1460-1468.
3. Wang W, Li HL, Wang DX, et al. Haloperidol prophylaxis decreases delirium incidence in elderly patients after noncardiac surgery: a randomized controlled trial*. *Crit Care Med*. 2012;40:731-739.
4. Su X, Meng ZT, Wu XH, et al. Dexmedetomidine for prevention of delirium in elderly patients after non-cardiac surgery: a randomised, double-blind, placebo-controlled trial. *Lancet*. 2016;388:1893-1902.
5. van den Boogaard M, Slooter AJC, Bruggemann RJM, et al. Effect of haloperidol on survival among critically ill adults with a high risk of delirium: the reduce randomized clinical trial. *JAMA*. 2018;319:680-690.
6. Needham DM, Colantuoni E, Dinglas VD, et al. Rosuvastatin versus placebo for delirium in intensive care and subsequent cognitive impairment in patients with sepsis-associated acute respiratory distress syndrome: an ancillary study to a randomised controlled trial. *Lancet Respir Med*. 2016;4:203-212.
7. Barnes-Daly MA, Phillips G, Ely EW. Improving hospital survival and reducing brain dysfunction at seven california community hospitals: implementing PAD guidelines via the ABCDEF bundle in 6,064 patients. *Crit Care Med*. 2017;45:171-178.
8. Skrobik Y, Duprey MS, Hill NS, Devlin JW. Low-dose nocturnal dexmedtomidine prevents ICU delirium. A randomized, placebo-controlled trial. *Am J Respir Crit Care Med*. 2018;197:1147-1156.

# 9

# CLINICAL SYNDROMES

Archit Sharma and Alex T Suginaka

1. You are called to evaluate a 64-year-old man who is 3 days into his postoperative course from a heart transplant. The patient's spouse is at bedside and describes 2 minutes of seizurelike activity, followed by persistent confusion. Vital signs are unremarkable, and a neurologic examination reveals left hemianopsia but otherwise no focal deficits. Reviews of basic laboratory studies from the day are also unremarkable. Magnetic resonance imaging (MRI) of the brain is obtained and resulted below.

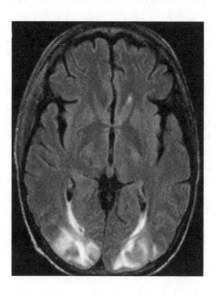

Which of the following is the most likely diagnosis?

A. Hypomagnesemia
B. Posterior reversible encephalopathy syndrome
C. Subarachnoid hemorrhage
D. Progressive multifocal leukoencephalopathy
E. Viral encephalitis

**2.** A 42-year-old woman is transferred to the intensive care unit (ICU) from the floor. The primary team was concerned about deteriorating mental status and the potential for loss of airway protection. Her records show that she was admitted two days prior with diffuse abdominal swelling. Computed tomography (CT) demonstrated ascites, as well as an ovarian mass concerning for malignancy. On initial examination, she is visibly irritable but appropriately responsive to voice. Vital signs reveal a temperature of 38.8°C, heart rate of 124 bpm, blood pressure (BP) of 135/75 mm Hg, respiratory rate (RR) of 20 breaths/min, and pulse oximetry of 98% on room air. Further history obtained from her husband reveals a 2-week history of hallucinations and lip smacking leading up to admission. She takes only sertraline for depression. Which of the following are the most appropriate next step in management?

    **A.** Baseline transthoracic echocardiogram, initiation of doxorubicin
    **B.** Therapeutic paracentesis, initiation of lactulose
    **C.** Administer haloperidol, discontinue sertraline
    **D.** Lumbar puncture, initiation of methylprednisolone

**3.** A 32-year-old man presents to the ICU after coiling of the anterior communicating artery aneurysm for subarachnoid hemorrhage. He is placed on cefazolin for external ventricular drain prophylaxis. On the sixth postoperative day he develops frequent loose stools and a temperature of 38.8°C. Which of the following is INCORRECT regarding fever?

    **A.** Early administration of acetaminophen to treat fever due to probable infection reduces the number of ICU-free days
    **B.** Fever may enhance immune cell function, inhibit pathogen growth, and increase the activity of antimicrobial drugs
    **C.** The ability to develop fever in older adults is impaired, and baseline temperature in older adults is lower than in younger adults
    **D.** For every increase of one degree above 37°C, there is a 13% increase in $O_2$ consumption
    **E.** Acetaminophen is oxidized in the brain by the p450 cytochrome system, and the oxidized form inhibits cyclooxygenase activity

**4.** A 50-year-old man was involved in a motorcycle accident over July 4th weekend. He received cardiopulmonary resuscitation (CPR) on the scene until arrival of emergency medical services, with return of spontaneous circulation in transit to the hospital. He underwent decompressive craniectomy and subdural hematoma evacuation for which he has been recovering in the intensive care unit for 2 weeks. He remains intubated and under continuous electroencephalography (EEG) monitoring. Despite being off sedative medications, he has yet to regain consciousness. The neurologist consulted is leaving for vacation and asks you to perform an examination and document an assessment for coma today. The patient intermittently opens his eyes, moves bilateral upper extremities without purpose, and has a strong cough and gag reflex. EEG demonstrates delta waves with no evidence of sleep patterns. Which of the following is the most likely diagnosis?

    **A.** A. General anesthesia
    **B.** Coma
    **C.** Brain death
    **D.** Vegetative state
    **E.** Minimally conscious state

**5.** A 71-year-old woman presents with a 2-week history of progressive numbness, tingling, and weakness in bilateral lower extremities. An MRI is obtained and reveals the findings below.

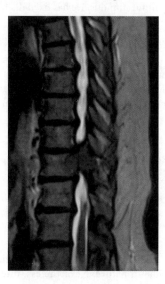

Which of the following regarding diagnosis and treatment of this lesion is TRUE?

**A.** Dexamethasone reduces neurologic impairment and spinal pain
**B.** Radiotherapy is very effective for renal, thyroid, non–small-cell lung, and gastrointestinal cancers
**C.** Surgery is contraindicated in the presence of spinal instability
**D.** CT myelography should be performed if allergy to gadolinium is present
**E.** Cervical segments are most commonly involved with cord compression due to spinal metastasis

**6.** Medical assistance is called for overhead during your flight to Hawaii. A 75-year-old man has fallen in the aisle after attempting to walk back to the restrooms. History is obtained from the son who accompanies him. He recalls a history of diabetes and hypothyroidism. The patient is returning home after visiting family and is being evaluated by a prominent dementia specialist. The son cannot name a diagnosis but remembers that a recent MRI revealed "enlarged chambers." The patient is mumbling about having successfully made it to the restroom five times during this flight. Which of the following is the most likely diagnosis?

**A.** Alcohol intoxication
**B.** Alzheimer dementia
**C.** Normal pressure hydrocephalus (NPH)
**D.** Diabetic peripheral neuropathy
**E.** Parkinson disease

**7.** A 49-year-old woman requires endotracheal intubation for declining neurologic status. Airway is secured promptly with a rapid sequence induction of ketamine 150 mg and succinylcholine 140 mg. The neurosurgeon on call is on the phone wanting an explanation of why the intracranial pressure (ICP) has elevated to 27 mm Hg. What are the anticipated physiologic effects of ketamine?

| | CEREBRAL BLOOD FLOW (CBF) | INTRACRANIAL PRESSURE (ICP) | MEAN ARTERIAL PRESSURE (MAP) |
|---|---|---|---|
| A. | Increase | No change | Increase |
| B. | Increase | Increase | Increase |
| C. | Decrease | Decrease | Decrease |
| D. | No change | Increase | No change |

8. A 34-year-old man suffers blunt head trauma during a basketball game in prison. Imaging reveals large right suboral hematoma with 8 mm midline shift. The patient is intubated; his eyes do not open to stimulus; he has no verbal response; and limbs extend to painful stimulus. He has fixed dilated pupils. Which of the following regarding uncal herniation is TRUE?

   A. The Cushing triad is often present (papilledema, hypertension, bradycardia)
   B. Contralateral pupil reactivity remains intact with midbrain involvement
   C. Pupil dilation, downward and outward eye deviation reflects ipsilateral cranial nerve III palsy
   D. Hemiplegia due to compression of spinothalamic tract in the midbrain can occur
   E. Vestibulo-ocular reflexes are absent in early transtentorial herniation

# Chapter 9 ▪ Answers

**1.** Correct Answer: B

**Rationale:**

Posterior reversible encephalopathy syndrome (PRES) is a neurological disorder that presents with a range of signs and symptoms that are reversible in nature. Nevertheless, intensive care monitoring and treatment are commonly required because of dreaded complications such as intracranial hypertension, cerebral hemorrhage, ischemia, or status epilepticus. Diagnosis is aided by the characteristic finding of vasogenic edema on neuro-imaging. Frequently, this is a symmetric distribution in the parieto-occipital regions of the brain, as seen in the fluid-attenuated inversion recovery (FLAIR) sequence above.

    PRES more commonly presents in the setting of hypertensive emergency; however, in 30% of cases, the BP is normal or only slightly elevated. Exogenic toxins can precipitate endothelial dysfunction predisposing to the syndrome. Immunosuppressive medications in the setting of solid organ transplantation and calcineurin inhibitors such as tacrolimus have been implicated in the development of PRES.

    Hypomagnesemia (A) is commonly seen in PRES; however, it is not likely to have precipitated this patient's event given normal labs. Although his presentation could be consistent with subarachnoid hemorrhage (C), the MRI does not support this diagnosis. Progressive multifocal leukoencephalopathy (D) is a rare syndrome caused by the JC virus in an immunocompromised patient, where MRI may reveal diffuse areas of white matter demyelination. This would be a less likely etiology in the immediate postoperative period. Finally, viral encephalitis (E) can also produce demyelinating lesions on MRI that are localized to different areas of the brain depending on viral etiology with herpes simplex virus (HSV) classically involving the temporal lobe. However, the clinical scenario does not suggest a viral prodrome or infectious presentation.

References
1. Gao B, Lyu C, Lerner A, et al. Controversy of posterior reversible encephalopathy syndrome: what have we learnt in the last 20 years? *J Neurol Neurosurg Psychiatry*. 2018;89:14-20.
2. Fischer M, Schmutzhard E. Posterior reversible encephalopathy syndrome. *J Neurol*. 2017;264:1608-1616.
3. Fugate JE, Rabinstein AA. Posterior reversible encephalopathy syndrome: clinical and radiological manifestations, pathophysiology, and outstanding questions. *Lancet Neurol*. 2015;14(9):914-925.

**2.** Correct Answer: D

**Rationale:**

Anti-NMDAR (NMDA receptor) encephalitis is the most common form of autoimmune encephalitis. It typically presents as a paraneoplastic syndrome with psychotic features including behavioral changes such as agitation, hallucinations, delusions, and catatonia. Patients can also develop abnormal movements of the face and limbs, speech and memory problems, reduced level of consciousness, and autonomic instability. Antibodies are formed against the glutamate NR1 subunit of NMDAR. The association with ovarian teratoma is strong with 58% of affected young women having the diagnosis. Antibodies can be detected in the cerebrospinal fluid (CSF) to make the diagnosis. Initial therapy includes systemic glucocorticoids, intravenous immunoglobulin, and plasma exchange.

    Ultimate therapy for this patient would be removal of the tumor. Although transthoracic echocardiogram would be indicated before starting doxorubicin (A) due to concerns of developing cardiomyopathy, this would not be an acute solution for a patient with psychosis. The ascites here is most likely secondary to the malignant process and not hepatic in origin (B), thus eliminating lactulose as a great treatment option. She does demonstrate features of tardive dyskinesia; however, a selective serotonin reuptake inhibitor (SSRI) such as sertraline would not contribute to this. Treatment with haloperidol (C) would likely further exacerbate symptoms of tardive dyskinesia.

References
1. Dalmau J, Graus F. Antibody-mediated encephalitis. *N Engl J Med.* 2018;378:840-851.
2. Ropper AH, Lieberman JA, First MB. Psychotic disorders. *N Engl J Med.* 2018;379(3):270-280.
3. Titulaer MJ, McCracken L, Gabilondo I, et al. Treatment and prognostic factors for long-term outcome in patients with anti-NMDA receptor encephalitis: an observational cohort study. *Lancet Neurol.* 2013;12:157-165.

**3.** Correct Answer: A

**Rationale:**

Early administration of acetaminophen to treat fever due to probable infection does not affect the number of ICU-free days. A study published in 2015 by Young et al randomized febrile ICU patients with known or suspected infection to receive 1 g intravenous acetaminophen or placebo every 6 hours until discharge, fever resolution, antibiotic discontinuation, or death. Primary outcome was ICU-free days from randomization to day 28. There was no significant difference between groups. Despite this, there is evidence to support that early treatment of fever leads to reduction of vasopressor dose and reduced mortality in septic patients requiring mechanical ventilation.

Fever has many pathophysiologic effects including increased oxygen consumption (D), enhanced immune function, increased antimicrobial activity, and decreased pathogen growth (B). Older adults have a lower baseline temperature and impaired ability to develop fever (C). Acetaminophen is the mainstay of therapy and works by inhibiting cyclooxygenase. The oxidized form is active in the brain after metabolization by the p450 system (E).

References
1. Dinarello CA. Infection, fever, and exogenous and endogenous pyrogens: some concepts have changed. *J Endotoxin Res.* 2004;10:201.
2. Flower RJ, Vane JR. Inhibition of prostaglandin synthetase in brain explains the anti-pyretic activity of paracetamol (4-acetamidophenol). *Nature.* 1972;240:410.
3. Young P, Saxena M, Bellomo R, et al. Acetaminophen for fever in critically ill patients with suspected infection. *N Engl J Med.* 2015;373:2215-2224.

**4.** Correct Answer: D

**Rationale:**

The table that follows outlines key features and differences in the stages of recovery from coma and general anesthesia.

| | EYES | MOVEMENT | VENTILATORY SUPPORT | BRAINSTEM REFLEXES | EEG |
|---|---|---|---|---|---|
| Minimally conscious state | Tracking | Purposeful | None | Present | Sleep-wake |
| Vegetative state | Cycling open/closed | Nonpurposeful | None (usually) | Present | Delta-theta |
| Coma | No | No | Mechanical | Present | Delta-theta-alpha, possibly burst |
| Brain death | No | No | Mechanical | Absent | Isoelectric |
| General anesthesia | No | No | Mechanical | Present | Range from delta to burst |

This patient demonstrates brainstem reflexes and EEG activity inconsistent with brain death (C). The presence of eye movements eliminates general anesthesia and coma (A, B). Although he is intubated, we cannot infer about ventilator dependence based on the information provided. The presence of nonpurposeful movements, coupled with the absence of sleep-wake activity on EEG, eliminates minimally conscious state as a diagnosis (E). This clinical picture is most consistent with vegetative state.

References
1. Brown EN, Lydic R, Schiff ND. General anesthesia, sleep, and coma. *N Engl J Med.* 2010;363:2638-2650.
2. Edlow BL. Giacino JT, Wu O. Functional MRI and outcome in traumatic coma. *Curr Neurol Neurosci Rep.* 2013;13(9):375.
3. Laureys S, Owen AM, Schiff ND. Brain function in coma, vegetative state, and related disorders. *Lancet Neurol.* 2004;3:537.

**5.** Correct Answer: A

**Rationale:**

Spinal metastases frequently occur in cancer and compression of the spinal cord can occur when tumor extends into the epidural space. Diagnosis is confirmed by imaging, and MRI with gadolinium is the gold standard modality with up to 100% sensitivity in detection of cord compression. When contrast is not used, tumor may still be detected (D). For patients who cannot undergo MRI, CT myelography is the next best option. Compression occurs in the thoracic, lumbar, and cervical segments in 60%, 25%, and 15% of cases, respectively (E).

Treatment of malignant cord compression is directed toward palliation and cure. Glucocorticoids have been demonstrated to reduce neurologic impairment and pain (A). Radiotherapy is a good option for hematologic tumors such as lymphoma and myeloma which are characteristically radiosensitive. On the contrary, non–small-cell lung cancer and renal, thyroid, and gastrointestinal cancers, as well as sarcoma and melanoma, are relatively radioresistant and are generally treated with surgery (B). Radiotherapy is not an effective treatment for spinal instability, thus surgical correction should be pursued (C).

References

1. Loblaw DA, Mitera G, Ford M, Laperriere NJ. A 2011 updated systematic review and clinical practice guideline for the management of malignant extradural spinal cord compression. *Int J Radiat Oncol Biol Phys*. 2012;84:312-317.
2. Ropper AE, Ropper AH. Acute spinal cord compression. *N Engl J Med*. 2017;376(14):1358-1369.
3. Switlyk MD, Hole KH, Skjeldal S, et al. MRI and neurological findings in patients with spinal metastases. *Acta Radiol*. 2012;53:1164-1172.

**6.** Correct Answer: C

**Rationale:**

Limited information is provided in the stem to make a definitive diagnosis. Key pieces include presumed dementia, gait instability, frequent urination, and an MRI suggestive of ventriculomegaly. These fit the classic triad of NPH (C). Diagnosis is usually aided by cognitive evaluation, MRI, lumbar puncture, and ruling out other causes of gait and urinary dysfunction. Peripheral neuropathy may explain gait and urinary problems with his history of diabetes but likely would not explain the MRI and cognitive findings (D). Alcohol intoxication may explain frequent trips to the restroom and an unstable gait; however, this would be an unlikely explanation for his chronic problems (A).

The differential for dementia should include Alzheimer and Parkinson disease. In fact, Alzheimer dementia is more common than NPH overall. Gait impairment and urinary incontinence can coexist in patients with Alzheimer disease; however, they are usually explained by other causes. Characteristically, dementia precedes these findings in Alzheimer disease (B). Parkinson disease can present with dementia later in the disease course. Distinguishable motor findings are typically present including tremor, bradykinesia, and rigidity but can manifest as gait instability and urinary incontinence (E). Again, the presence of ventriculomegaly makes NPH more likely than these causes of dementia.

References

1. Espay AJ, Da Prat GA, Dwivedi AK, et al. Deconstructing normal pressure hydrocephalus: ventriculomegaly as early sign of neurodegeneration. *Ann Neurol*. 2017;82:503.
2. Klassen BT, Ahlskog JE. Normal pressure hydrocephalus: how often does the diagnosis hold water? *Neurology*. 2011;77:1119-1125.
3. Nassar BR, Lippa CF. Idiopathic normal pressure hydrocephalus: a review for general practitioners. *Gerontol Geriatr Med*. 2016;2:2333721416643702.

**7.** Correct Answer: B

**Rationale:**

Ketamine is an NMDA receptor antagonist that provides dissociative effects and can be used to provide rapid anesthesia in intubation scenarios, with dosing typically 1 to 2 mg/kg IV. When used as a sole induction agent, it may increase cerebral blood flow and ICP by virtue of sympathetic stimulation (B). This effect has traditionally warranted the use of other anesthetics in patients with concern for intracranial hypertension. Sympathetic stimulation also preserves or increases mean arterial pressure following induction, provided that the patient's catecholamine stores are not depleted. Other notable effects include bronchodilation and unpleasant dreams.

References

1. Bucher J, Koyfman A. Intubation of the neurologically injured patient. *J Emerg Med*. 2015;49:920.
2. Himmelseher S, Durieux ME. Revising a dogma: ketamine for patients with neurological injury? *Anesth Analg*. 2005;101:524.
3. Miller M, Kruit N, Heldreich C, et al. Hemodynamic response after rapid sequence induction with ketamine in out-of-hospital patients at risk of shock as defined by the shock index. *Ann Emerg Med*. 2016;68:181.

**8.** Correct Answer: C

**Rationale:**

Expanding mass lesions in the brain can lead to lateral and downward displacement of the brain. Horizontal shifts of midline structures >8 mm are associated with impaired consciousness and shifts >11 mm are typically consistent with coma. In uncal herniation syndrome, lateral forces lead to asymmetric herniation of the temporal uncus. The ipsilateral oculomotor nerve (CN III) is displaced and stretched, leading to pupillary dilation, downward and outward eye deviation (C).

Subsequently, contralateral pupil reactivity may be lost with midbrain damage (B). Hemiplegia occurs with compression of the corticospinal tract, not the spinothalamic tract (D). Vestibulo-ocular reflexes are present and normal early until brainstem compression occurs (E). Clinically, these patients develop signs of elevated ICP as identified in the Cushing triad (hypertension, bradycardia, irregular respirations). Papilledema is consistent with ICP elevation but not a part of the triad (A).

References

1. Edlow JA, Rabinstein A, Traub SJ, Wijdicks EF. Diagnosis of reversible causes of coma. *Lancet.* 2014;384:2064.
2. Simonetti F, Uggetti C, Farina L, et al. Uncal displacement and intermittent third nerve compression. *Lancet.* 1993;342:1431.
3. Wijdicks EF, Giannini C. Wrong side dilated pupil. *Neurology.* 2014;82:187.

# 10

# INFLAMMATORY AND DEMYELINATING

Minh Hai Tran, Brian P. Lemkuil, and Ulrich Schmidt

1. A 21-year-old male presents to the emergency department with a history of fevers to 100.4°F, headache, nausea, and vomiting for the last 48 hours. He has a history of tonic-clonic seizures for which he takes phenytoin. He has recently started taking ibuprofen for his headaches. He has no allergies. He has not had his flu shot this year, and no one else is unwell in his family. On examination, he is lying down in a dark room and requests for you to avoid turning on the light. He is somnolent but has no focal weakness. He is unable to flex his neck without discomfort.

   The emergency room physician had empirically started ceftriaxone and vancomycin and performed a lumbar puncture with the following results.

| CSF | NORMAL RANGES | RESULTS |
| --- | --- | --- |
| Color | Clear | Clear |
| WBC | <5 cells/mm³ | 110 cells/mm³ |
| RBC | 0 cells/mm³ | 100 cells/mm³ |
| Protein | <50 mg/dL | 64 mg/dL |
| Glucose | >0.67 CSF/serum glucose ratio | 0.73 |
| Gram stain | Negative | Negative |

CSF, cerebrospinal fluid.

   What is the **MOST LIKELY** cause of his symptoms?

   A. Bacterial meningitis
   B. Recent seizure
   C. Herpes simplex virus meningitis
   D. Ibuprofen

2. A 41-year-old African American female presents with progressive left-sided upper and lower facial muscle weakness and headaches over the last 3 months. She reports polyuria and polydipsia with >10 L of urine output per day. Lumbar puncture reveals clear cerebrospinal fluid (CSF) with WBC count 22 cells/mm$^3$, protein 280 mg/dL, and glucose 25 mg/dL. The gram stain and culture were negative. A slice of her MRI brain imaging showing leptomeningeal enhancement (arrows) is shown in the following figure.

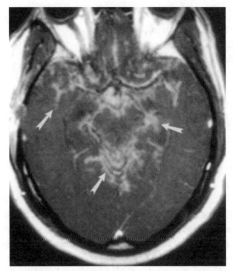

(Image courtesy of Smith JK, Matheus MG, Castillo M. Imaging Manifestations of Neurosarcoidosis. *Am J Roentgenol.* 2004;182(2):289-295.)

Which test would be **MOST LIKELY** to assist with the diagnosis of her condition?

A. Tensilon test
B. Chest computed tomography
C. Synacthen test
D. 24-hour urinary electrolytes

3. A homeless 35-year-old alcoholic male with a body mass index of 18 kg/m$^2$ is admitted for seizures, encephalopathy, and dysarthria. On presentation, he had a serum sodium of 108 mmol/L, potassium 2.4 mmol/L, chloride 98 mmol/L, alanine aminotransferase 356 IU/L, aspartate aminotransferase 450 IU/L, and gamma-glutamyl transpeptidase 1200 IU/L. He was started on lactulose, thiamine replacement, and saline infusions. CT scan of brain was unremarkable. He recovered within 36 hours, coincident with a sodium correction to 130 mmol/L. The patient then deteriorated on day 6 to a catatonic state with flaccid paralysis of all extremities. Which of the following **MOST LIKELY** caused his deterioration?

A. Administration of thiamine before glucose
B. Nonconvulsive status epilepticus
C. Aggressive nutritional support and elevated phosphate
D. Saline infusion

4. A 22-year-old Scandinavian female presents with acute symptoms of vision loss, headaches, fatigue, and leg weakness. She reports that her mother has a history of multiple sclerosis (MS). MRI demonstrates inflammatory lesions of the same age found in multiple areas. Despite various treatment modalities, the patient progressed to death 6 months later.

Which of the following MS variant diseases is **MOST** likely?

A. Balo concentric sclerosis
B. Marburg variant
C. Schilder disease
D. Devic disease

**5.** A 5-year-old male presents with irritability, ataxia, headaches, and progressive somnolence. His mother reports fevers after receiving his vaccinations for measles, mumps, and rubella, 3 weeks ago. The pediatrician is highly concerned for acute disseminated encephalomyelitis (ADEM). The mother believes that the recent vaccinations are the cause of the child's symptoms.

Which of the following statements is **LEAST** true?

**A.** The disease is typically monophasic.
**B.** Recovery can occur in 50% to 75% of cases.
**C.** Vaccines have been linked to ADEM.
**D.** First-line therapy is plasmapheresis.

# Chapter 10 ▪ Answers

**1.** Correct Answer: C

**Rationale:**

Aseptic meningitis refers to the patient population that have negative CSF gram stain and cultures but laboratory and clinical evidence of meningeal irritation. The most common causes are the enteroviruses such as coxsackie virus and echovirus. Additional etiologies form a fairly extensive list which includes other infections (mycobacteria, fungi, spirochetes), parameningeal infections (HIV, herpes simplex, varicella zoster, Epstein-Barr virus, cytomegalovirus, human herpes virus-6, and adenoviruses), medications (ibuprofen), and malignancies (lymphoma).

CSF from bacterial meningitis would have positive gram stains, greatly elevated WBCs >150 cells/mm$^3$, high protein, and reduced glucose levels. Seizures may be associated with CSF pleocytosis and transiently elevated CSF protein levels, however, the clinical presentation does not fit this. Drug-induced aseptic meningitis is primarily a diagnosis of exclusion and unlikely to have elevated WBCs and RBCs. A fungal infection would be a very rare cause of aseptic meningitis in an immunocompetent individual; however, HIV testing would likely be warranted in this diagnostic workup.

## References

1. Connolly KJ, Hammer SM. The acute aseptic meningitis syndrome. *Infect Dis Clin North Am.* 1990;4(4):599.
2. Jarrin I, Sellier P, Lopes A, et al. Etiologies and management of aseptic meningitis in patients admitted to an internal medicine department. *Medicine.* 2016;95:e2372.
3. Chatzikonstantinou A, Ebert AD, Hennerici MG. Cerebrospinal fluid findings after epileptic seizures. *Epileptic Disord.* 2015;17(4):453-459.
4. Kupila L, Vuorinen T, Vainionpää R, Hukkanen V, Marttila RJ, Kotilainen P. Etiology of aseptic meningitis and encephalitis in an adult population. *Neurology.* 2006;66(1):75.

**2.** Correct Answer: B

**Rationale:**

Sarcoidosis is a rare multisystem noncaseating granulomatous disease, which affects 3 to 10 per 100 000 among Caucasians and 35 to 80 per 100 000 among African Americans. 5% to 10% of patients with systemic sarcoidosis will have neurological involvement whereas only 17% of patients will solely present with neurosarcoidosis. Any component of the central or peripheral nervous system can be affected. Cranial mononeuropathies are common, in particular, the peripheral facial nerve is affected in 25% to 50% of neurosarcoidosis cases. Neuroendocrine dysfunction may manifest as polyuria or disturbances in temperature, libido, or appetite due to hypothalamic inflammation. Diabetes insipidus may either be central from hypopituitarism or nephrogenic from activated macrophage calcitriol causing hypercalcemia. Lung parenchyma and mediastinal lymph nodes are the most common sites affected peripherally with reported involvement in 24% to 68% of individuals presenting with neurologic sarcoidosis. The diagnosis is based on clinical symptoms, CSF evidence of inflammation (pleocytosis, elevated CSF protein), and/or MRI imaging demonstrating leptomeningeal enhancement especially around the base of the brain (arrows); however, neurosarcoidosis can involve the bone, dura mater, nerve roots, and brain parenchyma. Confirmation of systemic sarcoidosis may occur either through positive histology or two indirect indicators (gallium scan imaging, chest imaging demonstrating enlarged lymphadenopathy, or elevated angiotensin-converting enzyme [ACE] levels). Corticosteroids remain the mainstay of initial treatment followed by immunomodulatory therapy.

Chest CT scan with evidence of hilar adenopathy or parenchymal changes is consistent with sarcoidosis and may also guide a tissue biopsy diagnosis, and thus is the correct answer. Tensilon test is useful in diagnosis of myasthenia gravis and is performed by administering edrophonium which prevents acetylcholine breakdown causing improvement in symptoms. Synacthen test (or cosyntropin test) uses adrenocorticotropin hormone (ACTH) to evaluate adrenal gland function. 24-hour urinary electrolytes may help confirm suspicion of diabetes insipidus but would not assist with the diagnosis of neurosarcoidosis.

### References

1. Burns TM. Neurosarcoidosis. *Arch Neurol.* 2003;60(8):1166.
2. Joseph FG, Scolding NJ. Neurosarcoidosis: a study of 30 new cases. *J Neurol Neurosurg Psychiatry.* 2009;80(3):297.
3. Stuart CA, Neelon FA, Lebovitz HE. Disordered control of thirst in hypothalamic-pituitary sarcoidosis. *N Engl J Med.* 1980;303(19):1078.
4. Smith JK, Matheus MG, Castillo M. Imaging manifestations of neurosarcoidosis. *Am J Roentgenol.* 2004;182:289-295.
5. Pawate S, Moses H, Sriram S. Presentations and outcomes of neurosarcoidosis: a study of 54 cases. *Q J Med.* 2009;102:449-460.

### 3. Correct Answer: D

**Rationale:**

Rapid correction of serum sodium with saline infusions (or hypertonic saline) in patients with chronic hyponatremia can cause central pontine myelinolysis (CPM) or osmotic demyelination syndrome. CPM was originally described in 1959 as a disease associated with malnourished alcoholics. Extrapontine myelinolysis was recognized in 1962, and the link with rapid correction of hyponatremic patients was found in 1982. It remains a rare disease with a biphasic presentation. Patients typically are encephalopathic or seizing upon presentation. Laboratory testing usually reveals profound hyponatremia (Na <120 mmol/L). The rapidity of sodium correction is thought to cause the damage to the myelin sheath. There is an initial period of symptom improvement before deterioration which may include corticobulbar fiber involvement (dysarthria and dysphagia), corticospinal tract involvement (flaccid quadriparesis followed by spasticity), and pupillary or oculomotor changes from tegmentum/pontine extension. The appearance of "locked-in syndrome" may also occur. Extrapontine involvement may be characterized by psychiatric, behavioral, parkinsonism, dystonia, catatonia, mutism, and movement disorders.

There is no absolute "safe" limit for rate of sodium correction. A 10 mmol/L rise per 24 hours was previously recommended; however, now experts recommend a correction rate of <8 mmol/L per 24 hours. Clinical improvement or stability should not be considered evidence that sodium correction has not occurred too rapidly. Clinical symptoms of CPM, which are usually irreversible, most commonly occur 2 to 6 days following rapid sodium correction.

Hypophosphatemia rather than hyperphosphatemia is the hallmark and primary etiology of refeeding syndrome that can occur in severely malnourished patients following initiation of nutritional support. Refeeding syndrome most commonly involves multiorgan dysfunction and can result in neurologic symptoms due to electrolyte abnormalities and fluid shifts. Thiamine deficiency can result in a Wernicke encephalopathy and is associated with chronic alcoholics. Clinical manifestations include encephalopathy, ataxia, and oculomotor deficits.

### References

1. Martin RJ. Central pontine and extrapontine myelinolysis: the osmotic demyelination syndromes. *J Neurol Neurosurg Psychiatry.* 2004;75(suppl 3):iii22-iii28.
2. Jonathan Graff-Radford JEF, Kaufmann TJ, Mandrekar JN, Rabinstein AA. Clinical and radiologic correlations of central pontine myelinolysis syndrome. *Mayo Clin Proc.* 2011;86:1063-1067.
3. Gautam D, Khan SA. Current concepts in pontine myelinolysis: review of literature. *Transl Biomed.* 2015;4.
4. Dhrolia MF, Akhtar SF, Ahmed E, Naqvi A, Rizvi A. Azotemia protects the brain from osmotic demyelination on rapid correction of hyponatremia. *Saudi J Kidney Dis Transpl.* 2014;25:558-566.

### 4. Correct Answer: B

**Rationale:**

MS is an autoimmune central nervous system (CNS) demyelinating disease with a prevalence of 15 to 250 per 100 000 people. It is more common in females, especially of Scandinavian descent, with increased prevalence associated with geographical latitude extremes. MS typically has a relapsing and remitting course separated in time and CNS location. A number of MS variant diseases has been described. The Marburg variant is a fulminant form of MS, typically characterized as monophasic with widespread involvement at onset with rapid progression to death usually within weeks to months. Balo concentric sclerosis is a demyelinating disease that affects the white matter of the brain involving alternating concentric rings of myelin loss and preservation. Initially the prognosis was considered similar to Marburg variant, but now there are reports of patients surviving and even having spontaneous remissions.

Neuromyelitis optica or Devic disease is a heterogenous inflammatory and demyelinating condition of the optic nerve and spinal cord. It has a relapsing and remitting course however with the discovery of a specific autoantibody NMO-IgG which targets astrocyte aquaporin-4, and it is now considered distinct from MS. Schilder disease or diffuse myelinoclastic sclerosis presents as pseudotumoral demyelinating lesions usually affecting children 5 to 14 years old. These intracranial lesions are often mistaken for tumors or abscess.

### References

1. Karussis D. The diagnosis of multiple sclerosis and the various related demyelinating syndromes: a critical review. *J Autoimmun.* 2014;48-49:134-142.
2. Karaarslan E, Altintas A, Senol U, et al. Balo's concentric sclerosis: clinical and radiologic features of five cases. *AJNR Am J Neuroradiol.* 2001;22:1362-1367.
3. Nunes JC, Radbruch H, Walz R, et al. The most fulminant course of the Marburg variant of multiple sclerosis-autopsy findings. *Mult Scler.* 2015;21:485-487.
4. Morrow MJW. Dean neuromyelitis optica. *J Neuroophthalmol.* 2012;32:154-166.
5. Garell PC, Menezes AH, Baumbach G, et al. Presentation, management and follow-up of Schilder's disease. *Pediatr Neurosurg.* 1998;29:86-91.

**5.** Correct Answer: D

**Rationale:**

ADEM which affects 0.8 per 100 000 people can clinically appear similar to other demyelinating inflammatory conditions such as MS. It is however much more common in children ages 5 to 9 years old, is typically monophasic rather than having a relapsing and remitting course (although this has rarely been reported), and is usually temporally associated with a recent infection or up to 3 months following vaccination. Decreased level of consciousness with progression to coma and death is more a hallmark of ADEM than MS. MRI may demonstrate reversible ill-defined white matter lesions of the brain and spinal cord with frequent involvement of thalami and basal ganglia. CSF may have a mild pleocytosis and elevated protein but is usually negative for oligoclonal IgG bands. Measles vaccination has been linked to ADEM. However, the incidence of postimmunization ADEM for live measles vaccine is 1 to 2 cases per million vaccinations, which is much lower than the incidence of postinfectious ADEM caused by measles infection itself (1 in 1000). Since, there is no specific biomarker for ADEM, the diagnosis is usually one of exclusion. The treatment of choice is steroids. Plasmapheresis and cytotoxic medications are used as second-line therapy. Recovery has been reported in up to 75% of patients.

### References

1. Garg RK. Acute disseminated encephalomyelitis. *Postgrad Med J.* 2003;79:11-17.
2. Pohl D, Alper G, Van Haren K, et al. Acute disseminated encephalomyelitis updates on an inflammatory CNS syndrome. *Am Acad Neurol.* 2016;87.
3. Huynh W, Cordato DJ, Kehdi E, Masters LT, Dedousis C. Post-vaccination encephalomyelitis: literature review and illustrative case. *J Clin Neurosci.* 2008;15:1315-1322.

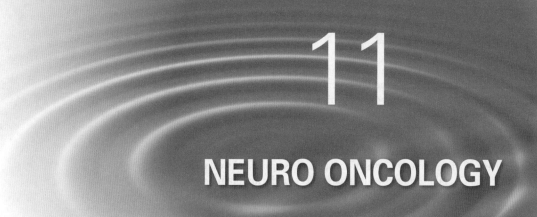

# NEURO ONCOLOGY

Milad Sharifpour and Ofer Sadan

1. A 29-year-old woman with no known past medical history is admitted to the ICU with status epilepticus. Her family reports that she complained of headaches, fevers, and myalgias that started a few days prior to presentation. On exam, you notice abnormal movements of her lips and mouth, but no evidence of seizure activity on EEG. A brain MRI is unremarkable. CSF obtained via lumbar puncture was notable for 14 WBCs, no RBC, mildly elevated protein, and normal glucose. CSF culture is negative and PCR for HSV is also negative. Anti-NMDA antibody in the CSF and serum is positive. What is the MOST appropriate next step to make a diagnosis?

   A. Repeat brain MRI to assess for progression of the disease
   B. Repeat CSF collection for cytology and flow cytometry to rule out CNS lymphoma
   C. Send serum for anti-ANA and anti-dsDNA antibodies to confirm the diagnosis of systemic lupus erythematosus (SLE)
   D. Pelvic ultrasound to rule out ovarian teratoma

2. A 52-year-old woman with past medical history of infiltrating lobular carcinoma of the breast status post left mastectomy and neoadjuvant chemotherapy is brought to the ER by her family, reporting a 3-day history of headaches, nausea, vomiting, diplopia, and a witnessed fall prior to presentation. Neurological examination is notable for medial deviation of the right eye and inability to completely close the eyes. Lumbar puncture is performed and while waiting for the results, a brain MRI is obtained, which is notable for diffuse leptomeningeal contrast enhancement of the cortical surface and the basal cisterns along the ventral surface of the brainstem. What is the CSF profile most consistent with this patient's presentation?

   A. Elevated protein, low glucose, lymphocytic pleocytosis
   B. Elevated protein, low glucose, neutrophilic pleocytosis
   C. Normal protein, normal glucose, lymphocytic pleocytosis
   D. Mildly elevated protein, normal glucose, normal WBC count

3. A 72-year-old man with past medical history of hypertension and prostate cancer status post radiation therapy is brought to ED after sustaining a witnessed mechanical fall. He denies loss of consciousness and reports that his head did not hit the floor. He reports a 3-week history of progressive lower back pain radiating down his left leg. The day before he experienced two episodes of fecal incontinence. A head CT is negative for any acute abnormalities. MRI spine shows collapsed $L_2$-$L_4$ lumbar vertebrae and a mass invading the spinal cord with surrounding vasogenic edema. What is the most appropriate next step in management?

   A. Stat consult to spine surgery for emergent surgery
   B. Stat consult to radiation oncologist for emergent radiation therapy
   C. Administer IV steroids
   D. Consult interventional radiology to obtain a biopsy

**4.** A 46-year-old patient with a history of known glioblastoma multiforme of the right temporal lobe has a witnessed seizure. He is now postical and lethargic. A head CT is performed which reveals a heterogeneous mass with hemorrhage into the tumor and a large amount of vasogenic edema leading to mass effect on the midbrain. After his postical period has resolved, which set of clinical findings would be most suggestive of uncal herniation?

A. Ipsilateral pupillary dilation, decreased level of consciousness
B. Ipsilateral pupillary dilation, decreased level of consciousness, contralateral weakness
C. Contralateral pupillary dilation, decreased level of consciousness, ipsilateral weakness
D. Ipsilateral pupillary dilation and imaging revealing mass effect on the midbrain

# Chapter 11 ▪ Answers

**1.** Correct Answer: D

**Rationale:**

The patient described has an anti-NMDA receptor antibody–mediated encephalitis. The usual presentation is subacute (3 months) progressive neurological symptoms, which could include new psychiatric symptoms, movement disorders, and new onset seizures. MRI will characteristically show T2 abnormalities, but these are not necessary for the diagnosis. Imaging is needed more for exclusion of other causes (option A is incorrect). The CSF profile could be consistent with primary CNS malignancies; however, CNS malignancies are usually accompanied by specific imaging findings, and not by a positive anti-NMDA receptor antibody (option B is incorrect). As part of the autoimmune encephalitis workup, it is important to rule out systemic autoimmune diseases. However, in this specific case, there are no other signs or symptoms of SLE, and the patient has marker for autoimmune encephalitis (option C is incorrect).

Anti-NMDA receptor encephalitis is the first specific autoantibody described for CNS paraneoplastic syndrome. The most common associated neoplasm, especially given the young age, is an ovarian teratoma (option D is correct).

References
1. Graus F, Titulaer MJ, Balu R, et al. A clinical approach to diagnosis of autoimmune encephalitis. *Lancet Neurol.* 2016;15(4):391-404.
2. Dalmau J, Gleichman AJ, Hughes EG, et al. Anti-NMDA-receptor encephalitis: case series and analysis of the effects of antibodies. *Lancet Neurol.* 2008;7(12):1091-1098.

**2.** Correct Answer: A

**Rationale:**

The patient in the aforementioned scenario is presenting with leptomeningeal carcinomatosis (LM). CSF findings are characterized by elevated protein count, low glucose count, and lymphocytic pleocytosis.

LM is defined by the spread of tumor to the arachnoid and pia mater (leptomeninges) as opposed to the dura mater and is diagnosed in 5% of patients with metastatic cancer. The most common solid tumors associated with LM are breast CA, lung CA, melanoma, and cancers of the GI tract.

Patients often present with multifocal neurological signs and symptoms, including headaches, nausea/vomiting, and neck pain or stiffness, etc., which may indicate increased intracranial pressure and/or meningeal irritation. Other symptoms may include diplopia, facial weakness, sensorineural hearing loss, and dysphagia or dysarthria, which indicate invasion of cranial nerves. Gait instability, falls, and dizziness can result from brainstem invasion.

LM is suspected in patients presenting with multilevel neurological findings and diagnosis is confirmed by brain MRI and CSF analysis. Brain MRI is notable for diffuse leptomeningeal contrast enhancement. Prominent CSF findings include elevated protein count, low glucose count, and lymphocytic pleocytosis (option A is correct). Elevated protein, low glucose, and neutrophilic pleocytosis are consistent with findings in patients with bacterial meningitis (option B is incorrect). Normal to elevated protein count, with normal glucose count, and lymphocytic pleocytosis is consistent with viral meningitis (option C is wrong). Mildly elevated protein, normal glucose, and normal WBC count is consistent with CSF finding in patients with multiple sclerosis (option D is wrong).

References
1. Grossman SA, Krabak MJ. Leptomeningeal carcinomatosis. *Cancer Treat Rev.* 2009;25(2):103-119.
2. Kaplan GJ, DeSouza TG, Farkash A, et al. Leptomeningeal metastases: comparison of clinical features and laboratory data of solid tumors, lymphomas, and leukemias. *J Neurooncol.* 1990;9:225.
3. Seehusen DA, Reeves MM, Fomin DA. Cerebrospinal fluid analysis. *Am Fam Physician.* 2003;68(6):1103-1109.
4. Freedman MS, Thompson EJ, Deisenhammer F, et al. Recommended standard of cerebrospinal fluid analysis in the diagnosis of multiple sclerosis. A concensus statement. *Arch Neurol.* 2005;62(6):865-870.

**3.** Correct Answer: C

**Rationale:**

The patient described in the scenario above has spinal cord compression due to metastatic disease and should receive steroids. In addition, analgesics should be administered and the patient should undergo rest and appropriate immobilization to protect vulnerable spine segments from further damage.

Vertebral metastases occur in up to 3% to 5% of patients with a diagnosis of cancer and can be the presenting symptom. Back pain is the most common feature and occurs in up to 95% of the patients with metastatic spinal cord compression syndrome. It is more commonly radicular in nature but can be localized, particularly to mid- and high thoracic spinal areas. While radiation therapy and/or surgical resection are considered definitive treatment, randomized trials support the use of steroids as beneficial adjunctive therapy in patients with myelopathy from spinal cord compression while planning for definitive therapy. Steroids are contraindicated in patients who are suspected to have lymphoma as the underlying cause of spinal cord compression.

References

1. Al-Qurainy R, Collis E. Metastatic spinal cord compression: diagnosis and management. *BMJ*. 2016;353:i2539
2. Levack P, Graham J, Collie D, et al. A prospective audit of diagnosis, management and outcome of malignant spinal cord compression. *Clin Resour Audit Group*. 2001.

**4.** Correct Answer: B

**Rationale:**

Compression (torquing) of the outer fibers of third cranial nerve, compression of ipsilateral corticospinal tract, and the resulting effects on the reticular activating system define brain herniation syndrome.

Uncal herniation is a dynamic process in which the uncus or a portion of the anterior temporal lobe prolapses into the hiatus encircled by the tentorium cerebelli. As the uncus herniates into this space, it compresses the midbrain first, resulting in ipsilateral third nerve palsy. When the lesion is cortical and unilateral, pupillary abnormalities manifest on the same side as the lesion. Contralateral weakness or hemiplegia occurs secondary to transtentorial herniation.

Option C is incorrect because it represents left-sided uncal herniation or a Kernohan notch syndrome (false localizing sign) from a right-sided lesion. Imaging is not required for diagnosis of the clinical syndrome, but it does provide supporting evidence.

Cerebral herniation is a "brain code"—life-threatening neurological emergencies indicating that intracranial compliance adaptive mechanisms have been overwhelmed. Cerebral herniation is initially treated with hyperventilation and osmotherapy. Additional therapeutic measures which might be considered for this case include administration of dexamethasone for vasogenic edema, CSF drainage to reduce intracranial pressure, pharmacological reduction of cerebral metabolic rate, decompressive hemicraniectomy, and intraoperative tumor debulking.

References

1. Maramattom BV, Wijdicks EF. Uncal herniation. *Arch Neurol*. 2005;62(12):1932-1935.
2. McKenna C, Fellus J, Barrett AM. False localizing signs in traumatic brain injury. *Brain Inj*. 2009;23(7):597-601.

# 12

# ANALGESIA, SEDATION AND NEUROMUSCULAR BLOCKADE

Daniel P Walsh and Somnath Bose

1. A 76-year-old female is admitted after falling on her stairs and fracturing multiple ribs. She is transferred to the intensive care unit (ICU) for increased oxygen requirement. She reports that her pain is very severe. Her breathing is rapid and shallow. Which of the following would be the MOST effective method of controlling her pain?

   A. Intravenous narcotic patient controlled analgesia
   B. Lidocaine patch over fracture area
   C. Epidural catheter with infusion of local anesthetic
   D. Acetaminophen
   E. Lorazepam

2. A patient in your ICU has rapid deterioration of their respiratory status and needs emergent intubation. You would like to use succinylcholine for neuromuscular blockade after your induction agent. Administering succinylcholine would be most appropriate in which of the following scenarios?

   A. The patient has a family history of malignant hyperthermia
   B. The patient has septic shock complicated by anuria, metabolic acidosis, and has a potassium of 6.7 mEq/L
   C. The patient has been in the ICU for three weeks
   D. The patient was admitted to the ICU 3 hours ago immediately after sustaining severe burns to the entire lower half of body
   E. The patient has a history of a large MCA stroke with profound residual hemiparesis

3. You have just intubated a patient for respiratory failure and will be initiating a sedation regimen. Which of the following would be the LEAST preferred choice for sedation?

   A. Midazolam
   B. Propofol
   C. Fentanyl
   D. Dexmedetomidine
   E. Hydromorphone

4. Which of these nonpharmacologic analgesic adjunct interventions are NOT suggested for routine use?

   A. Massage
   B. Music
   C. Cold Therapy
   D. Relaxation Techniques
   E. Hypnosis

5. Which of the following medications is recommended to use as a sleep aid for ICU patients?

   A. Melatonin
   B. Dexmedetomidine
   C. Propofol
   D. Midazolam
   E. None of the above

6. Which of the following neuromuscular blocking drugs do not depend on hepatic or renal function for clearance?

   A. Rocuronium
   B. Cisatracurium
   C. Vecuronium
   D. Pancuronium

7. Which of the statements is true regarding the choice of pharmacological agents for treatment of hypo- or hyperactive delirium in patients presenting with respiratory failure or shock?

   A. Use of Haloperidol is associated with shorter duration of delirium when compared with placebo
   B. Use of Ziprasidone is associated with shorter duration of delirium when compared with placebo
   C. Use of Haloperidol is associated with shorter duration of delirium when compared with Ziprasidone
   D. The use of either Haloperidol or Ziprasidone does not result in shorter duration of mechanical ventilation when compared to placebo

8. Sugammadex has the HIGHEST affinity for which of the following neuromuscular blocking agents?

   A. Rocuronium
   B. Mivacuriam
   C. Vecuronium
   D. Cisatracurium
   E. Atracurium

9. Which of the following would be the LEAST useful to use as an analgesic adjunct with the goal of reducing opioid consumption in the ICU?

   A. Dexmedetomidine
   B. Ketamine
   C. Acetaminophen
   D. Midazolam
   E. Gabapentin

10. Which of the following medications has the HIGHEST increase in context-sensitive half-life during a prolonged infusion?

    A. Ketamine
    B. Midazolam
    C. Propofol
    D. Dexmedetomidine
    E. Fentanyl

# Chapter 12 ▪ Answers

1. Correct Answer: C

   **Rationale:**
   Although epidural anesthesia has not definitively been shown to decrease mortality, pulmonary complications, or length of stay in patients with rib fractures, it has been shown to provide superior subjective pain control compared to intravenous narcotics. Lorazepam has no analgesic properties. Lidocaine patches and acetaminophen are good analgesia adjunctive therapies but would not be adequate to control this patient's pain when used as a primary agent.

Reference

1. Galvagno SM, Smith CE, Varon AJ, et al. Pain management for blunt thoracic trauma: A joint practice management guideline from the Eastern Association for the Surgery of Trauma and Trauma Anesthesiology Society. *J Trauma Acute Care Surg.* 2016;81(5):936-951.

---

**2.** Correct Answer: D

**Rationale:**

Succinylcholine can trigger malignant hyperthermia and thus contraindicated in patients with suspicion of or known history of malignant hyperthermia. Succinylcholine briefly but routinely increases potassium by 0.5 mEq/L after administration; it is therefore contraindicated in patients with concerningly high baseline potassium levels. The release of potassium can be unpredictably large in patients with upregulation of nicotinic acetylcholine receptors. Examples of conditions in which this can happen are patients with burns, stroke, prolonged immobility, or Guillain-Barré syndrome. It is considered safe to administer succinylcholine within 24 hours (possibly up to 48-72 hours) of these conditions; however, as it takes time for upregulation of the receptors. It is harder to quantify the extent of immobility in a long-term intensive care patient; one study suggests that after 16 days of ICU stay, the risk for greater hyperkalemic response increases markedly.

References

1. Miller RD. *Miller's Anesthesia.* 8th ed.; San Diego: Churchil Livingstone; Chap 29
2. Blanié A, Ract C, Leblanc PE, et al. The limits of succinylcholine for critically ill patients. *Anesth Analg.* 2012;115(4):873-879.

---

**3.** Correct Answer: A

**Rationale:**

The 2018 Society for Critical Care Medicine Clinical Practice Guidelines for management for pain and agitation/sedation recommend propofol or dexmedetomidine over benzodiazepines for sedation for shorter duration of mechanical ventilation. Benzodiazepine-based sedation regimens are strongly associated with ICU delirium and thus are the least preferred choice. The guidelines also recommend a protocol-based pain assessment for treating pain before assessing the need for sedation.

Reference

1. Devlin JW, Skrobik Y, Gélinas C, et al. Clinical practice guidelines for the prevention and management of pain, agitation/sedation, delirium, immobility, and sleep disruption in adult patients in the ICU. *Crit Care Med.* 2018;46(9):e825-e873.

---

**4.** Correct Answer: E

**Rationale:**

The 2018 Society for Critical Care Medicine Clinical Practice guidelines for pain and agitation/sedation suggest using music, massage, cold therapy, and relaxation techniques as nonpharmacologic adjuncts for reducing pain but do not suggest offering hypnosis.

Reference

1. Devlin JW, Skrobik Y, Gélinas C, et al. Clinical practice guidelines for the prevention and management of pain, agitation/sedation, delirium, immobility, and sleep disruption in adult patients in the ICU. *Crit Care Med.* 2018;46(9):e825-e873.

---

**5.** Correct Answer: E

**Rationale:**

The 2018 Society for Critical Care Medicine Clinical Practice guidelines for pain and agitation/sedation, delirium, and sleep do not suggest using any medications for sleep. The guidelines state there is currently insufficient evidence to recommend any medications to promote sleep in critically ill patients. There is low-quality evidence to suggest melatonin is helpful for improving sleep in critically ill patients. Although melatonin has a low side effect profile, there is no recommendation for or against its use as the current evidence is of very low quality. The guidelines do not suggest using propofol solely to improve sleep. Dexmedetomidine increases stage 2 sleep in critically ill patients but has not demonstrated reduction in sleep fragmentation, or an increase in deep or REM sleep. So, the guidelines do not recommend dexmedetomidine to promote sleep.

Reference

1. Devlin JW, Skrobik Y, Gélinas C, et al. Clinical practice guidelines for the prevention and management of pain, agitation/sedation, delirium, immobility, and sleep disruption in adult patients in the ICU. *Crit Care Med.* 2018;46(9):e825-e873

**6.** Correct Answer: B

**Rationale:**

Cisatracurium (and certain other benzylisoquinolinium derivatives such as atracurium and mivacurium) does not depend on renal or hepatic function for its metabolism. More than 75% of cisatracurium undergoes spontaneous degradation via Hofmann elimination. Atracurium undergoes both Hofmann degradation and ester hydrolysis by nonspecific esterases. However, alterations in physiologic pH or temperature can affect the rate of Hofmann elimination. On the other hand, aminosteroid compounds (vecuronium, rocuronium, pancuronium, etc) have hepatic and/or renal mechanisms of elimination.

Reference

1. Miller RD. *Miller's Anesthesia*. 8th ed.; San Diego: Churchill Livingstone; 2015:Chap 29

**7.** Correct Answer: D

**Rationale:**

The recently concluded MIND-ICU trial compared Ziprasidone and Haloperidol with placebo in the treatment of hypo- or hyperactive delirium in critically ill patients on mechanical ventilation. Of the patients, 90% had hypoactive delirium. There was no difference between the groups with regard to primary end points of delirium-free days. Secondary analyses revealed no difference between groups with regard to duration of mechanical ventilation, 30 or 90 day mortality, oversedation, or days to ICU discharge. Overall choice of antipsychotics Haloperidol or Ziprasidone did not improve outcomes when compared to placebo.

Reference

1. Girard TD, Exline MC, Carson SS, et al. Haloperidol and ziprasidone for treatment of delirium in critical illness. *N Engl J Med*. 2018;379:2506-2516

**8.** Correct Answer: A

**Rationale:**

Sugammadex binds aminosteroid neuromuscular blocking drugs such as rocuronium and vecuronium causing a quick reversal of their effects. Sugammadex has little to no affinity for nonsteroidal neuromuscular blocking agents such as mivacurium, atracurium, and cisatracurium. Although sugammadex does have significant affinity for vecuronium, it has a higher affinity for rocuronium.

Reference

1. Bom A, Hope F, Rutherford S, Thomson K. Preclinical pharmacology of sugammadex. *J Crit Care*. 2009;24(1):29-35.

**9.** Correct Answer: D

**Rationale:**

Benzodiazepines do not have analgesic properties. Acetaminophen, ketamine, and dexmedetomidine have generalized analgesic effects. Gabapentin is helpful in managing neuropathic pain symptoms.

References

1. Devlin JW, Skrobik Y, Gélinas C, et al. Clinical practice guidelines for the prevention and management of pain, agitation/sedation, delirium, immobility, and sleep disruption in adult patients in the ICU. *Crit Care Med*. 2018;46(9):e825-e873.
2. Habibi V, Kiabi FH, Sharifi H. The effect of dexmedetomidine on the acute pain after cardiothoracic surgeries: a systematic review. *Braz J Cardiovasc Surg*. 2018;33(4):404-417.
3. Jessen Lundorf L, Korvenius Nedergaard H, Møller AM. Perioperative dexmedetomidine for acute pain after abdominal surgery in adults. *Cochrane Database Syst Rev*. 2016;18(2):CD0103558.

**10.** Correct Answer: E

**Rationale:**

The context sensitive half-life is the time required for blood or plasma concentrations of a drug to decrease by 50% after discontinuation of the drug administered by infusion. It factors in the effects of a prolonged infusion on half-life of a drug. In the context of continuous infusions many drugs that are short acting after a single bolus have an increase in their half-life as their volume of distribution becomes saturated. The half-life of fentanyl increases to over 300 minutes after an infusion of 5 hours. The half-life of midazolam increases to between 50 and 75 minutes after an infusion of 5 hours. The half-life of dexmedetomidine increases to around 100 minutes after an infusion of 5 hours. The half-life of propofol and ketamine both increase slightly but are around 25 minutes after an infusion of 5 hours.

References

1. Miller RD. *Miller's Anesthesia*. 8th ed.; San Diego: Churchil Livingstone; 2015:Chap 29 & 30.
2. Iirola T, Ihmsen H, Laitio R, et al. Population pharmacokinetics of dexmedetomidine during long-term sedation in intensive care patients. *Br J Anaesth*. 2012;108(3):460-468.

# 13

# NEURO MONITORING AND DIAGNOSTIC MODALITIES

David P. Lerner, Noor Abdalla, and Saef Izzy

1.  A 49-year-old female is admitted to the medical intensive care unit with sepsis due to pyelonephritis and acute kidney injury. Prior urinary tract infections have been due to extended-spectrum B-lactamase *Escherichia coli*. Her initial pertinent lab values include creatinine 1.8 mg/dL, BUN 32 mg/dL, WBC 22.4 × 10⁹/L with elevated band percentage (24%). She was resuscitated with 6 L of IV fluids and started on norepinephrine to maintain a mean arterial pressure of 65. Empiric antibiotic therapy was started with imipenem and vancomycin. Over the course of 48 hours she has improvement in her lab values and vitals and was weaned from vasoactive medications. Despite improvement in the above, she has had ongoing alteration in her level of consciousness. She underwent a prolonged EEG monitoring (see figure that follows).

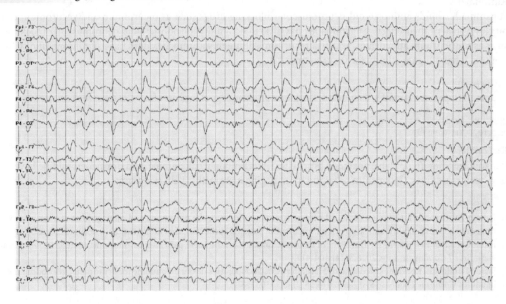

Standard 10 to 20 electrode placement. This is a standard "double banana" montage with left over right. EEG demonstrates broad, generalized periodic discharges right greater than left hemispheric involvement.

What is the next best step in management?

A.  Change of imipenem to different antibiotic given ongoing seizures
B.  Continue with supportive care and no change to medications
C.  Initiation of antiepileptic medication—levetiracetam 500 mg twice a day
D.  Benzodiazepine trial—lorazepam 1 mg IV once

2. A 36-year-old female presents with worsening dyspnea, double vision, and dysarthria over the course of the last 3 days, which was preceded by an upper respiratory tract infection that cleared without any treatment. On examination she has mild labial and palatal dysarthria, limited right eye elevation, and abduction with horizontal double vision on right lateral gaze. She is admitted to the neurology service for workup. A nerve conduction study is completed and demonstrates 50% decrement with rapid stimulation. Laboratory workup reveals positive MuSK (muscle specific kinase) antibody. What is the best treatment plan for this patient?

   **A.** Rapid therapy with IVIG and maintenance therapy with oral prednisone
   **B.** Rapid therapy with plasmapheresis and maintenance therapy with oral prednisone
   **C.** Rapid therapy with intravenous methylprednisolone and maintenance therapy with oral prednisone
   **D.** Rapid therapy with plasmapheresis and maintenance therapy with rituximab
   **E.** Rapid therapy with rituximab and maintenance therapy with rituximab

3. A 55-year-old female with lupus (on hydroxychloroquine) and hypertension was brought to the emergency department for obtundation. She was intubated in the field given agonal respirations. CT angiogram revealed diffuse subarachnoid hemorrhage and an anterior communicating artery aneurysm. The aneurysm was secured with endovascular coiling. On hospital day 8 the patient had worsening of her examination with weakness of the left face, arm, and leg, as well as mild dysarthria. Her transcranial Doppler ultrasound results are shown below. Angiography was done to evaluate for potential cerebral artery vasospasm. Mild-to-moderate right proximal anterior communicating artery vasospasm was found and treated with intra-arterial verapamil resulting in angiographic and clinical improvement of her symptoms.

| BLOOD VESSEL | TCD MEAN VELOCITY (CM/S) |
| --- | --- |
| R MCA | 63 |
| R ACA | 35 |
| R PCA | 45 |
| R vertebral | 36 |
| L MCA | 59 |
| L ACA | 49 |
| L PCA | 50 |
| L vertebral | 39 |
| Basilar | 31 |

Which of the comments is true regarding the use of transcranial Doppler ultrasound for cerebral artery vasospasm following aneurysmal subarachnoid hemorrhage?

   **A.** The most reliable blood vessels for evaluating vasospasm via transcranial Doppler ultrasound is the anterior cerebral artery and vertebral artery
   **B.** If there is vasospasm (defined as mean velocity >120 cm/s) present on transcranial Doppler, there will be clinical changes
   **C.** Lindegaard ratio can help evaluate the etiology of elevated mean velocities by comparing the middle cerebral artery and ipsilateral extracranial carotid artery velocities
   **D.** Following intra-aterial treatment with verapamil, transcranial Doppler velocities will typically increase due to hyperemia

4. A 73-year-old woman with schizophrenia on lithium was found unresponsive by her husband in the bathroom. EMS was called, and on arrival she was unresponsive, intubated in the field, and brought to the ED. Her initial vital signs were stable and within normal limits. Off sedation, her eyes remained closed, minimally reactive pupils, no corneal or cough but intact gag reflex, and no movement to painful stimulation. A head CT, and CTA head and neck were completed (see figures that follow).

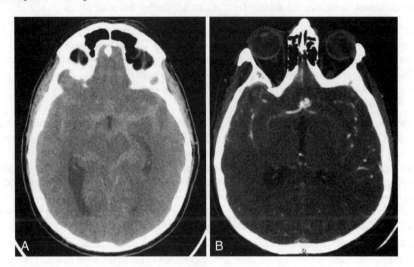

What is the patient's Hunt and Hess and modified Fisher grade?

A. Hunt and Hess score 0 and Fisher grade 1
B. Hunt and Hess score 5 and Fisher grade 4
C. Hunt and Hess score 5 and Fisher grade 3
D. Hunt and Hess score 0 and Fisher grade 4

5. A 68-year-old female is brought to the emergency department from home for increased confusion, nausea, and emesis. She was in her usual state of health until the morning of presentation. She was last known well at 9:15 AM when her husband saw her getting dressed. He heard a thud at 9:30 AM and found her on the ground in the bedroom confused. EMS was called and en route she had an episode of emesis. Her initial head CT demonstrated a cerebellar hemorrhage. A follow-up MRI was completed 5 days following admission (see figures that follow).

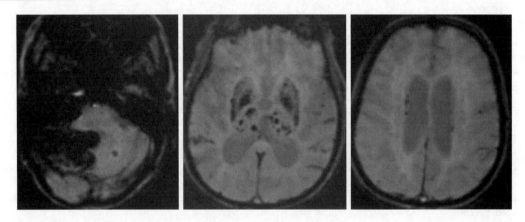

What is the most likely underlying etiology of her intraparenchymal hemorrhage?

A. Cerebral amyloid angiopathy
B. Hypertensive angiopathy
C. Autoimmune vasculitis
D. Infective endocarditis

**6.** A 48-year-old male with no past medical history was lifting weights at the gym when he felt a "pop" in the back of his head immediately followed by a 10/10 holocephalic headache. He was nauseated and had one episode of emesis but retained normal consciousness. He was brought to the emergency department via EMS, and on arrival his vitals were within normal limits. His neurologic examination was normal with the exception of nuchal rigidity. A head CT was completed shortly after arrival. The only abnormalities demonstrated on the head CT are shown in the figure that follows. A CTA was completed which was negative for an aneurysm or vascular malformation.

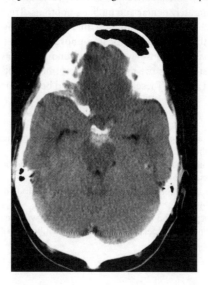

Which of the following is consistent with findings presented?

**A.** The location of the subarachnoid hemorrhage is more likely associated with an aneurysm than basilar subarachnoid hemorrhage

**B.** This particular subarachnoid hemorrhage most commonly results in hydrocephalus due to obstruction of the foramen of Magendie and Luschka

**C.** The location of this subarachnoid hemorrhage is thought to be due to venous hemorrhage rather than arterial hemorrhage

**D.** Because the CT angiogram was negative, there is no need for a digital subtraction angiogram

# Chapter 13 ■ Answers

**1.** Correct Answer: D

**Rationale:**
The EEG above demonstrates triphasic waves. The triphasic wave has a high-amplitude (>70 microV), positive transient followed by a negative deflection with an anterior-posterior gradient and anterior-posterior delay. Triphasic waves were initially described in hepatic encephalopathy but have been described in multiple metabolic derangements, and they can be associated with nonconvulsive seizures. Treatment of triphasic waves with benzodiazepine will result in improvement in the discharges, but it may not change the clinical picture of the patient. A trial of benzodiazepine might help in the diagnosis of nonconvulsive status. A positive benzodiazepine test if there is resolution of potentially ictal EEG pattern and improvement in clinical state or appearance of previously absent normal EEG pattern. If there is demonstration of the above, then treatment with an AED would be appropriate. Imipenem and other carbapenem medications have been associated with increased risk of seizures; with imipenem use, 4/1000 patients have seized.

References
1. Brigo F, Storti M. Triphasic waves. *Am J Electroneurodiagnostic Technol.* 2011;51:16-25.
2. Fountain NB, Waldman WA. Effects of benzodiazepines on triphasic waves: implications for non-convulsive status epilepticus. *J Clin Neurophysiol.* 2001;18:345-352.
3. Jirsch J, Hirsch LJ. Nonconvulsive seizures: developing a rational approach to the diagnosis and management in the critically ill population. *Clin Neurophysiol.* 2007;118:1660-1670.
4. Cannon JP, Lee TA, Clark NM, et al. The risk of seizures among the carbapenems: a meta-analysis. *J Antimicrob Chemother.* 2014;69:2043-2055.

**2.** Correct Answer: D

**Rationale:**

MuSK is a tyrosine kinase receptor found on muscle which is important in the maintenance of the neuromuscular junction. The repetitive stimulation presented in the question demonstrates the typical findings of myasthenia gravis, a decrement of >33% at 3 Hz cycling. Other findings on electrodiagnostic testing include increased jitter on single fiber electromyography. MuSK-positive myasthenia gravis can present with crisis as their initial presentation and typically have predominately ocular and bulbar symptoms. Treatment of crisis is the same as for other myasthenia gravis patients, which is initial treatment with a rapidly acting intervention, either IVIG or plasmapheresis, and concurrent or shortly after with chronic immunosuppressive therapy. MuSK positive myasthenia patients appear to have improved early response with 93% responding to plasmapheresis and only 61% responding to IVIG. Although initiation of steroids is the mainstay of treatment of other myasthenia gravis patients, MuSK antibody patients do not respond as well. These patients respond better to rituximab for chronic immunosuppressive therapy.

References

1. Hoch W, McConville J, Helms S, et al. Auto-antibodies to the receptor tyrosine kinase MuSK in patients with myasthenia gravis without acetylcholine receptor antibodies. *Nat Med.* 2001;7:365-368.
2. Schwartz MS, Stalberg E. Myasthenia gravis with features of the myasthenic syndrome. An investigation with electrophysiologic methods including single-fiber electromyography. *Neurology.* 1975;25:80-84.
3. Nuptial JT, Sanders DB, Evoli A. Anit-MuSK antibody myasthenia gravis: clinical findings and response to treatment in two large cohorts. *Muscle Nerve.* 2011;44:36-40.
4. Sanders DB, Guptill JT. Myasthenia gravis and Lambert-Eaton myasthenic syndrome. *Continuum.* 2014;20.
5. Nuptial JT, Sanders DB. Update on muscle-specific tyrosine kinase antibody positive myasthenia gravis. *Cure Opin Neurol.* 2010;23:530-535.

**3.** Correct Answer: C

**Rationale:**

Transcranial Doppler ultrasound (TCD) is a noninvasive, easily reproducible test that can be used to monitor for cerebral artery vasospasm following aneurysmal subarachnoid hemorrhage. It can be used for other disease evaluation including emboli detection, brain death evaluation, and sickle cell disease. TCD uses low-frequency (2 MHz) pulse Doppler to evaluate velocity of blood flow through the proximal intra- and extra-cranial arteries. Although a good screening tool, it has limited sensitivity (90%), specificity (70%), and positive predictive value (57%) when compared to digital subtraction angiography. Early studies using TCD evaluated the diameter of blood vessels and the mean velocity. Mean velocities >120 cm/s correlated with decrease in blood vessel diameter by 50%. The patient's transcranial Doppler ultrasounds are normal despite having angiographic and clinical vasospasm which can be seen given the sensitivity of the testing. More importantly, there are limitations in the ability to TCD to detect vasospasm in major blood vessels other than the middle cerebral and basilar arteries. Although not present here, elevated velocities may not be a sign of vasospasm. At times there can be hyperemia resulting in increased velocities throughout. The advent of the Lindegaard ratio can be used to further evaluate elevation in velocities by comparing the mean velocity in the middle cerebral artery with that of the ipsilateral extracranial internal carotid artery (MEANmca/MEANeica) with ratios of 3 to 6 consistent with mild spasm and >6 moderate spasm while a ratio of <3 meaning there is increased flow throughout the vascular system. Lindegaard ratio >3 and mean velocity >120 cm/s correlated with clinical vasospasm 85% and angiographic vasospasm 83.2%. There are many treatment options for angiographic vasospasm and verapamil works by blocking L-type calcium channels and results in relaxation of smooth muscle. Following treatment with verapamil mean TCD velocities will decrease rather than increase.

References

1. Purykayastha S, Sorond F. Transcranial Doppler ultrasound: technique and application. *Semin Neurol.* 2012;32:411-420.
2. White H, Venkatesh B. Application of transcranial Doppler in the ICU: a review. *Intensive Care Med.* 2006;32:981-994.
3. Kumar G, Shahripour RB, Harrrigan MR. Vasospasm on transcranial Doppler is predictive of delayed cerebral ischemia in aneurysmal subarachnoid hemorrhage: a systematic review and meta-analysis. *J Neurosurg.* 2016;124:1257-1264.
4. Lindegaard KF, Nornes H, Bakke SJ, et al. Cerebral vasospasm diagnosis by means of angiography and blood velocity measurements. *Acta Neurochir (Wien).* 1989;100:12-24.
5. Gonzalez NR, Boscardin WJ, Glenn T, et al. Vasospasm probability index: a combination of transcranial doppler velocities, cerebral blood flow and clinical risk factors to predict cerebral vasospasm after aneurysmal subarachnoid hemorrhage. *J Neurosurg.* 2007;107:1101-1112.
6. Sayama CM, Jiu JK, Caldwell WT. Update on endovascular therapies for cerebral vasospasm induced by aneurysmal subarachnoid hemorrhage. *Neurosurg Focus.* 2006;21:E12.

**4.** Correct Answer: C

**Rationale:**

The patient presents with a subarachnoid hemorrhage in the setting of a basilar tip aneurysm which is seen on the sagittal reformatted images shown. The description of the patient's presentation is best described by scales that have been previously developed that assist with long-term outcome as well as anticipated complications during the hospitalization. The Hunt and Hess score was developed as a tool for assessment of death. There are five grades with the lowest scores having better prognosis and higher having worse prognosis (Hunt and Hess Grade table). With the course of time and improved treatment strategies, the prognosis has improved, but those with the highest grade have a high mortality (71%). The Hunt and Hess grading system is based on the clinical exam of the patient. The second commonly used grading system for subarachnoid hemorrhage (SAH) is the modified Fisher scale (Modified Fisher Grade table). This is a radiographic-based scale which uses the thickness of subarachnoid blood and intraventricular extension to predict clinically relevant vasospasm. Vasospasm is a well-defined complication of subarachnoid hemorrhage which results in vasoconstriction of the cerebral vasculature through both calcium-dependent and calcium-independent pathways and results in cerebral ischemia.

## HUNT AND HESS GRADE

| GRADE | DESCRIPTION | MORTALITY (%) | FOLLOW-UP MORTALITY (%) |
|---|---|---|---|
| I | Asymptomatic or minimal headache and slight nuchal rigidity | 11 | 3 |
| II | Moderate or severe headache, nuchal rigidity, no neurologic deficit other than cranial nerve palsy | 26 | 3 |
| III | Drowsiness, confusion, or mild focal deficit | 37 | 9 |
| IV | Stupor, moderate to severe hemiparesis, possibly early decerebrate rigidity and vegetative disturbance | 71 | 24 |
| V | Deep coma, decerebrate posturing, moribund appearance | 100% | 71 |

## MODIFIED FISHER GRADE

| GRADE | DESCRIPTION | VASOSPASM (%) |
|---|---|---|
| 1 | Focal or diffuse thick SAH, without intraventricular hemorrhage | 24 |
| 2 | Focal or diffuse thin SAH, with intraventricular hemorrhage | 33 |
| 3 | Thick SAH without intraventricular hemorrhage | 33 |
| 4 | Thick SAH with intraventricular hemorrhage | 40 |

References

1. Hunt WE, Hess RM. Surgical risks as related to time of intervention in the repair of intracranial aneurysms. *J Neurosurg.* 1968;28:14-20.
2. Antigua H, Ortega-Gutierrez S, Schmidt JM, et al. Subarachnoid hemorrhage: who dies, and why? *Crit Care.* 2015;31;309-316.
3. Frontera JA, Claaassen J, Schmidt JM, et al. Prediction of symptomatic vasospasm after subarachnoid hemorrhage: the modified Fisher Scale. *Neurosurgery.* 2006;59:21-27.
4. Kolas AG, Sen J, Belli A. Pathogenesis of cerebral vasospasm following aneurysmal subarachnoid hemorrhage: putative mechanisms and novel approaches. *J Neurosci.* 2009;87:1-11.

**5.** Correct Answer: B

**Rationale:**

Given the findings on MRI, the most likely cause of her cerebellar hemorrhage is hypertension. This location is one of the common places for hypertensive bleeds (other being thalamus, basal ganglia, and pons). This is thought to be due to degeneration of the internal elastic lamina and resultant lipohyalinosis of the small vessels of the brain. The MRI of patients with hypertensive angiopathy will demonstrate areas of microhemorrhage within the same vascular regions as macrohemorrhages. Cerebral amyloid angiopathy is the most common cause of lobar intraparenchymal hemorrhage in older adults. This is the result of beta-amyloid protein deposition within the intima and media of the large and medium-sized intracranial vasculature. Autoimmune vasculitis is another important etiology of intraparenchymal hemorrhage. The typical imaging finding is both ischemic and hemorrhagic infarcts of varying age. The clinical presentation of autoimmune vasculitis can mimic the presentation above, but there is typically a prodromal phase with progressive symptoms. Lastly, infective endocarditis results in intraparenchymal hemorrhage from formation of mycotic aneurysms. Infected embolic material from the affected valve will embolize and can result in formation of microhemorrhages at the sites as well as macrohemorrhages if the aneurysms rupture. Vessel imaging with CT angiography, MR angiography, or digital subtraction arteriogram are best for evaluating an aneurysm.

References

1. Campbell GJ, Roach M. Fenestration in the internal elastic lamina at bifurcations of human cerebral arteries. *Stroke.* 1981;12:489-496.
2. Fisher CM. Pathologic Observations in hypertensive cerebral hemorrhage. *J Neuropathol Exp Neurol.* 1971;30:536-550.
3. Tsushima Y, Aoki J, Endo K. Brain microhemorrhages detected on T2*-weighted gradient-cheo MR images. *AJNR Am J Neuroradiol.* 2003;24(1):88-96.
4. Rosand J, Greenberg SM. Cerebral amyloid angiopathy. *Neurologist.* 2000;6:315-325.
5. Pomper MG, Miller TJ, Stone JH, et al. CNS vasculitis in autoimmune disease: MR imaging findings and correlation with angiography. *Am J Neuroradiol.* 1999;20:75-85.

**6.** Correct Answer: C

**Rationale:**

The differential diagnosis for subarachnoid hemorrhage is broad, including aneurysm, trauma, vascular tumors, dural arteriovenous fistula, and arteriovenous malformation. The head CT above demonstrates an isolated perimesencephalic subarachnoid hemorrhage. Although less common than the typical basilar subarachnoid hemorrhage, perimesecephalic subarachnoid hemorrhage can be the result of an arterial aneurysm (typically verterbrobasilar), but 95% are idiopathic despite extensive evaluation. Patients presenting with isolated perimesencephalic subarachnoid hemorrhage appear similar with thunderclap headache, nausea, emesis, but typically do not have a loss of consciousness or decreased level of consciousness. Despite CT angiograms being negative, they will undergo typically multiple digital subtraction angiograms to evaluate for an underlying vascular lesion and/or aneurysm. There is no standard of care practice on evaluation of perimesencephalic subarachnoid hemorrhage, but personal practice includes angiogram at the time of presentation and then at day 7 of hospitalization as small aneurysms may collapse at the time of rupture, and allowing for an extended time interval to pass it may reexpand. This type of subarachnoid hemorrhage has lower rates of complications than other subarachnoid hemorrhages including vasospasm and hydrocephalus. Although there is no definitive etiology for perimesencephalic subarachnoid hemorrhage, it is thought to be due to a venous tear and hemorrhage rather than arterial.

References

1. Boswell S, Thorell W, Gogela S, et al. Angiogram-negative subarachnoid hemorrhage: outcomes data and review of the literature. *J of Stroke and Cerebro Dis.* 2013;22:750-757.
2. Coelho LG, Costa JM, Silva EI. Non-aneurysmal spontaneous subarachnoid hemorrhage: perimesencephalic versus non-perimesencephalic. *Rev Bras Ter Intensiva.* 2016;28:141-146.
3. van Gijn J, van Dongen KJ, Vermeulen M, et al. Perimesencphalic hemorrhage: a nonaneurysmal and benign form of subarahnoid hemorrhage. *Neurology.* 1985;35:493-497.
4. Gupta SK, Gupta R, Khosla VK, et al. Nonaneurysmal nonperimesencephalic subarachnoid hemorrhage: is it a benign entity? *Surg Neurol.* 2009;71:571-572.
5. Jung JY, Kim YB, Lee JW, et al. Spontaneous subarachnoid haemorrhage with negative initial angiography: a review of 143 cases. *J Clin Neurosci.* 2006;13(10):1011-1017.
6. van der Schaaf IC, Velthuis BK, Gouw A, et al. Venous drainage in perimesencephalic hemorrhage. *Stroke.* 2004;35:1614-1618.

# 14

# MANAGEMENT STRATEGIES

Ofer Sadan and Milad Sharifpour

1. A 31-year-old man, with no past medical history, is admitted to the ICU with acute liver failure (ALF) following ingestion of an unknown herbal supplements. On initial examination, he is awake, oriented only to self, follows simple commands and has mild asterixis but no focal motor deficits. Notable laboratory test results include AST 1734, ALT 1567, T. Bilirubin 2.3, and Ammonia 110. On day 2 of ICU admission, he has a witnessed generalized tonic-clonic seizure. Two milligrams of lorazepam are administered intravenously and the convulsions are terminated. A Stat Head CT is performed, which shows diffuse cerebral edema and no ischemic or hemorrhagic changes. What is the MOST appropriate medication to administer at this time?

   **A.** Fosphenytoin
   **B.** Valproate
   **C.** Levetiracetam
   **D.** Midazolam infusion

2. A 76-year-old woman, with past medical history of hypertension, coronary artery disease, atrial fibrillation, and Parkinson disease is admitted to the ICU with progressively worsening mental status. She suffered a ground level fall 2 days before her admission. Her home medications are amlodipine, lisinopril, levodopa, and apixaban. On physical examination, she is somnolent, only opens her eyes to painful stimuli, pupils are equal in size and briskly reactive to light, does not vocalize, and withdraws from noxious stimuli in all four extremities. The patient is emergently intubated for airway protection and admitted to the ICU. On arrival to the ICU, a head CT is obtained (see figure that follows).

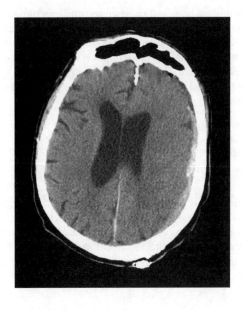

What will be the MOST appropriate next step in treatment?

A. Administer stat IV levetiracetam
B. Administer stat IV mannitol
C. Administer stat IV NaCl 3%
D. Neurosurgical consultation for hematoma evacuation

3. A 45-year-old woman, who is an active smoker and has history of untreated hypertension, presented following a sudden "thunderclap" headache. Head CT revealed (see figure that follows) subarachnoid hemorrhage of an anterior communicating artery aneurysm. She underwent successful endovascular coiling of the aneurysm, and an external ventricular drain was placed for hydrocephalus. Five days after presentation, she acutely became somnolent. Vital signs are T 37.4, HR 94, R 24, BP 124/75 (MAP 91), and $O_2$ saturation 95% on room air. On examination she is somnolent but easily arousable and follows simple commands with all four extremities, but there is a clear drift of the right hand and leg.

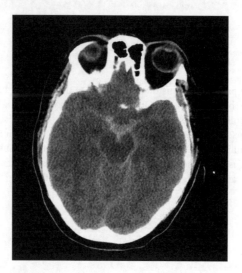

What is the **most** appropriate next step in management?

A. Administer stat IV Levetiracetam
B. Bolus 1 liter of fluid
C. Consult interventional radiology for stat angioplasty
D. Administer empiric IV Vancomycin and Ceftriaxone in meningitis doses.

4. A 57-year-old man, with past medical history of hypertension and hyperlipidemia, presented with an acute onset of slurred speech and right-sided weakness. He was diagnosed with an acute left middle cerebral artery (LMCA) stroke and IV tPA was administered. He was then admitted to the ICU for close monitoring. On day 3 poststroke, his focal deficits persist, and it is noted that one of his pupils is larger than the other. He subsequently becomes unresponsive and is emergently intubated and hyperventilated. Stat head CT demonstrated increasing cerebral edema and midline shift of 9.6 mm and uncal herniation without signs of cerebral hemorrhage. What is the **most** appropriate next step in treatment?

A. Transfuse to keep the hemoglobin>10 mg/dL
B. Administer IV dexamethasone
C. Administer hypertonic saline
D. Readminister IV tPA at half the original dose

5. A 76-year-old man with history of COPD and stage 3 chronic kidney disease underwent elective craniotomy for tumor resection. His postoperative course was complicated by the development of status epilepticus and respiratory failure. On postoperative day 5, he developed a fever of 38.7°C and his WBC increased from 12 000 to 19 500. Blood, urine, and respiratory cultures were obtained. A CSF sample revealed: Nucleated cells 230 cells/mL³, RBC: 1500 cells/mL³, Protein 220, and Glucose 34 mg/dL (systemic glucose 110 mg/dL). Which empiric antibiotic regimen is most appropriate to initiate at this time?

    **A.** Ceftazidime and vancomycin
    **B.** Ampicillin, ceftriaxone, and vancomycin
    **C.** Vancomycin, ceftriaxone, and metronidazole
    **D.** Cefepime and vancomycin

**6.** A 24-year-old woman, with history of recent upper respiratory infection, was admitted to the ICU with a week of progressive ascending weakness. On initial examination she was awake, alert, oriented, and cooperative. She had quadriparesis and areflexia. She subsequently developed respiratory distress and was intubated. Head and cervical spine CT are read as normal. A lumber puncture is performed, which reveals the following CSF profile: 0 WBCs, 0 RBCs, Protein 120 mg/dL, and Glucose 80 mg/dL. What is the next best step in management?

    **A.** Administer IV methylprednisolone
    **B.** Administer intravenous immunoglobulin
    **C.** Perform stat nerve conduction and electromyography studies
    **D.** Administer IV Acyclovir

**7.** A 38-year-old man suffers multisystem trauma and hemorrhagic shock after a motor vehicle accident. Initial CT imaging revealed a left-sided depressed skull fracture with underlying subdural hematoma (SDH) with contrecoup intracerebral hemorrhage, multiple bilateral rib fractures, lung contusions, and a splenic laceration. After initial damage control surgery, he was admitted to the ICU, where an increased intracranial pressure (ICP) monitor was placed. The patient remained sedated and ventilated, with limited neurological examination. On ICU day 2, he developed acute kidney injury with oliguria, and by day 3 he became anuric unresponsive to diuretic therapy. On the same day he had a sustained elevation in ICP to 27 mm Hg. Basic metabolic panel on day 3: Na 142; K 4.7; Cl 109, BUN 45, creatinine 3.5. What is the next most appropriate step to manage the ICP elevation?

    **A.** Administer IV mannitol
    **B.** Administer dexamethasone
    **C.** Administer NaCl 23.4%
    **D.** Neurosurgical consultation for an emergent decompressive hemicraniectomy

**8.** A 45-year-old man with a history poorly controlled hypertension is admitted to the ICU after elective endovascular repair of a descending thoracic aortic aneurysm. His intraoperative course was uneventful but on arrival in the ICU, he complains of lower limb weakness. His vital signs are within normal limits with blood pressure 110/65. On physical examination, he is awake, alert, and oriented. His cranial nerves and upper limb strength are intact. There is a clear nearly symmetric motor deficit in the bilateral lower limbs, with 3/5 weakness in the proximal muscles, and 2/5 in the distal ones. Tone is flaccid, and there is no Babinski sign or sensory deficit. In addition to increasing the blood pressure what is the MOST appropriate next step in management?

    **A.** Increase the blood pressure and insert a lumbar drain for CSF drainage
    **B.** Obtain a stat MRI brain and spine
    **C.** Initiate high-dose steroid treatment
    **D.** Obtain a stat angiogram of the lumbar vessels

**9.** A 78-year-old woman with past medical history of hypertension, COPD, and coronary artery disease is admitted to the ICU with respiratory failure due to community-acquired pneumonia. She is intubated and mechanically ventilated. Empiric antibiotic therapy for pneumonia was initiated following obtaining cultures. On the morning of her third ICU day, she his noted to be less arousable when sedation is decreased. On examination she does not follow commands, has a gaze preference to the left, and only moves her left side spontaneously. A stat head CT does not show any acute findings. The last documented normal neurological examination was at the shift change the day prior. The patient's home meds include a baby aspirin (81 mg) and a statin. What is the MOST appropriate intervention at this time?

    **A.** Administer stat IV tPA
    **B.** No acute intervention
    **C.** Administer stat fosphenytoin
    **D.** Obtain a stat CT angiogram and CT perfusion study for possible thrombectomy

**10.** A 32-year-old woman is admitted to the hospital with a 2-week course of progressively worsening confusion. She has no past medical history except for a mild upper respiratory infection two weeks before admission. On examination, she is awake, not oriented to time, place, or person and is only able to follow simple commands. There are no obvious focal neurological deficits. During the assessment, she develops a generalized tonic-clonic seizure. The seizure does not break despite three 2 mg doses of IV lorazepam and is emergently intubated and a propofol infusion is initiated, which terminates the convulsions. She is treated empirically with antibiotics for bacterial meningitis and acyclovir for viral encephalitis. EEG monitoring is notable for left temporal focal nonconvulsive status epilepticus, and fosphenytoin is administered with resolution of the seizures is administered. A head CT is obtained but does not show any acute abnormality. An MRI of the brain shows bitemporal T2 hyperintensities and no sign of a space occupying lesion, hemorrhage, or stroke. A lumbar puncture is performed, and CSF content shows 8 WBCs, 0 RBCs, Glucose 80 mg/dL (systemic 120 mg/dL), and protein 95 mg/dL. PCR for HSV 1&2, CMV, EBV, and VZV are negative, and acyclovir is discontinued. Gram stain and cultures are negative. What is the MOST appropriate therapeutic intervention at this time?

**A.** Administer methylprednisolone

**B.** Re-administer IV acyclovir

**C.** Administer valproic acid

**D.** Wean propofol to obtain a neurological examination

# Chapter 14 ▪ Answers

**1.** Correct Answer: C

**Rationale:**

The patient in this question suffers from ALF because of a toxic exposure. A common complication of ALF is cerebral edema and occasionally seizures. The patient responded to the first line treatment for the seizure (IV lorazepam) and now needs prophylaxis as the underlying cause of the seizure remains uncontrolled. When choosing an antiepileptic regimen, one should consider clearance and potential side effects. Fosphenytoin is primarily metabolized by the liver and could reach toxic levels in administered in the setting of ALF (Answer A is incorrect). Valporate is also metabolized by the liver and is known to induce hyperammonemia, even with normal functioning liver, and therefore it should not be used when hyperammonemia already exists (Answer B in incorrect). Levetiracetam is a relatively safe and effective medication, which is not primarily metabolized by the liver, and therefore the best from the above-stated options (Answer C is correct). Benzodiazepines, propofol, ketamine, etc, are indicated only if a patient fails treatment with other anti-epileptic drugs (Answer D is incorrect).

## References

1. Polsen J, Lee WM; American Association for the Study of Liver Disease. AASLD position paper: The management of acute liver failure. *Hepatology.* 2005;41:1179-1197.
2. Glauser T, Glauser T, Gloss D, et al. Evidence-based guidelines: treatment of convulsive status epilepticus in children and adults: report of the guideline committee of the American Epilepsy Society. *Epilepsy Curr.* 2016;16:48-61.
3. Lacerda G, Krummel T, Sabourdy C, Ryvlin P, Hirsch E. Optimizing therapy of seizures in patients with renal or hepatic dysfunction. *Neurology.* 2006;67:S28-S33.

**2.** Correct Answer: D

**Rationale:**

This patient has the classic presentation of SDH, with the gradual neurological deterioration after a fall. Imaging reveals a L. hemispheric SDH, primarily acute but probably with some chronic components (less-hyperintense areas). Head CT also demonstrates left-sided cerebral edema with left to right midline shift. Although seizures are very common in SDH patients, the description does not suggest a current seizure. It is common to administer prophylactic, not therapeutic doses of an antiepileptic medication (Answer A is incorrect). Although imaging does show significant cerebral edema with a midline shift, osmotherapy is generally avoided as it may cause further shrinkage of the brain tissue, which will expand the subdural space and exacerbate the bleed (Answers B and C are incorrect).

The correct answer is D: in an acute, symptomatic SDH, the solution is surgical evacuation. The patient requires a clot evacuation in the operating room as soon as possible.

## References

1. Fomchenko EI, Gilmore EJ, Matouk CC, et al. Management of subdural hematomas: part I. medical management of subdural hematomas. *Curr Treat Options Neurol.* 2018;20:28.
2. Fomchenko EI, Gilmore EJ, Matouk CC, et al. Management of subdural hematomas: part II. surgical management of subdural hematomas. *Curr Treat Options Neurol.* 2018;20:34.

**3.** Correct Answer: B

**Rationale:**

This patient has a classic presentation of symptomatic cerebral vasospasm and delayed cerebral ischemia after sub-arachnoid hemorrhage. She has several risk factors for vasospasm, including: sex, smoking history, and the blood pattern on the head CT (blood in the cistern and the presence of intraventricular blood). The highest incidence of vasospasm occurs between post-bleed days 4 to 10 (although it can occur up to three weeks post bleed). Although angioplasty is a definitive treatment for vasospasm, the first bedside intervention should be fluid administration to increase the mean arterial pressure (MAP) to improve cerebral perfusion. The description is not suggestive of a seizure and therefore choice A is incorrect. The description also does not suggest a new infection, and therefore Answer D is incorrect.

Reference

1. Francoeur CL, Mayer SA. Management of delayed cerebral ischemia after subarachnoid hemorrhage. *Crit Care*. 2016;20(91):277.

**4.** Correct Answer: C

**Rationale:**

The patient suffered an extensive MCA stroke and did not improve with IV thrombolytics. Brain edema and ICP are often associated with occlusion of large intracranial arteries. Edema of the brain begins to develop during the first 24 to 48 hours and reaches a maximum extent of 3 to 5 days from the occurrence of acute ischemic stroke. The presentation described is classic for uncal herniation secondary to increasing edema, with pressure on mid-brain causing a CN III palsy manifested by a blown pupil. Because post-stroke edema is cytotoxic in nature and vasogenic edema occurs secondarily (as opposed to perineoplastic changes), steroids are not beneficial (Option B is incorrect). In fact, it has been shown that steroid administration in the setting of acute stroke worsens outcomes. Although increasing cerebral edema could cause secondary cerebral ischemia by compressing healthy brain tissue, there is no indication to increase transfusion threshold (Option A is incorrect). Redosing tPA could be detrimental in the settings of a large stroke and should not be attempted (Option D is incorrect). Treatment of stroke-related cerebral edema is osmotherapy, such as hypertonic saline (Option C is correct) or mannitol. Following this initial intervention, the patient should be evaluated for possible hemicraniectomy.

References

1. Ayata C, Ropper AH. Ischaemic brain oedema. *J Clin Neurosci*. 2002;9(2):113-124.
2. Bar B, Biller J. Select hyperacute complications of ischemic stroke: cerebral edema, hemorrhagic transformation, and orolingual angioedema secondary to intravenous alteplase. *Expert Rev Neurother*. 2018;18(10):749-759.

**5.** Correct Answer: A

**Rationale:**

The patient presents with post craniotomy meningitis. According to the Infectious Diseases Society of America 2017 guidelines, coverage for gram-positive bacteria, and gram-negative bacteria including antipseudomonal coverage is required. Vancomycin should be aggressively dosed to achieve a trough concentration of 15 to 20 µg/mL. The recommendation for gram-negative coverage includes: cefepime, ceftazidime, or meropenem. Although cefepime is an option, there is increased risk of seizures associated with its use compared with other beta-lactams. The risk is especially significant in older patients with renal impairment. For these reasons it is preferable not to choose cefepime in this elderly patient with chronic kidney disease and seizures (option D is incorrect). Option B represents a common empiric coverage regimen for community acquired bacterial meningitis, which is not relevant for this patient. Option C does not cover pseudomonas. The correct answer is Option A: ceftazidime and vancomycin.

References

1. Tunkel AR, Hasbun R, Bhimraj A, et al. 2017 Infectious disease Society of America's clinical practice guidelines for healthcare associated ventriculitis and meningitis. *Clin Infect Dis*. 2017 64:e34-e65.
2. https://www.fda.gov/Drugs/DrugSafety/ucm309661.htm.

**6.** Correct Answer: B

**Rationale:**

The patient described has a classic presentation of Guillain-Barré syndrome. This disease often appears following a febrile illness or a gastrointestinal tract infection. Typical features include ascending flaccid paralysis and a CSF sample with no WBCs and high protein. Nerve conduction and electromyography studies can be helpful to confirm the diagnosis; however, they are usually not needed to initiate treatment (Option C is incorrect). High-dose steroid therapy is not effective for Guillain-Barré syndrome (Option A is incorrect). First line treatment includes intravenous immunoglobulin or plasma exchange (Option B is correct). The patient's clinical presentation is not suggestive of encephalitis as there are no clear signs of CNS involvement (no cortical deficits such as aphasia, or upper motor neuron pattern of injury) therefore Option D is incorrect.

Reference

1. Willison HJ, Jacobs BC, van Doorn PA. Guillain Barre syndrome. *Lancet*. 2016;388(10045):717-727.

**7.** Correct Answer: C

**Rationale:**

T Cerebral edema and ICP are complications of severe TBI, which occurred in this patient. Cerebral edema in the settings of TBI is mainly cytotoxic and not vasogenic; therefore, steroids are not indicated (Option B is incorrect). The fastest and most effective intervention to reduce increased ICP in patients with TBI is osmotherapy. Although surgery might be indicated, osmotherapy is the initial therapy of choice (Option D is incorrect). There is no difference in outcome between the use of mannitol and 23.4% hypertonic saline in patients with increased ICP. However because mannitol's effect is through diuresis, it may lead to systemic volume overload in an anuric patient. The correct answer is C. Hypertonic saline is the appropriate therapy to reduce intracranial pressure in a patient with TBI and ATN.

References

1. Winkler EA, Minter D, Yue JK, Manley GT. Cerebral edema in traumatic brain injury: pathophysiology and prospective therapeutic targets. *Neurosurg Clin N Am.* 2016;27:473-488.
2. Continuum: lifelong learning in neurology. *Neurocrit Care.* 2015;21:1299-1323.

**8.** Correct Answer: A

**Rationale:**

A devastating complication of thoracic aortic aneurysm repair is spinal cord ischemia. In open thoracic aortic aneurysm repair, cross clamping the aorta causes decreased blood flow to the spinal cord resulting in ischemia. In endovascular repair, such as in this vignette, there is no aortic cross-clamp, but the endostent deployed can occlude small collateral arteries that perfuse the anterior spinal cord, which can result in hypoperfusion and spinal ischemia. Because of the anatomic blood supply of the spinal cord, the anterior motor fibers are supplied primarily by a single anterior spinal artery commonly resulting in bilateral leg weakness.

Although there are no large randomized control trials, the common treatment aims at improving spinal cord perfusion by increasing MAP and inserting a lumbar drain for CSF removal. The result of these interventions is an increase in spinal cord perfusion pressure (SCPP), which is the difference between MAP and intraspinal pressure (ISP), i.e., SCPP=MAP-ISP. Although this treatment may be more effective when performed prophylactically before surgery, it may also be used as a rescue treatment when postoperative cord ischemia occurs (Option A is correct).

Obtaining an MRI may be important to rule out other causes of spinal cord ischemia, such as spinal cord hematoma but would not be the immediate next step (Answer B is incorrect). Steroids have no demonstrated role in spinal cord ischemia (Option C is incorrect). The mechanism of spinal cord ischemia in this case is due to the endo-stent occlusion of perfusing arteries resulting in decreased anterior spinal cord perfusion; therefore, IR-guided thrombectomy will not treat the underlying problem (Option D is incorrect).

References

1. Coselli JS, LeMaire SA, Köksoy C, et al. Cerebrospinal fluid drainage reduces paraplegia after thoracoabdominal aortic aneurysm repair: Results of a randomized controlled trial. *J Vasc Surg.* 2002;35:631-639.
2. Khan NR, Smalley Z, Nesvick CL, et al. The use of lumbar drains in preventing spinal cord injury following thoracoabdominal aortic aneurysm repair: an updated systematic review and meta-analysis. *J Neurosurg Spine.* 2016;25:383-393.

**9.** Correct Answer: D

**Rationale:**

The patient described in the vignette demonstrates evidence of an ischemic stroke, an infrequent but important complication in critically ill patients. Timely detection is challenging because physical examination can be limited by sedation, delirium, or other medications, which can make acute neurologic changes difficult to detect. The patient probably has a LMCA syndrome based on the description. Because her last known normal examination was over 4.5 hours before the diagnosis, she is out of the window for IV thrombolytic therapy (Answer A is incorrect). However, in the era of endovascular thrombectomy, there are still urgent interventions that could change the course and outcome. Although a seizure is in the differential when an acute neurological change occurs, the gaze deviation (to the left in this case) suggests that this is a stroke and not a seizure (Option C is incorrect).

According to the 2018 American Stroke Association, there is enough level I data to recommend pursuing a CT angiogram and CT perfusion study to assess the stroke burden even up to 24 hours from the time of last known normal examination. Several randomized controlled trials have shown the benefit of patient-selective approach to find the correct candidate for mechanical thrombectomy. Therefore, it is not necessarily too late for this patient to receive timely and potentially beneficial intervention (Option D is correct).

Reference

1. Powers WJ, Rabinstein AA, Ackerson T, et al. 2018 Guidelines for the early management of patients with acute ischemic stroke: a guideline for healthcare professionals from the American Heart Association/American Stroke Association. *Stroke.* 2018;49:e46-e99.

**10.** Correct Answer: A

**Rationale:**

The patient in this scenario presents with a clinical picture of autoimmune encephalitis. The subacute progressive process, new onset seizures, and the temporal findings on imaging, all point toward the diagnosis. As part of the workup, it is critical to rule out other causes including infections (viral and bacterial), neoplastic etiology, toxic metabolic syndromes, posterior reversible encephalopathy syndrome (PRES), and a central manifestation of a systemic autoimmune disease (SLE, Sjögren, Behçet, etc). Once other potential diagnoses are excluded, early treatment with high-dose steroids and plasma exchange or IVIg is recommended (Option A is correct).

Although it is possible to have an early false negative PCR for HSV, this patient has been symptomatic for two weeks, and therefore the chances of false negative PCR are low (Option B is incorrect).

The patient is treated with a second and third line agents to control her seizures (phenytoin and propofol), with a good response. There is no advantage at this point in adding another antiepileptic agent, particularly valproic acid because of the significant interactions it has with phenytoin (Option C is incorrect). As for seizure control, the aim is to control all seizures, focal or generalized, with medications, and one cannot "tolerate" focal status epilepticus to achieve other clinical goals such as an examination (Option D is incorrect).

References

1. Graus F, Titulaer MJ, Balu R, et al. A clinical approach to diagnosis of autoimmune encephalitis. *Lancet Neurol.* 2016;15:391-404.
2. Lancaster E. The diagnosis and treatment of autoimmune encephalitis. *J Clin Neurol.* 2016;12:1-13.
3. Perruca E. Clinically relevant drug interactions with antiepileptics. *Br J Clin Pharmacol.* 2006;61:246-255.

# CARDIOVASCULAR DISORDERS

# 15

# ACUTE CORONARY SYNDROME

Nino Mihatov and David M. Dudzinski

1. A 46-year-old man with atrial fibrillation, hypertension, hyperlipidemia, and diabetes is admitted with unstable angina. He undergoes coronary angiography which demonstrates a 90% stenosis of the mid left circumflex in a left dominant system. A single drug-eluting stent is deployed with an excellent angiographic result, and the patient is given aspirin and ticagrelor. The patient is admitted to the cardiac service and shortly after arriving to the floor reports new onset chest pain. A 12-lead electrocardiogram is performed:

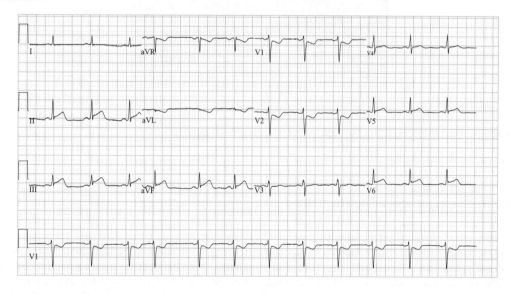

Which of the following is the next BEST step in management?

A. Intravenous nitroglycerin
B. Observation
C. Urgent repeat coronary angiography
D. Transthoracic echocardiogram (TTE)

2. A 55-year-old male with known coronary artery disease with prior percutaneous coronary intervention of the right coronary artery 2 years prior to presentation, hyperlipidemia, and hypertension presents to the emergency department with 2 days of exertional chest pain which culminated in acute onset of "stabbing" substernal chest pain radiating to the left shoulder. Vital signs on presentation are:

**Temperature: 36.3°F**
**Blood pressure: 200/89 mm Hg**
**Heart rate: 81 beats per minute**
**Respiratory rate: 18 per minute**
**Oxygen saturation: 93% on room air**
Laboratory studies are notable for a cardiac troponin-T that is undetectable.
A 12-lead electrocardiogram demonstrates normal sinus rhythm, Q-waves in inferior leads, and nonspecific ST segment changes.
A plain film chest radiograph is obtained (see figure that follow).

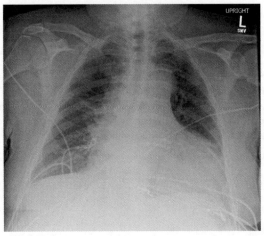

A bedside point-of-care ultrasound demonstrates a moderate-sized circumferential pericardial effusion.

Which of the following is the most appropriate next step in management?

A. Coronary angiography
B. Contrasted computed tomography (CT) of the chest
C. Pericardiocentesis
D. Transesophageal echocardiography (TEE)

3. A 66-year-old male with hypertension and hyperlipidemia presents with substernal chest pain. His presenting electrocardiogram demonstrates inferior ST elevations with reciprocal changes in the high lateral leads. Emergent coronary angiography is pursued with percutaneous coronary intervention undertaken on a subtotally occluded right coronary artery. Aspirin, ticagrelor, metoprolol, and atorvastatin are initiated. He is admitted to the intensive care unit for postintervention monitoring after repeat electrocardiogram shows resolution of previous ST segment elevations.

   Twelve hours later, the patient develops subacute significant shortness of breath following medication administration. The patient's oxygen saturation is 99% on room air and his physical exam is unremarkable. A repeat electrocardiogram is unchanged from postintervention. Contrasted computed tomography (CT) of the chest is negative for pulmonary embolism.

Which one of his medications is a potential culprit of his dyspnea symptoms?

A. Aspirin
B. Metoprolol
C. Ticagrelor
D. Atorvastatin

**4.** A 65-year-old female with hypertension and hyperlipidemia develops substernal chest pressure with dyspnea.

Physical exam is notable for the following:
Blood pressure: 126/62 mm Hg, pulse: 76 beats per minute, oxygen saturation of 97% on 4 L nasal cannula
General: Sitting up with increased work of breathing
Heart: Regular rate and rhythm. A III/VI holosystolic murmur is heard at the cardiac apex, which is nondisplaced on chest palpation
Lung: Posterior diffuse crackles
Abdomen: Soft, nontender, and nondistended
Extremities: Warm, without edema
12-lead electrocardiogram reveals the following:

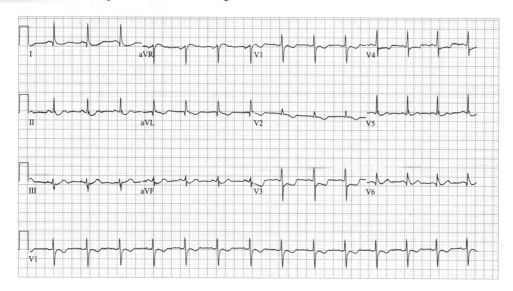

What is the most likely mechanism of this patient's dyspnea?

**A.** Pulmonary embolism
**B.** Mitral regurgitation
**C.** LV systolic dysfunction
**D.** Tamponade

**5.** A 96-year-old female is admitted to the intensive care unit for closer hemodynamic monitoring following uncomplicated deployment of a drug-eluting stent to the first obtuse marginal, via the left radial artery, in the context of a presentation consistent with an ST elevation myocardial infarction (STEMI). Four hours postprocedure, the patient develops acute hypotension necessitating vasopressor support.

A 12-lead electrocardiogram is performed.

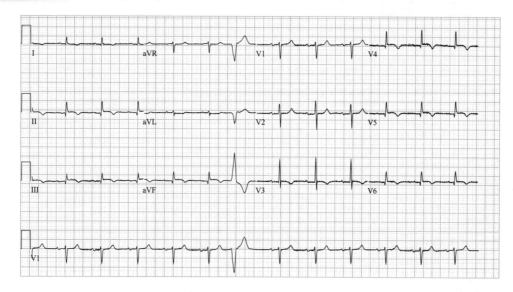

Compared to her postintervention electrocardiogram, ST segment elevations in leads II, III, aVF, V5, and V6 persist but are less prominent. Otherwise, there are no significant changes. Assessment of her left radial access site is unrevealing.

What is the best next step in management?
A. Repeat diagnostic coronary angiography
B. Urgent surface echocardiogram
C. Computed tomography imaging of the abdomen
D. Right heart catheterization

6. A 57-year-old male with a history of hyperlipidemia is admitted to the intensive care unit with hypotension necessitating vasopressor support. He had been in his usual state of health, but in the preceding 24 hours, he developed progressively worsening dyspnea, culminating in respiratory failure and necessitating intubation.

His admission electrocardiogram is shown here:

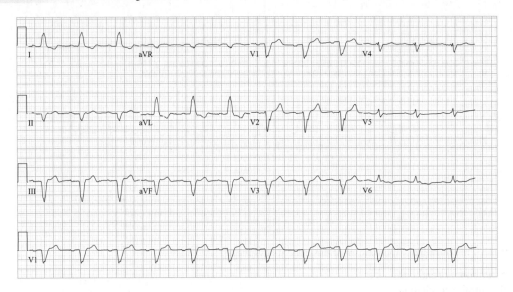

His presenting troponin-T is 2.52 ng/mL (reference <0.03 ng/mL).

Shortly after admission, the patient is witnessed to have repeated episodes of self-terminating ventricular tachycardia, the longest of which last up to 45 seconds.
An echocardiogram is performed and demonstrates severe biventricular dysfunction with an estimated left ventricular ejection fraction of 12%.
Which of the following would be the most appropriate next step in management?
A. Urgent coronary angiography with the intent to revascularize
B. Insertion of a percutaneous left ventricular assist device (LVAD)
C. Insertion of an intra-aortic balloon pump (IABP)
D. Cardiac biomarker panel

**7.** A 76-year-old female undergoes uncomplicated coronary angiography via the right femoral artery for evaluation of a newly diagnosed cardiomyopathy. She is found to be without obstructive coronary artery disease. The patient is admitted to the intensive care unit for further monitoring.

Her femoral angiogram is shown in the figure that follows.

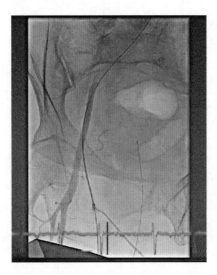

Two days following admission, the patient begins to cough. Shortly thereafter, she is observed to have sudden and rapid expansion of her right lower quadrant, with associated hypotension.

Which of the following is the most appropriate next step?
**A.** Computed tomography (CT) imaging of the abdomen without contrast
**B.** Initiation of a massive transfusion protocol
**C.** Manual pressure proximal to the angiography access site
**D.** Urgent surgical exploration

**8.** An 88-year-old male with complex coronary disease that includes prior three-vessel coronary artery bypass grafting and prior complete heart block necessitating dual chamber permanent pacemaker implantation presents with substernal chest pain identical in character to his past angina.

His presenting electrocardiogram is:

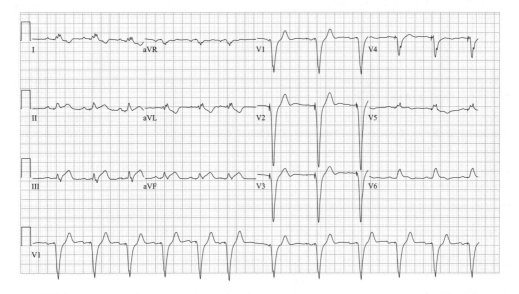

His presenting troponin-T is 0.54 ng/mL (reference <0.03 ng/mL).

Which of the following is the next best step in management?

**A.** Emergent coronary angiography with the intent to revascularize

**B.** Urgent (24-48 hours) coronary angiography with the intent to revascularize

**C.** Noninvasive risk stratification

**D.** Intravenous nitroglycerin

---

**9.** A 67-year-old man presents with 3 days of severe substernal chest pain.

His presenting electrocardiogram is:

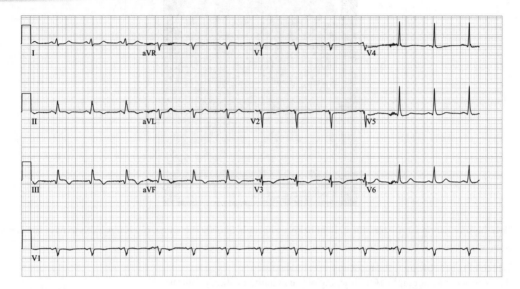

A surface echocardiogram reveals an estimated left ventricular ejection fraction of 22% with inferior and inferoseptal akinesis. A 1.5 cm ventricular septal defect at the junction of the inferior wall and septum is noted and is associated with bidirectional shunting.

Coronary angiography reveals a 50% narrowing of the ostium of the left main coronary artery, subtotal occlusion of the left anterior descending artery, and total occlusion of the right coronary artery with left to right collaterals. A plan for surgical revascularization, with patch repair of the ventricular septal defect, is formulated. Shortly thereafter, the patient develops progressive cardiogenic shock with ventricular tachycardia. Which of the following is the next BEST step in management?

**A.** Insertion of an intra-aortic balloon pump

**B.** Initiation of inotropic support

**C.** Percutaneous coronary intervention with drug-eluting stent deployment to the left anterior descending artery

**D.** Veno-arterial extracorporeal membrane oxygenation (ECMO) initiation

---

**10.** A 58-year-old with active tobacco use, hyperlipidemia, and hypertension presents with substernal chest pain that developed following snow shoveling.

Shortly following his presentation, he is observed to have a witnessed cardiac arrest with multiple episodes of ventricular fibrillation. He required 10 minutes of cardiopulmonary resuscitation with advanced cardiac life support and four defibrillator therapies.

Following return of spontaneous circulation (ROSC), the patient was noted to have the following laboratory data. His mental status is not determinable.

| Bicarbonate: 23 mmol/L | ALT: 506 U/L | Troponin-T 0.43 ng/mL (reference: |
| Creatinine: 1.03 mg/dL | AST: 658 U/L | <0.03 ng/mL) |

| Arterial pH: 6.93 | White blood cell: 19 000/µL | |
| Arterial $CO_2$: 59 | Hemoglobin: 14.1 g/dL | |
| | Platelet: 264 K/µL | |

His post-ROSC ECG is shown:

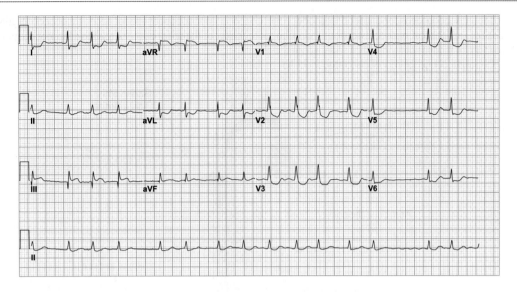

What is the MOST appropriate timing for coronary angiography?

**A.** Urgently post-ROSC
**B.** Within 24 to 48 hours of presentation
**C.** Following correction of metabolic derangement
**D.** Following establishment of a favorable neurologic prognosis

# Chapter 15 ▪ Answers

**1.** Correct Answer: C

**Rationale:**
The 12-lead electrocardiogram demonstrates an inferoposteroapical ST segment elevation myocardial infarction (STEMI) in the context of a recently deployed stent. Stent thrombosis is an uncommon but serious complication that accounts for less than 10% of cardiac deaths following stent placement. Most cases occur within the first 30 days of placement and are independent of the stent type. The presentation is often with myocardial injury, usually with ST segment elevation (mimicking the acute coronary syndrome), or death. Treatment includes urgent coronary angiography with repeat revascularization.

Although the most common cause for stent thrombosis is P2Y12 discontinuation, other risk factors include acute coronary syndrome presentation, diabetes mellitus, side-branch stenting, greater stent length, suboptimal stent apposition. The cumulative rate of stent thrombosis is approximately 2% at 2 years and is similar for both bare metal stents and first-generation drug-eluting stents. A high index of suspicion is key for successful recognition and management.

References
1. Stone GW, Moses JW, Ellis SG, et al. Safety and efficacy of sirolimus- and paclitaxel-eluting coronary stents. *N Engl J Med.* 2007;356(10):998-1008.
2. Palmerini T, Kirtane AJ, Serruys PW, et al. Stent thrombosis with everolimus-eluting stents: meta-analysis of comparative randomized controlled trials. *Circ Cardiovasc Interv.* 2012;5(3):357-364.
3. Werkum JW, van Heestermans AA, Zomer AC, et al. Predictors of coronary stent thrombosis: the dutch stent thrombosis registry. *J Am Coll Cardiol.* 2009;53(16):1399-1409.

**2.** Correct Answer: B

**Rationale:**
The constellation of presenting chest pain, hypertension, widened mediastinum, and pericardial effusion must prompt a consideration of acute aortic dissection, even in the context of a presenting syndrome suspicious for unstable angina. Known risk factors for aortic dissection include male sex, history of hypertension, and advanced age, as well as connective tissue disorders. Greater than 90% of patients presenting with a type A dissection (involving the ascending aorta) report chest pain, while only 47% of patients with a type A dissection report back pain.

The presenting signs for dissection include hypertension in approximately 49% of all aortic dissection presentations but only 36% of type A dissection. Plain film radiography of the chest can be suggestive but not diagnostic as only 62% of patients demonstrate a widened mediastinum.

Common complications of dissection include:

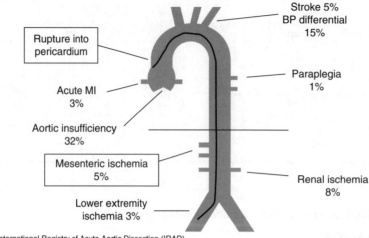

International Registry of Acute Aortic Dissection (IRAD)

A high index of suspicion for aortic dissection is required. On examination, an upper extremity pulse deficit and/or blood pressure differential should be evaluated, and so bilateral blood pressure should be measured. Imaging modalities to confirm the diagnosis include computed tomography angiography, magnetic resonance imaging angiography, transesophageal echocardiography, and aortography. While all modalities have >95% sensitivity and specificity, contemporary computed tomography angiography is reported to have a near 100% sensitivity and 98% specificity.

### References

1. Hagan PG, Nienaber CA, Isselbacher EM, et al. The International Registry of Acute Aortic Dissection (IRAD): new insights into an old disease. *JAMA*. 2000;283(7):897-903.
2. Shiga T, Wajima Z, Apfel CC, Inoue T, Ohe Y. Diagnostic accuracy of transesophageal echocardiography, helical computed tomography, and magnetic resonance imaging for suspected thoracic aortic dissection: systematic review and meta-analysis. *Arch Intern Med*. 2006;166(13):1350-1356.

---

**3.** Correct Answer: C

**Rationale:**

Ticagrelor, a reversible and direct-acting oral antagonist of the adenosine diphosphate receptor P2Y12, is an active drug and provides more consistent P2Y12 inhibition than pro-drug clopidogrel. Ticagrelor is associated with dose-related episodes of dyspnea, via an unknown mechanism, and ventricular pauses. As many as 14% of patients initiated on ticagrelor experience dose-dependent dyspnea which is described as "sudden and unexpected air hunger" or unsatisfied inspiration. Ticagrelor-related dyspnea typically begins within 1 week, but up to one-third may present within 24 hours. It is usually a diagnosis of exclusion after ruling out any other cardiopulmonary cause. This is especially challenging when presentation is soon after acute coronary syndrome. The symptoms resolve with cessation of ticagrelor therapy. Careful attention must be paid at the timing of cessation of ticagrelor and initiation of an alternative P2Y12 inhibitor such as clopidogrel or prasugrel.

### References

1. Wallentin L, Becker RC, Budaj A, et al. Ticagrelor versus clopidogrel in patients with acute coronary syndromes. *N Engl J Med*. 2009;361(11):1045-1057.
2. Angolillo DJ, Rollini F, Storey RF, et al. International expert consensus on switching platelet P2Y$_{12}$ receptor–inhibiting therapies. *Circulation*. 2017;136:1955.

---

**4.** Correct Answer: B

**Rationale:**

The patient presents with a clinical syndrome suggestive of an acute coronary syndrome (ACS). The 12-lead electrocardiogram demonstrates most notably ST segment depressions in the right precordial leads (V1-V3) with prominent R-waves. These findings could suggest a posterior myocardial infarction versus anterior subendocardial ischemia. The presence of prominent R-waves is suspicious for posterior pathologic Q-waves and makes the ST segment depressions more suggestive of infarction. Posterior leads, placed alongside the inferior border of the left scapula (at the same horizontal level as V6), could also be obtained to confirm suspicion of a transmural infarct. Portable echocardiography can be considered to clarify the diagnosis of ST elevation myocardial infarction (STEMI). Early recognition and revascularization are key to managing a posterior STEMI.

The mitral valve has two papillary muscles. The anterolateral papillary muscle receives dual blood supply from the left anterior descending artery and the left circumflex. The posteromedial papillary muscle is supplied only by the posterior descending artery which in most patients branches off the right coronary artery. In posterior myocardial infarctions, attention should be paid to the increased risk of papillary muscle ischemia leading to acute mitral regurgitation. Clinical exam may reveal a holosystolic murmur at the left sternal border with pulmonary edema that corroborates the diagnosis. A murmur, however, may not be heard in up to 50% of cases.

### References
1. Antman EM, Anbe DT, Armstrong PW, et al. ACC/AHA guidelines for the management of patients with ST-elevation myocardial infarction: a report of the American College of Cardiology/American Heart Association Task Force on Practice Guidelines (Committee to revise the 1999 guidelines for the management of patients with acute myocardial infarction). *Circulation*. 2004;110(9):e82-e292.
2. Casas RE, Marriott HJ, Glancy DL. Value of leads V7-V9 in diagnosing posterior wall acute myocardial infarction and other causes of tall R waves in V1-V2. *Am J Cardiol*. 1997;80(4):508-509.

---

**5.** Correct Answer: B

**Rationale:**

Complications of diagnostic coronary angiography and percutaneous coronary intervention that can cause hypotension include coronary perforation leading to cardiac tamponade, access site complications leading to bleeding, or intracoronary artery complications (dissection, stent thrombosis, stent migration) leading to left ventricular dysfunction and impaired cardiac output. In the absence of a clinical syndrome or electrocardiographic evidence of stent compromise, attention should be directed toward the access site which, particularly with radial access, can be visually inspected. In the absence of access site compromise, transthoracic echocardiography should be considered for evaluation of pericardial effusion and mechanical complications of myocardial infarction.

Coronary artery perforation is a rare complication occurring in less than 1% of treated lesions. Perforation can be caused by a wire exiting a vessel or by compromise of the vessel wall by a balloon, stent, or other intracoronary devices. Most cases of perforation are identified intraprocedurally but upward of 13% of cardiac tamponade instances can be delayed and occur within 24 hours after departure from the catheterization laboratory. Intraprocedural perforations can be managed with balloon occlusion of the perforated artery. If tamponade were to develop, emergent pericardiocentesis should be pursued. For delayed presentations, repeat angiography can be considered to identify active extravasation that may benefit from a trial of balloon occlusion or coil embolization.

### References
1. Stankovic G, Orlic D, Corvaja N, et al. Incidence, predictors, in-hospital, and late outcomes of coronary artery perforations. *Am J Cardiol*. 2004;93(2):213-216.
2. Ellis SG, Ajluni S, Arnold AZ, et al. Increased coronary perforation in the new device era. Incidence, classification, management, and outcome. *Circulation*. 1994;90(6):2725-2730.

---

**6.** Correct Answer: A

**Rationale:**

The patient presents with rapidly decompensating heart failure leading to cardiogenic shock. His 12-lead electrocardiogram reveals Q-waves consistent with old inferior, anteroseptal and anterior wall infarction, suggesting that ischemia may be related causally to the biventricular dysfunction. While consideration of ventricular support devices in this case is important, a univentricular support device, such as an IABP or percutaneous LVAD, would likely be inadequate in the presence of biventricular failure. Furthermore, there is minimal evidence in favor of IABP or PVAD in cardiogenic shock. His ventricular arrhythmias are likely a consequence of the acute decompensation on the background of severe biventricular cardiomyopathy.

Immediate diagnostic angiography with intent to perform revascularization is indicated in patients with non-ST elevation myocardial infarction (NSTEMI) who have refractory angina or hemodynamic or electrical instability. Acute myocardial infarction is the leading cause of cardiogenic shock and early revascularization is associated with improved mortality when compared to medical therapy. Mortality nevertheless remains high in this subset of patients. In patients for whom percutaneous coronary intervention may not be possible or for whom a mechanical complication of myocardial infarction is present, coronary artery bypass grafting can be considered.

### References
1. Amsterdam EA, Wenger NK, Brindis RG, et al. 2014 AHA/ACC guideline for the management of patients with non-ST-elevation acute coronary syndromes: a report of the American College of Cardiology/American Heart Association task force on practice guidelines. *J Am Coll Cardiol*. 2014;64(24):e139-e228.
2. Jeger RV, Urban P, Harkness SM, et al. Early revascularization is beneficial across all ages and a wide spectrum of cardiogenic shock severity: a pooled analysis of trials. *Acute Cardiac Care*. 2011;13(1):14-20.

**7.** Correct Answer: C

**Rationale:**

Routine diagnostic coronary angiography with percutaneous coronary intervention can be performed via the radial or femoral artery. The radial artery approach carries similar procedural success with lower rates of bleeding and vascular complications compared to the femoral artery. When femoral artery access is utilized, cannulation of the common femoral artery (CFA) should occur above the femoral artery bifurcation and below the internal epigastric artery. This target can be identified fluoroscopically by visualizing the femoral head, which typically lies above the CFA bifurcation and below the internal epigastric artery and permits easy compression of the common femoral artery following the procedure. In patients with a "high stick," that is a stick arterial puncture site at or above the superior border of the femoral head, there is an increased risk of retroperitoneal bleeding. Conversely, "low sticks" at or below the inferior border of the femoral head carry an increased risk of pseudoaneurysm formation.

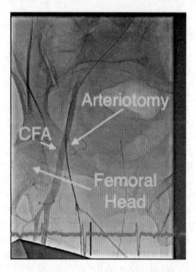

Access site bleeding should be suspected in postprocedural patients with hypotension, lower abdominal or back pain, or rapidly expanding hematoma. The first step in managing active hemorrhage centers on primary bleeding control with manual compression of the common femoral artery. Thereafter, anticoagulation should be reversed and blood products should be administered. Computed tomography of the abdomen can be utilized when the diagnosis is uncertain and hemodynamic parameters have stabilized. While most bleeding stops with manual pressure, surgical exploration can be considered following failure of manual compression.

References

1. Rao SV, Ou FS, Wang TY, et al. Trends in the prevalence and outcomes of radial and femoral approaches to percutaneous coronary intervention: a report from the National Cardiovascular Data Registry. *JACC Cardiovasc Interv.* 2008;1(4):379-386.
2. Mason PJ, Shah B, Tamis-Holland JE, et al. An update on radial artery access and best practices for transradial coronary angiography and intervention in acute coronary syndrome: a scientific statement from the American Heart Association. *Circ Cardiovasc Interv.* 2018;11:e000035.

**8.** Correct Answer: A

**Rationale:**

Early diagnosis of an ST elevation myocardial infarction (STEMI) remains key in determining management. Early diagnosis leads to earlier reperfusion which ultimately improves mortality. Diagnosis of STEMI necessitates the presence of new ST elevations in at least two contiguous leads (of ≥2 mm in men ≥40 years, ≥2.5 mm in men <40 years, or ≥1.5 mm in women in leads $V_2$-$V_3$ and/or ≥1 mm in other contiguous chest leads or limb leads).

The diagnosis of myocardial ischemia and infarction in the presence of conduction disturbances proves more challenging. Ischemic symptoms with a presumed new left bundle branch block (LBBB) or right bundle branch block (RBBB) that is not rate related is associated with adverse prognosis. In patients with an LBBB, ST segment elevation ≥1 mm concordant with the QRS complex in any lead may be an indicator of acute myocardial ischemia. Similar criteria can be used to diagnose acute myocardial infarction in the presence of right ventricular pacing as demonstrated in this patient's electrocardiogram. Because of the concordant QRS-ST changes apparent in the inferior leads of this patient's electrocardiogram, angiography should be pursued.

References

1. Thygesen K, Alpert JS, Jaffe AS, et al; Executive Group on behalf of the Joint European Society of Cardiology (ESC)/American College of Cardiology (ACC)/American Heart Association (AHA)/World Heart Federation (WHF) Task Force for the Universal Definition of Myocardial Infarction. Fourth universal definition of myocardial infarction (2018). *Circulation.* 2018;138(20):e618-e651.
2. Wang TY, Nallamothu BK, Krumholz HM, et al. Association of door-in to door-out time with reperfusion delays and outcomes among patients transferred for primary percutaneous coronary intervention. *JAMA.* 2011;305(24):2540-2547.

**9.** Correct Answer: A

**Rationale:**

Mechanical complications of myocardial infarction include rupture of the ventricular free wall, rupture of the interventricular septum, and rupture of the papillary muscle with acute mitral regurgitation; these can occur within the first 24 hours post–myocardial infarction or as late as 2 weeks. With mainstream revascularization therapies, the incidence of rupture of the interventricular septum occurs in 0.2% of myocardial infarctions. Infarction related to the left anterior descending artery appears to have the highest risk of rupture of the interventricular septum.

Definitive management of a post–myocardial infarction ventricular septal rupture necessitates closure. In patients with cardiogenic shock, urgent surgical intervention is necessary. Temporary hemodynamic support can be provided by afterload reduction with vasodilators and intra-aortic balloon pump counterpulsation. This minimizes the degree of left to right shunting. Veno-arterial extracorporeal membrane oxygenation (ECMO) could result in a prohibitively high increase in ventricular afterload which would worsen left to right shunting. Inotropes alone may not achieve the goal of afterload reduction.

References

1. Hayashi T, Hirano Y, Takai H, et al. Usefulness of ST-Segment elevation in the inferior leads in predicting ventricular septal rupture in patients with anterior wall acute myocardial infarction. *Am J Cardiol.* 2005;96(8):1037-1041.
2. Crenshaw BS, Granger CB, Birnbaum Y, et al. Risk factors, angiographic patterns, and outcomes in patients with ventricular septal defect complicating acute myocardial infarction. GUSTO-I (global utilization of streptokinase and TPA for occluded coronary arteries) trial investigators. *Circulation.* 2000;101(1):27-32.

**10.** Correct Answer: A

**Rationale:**

The timing of coronary angiography in patients with cardiac arrest and unknown mental status is controversial. Coronary angiography should be performed emergently for cardiac arrest patients with suspected cardiac etiology of arrest and ST segment elevation on ECG. Patients with ventricular fibrillation or pulseless ventricular tachycardia should be considered at high risk for coronary event, for which urgent angiography should be considered. Emergency coronary angiography is reasonable for select (eg, electrically or hemodynamically unstable) adult patients who are comatose after out-of-hospital cardiac arrest of suspected cardiac origin even without ST elevation on ECG.

There are no guideline consensus statements on the timing of angiography in the absence of ST elevations. There is additional evidence that in those patients with out-of-hospital cardiac arrest and a nonshockable rhythm, early coronary angiography (within 24 hours) was associated with improved mortality. Thus, many argue in favor of early coronary angiography.

Neurologic prognosis is difficult to reliably determine immediately following resuscitation. Thus, the decision with regard to cardiovascular intervention should be made independent of perception of neurologic prognosis.

References

1. Callaway CW, Donnino MW, Fink EL, et al. Part 8: post-cardiac arrest care: 2015 American Heart Association guidelines update for cardiopulmonary resuscitation and emergency cardiovascular care. *Circulation.* 2015;132 (18 suppl 2):S465-S482.
2. Yannopoulos D, Bartos JA, Aufderheide TP, et al. The evolving role of the cardiac catheterization laboratory in the management of patients with out-of-hospital cardiac arrest: a scientific statement from the American Heart Association. *Circulation.* 2019;139(12):e530-e552. doi:10.1161/CIR0000000000000630.

# 16

# ARRHYTHMIAS AND PACEMAKER

Christoph G. S. Nabzdyk and Yvonne Lai

1. You are being emergently called bedside to a 52-year-old otherwise healthy female who underwent a thoracotomy for left lower lobectomy for non–small-cell lung cancer one day ago. According to the nurse, the patient received a 2 mg intravenous hydromorphone bolus 15 minutes ago. You find a somnolent patient, with a respiratory rate of 9/min, stable oxygen saturation of 97% on room air. The patient's heart rate is 167 beats/min and irregular, blood pressure 73/34 mm Hg. An electrocardiogram (ECG) confirms the new diagnosis of atrial fibrillation (AF). The nurse states that the tachycardia started about 5 minutes ago.

   Which would be the MOST appropriate next step?

   A. Amiodarone 150 mg IV bolus
   B. Synchronized cardioversion
   C. Naloxone 0.04 mg IV x1, with possible repeat boluses as indicated
   D. Procainamide 10 mg/kg IV bolus over 5 minute
   E. Metoprolol 5 mg IV bolus

2. A 46-year-old male with Epstein anomaly, hypertension, coronary artery disease, and chronic obstructive pulmonary disease underwent an uncomplicated laminectomy but reports severe pain in the postanesthesia recovery unit. His pain eventually improved after repeated intravenous opioid boluses. However, an ECG reveals new-onset AF with a widened QRS complex and a heart rate between 130 and 140 beats/min. The patient's blood pressure is stable at 110/50 mm Hg, respiratory rate 17/min,
   $O_2$ saturation 98% while receiving 3 L oxygen/min via nasal cannula. The patient is otherwise asymptomatic. The heart rate and rhythm have not changed for the last hour. The patient was in sinus rhythm leading up to this event.

   Which next intervention is MOST appropriate?

   A. Synchronized cardioversion
   B. Amiodarone 150 mg IV bolus
   C. Metoprolol 5 mg IV bolus
   D. Procainamide 10 mg/kg IV bolus over 5 minute
   E. Digoxin 0.25 mg IV bolus

3. A 51-year-old male underwent an uncomplicated triple-vessel coronary artery bypass grafting 4 weeks ago and now presents to the emergency department with chest pain, a friction rub on auscultation, and diffuse ST-segment elevations on ECG. While blood samples are drawn for analysis, the patient states that he "feels lightheaded". A noninvasive blood pressure obtained is recorded to be 62/36 mm Hg. An ECG reveals a heart rate of 33/min with narrow complex QRS complexes. The patient is quickly given three boluses of 1 mg atropine IV with no response in heart rate.

   While you are waiting for the transcutaneous pacing (TCP) equipment to arrive, which of the following interventions is MOST appropriate?

A. Administer more atropine
B. Administer norepinephrine
C. Administer dopamine
D. Administer dobutamine
E. Administer isoproterenol

4. A 95-year-old female develops bradycardia in the postanesthesia care unit shortly after having undergone a transcatheter aortic valve replacement (TAVR). ECG shows a heart rate of 41, and a third-degree atrioventricular block (AVB) is noted. A preoperative ECG showed normal sinus rhythm, right bundle branch block (RBBB), and signs of left ventricular hypertrophy. Her blood pressure up to this point had been normal but now is 93/53 mm Hg. She does report mild dizziness but appears otherwise neurologically intact.

   Which of the following statements is TRUE?

   A. Most of the patients after TAVR require a lifelong permanent pacemaker (PPM).
   B. Immediate TCP is indicated for TAVR-induced third-degree AVB.
   C. A preoperative RBBB in patients undergoing TAVR is associated with worse outcomes.
   D. Dopamine and isoproterenol are not efficacious in this situation.
   E. Aminophylline is recommended for this patient with a third-degree AVB.

5. A 65-year-old patient with extensive adenocarcinoma of the lung is scheduled to undergo thoracotomy, left lower lobectomy, pericardiectomy, and pleurectomy. The patient has a medical history of hypertension, coronary artery disease, poorly controlled type II diabetes mellitus, a PPM due to a Mobitz type II AVB, and congestive heart failure with a left ventricular ejection fraction (LVEF) of 40% and mild diastolic dysfunction. Unfortunately, the available medical record does not contain any information about the PPM and the patient states that he had not seen a cardiologist in a few years. No pacing spikes are seen on the ECG.

   Which of the following is the MOST appropriate way to proceed?

   A. Obtain electrophysiology (EP) consult and ask for the PPM to be set to AAI with a backup rate at 60 bpm
   B. Apply a magnet at the beginning of the case and convert PPM to VOO at a rate of 60 bpm
   C. Obtain EP consult and ask for the PPM to be set to VVI at a rate of 60 bpm
   D. Obtain EP consult and ask for the PPM to be set to AOO at a rate of 60 bpm
   E. Obtain EP consult and ask for the PPM to be set to DOO at a rate of 60 bpm

6. A 67-year-old man with peripheral vascular disease is about to undergo transmetatarsal amputation and lower extremity skin grafting. The patient had a recent diagnosis of ischemic cardiomyopathy (LVEF 25%) and a latest generation implantable cardioverter defibrillator (ICD) placed a few months ago. The patient is pacemaker dependent 99% of the time according to the recent outpatient ICD interrogation. The surgeon is urging you to quickly bring the patient into the operating room, not worry about the ICD, and promises to avoid any electrocautery.

   Which of the following statements is MOST correct?

   A. Applying a magnet for the duration of the case or obtaining an EP consultation before the case is the standard of care for all surgical patients.
   B. Proceed with the case as requested, ensure that a magnet and TCP equipment are readily available, and insist that only brief bipolar electrocautery bursts are used if any.
   C. Use of harmonic scalpel confers a similar risk of electromagnetic interference as monopolar and bipolar electrocautery.
   D. A magnet application onto the ICD will reliably deactivate antitachycardia pacing and defibrillation.
   E. A magnet application onto the ICD will reliably switch the pacemaker into an asynchronous mode.

7. A 75-year-old male suffered an acute myocardial infarction (AMI) while driving his car resulting in a head-on collision with an incoming driver. He suffered multiple rib fractures causing a pneumohemothorax and pericardial tamponade and is he being rushed in the operating room for exploration. In the operating room, you note that the patient has intermittent sinus arrest. The surgeon is placing atrial and ventricular pacing wires and is asking you how you would like to pace the patient now that the surgical portion of the case is over.

   Which of the following statements is MOST accurate?

**A.** VOO is the preferred pacing mode for this patient.

**B.** DOO confers less risk of R-on-T phenomenon compared with VOO.

**C.** R-on-T phenomenon is impossible in VVI pacing.

**D.** R-on-T phenomenon is impossible in DDD pacing.

**E.** AAI is a reasonable pacing mode for this patient.

---

**8.** You are called to bedside in the ICU to a 73-year-old female admitted with urosepsis and non-ST elevation myocardial infarction for evaluation of arrhythmia on telemetry. Her 12-lead ECG reveals intermittent torsades de pointes (TdP) and the patient is hemodynamically stable.

Which of the following statements is MOST correct?

**A.** Magnesium sulfate is the first-line agent in sustained TdP.

**B.** Amiodarone prolongs QT interval and is considered low risk for TdP.

**C.** Sotalol and verapamil are safe nodal blocking agents for patients at risk for TdP.

**D.** Haloperidol, methadone, erythromycin, and procainamide are safe in patients at risk for TdP.

**E.** Hyperkalemia is a risk factor for TdP.

---

**9.** A 75-year-old male with AMI was admitted to the intensive care unit (ICU). Initially hemodynamically and respiratory stable, the patient's heart rhythm suddenly changed into what appears to be a supraventricular tachycardia with a heart rate of 180 beats/min. The resident asks for your help and suggests administering lidocaine for the patient's arrhythmia. As you discuss the plan at the bedside, the patient suddenly becomes unresponsive and ventricular tachycardia (VT) is noted on the telemetry.

Which of the following statements is MOST correct regarding the next steps in the patient's management?

**A.** Amiodarone use improves survival of in-hospital cardiac arrest.

**B.** Prophylactic lidocaine and high-dose amiodarone administration for the prevention of VT after AMI may increase mortality.

**C.** Lidocaine administration is associated with increased survival when given prophylactically after return of spontaneous circulation in adults with ventricular fibrillation/pulseless ventricular tachycardia (VF/pVT) cardiac arrest.

**D.** Lidocaine for VF/pVT leads to worse long-term survival when compared with amiodarone.

**E.** Lidocaine administration is efficacious for the treatment of supraventricular tachycardia.

---

**10.** An 83-year-old male with a history of ischemic cardiomyopathy, systolic heart failure (LVEF 24%), and combined pacemaker and ICD for cardiac synchronization therapy (CRT-D) underwent coronary artery bypass graft (CABG) surgery three days ago. He still has atrial and ventricular epicardial pacing wires in place. He is now urgently admitted to the ICU with acute decompensation of his heart failure and volume overload. On transthoracic echocardiogram, his LVEF is reduced to 15% and the patient's heart rhythm shows frequent alternating runs of AF/atrial flutter (HR 110s) and monomorphic VT (HR 100s). During these episodes, the patient becomes lightheaded because of mild hypotension.

Which of the following statements about the next steps in management is MOST accurate?

**A.** Overdrive pacing is not efficacious for breaking postoperative atrial flutter in patients that underwent heart surgery.

**B.** Biatrial but not right atrial pacing reduces the incidence of AF after CABG.

**C.** Epicardial overdrive pacing is contraindicated in patients with monomorphic VT.

**D.** Procainamide is recommended as initial treatment of patients with stable sustained monomorphic VT.

**E.** Verapamil and diltiazem are safe choices for patients with VTs and myocardial dysfunction.

# Chapter 16 ▪ Answers

**1.** Correct Answer: B

**Rationale:**

Postoperative AF is common after thoracic procedures. Hemodynamic instability in patients with tachycardia secondary to AF/atrial flutter and preexcitation warrants emergent cardioversion. In hemodynamically stable patients with AF/atrial flutter, the use of a beta-blocker or nondihydropyridine calcium channel antagonist is recommended to achieve rate control. In critically ill patients with AF/atrial flutter without preexcitation, intravenous amiodarone may be used to control heart rate. Intravenous procainamide is recommended for hemodynamically stable patients with preexcited AF and rapid ventricular response. While this patient did appear somnolent after the hydromorphone administration, there is little evidence to suggest that the patient was severely respiratory compromised.

Reference
1. January CT, Wann LS, Alpert JS, et al. 2014 AHA/ACC/HRS guideline for the management of patients with atrial fibrillation: a report of the American College of Cardiology/American Heart Association task force on practice guidelines and the Heart Rhythm Society. *J Am Coll Cardiol.* 2014;64:e1-e76.

**2.** Correct Answer: D

**Rationale:**

This patient has Wolff-Parkinson-White (WPW) syndrome, possibly as a result of his Epstein anomaly. Epstein anomaly is a congenital heart defect with apical displacement of the tricuspid valve and represents a known cause of WPW. Use of nodal blocking agents in patients with WPW is potentially harmful because these drugs accelerate the ventricular rate via the excitatory pathway and even may cause ventricular fibrillation.

Procainamide or ibutilide is the recommended agent to achieve sinus rhythm or ventricular rate control in hemodynamically stable patients with preexcited AF and rapid ventricular response. Synchronized cardioversion is recommended for patients with AF, WPW, and rapid ventricular response who are hemodynamically unstable.

References
1. January CT, Wann LS, Alpert JS, et al. 2014 AHA/ACC/HRS guideline for the management of patients with atrial fibrillation: a report of the American College of Cardiology/American Heart Association task force on practice guidelines and the Heart Rhythm Society. *J Am Coll Cardiol.* 2014;64:e1-e76.
2. Kim RJ, Gerling BR, Kono AT, et al. Precipitation of ventricular fibrillation by intravenous diltiazem and metoprolol in a young patient with occult Wolff-Parkinson-White syndrome. *Pacing Clin Electrophysiol.* 2008;31:776-779.
3. Simonian SM, Lotfipour S, Wall C, et al. Challenging the superiority of amiodarone for rate control in Wolff-Parkinson-White and atrial fibrillation. *Intern Emerg Med.* 2010;5:421-426.
4. Boriani G, Biffi M, Frabetti L, et al. Ventricular fibrillation after intravenous amiodarone in Wolff-Parkinson-White syndrome with atrial fibrillation. *Am Heart J.* 1996;131:1214-1216.

**3.** Correct Answer: C

**Rationale:**

Atropine is an anticholinergic, which is a muscarinic acetylcholine receptor antagonist. The Advanced Cardiovascular Life Support guidelines suggest a maximum dose of up to 3 milligram in the setting of symptomatic sinus bradycardia. If atropine does not yield a sufficient heart rate increase, TCP is recommended. Should TCP not be available or require time to be obtained, it is reasonable to start either an epinephrine or dopamine infusion. Norepinephrine has a nonlinear effect on heart rate; at lower doses, norepinephrine may cause reflex bradycardia, whereas at higher doses, it causes an increase in heart rate. Dobutamine and isoproterenol are strong chronotropes. Because of their isolated beta activities, their administration is associated with hypotension due to vasodilation, which would be deleterious in this patient. Dopamine and epinephrine are the preferred chronotropes should atropine fail and TCP not be immediately available. Although isoproterenol is a possible third alternative chronotrope, the known hypotensive effects are of particular concern in this patient.

References
1. Rigaud M, Boschat J, Rocha P, et al. Comparative haemodynamic effects of dobutamine and isoproterenol in man. *Intensive Care Med.* 1977;3:57-62.
2. Tuttle RR, Mills J. Dobutamine: development of a new catecholamine to selectively increase cardiac contractility. *Circ Res.* 1975;36:185-196.
3. Neumar RW, Shuster M, Callaway CW, et al. Part 1: executive summary: 2015 American Heart Association guidelines update for cardiopulmonary resuscitation and emergency cardiovascular care. *Circulation.* 2015;132:S315-S367.

4. Goldstein DS, Zimlichman R, Stull R, et al. Plasma catecholamine and hemodynamic responses during isoproterenol infusions in humans. *Clin Pharmacol Ther*. 1986;40:233-238.
5. VanValkinburgh D, McGuigan JJ. *Inotropes and Vasopressors*. Treasure Island, FL: StatPearls; 2018.
6. Kusumoto FM, Schoenfeld MH, Barrett C, et al. 2018 ACC/AHA/HRS guideline on the evaluation and management of patients with bradycardia and cardiac conduction delay: a report of the American College of Cardiology/American Heart Association task force on clinical practice guidelines and the Heart Rhythm Society. *Heart Rhythm*. 2018. doi:10.1016/j.hrthm.2018.10.037.

**4.**  Correct Answer: C

**Rationale:**

Conduction system abnormalities are common after TAVR. A new-onset left bundle branch block occurs in 19% to 55% and a new high-degree AVB in approximately 10% of patients. Up to 50% of these new-onset conduction disturbances resolve before discharge. Further, only 50% of patients with a new PPM after TAVR will be pacer dependent at 6 to 12 months. In older studies, up to 51% of patients received PPM implant after TAVR, but owing to evolving technology, there has been a significant decrease in the need for pacemaker implantation after TAVR.

Although it is imperative to place TCP pads on this patient, this patient appears hemodynamically and neurologically fairly intact and thus an attempt at chemical pacing is reasonable. Hemodynamic instability and bradycardia refractory to medical therapy (including atropine and sympathomimetics) warrant transcutaneous or transvenous pacing. Preprocedural conduction abnormalities, particularly RBBB is associated with increased risk of PPM and death after TAVR.

Beta-adrenergic agonists such as isoproterenol, dopamine, dobutamine, and epinephrine enhance atrioventricular nodal and His-Purkinje conduction, and automaticity of atrioventricular junctional and ventricular pacemakers in the setting of a complete AVB. Clinical efficacy of dopamine was shown to be equivalent to TCP in patients with unstable bradycardia unresponsive to atropine. Isoproterenol was able to elicit an escape rhythm in the majority of pacemaker-dependent patients. Use of aminophylline is reasonable for patients with a second- or third-degree AVB associated with acute inferior myocardial infarction.

## References

1. Kusumoto FM, Schoenfeld MH, Barrett C, et al. 2018 ACC/AHA/HRS Guideline on the evaluation and management of patients with bradycardia and cardiac conduction delay: a report of the American College of Cardiology/American Heart Association task force on clinical practice guidelines and the heart rhythm society. *Heart Rhythm*. 2018. doi:10.1016/j.hrthm.2018.10.037.
2. Piazza N, Onuma Y, Jesserun E, et al. Early and persistent intraventricular conduction abnormalities and requirements for pacemaking after percutaneous replacement of the aortic valve. *JACC Cardiovasc Interv*. 2008;1:310-316.
3. Auffret V, Webb JG, Eltchaninoff H, et al. Clinical Impact of baseline right bundle branch block in patients undergoing transcatheter aortic valve replacement. *JACC Cardiovasc Interv*. 2017;10:1564-1574.
4. Gonska B, Seeger J, Kessler M, et al. Predictors for permanent pacemaker implantation in patients undergoing transfemoral aortic valve implantation with the Edwards Sapien 3 valve. *Clin Res Cardiol*. 2017;106:590-597.

**5.**  Correct Answer: E

**Rationale:**

Although applying a magnet may convert a PPM to an asynchronous mode (such as DOO or VOO), this would not be guaranteed in this case as little is known about the model of the PPM, the patient's degree of dependence on the PPM, and the PPM's battery function. Given that the patient had not seen a cardiologist in years, the least that should be done is to obtain an EP consult for PPM interrogation before this elective surgery. AAI and AOO are not ideal pacing modes for this patient given his high risk of progression to third-degree AV block. Both modes require intact AV conduction for proper functioning. Given the close proximity to the heart, electrocautery may inhibit PPM function in AAI and VVI modes.

DOO provides asynchronous atrial and ventricular pacing and thus atrioventricular coupling when compared with VOO. This confers hemodynamic benefits especially for patients with mild diastolic dysfunction (impaired relaxation) in whom left ventricular filling is more dependent on atrial contraction than in patients with normal diastolic function or severe diastolic dysfunction. Both asynchronous modes (DOO and VOO) can cause an R-on-T phenomenon and trigger malignant ventricular tachyarrhythmias.

## References

1. Ghio S, Marinoni G, Broglia P, et al. Hemodynamic benefits of sequential atrioventricular pacing. *G Ital Cardiol*. 1991;21:957-964.
2. Hartzler GO, Maloney JD, Curtis JJ, et al. Hemodynamic benefits of atrioventricular sequential pacing after cardiac surgery. *Am J Cardiol*. 1977;40:232-236.
3. Crossley GH, Poole JE, Rozner MA, et al. The Heart Rhythm Society (HRS)/American Society of Anesthesiologists (ASA) expert consensus statement on the perioperative management of patients with implantable defibrillators, pacemakers and arrhythmia monitors: facilities and patient management this document was developed as a joint project with the American Society of Anesthesiologists (ASA), and in collaboration with the American Heart Association (AHA), and the Society of Thoracic Surgeons (STS). *Heart Rhythm*. 2011;8:1114-1154.

**6.** Correct Answer: B

**Rationale:**

The 2011 Heart Rhythm Society/American Society of Anesthesiologists expert consensus statement notes that a single recommendation for all patients with cardiovascular implantable electronic devices (CIEDs) is not appropriate. It further states that in some circumstances, remote or perioperative CIED interrogation or reprogramming (including changing pacing to an asynchronous mode and/or inactivating ICD tachytherapies), application of a magnet over the CIED with or without postoperative CIED interrogation or use of no perioperative CIED interrogation or intervention may be necessary. This decision should be made depending on the nature and location of the operative procedure, likelihood of use of monopolar electrocautery, type of CIEDs (ie, pacemaker vs ICD), and dependence of the patient on cardiac pacing. It is further recommended to inactivate the ICD for all surgeries above the umbilicus implying that it was unnecessary to do so for surgeries below the umbilicus. It was argued that the risk of electromagnetic interference being detected, and hence of discharge of the device, was very low. It will take 3 to 4 seconds to detect the ventricular fibrillation and another 5 to 10 seconds for the ICD to charge before the shock can be delivered.

Application of a magnet in patients with ICD, who are not pacemaker-dependent and are undergoing infraumbilical surgery, is thus not universally necessary. Application of a magnet will generally deactivate both modes, antitachycardic pacing and defibrillation, even though some ICD models (Boston Scientific and St. Jude Medical) can be programmed to ignore the magnet. If the magnet deactivates both modes on magnet application, removal of the magnet generally reactivates both modes.

Applying a magnet onto an ICD will **not** affect the pacemaker function of the ICD. This is distinctly different when compared with the application of a magnet onto a simple pacemaker, which generally switches the pacemaker into an asynchronous mode (DOO, VOO). Harmonic scalpel and bipolar electrocautery as opposed to monopolar electrocautery confer minimal risk of electromagnetic interference.

References

1. Crossley GH, Poole JE, Rozner MA, et al. The Heart Rhythm Society (HRS)/American Society of Anesthesiologists (ASA) expert consensus statement on the perioperative management of patients with implantable defibrillators, pacemakers and arrhythmia monitors: facilities and patient management this document was developed as a joint project with the American Society of Anesthesiologists (ASA), and in collaboration with the American Heart Association (AHA), and the Society of Thoracic Surgeons (STS). *Heart Rhythm*. 2011;8:1114-1154.
2. Bruce Kleinman JM, Loo J, Radzak J, Cytron J,Streckenbach S. Unintended discharge of an icd in a patient undergoing total knee replacement. *APSF Newsletter*. 2017;32.
3. Fleisher LA, Fleischmann KE, Auerbach AD, et al. 2014 ACC/AHA guideline on perioperative cardiovascular evaluation and management of patients undergoing noncardiac surgery: executive summary: a report of the American College of Cardiology/ American Heart association task force on practice guidelines. *Circulation*. 2014;130:2215-2245.

**7.** Correct Answer: E

**Rationale:**

VOO and DOO are asynchronous modes that both can cause an R-on-T phenomenon. Although VVI and DDD modes should be safer with regards to R-on-T phenomenon because of ventricular sensing, there have been case reports of R-on-T phenomenon in patients paced in a VVI mode as a result of pacemaker undersensing. Another study reported two other cases of undersensing of demand pacemakers in patients with AMI rendering the patients effectively paced in an asynchronous mode. Given that the patient appears to have an intact atrioventricular conduction system, AAI would be a reasonable pacing mode for this patient at this point. Should the patient develop a higher degree of atrioventricular conduction delay (eg Mobitz II or third-degree AVB), DDD would be a reasonable pacing mode.

References

1. Treese N, Kasper W, Meinertz T, et al. Undersensing of demand pacemakers in acute myocardial infarction. *Klin Wochenschr*. 1980;58:1319-1321.
2. Beiras Torrado X, Crespo Carazo N, Amorin Ferreiro F, et al. Sensing anomalies with the VVI pacemaker. Clinical study by Holter. *Rev Esp Cardiol*. 1990;43(suppl 2):48-51.
3. Chemello D, Subramanian A, Kumaraswamy N. Cardiac arrest caused by undersensing of a temporary epicardial pacemaker. *Can J Cardiol*. 2010;26:e13-e14.
4. Nakamori Y, Maeda T, Ohnishi Y. Reiterative ventricular fibrillation caused by R-on-T during temporary epicardial pacing: a case report. *JA Clin Rep*. 2016;2:3.

**8.** Correct Answer: B

**Rationale:**

Torsades de pointes (TdP) is a specific form of polymorphic VT characterized by a pattern of twisting points and is considered the acquired form of drug-induced long-QT syndrome (LQTS). Amiodarone prolongs QT interval, but it is considered to have a low risk for triggering TdP. Direct current cardioversion is the treatment of choice for sustained TdP or TdP that progressed to ventricular fibrillation. Verapamil is considered safe for patients with TdP, however sotalol has been associated with TdP and is listed as a drug that raises the risk of TdP. Likewise, haloperidol, methadone, erythromycin, and procainamide are known to increase the risk for TdP occurrence. Hypokalemia is a risk factor for TdP and should be corrected to a potassium level of 4.5 to 5.0 mmol/L in patients with TdP. Magnesium sulfate (2 g) can be infused to terminate TdP irrespective of the serum magnesium level, and repeat doses may be necessary.

### References
1. Banai S, Tzivoni D. Drug therapy for torsade de pointes. *J Cardiovasc Electrophysiol*. 1993;4:206-210.
2. Zipes DP, Camm AJ, Borggrefe M, et al. ACC/AHA/ESC 2006 guidelines for management of patients with ventricular arrhythmias and the prevention of sudden cardiac death: a report of the American College of Cardiology/American Heart Association task force and the European Society of Cardiology Committee for practice guidelines (writing committee to develop guidelines for management of patients with ventricular arrhythmias and the prevention of sudden cardiac death): developed in collaboration with the European Heart Rhythm Association and the Heart Rhythm Society. *Circulation*. 2006;114:e385-e484.
3. Drew BJ, Ackerman MJ, Funk M, et al. Prevention of torsade de pointes in hospital settings: a scientific statement from the American Heart Association and the American College of Cardiology Foundation. *J Am Coll Cardiol*. 2010;55:934-947.

---

**9.** Correct Answer: B

### Rationale:

There is no randomized controlled trial (RCT) suggesting that use of amiodarone or lidocaine improves survival of in-hospital cardiac arrest. A recent, large RCT evaluating amiodarone versus lidocaine versus placebo suggests that in the setting of out-of-hospital cardiac arrest, amiodarone and lidocaine are superior to placebo with regards to survival to hospital and there was no difference between the two drugs. Unfortunately, there was no difference in the rate of survival-to-hospital discharge or favorable neurologic outcomes across all three groups in out-of-hospital cardiac arrest caused by VF/pVT. A prior, smaller RCT suggested that amiodarone administration would increase survival to hospital admission when compared with lidocaine administration. Lidocaine may suppress VF/pVT, however, may adversely affect mortality rates after AMI. The ACC/AHA guidelines further state that in patients with suspected AMI, prophylactic administration of lidocaine or high-dose amiodarone for the prevention of VT is potentially harmful. Amiodarone, but not lidocaine, should be considered as possible second- or third-line therapy for supraventricular tachycardia. Lidocaine has no role in treatment of supraventricular tachycardia, according to the AHA/ACC guidelines.

### References
1. Teo KK, Yusuf S, Furberg CD. Effects of prophylactic antiarrhythmic drug therapy in acute myocardial infarction. An overview of results from randomized controlled trials. *JAMA*. 1993;270:1589-1595.
2. Panchal AR, Berg KM, Kudenchuk PJ, et al. 2018 American Heart Association focused update on advanced cardiovascular life support use of antiarrhythmic drugs during and immediately after cardiac arrest: an update to the American Heart Association guidelines for cardiopulmonary resuscitation and emergency cardiovascular care. *Circulation*. 2018;138:e740-e749.
3. Page RL, Joglar JA, Caldwell MA, et al. 2015 ACC/AHA/HRS guideline for the management of adult patients with supraventricular tachycardia: executive summary: a report of the American College of Cardiology/American Heart Association task force on clinical practice guidelines and the heart rhythm society. *Circulation*. 2016;133:e471-e505.
4. Al-Khatib SM, Stevenson WG, Ackerman MJ, et al. 2017 AHA/ACC/HRS guideline for management of patients with ventricular arrhythmias and the prevention of sudden cardiac death. *Circulation*. 2018;138:e272-e391.

---

**10.** Correct Answer: D

### Rationale:

Overdrive pacing has been shown to terminate postoperative atrial flutter in the vast majority of patients that underwent heart surgery. According to the AHA/ACC guidelines, rapid atrial pacing is useful for acute conversion of atrial flutter in patients who have pacing wires in place as part of a PPM or implantable cardioverter-defibrillator or for temporary atrial pacing after cardiac surgery. Both, temporary right atrial or biatrial pacing after CABG and other cardiac surgeries decreased the incidence of postoperative AF in the majority of the studies.

Procainamide is considered reasonable as an initial treatment modality for patients with stable sustained monomorphic VT. Direct-current cardioversion is recommended in patients with hemodynamically unstable, sustained monomorphic VT.

AHA/ACC/ESC guidelines support the use of overdrive pacing in patients with refractory, slower VTs. However, electrical cardioversion/defibrillation should be immediately available, because acceleration of VT and degeneration to ventricular fibrillation are well-described complications. Intravenous amiodarone can be beneficial in patients with hemodynamically unstable, sustained monomorphic VT that was refractory to cardioversion or procainamide/other antiarrhythmic drugs.

The AHA/ACC/ESC guidelines warn against the use of calcium channel blockers such as verapamil and diltiazem in patients with myocardial dysfunction for the purpose of terminating wide-QRS-complex tachycardias.

## References

1. Page RL, Joglar JA, Caldwell MA, et al. 2015 ACC/AHA/HRS guideline for the management of adult patients with supraventricular tachycardia: executive summary: a report of the American College of Cardiology/American Heart Association Task force on clinical practice guidelines and the heart. *Circulation*. 2016;133:e471-e505.

2. Daoud EG, Snow R, Hummel JD, et al. Temporary atrial epicardial pacing as prophylaxis against atrial fibrillation after heart surgery: a meta-analysis. *J Cardiovasc Electrophysiol*. 2003;14:127-132.

3. Priori SG, Blomstrom-Lundqvist C. 2015 European Society of cardiology guidelines for the management of patients with ventricular arrhythmias and the prevention of sudden cardiac death summarized by co-chairs. *Eur Heart J*. 2015;36:2757-2759.

4. Zipes DP, Camm AJ, Borggrefe M, et al. ACC/AHA/ESC 2006 guidelines for management of patients with ventricular arrhythmias and the prevention of sudden cardiac death–executive summary: a report of the American College of Cardiology/American Heart Association Task Force and the European Society of Cardiology committee for practice guidelines (writing committee to develop guidelines for management of patients with ventricular arrhythmias and the prevention of sudden cardiac death) developed in collaboration with the European Heart Rhythm Association and the Heart Rhythm Society. *Eur Heart J*. 2006;27:2099-2140.

# 17

# HEART FAILURE

Christoph G. S. Nabzdyk and Yvonne Lai

1. An 82-year-old obese male with a long-standing history of diabetes mellitus presents to the emergency department with dyspnea, cough, mild fever, and tachycardia (heart rate 105 bpm). The patient's blood pressure is 93/58 mm Hg. The patient reports having had a cold for the past few days and noticed a sudden-onset shortness of breath yesterday. A chest x-ray reveals diffuse opacification of the right lung. Heart and lung sounds are difficult to auscultate. Empiric antibiotics for community-acquired pneumonia are started, and supplemental $O_2$ via nasal cannula is given. His respiratory rate is 18 breaths/min and oxygen saturation is 97% while receiving 4 L/min of $O_2$ supplementation.

   Which of the following actions is most appropriate?

   A. Initiate biphasic positive airway pressure (BIPAP) to improve pulmonary edema
   B. Start high-flow nasal cannula to decrease work of breathing and eliminate $CO_2$
   C. Obtain CT scan of the chest to further evaluate the right lung process
   D. Obtain transthoracic echocardiogram
   E. Start phenylephrine to increase blood pressure and improve coronary blood flow

2. An 81-year-old woman with a body mass index of 36 kg/m$^2$ and long-standing congestive heart failure, hypertension, atrial fibrillation, and chronic obstructive pulmonary disease is admitted to the intensive care unit with exacerbation of heart failure. The patient presented with severe shortness of breath, diffuse bilateral pulmonary edema on chest x-ray, elevated brain natriuretic peptide levels of 13 187 pg/mL, and an elevated creatinine of 2.13 mg/dL. Echocardiogram reveals a left ventricular ejection fraction of 55%.

   Which statement with regards to this patient is most accurate?

   A. Beta-blocker therapy yields equal reduction in mortality in diastolic heart failure versus systolic heart failure patients.
   B. Ischemic heart disease is the major mechanism leading to diastolic heart failure.
   C. Diastolic heart failure is characterized by eccentric ventricular hypertrophy.
   D. Diastolic pulmonary gradient is a poor predictor of mortality in patients with pulmonary hypertension due to left heart disease.
   E. Patients with diastolic heart failure have a lower 5-year survival than patients with systolic heart failure.

3. A 79-year-old male with acutely decompensated systolic heart failure is admitted from the emergency department with respiratory failure and acute anuric renal failure. The patient is bradycardic and hypotensive. At home, the patient has been taking atenolol, digoxin, hydrochlorothiazide, and lisinopril. A milrinone infusion is started for inotropic support. The patient's renal function did not improve over the following days ultimately requiring renal continuous veno-venous hemofiltration (CVVH).

   Which of the statements regarding the medical therapy is CORRECT?

   A. Milrinone metabolism is highly dependent on hepatic function.
   B. Milrinone's terminal elimination halflife is approximately 2 hours in patients with normal renal function.
   C. Milrinone can safely be used in patients requiring CVVH.
   D. CVVH clears digoxin from the patient's plasma.
   E. Atenolol metabolism is independent of renal function.

4. A 72-year-old male with coronary artery disease presents 5 days after experiencing chest pain complaining of dyspnea. He is in the emergency department with heart rate 87 beats/min and blood pressure 86/42 mm Hg, oxygen saturation 91% on 50% oxygen via facemask. You do a bedside echocardiogram and find that he has a depressed ejection fraction and severe mitral regurgitation. A formal echocardiogram was performed and a ruptured papillary muscle identified. His other lab values are significant for lactate 5.6 mmol/L and creatinine 2.01 mg/dL. You place him on BIPAP to improve oxygenation and inotropes to augment perfusion. Despite these measures, he continues to have worsening metabolic acidosis and now LFTs are rising. An intra-aortic balloon pump (IABP) is placed and the patient is being prepared to go to the operating room. Which of the following is **NOT** true regarding IABP?

 A. IABP is the most commonly used mechanical support device.
 B. It has been shown to improve mortality in patients with cardiogenic shock.
 C. It has been indicated for patients with mechanical complications from myocardial infarction such as a ventricular septal defect and mitral regurgitation.
 D. It is contraindicated in a patient with aortic insufficiency.
 E. Helium is used to inflate the balloon.

5. A 64-year-old female with longstanding hypertension and mild aortic stenosis and subsequent left ventricular hypertrophy is in septic shock requiring vasopressors. You do a bedside echocardiogram, and left ventricular function is within normal limits. You decide to continue volume resuscitation, and she becomes more hypoxic requiring supplemental oxygen. You suspect heart failure with preserved ejection fraction (HFpEF). Which of the following is **NOT** true regarding diastolic function?

 A. Atrial fibrillation is tolerated poorly.
 B. End-stage renal disease is associated with diastolic dysfunction.
 C. Lusitropy is a determinant of the effectiveness of early diastole.
 D. Diastolic dysfunction can be a component of septic cardiomyopathy.
 E. Ventricular relaxation is only a passive process.

# Chapter 17 ▪ Answers

**1.** Correct Answer: D

**Rationale:**
Sudden onset of shortness of breath and asymmetric pulmonary edema can be the presenting symptoms of acute severe mitral regurgitation. This patient's body habitus could make it difficult to appreciate a systolic murmur that is associated with severe mitral regurgitation. Acute severe mitral regurgitation has been described in the setting of (1) papillary muscle rupture after myocardial infarction, (2) papillary muscle dysfunction due to coronary vasospasm and slow-flow phenomenon, (3) permanent pacemakers (right ventricular pacing), (4) bacterial endocarditis, and (5) spontaneous peripartum chordae tendineae rupture. This patient's diabetes mellitus and often associated small-fiber polyneuropathy may have masked the angina from myocardial infarction.

   Asymmetric pulmonary edema and a sudden onset of shortness of breath in patients at risk for ischemic mitral valve disease should trigger an immediate echocardiographic evaluation of the heart. Confirmation of the diagnosis may warrant urgent cardiologic or cardiac surgical intervention. The indiscriminate use of phenylephrine in this patient could worsen the mitral regurgitation, and it may not be warranted, given a normal mean arterial pressure and appropriate mentation.

References
1. Young AL, Langston CS, Schiffman RL, et al. Mitral valve regurgitation causing right upper lobe pulmonary edema. *Tex Heart Inst J.* 2001;28:53-56.
2. Ternus BW, Mankad S, Edwards WD, et al. Clinical presentation and echocardiographic diagnosis of postinfarction papillary muscle rupture: a review of 22 cases. *Echocardiography.* 2017;34:973-977.
3. Birnbaum Y, Chamoun AJ, Conti VR, et al. Mitral regurgitation following acute myocardial infarction. *Coron Artery Dis.* 2002;13:337-344.

**2.** Correct Answer: D

**Rationale:**
Although obesity, coronary artery disease, diabetes mellitus, atrial fibrillation, and hyperlipidemia are highly prevalent in patients with HFpEF, hypertension is the most important cause of HFpEF. It is associated with concentric ventricular hypertrophy and increased ventricular mass. The prevalence of HFpEF has increased

over a study period of 15 years, whereas survival remained unchanged during the interval. Survival of patients with HF*p*EF has been reported to be higher or similar to that of patients with reduced ejection fraction. While beta-blocker, diuretics, and ACE-inhibitors are frequently used in patients with HF*p*EF; results from randomized controlled trials evaluating these regimens in patients with HF*p*EF have been disappointing. Several beta-blockers proved to be effective in reducing the risk of death in patients with chronic heart failure with reduced ejection fraction (HF*r*EF). According to the 2013 ACC/AHA guidelines on heart failure management, the randomized controlled trials mostly enrolled patients with HF*r*EF, and it is only in these patients that efficacious therapies have been demonstrated; ie, no efficacious therapies for HF*p*EF patients have been identified to date. In a retrospective study of 1236 patients with cardiomyopathy and pulmonary hypertension due to left heart disease, an elevated diastolic pulmonary gradient was not associated with worse survival. Other studies also confirmed that diastolic pulmonary gradient is a poor predictor of mortality in patients with pulmonary hypertension due to left heart disease.

### References

1. Zile MR, Brutsaert DL. New concepts in diastolic dysfunction and diastolic heart failure: part II: causal mechanisms and treatment. *Circulation*. 2002;105:1503-1508.
2. Zile MR, Brutsaert DL. New concepts in diastolic dysfunction and diastolic heart failure: part I: diagnosis, prognosis, and measurements of diastolic function. *Circulation*. 2002;105:1387-1393.
3. Yancy CW, Jessup M, Bozkurt B, et al. 2013 ACCF/AHA guideline for the management of heart failure: a report of the American College of Cardiology Foundation/American Heart Association Task Force on Practice Guidelines. *J Am Coll Cardiol*. 2013;62:e147-e239.
4. Tampakakis E, Leary PJ, Selby VN, et al. The diastolic pulmonary gradient does not predict survival in patients with pulmonary hypertension due to left heart disease. *JACC Heart Fail*. 2015;3:9-16.

**3.** Correct Answer: B

**Rationale**

While up to 15% of milrinone undergoes hepatic metabolism (glucuronidation), the vast majority of milrinone is excreted unchanged via the kidneys. Milrinone's terminal elimination half-life is approximately 2 hours in patients with normal renal function. There appears to exist a linear relationship between creatinine clearance and the renal clearance of milrinone. The terminal elimination half-life of milrinone in subjects receiving CVVH is longer compared with that in subjects with normal renal function (up to 20 hours have been reported). Digoxin metabolism is dependent on renal function. Dialysis does not eliminate digoxin from the patient's plasma. Digoxin-specific Fab-antibody fragments are the antidote for digoxin overdose. Hypokalemia as oppose to hyperkalemia increases digoxin toxicity because of increased binding of digoxin to the Na/K-ATPase (digoxin competes with potassium for the binding at the Na/K-ATPase), thus the combination of dialysis and digoxin confers the risk of inducing digoxin toxicity. Likewise, atenolol metabolism is dependent on renal function while other beta-blockers, such as metoprolol and carvedilol, are not.

### References

1. Thiemann DR. Digitalis and hemodialysis is a bad combination. *J Am Soc Nephrol*. 2010;21:1418-1420.
2. Taniguchi T, Shibata K, Saito S, et al. Pharmacokinetics of milrinone in patients with congestive heart failure during continuous venovenous hemofiltration. *Intensive Care Med*. 2000;26:1089-1093.
3. Hartmann B, Czock D, Keller F. Drug therapy in patients with chronic renal failure. *Dtsch Arztebl Int*. 2010;107:647-655; quiz 655-646.

**4.** Correct Answer: B

**Rationale:**

The IABP is the most commonly used mechanical circulatory support device. Indications for IABP include cardiogenic shock, postmyocardial infarction, cardiomyopathy, and complications of acute myocardial infarction such as acute ventricular septal defect and mitral regurgitation. The IABP-SHOCK II trial randomized 600 patients with cardiogenic shock from myocardial infarction to receive IABP or not. It showed no difference in mortality, length of stay in the intensive care unit, renal function, sepsis, stroke, or peripheral ischemic complications. Some contraindications for IABP insertion include aortic dissection, severe aortic insufficiency, severe coagulopathy, and tachyarrhythmias. Helium is used to inflate the balloon because of its low viscosity and quick elimination if the balloon ruptures.

### References

1. Gold HK, Leinbach RC, Sanders CA, et al. Intraaortic balloon pumping for ventricular septal defect or mitral regurgitation complicating acute myocardial infarction. *Circulation*. 1973;47:1191.
2. Ibanez B, James S, Agewall S, et al. 2017 ESC guidelines for the management of acute myocardial infarction in patients presenting with ST-segment elevation: the task force for the management of acute myocardial infarction in patients presenting with ST-segment elevation of the European Society of Cardiology (ESC). *Eur Heart J*. 2018;39:119.

**5.** Correct Answer: E

**Rationale:**

Heart failure with preserved ejection fraction is typically associated with hypertension, old age, coronary artery disease, diabetes mellitus, obstructive sleep apnea, and kidney disease. Left ventricular filling is dependent on myocardial relaxation (an active process requiring metabolic energy) and ventricular compliance (which is a passive process). Lusitropy is defined as the rate of myocardial relaxation, which is a cAMP-dependent pathway. Atrial fibrillation is not tolerated well because lack of atrial kick reduces ventricular filling, thereby limiting stroke volume. Septic cardiomyopathy causes both systolic and diastolic dysfunction.

References

1. Little WC. Diastolic dysfunction beyond distensibility: adverse effects of ventricular dilatation. *Circulation.* 2005;112:2888.
2. Zakeri R, Chamberlain AM, Roger VL, Redfield MM. Temporal relationship and prognostic significance of atrial fibrillation in heart failure patients with preserved ejection fraction: a community-based study. *Circulation.* 2013;128:1085.

# 18

# VASCULAR DISORDERS

Kristen Holler and Mariya Geube

1. A 56-year-old male is admitted to the intensive care unit (ICU) with a diagnosis of an acute descending thoracic aortic dissection. Which of the following echocardiographic findings is MOST helpful when distinguishing the true lumen from the false lumen?

   A. The false lumen is usually smaller than the true lumen
   B. The false lumen expands during systole
   C. Intimal remnants (cobwebs) can often be seen in the true lumen
   D. Color-flow Doppler pattern is in-phase with the cardiac cycle in the true lumen

2. A patient presents to the hospital for elective abdominal aortic aneurysm (AAA) repair. Which of the patients would MOST likely benefit from surgical intervention?

   A. A 60-year-old male patient with asymptomatic 5.3-cm aneurysm discovered during abdominal computer tomography (CT) scan for colon cancer staging
   B. A 46-year-old male patient with a 5.2-cm aneurysm with back pain
   C. A 52-year-old female patient with a 4.9-cm aneurysm awaiting kidney transplant
   D. A 40-year-old female patient with a known aneurysm measuring 5.1-cm on follow-up imaging with prior study demonstrating a size of 5.0 cm 2 years ago

3. A 78-year-old female with a previous history of a thoracic endovascular aortic repair (TEVAR) complicated by endoleak presents to the ICU after undergoing additional endovascular graft placement for extension of the original repair. Which of the following IS NOT a risk factor for postoperative spinal cord ischemia (SCI)?

   A. History of prior aneurysm repair
   B. Extension of the repair to include coverage of the left subclavian artery
   C. Mild intraoperative hypothermia
   D. Pre-existing chronic renal insufficiency

4. A 56-year-old male is diagnosed with a contained rupture of a thoracic aortic aneurysm and was emergently taken to the operating room for thoracic endovascular aortic repair. On postoperative day 1, he begins to complain of loss of motor function in his lower extremities. When reviewing the patient's medication history, which of the following would place him at highest risk of developing a spinal hematoma after spinal drain placement?

   A. Aspirin 81 mg taken the morning of surgery
   B. Apixaban stopped 3 days before placement
   C. Dabigatran stopped 4 days before placement
   D. Enoxaparin DVT prophylaxis 14 hours before placement

5. A 59-year-old female with a past medical history of hypertension, chronic kidney disease, and heart failure with preserved ejection fraction underwent repair of AAA. Which of the following interventions and goals is MOST likely to reduce her risk of postoperative acute kidney injury?

A. Furosemide to maintain urine output >/= 0.5 mL/kg/hr
B. Bicarbonate containing IV fluid to maintain pH >7.3
C. Volume expansion to maintain CI >2.0
D. Mannitol 0.5 g/kg before aortic cross clamp

6. A 64-year-old male with a past medical history significant for hypertension, heart failure with reduced ejection fraction, myocardial infarction 2 years prior, and chronic kidney disease presents to the ICU following open AAA repair. He was restarted on his home medications on postoperative day 1. Three days later, his vitals and pertinent laboratory values include: blood pressure 150/100 mm Hg, heart rate 94 bpm, potassium 2.9 mmol/L, serum creatinine 2.6 mg/dL. The following electrocardiogram is obtained 24 hours after admission:

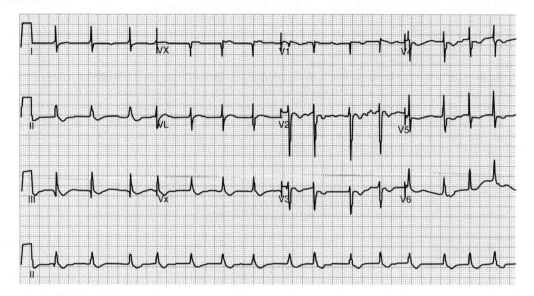

Which of the following medications was the patient most likely taking before surgery?

A. Atenolol
B. Digoxin
C. Lisinopril
D. Furosemide

7. Which of the following findings on physical examination are most likely observed in post-thoracic aortic aneurysm repair spinal cord infarction?

A. Bilateral loss of proprioception in lower extremities
B. Inability to flex the knee but maintained motor function of ankle and feet bilaterally
C. Loss of sensation, motor function, and dorsalis pedis pulse in the right lower extremity
D. Flaccid paralysis at T8 level with complete loss of sensory and motor function

8. Which of the following potential complications IS NOT paired correctly with the corresponding classification of aortic dissection?

A. Elevated lactate, elevated INR and AKI—DeBakey Type II
B. Elevated troponin—Stanford Type A
C. New onset diastolic murmur heard at the right second intercostal space—DeBakey Type III
D. New onset right hemiplegia—DeBakey Type I

9. A 65-year-old male is admitted to the ICU with confusion, headache, nausea, vomiting, and hypertension. He underwent right carotid endarterectomy 8 hours ago. The first set of vital signs obtained in the ICU showed blood pressure 171/94 mm Hg, heart rate 84 bpm, respiratory rate 22 per minute, and oxygen saturation 96% on room air. Which of the following IS NOT recommended as treatment for his complication?

A. Hypertonic saline
B. Mannitol
C. Labetalol
D. Levetiracetam

# Chapter 18 ▪ Answers

**1.** Correct Answer: D

**Rationale:**

It is important to distinguish the true from the false lumen in an acute aortic dissection, especially when the dissection involves the ascending aorta, as there is a potential in compromising the patency of the coronaries and head and neck vessels, or distally, the visceral arteries as these may originate from the false lumen. Additionally, identification of the true lumen is critical to guide aortic wire placement during interventions.

There are certain characteristics that help to identify the true lumen on echocardiography. In the descending aorta, the true lumen is usually smaller than the false lumen (A) and expands during systole (B). In the ascending aorta, the true lumen tends to be larger than the false lumen because proximal aortic pressures (closer to the left ventricle) are higher and thus keep the true lumen pressurized. The false lumen has a concave appearance compared to the convex appearance of the true lumen in systole. Echo findings of cobwebs (fibrinous remnants sheared from the intima during separation from media) are 100% specific for the false lumen in acute aortic dissection (C). Color-flow Doppler pattern is always in-phase with the cardiac cycle as opposed to the out-of-phase pattern in the false lumen (D).

Echocardiographic features of true and false lumen are important to recognize compression of the true lumen, which may result in organ malperfusion to identify the origin of important aortic branches (if they originate from the true vs false lumen) and provide live guidance for cannula placement in the true lumen.

References

1. Evangelista A, Frank A, Erbel R, et al. Echocardiography in aortic diseases: EAE recommendations for clinical practice. *Eur J Echocardiogr*. 2010;11(8):645-658. doi:10.1093/ejechocard/jeq056.
2. Armstrong WF, Ryan T. *Feigenbaum's Echocardiography*. Lippincott Williams & Wilkins; 2010:646-653.

**2.** Correct Answer: B

**Rationale:**

Based on the 2018 Society for Vascular Surgery practice guidelines, the strongest level recommendation is to pursue elective surgical repair in patients with AAA >5.5 cm, saccular aneurysms, and any aneurysm that is symptomatic (B) (back pain, abdominal pain), as these incur the highest risk of rupture. Likewise, strong evidence exists to serially monitor aortic dilation <4.0 cm, as the risk of rupture is low. However, a gray area exists for patients with aneurysms 5.0 to 5.4 cm. Several studies did not show statistically significant improvement in the clinical outcomes when comparing early intervention to surveillance for both endovascular and open repair. Weak evidence suggests that young patients, especially women, may benefit from earlier intervention (D). Similarly low-level recommendation suggests that repair for patients with smaller aneurysms who will require chemotherapy, radiation therapy, or solid organ transplant may be considered (C).

Ultrasonography is the standard method for screening and serially monitoring AAAs. Ultrasonography has a nearly 100% sensitivity in the diagnosis of AAAs and is preferred because of its relatively low cost, widespread availability, and noninvasive nature. It is accurate to within ~0.3 cm aneurysm diameter and is highly reproducible with different operators. However, it is limited by potentially suboptimal imaging in obese patients and disruption from bowel gas, and it cannot identify proximal and distal extent of the aneurysm. CT is the imaging modality of choice when ultrasound images are suboptimal. It also provides additional information regarding the extent of the aneurysm and its relationship to surrounding structures.

Strong evidence suggests elective surgical intervention for patients with AAA >5.5 cm, symptomatic aneurysms, and saccular aneurysms, as these carry the highest risk of rupture.

References

1. Gloviczki P, Lawrence PF, Forbes TL. Update of the Society for Vascular Surgery abdominal aortic aneurysm guidelines. *J Vasc Surg*. 2018;67(1):1. doi:10.1016/j.jvs.2017.11.022.
2. Filardo G, Powell JT, Martinez MA, Ballard DJ. Surgery for small asymptomatic abdominal aortic Aaneurysms. *Cochrane Database Syst Rev*. 2015;(2):CD001835. doi:10.1002/14651858.cd001835.pub4.

**3.** Correct Answer: C

**Rationale:**

The risk of SCI following thoracic endovascular aortic repair (TEVAR) is ~10%. Early identification and treatment of this devastating complication is critical in preventing permanent neurologic deficit. Prior aneurysm repair (A), magnitude of the repair, coverage of the left subclavian artery (B), and pre-existing chronic renal insufficiency (D) have all been shown to have higher incidences of SCI post TEVAR.

Spinal cord perfusion is dependent on one anterior and two posterior spinal arteries as well as a cervical vascular network proximally and pelvic vascular network distally. Proximal supply to the cervical vascular network is via the subclavian arteries that give rise to the vertebral arteries and then the anterior spinal artery. Thus, left carotid subclavian artery bypass should be considered before TEVAR when the proximal stent graft is expected to cover the origin of the left subclavian artery. The distal spinal cord is supplied by a pelvic vascular network, which arises from the lumbar and sacral arteries and forms a collateral network with branches of the inferior mesenteric and hypogastric arteries. Disruptions of either the proximal or distal collateral networks can place watershed areas of the spinal cord at risk of ischemia.

Strategies that increase spinal cord perfusion pressure (mean arterial pressure minus cerebrospinal fluid [CSF] pressure) as well as decrease metabolism and oxygen demand can reduce SCI post repair. Mild hypothermia (C) decreases metabolism and oxygen demand and would therefore be protective rather than a risk factor for developing postoperative ischemia.

CSF drainage is one intervention that can increase spinal cord perfusion pressure and potentially decrease the incidence of SCI after TEVAR. A recent Cochrane review in 2012 based on three randomized controlled trials of 287 patients examined the role perioperative drainage of cerebrospinal fluid in patients undergoing thoracoabdominal and thoracic aortic aneurysm repair. It is the mainstay of neuroprotection along with additional strategies that increase spinal cord perfusion pressure and oxygen delivery, such as augmentation of the mean arterial pressure and correction of severe anemia.

Postoperative SCI is a potentially devastating complication following TEVAR. Maintaining or augmenting spinal perfusion pressure and reducing metabolic demands are the mainstays of therapy for both prevention and treatment.

### References

1. Ullery BW, Cheung AT, Fairman RM, et al. Risk factors, outcomes, and clinical manifestations of spinal cord ischemia following thoracic endovascular aortic repair. *J Vasc Surg*. 2011;54(3):677-684.
2. Feezor R, Martin T, Hess P, et al. Extent of aortic coverage and incidence of spinal cord ischemia after thoracic endovascular aneurysm repair. *Ann Thorac Surg*. 2008;86:1809-1814.

**4.** Correct Answer: C

**Rationale:**

Consideration should be given with regard to preoperative placement of prophylactic lumbar spinal drain in patients at high risk for postoperative SCI; however, in patients who present for emergency repair of aortic aneurysm or dissection, a drain may not be placed because of time constraints. Postoperative rescue management of SCI includes therapies aimed at optimizing spinal cord perfusion pressure (the difference between the mean arterial pressure and either CSF pressure or central venous pressure, whichever is higher). This includes drainage of CSF via a subarachnoid drain, augmenting arterial pressure, and reducing central venous pressure or a combination of the three.

The American Society of Regional Anesthesia and Pain Medicine (ASRA) published updated guidelines in 2018 for anticoagulation interruption before performing neuraxial techniques, which includes newer oral anticoagulation agents.

The table that follows includes recommendations from the most updated ASRA guidelines as of 2018.

| | MINIMUM TIME BETWEEN LAST DOSE OF ANTICOAGULAND AND NEURAXIAL PROCEDURE |
|---|---|
| **Traditional Anticoagulants** | |
| Warfarin | when INR <1.5 |
| Heparin IV | when aPTT <40 |
| Heparin 5000 sq bid | 12 h and assess aPTT |
| Heparin 5000 sq tid | 4-6 h |
| Fondaparinux | Unknown/ avoid neuraxial procedure |
| Enoxaparin 1 mg/kg sq | 24 h |
| Enoxaparin 40 mg sq qd | 12 h |
| **Direct Thrombin Inhibitors** | |
| Argatroban | Unknown/ avoid neuraxial procedure |
| Bivalirudin | |
| Dabigatran | 5 d |

| | MINIMUM TIME BETWEEN LAST DOSE OF ANTICOAGULAND AND NEURAXIAL PROCEDURE |
|---|---|
| **Oral Antiplatelet Agents** | |
| Aspirin/NSAIDs | No restrictions |
| Clopidogrel | 5-7 d |
| Prasugrel | 7-10 d |
| Ticlopidine | 10 d |
| **GPIIB/IIIA Inhibitors** | |
| Abciximab | 2 d |
| Tirofiban | 4-8 h |
| **Direct Factor Xa Inhibitors** | |
| Rivaroxaban . | 3 d |
| Apixaban | 3 d |

In situations where the potential benefits outweigh the risks of neuraxial interventions such as lumbar spinal drain placement, clinical judgment as well as knowledge of the guidelines should be used.

### Reference

1. Regional anesthesia in the patient receiving antithrombotic or thrombolytic therapy. *Reg Anesth Pain Med.* 2018;43(5):566.

---

**5.** Correct Answer: C

**Rationale:**

Postoperative acute kidney injury is a common complication following aortic surgery, which increases hospital length of stay and is associated with significant increases in morbidity and mortality. The incidence varies widely, 18% to 47%, with endovascular repair being associated with a lower incidence as compared to that of an open repair.

The risk factors associated with acute kidney injury after aortic aneurysm repair include pre-existing renal dysfunction, increased age, involvement of the renal arteries in the aneurysm, preoperative exposure to radiocontrast, high complexity, prolonged procedure time, emergency surgery, and perioperative hypotension. These risk factors are related to larger doses of intraoperative contrast, renal microemboli, and inflammatory response. Strategies to prevent kidney injury include adequate perioperative hydration and planning for surgery at least several days from prior contrast administration if feasible. Intravascular ultrasound use intraoperatively can also reduce the dose of contrast needed.

Various strategies of perioperative renal protection have been proposed including: diuretics; furosemide and mannitol (A, D); calcium channel blockers; N acetylcysteine; bicarbonate; angiotensin-converting enzyme inhibitors; and renal vasodilators, fenoldopam, and dopamine. A 2013 Cochrane review did not support any of these pharmacologic interventions. However, a meta-analysis of studies conducted investigating volume expansion alone or in combination with an inotrope to maintain a cardiac index in the normal range (>2.0 L/min/m$^2$) (C) did show a reduction in postoperative acute kidney injury.

Both the Cochrane review and meta-analysis caution that many of the included studies are subject to small sample size and possible biases that make interpretation of the results challenging.

More evidence is needed to support pharmacologic interventions for perioperative renal protection. Currently available literature support individualized hemodynamic optimization utilizing fluids and inotropes as needed to maintain a cardiac index within the normal range.

### References

1. Brienza Ni, Giglio MT, Marucci M, Fiore T. Does perioperative hemodynamic optimization protect renal function in surgical patients? A meta-analytic study. *Crit Care Med.* 2009;37(6):2079-2090.
2. Canet E, Bellomo R. Perioperative renal protection. *Curr Opin Crit Care.* 2018;24:1. doi:10.1097/mcc.0000000000000560.
3. Zacharias M, Mugawar M, Herbison GP, et al. Interventions for protecting renal function in the perioperative period. *Cochrane Database Syst Rev.* 2013;9:CD003590. doi:10.1002/14651858.cd003590.pub4.

**6.** Correct Answer: B

**Rationale:**

Digoxin is one of the oldest medications used to treat heart failure with reduced ejection fraction. Digoxin should be used with caution secondary to its narrow therapeutic window and significant risk of toxicity.

Digoxin binds to the K+ site of the Na+/K+ adenosine triphosphate-ase pump and inhibits the ion transport, thus secondarily increasing intracellular calcium resulting in an ionotropic effect. Digoxin also has a stimulating effect on both sympathetic and parasympathetic tone with the latter being responsible for its chronotropic effects. Hypokalemia increases the risk of digoxin toxicity secondary to its interaction with the Na+/K+ ATPase pump. A number of other factors can also increase the risk of digoxin toxicity including hypomagnesaemia, hypercalcaemia, myocardial ischemia, hypoxemia, and acid-base disturbances. In addition, renal impairment can prolong the half life of digoxin, therefore increasing the risk of toxicity.

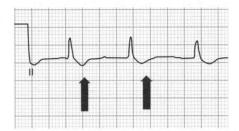

The electrocardiogram above shows characteristic ST segment downsloping depression as well as a shortened QT interval. However, a number of atrial and ventricular arrhythmias are possible with digoxin toxicity. Increased automaticity (atrial fibrillation/ flutter) with AV block, ventricular tachycardia, fibrillation and ectopy, and bradycardia can be seen.

Symptoms of acute digoxin toxicity include nausea, vomiting, diarrhea, hyperkalemia, lethargy, and confusion. The initial GI symptoms occur early at 2 to 4 hours post ingestion, with cardiovascular complications occuring later at 8 to 12 hours. Chronic digoxin toxicity typically has a more insidious onset and is often related to concurrent illness i.e. impaired renal function. The features are similar to acute toxicity with the addition of visual disturbances (reduced vision, yellow halos, and altered color perception)

The treatment of digoxin toxicity is with Digoxin-specific Fab antibody fragments, which bind to molecules of digoxin, making them unavailable for binding at their site of action.

Digoxin has a narrow therapeutic index and patients must be monitored closely to detect signs of toxicity in the setting of electrolyte, acid-base disturbances, and in renal impairment.

References

1. Bauman JL, DiDomenico RJ, Galanter WL. Mechanisms, manifestations, and management of digoxin toxicity in the modern era. *Am J Cardiovasc Drugs*. 2006;6(2):77-86. doi:10.2165/00129784-200606020-00002.
2. Mladěnka P, Applová L, Patočka J, et al. Comprehensive review of cardiovascular toxicity of drugs and related agents. *Med Res Rev*. 2018;38(4):1332-1403. doi:10.1002/med.21476.

**7.** Correct Answer: D

**Rationale:**

The most common clinical presentation of a spinal cord infarction is anterior spinal artery syndrome. The anterior spinal cord is at higher risk of ischemia because of its vascular anatomy; it is supplied by a single artery with few collaterals unlike the posterior cord, which is supplied by two arteries. An infarct of the anterior spinal cord presents as loss of motor function and pain/ temperature sensation, with sparing of proprioception and vibratory sense below the level of the lesion. The acute stages are characterized by flaccidity and loss of deep tendon reflexes; spasticity and hyperreflexia develop over ensuing days and weeks. In rare cases, the paralysis may affect one leg more than the other and may be asymmetric, depending on the collateral network integrity.

It is important to distinguish spinal cord infarction from other etiologies of postoperative neurologic deficits. Vascular occlusion (C) is a surgical emergency. It presents with lack of peripheral pulse, severe pain, and temperature change in addition to the motor deficit. The patient complains of paresthesia, which is not characteristic for anterior spinal cord syndrome. Spinal cord compression from hematoma or abscess is an important category to exclude as these often require prompt diagnosis and emergent surgical decompression (D). The clinical presentation can occur abruptly and mimic SCI. This diagnostic consideration mandates urgent magnetic resonance imaging of the spinal cord in all patients presenting with possible spinal cord infarct.

It is important to identify the cause of a postoperative neurologic deficit to avoid delay in treatment for etiologies requiring urgent intervention such as spinal cord compression or vascular occlusion.

Reference

1. Mullen M, McGarvey M. *Spinal Cord Infarction: Clinical Presentation and Diagnosis*. UpToDate; January 09, 2018.

**8.** Correct Answer: A

**Rationale:**

There are two main classification systems for thoracic aortic dissections, the Stanford classification and the DeBakey classification. Stanford Type A includes all dissections involving the ascending aorta regardless of the extent or site of origin. Stanford Type B includes all dissections distal from the left subclavian artery.

Stanford classification is focused on anticipated treatment of the dissection. Type A dissection accounts for about 60% of all dissections and mandates early surgical repair, as any delay carries a 2% increase in mortality for every hour delayed. Additionally, postponing repair increases the risk for developing life-threatening complications of proximal dissection, which include rupture into the pericardial sac with resulting cardiac tamponade, severe aortic regurgitation, and coronary artery occlusion from extension of the dissection flap into the coronary arteries with subsequent myocardial infarction. Type B dissections account for about 40% of aortic dissections and require medical management focused on decreasing the shear stress on the aortic wall, via reduction in both heart rate and arterial pressure. Surgical repair is indicated if there is severe compression of the true lumen or critical branches arising from the false lumen with signs of hypoperfusion to the lower extremities, visceral organs, and/ or kidneys.

The DeBakey classification takes into account the site of origin of the dissection and the extent of the dissection distally. Type I originated in the ascending aorta and propagates to the descending aorta. Type II originates within and is confined to the ascending aorta. Type III originates below the left subclavian artery and extends distally or, more rarely, retrogrades into the arch and ascending aorta.

| DEBAKEY TYPE I | DEBAKEY TYPE II | DEBAKEY TYPE III |
|---|---|---|
| Ascending and descending aorta | Ascending aorta only | Descending aorta only |
| Stanford A | | Stanford B |

By understanding these classification systems, the potential branch vessels that could be compromised by a dissection flap can be identified. Ischemic bowel is due to occlusion of visceral vessels branching off of the descending aorta and thus would not be affected in a DeBakey type II dissection, which is limited to the ascending aorta (A). Acute myocardial infarction can result from intimal flap dissection into a coronary artery. Cerebrovascular accident is a potential complication of dissections involving the carotid arteries. The aortic valve can also be compromised when a proximal dissection flap prolapses through the valve in diastole.

There is an uncommon form of aortic dissection, which originates as type III DeBakey, with subsequent retrograde (proximal) propagation to the aortic arch and ascending aorta. This scenario is not appropriately addressed by the DeBakey and Stanford classification systems. If the proximal propagation is confined within the aortic arch, then it is still considered type B. If the dissection involves the aorta proximal to the brachiocephalic trunk, then it is Stanford Type A.

There are two main systems for classifying aortic dissections; it is important to understand the dissection type as the complications vary. Beyond identifying branch vessels at risk of compromise based on dissection type, determining site of origin and propagation of the dissection is important as it effects management.

References

1. Nienaber CA, Eagle KA. Aortic dissection: new frontiers in diagnosis and management. *Circulation*. 2003;108(6):772-778. doi:10.1161/01.cir.0000087400.48663.19.
2. Emmett M. Predicting death in patients with acute type A aortic dissection. *Circulation*. 2002;106(25):e224. doi:10.1161/01.cir.0000043546.26296.d2.

**9.** Correct Answer: D

**Rationale:**

Cerebral hyperperfusion syndrome is relatively a rare following carotid endarterectomy or carotid stenting (incidence 0.74%-1.16%).

The pathophysiology of hyperperfusion injury is not completely understood, but it is believed that impaired autoregulation due to baroreceptor dysfunction, hypertension, and increased blood flow to the ipsilateral hemisphere play a significant role. It is reversible if recognized early but can progress to unilateral cerebral edema or intracerebral hemorrhage, which significantly increases morbidity and mortality.

Several imaging modalities are useful in the identification of cerebral hyperperfusion syndrome. Transcranial Doppler is noninvasive and provides real-time information. It will demonstrate increased flows when compared to preoperative values. CT or magnetic resonance imaging can detect areas of ischemia, edema, and intracerebral hemorrhage. Magnetic resonance perfusion study measures cerebral blood flow and may demonstrate interhemispheric differences in flow/ volume.

The mainstay of treatment is strict blood pressure control postoperatively (C). Hyperperfusion can be seen even in the setting of normotension in some patients. Medication selection is important as those with vasodilatory effects, which further increase cerebral blood flow, can worsen outcomes. Thus, antihypertensive agents that possess negative inotropic effects would be an appropriate first line therapy.

There is no indication for prophylactic use of antiepileptic medications in cerebral hyperperfusion syndrome (D).

Although their benefit for treating cerebral hyperperfusion syndrome specifically is unclear, osmotic agents such as hypertonic saline and mannitol should be considered in the setting of symptomatic cerebral edema (A/B).

Cerebral hyperperfusion syndrome is an uncommon but potentially serious complication following carotid endarterectomy and stenting. Care should be taken to minimize precipitating factors such as uncontrolled hypertension.

### Reference

1. Farooq MU, Goshgarian C, Min J, Gorelick PB. Pathophysiology and management of reperfusion injury and hyperperfusion syndrome after carotid endarterectomy and carotid artery stenting. *Exp Transl Stroke Med.* 2016;8(1):7. doi:10.1186/s13231-016-0021-2.

# 19

# VALVULAR HEART DISEASE

Brett J Wakefield and Mariya Geube

1. An 86-year-old female presents with lower gastrointestinal hemorrhage requiring massive transfusion. The bleeding subsides without additional intervention; however, persistent hypotension is encountered. Coagulation studies are normal except for a slightly prolonged activated partial thromboplastin time (aPTT). Echocardiography from 6 months ago demonstrates peak/mean aortic valve gradient of 80/40 mm Hg, with an estimated aortic valve area of 0.8 cm$^2$ and reduced left ventricular function. Which coagulation abnormality should be expected?

   A. Disseminated intravascular coagulation
   B. Willebrand disease
   C. Vitamin K deficiency
   D. Hemophilia A

2. A 68-year-old female with severe chronic obstructive pulmonary disease experienced a syncopal event while climbing the stairs at home. She presented to the emergency department with multiple rib and upper extremity fractures as well as a displaced hip fracture. Following an urgent hip fracture repair, she arrives to the ICU intubated and sedated. On physical examination, she has a laterally displaced point of maximal impulse with a systolic murmur heard best at the left sternal border. Which transthoracic echocardiographic view would best aid in diagnosis and grading of severity?

   A. Apical 4-chamber
   B. Suprasternal
   C. Apical 3-chamber
   D. Parasternal basal short axis

3. A 46-year-old female with a history of hepatitis C and intravenous drug abuse presents to the emergency department with fevers, rigors, confusion, and acute shortness of breath. The vital signs are as follows: heart rate 105 bpm; blood pressure 120/70 mm Hg; temperature 39.4 C; arterial saturation 85%. Chest radiograph shows diffuse pulmonary edema. Echocardiography demonstrates a vegetation on the noncoronary cusp of the aortic valve with severe aortic regurgitation. Although awaiting surgery, the patient is admitted to the cardiology ICU. Which intervention in the most appropriate next step?

   A. Nitroprusside
   B. Epinephrine
   C. Norepinephrine
   D. Furosemide

4. A 78-year-old male presents to the ICU with chest pain, shortness of breath, and respiratory distress requiring urgent intubation. The chest radiograph shows diffuse pulmonary edema, worse in the lower lung lobes. His vital signs are as follows: heart rate 114 bpm, blood pressure 90/50 mm Hg, pulse oxymetry 87%. The patient's electrocardiogram demonstrates ST-segment elevation in lead II, III, and aVF with reciprocal changes in leads I and aVL. On physical examination, he has a systolic murmur, bilateral crackles on lung auscultation, and cold and clammy extremities. Cardiac enzymes are pending. What interventions should be considered?

    **A.** Intra-aortic balloon pump

    **B.** Norepinephrine

    **C.** Inhalational epoprostenol

    **D.** Milrinone

**5.** A 46-year-old female with a history of hypertension, intracranial arteriovenous malformation, and previous mechanical mitral valve replacement is admitted to cardiology ICU with new onset of atrial fibrillation, shortness of breath, tachypnea, and crackles at both lung bases on auscultation. The patient has a heart rate of 137 bpm, blood pressure of 87/66 mm Hg, cold and clammy extremities, urine output of 10 mL/h, and potassium of 5.6 mmol/L. International normalized ratio (INR) is 1.8. Transesophageal echocardiography demonstrates the following image of the bioprosthetic mitral valve (red arrows) in the midesophageal two-chamber view. The mean transmitral gradient was measured 12 mm Hg with continuous wave Doppler.

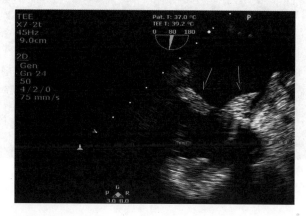

    What is the next step in management?

    **A.** Heparin infusion and nitroglycerin infusion for afterload reduction

    **B.** Heparin infusion and thrombolytic therapy

    **C.** Heparin infusion and urgent mitral valve replacement

    **D.** Heparin infusion and metoprolol for rate control and improved flow through the stenotic mitral valve

**6.** A 38-year-old female with a history of mitral valve prolapse presents to the cardiac ICU following a mitral valve repair. The intraoperative course was significant for two periods of cardiopulmonary bypass because of a failed first repair. The patient's hemodynamics is supported with a low-dose norepinephrine infusion. Following turning the patient in bed, there is an acute decrease in blood pressure refractory to treatment with multiple boluses of norepinephrine and phenylephrine. Emergent transthoracic echocardiography at the bedside demonstrates severe right ventricular dysfunction, in addition to new onset inferior and inferoseptal wall motion abnormalities. What is the most appropriate next step in management?

    **A.** Left-heart catheterization

    **B.** Preload reduction with nitroglycerin

    **C.** Intra-aortic balloon pump

    **D.** Epinephrine infusion

**7.** A 34-year-old female with a history of rheumatic heart disease presents for mitral valve replacement. Preoperative echocardiography demonstrates a transmitral gradient of 14 mm Hg, a mitral valve area of 0.9 cm², and an underfilled left ventricle with normal function. Electrocardiogram shows atrial fibrillation. What is the most likely finding on postoperative transesophageal echocardiography following mitral valve replacement in this patient?

    **A.** Decreased right ventricular function

    **B.** Increased transpulmonary pressure gradient

    **C.** Decreased left ventricular systolic function

    **D.** Worsened tricuspid regurgitation

**8.** A 48-year-old male with a history of hypertension, patent foramen ovale, coronary artery disease, and diabetes mellitus presents with increasing shortness of breath, wheezing, peripheral edema, diarrhea, and headache. Transthoracic echocardiography shows severe tricuspid regurgitation, severe mitral regurgitation, and evidence of right ventricular failure. The subvalvular apparatus of the tricuspid and mitral valves appear thickened. What is the likely etiology?

   A. Carcinoid heart disease
   B. Endocarditis
   C. Rheumatic heart disease
   D. Acute inferior myocardial infarction

9. A 78-year-old female presents with a femur fracture following a fall. She is persistently hypotensive in the ICU before surgery for open reduction internal fixation. Transthoracic echocardiography demonstrates the following continuous wave Doppler waveform:

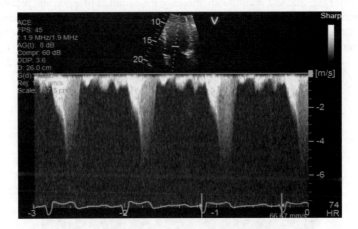

What is the most likely diagnosis?

   A. Aortic stenosis
   B. Subaortic membrane
   C. Aortic insufficiency
   D. Hypertrophic cardiomyopathy

10. A 78-year old female with severe aortic stenosis presents to the ICU following a transcatheter aortic valve replacement (TAVR). Preprocedural transthoracic echocardiography demonstrated severe aortic stenosis with left ventricular hypertrophy and an asymmetric septal bulge. Left ventricular wall thickness in the parasternal short axis view is 1.6 cm with a small cavity. Postoperatively, the patient develops sudden onset hypotension requiring vasopressor support; however, blood pressure continues to decrease despite escalating doses of norepinephrine. The vital signs are heart rate 94 bpm, blood pressure 85/54 mm Hg, respiratory rate 18/min. Transthoracic echocardiography demonstrates an underfilled left ventricle with midventricular obstruction. What is the most appropriate next step in management?

   A. Discontinue norepinephrine and start phenylephrine infusion
   B. Discontinue norepinephrine and start epinephrine
   C. Discontinue norepinephrine and start esmolol infusion
   D. Discontinue norepinephrine and administer fluid bolus

# Chapter 19 ▪ Answers

1. Correct Answer: B

**Rationale:**
This patient has severe aortic stenosis and has developed cardiogenic shock in the setting of acute gastrointestinal hemorrhage. Gastrointestinal bleeding in patients with severe aortic stenosis is not uncommon. Heyde syndrome refers to the triad of aortic stenosis, gastrointestinal angiodysplasia, and an acquired type IIA von Willebrand disease. von Willebrand factor serves as the major adhesion molecule that attaches platelets to exposed endothelium. In addition, von Willebrand factor binds factor VIII, extending its half-life in circulation. High shear stress caused by severe aortic stenosis leads to platelet aggregation and induction of von Willebrand factor–cleaving metalloproteinase. This metalloproteinase reduces the high molecular weight multimers of von Willebrand factor resulting in type IIA von Willebrand disease.

The coagulation panel of patients with von Willebrand disease is nonspecific. The aPTT may be normal or elevated. The concentration of von Willebrand factor (vWF:Ag) and the activity of von Willebrand factor (vWF:RCo) can diagnose the disease, help classify the subtype, and direct therapy. There are three primary classifications of von Willebrand disease. Type I is the most common and results from a quantitative decrease in functional von Willebrand factor. Type II results from functional deficits in von Willebrand factor and is divided into four subtypes—A, B, M, N. Acquired type IIA von Willebrand disease, as seen in this patient, results in loss of intermediate and high molecular weight von Willebrand multimers. Type III von Willebrand disease describes patients with no von Willebrand factor and extremely low levels of factor VIII.

In acquired von Willebrand disease due to aortic stenosis, the coagulation abnormalities will return to normal following aortic valve replacement. Before correction, the mainstay of treatment is 1-deamino-8-D-arginine vasopressin (DDAVP), which promotes the release of von Willebrand factor and factor VIII from endothelial cells. Intravenous DDAVP can be given as a 0.3 mcg/kg bolus with a peak effect at 30 minutes. The most common side effect is hyponatremia due to the medication's effect on free water clearance. Concentrated von Willebrand factor can be administered to patients with life-threatening bleeding or type III disease.

### References
1. Mital A. Acquired von Willebrand syndrome. *Adv Clin Exp Med*. 2016;25:1337-1344.
2. Loscalzo J. From clinical observation to mechanism–Heyde's syndrome. *N Engl J Med*. 2012;367:1954-1956.

**2.** Correct Answer: C

**Rationale:**

Given the physical examination findings, this patient likely has aortic stenosis. The degree of aortic stenosis is best evaluated in the apical 5-chamber and 3 chamber views. The apical 5-chamber view is obtained by tilting the probe anterior from the apical 4-chamber view until the left ventricular outflow tract and aortic valve come into view. The apical 3-chamber view is obtained rotating the probe counterclockwise at 60° from the apical 4-chamber view until the left atrium, left ventricle, left ventricular outflow tract, and aortic valve appear. Utilizing these views, continuous wave Doppler can be applied to obtain the velocity and gradient across the aortic valve. Valvular hemodynamic parameters classifying the degree of aortic stenosis are presented in the table that follows.

|  | MAXIMUM AORTIC JET VELOCITY (m/s) | MEAN PRESSURE GRADIENT (mm Hg) | AORTIC VALVE AREA (cm²) |
|---|---|---|---|
| Mild | 2.0-2.9 | <20 | 1.5-2.0 |
| Moderate | 3.0-3.9 | 20-39 | 1.0-1.5 |
| Severe | ≥4.0 | ≥40 | ≤1.0 |

Aortic stenosis increases both the systolic and diastolic pressures of the left ventricle. Gradually increased systolic pressure leads to concentric left ventricular hypertrophy and myocardial remodeling. According to the Law of LaPlace ($S = Pr/h$; S = systolic wall stress, P = pressure, r = ventricular radius, and h = ventricular thickness), left ventricular hypertrophy results in increased wall thickness and therefore decreased wall stress. This hypertrophy can displace the point of maximal impulse laterally and may lead to the development of a fourth heart sound, $S_4$. Furthermore, the left ventricular ejection time is increased, which decreases the time spent in diastole. Increased left ventricular diastolic pressure combined with a decreased time in diastole will decrease coronary perfusion and promote myocardial ischemia.

The definitive management of patients with aortic stenosis is aortic valve replacement. ICU management focuses on the following hemodynamic goals: correction of hypovolemia (decreased preload), avoidance of tachycardia, normal but not augmented inotropy and aggressive treatment of hypotension (maintaining afterload). Maintaining left ventricular filling pressure is vital to promote ejection in the setting of high transvalvular gradients. Reduced afterload should be aggressively treated and counteracted to increase diastolic blood pressure and restore coronary perfusion pressure. It is also important to avoid increases in myocardial oxygen demand such as pain, tachycardia, and other increases in sympathetic drive. In summary, the main hemodynamic goals in patients with severe aortic stenosis are to maintain adequate preload, increase afterload, avoid tachycardia, and maintain normal contractility.

### References
1. Lindman BR, Clavel MA, Mathieu P, et al. Calcific aortic stenosis. *Nat Rev Dis Primers*. 2016;2:16006.
2. Baumgartner H, Hung J, Bermejo J, et al. Recommendations on the echocardiographic assessment of aortic valve stenosis: a focused update from the european association of cardiovascular imaging and the american society of echocardiography. *J Am Soc Echocardiogr*. 2017;30:372-392.

**3.** Correct Answer: A

**Rationale:**

Acute aortic regurgitation can lead to rapid cardiovascular and respiratory deterioration. The left ventricle cannot accommodate the acute rise in left ventricular preload, and as a result, stroke volume decreases. Left ventricular diastolic pressure rises rapidly causing premature closure of the mitral valve in diastole. Further increases in left ventricular pressure may cause a phenomenon known as diastolic mitral regurgitation, which increases the pressures in the left atrium and pulmonary circulation. Patients with acute aortic regurgitation may present with tachycardia, hypotension, and pulmonary edema. Cardiogenic shock in the setting of acute aortic regurgitation is an indication for emergent aortic valve replacement. Inotropic agents (dobutamine) and/or vasodilators (nitroprusside) may be required to temporize the hemodynamics before the procedure. Nitrodilators cause venous and arterial vasodilation resulting in decreased preload and afterload. Addition of dobutamine may also improve cardiopulmonary function by increasing inotropy and decreasing systemic vascular resistance and thus afterload. Patients with severe aortic regurgitation have wide pulse pressure due to the rapid aortic run off. Decreasing left ventricular afterload helps to decrease the gradient between the aorta and the left ventricle in diastole, thus reducing the regurgitant volume.

Chronic aortic regurgitation, on the other hand, results in myocardial remodeling, which tolerates increased preload to a much greater extent than acute aortic regurgitation. In chronic aortic regurgitation, gradually increased left ventricular diastolic pressures result in eccentric left ventricular hypertrophy. Because of the eccentric hypertrophy, the increased preload can increase stroke volume and cause increased systolic pressures. This in turn increases left ventricular ejection time and thus decreases diastolic time resulting in decreased coronary perfusion. However, according to the law of Laplace, left ventricular dilation (increased radius) leads to increased wall tension and thus increased afterload. Thus, chronic aortic regurgitation represents a state of both increased preload and increased afterload.

### References
1. Hamirani YS, Dietl CA, Voyles W, Peralta M, Begay D, Raizada V. Acute aortic regurgitation. *Circulation*. 2012;126:1121-1126.
2. Stout KK, Verrier ED. Acute valvular regurgitation. *Circulation*. 2009;119:3232-3341.

**4.** Correct Answer: A

**Rationale:**

This patient developed flash pulmonary edema secondary to an acute posteromedial papillary muscle rupture in the setting of an inferior wall ST-elevation myocardial infarction. Papillary muscles are vulnerable to myocardial ischemia because they are perfused by the terminal portion of the coronary arteries. This can result in transient papillary muscle dysfunction or frank rupture. The posteromedial papillary muscle is more frequently involved because it is supplied by the posterior descending branch of the right coronary artery, whereas the anterolateral papillary muscle has a dual blood supply including the diagonal branches of the left anterior descending artery and the marginal branches of the left circumflex artery. Acute mitral regurgitation can occur because of infective endocarditis, myocardial ischemia, papillary muscle or chordae rupture, and prosthetic valve malfunction. Mitral regurgitation causes an abrupt increase in left ventricular end diastolic volume (preload) and a reduction in forward stroke volume. An important hemodynamic difference between acute and chronic mitral regurgitation is left atrial compliance. In chronic mitral regurgitation, the left atrium dilates with time and compliance increases gradually as the regurgitant volume increases. In acute mitral regurgitation, normal or decreased left atrial compliance cannot tolerate an abrupt increase in volume. This leads to pulmonary edema, pulmonary hypertension, and right ventricular failure.

Emergency surgery is indicated in patients with acute left ventricular failure due to ruptured papillary muscles. Placement of intra-aortic balloon pump may exert some beneficial physiologic effects in the setting of acute mitral regurgitation. These include improved coronary perfusion, decreased left ventricular afterload, and improved cardiac index. Afterload reduction with vasodilators such as nitroprusside will also improve forward flow; however, if the patient is in cardiogenic shock, this may not be tolerated. If hypotensive, increased inotropy with dobutamine is preferable to norepinephrine. Increased alpha-1 stimulation will increase afterload and may worsen the regurgitant volume and increase pulmonary pressures. Increased inotropy combined with afterload reduction can promote forward flow and decrease regurgitant fraction, while increasing blood pressure. Inhaled epoprostenol decreases pulmonary vascular resistance and is indicated in patients with an increased transpulmonary gradient (mean pulmonary artery pressure minus left atrial pressure); however, it has no role in case of left ventricular failure. Inhaled epoprostenol causes pulmonary arterial vasodilation, which may in fact increase the gradient between the pulmonary venous to pulmonary arterial circulation and worsen the venous congestion.

### Reference
1. Kutty RS, Jones N, Moorjani N. Mechanical complications of acute myocardial infarction. *Cardiol Clin*. 2013;31:519-531, vii-viii.

**5.** Correct Answer: C

**Rationale:**

Prosthetic valve thrombosis should be suspected in the setting of new onset heart failure, thromboembolism, or valve dysfunction in a patient with a mechanical valve. The incidence is estimated to be 0.3% to 1.3% per year. Thrombosis is more common on right-sided valves versus left-sided valves, the mitral valve versus aortic valve, and mechanical valves versus bioprosthetic valves. Anticoagulation therapy for all patients with a valve replacement includes daily aspirin with or without a vitamin K antagonist. The presence of a mechanical mitral valve requires lifelong vitamin K antagonist therapy with INR targets 2.5 to 3.5. This patient has an INR of 1.8 and is therefore subtherapeutic and at increased risk for prosthetic valve thrombosis. INR targets after mechanical aortic valve replacement require an INR of 2.0 to 3.0 because the higher velocity of flow through the valve helps to prevent blood stasis. Treatment of prosthetic valve thrombosis includes systemic anticoagulation, thrombolytic therapy, and/or surgery. Patients with subtherapeutic anticoagulation should receive intravenous heparin therapy. The 2014/2017 American College of Cardiology/American Heart Association guidelines recommend emergent surgery or low-dose thrombolytic therapy for patients with left-sided prosthetic valve thrombosis and signs of valve obstruction or heart failure. Patients with right-sided thrombosis are candidates for thrombolytic therapy. This patient has a history of an intracranial arteriovenous malformation, which is an absolute contraindication to thrombolytic therapy; therefore, urgent surgery should be pursued. Other absolute contraindications to thrombolysis include active internal bleeding, recent history of stroke, intracranial or spinal surgery, serious head trauma, intracranial neoplasm or aneurysm, and severe uncontrolled hypertension.

References

1. Nishimura RA, Otto CM, Bonow RO, et al. 2017 AHA/ACC focused update of the 2014 AHA/ACC guideline for the management of patients with valvular heart disease: a report of the American College of Cardiology/American Heart Association Task Force on Clinical Practice Guidelines. *J Am Coll Cardiol.* 2017;70:252-289.
2. Nishimura RA, Otto CM, Bonow RO, et al. 2014 AHA/ACC guideline for the management of patients with valvular heart disease: a report of the American College of Cardiology/American Heart Association Task Force on Practice Guidelines. *J Thorac Cardiovasc Surg.* 2014;148:e1-e132.
3. Dangas GD, Weitz JI, Giustino G, Makkar R, Mehran R. Prosthetic heart valve thrombosis. *J Am Coll Cardiol.* 2016;68:2670-2689.

**6.** Correct Answer: D

**Rationale:**

During cardiopulmonary bypass for operations that involve opening to left atrium, air is introduced into the left-sided cardiac chambers. On separation from cardiopulmonary bypass, transesophageal echocardiography can be used to ensure adequate de-airing of the left-sided structures. Air is typically found near the pulmonary veins, left atrial appendage, along the atrial septum, and near the left ventricular apex. If the cardiac chambers are not adequately de-aired, air can enter the aorta and subsequently embolize to the coronary, cerebral, or systemic circulations causing ischemic complications. If air enters the coronary circulation while the patient is in the supine position, air preferentially enters the right coronary circulation because it has the most anterior coronary ostia. In addition, air may enter saphenous vein grafts because they are typically anastomosed to the anterior portion of the aorta. Although this is most likely to occur in the operating room, residual air can dislodge during transport or even in the ICU, particularly with a change in body position or turning. This 38-year-old patient likely does not have significant coronary artery disease, and a left-sided heart catheterization would not be the immediate next step in management. The most likely explanation is residual intracardiac air embolizing to the right coronary artery circulation. Intracoronary air can range from asymptomatic to complete hemodynamic deterioration and cardiac arrest, depending on the amount of air. Inotropic and vasopressor agents should be used to augment the blood pressure and cardiac output, thus flushing the air through the coronary circulation while monitoring ST segments for resolution. If resolution does not occur, other causes of postoperative ST-segment elevation should be evaluated.

Another unique cause of ST-segment elevation following mitral valve surgery involves surgical occlusion of the left circumflex artery. The left circumflex artery lies within the left atrioventricular groove and courses along the posterior border of the mitral valve. In left dominant circulation when the left circumflex gives rise to the posterior descending artery, the circumflex courses even closer and along the entire posterior annulus of the mitral valve. Owing to this anatomic relationship, the surgical sutures may cross through the circumflex artery and cause iatrogenic ischemic injury. EKG and hemodynamic changes postoperatively will depend on the level of obstruction. Proximal circumflex injuries may lead to lateral and inferior wall ischemia; however, a distal circumflex injury in a patient with a left dominant circulation may present with only inferior wall ischemia.

References

1. Orihashi K, Matsuura Y, Hamanaka Y, et al. Retained intracardiac air in open heart operations examined by transesophageal echocardiography. *Ann Thorac Surg.* 1993;55:1467-1471.
2. Ender J, Selbach M, Borger MA, et al. Echocardiographic identification of iatrogenic injury of the circumflex artery during minimally invasive mitral valve repair. *Ann Thorac Surg.* 2010;89:1866-1872.

**7.** Correct Answer: C

**Rationale:**

Left ventricular preload (left ventricular end diastolic volume) is decreased in chronic mitral stenosis leading to deconditioning of left ventricle with time. Following mitral valve replacement, the abrupt increase in preload frequently unmasks left ventricular dysfunction requiring temporary postoperative inotropic support. The transpulmonary gradient is the difference between the mean pulmonary artery pressure and the left atrial pressure. Following mitral valve replacement, both values drop (mean pulmonary artery pressure decreases more than the left atrial pressure), thus the transpulmonary gradient decreases. Right ventricular function will typically improve because of the decreased transpulmonary gradient. This may reduce the degree of tricuspid regurgitation (typically due to right ventricular dilation). In the presence of a prosthetic mitral valve, the transmitral gradient is typically less than 6 mm Hg. A higher gradient is concerning patient prosthesis mismatch (the prosthetic valve is too small for the size of the patient).

Mitral stenosis is typically secondary to rheumatic heart disease. In approximately 40% of patients, mitral stenosis occurs with mitral regurgitation. The second most common valve affected is the aortic valve followed by the tricuspid valve. The time course between rheumatic fever and obstructive mitral valve disease can vary from a couple years to more than 20 years. Rheumatic heart disease causes characteristic changes in the mitral valve including leaflet-edge thickening, chordal shortening and fusion, and commissural fusion. The normal mitral valve area is 4 to 6 cm². Mild mitral stenosis occurs as the mitral valve area drops below 2 cm², and stenosis is severe with a mitral valve area of less than 1 cm². Mitral stenosis leads to increased left atrial pressures, left atrial dilation, and increased pulmonary venous, capillary, and ultimately arterial pressures. Anything that increases blood flow across the stenotic mitral valve (tachycardia due to exercise, anemia, infection) will increase the pressure gradient (modified Bernoulli equation: pressure gradient = $4 \times \text{velocity}^2$) and worsen pulmonary congestion. Atrial fibrillation reduces cardiac output by eliminating the atrial contribution to diastolic filling leading to increased left atrial pressure and worsened pulmonary congestion. Atrial fibrillation in patients with mitral stenosis begins intermittently and progresses to persistent atrial fibrillation overtime as the left atrium continues to dilate.

### References

1. Chandrashekhar Y, Westaby S, Narula J. Mitral stenosis. *Lancet.* 2009;374:1271-1283.
2. Kaul TK, Bain WH, Jones JV, et al. Mitral valve replacement in the presence of severe pulmonary hypertension. *Thorax.* 1976;31:332-336.

**8.** Correct Answer: A

**Rationale:**

Neuroendocrine tumors are rare tumors arising primarily in the gastrointestinal tract (67.5%) and the bronchopulmonary system (25.3%). These tumors may secrete many different products, including 5-hydroxytryptamine (5-HT, serotonin), prostaglandins, histamine, substance P, and transforming growth factor-β. These vasoactive substances are typically metabolized in the liver; however, when metastasis form and bypass this metabolism, systemic symptoms can develop. Approximately half of patients with neuroendocrine tumors will develop carcinoid syndrome, characterized by cutaneous flushing, diarrhea, and bronchospasm, and only 20% to 30% of those patients will develop carcinoid heart disease. The neuroendocrine products cause deposition of plaques along the endocardial surfaces of the valve leaflets, chordae tendinae, papillary muscles, and walls of the heart. These deposits primarily form on the ventricular aspect of the valves. The most common valve involved is the tricuspid valve because of the metabolism of the products in the pulmonary circulation. This can result in tricuspid regurgitation or a combination of tricuspid regurgitation and stenosis. The mitral valve can be involved in the setting of a patent foramen ovale, in which case the vasoactive substances bypass the lung. Carcinoid heart disease can present with signs and symptoms of right ventricular failure including dyspnea, peripheral edema, and liver disease; however, not all patients with carcinoid heart disease present with symptoms. The most common cause of death in these patients is right ventricular failure, and the second most common cause is tumor progression.

Mild tricuspid regurgitation is common in patients with a normal right ventricle and tricuspid valve. However, various pathologies can contribute to an increased severity of tricuspid regurgitation. The most common cause of tricuspid regurgitation is right ventricular dilation, which causes dilation of the tricuspid annulus (secondary/functional tricuspid regurgitation). Typically, a right ventricular systolic pressure of 55 mm Hg or greater will cause functional tricuspid regurgitation. Other causes include rheumatic and carcinoid heart disease, endocarditis, Ebstein anomaly, connective tissue disease (Marfan), and rheumatoid arthritis. Tricuspid regurgitation is well tolerated in patients with no evidence of pulmonary hypertension or right ventricular failure; however, tricuspid regurgitation in the setting of pulmonary hypertension can lead to heart failure and is associated with poor survival.

Management of carcinoid heart disease involves diuretics and salt and water restriction. When severe, tricuspid valve replacement is the operation of choice. Because of the tricuspid valve restriction in addition to the calcified and diseased subvalvular apparatus, a tricuspid valve repair is not an option.

### Reference

1. Hassan SA, Banchs J, Iliescu C, Dasari A, Lopez-Mattei J, Yusuf SW. Carcinoid heart disease. *Heart.* 2017;103:1488-1495.

**9.** Correct Answer: D

**Rationale:**

The left ventricular outflow tract gradient of hypertrophic cardiomyopathy is characteristically dagger-shaped. The waveform has a convex to the left orientation initially, which switches to concave to the left on the initiation of obstruction. This concave to the left orientation occurs because of the increased acceleration across the outflow tract, which is progressively narrowing (outflow obstruction). This increased acceleration does not occur with a subaortic membrane because the subaortic membrane causes a fixed and not dynamic obstruction. The gradient waveform through the aortic valve in patients with aortic stenosis is symmetric and demonstrates a convex to the left formation until the peak velocity. Severe aortic insufficiency may cause increased gradients as well, because of the increased flow through the aortic valve, which is the sum of the flow from the left atrium and the regurgitant flow from the aortic valve. According to the modified Bernoulli principle ($4V^2$, where V is peak velocity), this increased velocity will increase the transvalvular pressure gradient.

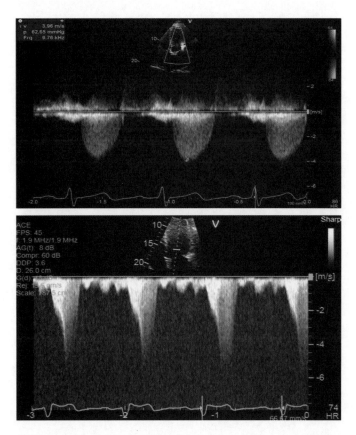

Transthoracic apical 5-chamber view with continuous wave Doppler. Difference between fixed obstruction of the left ventricular outflow tract due to aortic stenosis and dynamic obstruction of left ventricular outflow tract in left ventricular obstructive hypertrophy.

**Reference**

1. Sherrid MV, Wever-Pinzon O, Shah A, Chaudhry FA. Reflections of inflections in hypertrophic cardiomyopathy. *J Am Coll Cardiol.* 2009;54:212-219.

**10.** Correct Answer: D

**Rationale:**

Hypotension following TAVR can be due to hypovolemia, acidosis, bleeding, myocardial infarction, acute heart failure, cardiac tamponade, aortic root injury, severe paravalvular leak, or dynamic intracavitary gradients. The abrupt release of the fixed aortic obstruction following TAVR can result in improvement in ventricular function. This increased inotropy can precipitate hypertrophic cardiomyopathy–like physiology in these severely hypertrophied ventricles. Patients with small left ventricular end diastolic diameters, asymmetric hypertrophy, high-valve gradients, and increased ejection fraction have an increased risk of dynamic intracavitary gradients. When these gradients are associated with acute hypotension and cardiovascular collapse, the term "suicide left ventricle" has been used. Treatment mirrors the treatment for the left ventricular outflow tract obstruction seen in hypertrophic cardiomyopathy.

The most appropriate first choice in this patient's management is correction of hypovolemia with fluid bolus administration. If hypotension persists despite increased preload, the catecholamine agents should be avoided and noncatecholamine vasopressors (phenylephrine, vasopressin) should be used. Beta blockers may be useful as well to decrease inotropy and allow ventricular filling, in the absence of hypotension.

### References

1. Suh WM, Witzke CF, Palacios IF. Suicide left ventricle following transcatheter aortic valve implantation. *Catheter Cardiovasc Interv*. 2010;76:616-620.
2. Tomey MI, Gidwani UK, Sharma SK. Cardiac critical care after transcatheter aortic valve replacement. *Cardiol Clin*. 2013;31:607-618, ix.

# 20

# PERICARDIAL DISEASES

Hasan Khalid Siddiqi and David M. Dudzinski

1. A 35-year-old male with no significant past medical history presents to the Emergency Department with one day of worsening chest pain. The chest pain was abrupt in onset, is described as "sharp" in nature, and worsens with inspiration. It is primarily centered in the center of his chest but occasionally radiates to the left upper back. He feels that the pain worsens when he lays down. Vital signs are unremarkable including equal bilateral upper extremity blood pressures and radial pulses. On physical examination, he is febrile to 38.2°C. A triphasic "scratching" sound in time with the cardiac cycle is auscultated at the left lower sternal border. Initial laboratory studies show a negative troponin T and mild elevations in white blood cell count and the C-reactive protein. His ECG is shown below:

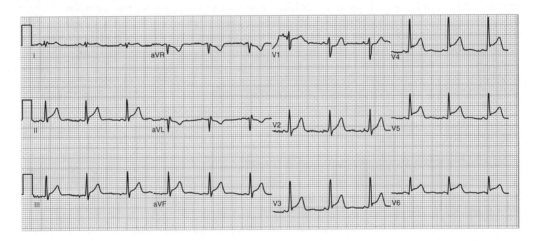

Which of the following is the most appropriate next step:

A. Heparin bolus and drip
B. High-dose aspirin and colchicine
C. Corticosteroids
D. Computed tomography angiography of the chest
E. Coronary angiography

2. A 51-year-old male with a recent history of acute pericarditis 6 weeks ago now resents with new onset chest pain. He stopped high-dose ibuprofen 4 weeks ago and has been feeling well since then. The chest pain started 12 hours ago, is very sharp, substernal, and pleuritic in nature. The symptoms are similar to his prior episode of pericarditis. He denies palpitations, lightheadedness, orthopnea, shortness of breath, and lower extremity edema. On physical examination, he is afebrile, with a pulse of 104 beats per minute, blood pressure 134/68 mm Hg, and a room air oxygen saturation of 99%. He has an audible friction rub. Kussmaul sign and jugular venous distension are absent. Laboratory evaluation reveals two negative serial troponin values, normal white blood cell count and creatinine, and mildly elevated C-reactive protein. ECG has nonspecific changes without ST-segment elevation. Echocardiogram shows normal biventricular function, no wall motion abnormalities, and a trace pericardial effusion that was previously visualized as well.

What is the most appropriate next therapy?

**A.** Heparin bolus and drip
**B.** Corticosteroids
**C.** Broad spectrum antibiotics
**D.** High dose ibuprofen and colchicine
**E.** Anakinra

3. A 62-year-old woman with a history of acute pericarditis 4 years ago that was treated with nonsteroidal anti-inflammatory drug (NSAID) to complete resolution presents with 8 weeks of insidiously worsening fatigue, bilateral lower extremity edema, breathlessness, and a feeling of abdominal fullness. She denies any fevers, chest pain, palpitations, or light-headedness. Physical examination is remarkable for 2+ pitting bilateral lower extremity edema, elevated jugular venous pressure with a rapid y descent, and an early diastolic sound best heard at the apex. Echocardiography shows normal right and left ventricular systolic function, a thickened pericardium without pericardial effusion, moderate left-sided pleural effusion, inspiratory ventricular septal motion toward the left ventricle, along with marked dilatation and absent respirophasic collapse of the inferior vena cava and hepatic veins.

The therapy most likely to yield relief of the patient's symptoms is:

**A.** High-dose NSAIDs and colchicine
**B.** Corticosteroids
**C.** Percutaneous coronary intervention
**D.** Pericardiectomy
**E.** Reassurance

4. A 44-year-old woman with a past medical history of asthma presents with acute onset chest pain of 2 hours duration. She reports being in her usual state of health until the morning, when she had acute onset of sharp substernal chest pain. The pain is sharp, does not radiate, and has an intensity of 8/10. It is worse when she leans forward. She does not have any associated shortness of breath, nausea, palpitations, or light-headedness. She denies any recent long car rides or airplane trips. Her son is recovering from an upper respiratory infection. Vital signs include temperature of 38.1°C, heart rate of 105 beats per minute, blood pressure of 124/72 mm Hg, and a room air oxygen saturation of 99%. On physical examination, she has normal heart sounds without any murmurs, friction rub, or S3 or S4. There is no jugular venous distension. Laboratory findings are remarkable for a troponin T of 0.03 ng/dL (normal <0.01), D-dimer <500 ng/mL, leukocytosis to 14,000/ μL, creatinine 0.78 mg/dL, and CRP 3.5 mg/L. ECG shows nonspecific changes without evidence of active ischemia. Echocardiography shows a small pericardial effusion and normal biventricular function without wall motion abnormalities.

What is the best next step in the management of this patient?

**A.** Send home with close follow-up with primary care physician
**B.** Admit to hospital for heparin bolus and drip
**C.** Admit to hospital for observation, high-dose NSAIDs, and colchicine
**D.** Activate cardiac catheterization laboratory for coronary angiography immediately
**E.** Admit to hospital for exercise stress testing

5. A 67-year-old male with history of former smoking, hypertension, diabetes, and stage III small cell lung cancer (on chemotherapy) presents to the Emergency Department with 3 days of progressive shortness of breath and an episode of syncope. Vital signs show a temperature of 36.6°C, regular heart rate of 130 beats per minute, and room air oxygen saturation of 94%. Blood pressure at rest is 96/54 mm Hg at end inspiration and drops to 82/50 mm Hg with inspiration. Physical examination reveals a pale cachectic and uncomfortable appearing male with cool extremities, muffled heart sounds, and jugular venous pressure of 14 cm $H_2O$. Laboratory studies are remarkable for creatinine 2.5 mg/dL (baseline 1.0), hemoglobin 7.5 g/dL (baseline 8.0), platelets 120,000/μL, white blood cell count 13,000/μL, CRP 4.2 mg/L, troponin T 0.1 ng/dL, NT pro-BNP 8,000 pg/mL (no known baseline). Precordial leads from his ECG are shown in the figure that follows:

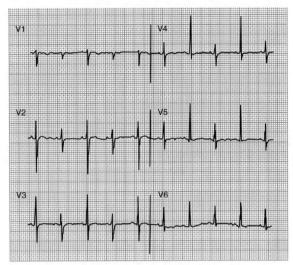

(Figure courtesy of Ary Goldberger, MD. From Hoit B. Diagnosis and treatment of pericardial effusion. In: Downey BC. UpToDate. Waltham, Mass: UpToDate; 2019. www.uptodate.com. Accessed April 2, 2019.)

What is the appropriate next diagnostic step?

**A.** Limited echocardiogram
**B.** CTA of the chest and abdomen (arterial phase)
**C.** Coronary angiography
**D.** CT chest pulmonary embolism protocol
**E.** Cardiac MRI

# Chapter 20 ▪ Answers

**1.** Correct Answer: B

**Rationale:**
This patient's presentation is consistent with acute pericarditis. The majority of cases of acute pericarditis in developed countries are either due to viral or idiopathic causes. However, in developing nations, tuberculosis is a leading cause of pericarditis. Typical symptoms include acute onset, severe, and often sharp chest pain that is usually retrosternal, but occasionally in the left chest. The classic pattern of pericarditis pain is radiation to the trapezius ridge in the back. The pain in pericarditis is often pleuritic in nature. Additionally, it can be positional, with worsening pain with reclining and palliation with leaning forward. A low-grade fever and sinus tachycardia may be present. On physical examination a pericardial friction rub may be present and is classically heard as a triphasic scratching sound in the precordium, best heard with the patient leaning forward. However, there may be only monophasic or biphasic rub. Muffled heart sounds or elevation of the jugular venous pressure should raise immediate suspicion for a large pericardial effusion and possible tamponade physiology.

Diagnosis of acute pericarditis is a clinical decision made based on having two or more of the following: chest pain; pericardial friction rub; ECG changes with typical concave ST segment elevation spanning multiple coronary territories and/or PR depression; pericardial effusion. In addition, other morbid conditions such as acute myocardial infarction, aortic dissection, and pulmonary embolism should be considered in the differential diagnosis and excluded by appropriate clinical judgment or targeted testing. This patient has three out of four of the listed criteria and several signs and symptoms consistent with acute pericarditis.

First line treatment of the first episode of acute pericarditis thought to be secondary to viral or idiopathic causes consists of high-dose NSAIDs and weight-based colchicine dosing. The usual NSAID regimen consists of aspirin 750 to 1,000 mg every 8 hours or ibuprofen 600 to 800 mg every 8 hours for 1 to 2 weeks, followed by tapering to discontinuation over 2 to 3 weeks. Colchicine (0.5-0.6 mg every 12 hours for patients weighing >70 kg, or 0.5-0.6 mg once daily for patients weighing <70 kg) should be continued for 3 months, and then discontinued without tapering. The use of colchicine improves response to NSAID and reduces the risk of recurrent pericarditis by half.

The clinical history and ECG with concave ST-segment elevations spanning multiple coronary territories are highly suggestive of acute pericarditis, and unlikely to reflect acute coronary syndrome. Therefore, initiation of heparin in this patient is not the best next step, especially as there is a theoretical risk of hemorrhagic conversion in the setting of acute pericarditis. Corticosteroids are not the first line therapy for acute pericarditis (viral or idiopathic) unless the patient cannot tolerate NSAIDs or colchicine, or if there is another indication for corticosteroids, such as an autoimmune pericarditis. Imaging studies such as CTA and coronary angiography are not as necessary at this time because acute coronary syndrome and aortic dissection are less likely given the clinical picture of pericarditis, negative troponin, ECG, and equal bilateral blood pressures.

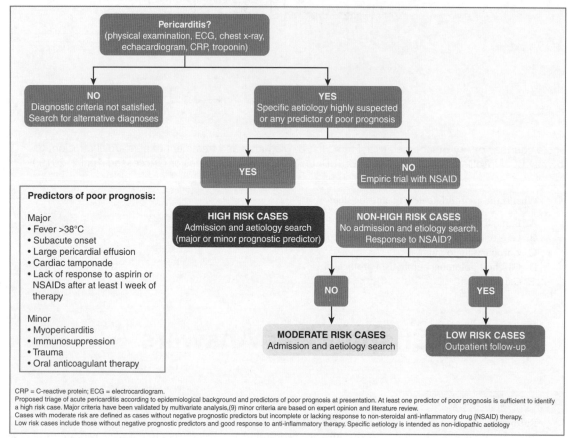

(Figure from Adler Y, Charron P, Imazio M, et al. 2015 ESC guidelines for the diagnosis and management of pericardial diseases: the task force for the diagnosis and management of pericardial diseases of the European Society of Cardiology (ESC). Eur Heart J. 2015;36:2921.)

## References

1. Adler Y, Charron P, Imazio M, et al. 2015 ESC guidelines for the diagnosis and management of pericardial diseases: the task force for the diagnosis and management of pericardial diseases of the European Society of Cardiology (ESC). *Eur Heart J*. 2015;36:2921.
2. LeWinter MM. Clinical practice. Acute pericarditis. *N Engl J Med*. 2014;371:2410.
3. Imazio M, Gaita F. Diagnosis and treatment of pericarditis. *Heart*. 2015;101:1159.
4. Imazio M, Gaita F, LeWinter M. Evaluation and treatment of pericarditis: a systematic review. *JAMA*. 2015;314:1498.
5. Dudzinski DM, Mak GS, Hung JW. Pericardial diseases. *Curr Probl Cardiol*. 2012;37:75.

**2.** Correct Answer: D

**Rationale:**

Approximately 15% to 30% of patients with idiopathic acute pericarditis will have a recurrence. Recurrent pericarditis is diagnosed with new symptoms of pericarditis after resolution of prior symptoms, signs of persistent pericardial inflammation (ECG changes, elevation of CRP, friction rib, new or worse pericardial effusion) after a symptom-free period of 4 weeks or more from the prior episode of pericarditis.

This patient has a history of pericarditis and presents with acute onset chest pain similar to his prior episode of pericarditis. A nonspecific ECG and negative troponins with 12 hours of chest pain decreases the likelihood of acute coronary syndrome, and thus heparin not indicated. The similarity of symptoms to prior pericarditis, friction rub, and elevated CRP occurring 4 weeks after stopping ibuprofen all point toward recurrent pericarditis as the cause of his chest pain.

First line therapy for recurrent pericarditis consists of reinitiating high-dose NSAIDs along with colchicine. NSAID therapy should be continued until complete resolution of symptoms and objective signs of pericarditis (CRP normalization, etc.), and then tapered. Colchicine should be continued for the duration of NSAID therapy. It improves response to NSAID and reduces the risk of recurrence by half. Proton pump inhibitor should be prescribed for gastric protection from NSAIDs. Exercise restriction is also reinstated until resolution of symptoms and normalization of CRP.

In the presence of contraindications to NSAIDs and colchicine, or recurrence of pericarditis during NSAID/colchicine therapy, low-dose corticosteroids can be considered as second line therapy, after exclusion of infectious causes. Prednisone at doses of 0.2 to 0.5 mg/kg/d (or equivalent other steroid dosing) may be considered for at least 2 to 4 weeks, and until symptoms and signs resolve. Once remission has been achieved, the steroids should be gradually tapered over 2 to 4 weeks. Next line therapies include immunosuppressive medications such as azathioprine, anakinra (a recombinant anti-interleukin-1 receptor antagonists), and intravenous immunoglobulin infusions.

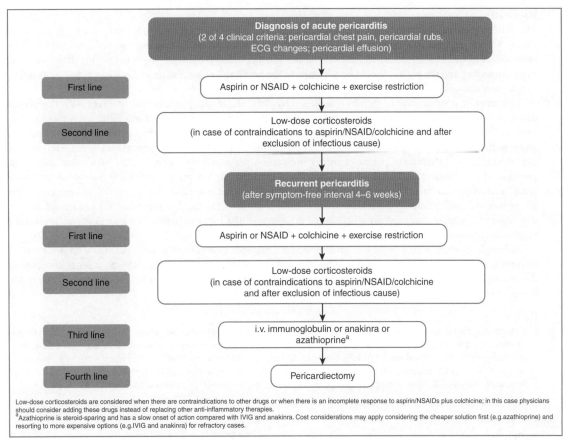

(Figure from Adler Y, Charron P, Imazio M, et al. 2015 ESC guidelines for the diagnosis and management of pericardial diseases: the task force for the diagnosis and management of pericardial diseases of the European Society of Cardiology (ESC). Eur Heart J. 2015;36:2921.)

### References
1. Lilly LS. Treatment of acute and recurrent idiopathic pericarditis. *Circulation*. 2013;127:1723-1726.
2. Zipes DP, Libby P, Bonow RO, Mann DL, Tomaselli GF, Braunwald E. *Braunwald's Heart Disease: A Textbook of Cardiovascular Medicine*. 11th ed. Philadelphia, PA: Elsevier/Saunders; 2018.

---

**3.** Correct Answer: D

**Rationale:**

This patient's clinical picture, along with signs on physical examination and diagnostic testing, are most consistent with constrictive pericarditis. The definitive treatment of constrictive pericarditis is surgical pericardiectomy.

Constrictive pericarditis is the result of inflammatory injury to the pericardium arising from a plethora of causes. The risk of progressing to constrictive pericarditis is very low with most etiologies of pericardial disease, ranging from 1% in viral and idiopathic pericarditis, but up to 20% to 30% in bacterial and purulent pericarditis. Tuberculosis is a major cause of constrictive pericarditis in the developing world.

The clinical presentation of constrictive pericarditis is due to manifestations of impaired diastolic filling of both ventricles. The rigid pericardium lacks compliance, and as a result, leads to diastolic constraint on the heart with preserved ventricular function; accordingly, constrictive pericarditis is on the differential diagnosis for a heart failure with preserved ejection fraction syndrome. Signs and symptoms of right heart failure are the most prominent manifestations of constrictive pericarditis. This includes venous and hepatic congestion, hepatomegaly, and ascites. There can be significant tricuspid regurgitation present. Pleural effusions may also be seen.

### References

1. Imazio M, Brucato A, Maestroni S, et al. Risk of constrictive pericarditis after acute pericarditis. *Circulation.* 2011;124:1270-1275.
2. Welch TD, Ling LH, Espinosa RE, et al. Echocardiographic diagnosis of constrictive pericarditis: mayo clinic criteria. *Circ Cardiovasc Imaging.* 2014;7:526-534.
3. Biçer M, Özdemir B, Kan İ, et al. Long-term outcomes of pericardiectomy for constrictive pericarditis. *J Cardiothorac Surg.* 2015;10:177.

## 4. Correct Answer: C

**Rationale:**

The patient presents with symptoms of positional chest pain after being exposed to a family member with a viral illness. She has evidence of mild myocardial injury with a very mildly elevated troponin, and echocardiogram shows no evidence of wall motion abnormalities but reveals a small pericardial effusion. The best unifying diagnosis here is myopericarditis, and the patient should be admitted to the hospital for observation and treatment with anti-inflammatory medications.

The term myopericarditis or perimyocarditis refers to inflammatory injury that involves both the pericardium and myocardium. Myopericarditis indicates a primarily pericarditic syndrome, with symptoms of pericarditis (chest pain, often pleuritic and positional, nonspecific or widespread ECG changes, CRP elevations) along with elevation in cardiac injury biomarkers (troponin, CK-MB) without new global or focal left ventricular dysfunction. In contrast, perimyocarditis indicates a predominantly myocarditic syndrome with minor pericardial involvement and presents with new focal or diffuse left ventricular dysfunction along with some symptoms of pericarditis. Etiologies for both are similar and include cardiotropic viral illnesses, connective tissue diseases, inflammatory bowel diseases, radiation-induced myocardial injury, or drug-induced myocardial injury. The most common presentation of myopericarditis involves a preceding viral gastrointestinal or respiratory illness.

Although myocarditis may require an endomyocardial biopsy for confirmation, most patients with myopericarditis have a benign prognosis and self-limited illness, and therefore biopsy is not necessary in the absence of ventricular dysfunction or heart failure. Mainstay for treatment is similar to pericarditis when ventricular function is preserved and consists of high-dose anti-inflammatory agents and exercise restriction.

### References

1. Caforio AL, Pankuweit S, Arbustini E, et al. European Society of CardiologyWorking Group on Myocardial and Pericardial Diseases. Current state of knowledge on etiology, diagnosis, management, and therapy of myocarditis: a position statement of the European Society of Cardiology Working Group on Myocardial and Pericardial Diseases. *Eur Heart J.* 2013;34:2636-2648.
2. Imazio M, Cooper LT. Management of myopericarditis. *Expert Rev Cardiovasc Ther.* 2013;11:193-201.
3. Imazio M, Trinchero R. Myopericarditis: etiology, management, and prognosis. *Int J Cardiol.* 2008;127:17-26.

## 5. Correct Answer: A

**Rationale:**

This patient is presenting with evolving cardiogenic shock (hypotension, cool extremities, syncope, and evidence of organ dysfunction with acute kidney injury), likely due to pericardial tamponade. The next appropriate step is emergent limited echocardiography, to accompany emergent pericardiocentesis.

Pericardial tamponade is a life-threatening emergency in which pressure in the pericardial space rises due to a variety of possible reasons, leading to compression of the heart, ultimately impairing cardiac output and leading to shock or death. Causes of pericardial tamponade are similar to those that cause pericardial effusions and are listed in the table that follows. In the case of this patient, his history of progressive lung cancer makes a malignant effusion most likely.

Pulsus paradoxus is an important physical finding in cardiac tamponade. Pulsus paradoxus refers to an abnormally large reduction in both the stroke volume and the systemic blood pressure with inspiration, which in pericardial tamponade is due to the extrinsic constraint on cardiac chamber expansion leading to enhanced ventricular interdependence. Transthoracic echocardiogram is the imaging modality of choice in diagnosing and guiding management of cardiac tamponade. Cardiac CT and MRI can be utilized to better understand the pericardium and help understand the cause of tamponade, but are rarely indicated in the acute setting.

Here, the patient is in cardiogenic shock and needs urgent imaging of the pericardium with a limited echocardiogram to guide treatment. Cardiac MRI, CTA chest, and CT chest would not add to the immediate management of this patient, as aortic dissection and pulmonary embolism are less likely based on clinical presentation. Coronary angiography is not warranted because there is no evidence of acute coronary syndrome. The troponin elevation, in this case, is explained by damage from cardiogenic shock rather than acute plaque rupture.

**Common causes:**

- Pericarditis

- Tuberculosis

- Iatrogenic (invasive procedure-related, postcardiac surgery)

- Trauma

- Neoplasm/malignancy

**Uncommon causes:**

- Collagen vascular diseases (systemic lupus erythematosus, rheumatoid arthritis, scleroderma)

- Radiation-induced

- Postmyocardial infarction

- Uraemia

- Aortic dissection

- Bacterial infection

- Pneumopericardium

Causes of cardiac tamponade

Table from Adler Y, Charron P, Imazio M, et al. 2015 ESC guidelines for the diagnosis and management of pericardial diseases: the task force for the diagnosis and management of pericardial diseases of the European Society of Cardiology (ESC). Eur Heart J. 2015;36:2921.

## References

1. Zipes DP, Libby P, Bonow RO, Mann DL, Tomaselli GF, Braunwald E. *Braunwald's Heart Disease: A Textbook of Cardiovascular Medicine.* 11th ed. Philadelphia, PA: Elsevier/Saunders; 2018.

2. Adler Y, Charron P, Imazio M, et al. 2015 ESC guidelines for the diagnosis and management of pericardial diseases: the task force for the diagnosis and management of pericardial diseases of the European Society of Cardiology (ESC). *Eur Heart J.* 2015;36:2921.

# 21

# MYOCARDIAL DISEASE

Rachel C. Frank and David M. Dudzinski

1. A 22-year-old male is admitted to the intensive care unit (ICU) after sustaining a cardiac arrest while playing soccer in a rural area. Cardiopulmonary resuscitation was performed, but no automatic external defibrillator was available; he was intubated in the field because of poor mental status. He is transferred to your tertiary care ICU. Examination reveals an ejection systolic murmur, and he followed commands when sedation was lightened. Transthoracic echocardiography reveals discrete upper septal hypertrophy measuring 18 mm and an elevated left ventricular outflow velocity. He successfully passes a spontaneous awakening trial and spontaneous breathing trial. Unfortunately, at that time, he develops atrial fibrillation, became hypotensive to blood pressures of 94/52, and $FiO_2$ was increased from 0.4 to 0.6 in response to desaturations to the low 80s.

The best treatment for this patient's atrial fibrillation is:

   A. Sotalol
   B. Digoxin
   C. IV metoprolol
   D. Amiodarone
   E. Norepinephrine

2. A 75-year-old female with prior history of hypertension and hyperlipidemia presents with acute onset chest pain and dyspnea for last 4 hours ago. Physical examination revealed bilateral rales, cool extremities, and diaphoresis. She had no murmurs on auscultation. ECG revealed 1.5-mm ST segment elevations throughout the precordial leads. High-sensitivity troponin was elevated at 100 ng/L. Left coronary angiogram reveals nonobstructive coronary disease and ventriculography shows apical ballooning with sparing of base as well as globally reduced ejection fraction.

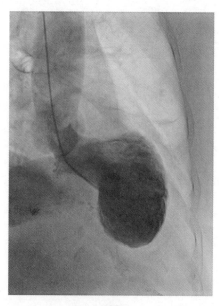

Left ventriculography on cardiac catheterization.

On arrival to the ICU she has bibasilar rales with oxygen requirement of 6 L/min via nasal cannula. Blood pressure is 95/48 mm Hg and HR is 122 beats per minute.

Which of the following medications should be avoided at this stage?

A. Diuretics
B. Beta blockers
C. Nitrates
D. Levosimendan

3. A 44-year-old female, G1P0, at 36 weeks gestation presents with worsening shortness of breath, lower extremity edema, and fatigue. Vital signs are notable for blood pressure of 84/58 mm Hg, heart rate of 144 beats per minute, respiratory rate 38 breaths per minute, and oxygen saturation of 92% while breathing room air. Examination is notable for 2+ bilateral lower-extremity pitting edema and bibasilar rales extending one-third of the way up bilateral lung fields. Urinalysis shows no protein and indices of renal and hepatic function are normal. Diuretics and afterload reduction with hydralazine and nitrates are started. Echocardiography shows left ventricular dilatation and severe left ventricular dysfunction with ejection fraction of 15%. Cesarean section delivery is performed, but her hemodynamics continue to worsen. Further diagnostic testing including coronary angiography at time of pulmonary artery catheter placement does not reveal alternate etiology, but she is noted to have a cardiac output of 2.1 L/min (cardiac index of 1.3 L/min/m$^2$). Unfortunately, her clinical condition worsens and she develops progressive cardiogenic shock refractory to medical therapy including norepinephrine, milrinone, and epinephrine.

The most appropriate next step in management is:

A. Phenylephrine
B. Continue medical management only
C. Urgent mechanical circulatory support
D. Heart transplantation

4. A 22-year-old male with no known medical history presents with insidious fatigue, nonproductive cough, and shortness of breath with exertion over the prior 3 weeks. His laboratory test results are notable for an elevated high sensitivity troponin to 60 ng/L, and an NT-proBNP elevated to 2,400 pg/mL. Ejection fraction on transthoracic echocardiogram is noted to be 15% but a normal LV dimension and wall thickness, with no other structural abnormality. He is admitted to the Cardiac ICU for further monitoring and management. You are suspicious for myocarditis. He exhibits no dysrhythmia on telemetry. His symptoms improve with medical management.

The next best test to confirm a diagnosis is:

A. Viral serologies
B. Endomyocardial biopsy
C. Cardiac MRI
D. Cardiac PET scan

5. A 48-year-old male with no known medical history came to the emergency room reporting worsening dyspnea on exertion. ECG is without ischemic changes and high-sensitivity troponin is modestly elevated at 68 ng/L. He is quickly admitted to the cardiac intensive care unit in advanced cardiogenic shock and with recurrent ventricular tachycardia despite diuretics, inodilators, lidocaine, and amiodarone. Emergent myocardial biopsy at time of initiation of mechanical support reveals lymphocytes and multinucleated giant cells.

Which of the following agents is an appropriate treatment?

A. Azathioprine, cyclosporine, and corticosteroids
B. IVIG
C. Corticosteroid monotherapy
D. NSAIDs

# Chapter 21 ▪ Answers

**1.** Correct Answer: D

**Rationale:**
Hypertrophic cardiomyopathy (HCM) is defined as left ventricular wall thickness >15 mm not explained by loading conditions including hypertension or aortic valve stenosis. Patients with HCM are at risk for lethal ventricular arrhythmias, and cardiac arrest may be the initial presentation, whereas other patients may experience dyspnea, palpitations, chest pain, or syncope as presenting symptoms. However, the most common arrhythmia experienced by patients with HCM is atrial fibrillation that occurs in approximately 20% to 25%.

HCM may cause obstruction to left ventricular outflow, caused by systolic anterior motion of the anterior mitral valve leaflet. Conditions that worsen the obstruction include hypotension and tachycardia. Atrial fibrillation can cause both of these. Also, patients with HCM are markedly dependent on the "atrial kick" for adequate ventricular filling. These conditions can worsen left ventricular outflow tract obstruction resulting in flash pulmonary edema and hemodynamic collapse.

As such, any patient with hypertrophic obstructive cardiomyopathy experiencing hemodynamic stressors with acute changes to preload or afterload, such as intubation or extubation, should have close monitoring and titration of hemodynamics. Avoiding hypotension by maintaining preload and afterload, preventing a hyperdynamic state, and maintenance of sinus rhythm are essential to optimize hemodynamics.

Digoxin and norepinephrine should be avoided in this patient population as it can increase contractility and thereby worsen left ventricular outflow tract obstruction. In patients with HCM who develop atrial fibrillation, AHA/ACC guidelines recommend amiodarone or disopyramide combined with beta blocker or nondihydropyridine calcium channel blocker as first line medications. Although beta blocker can help reduce left ventricular outflow tract obstruction, these could possibly exacerbate hypotension and thus not the best initial choice. In the setting of moderate hypotension, amiodarone bolus and load is the best initial choice for medical management. Should the hypotension be profound, immediate cardioversion would be the best step in management.

### References

1. Elliot P, Anastasakis A, Borger MA, et al. 2014 ESC guidelines on diagnosis and management of hypertrophic cardiomyopathy: the task force for the diagnosis and management of hypertrophic cardiomyopathy of the European Society of Cardiology (ESC). *Eur Heart J.* 2014;35:2733-2779.
2. January CT, Wann LS, Alpert JS, et al. 2014 AHA/ACC/HRS guidelines for the management of patients with atrial fibrillation. *JACC.* 2014;64:E1-E76.

**2.** Correct Answer: B

**Rationale:**
Patients with Takotsubo cardiomyopathy often have a clinical presentation that is similar to those patients presenting with acute coronary syndrome. The wall motion abnormalities seen in Takotsubo cardiomyopathy extend beyond a single vascular territory, but multivessel coronary lesions must be excluded. Diagnostic modality of choice is coronary angiography. When obstructive coronary artery disease is seen in one vessel, but the wall motion abnormalities extend beyond one vascular territory, the diagnosis of Takotsubo cardiomyopathy may be suggested. The most classic phenotype of Takotsubo cardiomyopathy is the apical ballooning with basilar sparing, seen on left ventricular catheterization or on transthoracic echocardiography. Other morphologies include midventricular, biventricular, and an "inverted" form with basal hypokinesis. The underlying pathophysiology is thought to be related to catecholamine surge resulting in myocardial myocyte dysfunction.

Takotsubo cardiomyopathy is more likely to affect women than men and often occurs in postmenopausal women who experienced a hemodynamic, physical, or emotional stressor. It can occur secondary to medical conditions including sepsis, subarachnoid hemorrhage, and pheochromocytoma. Mortality is similar to that of STEMI in the acute phase for hospitalized patients, 4% to 5%. Complications of Takotsubo cardiomyopathy include cardiogenic shock, severe mitral regurgitation, arrhythmias, pulmonary edema, and left ventricular outflow tract obstruction (particularly in patients with preexisting left ventricular upper septal hypertrophy).

Studies have reported increased mortality in Takotsubo cardiomyopathy with catecholamines. However, a calcium sensitizer called levosimendan may theoretically be used in place of inotropes and vasopressors, though this medication is not available in the United States. ACE inhibitors may help with recovery of cardiac function but should be avoided in the early phase of cardiogenic shock. Beta blockers have not shown benefit in Takotsubo cardiomyopathy and are contraindicated in cardiogenic shock or decompensated heart failure. Management is guided by standard heart failure measures, including afterload reduction and diuresis.

References

1. Pelliccia F. Pathophysiology of takotsubo syndrome. *Circulation*. 2017;135:2426-2441.
2. Santoro F, Ieva R, Ferraretti A, et al. Safety and feasibility of levosimendan administration in takotsubo cardiomyopathy: a case series. *Cardiovasc Ther*. 2013;31:e133-e137.

**3.** Correct Answer: C

**Rationale:**

Peripartum cardiomyopathy is a condition that can occur from 1 month before delivery up to 5 months following delivery and is characterized by left ventricular ejection fraction <45%, and no prior history of cardiac disease. Peripartum cardiomyopathy is a diagnosis of exclusion and other causes of heart failure must be exonerated. Diagnostic testing should be driven by an interdisciplinary team and often includes transthoracic echocardiography, as well as cardiac MRI, endomyocardial biopsy, and coronary angiography. Cardiac workload increases during pregnancy as a result of increased circulating volume, heart rate, and stroke volume. This results in a net increase in cardiac output of approximately 20% to 50%. Vascular resistance decreases by about 20% but rises in the third trimester.

Management of peripartum cardiomyopathy is similar to management of other etiologies of heart failure, but with mindfulness regarding teratogenicity of medications. During the gravid period, beta blockers and hydralazine may be used for medical afterload reduction under close monitoring to avoid decreases in uretoplacental perfusion. The main stays in medical management following delivery are ACE inhibitors and beta blockers. Optimization of volume status and management of anemia are additional considerations in management. Peripartum cardiomyopathy is associated with atrial and ventricular arrhythmias, the most common of which is atrial fibrillation.

As with other cardiomyopathies, management of patients with shock and clinical instability should include vasopressors and inotropes. However, phenylephrine should be avoided as it primarily increases afterload without providing inotropy. Appropriate consideration of mechanical circulatory support includes ventricular assist devices and extracorporeal membrane oxygenation, whether as a bridge to recovery or transplantation. For patients with hemodynamic instability, cesarean delivery is preferred to minimize hemodynamic stressors of vaginal birth. Over 50% of women with peripartum cardiomyopathy eventually recover ejection fraction. However, some will require mechanical support as a bridge to transplant or recovery. Those requiring mechanical support have better survival than women with other nonischemic or ischemic cardiomyopathies.

References

1. Arany Z. Peripartum cardiomyopathy. *Circulation*. 2016;133:1397-1409.
2. Hilfiker-Kleiner D. Peripartum cardiomyopathy: current management and future perspectives. *Eur Heart J*. 2015;36:1090-1097.

**4.** Correct Answer: C

**Rationale:**

Viral myocarditis is one of the most common causes of myocarditis. It may be caused by a variety of viral infections including hepatitis C, HIV, and enteroviruses among others, as well as bacterial and parasitic infections. Viral myocarditis may be preceded by upper respiratory tract symptoms, gastroenteritis, fatigue, fevers, and myalgias, followed by the onset of heart failure symptoms. Presentation can vary from occult heart failure to cardiovascular collapse or complex ventricular arrhythmias. With advances in imaging, cardiac MRI has been particularly useful in diagnosis of myocarditis. In myocarditis, cardiac MRI may show late gadolinium enhancement and relative myocardial enhancement compared to skeletal muscle, indicating damage, scaring, edema, and increased capillary permeability.

Once MRI suggests myocarditis, endomyocardial biopsy is useful as it may exonerate other infiltrative etiologies including sarcoidosis, amyloidosis, and hemochromatosis. Biopsy is still considered the gold standard for diagnosis. However, the biopsy of the native heart is not without risks, such as ventricular perforation, valvular damage, and vascular injury. Thus, endomyocardial biopsy may be useful in select patients after cardiac MRI or when hemodynamic instability or need for rapid tissue diagnosis requires expeditious biopsy. Although cardiac PET scans can also assist in confirming the diagnosis of myocarditis, they are not easily available and needs preparation before testing and thus not the diagnostic modality of choice. Although viral serologies may be positive in a select number of patients, the overall sensitivity is poor, and thus these results are unlikely to change management. In this patient, with clinical improvement on medical management, cardiac MRI may be the next best test, to avoid risks of endomyocardial biopsy while assisting in assessment of a diagnosis, with biopsy considered only if there is no definitive diagnosis made by cardiac MRI and or concerning clinical trajectory.

References

1. Dennert R. Crijns HJ, Heymans S, et al. Acute viral myocarditis. *Eur Heart J*. 2008;29:2073-2082.
2. Friedrich MG, Marcotte F. Cardiac magnetic resonance assessment of myocarditis. *Circ Cardiovasc Imaging*. 2013;6:833-839.

**5.** Correct Answer: A

### Rationale:

Giant cell myocarditis is a type of myocarditis characterized by cardiovascular collapse, with frequent ventricular arrhythmias and/or advanced atrioventricular heart block. The gold standard for diagnosis is endomyocardial biopsy. Although given the potential for sampling bias, a negative first biopsy with a high clinical suspicion should warrant consideration for repeat biopsy. Cardiac MRI and cardiac PET scan can help identify affected areas and can assist with biopsy planning, increasing the yield. In giant cell myocarditis, pathology reveals lymphocytic infiltrate with multinucleated giant cells. Beyond the initial presentation, patients with giant cell myocarditis are at high risk for malignant ventricular arrhythmias.

Therapeutically, there is no clear mortality benefit for the use of IVIG in patients with giant cell myocarditis. Literature suggests improved survival in patients receiving immunosuppresive therapy with multiple agents: azathioprine, cyclosporine, antithymocyte globulin, methotrexate, mycophenolate mofetil, and glucocorticoids. IVIG or glucocorticoids alone is less effective. NSAIDs are not helpful in myocarditis and may worsen heart failure. The patient with giant cell myocarditis should also be evaluated for mechanical circulatory support.

### References

1. Kindermann I, Barth C, Mahfoud F, et al. Update on myocarditis. *JACC.* 2012;59:779-792.
2. Kandolin R, Lehtonen J, Salmenkivi K, et al. Diagnosis, treatment, and outcome of giant-cell myocarditis in the era of combined immunosuppression. *Circ Heart Fail.* 2013;6:15-22.

# 22

# CONGENITAL HEART DISEASE IN ADULTS

Archit Sharma and Aaron C. Tyagi

1. A 36-year-old female with known Eisenmenger syndrome (ES) is admitted to the ICU after 2-day hospital course for worsening hypoxia. She is followed as an outpatient in the cardiology clinic, and it is noted that her oxygen levels are usually low. Her vital signs show a heart rate of 95 bpm, oxygen saturation of 86% on noninvasive positive pressure ventilation, blood pressure of 116/80 mm Hg, and a respiratory rate of 18. On examination, you note the female in mild respiratory distress with signs of cyanosis. Chest X-ray showed mild pleural effusions bilaterally but no concern for pulmonary edema. Transthoracic echocardiography done the prior day showed concern for biventricular dysfunction. What is the next best step to confirm this patient's diagnosis?

    A. Transesophageal echocardiography
    B. CTA of the chest
    C. Cardiac catheterization
    D. Repeat CXR

2. You are posted in the Neonatal intensive care unit of the hospital. You get an emergency page that a pregnant patient has just delivered in the Emergency Department, and the child has a congenital cardiac condition for which he will need a Fontan procedure. The Fontan surgery, which involves the anastomosis of the right atrium to the pulmonary artery, is a useful surgical treatment for each of the following congenital cardiac defects EXCEPT

    A. Tricuspid atresia
    B. Hypoplastic left heart syndrome
    C. Pulmonary valve stenosis
    D. Truncus arteriosus
    E. Pulmonary artery atresia

3. A 15-year-old male patient was admitted to the ICU with a diagnosis of stroke after he got some accidental air bubbles injection while receiving IV fluid resuscitation in the emergency department, where he was seen for a viral prodrome. The patient's family mentions that he has a known cardiac condition from birth, even though they do not know the name. Accidental injection of air into a peripheral vein would be LEAST likely to result in arterial air embolism in the patient with which of the following anatomic cardiac defects?

    A. Patent ductus arteriosus
    B. ES
    C. Teratology of Fallot
    D. Pulmonary atresia with ventricular septal defect
    E. Tricuspid atresia

4. A patient with known pulmonary arterial hypertension (PAH) from congenital heart disease has recently been diagnosed with ES. What is the most appropriate treatment that should be initiated in this patient?

    A. Digoxin
    B. Beta blocker therapy
    C. Calcium channel blocker therapy
    D. Bosentan

**5.** A 23-year-old male presents to the emergency department after collapsing during a pick-up basketball game. On examination you find a young male in no apparent distress. He exhibits a harsh, systolic crescendo-decrescendo murmur. His EKG is an unremarkable save for short, sharp Q-waves in the lateral leads. Which of the following is most strongly associated with this diagnosis?

**A.** Family history
**B.** Smoking
**C.** Drug use
**D.** Alcohol use

# Chapter 22 ▪ Answers

**1.** Correct Answer: B

**Rationale:**
This patient is exhibiting signs of acute respiratory distress leading to respiratory failure with a known history of ES. Given this history, she likely is suffering from pulmonary arterial thrombosis and requires a CTA of her chest to confirm the diagnosis. ES is a consequence of severe PAH, more commonly as a result of congenital heart disease. It is most commonly associated with atrial and/or ventricular septal defects. The primary pathophysiology results in left to right shunting. This leads to shearing forces and stress on the pulmonary vasculature, resulting in endothelial dysfunction, release of inflammatory mediators, and vascular remodeling. The increase in pulmonary vascular resistance causes a right-to-left shunt that leads to cyanosis, which completes the picture of ES. TEE will only show the shunting and might not reveal the thrombosis (A). Cardiac catheterization will reveal the elevated pulmonary pressures but will not be diagnostic for a pulmonary venous thrombosis (C). Because the patient has only mild pleural effusions, a chest radiograph will not be very useful either (D).

Patients with ES are at risk for multiple comorbidities, including pulmonary arterial thrombosis (~20%). Risk factors that further increase this risk include biventricular dysfunction, female sex, dilation of the pulmonary arteries, and decreased pulmonary blood flow.

References
1. Beghetti M, Galie N. Eisenmenger's syndrome. *J Am Coll Cardiol.* 2009;53(9):733-740. doi:10.1016/j.jacc.2008.11.025.
2. Broberg CS, Ujita M, Prasad S, et al. Pulmonary arterial thrombosis in eisenmenger syndrome is associated with biventricular dysfunction and decreased pulmonary flow velocity. *J Am Coll Cardiol.* 2007;50(7):634-642.
3. Silversides CK, Granton JT, Konen E, Hart MA, Webb GD, Therrien J. Pulmonary thrombosis in adults with eisenmenger syndrome. *J Am Coll Cardiol.* 2003;42(11):1982-1987.

**2.** Correct Answer: D

**Rationale:**
Truncus arteriosus occurs when there is presence of a single arterial trunk, overriding both ventricles (which are connected via a ventricular septal defect). This trunk gives rise to both the aorta and pulmonary artery. Surgical treatment of this defect includes banding of the left and right pulmonary arteries and enclosure of the associated VSD, and hence the Fontan would not be employed in this situation.

The Fontan procedure (usually modified Fontan) refers to the anastomosis of the right atrial appendage (or the superior and inferior vena cava) to the pulmonary artery. Because this procedure leads to an increase in pulmonary blood flow, it as the treatment of choice for treatment of congenital cardiac defects, which decrease the pulmonary artery blood flow (eg, pulmonary atresia and stenosis [C and E] and tricuspid atresia[A]). The Fontan procedure is also used to divert systemic venous return to pulmonary artery when it is necessary to surgically convert the right ventricle to a systemic ventricle (eg, hypoplastic left heart syndrome[B]).

References
1. Fontan F, Baudet E. Surgical repair of tricuspid atresia. *Thorax.* 1971;26(3):240-248.
2. Gewillig M, Brown SC. The Fontan circulation after 45 years: update in physiology. *Heart.* 2016;102(14):1081-1086.
3. Fontan F, Deville C, Quaegebeur J, et al. Repair of tricuspid atresia in 100 patients. *J Thorac Cardiovasc Surg.* 1983;85(5):647-660.

**3.** Correct Answer: A

**Rationale:**

Patent ductus arteriosus (A) causes left to right shunting and, hence, has the least risk of causing arterial air embolism. The anesthetic management of patients with congenital heart disease requires thorough knowledge of the pathophysiology of the cardiac defect. They can be categorized into defects causing left to right intracardiac shunts (acyanotic) and right to left shunts (cyanotic). The common congenital heart defects that result in right to left shunting include tetralogy of Fallot(C), Ebstein malformation of the tricuspid valve, pulmonary atresia with a ventricular septal defect (D), ES (B), tricuspid atresia (E), and patent foramen ovale. Meticulous care must be taken to avoid infusion of air via intravenous solutions because this can lead to arterial air embolism. Patients with congenital defects that result in left to right intracardiac shunting, such as patent ductus arteriosus, are at minimal risk for arterial air embolism because blood flow through the shunt is primarily from the systemic to the pulmonary system.

References

1. Hopkins WE, Ochoa LL, Richardson GW, Trulock EP. Comparison of the hemodynamics and survival of adults with severe primary pulmonary hypertension or eisenmenger syndrome. *J Heart Lung Transplant*. 1996;15(1 Pt 1):100-105.
2. Apitz C, Webb GD, Redington AN. Tetralogy of fallot. *Lancet*. 2009;374(9699):1462-1471.
3. Blalock A, Taussig HB. The surgical treatment of malformations of the heart: in which there is pulmonary stenosis or pulmonary atresia. *J Am Med Assoc*. 1945;128(3):189-202.

**4.** Correct Answer: D

**Rationale:**

Patients with congenital heart disease are at increased risk and incidence of development of PAH. The mortality remains high among these patients if left untreated. More recently, safe and effective drug therapy (disease targeted therapy) has become available for the treatment of PAH, which includes endothelin receptor antagonists, phosphodiesterase-5 inhibitors, and prostanoids. Disease-targeted therapies such as sildenafil and bosentan have been associated with improved survival at 10 years as shown in the BREATH-5 Trial. It has been shown that disease-targeted therapies for PAH results in better survival when comparted to traditionally used drugs such as digoxin, beta blockers, and calcium channel blockers. And disease-targeted therapies are the mainstay of treating PAH. Patients with PAH due to ES has a better survival than patient's with primary PAH. This may be due to the fact that right ventricular function in patients with ES, and resultant PAH is better than those with idiopathic PAH.

References

1. Gali N, Beghetti M, Gatzoulis MA, et al. Bosentan therapy in patients with eisenmenger' syndrome: a multicenter, double-blind, randomized, placebo-controlled study. *Circulation*. 2006;114:48-54.
2. Beghetti M, Galie N. Eisenmenger's syndrome. *J Am Coll Cardiol*. 2009;53(9):733-740. doi:10.1016/j.jacc.2008.11.025.
3. Diller G-P, Körten MA, Bauer UM, et al. Current therapy and outcome of eisenmenger syndrome: data of the German National Register for Congenital Heart Defects. *Eur Heart J*. 2016;37(18):1449-1455.

**5.** Correct Answer: A

**Rationale:**

This patient's history strongly suggests hypertrophic obstructive cardiomyopathy (HOCM). Of the listed options, family history has the strongest risk association with sudden death from HOCM. HOCM is an autosomal dominant genetic disorder that affects the beta-myosin chains leading to asymmetric septal wall hypertrophy. This leads to a left-ventricular outflow obstruction and the subsequent symptoms. Symptoms are typically effort related, including exertional angina, dyspnea, syncope, and sudden death. Heart failure can develop over time because of stiffening of the left ventricle and development of left-ventricular hypertrophy. EKG findings include LVH as well as a "pseudo infarction pattern" evidenced by "dagger-like" Q waves in the lateral or inferior leads. These pathognomonic findings are not associated with smoking, drugs, or alcohol use (B, C, and D). Treatment includes beta-blockers or calcium channel blockers, surgical myectomy, or cardiac ablation of portions of the septum.

References

1. Colledge NR, Walker BR, Ralston S, Davidson S. *Davidson's Principles and Practice of Medicine*. Edinburgh: Churchill Livingstone/Elsevier; 2010.
2. Gersh BJ, Maron BJ, Bonow RO, et al. 2011 ACCF/AHA guideline for the diagnosis and treatment of hypertrophic cardiomyopathy: executive summary: a report of the American College of Cardiology Foundation/American Heart Association Task Force on Practice Guidelines. *Circulation*. 2011;124:2761.
3. Faber L. Percutaneous septal ablation in hypertrophic obstructive cardiomyopathy: from experiment to standard of care. *Adv Med*. 2014;2014:464851. doi:10.1155/2014/464851.

# 23

# SHOCK STATES

Jason H. Maley and Kathryn A. Hibbert

1. A 55-year-old man with a history of chronic obstructive pulmonary disease (COPD) (no home $O_2$, $FEV_1$ 67% predicted) presents to the emergency department with shortness of breath and lightheadedness that started suddenly 4 hours prior. He underwent a right knee replacement 6 months prior but otherwise has not been in the hospital recently and has felt well. His only current medication is an albuterol inhaler. He has no other past medical history. His vitals are temperature 99°F, heart rate (HR) 90 beats/min, blood pressure (BP) 85/55 mm Hg, respiratory rate 20/min, and pulse oximetry 90% breathing ambient air. On examination, he is anxious, with clear lung fields and cold extremities and mottled skin. A chest radiograph does not reveal any acute process, and a chest computed tomography (CT) with pulmonary angiography demonstrates bilateral segmental pulmonary emboli. He is given 2 L of intravenous (IV) lactated ringers (LR) solution and is complaining of dizziness and noted to be confused. His repeat vitals are HR 105 beats/min, BP 70/40 mm Hg, respiratory rate 20/min, and $SpO_2$ 88% on room air. In addition to supportive care and appropriate triage, what is the most appropriate next step?

   A. Administer an additional 1 L of LR
   B. Begin IV heparin infusion without bolus
   C. Begin IV heparin infusion with bolus
   D. Administer systemic thrombolytic therapy at full dose
   E. Administer systemic thrombolytic therapy at half dose

2. A 65-year-old woman with acute myeloid leukemia is undergoing induction chemotherapy as an inpatient. On hospital day 4, she is noted to be hypotensive, febrile, and rigoring. Lactic acid is measured at 5 mmol/L. She is transferred to the intensive care unit (ICU) and her laboratory results from that morning are reviewed. They are notable for an absolute neutrophil count of 120/μL and a creatinine that is elevated to 3 mg/dL from a baseline of 1.2 mg/dL. Which of the following interventions have been demonstrated to improve mortality for this patient population?

   A. Early initiation of renal replacement therapy
   B. Early administration of antibacterial agents
   C. Procalcitonin-guided antibiotic administration
   D. Early administration of systemic antifungal therapy
   E. Fluid administration guided by lactic acid

3. A 56-year-old man with diffuse large B-cell lymphoma develops shortness of breath, wheezing, and hypotension while in the chemotherapy infusion center. His second infusion of rituximab treatment was initiated several minutes before the start of his symptoms. He was otherwise asymptomatic at the time of arrival to the infusion appointment. His vitals signs are T 98.8, HR 120 beats per minute, BP 100/60 mm Hg, respiratory rate 22 breaths per minute, and $SpO_2$ 98% on room air. On examination, he is in acute distress with diffuse wheezing and urticaria are noted on his abdomen and chest. What is the immediate first-line management?

   A. Administer 50 mg diphenhydramine IV
   B. Administer up to 5 mL of 1:1000 dilution epinephrine IM
   C. Administer up to 5 mL of 1:1000 dilution epinephrine IV
   D. Administer up to 0.5 mL of 1:10 000 dilution epinephrine IV
   E. Administer up to 0.5 mL of 1:1000 dilution epinephrine IM

4. A 65-year-old woman with a history of nonischemic cardiomyopathy is admitted for dyspnea and progressive edema to the medical ward. On admission, her medications include lisinopril, carvedilol, and aspirin. She receives 80 mg of IV furosemide and makes a total of 30 mL of urine over the next 8 hours. Her creatinine is increased from a baseline of 1.2 to 2.5 mg/dL, her lactate is elevated at 4 mmol/L, and her hemoglobin is stable at 12 mg/dL. Her nurse reports progressive disorientation and somnolence. On examination, her vitals are temperature 98°F, HR 80 beats per minute, BP 95/75 mm Hg, respiratory rate 14/min, and $SpO_2$ 94% breathing ambient air. Her extremities are edematous and cool, pulses are weak, and an S3 is auscultated. An electrocardiogram (EKG) does not show any changes compared with baseline. Beside echocardiogram reveals severe diffuse left ventricular (LV) hypokinesis without evidence of effusion or significant right ventricular dysfunction. She is transferred to the ICU. A central venous catheter is placed, and her central venous oxygen saturation ($CVO_2$) is 30%. What is the best next step in management?

   A. Administration of 1 liter of IV 0.9% NaCl solution
   B. Initiate heparin infusion with a bolus
   C. Administration of dobutamine infusion
   D. Reversal of beta-blockers with glucagon administration
   E. Repeat administration of Lasix 80 mg IV

5. A 65-year-old man with a history of heavy alcohol use presents to the emergency department with severe abdominal pain and is diagnosed with alcoholic pancreatitis. He is noted to have a BP of 70/40 mm Hg after receiving 3 L of IV normal saline and is admitted to the ICU for management of severe pancreatitis and shock. On ICU day 1 and 2, his blood glucose levels are noted to be greater than 250 mg/dL on multiple consecutive measurements. Which of the following statements regarding glycemic control in critically ill adults is correct?

   A. Hyperglycemia is associated with better clinical outcomes compared with normoglycemia.
   B. Insulin therapy to achieve blood glucose of <110 mg/dL is recommended.
   C. Insulin therapy to achieve blood glucose of 140 to 180 mg/dL is recommended.
   D. Seizure is the most common adverse effect of intensive insulin therapy.
   E. Hypoglycemia is associated with better clinical outcomes than normoglycemia.

6. A 54-year-old man with ischemic cardiomyopathy (last known ejection fraction 0.4) and coronary artery disease status post prior three-vessel coronary artery bypass grafting presents to his primary care doctor with fatigue and is found to be hypotensive with BP 85/55 mm Hg. He is triaged to the emergency department where he remains hypotensive with initial BP 90/48 mm Hg and is found to be febrile with temperature 39°C with HR 110 beats per minute. He reports fevers at home over the last 48 hours with one episode of rigors. He receives 2 L of IV fluids and is started on norepinephrine.

   Which of the following is most accurate regarding placement of a pulmonary artery (PA) catheter in this patient?

   A. Use of PA catheters is associated with improved outcomes in cardiogenic shock.
   B. Use of PA catheters is associated with improved outcomes in septic shock.
   C. PA catheters are demonstrated to be useful in early goal-directed therapy for sepsis.
   D. PA catheters are useful in distinguishing cardiogenic shock and vasodilatory shock.
   E. The most frequent complication of PA catheters is significant bleeding.

7. A 23-year-old man is transferred from another hospital with refractory cardiogenic shock and a diagnosis of fulminant viral myocarditis with an echocardiogram that demonstrated biventricular systolic dysfunction with estimated ejection fraction of 0.15. On arrival to the ICU, he has a PA catheter in place with PA pressures 54/30 mm Hg, a pulmonary capillary wedge pressure of 30 mm Hg, cardiac index 1.8 L/min/m², and mixed venous saturation ($MVO_2$) of 40%. He has been treated with inotropic support with dobutamine up to a dose of 20 μg/kg/min and diuresis with a continuous high-dose IV furosemide infusion without improvement. His labs are significant for a lactate of 4 mmol/L and a creatinine that has increased from a baseline of 0.8 to 2.6 mg/dL. On examination, his extremities are cold and mottled. Which of the following is the next best step in managing this patient?

   A. Addition of milrinone infusion
   B. Placement of a percutaneous mechanical circulatory support device
   C. Initiation of a workup for a heart transplant
   D. Transition from furosemide to bumetanide
   E. Addition of neosynephrine infusion

8. A 34-year-old with quadriplegia secondary to a motor vehicle accident that has been complicated by neurogenic bladder and recurrent urinary tract infections presents to the emergency department with fever, chills, and purulent urine with intermittent straight cath. He is found on presentation to have T 38.8 C, HR 124 beats per minute, BP 88/54 mm Hg, and respiratory rate 18 breaths per minute. He receives a total of 2500 mL of IV fluids (30 mL/kg) but remains hypotensive. His laboratory tests are notable for a leukocytosis to 18 000/μL with 70% neutrophils and 15% bands. Blood and urine cultures are ordered. Which of the following is most accurate regarding management of his septic shock?

   A. IV fluids should be given to a target central venous pressure of 8 to 12 cm $H_2O$.
   B. A central venous catheter should be placed to guide further management.
   C. Lactate should be drawn within 3 hours of presentation.
   D. Antibiotics should be given immediately.
   E. He should receive an additional 2500 mL of IV fluid.

9. A 40-year-old woman with idiopathic pulmonary arterial hypertension on continuous treprostinil has worsening shortness of breath and weight gain of 8 kg in the setting of nonadherence to her home diuretic regimen. On evaluation in the emergency department, she is found to have T 37°C, BP 90/62 mm Hg, HR 126 beats per minute, respiratory rate 40 breaths per minute, and $SpO_2$ 74% that improves to 84% on high-flow nasal cannula at 60 L/min and $FiO_2$ 0.6. While undergoing other workup, the patient's respiratory status worsens and the decision is made to intubate her. Which of the following is most accurate regarding her physiology?

   A. She should receive an IV fluid bolus before induction to maintain preload.
   B. Vasopressin may help preserve right ventricular systolic function during intubation.
   C. She should receive high minute ventilation with a high positive end-expiratory pressure to maintain her oxygenation during intubation.
   D. There is evidence that norepinephrine is the best medication for hemodynamic support in this situation.
   E. Propofol is the preferred agent for induction in this patient.

10. A 68-year-old woman with hypertension and hyperlipidemia is admitted with septic shock due to urinary tract infection and gram-negative rod bacteremia. She is treated with 6 L of IV fluids, antibiotics, and norepinephrine up to a dose of 1.5 μg/kg/min. She develops worsening end-organ dysfunction including acute kidney injury requiring renal replacement therapy, acute respiratory failure with hypoxemia requiring intubation, and disseminated intravascular coagulation. On day 3 of her critical illness, she remains on high-dose norepinephrine and mean arterial pressure of 55 mm Hg. In addition to ensuring adequate source control, what is the next best step in her management?

   A. Addition of continuous vasopressin infusion
   B. A cosyntropin stimulation test to determine if she has adrenal insufficiency
   C. Volume resuscitation with 30 mL/kg of IV fluids
   D. Early initiation of parenteral nutrition
   E. Liberal tidal volumes to allow her to regulate her acid-base status

# Chapter 23 ■ Answers

1. Correct Answer: D

**Rationale:**
This patient presents with obstructive shock from pulmonary embolism (PE). PE may be categorized as "massive" based on the presence of sustained hypotension (systolic BP <90 mm Hg for at least 15 minutes or requiring inotropic support, not because of a cause other than PE, such as arrhythmia, hypovolemia, sepsis, or LV dysfunction), pulselessness, or persistent profound bradycardia (HR <40 beats/min with signs or symptoms of shock). In the setting of massive PE, clinical guidelines recommend administration of systemic thrombolytic therapy based on evidence demonstrating improved mortality. Thrombolysis may be contraindicated if patients have a high-bleeding risk, including having undergone major surgery within 3 weeks or presentation, however our patient's distant surgery and lack of other risk factors make him a good candidate for full-dose systemic thrombolysis (answer D is correct). Systemic thrombolysis at half dose has been examined in patients at increased bleeding risk and in the treatment of submassive PE. Data are not conclusive about the benefit of this strategy over others in submassive PE, and full-dose systemic thrombolysis would be most appropriate in massive PE.

IV heparin infusion will ultimately be necessary for this patient, but alone is insufficient; heparin stabilizes the clot while the endogenous fibrinolytic system reduces the clot size over the course of days to months (answer C is incorrect). When administered in PE, a bolus should be performed as it allows a therapeutic level of anticoagulation to be achieved at a faster rate (answer B is incorrect).

Administration of additional IV crystalloid targets suspected intravascular volume depletion. However, the patient has worsened despite receiving 1L of IV fluids. In addition to the fact that fluids do not correct the underlying disease, in acute right heart failure, aggressive volume repletion can worsen interventricular dependence and decrease LV cardiac output.

### References

1. Jaff MR, McMurtry MS, Archer SL, et al. Management of massive and submassive pulmonary embolism, iliofemoral deep vein thrombosis, and chronic thromboembolic pulmonary hypertension: a scientific statement from the American Heart Association. *Circulation*. 2011;123(16):1788-1830.
2. Kearon C, Akl EA, Ornelas J, et al. Antithrombotic therapy for VTE Disease: CHEST guideline and expert panel report. *Chest*. 2016;149(2):315-352.

---

**2.** Correct Answer: B

**Rationale:**

This patient is presenting with neutropenic septic shock, a form of distributive shock incited by an infectious etiology. Patients with neutropenic septic shock are at high risk for infection with both resistant gram-negative and gram-positive organisms. Patients in septic shock experience mortality benefit from early administration of appropriate antibiotic therapy (answer B is correct). In the initial 6 hours following the onset of hypotension, every 1-hour delay in antibiotic therapy may be associated with an increase in mortality of greater than 7% in a broad septic shock population.

Timing of renal replacement therapy in septic shock has been examined in several large randomized trials. Routine early renal replacement therapy does not appear to improve outcomes and leads to an increased rate of renal replacement therapy when compared with the later initiation of renal replacement therapy guided by clinical indications (answer A is incorrect). Procalcitonin has been investigated to guide de-escalation of antibiotics in the emergency department and inpatient setting, however does not impact mortality in septic shock (answer C is incorrect). Similarly systemic antifungals are not recommended as first line in septic shock, and their early administration has not been shown to improve mortality (answer D is incorrect). Finally, multiple large multinational randomized trials failed to demonstrate that fluid administration guided by specific biomarkers or resuscitation protocols improved mortality when compared with usual care (answer E is incorrect).

### References

1. Kumar A, Roberts D, Wood KE, et al. Duration of hypotension before initiation of effective antimicrobial therapy is the critical determinant of survival in human septic shock. *Crit Care Med*. 2006;34(6):1589-1596.
2. Barbar SD, Clere-Jehl R, Bourredjem A, et al. Timing of renal-replacement therapy in patients with acute kidney injury and sepsis. *N Engl J Med*. 2018;379(15):1431-1442.
3. Rowan KM, Angus DC, Bailey M, et al. Early, goal-directed therapy for septic shock – a patient-level meta-analysis. *N Engl J Med*. 2017;376(23):2223-2234.

---

**3.** Correct Answer: E

**Rationale:**

The patient is experiencing anaphylaxis secondary to a rituximab infusion, as evidenced by bronchospasm, urticaria, and hypotension following the initiation of his second exposure to the medication. Epinephrine should be injected by the intramuscular (IM) route up to a dose of 0.5 mg as soon as anaphylaxis is recognized. This route achieves peak plasma concentrations quickly and reliably. Epinephrine has historically been labeled based on dilution, leading to confusion among providers. A dilution of 1:1000 refers to 1 mg/mL concentration. Therefore, to administer 0.5 mg, one administers 0.5 mL IM (answer E is correct; answers B, C, and D are incorrect). Intravenous epinephrine is reserved for refractory shock despite initial treatment and aggressive fluid administration. As anaphylaxis induces rapid vasoplegia and vascular leak, aggressive IV crystalloid resuscitation should be administered in the hypotensive patient. Diphenhydramine, H2 histamine antagonists, glucocorticoids, and inhaled beta-2 agonists are adjunctive therapies for anaphylaxis (answer A is incorrect).

### Reference

1. Simons FE, Ardusso LR, Dimov V, et al. World allergy organization anaphylaxis guidelines: 2013 update of the evidence base. *Int Arch Allergy Immunol*. 2013;162(3):193-204.

---

**4.** Correct Answer: C

**Rationale:**

This patient is in cardiogenic shock as evidenced by clinical examination, evidence of progressive end-organ dysfunction, hypotension, and low $CVO_2$. Her bedside echocardiogram supports this diagnosis and notably lowers the probability of other low output states including tamponade or right heart failure from PE. Her clinical examination and laboratory values do not support hypovolemia or hemorrhage. The goals of therapy for this patient include increasing cardiac contractility, decreasing systemic vascular, and relieving volume overload. The initial management in the setting of shock should focus on the immediate restoration of end-organ perfusion, which is facilitated with inotropic support with dobutamine, a B1 receptor agonist, or milrinone, a phosphodiesterase 3 inhibitor (answer C is correct). Administration of IV fluid will not improve the cardiac output for this patient and will result in further evidence of hydrostatic edema including pulmonary edema (answer A is incorrect). Heparin is indicated in acute coronary syndromes and venous thrombosis, neither of which is apparent in this patients evaluation (answer B is incorrect). In cases of bradyarrhythmia from beta-blocker overdose, glucagon may be used for reversal; however, the patient's HR of 80 beats per minute is unlikely to be the cause of cardiogenic shock (answer D is incorrect). Loop diuretic efficacy depends on delivery to the site of action within the ascending limb of the loop of Henle. When cardiogenic shock results in a decreased glomerular filtration rate (assumed to be approaching zero in an oliguric patient), drug delivery is significantly decreased. In conjunction with inotropic support and afterload reduction, higher doses of diuretic medications will be required to achieve adequate concentration at the drug target but are unlikely to be effective in isolation (answer E is incorrect).

### Reference

1. van Diepen S, Katz JN, Albert NM, et al. Contemprorary management of cardiogenic shock: a scientific statement from the American Heart Association. *Circulation*. 2017;136:e232-e268.

---

**5.** Correct Answer: C

**Rationale:**

Both hyperglycemia and hypoglycemia are associated with worse clinical outcomes in critically ill patients based on the results of multiple prospective randomized trials and retrospective data. Hyperglycemia is variably defined as glucose measurements greater than 180 mg/dL or 200 mg/dL. Hypoglycemia is typically a blood glucose less than 80 mg/dL. Literature on hyperglycemia is mainly retrospective and describes an association with increased mortality in a variety of patient populations including critically ill medical and surgical patients. Multiple prospective randomized controlled trials have examined intensive insulin therapy to target strict glucose control, typically 81 to 110 mg/dL, compared with conventional glucose control. These studies have demonstrated that intensive insulin therapy results in a higher rate of hypoglycemia, which is the most common adverse effect, and thereby increased mortality. Currently, it is recommended to maintain blood glucose of 140 to 180 mg/dL to avoid dangerous hypoglycemia or hyperglycemia (answer C is correct).

### References

1. Finfer S, Chittock DR, Su SY, et al. Intensive versus conventional glucose control in critically ill patients. *N Engl J Med*. 2009;360(13):1283-1297.
2. Falciglia M, Freyberg RW, Almenoff PL, D'Alessio DA, Render ML. Hyperglycemia-related mortality in critically ill patients varies with admission diagnosis. *Crit Care Med*. 2009;37(12):3001-3009.
3. Jacobi J, Bircher N, Krinsley J, et al. Guidelines for the use of an insulin infusion for the management of hyperglycemia in critically ill patients. *Crit Care Med*. 2012;40(12):3251-3276.
4. Rhodes A, Evans LE, Alhazzani W, et al Surviving sepsis campaign: international guidelines for management of sepsis and septic shock 2016. *Crit Care Med*. 2017;45(3):486-552.

---

**6.** Correct Answer: D

**Rationale:**

Multiple trials have shown no benefit to use of PA catheters in patients with shock; retrospective study data in patients with cardiogenic shock is conflicting with respect to association between PA catheter use and outcomes (answers A and B are incorrect). Additionally, although the early goal-directed therapy was first developed using a PA catheter, there has been no trial that demonstrates that PA catheters increase the likelihood of meeting resuscitation goals in sepsis (answer C is incorrect). However, PA catheters are useful in distinguishing between cardiogenic and vasodilatory shock and are recommended in the management of cardiogenic shock when a vasodilatory or septic component is suspected (answer D is correct). Bleeding complications from PA catheters are uncommon even in critically ill patients (answer E is incorrect).

### References

1. Richard C, Warszawski J, Anguel N, et al; French Pulmonary Artery Catheter Study Group. Early use of the pulmonary artery catheter and outcomes in patients with shock and acute respiratory distress syndrome: a randomized controlled trial. *JAMA*. 2003;290:2713-2720.
2. Connors AF Jr, Speroff T, Dawson NV. et al. The effectiveness of right heart catheterization in the initial care of critically ill patients. SUPPORT investigators. *JAMA*. 1996;276:889-897.
3. Rossello X, Vila M, Rivas-Lasarte M, et al. Impact of pulmonary artery catheter use on short- and long-term mortality in patients with cardiogenic shock. *Cardiology*. 2017;136:61-69.
4. van Diepen S, Katz JN, Albert NM, et al. Contemprorary management of cardiogenic shock: a scientific statement from the American Heart Association. *Circulation*. 2017;136:e232-e268.

**7.** Correct Answer: B

**Rationale:**

This patient has acute decompensated systolic heart failure and severe cardiogenic shock that has not responded to IV inotrope infusion and diuresis. There are no clear data that one inotrope is superior to another, and because the patient has failed to respond to high doses of dobutamine, it is unlikely that milrinone will have a significantly greater effect (answer A is incorrect). Similarly, although oral bioavailability of bumetanide is more reliable than that of furosemide, there is no evidence that patients with severe cardiogenic shock who have failed to respond to furosemide will have a greater response to bumetanide (answer D is incorrect). This patient does not have evidence of a low systemic vascular resistance, and addition of neosynphrine will simply increase LV afterload and therefore may worsen cardiac function and should be avoided (answer E is incorrect). Although a heart transplant may be considered in nonresolving cardiogenic shock, this patient has a potentially reversible cause of heart failure and needs immediate hemodynamic support (answer C is incorrect). The next best step is therefore initiation of percutaneous mechanical circulatory support to increase cardiac output and improve tissue perfusion (answer B is correct). There are no data to support the use of one mechanical support device over the other, and the support device should be chosen based on local expertise and availability.

Reference

1. van Diepen S, Katz JN, Albert NM, et al. Contemprorary management of cardiogenic shock: a scientific statement from the American Heart Association. *Circulation*. 2017;136:e232-e268.

**8.** Correct Answer: C

**Rationale:**

This patient is presenting with septic shock, defined as severe sepsis with persistent hypotension. He has received an initial fluid challenge of 30 mL/kg, and trials that attempted to replicate the improved outcomes originally seen with a central venous target of 8 to 12 cm $H_2O$ have failed to demonstrate a benefit (answer A is incorrect). Additionally, if patients with septic shock are randomized to receive a central venous line or not, there does not appear to be a benefit to the placement of a central line. It is recommended that patients with septic shock have an initial lactate drawn within 3 hours of presentation; if the lactate is elevated, it should be repeated within 6 hours of presentation (answer C is correct). Elevated lactate is associated with worse outcomes in septic shock and therefore has prognostic utility. In addition, adherence to checking lactate is associated with better care of sepsis patients, likely because it is a marker for recognition of sepsis. Although the patient should receive prompt antibiotics, it is recommended that blood cultures be drawn before antibiotic administration if it can be done without significantly delaying antibiotics. After initial fluid resuscitation, a repeat evaluation of intravascular volume status and hemodynamics is recommended (answer E is incorrect).

References

1. The ProCESS Investigators. A randomized trial of protocol-based care for early septic shock. *N Engl J Med*. 2014;370:1683-1693.
2. Rhodes A, Evans LE, Alhazzani W, et al Surviving sepsis campaign: international guidelines for management of sepsis and septic shock 2016. *Crit Care Med*. 2017;45(3):486-552.
3. Mikkelsen ME, Miltiades AN, Gaieski DF, et al. Serum lactate is assocaited with mortality in severe sepsis independent of organ failure and shock. *Crit Care Med*. 2003;37(5):1670-1677.
4. Centers for Medicare and Medicaid Services, The Joint Commission. *Specifications Manual for National Hospital Inpatient Quality Measures Discharges 10-01-15 (4Q15) Through 06-30-16 (2Q16)*. http://www.jointcommission.org/assets/1/6/IQRManualRelease Notes_V5_01.pdf.

**9.** Correct Answer: B

**Rationale:**

Patients with right heart failure and cardiogenic shock have very tenuous hemodynamics, and intubation presents a uniquely dangerous challenge in this patient population. The combination of induction medications and mechanical ventilation with increased intrathoracic pressures acutely decreases preload to the right ventricle and can increase afterload via an increase in pulmonary vascular resistance with overdistention of the lungs. In addition to avoiding intubation whenever possible, strategies can be undertaken to minimize risk if intubation is unavoidable. Vasopressor support is recommended, and both neosynephrine and vasopressin can preserve right ventricular systolic function by preserving cardiac preload in the setting of vasodilatory induction drugs and by preserving perfusion to the right ventricle and preventing worsening ischemia (answer B is correct). Norepinephrine provides additional inotropic support and is commonly used but there is no high-quality evidence that shows that norepinephrine is superior to other agents (answer D is incorrect). Although hypercarbia is poorly tolerated, aggressive ventilation with high tidal volumes, high respiratory rate, and high positive end-expiratory pressures can worsen right ventricular afterload by increasing pulmonary vascular resistance, which is lung volume dependent (answer C is incorrect). Propofol is vasodilatory, therefore decreasing preload, and has a potential negative inotropic effect and for those reasons is not a preferred agent in this setting (answer E is incorrect). Etomidate is often recommended, given its smaller effect on hemodynamics. Although an acute decrease in preload is a concern, this patient is already volume overloaded and additional IV fluids are not recommended (answer A is incorrect).

### References

1. Price LC, Wort SJ, Finney SJ, et al. Pulmonary vascular and right ventricular dysfunction in adult critical care: current and emerging options for management: a systematic literature review. *Crit Care.* 2010;14(5):R169.
2. Maxwell BG, Pearl RG, Kudelko KT, et al. Case 7-2012 airway management and perioperative decision making in the patient with severe pulmonary hypertension who requires emergency noncardiac surgery. *J Cardiothorac Vasc Anesth.* 2012;26(5):940-944.
3. Green EM, Givertz MM. Management of acute right ventricular failure in the intensive care unit. *Curr Heart Fail Rep.* 2012;9(3):228-235.

**10.** Correct Answer: A

**Rationale:**

This patient has ongoing septic shock with multiorgan failure despite initial fluid resuscitation and antibiotic therapy. In this setting, the addition of vasopressin to either achieve a mean arterial pressure goal of 65 mm Hg or to reduce the dose of norepinephrine is recommended. Although the trial data are conflicting, empiric addition of corticosteroids in refractory septic shock is recommended. However, cosyntropin stimulation testing has not been demonstrated to identify patients who will benefit from steroids (answer B is incorrect). Although an initial fluid resuscitation with 30 mL/kg of IV fluids is recommended, there are no data for later goal-directed therapy multiple days into a critical illness (answer C is incorrect). Although early hypocaloric enteral nutrition is recommended for patients with sepsis and septic shock, parenteral nutrition either alone or in combination with enteral nutrition is not recommended in patients who can tolerate enteral feeding (answer D is incorrect). Patients with septic shock are at increased risk of acute respiratory distress syndrome and are recommended to receive low tidal volume and lung protective ventilation (answer E is incorrect).

### References

1. Rhodes A, Evans LE, Alhazzani W, et al Surviving sepsis campaign: international guidelines for management of sepsis and septic shock 2016. *Crit Care Med.* 2017;45(3):486-552.
2. Sprung CL, Annane D, Keh D, et al. Hydrocortisone therpy for patients with septic shock. *N Engl J Med.* 2008;358:111-124.

# 24

# MECHANICAL CIRCULATORY SUPPORT AND THE TRANSPLANTED HEART

Annie van Beuningen and David M. Dudzinski

1. A 60-year-old male with a history of nonischemic dilated cardiomyopathy is admitted to the intensive care unit (ICU) after presenting to the emergency department with several days of progressive dyspnea and lower-extremity swelling. He is found to be hypotensive and tachycardic and on examination is noted to be confused with edematous, cool extremities. A 12-lead ECG shows rapid atrial fibrillation with nonspecific ST-segment changes. His last transthoracic echocardiogram performed 1 year ago showed a severely dilated LV cavity with a left ventricular ejection fraction of 28%, severe mitral regurgitation, moderate aortic insufficiency, and severe tricuspid regurgitation. In this patient, which of the following represents a contraindication to the use of an intra-aortic balloon pump (IABP)?

   A. Atrial fibrillation
   B. Severe LV cavity dilatation
   C. Moderate aortic insufficiency
   D. Severe mitral regurgitation
   E. Severe tricuspid regurgitation

2. A 78-year-old male is admitted to the ICU to undergo evaluation for urgent coronary artery bypass grafting after a coronary angiography revealed critical left main artery stenosis. During the catheterization procedure, an IABP was placed via the left common femoral artery because of ongoing chest pain. Chest pain abated after the IABP was placed. After several hours in the ICU, the patient complains of mild recurrent chest pain, and his nurse reports that there is new blood that can be seen in the IABP catheter that is connected to the console. Which of the following is the most appropriate next step in the management of this patient?

   A. Chest X-ray to confirm IABP placement
   B. Urgent transthoracic echocardiogram
   C. Repeat coronary angiography
   D. Removal of the IABP
   E. Abdominal CT scan

3. A 43-year-old woman is admitted to the ICU with palpitations and dyspnea because she is 10 weeks from successful orthotopic heart transplantation for severe idiopathic dilated cardiomyopathy. Her posttransplant course has been uneventful thus far. On admission her blood pressure is 107/62, heart rate is 113, oxygen saturation is 88% on room air, and temperature is 37.9°C. Her physical examination is notable for bibasilar rales, an elevated jugular venous pressure, and mild pitting pedal edema. Her cardiac examination reveals a rapid, irregularly irregular heart rate and a II/VI holosystolic murmur loudest at the right lower sternal border. A 12-lead ECG shows rapid atrial fibrillation. Which of the following is the next best diagnostic test to obtain in the management of this patient?

A. Endomyocardial biopsy
B. Two sets of sterile blood cultures
C. Transesophageal echocardiogram
D. Coronary angiography
E. Cardiac MRI

4. A 64-year-old man with a history of coronary artery disease and severe ischemic cardiomyopathy is brought to the hospital by his wife, who found him at home confused and lethargic. He has a durable continuous flow left ventricular assist device (LVAD) that was surgically implanted 1 year ago as destination therapy for his end stage heart failure. On arrival he is arousable but somnolent. His blood pressure is unable to be obtained with a manual cuff; however, a reading obtained with a Doppler ultrasound is 54 mm Hg. His heart rate is 119 beats per minute, respirations are 26 per minute, and his temperature is 38.0°C. On examination, his jugular venous pressure is 5 mm Hg, his cardiac examination reveals a continuous hum, his peripheral pulses are not palpable, and his extremities are warm without significant edema. Interrogation of his LVAD shows high flow with normal power. Which of the following would NOT be an appropriate intervention in the acute management of this patient?

A. Placement of an arterial line
B. Administration of IV norepinephrine
C. Initiation of broad spectrum antibiotics
D. Administration of IV dobutamine
E. Obtaining two sets of sterile blood cultures

5. A 32-year-old female with no prior medical history presents with several days of fevers, chills, myalgias, and progressive shortness of breath. She is found to have a blood pressure of 84/70, heart rate of 123, and oxygen saturation of 84% on room air. She is admitted to the ICU and an urgent echocardiogram shows a left ventricular ejection fraction of 15%, normal left ventricular end diastolic diameter, and severe right ventricular systolic dysfunction. She is started on intravenous norepinephrine and dobutamine, given intravenous furosemide and is intubated for progressive hypoxia; however, she remains persistently hypotensive with poor urine output despite escalating doses of intravenous therapy and diuretics. Which of the following would be the most appropriate choice for mechanical circulatory support in this patient?

A. Veno-arterial extracorporeal membrane oxygenation (VA-ECMO)
B. Percutaneous LVAD
C. IABP
D. Durable, surgically implanted LVAD
E. Veno-venous (VV) ECMO

6. A 53-year-old woman is recovering in the ICU on postoperative day 2 after undergoing LVAD implantation. Over the course of several hours she is noted to become progressively hypotensive with her mean arterial pressure dropping from 75 to 53 mm Hg as measured by a radial arterial line. Her LVAD monitor shows multiple power spikes in the last 2 hours. Her nurse additionally notes that the patient's urine has become much darker in color over the last several hours. Which of the following is the next best step in management?

A. Complete transthoracic echocardiogram
B. Transesophageal echocardiogram
C. Echocardiographic ramp study
D. CT angiography of the chest and abdomen

7. A 49-year-old male is admitted to the ICU following a witnessed cardiac arrest and successful resuscitation. His postarrest ECG showed anteroseptal ST elevations, and he underwent emergent coronary angiography and revascularization of a thrombotically occluded left anterior descending artery. He was placed on VA-ECMO for ongoing cardiogenic shock during the procedure. Several hours after admission to the ICU, the pulsatility of his arterial waveform begins to decrease, and increasing amounts of frothy secretions are being suctioned from his endotracheal tube. An echocardiogram shows a markedly dilated left ventricle with an ejection fraction of 10%. Which of the following would NOT be an appropriate intervention in the management of this patient?

A. Initiation of IV dobutamine
B. Placement of an IABP
C. Transfusion of packed red blood cells
D. Insertion of a left ventricular drainage catheter
E. Placement of a percutaneous ventricular assist device

**8.** A 52-year-old female is recovering in the ICU after undergoing an uncomplicated orthotopic heart transplant 12 hours earlier. For the last 5 hours her urine output has been decreasing, and she has been requiring increasing doses of inotropes to maintain a median arterial blood pressure of 65 mm Hg or greater. Though the intraoperative TEE showed hyperdynamic function in the transplanted heart, now a transthoracic echocardiogram shows LV systolic dysfunction with an ejection fraction of 30%, with normal right ventricular size and function. Which of the following is the most likely diagnosis?

**A.** Coronary allograft vasculopathy
**B.** Primary graft dysfunction
**C.** Infectious myocarditis
**D.** Recurrent myocardial disease

# Chapter 24 ▪ Answers

**1.** Correct Answer: C

**Rationale:**

IABP counterpulsation is a commonly used form of mechanical circulatory support that involves placement of a catheter with a helium-filled balloon into the proximal descending aorta via the common femoral artery under fluoroscopic guidance. The balloon is inflated just after the aortic valve closes and deflates before the opening of aortic valve. This results in blood displacement toward the proximal aorta during diastole while the balloon is inflated, and a suction effect in the aorta during systole when the balloon is rapidly deflated. The resulting hemodynamic changes include a reduction in systolic blood pressure (to reduce myocardial wall stress and work), an increase in diastolic blood pressure, and an increase in the mean arterial pressure. Some studies have shown that IABP counterpulsation results in an increase in total coronary blood flow.

Contraindications to the use of IABP counterpulsation include severe peripheral arterial disease, aortic dissection or significant aortic aneurysm, and severe coagulopathy. IABP is contraindicated in moderate or greater aortic insufficiency, as inflation of the balloon during diastole will increase regurgitant flow across the aortic valve and worsen heart failure. Atrial fibrillation is not a contraindication to using IABP. IABP counterpulsation decreases preload and thus is beneficial in LV dilation, mitral regurgitation, and tricuspid regurgitation.

**Reference**

1. Santa-Cruz RA, Cohen MG, Ohman EM. Aortic counterpulsation: a review of the hemodynamic effects and indications for use. *Catheter Cardiovasc Interv.* 2006;67:68.

**2.** Correct Answer: D

**Rationale:**

Although the IABP is a widely used tool in the management of a variety of acute cardiac conditions, it is associated with complications occasionally. The presence of blood in the IABP catheter indicates balloon rupture, and the device should be immediately removed. Rarely, balloon rupture can result in thrombosis or balloon entrapment within the arterial tree and may require surgical exploration for safe removal. Blood in the IABP catheter is clearly indicative of balloon rupture, and no other investigations are necessary for diagnosis. Other important complications of IABP use include limb ischemia, vascular laceration, and hemorrhage. In one large review of 17,000 patients who underwent IABP placement, 7% of patients had at least one complication, whereas 2.6% suffered a major complication (acute limb ischemia, balloon rupture, significant bleeding, or death related directly to the IABP).

**References**

1. Ferguson JJ III, Cohen M, Freedman RJ Jr, et al. The current practice of intra-aortic balloon counterpulsation: results from the Benchmark Registry. *J Am Coll Cardiol.* 2001;38:1456.
2. Mihatov N, Dudzinski DM. Intraaortic balloon pump rupture. *J Invasive Cardiol.* 2015;27(9):E203.

**3.** Correct Answer: A

**Rationale:**

This patient is presenting with new atrial fibrillation as well as signs and symptoms of heart failure, which in a patient with a recent cardiac transplant is highly concerning for acute cardiac allograft rejection. Any suspicion for acute rejection should prompt an urgent evaluation with an endomyocardial biopsy to try and establish the diagnosis. Echocardiography is not specific for diagnosing rejection. Although cardiac MRI may be used as a screening tool, endomyocardial biopsy still remains the gold standard for diagnosis of allograft rejection. Coronary allograft vasculopathy or coronary artery disease may be diagnosed with coronary angiography but typically occurs years after transplantation.

The incidence of any rejection in the first year after transplant reaches 25%, and the incidence of rejection requiring treatment is reported to be about 13%. The risk of developing acute rejection is much higher early after transplant, peaking at one month posttransplant and declining thereafter. Clinical symptoms of acute rejection are typically related to left ventricular systolic dysfunction and can include dyspnea, orthopnea, paroxysmal nocturnal dyspnea, peripheral edema, and gastrointestinal symptoms. Importantly, acute cellular rejection can present with atrial arrhythmias including both atrial fibrillation and atrial flutter. Once a diagnosis is made, the type of treatment varies based on histologic criteria as well as the presence of symptoms and/or hemodynamic compromise. In general, oral or intravenous corticosteroids and antithymocyte globulin are the mainstays of acute rejection therapy.

### Reference
1. Lund LH, Edwards LB, Kucheryavaya AY, et al. The registry of the International Society for Heart and Lung Transplantation: thirty-first official adult heart transplant report–2014; focus theme: retransplantation. *J Heart Lung Transplant*. 2014;33:996.

---

**4.** Correct Answer: D

**Rationale:**

This patient is presenting with clinical features consistent with sepsis and should be treated with aggressive early intervention based on surviving sepsis guidelines, including fluid resuscitation, blood cultures, broad-spectrum antibiotics, and vasopressor therapy to maintain a mean arterial pressure of 70 to 80 mm Hg. An arterial line is necessary in this patient, to monitor blood pressure, because a noninvasive blood pressure device might not pick up blood pressure in the absence of pulsatile flow. Dobutamine is an inodilator that would likely worsen this patient's hypotension.

A rapid clinical assessment of patients with continuous flow LVADs can be challenging, as it is often not possible to obtain a reliable noninvasive blood pressure measurement, as these patients often do not have palpable peripheral pulses or audible heart sounds. Doppler ultrasonography can be used to obtain a single blood pressure reading; in patients with pulsatility, this more accurately approximates the systolic blood pressure, but in patients with no pulsatility Doppler measurements more closely approximate the mean arterial pressure. However an arterial line should be placed for continuous blood pressure monitoring in unstable patients.

Checking the LVAD monitor for flow, power and pulsatility index can also be useful in elucidating the etiology of a patient's hypotension. In hypotensive patients with low flow, the differential diagnosis includes hypovolemia (hemorrhage, overdiuresis), ventricular arrhythmias, RV dysfunction, cardiac tamponade, and improper pump settings. Sepsis should be suspected in hypotensive patients with high flow and normal power, whereas high power and low flow could indicate pump thrombosis.

### References
1. Peberdy M, Guck J, Ornato J, et al. Cardiopulmonary resuscitation in adults and children with mechanical circulatory support: a scientific statement from the American Heart Association. *Circulation*. 2017;135:e1115.
2. Feldman D, Pamboukian SV, Teuteberg JJ, et al. The 2013 International Society for Heart and Lung Transplantation Guidelines for mechanical circulatory support: executive summary. *J Heart Lung Transplant*. 2013;32:157.
3. Slaughter MS, Pagani FD, Rogers JG, et al. Clinical management of continuous-flow left ventricular assist devices in advanced heart failure. *J Heart Lung Transplant*. 2010;29:S1.

---

**5.** Correct Answer: A

**Rationale:**

VA-ECMO is the best choice for mechanical circulatory support for this patient given the need for both cardiac and respiratory support. Indications for VA-ECMO include refractory cardiogenic shock, cardiac arrest, massive pulmonary embolism, and failure to wean from cardio-pulmonary bypass after cardiac surgery. In the setting of biventricular failure with both severe right and left ventricular dysfunction, a LVAD (either percutaneous or surgical) alone is insufficient and can often worsen right ventricular function when placed for isolated left ventricular failure. Although there are no contraindications to IABP placement in this setting, it would be unlikely to provide sufficient hemodynamic support given her refractory cardiogenic shock, and would not directly support oxygenation. VV ECMO would only provide oxygenation, but no hemodynamic support, and thus not useful in this patient.

### Reference
1. The Registry of the Extracorporeal Life Support Organization. www.elso.org. Accessed October 25, 2018.

**6.** Correct Answer: C

**Rationale:**

In this patient with a recently implanted LVAD, hypotension in conjunction with power spikes on the LVAD and clinical signs of hemolysis is strongly suggestive of pump thrombosis, which can be seen as both an early and late complication of VAD therapy. Pump thrombosis that results in pump obstruction is associated with high mortality and requires prompt diagnosis and management. The diagnosis is here suggested by changes in pump performance, most commonly surges in power, along with clinical signs of hemolysis (hemoglobinuria). In addition to laboratory markers of hemolysis, echocardiographic ramp studies during which left ventricular parameters are measured at varying pump speeds have been shown to be both sensitive and specific for pump thrombosis. Early pump thrombosis generally requires urgent surgical pump exchange or heart transplantation, whereas late pump thrombosis can sometimes be managed with intensified anticoagulation. Echocardiogram without a ramp study is not helpful in diagnosing pump thrombosis. CT angiography is reserved for selected patients when the diagnosis is challenging after echocardiographic ramp study.

References

1. Potapov EV, Stepanenko A, Krabatsch T, Hetzer R. Managing long-term complications of left ventricular assist device therapy. *Curr Opin Cardiol.* 2011;26:237.
2. Stainback RF, Estep JD, Agler DA, et al. Echocardiography in the management of patients with left ventricular assist devices: recommendations from the American Society of Echocardiography. *J Am Soc Echocardiogr.* 2015;28:853.
3. Estep JD, Vivo RP, Cordero-Reyes AM, et al. A simplified echocardiographic technique for detecting continuous-flow left ventricular assist device malfunction due to pump thrombosis. *J Heart Lung Transplant.* 2014;33:575.

**7** Correct Answer: C

**Rationale:**

VA-ECMO is an effective strategy to support patients with refractory cardiogenic shock after an acute myocardial infarction; however, ECMO directly increases afterload on the left ventricle, which can worsen left ventricular function. Frequent monitoring of LV size and function with echocardiography and close attention to the pulsatility of the arterial waveform are both critical to identify an overloaded left ventricle. Strategies to improve LV unloading include administration of inotropes (dobutamine, milrinone) to improve inherent native LV ejection, IABP counterpulsation, or a left ventricular "vent" by either percutaneous (percutaneous LVAD) or surgical methods (left ventricular drainage catheter placed via left superior pulmonary vein).

References

1. Ortega-Deballon I, Hornby L, Shemie SD, et al. Extracorporeal resuscitation for refractory out-of-hospital cardiac arrest in adults: a systematic review of international practices and outcomes. *Resuscitation.* 2016;101:12.
2. Meani P, Gelsomino S, Natour E, et al. Modalities and effects of left ventricle unloading on extracorporeal life support: a review of the current literature. *Eur J Heart Fail.* 2017;19(suppl 2):84-91.

**8.** Correct Answer: B

**Rationale:**

Primary graft dysfunction is left ventricular, right ventricular, or biventricular dysfunction that occurs within 24 hours of cardiac transplantation that is not due to an identifiable cause such as hyperacute rejection, pulmonary hypertension, or surgical complications. The cause of primary graft dysfunction is poorly understood, but donor, recipient, and surgical procedural factors all appear to play a role. Treatment involves aggressive pharmacologic and mechanical circulatory support, as well as re-transplantation in select patients. Coronary allograft vasculopathy, infectious myocarditis, and recurrent myocardial disease may be potential causes months to years after transplantation.

Reference

1. Kobashigawa J, Zuckermann A, Macdonald P, et al. Report from a consensus conference on primary graft dysfunction after cardiac transplantation. *J Heart Lung Transplant.* 2014;33:327.

# 25

# CALCULATED CARDIOVASCULAR PARAMETERS

Revati Nafday, Steven Hur, and Lundy Campbell

1. A 52-year-old female with a history of nonischemic cardiomyopathy and reduced ejection fraction undergoes emergent spine surgery after being involved in a motor vehicle collision. There is significant blood loss during the case requiring transfusion of blood products. The patient arrives to the ICU intubated, sedated, and requiring vasopressor support.

   A pulmonary artery catheter is placed to guide management and the mixed venous oxygen saturation is noted to be low. Which of the following is not a potential cause of decreased oxygen delivery in this patient?

   **A.** Acute blood loss anemia
   **B.** Low cardiac output (CO) state
   **C.** Shivering due to hypothermia
   **D.** Transfusion-related acute lung injury

2. A 56-year-old male with acute on chronic systolic heart failure and septic shock from pneumonia is admitted to the ICU. A recent transthoracic echo reveals moderate tricuspid regurgitation and an ASD with significant left to right shunting. A pulmonary artery catheter is placed to guide hemodynamic management. Which of the following would most consistently underestimate CO if measured by thermodilution?

   **A.** Left to right intra cardiac shunt
   **B.** Right to left intra cardiac shunt
   **C.** Right-sided valvular lesions
   **D.** Injectate larger than programmed input volume
   **E.** Injectate warmer than programmed input temperature

3. An 80-year-old female was admitted to the ICU from the emergency department with the diagnosis of septic shock secondary to urosepsis. She was noted to be in her usual state of good health 12 hours earlier, but was then found at home lying in bed with altered mental status by her daughter. In the emergency department she was found to be hypotensive with a mean arterial blood pressure (MAP) of 45, lethargic, and was mostly incoherent on physical examination. She was given 2 L of IV fluids with improvement in her BP and mental status. Blood cultures were obtained and a urinalysis revealed *E. coli* in her urine. She was started on broad-spectrum antibiotics and was admitted to the ICU for further management of her urosepsis.

   The resident has seen the patient on admission and is concerned because she continues to require aggressive volume resuscitation to maintain her pressures and is now on a norepinephrine infusion at high doses. On physical examination she is cold to the touch, quite pale, and has a moderately distended abdomen. Your resident is concerned that her initial diagnosis may be incorrect, is worried about a retroperitoneal hemorrhage causing hypovolemic shock, and elects to place a pulmonary artery catheter to help further elucidate the etiology of her shock.

   Which of the following hemodynamic parameters obtained from the pulmonary artery catheter would be most helpful in distinguishing hypovolemic shock from septic shock?

    **A.** CO
    **B.** Central venous pressure
    **C.** Pulmonary capillary wedge pressure
    **D.** Systemic vascular resistance (SVR)

**4.** A 52-year-old female undergoes spine fusion surgery with 2 L of intraoperative blood loss. On POD#3 she develops new onset atrial fibrillation with plans to undergo transesophageal echocardiography (TEE) before cardioversion. After topicalization with 20% benzocaine spray, sedation with fentanyl and versed, the TEE rules out clot and confirms otherwise normal heart function. Electrical cardioversion is successful, but shortly afterward the patient becomes dyspneic and cyanotic. Despite adequate spontaneous ventilation with a non-rebreather mask, the patient remains cyanotic with a pulse oximetry saturation of 85%. Which study would be most helpful in confirming the diagnosis?

    **A.** CBC
    **B.** Bedside Ultrasound
    **C.** Chem Panel
    **D.** Arterial Blood Gas with Co-oximetry
    **E.** EEG

**5.** As part of a clinical study, you are measuring oxygen consumption using indirect calorimetry in a ventilated patient in the ICU and want to compare your measurements to a calculated value. Radial artery and pulmonary artery catheters are placed, and the following measurements are obtained:

$Hb = 11.7$ g/dL

$SaO_2 = 97\%$

$SvO_2 = 72\%$

CO (thermodilution): 5.1 L/min

Assuming minimal contribution from dissolved oxygen, what is the patient's calculated oxygen consumption?

    **A.** 0.2 L/min
    **B.** 0.76 L/min
    **C.** 1.3 L/min
    **D.** D. 20 L/min

# Chapter 25 ▪ Answers

**1.** Correct Answer: C

**Rationale:**
The mixed venous oxygen saturation is the oxygen saturation of blood sampled at the proximal pulmonary artery and reflects the balance between global delivery and global uptake of oxygen. Oxygen delivery is the product of arterial oxygen content and CO:

$$DO_2 = CaO_2 \times CO$$

In blood, oxygen is carried in two forms: the majority bound to hemoglobin and the remainder dissolved in plasma. Therefore, the arterial content of oxygen is expressed by the following equation representing both components:

$$CaO_2 = 1.34 \times Hb \times SaO_2 + 0.003 \times PaO_2$$

$$CaO_2 = mL \text{ of } O_2 \text{ per } 100\,mL \text{ blood}$$

Oxygen-combining capacity: 1.34 mL of $O_2$ per gram of hemoglobin
Hb = grams of hemoglobin per 100 mL blood
$SaO_2$ = fraction of Hb saturated with $O_2$
$PaO_2$ = oxygen tension
Solubility: 0.003 mL of $O_2$ per 100 mL plasma for each mm Hg $PaO_2$

Factors that will decrease oxygen delivery include decreased hemoglobin (A), decreased CO due to heart failure or hypovolemia (B), hypoxia (D), and abnormalities such as carbon monoxide poisoning or methemoglobinemia that affect the oxygen-carrying capacity of hemoglobin. Shivering (C) could potentially decrease mixed venous oxygen saturation through increased metabolic demand and oxygen uptake but should not affect oxygen delivery.

### Reference

1. Miller RD. *Miller's Anesthesia*. 8th ed. Philadelphia, PA: Elsevier Churchill Livingstone; 2015.

## 2. Correct Answer: D

**Rationale:**

CO measurement using thermodilution is the gold standard in current practice owing to its ease of use, safety, and reproducibility over time. To run thermodilution CO, 10 mL of saline cooler than blood is rapidly injected into the RA, and the change in temperature after injection is measured by a thermistor in the PA and is integrated over time. The area under the curve of this injectate is inversely proportional to CO. To provide a more reliable measurement, the test is run three times and values within 10% of each other are averaged. An initial steep positive deflection with high amplitude represents rapid delivery of the cold injectate to the thermistor causing a rapid maximal change in temperature. A steep negative deflection with prompt return to baseline represents forward flow and resolution of temperature change.

Low CO states demonstrate an attenuated rise and fall and overall larger area under the curve. Left to right shunting may overestimate CO by diluting out the injectate, whereas right to left shunting overestimates CO by allowing the injectate to quickly bypass the pulmonary circulation. Right-sided valvular lesions can also overestimate or underestimate CO making thermodilution unreliable. A larger than programmed injectate would cause a larger area under the curve than expected and thus underestimates actual CO. Warmer than programmed injectate would cause a smaller area under the curve than expected and thus overestimates actual CO. Injectate that is warmer than programmed into the computer would be the only answer that would consistently overrestimate CO.

Other sources of error include extremely low flow states causing injectate heat loss from slow transit, rapid fluid administration causing temperature fluctuation, improper injection technique, improper placement, and thermistor clot.

### References

1. Greenberg SB, Murphy GS, Vender JS. Current use of the pulmonary artery catheter. *Curr Opin Crit Care*. 2009;15(3):249-253.
2. Marino PL *Marino's the ICU Book* Philadelphia Wolters Kluwer Health/Lippincott Williams & Wilkins. 2014
3. Nishikawa T, Dohi S. Errors in the measurement of cardiac output by thermodilution. *Can J Anaesth*. 1993;40(2):142-153.
4. Tuman KJ, Carroll GC, Ivankovich AD. Pitfalls in interpretation of pulmonary artery catheter data. *J Cardiothorac Anesth*. 1989;3:625-641.

## 3. Correct Answer: D

**Rationale:**

Shock is the physiologic state that results from cell dysfunction or death due to inadequate oxygen delivery or uptake. There are multiple causes of shock, including low circulatory volume (hypovolemic shock), severe vasodilation (septic or anaphylactic shock), low CO from heart failure (cardiogenic shock), or obstruction to forward blood flow (obstructive shock). In all cases, shock is manifested by low MAP. The diagnosis of the type of shock may be challenging, but it is important as the treatment of shock differs between the various etiologies. The hallmark of septic shock is low blood pressure due to profound vasoplegia from bacterial endotoxin. Early septic shock is characterized by high CO, low circulating volume, and low SVR due to vasoplegia, low cardiac filling pressures (CVP and PCWP), and an elevated mixed venous oxygen content due to the inability of cells to utilize delivered oxygen due to poisoning from the bacterial infection.

The hallmark of hypovolemic shock, in contrast, is low MAP due to low effective circulating volume only. In this case, the body's usual homeostatic mechanisms to increase blood pressure by increasing both CO and SVR are intact, and both of these numbers will be elevated. Owing to volume loss, the cardiac filling pressures (CVP and PCWP) will all be low. Therefore, the greatest contrast to septic shock is an elevated SVR.

Note that MAP = CO × SVR. Raising both CO and SVR will work to raise blood pressure back toward normal. In septic shock the primary problem is low SVR, so the body has no way to raise vascular resistance and can only rely on increased CO to move MAP toward a more normal value. Because of this difference, patients in septic shock will usually feel warm to the touch, whereas patients in hypovolemic shock will usually feel cold to the touch because of the high SVR state.

Of note, the use of a pulmonary artery catheter has never been shown to improve survival in randomized controlled clinical trials of patients in shock.

### References

1. Vincet JL, De Backer D. Circulatory shock. *NEJM*. 2013;369:1726-1734.
2. Harvey S, Harrison DA, Singer M, et al. Assessment of the clinical effectiveness of pulmonary artery catheters in management of patients in intensive care (PAC-Man): a randomized controlled trial. *Lancet*. 2005;366:472-477.
3. Shah MA, Hasselblad V, Stevenson LW, et al. Impact of the pulmonary artery catheter in critically ill patients. Meta-analysis of randomized clinical trials. *JAMA*. 2005;294:1664-1670.

### 4. Correct Answer: D

**Rationale:**

Acquired methemoglobin is a form of hemoglobin where heme is oxidized to the ferric $Fe^{3+}$ state. Affected hemoglobin is unable to reversibly bind oxygen causing a functional anemia. Normally, hemoglobin displays increased affinity to oxygen causing a left shift in the hemoglobin dissociation curve. Classic features of methemoglobinemia include cyanosis with a normal $PaO_2$, decreased $SaO_2$, and "chocolate brown blood." Symptomatic methemoglobinemia usually occurs when levels exceed 10% of total hemoglobin. Patients with anemia are typically more sensitive to the effects of methemoglobinemia. Common acquired causes of methemoglobinemia are drugs such as dapsone, lidocaine, prilocaine, benzocaine, metoclopramide, nitroglycerin, and sulfonamides. Other substances such as antifreeze, aniline dyes, hydrogen peroxide, nitrates, nitrites, paraquat, and resorcinol can also cause this.

Deoxyhemoglobin absorbs more red light and oxyhemoglobin absorbs more infrared light. Pulse oximetry works by emitting these two wavelengths and then calculates how much of each is absorbed, thus determining the percent saturation. Methemoglobin, however, absorbs both red and infrared light equally making pulse oximetry inaccurate. At increasing levels, pulse oximetry reading will approximate 85%. Co-oximetry measures the absorbance of additional wavelengths specific to other dyshemoglobins such as methemoglobin and carboxyhemoglobin.

Methylene blue is the preferred treatment. Methylene blue has a potent, reversible inhibitory effect on MAO, so consideration of an alternative treatment like Vitamin C should be given if patients are at risk for serotonin syndrome. Given this patient's high suspicion for methemoglobinemia based on sequence of events and clinical signs, blood gas with co-oximetry is most helpful with diagnosis. CBC, ultrasound, chemistry panel, and EEG may help rule out other less likely contributors but will not confirm the diagnosis.

### References

1. Ash-Bernal R, Wise R, Wright SM. Acquired Methemoglobinemia: a retrospective series of 138 cases at 2 teaching hospitals. *Medicine (Baltimore)*. 2004;83(5):265-273.
2. Barker SJ, Tremper KK, Hyatt J. Effects of methemoglobinemia on pulse oximetry and mixed venous oximetry. *Anesthesiology*. 1989;70(1):112.
3. Kane GC, Hoehn SM, Behrenbeck TR, Mulvagh SL. Benzocaine-induced methemoglobinemia based on the Mayo Clinic experience from 28 478 transesophageal echocardiograms: incidence, outcomes, and predisposing factors. *Arch Intern Med*. 2007;167(18):1977.
4. Rino PB, Scolnik D, Fustiñana A, Mitelpunkt A, Glatstein M. Ascorbic acid for the treatment of methemoglobinemia: the experience of a large tertiary care pediatric hospital. *Am J Ther*. 2014;21(4):240-243.

### 5. Correct Answer: A

**Rationale:**

The Fick equation relates CO, oxygen consumption, and the arteriovenous oxygen content difference as follows:

$$CO = VO_2 / (CaO_2 - CvO_2)$$

Rearrange to solve for oxygen consumption yields:

$$VO_2 = CO \times (CaO_2 - CvO_2)$$

Oxygen content of arterial or venous blood is given by the equation:

$$C_{a/v}O_2 = 1.34 \times Hb \times S_{a/v}O_2 + 0.003 \times P_{a/v}O_2$$

Excluding the dissolved oxygen term, $CaO_2$ and $CvO_2$ can be calculated from the information given:

$$CaO_2 = 1.34 \times 11.7 \times 0.97 = 15.2 \, mL \, O_2 / 100 \, mL \, blood$$

$$CvO_2 = 1.34 \times 11.7 \times 0.72 = 11.3 \, mL \, O_2 / 100 \, mL \, blood$$

Therefore, $VO_2 = 5100 \, mL \, blood / min \times (15.2 - 11.3 \, mL \, O_2 / 100 \, mL \, blood) = 199 \, mL \, O_2 / min$, or approximately 0.2 L/min (A).

### References

1. Bizouarn P, Blanloeil Y, Pinaud M. Comparison between oxygen consumption calculated by Fick's principle using a continuous thermodilution technique and measured by indirect calorimetry. *Br J Anaesth*. 1995;75:719-723.
2. Miller RD. *Miller's Anesthesia*. 8th ed. Philadelphia, PA: Elsevier Churchill Livingstone; 2015.

# 26
# LIFE SUPPORT AND RESUSCITATION

Yuk Ming Liu and John Andre

1. A patient presents to the emergency department (ED) with acute-onset chest pain radiating to his jaw and down his left arm. During evaluation he becomes unresponsive and pulseless. His ECG demonstrated wide complex tachycardia.

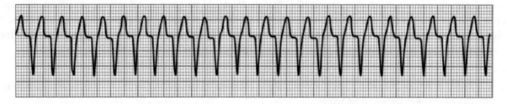

Which of the following answer choices is most correct regarding the underlying rhythm and coinciding appropriate treatment for this patient?

A. Pulseless electrical activity (PEA), synchronized cardioversion with biphasic 120 J
B. Pulseless ventricular tachycardia, synchronized cardioversion with monophasic 360 J
C. Ventricular fibrillation, unsynchronized cardioversion with biphasic 120 J
D. PEA, unsynchronized cardioversion with biphasic 200 J
E. Pulseless ventricular tachycardia, unsynchronized cardioversion with biphasic 120 J

2. A 70-year-old man with history of coronary artery disease has a witnessed cardiac arrest. He undergoes 10 minutes of resuscitation with return of spontaneous circulation (ROSC) but remains comatose. Which of the following treatments for postresuscitation care is most likely to improve outcome for this patient?

A. 100% $FiO_2$ for at least 24 hours
B. Permissive hypotension to avoid using vasopressors
C. Hypothermia between 32°C and 36°C for 24 hours
D. Glycemic control with goal range 120 to 180 mg/dL
E. Normocarbia with a $PaCO_2$ between 35 and 45 mm Hg

3. A 23-year-old man presents to the ED after being a passenger in a high-speed motor vehicle accident. He was restrained and there was airbag deployment. Upon initial presentation to the ED, he was conversant, oriented, and following commands. However 20 minutes later, he is lethargic, only opening his eyes to painful stimuli, is making incomprehensible sounds, and only withdraws to pain. What are the initial and subsequent Glasgow Coma Scores (GCS) for this patient?

A. 15, 8
B. 15, 4
C. 13, 8
D. 10, 4

4. A 33-year-old morbidly obese man presents to the ED after being an unrestrained passenger in a high-speed motor vehicle accident. On evaluation, it is noted that he has distended neck veins, difficulty breathing, and hyperresonance to percussion on the right. Breath sounds are difficult to auscultate. What is the MOST likely diagnosis and appropriate treatment for this patient?

   A. Cardiac tamponade, pericardiocentesis
   B. Cardiac tamponade, resuscitative thoracotomy
   C. Tension pneumothorax (TPX), tube thoracostomy
   D. TPX, needle decompression with 14G angiocath

5. A 4-year-old girl presents to the ED after being struck by a vehicle while riding her bike. She was awake and complaining of neck pain immediately after the accident but is somnolent with sonorous respirations on your examination in the ED. Her oxygen saturation is 89% and her heart rate (HR) is 50 beats/min. According to the Pediatric Acute Life Support guidelines, what are the MOST appropriate initial steps in assessment and management for this patient?

   A. First impression; cardiopulmonary resuscitation (CPR)
   B. First impression; focused assessment with sonography for trauma (FAST) examination to evaluate for pericardial fluid
   C. Evaluate-identify-intervene; STAT head CT
   D. Evaluate-identify-intervene; intubation

6. A 2-year-old, 12 kg child requires CPR. Which of the following steps is most appropriate for this patient?

   A. A compression depth of 2.5 cm
   B. Initial energy for defibrillation of 24 J
   C. Epinephrine administration of 1 mg/dose
   D. Avoid amiodarone which is contraindicated in pediatric patients

7. A 23-year-old man is brought to the ED after sustaining a gunshot wound to the leg. When emergency medical services (EMS) arrived at the scene with pulsatile bleeding from the leg, they placed a tourniquet with good effect. Upon initial evaluation of the patient, he is arousable to pain but confused. His vital signs are T 36.2, HR 120, respiratory rate (RR) 20, and blood pressure (BP) 80/60. Laboratory data reveal a hemoglobin of 12 mg/dL and a base deficit of −8 mEq/L. What class of hemorrhagic shock is most consistent with the patient's clinical examination and laboratory findings?

   A. Class I
   B. Class II
   C. Class III
   D. Class IV

8. A 25-year-old patient is hypotensive (BP 87/54) and tachycardic (HR 110) after sustaining a stab wound to the right thigh. Based on his vital signs, he would be expected to have lost approximately what percentage of his total circulating blood volume?

   A. 5%
   B. 10% to 15%
   C. 15% to 30%
   D. >30%

# Chapter 26 ▪ Answers

1. Correct Answer: E

   **Rationale:**
   A successful resuscitation effort is determined by high-quality CPR in addition to timely defibrillation, if amenable.
   Recognizing the difference between shockable and nonshockable rhythms is key to resuscitation efforts. The patient in this question has pulseless ventricular tachycardia, which should be treated with biphasic unsynchronized cardioversion

starting at 120 J. This cardioversion continues during the process of advanced cardiac life support (ACLS) until ROSC occurs or the patient becomes asystolic or develops PEA. If using a monophasic defibrillator, then a single unsynchronized 360-Joule dose should be administered.

### Reference

1. Link MS, Berkow LC, Kudenchuk PJ, et al. Part 7: adult advanced cardiovascular life support: 2015 American Heart Association guidelines update for cardiopulmonary resuscitation and emergency cardiovascular care. *Circulation.* 2015;132(18 suppl 2):S444-S464.

---

**2.** Correct Answer: C

**Rationale:**

The tenets of postcardiac arrest care include targeted temperature management (TTM), hemodynamic and ventilation optimization, immediate coronary reperfusion with percutaneous coronary intervention (PCI, if amenable), glycemic control, and neurologic care.

The 2015 ACLS guidelines recommend that all comatose (ie, lacking meaningful response to verbal commands) adult patients with ROSC after cardiac arrest should undergo TTM, with a target temperature between 32°C and 36°C maintained constantly for at least 24 hours. This recommendation is based on studies of TTM which compared cooling to temperatures between 32°C and 34°C with no well-defined TTM and found improvement in neurologic outcome for those in whom hypothermia was induced. A more recent high-quality study compared temperature management at 36°C and at 33°C and found outcomes to be similar for both. Taken together, the initial studies suggest that TTM is beneficial, so the recommendation remains to select a single target temperature within the 32°C and 36°C range.

There are multiple goals when it comes to hemodynamic and ventilation optimization in postcardiac arrest patients. Based on the 2015 ACLS guidelines, patients should receive the lowest possible $FiO_2$ to maintain an $SpO_2$ of 94% or greater. The patients' associated comorbidities and current medical problems will ultimately dictate the goal $PaCO_2$ in the postcardiac arrest patient. Permissive hypercapnia may be most appropriate in patients with acute lung injury while maintenance of normocarbia is warranted in patients with cerebral edema. With regards to hemodynamics goals, the ACLS guidelines recommend maintaining a mean arterial pressure of 65 mm Hg or greater. In patients who have suspected coronary artery occlusion as the source of the cardiac arrest, coronary reperfusion is warranted after return of spontaneous circulation.

The *2015 AHA Guidelines* do not recommend a specific target range for glucose management in the postcardiac arrest patient. Variability in glucose levels in this patient population is common and often time-dependent. Stress-induced hyperglycemia is commonly found in the earlier phase of a postcardiac arrest patient while hypoglycemia is commonly seen during the rewarming process after 24 hours of hypothermia. Despite numerous studies looking at glycemic control in postcardiac arrest patients, the optimal target range still remains unknown. Given the variability of blood glucose levels in these patients, frequent monitoring should be performed to avoid hypoglycemia and hyperglycemia.

### References

1. Link MS, Berkow LC, Kudenchuk PJ, et al. Part 7: adult advanced cardiovascular life support: 2015 American Heart Association guidelines update for cardiopulmonary resuscitation and emergency cardiovascular care. *Circulation.* 2015;132(18 suppl 2):S444-S464.
2. Beiser DG, Carr GE, Edelson DP, Peberdy MA, Hoek TL. Derangements in blood glucose following initial resuscitation from in-hospital cardiac arrest: a report from the national registry of cardiopulmonary resuscitation. *Resuscitation.* 2009;80:624-630.
3. Lee BK, Lee HY, Jeung KW, Jung YH, Lee GS, You Y. Association of blood glucose variability with outcomes in comatose cardiac arrest survivors treated with therapeutic hypothermia. *Am J Emerg Med.* 2013;31:566-572.
4. Nakashima R, Hifumi T, Kawakita K, et al. Critical care management focused on optimizing brain function after cardiac arrest. *Circ J* 2017;81:427-439.

---

**3.** Correct Answer: A

**Rationale:**

The GCS (see figure that follows) is a reliable and objective way of recording the initial and subsequent level of consciousness in a person after a traumatic injury. The scale assesses patients according to three aspects of responsiveness: eye-opening, motor, and verbal responses. The levels of response in the components of the GCS are "scored" from 1, for no response, up to normal values of 4 (eye-opening response), 5 (verbal response), and 6 (motor response). The total Coma Score thus has values between 3 and 15, 3 being the worst and 15 being the highest. The findings in each component of the scale can aggregate into a total GCS, which gives a less detailed description but can provide a useful "shorthand" summary of the overall severity. Based on the question, the patient had a GCS of 15 (4+5+6) at presentation, which later decreased to 8 (2+2+4).

| EYE-OPENING RESPONSE | VERBAL RESPONSE | MOTOR RESPONSE |
| --- | --- | --- |
| Spontaneous – 4 points | Oriented – 5 points | Obeys commands – 6 points |
| To verbal stimuli – 3 | Confused – 4 | Localizes pain – 5 |
| To pain only – 2 | Inappropriate words – 3 | Withdraws pain – 4 |
| No response – 1 | Incomprehensible sounds – 2 | Decorticate – 3 |
| | No response –1 | Decerebrate – 2 |
| | | No response – 1 |

From Teasdale G, Jennett B. Assessment of coma and impaired consciousness. A practical scale. *Lancet*. 1974;2(7872):81-84.

### References

1. Merrick C. *Advanced Trauma Life Support*. Chicago, IL: American College of Surgeons. 2018. Print.
2. Jain S, Teasdale GM, Iverson LM. *Glasgow Coma Scale*. *StatPearls* [Internet]. Treasure Island (FL): StatPearls Publishing; 2019 Jan-. 2019 Mar 3.

---

**4.** Correct Answer: C

**Rationale:**

The primary survey is designed to rapidly assess and treat any life-threatening injuries. Major causes of death in trauma patients are airway obstruction, respiratory failure, shock from hemorrhage, and brain injuries. Specific injuries which are immediately life-threatening include:

- Airway obstruction
- Tension pneumothorax
- Massive internal or external hemorrhage
- Open pneumothorax
- Flail chest
- Cardiac tamponade.

The patient's clinical signs and symptoms are most consistent with TPX which should be treated with immediate decompression.

TPX results from the trapping of air within the pleural space which does not have a way to escape. Progressive build-up of pressure in the pleural space pushes the mediastinum to the opposite hemithorax and obstructs venous return to the heart. This leads to circulatory instability and may result in traumatic arrest.

Classic signs of a TPX include deviation of the trachea away from the side with the tension, absent breath sounds, hyperresonance to percussion, deviated trachea, and distended neck veins. However these classic signs may be absent and more commonly the patient is tachycardic and tachypneic, and may be hypoxic.

Treatment of TPX is decompression. This will allow the mediastinum and associated organs to return to their normal positions and relieve the pressure. Whether the initial decompression is with a chest tube versus a needle is dependent on the clinician's skill set, available equipment, and the urgency of the need for decompression. Of note, a standard 14 gauge angiocatheter cannot penetrate the chest wall and reach the pleural space in up to one-third of trauma patients. A 10-gauge, 7.5 cm (3 inch) armored angiocatheter is able to penetrate the pleural space in most instances. If needle decompression is performed, it should be followed immediately by tube thoracostomy.

Cardiac tamponade is most commonly caused by penetrating injuries, such as gunshot or stab wounds, which cause blood to pool in the fixed, fibrous pericardial sac that leads to decreased venous return to the heart and resultant decreased cardiac output. Cardiac tamponade is a clinical diagnosis based on physical findings of muffled heart sounds, dilated neck veins, and hypotension which is known as "Beck triad." Cardiac tamponade can lead to Kussmaul sign (increased venous pressure with inspiration) and can progress to pulseless electrical activity. Treatment varies on the patient's clinical situation, ranging from pericardiocentesis to resuscitative thoracotomy. Differentiating between TPX and cardiac tamponade may be challenging as both can result in hemodynamic compromise or cardiac arrest. Asymmetric absence of breath sounds, hyperresonance to percussion, and tracheal deviation are signs of TPX that are not seen in cardiac tamponade. An ultrasound exam utilizing FAST protocol, if available, can be valuable in diagnosing and differentiating between these conditions.

### References

1. Merrick C. *Advanced Trauma Life Support*. Chicago, IL: American College of Surgeons. 2018. Print.
2. Zengerink I, Brink PR, Laupland KB, et al. Needle thoracostomy in the treatment of a tension pneumothorax in trauma patients: what size needle? *J Trauma*. 2008;64:111-114.

**5.** Correct Answer: A

**Rationale:**

Pediatric Advanced Life Support (PALS), similar to both ACLS and advanced trauma life support (ATLS), follows a systematic approach. First Impression followed by evaluate-identify-intervene (which includes primary assessment, secondary assessment, and diagnostic tests) constitutes the steps in the PALS algorithm.

The algorithm starts with a first impression to help determine whether or not the patient is in imminent danger, either of cardiac or respiratory failure. Patients who are conscious or unconscious, but breathing can progress to the evaluate-identify-intervene step in the algorithm. Patients who are not breathing adequately but have a pulse greater than 60 beats/min should undergo rescue breathing. Patients with a pulse less than 60 beats/min should undergo CPR.

The second step of the algorithm is evaluate-identify-intervene. This is an ongoing cycle, in which the clinician is repeatedly reevaluating the patient and performing interventions based on the findings. Throughout the process, if the patient stops breathing or has a pulse less than 60 beats/min, then the clinician should begin rescue breathing or CPR, respectively. If the patient remains breathing and has a pulse greater than 60 beats/min, then the clinician should progress to the next steps in the algorithm.

Evaluate-identify-intervene are components of the primary assessment and secondary assessment, and guide the choice of diagnostic testing. The primary assessment follows the primary survey in ATLS: Airway, Breathing, Circulation, Disability, Exposure.

An oxygen saturation that is less than 90% indicates that respiratory support is needed. In the pediatric patient population, a heart rate less than 60 beats/min suggests cardiac failure, and CPR should be initiated.

Reference

1. Chameides L, et al. *Pediatric Advanced Life Support*. Dallas, TX: American Heart Association. 2015. eBook.

**6.** Correct Answer: B

**Rationale:**

PALS program provides a structured approach to the assessment and treatment of the critically ill pediatric patient. While there are similarities between the PALS and adult algorithms, important differences also exist.

Compression depth for adults is a minimum of 5 cm/2 in. Compression depth for a child is at least one-third the depth of the chest size, or 5 cm for a child and 4 cm for an infant.

For pediatric patients noted to be in ventricular fibrillation or pulseless ventricular tachycardia, an unsynchronized shock should be administered starting at 2 J/kg. The PALS algorithm continues with subsequent shocks of 4 J/kg administered if needed.

Whereas adults receive 1 mg of epinephrine during ACLS, pediatric patients receive a weight-based dose at 0.01 mg/kg.

As in adults, amiodarone is recommended in pediatric patients for the management of ventricular fibrillation or pulseless ventricular tachycardia with the pediatric dosage of 5 mg/kg IV/IO/bolus dose.

Reference

1. Chameides L, Ralston M. *Pediatric Advanced Life Support*. Dallas, TX: American Heart Association. 2015. eBook.

**7.** Correct Answer: C

**Rationale:**

Hemorrhagic shock can be rapidly fatal. The primary goal is to stop the bleeding. Resuscitation may well depend on estimated severity of hemorrhage. The severity of hemorrhagic shock is commonly subdivided into four classes based on alterations in vital signs, urine output, GCS, and base deficit (see table that follows).

## ATLS CLASSIFICATION OF HEMORRHAGIC SHOCK

|  | CLASS I | CLASS II | CLASS III | CLASS IV |
| --- | --- | --- | --- | --- |
| Blood loss (%) | <15 | 15–30 | 30–40 | >40 |
| Pulse (beats/min) | <100 | 100–120 | 120–140 | >140 |
| Blood pressure (mm Hg) | Normal | Normal | Decreased | Much decreased |
| Pulse pressure | Normal or increased | Decreased | Decreased | Decreased |
| Respiratory rate (breaths/min) | 14–20 | 20–30 | 30–40 | >40 |
| Mental status | Slightly anxious | Mildly anxious | Anxious, confused | Confused, lethargic |
| Urine output (mL/hr) | >30 | 20–30 | 5–15 | Minimal |

The patient has tachycardia, mild hypotension with narrowed pulse pressure, a reduced GCS, and a base deficit most consistent with class III hemorrhagic shock.

A patient's age, severity of injury, time between injury and resuscitation, prehospital resuscitation efforts, and the patient's medical history (including medications) will all impact the patient's clinical presentation. Given this, it is essential that volume and blood resuscitation happen promptly and appropriately. The clinician should not wait until the patient fits a certain class of shock before initiating resuscitation.

### Reference

1. Merrick C. *Advanced Trauma Life Support*. Chicago, IL: American College of Surgeons. 2018. Print.

---

**8.** Correct Answer: D

**Rationale:**

Predicting blood loss is important to determine treatments of patients with traumatic injury, which can cause death by hypovolemic hemorrhagic shock. Hemorrhagic deaths typically occur very early, usually within the first 6 hours of admission, and early hypoperfusion or shock has been demonstrated to promote coagulopathy The ATLS guidelines suggest four classes of hypovolemic shock based on the percentage of estimated blood loss and include recommendations for appropriate treatment according to the classes. The importance of diagnosing hemorrhage at initial patient contact by first responders has been greatly emphasized, as more accurate diagnosis of hemorrhage severity and shock has been shown to lead to better treatment for these patients.

Based on the presence of tachycardia and hypotension, this patient would be expected to have lost more than 30% of his circulating blood volume.

### Reference

1. Mrrick C. *Advanced Trauma Life Support*. Chicago, IL: American College of Surgeons. 2018. Print.

# 27
# IMAGING AND DIAGNOSTIC MODALITIES

Sneha Kannan and David M. Dudzinski

1. A 35-year-old-patient with no past medical history comes to the Emergency Department with complaints of several days of fatigue and constant chest pain that is substernal but not radiating, "sharp," and worsened with inspiration, but seems to improve with sitting forward. He has noticed a 10 lbs unintentional weight gain over the past 2 weeks and significant fatigue. He reports only local travel in the last 2 months and otherwise had a "cold a few weeks ago." His family history is negative for ischemic heart disease, and he is a nonsmoker and has never used any substances such as cocaine, marijuana, or amphetamines. Examination in the Emergency Department reveals tachycardic heart without gallop or rub, and symmetric 2+ pitting edema to his calves. Initial laboratory test results are notable for an elevated troponin-T and the following ECG:

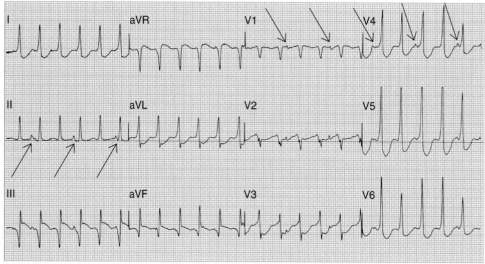

Image from Wagner GS, Strauss DG, eds. *Marriott's Practical Electrocardiography*. 12th ed. Philadelphia, PA: Wolters Kluwer; 2013:401.

Which of the following is the BEST imaging modality to diagnose the etiology of his underlying disease?

A. CT Coronary Angiography
B. Cardiac MRI
C. Transesophageal Echocardiogram
D. Cardiac catheterization with ventriculography

2. A 65-year-old male presents to the Emergency Department with cough, malaise, and fevers to 39°C. His past medical history is notable for hypertension, diabetes, and a drug-eluting stent placed into his distal right coronary artery 5 years before angina. He has no anginal symptoms at rest. He takes aspirin, atorvastatin, metoprolol, lisinopril, and metformin. Testing with viral panel in the Emergency Department resulted in positive PCR for Influenza A. Electrocardiogram shows sinus rhythm, normal QRS, and no ischemic changes, and a Troponin-T is <0.01 ng/mL. Over the course of the first 2 hours after presentation, he becomes increasingly hypoxemic, ultimately transferred to the ICU after intubation. His chest radiograph before intubation shows bilateral infiltrates. Oxygenation slowly improves over the next 12 hours. The morning after admission, he is noted to have a short run of wide complex tachycardia. Electrocardiogram shows new left bundle branch block (LBBB). He then continues to have frequent regular wide complex tachycardias, causing hemodynamic instability. Troponin-T now increases to 0.48 ng/mL. Which of the following is the BEST next step in managing his cardiac status?

   A. Cardiac catheterization
   B. Cardiac MRI
   C. Transthoracic echocardiogram and serial biomarkers
   D. CT Pulmonary Angiogram

3. A 68-year-old male with a past medical history of hypertension arrives at the Emergency Department with crushing chest pain. The pain started 1 hour ago and is substernal with radiation to his left shoulder. He is mildly diaphoretic and dyspneic. Vital signs on presentation are notable for a blood pressure of 110/65 mm Hg, heart rate of 100 beats per minute, and oxygen saturation of 99% on room air. His initial ECG is shown in the figure that follows:

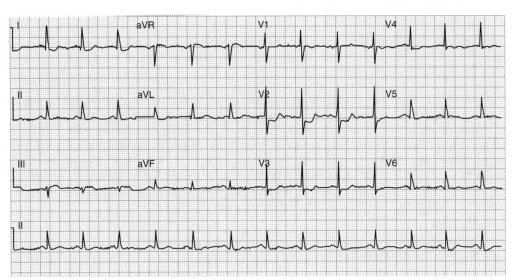

(Figure from van Gorselen EO, Verheugt FW, Meursing BT, Oude Ophius AJ. Posterior myocardial infarction: the dark side of the moon. Neth Heart J. 2007;15(1):16-21.)

Which of the following is the next BEST step to evaluate the extent of cardiac damage in this patient?

   A. Troponin
   B. CK-MB
   C. Right-sided ECG leads
   D. Posterior ECG leads
   E. Right-sided heart catheterization

4. A 75-year-old male is brought to the Emergency Department with severe hypotension. He has a past medical history of heart failure with reduced ejection fraction (last EF 24%) and has not been compliant with his diuretics or diet. He has been admitted multiple times in the past year for heart failure exacerbations. On arrival to the Emergency Department, he is cool and minimally responsive with an initial blood bilateral pressure of 70/40 mm Hg. He is started on dobutamine and norepinephrine. On arrival to the ICU, the patient has a right radial arterial line placed without complication. The monitor reports a blood pressure of 65/55 mm Hg. The blood pressure is immediately rechecked manually, and a reading of 80/40 mm Hg is obtained. Which of the following is the MOST likely reason for this discrepancy?

   A. Failure to adequately prime arterial line
   B. Patient has severe aortic regurgitation
   C. Patient has severe peripheral vascular disease
   D. Patient has concurrent sepsis

5. A 70-year-old male with past medical history of mild-moderate mitral regurgitation and moderate-severe tricuspid regurgitation, COPD, and secondary pulmonary hypertension presents to the Emergency Department with a fever and new cough. Vitals on presentation are notable for a blood pressure of 80/43, temperature of 38.7°C, and oxygen saturation of 80% on room air, which improves modestly with 6 L oxygen by nasal cannula. Chest radiograph shows multifocal airspace opacities suggestive of pneumonia, but not pulmonary edema. He is transferred to the ICU for intubation. Examination is also notable for cool extremities with +1 symmetric lower extremity edema. In determining whether to administer fluids to this patient to augment his mean arterial pressure, which of the following techniques would be LEAST helpful?

   A. Pulmonary Arterial Catheter (PAC)
   B. Central Venous Pressure (CVP)
   C. Pulse pressure variation
   D. Passive leg raise

6. A 68-year-old male with a past medical history of coronary artery disease and myocardial infarction requiring three drug-eluting stents presents to the Emergency Department with exertional chest pain. He describes the pain as substernal pressure, without radiation. After his past stents, he attended cardiac rehab and he now walks a few miles per week for exercise. He does not have pain at rest, but over the past months is only able to walk a few minutes when he notices the chest pain with mild dyspnea. The pain resolves when he sits down for a few minutes. He is not able to walk more than half a mile without having significant pain. He feels this is similar to the pain he had before his stents were placed. His ECG is unchanged. His last ECG exercise stress test was 10 years ago, before his stent placements. In evaluating his pain, which of the following is the most appropriate test?

   A. Cardiac MRI
   B. Transthoracic Echocardiography
   C. Technitium-99 Sestamibi Scan
   D. Exercise ECG Stress Test

7. A 79-year-old female with a past medical history of rheumatoid arthritis, heart failure with reduced ejection fraction (EF 30%), and severe pulmonary hypertension presents to the Emergency Department with fever and dysuria. Vitals on arrival are notable for a blood pressure of 70/48 mm Hg, heart rate of 105 beats per minute, and oxygen saturation of 89% on room air. She has cool extremities, crackles, and significant lower extremity edema. Urinalysis shows significant pyuria with positive nitrite and leukocyte esterase, and significant bacteriuria, and she is started on broad spectrum antibiotics. Laboratory studies are also notable for an NT-proBNP elevated to three times of recent baseline. She is placed on oxygen and her MAP rise to 66 on three vasopressors. Echocardiogram shows a similar EF, with estimated RVSP is 92 mm Hg. Her peripheral O2 venous saturation is 93% on 4 L of nasal cannula. The intensivist decides to place a PAC via the right internal jugular vein. Due to her medical history, which among the following complications is she at the GREATEST risk for?

   A. Complete heart block
   B. Thromboembolism
   C. Misplacement of the catheter into the LA
   D. Pulmonary artery rupture

**8.** A 70-year-old female with a past medical history of iron-deficiency anemia, pulmonary hypertension, and diastolic heart failure presents to the Emergency Department with fever and productive cough. She has also noticed a 10 lb weight gain in the last 2 weeks. Vitals on presentation are notable for a blood pressure of 69/40 mm Hg, a temperature of 39.0°C, a heart rate of 130 beats/min, and an oxygen saturation of 85% on room air. Her laboratory test results are notable for an NT-proBNP three times her baseline and a WBC count of 11,000 cells/μL. She is immediately started on broad spectrum antibiotics and transferred to the ICU for mixed shock. Her MAPs remain in the 50s, and she is started on pressor support with limited improvement. Her oxygenation remains poor, and she is intubated for hypoxemic respiratory failure and sedated with propofol. The decision is made to place a pulmonary artery catheter to further guide management. In interpreting her pulmonary artery catheter readings, which of the following in her presentation would lead to an INCREASE in her measured mixed venous oxygen saturation?

**A.** Fever
**B.** Tachycardia
**C.** Anemia
**D.** Sedation with propofol

# Chapter 27 ▪ Answers

**1.** Correct Answer: B

**Rationale:**
The presentation is most consistent with viral myocarditis. Diagnosis of myocarditis is multimodal, though the gold standard is considered to be endomyocardial biopsy (EMBx). However, because of the morbidity associated with an EMBx, the diagnosis is typically a combination of noninvasive diagnostic imaging, serology, and clinical presentation.

The patient is a young male with no risk factors for premature coronary artery disease and his clinical presentation is more consistent with a viral myopericarditis, with low concern for coronary ischemia, and thus would be a good candidate for Cardiac MRI. CT Coronary Angiography would not be the most appropriate test given low concern for coronary artery disease and a clinical picture highly consistent with viral myocarditis. Echocardiography would definitely provide information about cardiac function, but Cardiac MRI is a superior test for this scenario because it can provide ancillary information about findings suggestive of myocarditis such as myocardial edema and gadolinium enhancement. Transesophageal echocardiography as a test is rarely indicated in myocarditis. Invasive ventriculography can be performed with a left heart catheterization but should be reserved for when left ventricular function is unknown, and there is an indication for invasive catheterization. Thus, cardiac MRI would be the best first choice.

References
1. Friedrich MG, Sechtem U, Schulz-Menger J, et al. Cardiovascular magnetic resonance in myocarditis: a JACC white paper. *J Am Coll Cardiol.* 2009;53(17):1475-1487.
2. Goenka AH, Flamm SD. Cardiac magnetic resonance imaging for the investigation of cardiovascular diss. Part 1: current applications. *Tex Heart Inst J.* 2014;41(1):7-20.

**2.** Correct Answer: A

**Rationale:**
The recurrent tachyarrhythmias that appear to be ventricular in origin in association with hemodynamic instability and rising troponin-T is concerning for active myocardial ischemia. This supports performing cardiac catheterization for diagnosis and potential reperfusion. In the absence of hemodynamic instability, a more conservative approach with echocardiogram and serial troponin-T would be a reasonable alternative. However, LBBB would cause paradoxical septal motion on echocardiography, which may confound assessment of focal wall motion abnormalities as part of the ischemic evaluation.

Though prior guidelines associate a new LBBB with ischemia, recent studies have questioned this assumption. Studies show that a new LBBB is rarely caused by acute transmural ischemia. Thus, the 2013 ST elevation myocardial infarction guidelines urge a more holistic assessment based on cardiac biomarkers, ECG criteria for myocardial infarction, and clinical scenario.

Though cardiac MRI is being evaluated as an alternate diagnostic modality for ischemia, it currently has no role in a hemodynamically unstable patient. A CT Pulmonary Angiogram would be useful if pulmonary embolism was being considered but is unlikely based on this patient's clinical presentation.

### References

1. Neeland IJ, Kontos MC, de Lemos JA. Evolving considerations in the management of patients with left bundle branch block and suspected myocardial infarction. *J Am Coll Cardiol*. 2012;60:96-105.
2. O'Gara PT, Kushner FG, Ascheim DD, et al. 2013 ACCF/AHA guideline for the management of ST-elevation myocardial infarction: a report of the American College of Cardiology Foundation/American Heart Association Task Force on Practice Guidelines. *J Am Coll Cardiol*. 2013;61:e78-e140.

**3.** Correct Answer: D

**Rationale:**

This patient has ST segment depressions in the anteroseptal leads (V2-V4), and early R wave progression. The ST segment changes may be interpreted as anterior ischemia in the context of a non-ST segment elevation myocardial infarction, posterior STEMI is an important differential. The early R wave progression here indicates the evolution of Q waves in the posterior wall of the heart. Posterior MI accompanies ~15%-20% of STEMIs, most commonly inferior or lateral STEMI due to perfusion of these territories and the posterior territory usually by the right coronary artery. The next most important test that can be done at bedside is to better characterize this is posterior ECG leads (V7-V9). The posterior MI leads are located in the same horizontal plane as V6, located at the posterior axillary line (V7) and paraspinal (V9), with V8 in between. If posterior leads confirm ST segment elevation, noting that the AHA/ACC guideline requires only 0.5 mm of ST segment elevation in these posterior leads, then the patient should be triaged for emergent coronary angiography.

Ultimately troponins and CK-MB are important in characterizing myocardial damage and impacting treatment and prognostication, but the first step should be to exclude a STEMI in a patient with this pattern on ECG. A right-sided ECG would be important in a patient presenting with an inferior MI to evaluate for RV infarction.

### References

1. van Gorselen EO, Verheugt FW, Meursing BT, Oude Ophius AJ.Posterior myocardial infarction: the dark side of the moon. *Neth Heart J*. 2007;15(1):16-21.
2. Thygesen K, Alpert JS, Jaffe AS, et al; Executive Group on behalf of the Joint European Society of Cardiology (ESC)/American College of Cardiology (ACC)/American Heart Association (AHA)/World Heart Federation (WHF) Task Force for the Universal Definition of Myocardial Infarction. Fourth universal definition of myocardial infarction (2018). *Circulation*. 2018;138:e618-e651. doi:10.1161/CIR.0000000000000617.

**4.** Correct Answer: A

**Rationale:**

Arterial lines are useful to receive quick and real-time information about a patient's hemodynamics. An arterial line has a catheter (inserted into the patient) that transmits the pressure wave to the fluid-filled tubes of the monitoring system. The tubing system carries the impulse of the pressure wave to the transducer, which converts the mechanical pressure signal to an electrical signal that is then presented on the monitor as a waveform. There are three steps in the calibration of an arterial pressure line:

1. Priming—the air is removed out of the pressure tubing system
2. Leveling—the pressure transducer is kept at the level of the heart to most accurately capture the mean arterial pressure/aortic pressure without further effects of gravity
3. Zeroing—the pressure transducer is calibrated to atmospheric pressure as the zero point to better allow for interpretation of the arterial line blood pressures

If the arterial line system is not primed, an air bubble is introduced into what should be a fluid-filled tubing system. Air dampens pressure signals more than fluid does, so if an air bubble is introduced into the system, the waveform amplitude reflects serious dampening and reads systolic pressures as lower than actual and diastolic pressures higher than actual.

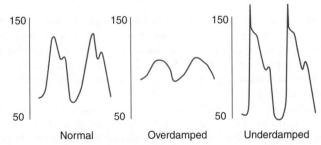

Underdamping can be caused by aortic regurgitation or hyperdynamic states such as sepsis (that would cause a widened pulse pressure). Disappearance of the diastolic waveform can be seen in patients with significant peripheral vascular disease.

References

1. Barash PG, Cullen BF, Stoelting RK, et al. Clinical anesthesia. *Chapter 25: Commonly Used Monitoring Techniques*. Philadelphia: Lippincott, Williams & Wilkins; 2013.
2. https://www.aic.cuhk.edu.hk/web8/haemodynamic%20monitoring%20intro.htm.

**5.** Correct Answer: B

**Rationale:**

Measures of fluid responsiveness can be separated into static and dynamic measures. The static measures include: CVP, pulmonary capillary wedge pressure, and clinical static endpoints (heart rate, blood pressure, etc). Dynamic measures include: pulse pressure variation, stroke volume variation, IVC collapsibility, and response to passive leg raise. Each of these has their own strengths and weaknesses, with dynamic measures generally thought to perform better than static measures. The 2016 surviving sepsis guidelines recommend using dynamic indices of volume responsiveness to guide volume resuscitation in sepsis.

The patient in the question has pulmonary hypertension and significant tricuspid regurgitation, which would confound interpretation of CVP measurements, if the CVP were to be used as a proxy for RV preload. However in patients with RV failure or severe TR, the CVP is falsely elevated and does not give an accurate representation of preload. The other measures of fluid status such as pulmonary artery wedge pressure (measure through a pulmonary artery catheter) measures left ventricular preload and thus a better representation of systemic preload than CVP. Dynamic indices such as pulse pressure variation, stroke volume variation, and passive leg raise have been shown to be superior measures for determining volume responsiveness.

References

1. Marik PE, Lemson J. Fluid responsiveness: an evolution of our understanding. *Br J Anaesth.* 2014;112(4):617-620.
2. Marik PE, Cavallazzi R, Vasu T, Hirani A. Dynamic changes in arterial waveform derived variables and fluid responsiveness in mechanically ventilated patients: a systematic review of the literature. *Crit Care Med.* 2009;37(9):2642-2647.

**6.** Correct Answer: C

**Rationale:**

There are numerous tests to assess cardiac perfusion. The patient in the question has a pattern of stable angina and has a history of prior revascularizations. Per the 2012 AHA/ACC guidelines for stable ischemic heart disease, the patient should proceed to nuclear imaging. The next step is to have a cardiac imaging study. The patient is able to exercise to some capacity; however, he has had prior revascularizations, therefore an imaging study would be the most appropriate. Had he not had prior revascularizations and were he able to exercise, an ECG stress test would be appropriate. A rest transthoracic echocardiogram would not provide information about myocardial perfusion. Cardiac MRI is being evaluated as a tool to evaluate myocardial perfusion in patients with ischemic heart disease but is not the test of choice currently.

Reference

1. Fihn SD, Gardin JM, Abrams J, et al. 2012 ACCF/AHA/ACP/AATS/PCNA/SCAI/STS Guideline for the diagnosis and management of patients with stable ischemic heart disease: a report of the American College of Cardiology Foundation/American Heart Association Task Force on Practice Guidelines, and the American College of Physicians, American Association for Thoracic Surgery, Preventive Cardiovascular Nurses Association, Society for Cardiovascular Angiography and Interventions, and Society of Thoracic Surgeons. *J Am Coll Cardiol.* 2012;60(24):e44-e164.

**7.** Correct Answer: D

**Rationale:**

The PAC is a tool that can be used to provide more information about a patient's hemodynamics by measuring the central venous, right ventricle, pulmonary artery, and pulmonary capillary wedge pressures. Using thermodilution, the PAC can also be used to estimate the cardiac output, and this value can be used to calculate both systemic and pulmonary vascular resistances; measurement of the oxygen saturation in the pulmonary artery (mixed venous saturation) can also be used to infer cardiac output. PACs have very discrete clinical scenarios in which they can be helpful. Notably the ESCAPE trial in 2005 found that PAC placement did not improve outcomes or mortality in patients hospitalized with heart failure. However the trial was designed to exclude patients in shock (cardiogenic or mixed), in whom PAC placement may be needed urgently. In this patient with mixed septic and cardiogenic shock phenotypes, PAC might help assess type of shock and guide therapy.

There are many complications that can arise from PAC placement. The patient's pulmonary hypertension puts her at risk for pulmonary artery rupture, a rare but severe and often fatal complication of PAC placements. Though the other choices are also possible complications, they are less likely associated with this patient's medical history. Thromboembolism is more common in patients with a predisposing thrombophilia or suspicion for atrial clots that could be dislodged by the PAC. Complete heart block is a risk factor for patients with underlying conduction disease (typically a LBBB, which could progress to complete heart block if there was injury to the right-sided conduction system during PAC placement). Misplacement of the catheter into the LA could happen in a patient with a patent foramen ovale or an atrial septal defect.

### References

1. Bossert T, Gummert JF, Bittner HB, et al. Swan-Ganz catheter-induced severe complications in cardiac surgery: right ventricular perforation, knotting, and rupture of a pulmonary artery. *J Card Surg.* 2006;21(3):292-295.
2. Binanay C, Califf RM, Hasselblad V, et al. Evaluation study of congestive heart failure and pulmonary artery catheterization effectiveness: the ESCAPE trial. *JAMA.* 2005;294(13):1625-1633.

## 8. Correct Answer: D

**Rationale:**

The oxygen saturation in the pulmonary artery is called mixed venous oxygen saturation and is measured using a pulmonary artery catheter. It is influenced by oxygen delivered to the tissue and the oxygen extracted by the tissues. Any physiologic parameter that increases the body's metabolic rate increases tissue oxygen consumption and thereby decreases the mixed venous oxygen saturation. Thus fever and tachycardia decreases mixed venous oxygenation. Oxygen delivery to the tissues is affected by cardiac output, hemoglobin, and oxygen content of arterial blood. Anemia reduces peripheral tissue oxygen delivery and as a result decreases mixed venous oxygen saturation. Sedation with propofol reduces the body's metabolic rate and thereby decreases tissue oxygen consumption, causing an increase in mixed venous oxygen saturation.

### Reference

1. Shepherd S, Pearse RM. Role of central and mixed venous oxygen saturation measurement in perioperative care. *Anesthesiology.* 2009;111(3):649-656.

# 28

# IMAGING (ULTRASOUND)

Thomas J. Krall and Kevin C. Thornton

1. A 34-year-old man with primary sclerosing cholangitis underwent orthotopic liver transplantation 6 hours ago. His other medical history includes obesity treated with sleeve gastrectomy 6 years ago, esophageal diverticulum, and peptic ulcer disease with remote gastrointestinal bleeding. He remains intubated and sedated in the ICU with current vital signs of T: 36.2°C, HR: 128 beats per minute, BP: 72/40 mm Hg, RR: 22 on the mechanical ventilator. He is currently receiving infusions of norepinephrine at 30 mcg/min and vasopressin at 0.04 units/min. He remains hypotensive despite rapid blood transfusion. An attempt at transthoracic cardiac ultrasound revealed no adequate windows. In deciding whether to perform a transesophageal echocardiogram (TEE) to work up his refractory shock, which of his medical problems would most likely be considered an absolute contraindication to TEE probe placement?

   A. Esophageal varices
   B. Prior gastric sleeve
   C. History of bleeding peptic ulcer
   D. Esophageal diverticulum

2. A 55-year-old man underwent bilateral lung transplantation for idiopathic pulmonary fibrosis with intraoperative central veno-arterial ECMO support. After implantation of the second lung, the team is unable to wean the patient off the ECMO circuit despite dobutamine and norepinephrine infusions. TEE images of the mid-esophageal long axis view at end-diastole (A) and mid-systole (B) are shown in the figures that follow. Based on the TEE findings, which of the following is the next best step in management?

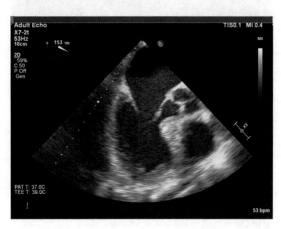

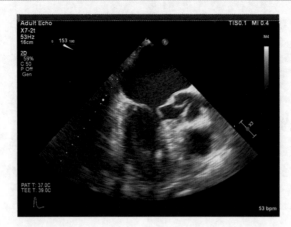

A. Add epinephrine infusion
B. Insert an intra-aortic balloon pump
C. Discontinue dobutamine
D. Perform aortic valve replacement

3. A 42-year-old woman with Crohn's disease is admitted to the ICU following laparotomy for small bowel obstruction. She is persistently hypotensive despite vasopressor and volume administration. She is breathing spontaneously on high-flow nasal cannula. Ultrasound imaging of her IVC reveals a 1.5 cm vessel diameter and >50% decrease in vessel diameter during inhalation. The critical care fellow concludes that these findings indicate the patient would increase her cardiac output with intravascular volume administration. Which of the following, if present, would confound that conclusion?

A. Pneumothorax
B. Pericardial effusion
C. Abdominal compartment syndrome
D. Deep venous thrombosis of the right femoral vein

4. A 54-year-old man is admitted to the ICU following Impella placement for cardiogenic shock. Routine screening ultrasound for Impella position shows the following parasternal long axis image. The distance between the calipers is 2 cm.

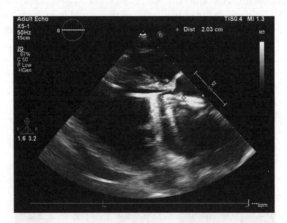

Which of the following is the best next step in management?

A. Advance the Impella 1.5 cm
B. Advance the Impella 3 cm
C. Remeasure from the end of the pigtail to the aortic annulus
D. Leave the Impella in its current position

5. Use of pulsed-wave Doppler in which of the following views allows for calculation of cardiac output?

A. Transesophageal mid-esophageal 4-chamber
B. Transthoracic apical 5-chamber
C. Transthoracic parasternal long axis
D. Transesophageal mid-esophageal long axis

6. A 54-year-old woman with a history of mechanical mitral valve replacement for endocarditis is brought to the emergency department for dyspnea. She reports 2 weeks of progressive fatigue, exertional dyspnea, and orthopnea. A CT angiogram of the chest shows diffuse ground-glass opacities and interstitial thickening and is negative for pulmonary embolism. A bedside cardiac ultrasound is performed, and the parasternal short axis view is shown in the figure that follows.

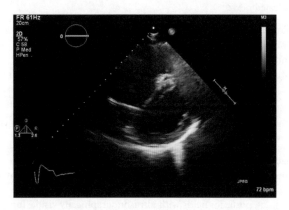

Which of the following assessments will likely lead to the diagnosis in this case?

A. Doppler ultrasound of the lower extremity veins
B. Color Doppler of the main pulmonary artery
C. Measurement of the IVC diameter in a subcostal view
D. Continuous-wave Doppler across the mitral valve in the apical 4-chamber view

7. In ultrasound assessment of a pericardial effusion, which of the following findings is most specific for cardiac tamponade?

A. IVC diameter >2 cm
B. RA collapse during >1/3 of the cardiac cycle
C. Inspiratory variation in transtricuspid inflow >30%
D. End-diastolic pericardial effusion width of >1.5 cm

8. An 85-year-old woman underwent a transapical transcatheter aortic valve replacement (TAVR) for severe symptomatic aortic stenosis. After an uneventful procedure, she is brought to the ICU intubated and sedated. In the 30 minutes after arrival to the ICU she develops progressive tachycardia and hypotension, which prompts the placement of a TEE probe. The mid-esophageal 4-chamber view is shown in the figure that follows.

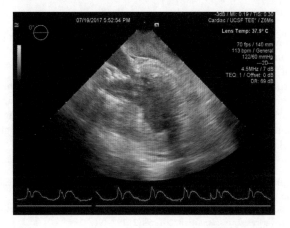

Based on the findings in the image, what is the most appropriate next step in management?

A. Left-sided chest tube placement
B. Emergent surgical pericardial evacuation
C. Pericardial drain placement
D. CT angiography of the chest

9. A 35-year-old woman with no prior medical history presents to your hospital's emergency department with a complaint of dyspnea that started acutely 2 hours ago. She appears moderately distressed and has a room air oxygen saturation of 85%, so you are consulted for possible ICU admission. Bedside cardiac ultrasound reveals grossly normal biventricular size and function. Thoracic ultrasound shows lung sliding and A lines in all fields bilaterally. There is no evidence of B lines, consolidated lung, or pleural effusion. Which of the following ultrasound examinations is most indicated next?

   A. Compression and color Doppler of the femoral and popliteal veins
   B. Focused assessment of the mitral valve with color Doppler
   C. Abdominal ultrasound to assess for the presence of free fluid
   D. Tissue Doppler quantification of diaphragmatic contraction velocity to assess for the risk of imminent respiratory failure

10. Which of the following thoracic ultrasound patterns will most likely be present in severe ARDS?

   A. B lines in all fields
   B. Large hypoechoic spaces in bilateral subpleural regions
   C. Absence of lung sliding anteriorly, with an area of lung sliding moving in and out of the frame through the respiratory cycle
   D. Anterior fields with B lines, posterior fields with ultrasonographically visible lung containing patchy areas of hyperechogenicity

# Chapter 28 ▪ Answers

1. Correct Answer: D

**Rationale:**
Bedside cardiac ultrasound is indicated in critically ill patients when unexplained hypotension is present. If TEE views are not adequate, then a TEE examination is indicated. This patient has unexplained hypotension following liver transplantation despite high doses of vasopressors and has not demonstrated volume responsiveness. Cardiac ultrasound is required to rule out pathology such as right or left ventricular dysfunction, acute valvular disorders, and hemodynamically significant pericardial effusion. Because no transthoracic views could be obtained, transesophageal echocardiography would offer insight into cardiac function.

According to the ASE/SCA Guidelines for Performing a Comprehensive Transesophageal Echocardiographic Examination, the absolute contraindications for TEE probe placement include:
- Perforated viscus
- Esophageal stricture
- Esophageal tumor
- Esophageal perforation, laceration
- Esophageal diverticulum
- Active upper GI bleed

The esophageal diverticulum would represent the absolute contraindication in this patient. The remainder of the patient's pathology falls under relative contraindications. Of note, at many centers transesophageal echocardiography is a standard monitor during liver transplantation, even in patients with nonbleeding esophageal varices. A series of small studies has shown relatively good safety of TEE in patients with varices, though the risk of bleeding is higher than in the general population.

References
1. Dalia AA, Flores A, Chitilian H, Fitzsimons MG. A comprehensive review of transesophageal echocardiography during orthotopic liver transplantation. *J Cardiothorac Vasc Anesth*. 2018;32(4):1815-1824.
2. Burger-Klepp U, Karatosic R, Thum M, et al. Transesophageal echocardiography during orthotopic liver transplantation in patients with esophagoastric varices. *Transplantation*. 2012;94(2):192-196.
3. Spier BJ, Larue SJ, Teelin TC. et al. Review of complications in a series of patients with known gastro-esophageal varices undergoing transesophageal echocardiography. *J Am Soc Echocardiogr*. 2009;22(4):396-400.
4. Hahn RT, Abraham T, Adams MS, et al. Guidelines for performing a comprehensive transesophageal echocardiographic examination: recommendations from the American Society of Echocardiography and the society of cardiovascular anesthesiologists. *J Am Soc Echocardiogr*. 2013;26(9):921-964.

**2.** Correct Answer: C

**Rationale:**

The diastolic picture shows a mid-esophageal long axis view of the left atrium, left ventricle, mitral valve, and aortic valve. The basal septum appears disproportionately thick, but without more information one cannot distinguish between disproportionate upper septal thickening and hypertrophic cardiomyopathy (HCM). In the systolic frame, one can see several abnormalities. The anterior leaflet of the mitral valve has moved into the left ventricular outflow tract (LVOT). A visible space is seen between the anterior and posterior mitral leaflets, which should have a tight coaptation point in systole. The aortic valve, which should be widely open during systole, appears only partially open. Taken together these findings lead to the diagnosis of systolic anterior motion (SAM) of the mitral valve. In SAM, the mitral valve moves into the LVOT during systole, creating an outflow tract obstruction. The force of the blood moving through the LVOT may pull the anterior mitral leaflet away from the posterior leaflet, leading to mitral regurgitation. The interrupted systolic ejection can lead to early aortic valve closure or partial opening in systole.

SAM is most commonly seen in HCM or after mitral valve repair. However, it can also be seen in hyperdynamic or hypovolemic states, when small LV size combined with excessive inotropy can lead to SAM in otherwise normal hearts.

Medical management of SAM hinges around volume loading, reducing inotropy, and increasing peripheral resistance. Therefore, stopping the dobutamine infusion would be the first step of the options provided. Adding epinephrine would likely worsen the SAM through increased inotropy and reduced diastolic filling time. An intra-aortic balloon pump reduces LV afterload and would not be beneficial here. Finally, the aortic valve likely has no pathology and only opens incompletely due to a small stroke volume (SV). Valve replacement is not indicated.

Reference

1. Ibrahim M, Rao C, Ashrafian H, Chaudhry U, Darzi A, Athanasiou T. Modern management of systolic anterior motion of the mitral valve. *Eur J Cardiothorac Surg.* 2012;41(6):1260-1270.

**3.** Correct Answer: C

**Rationale:**

Ultrasound assessment of the retro-hepatic IVC can provide insights into a patient's volume status. The assessment hinges around changes in intrathoracic pressure throughout the respiratory cycle being transmitted to the IVC via the right atrium. As a nonmechanically ventilated patient inhales, pressure in the thorax is reduced. This pressure reduction is transmitted to the thin-walled right atrium and then to the IVC.

Patients who are volume-responsive tend to have low right-sided filling pressures and an IVC that has not reached its maximum distensibility. When the right atrial pressure decreases during inspiration, the IVC luminal pressure decreases relative to the intra-abdominal pressure and the vessel collapses. In patients who are not volume responsive, the right-sided filling pressures are higher relative to the changes in thoracic pressure and the vessel size changes less.

The exact cutoff of IVC diameter change for predicting volume responsiveness is not well defined. Some studies identify >40% to 45% collapse during tidal breathing as a cutoff for volume responsiveness in spontaneously breathing nonventilated patients. However, these studies exclude many patients where the technique is prone to drawing the wrong conclusion. If the intra-abdominal pressure is elevated, as in choice C, then the IVC may collapse even in a patient who would not be volume responsive. This would call the fellow's conclusion into question and makes choice C the correct answer.

Both a hemodynamically significant pneumothorax and pericardial effusion would increase the right atrial pressure without changing the abdominal pressure, leading to a distended IVC even if a patient would indeed be volume responsive. A unilateral DVT would not alter venous return enough to be the correct answer in this case.

References

1. Preau S, Bortolotti P, Colling D, et al. Diagnostic accuracy of the inferior vena cava collapsibility to predict fluid responsiveness in spontaneously breathing patients with sepsis and acute circulatory failure. *Crit Care Med.* 2017;45(3).
2. Muller L, Bobbia X, Toumi M, et al. Respiratory variations of inferior vena cava diameter to predict fluid responsiveness in spontaneously breathing patients with acute circulatory failure: need for a cautious use. *Critical Care.* 2012;16(5):R188.
3. Zhang Z, Xu X, Ye S, Xu L. Ultrasonographic measurement of the respiratory variation in the inferior vena cava diameter is predictive of fluid responsiveness in critically ill patients: systematic review and meta-analysis. *Ultrasound Med Biol.* 2014;40(5):845-853.
4. Zhang J, Critchley LAH. Inferior vena cava ultrasonography before general anesthesia can predict hypotension after induction. *Anesthesiology.* 2016;124(3):580-589.
5. Airapetian N, Maizel J, Alyamani O, et al. Does inferior vena cava respiratory variability predict fluid responsiveness in spontaneously breathing patients? *Critical Care.* 2015;19(1):1-8.

**4. Correct Answer: A**

**Rationale:**

The image in this case demonstrates the utility of cardiac ultrasound in assessing placement of percutaneous left ventricular assist devices. The devices are frequently placed under fluoroscopy in the cardiac catheterization laboratory, but fluoroscopy is rarely available in the ICU.

A parasternal long axis view shows the Impella crossing the aortic valve and entering the LV. The device draws blood from the LV inflow port and pumps it into the aortic root via the outflow port. The inflow port should be positioned 3.5 to 4 cm beyond the aortic valve. Thus, in this case, the device should be advanced by 1.5 cm. It is important that the pigtail portion of the device is not included in the measurement.

If the device is pulled back into the aorta too far, both the inflow and outflow ports will be on the same side of the aortic valve and the device will not provide hemodynamic support. Additionally, turbulence from the aortic valve interfering with blood inflow can lead to hemolysis.

If the device is advanced too far into the LV, the papillary muscles and aortic valve can interfere with inflow and outflow, respectively, leading to hemolysis. The pigtail can tangle with the mitral apparatus, leading to worsening mitral regurgitation.

### Reference

1. Stainback RF, Estep JD, Agler DA, et al. Echocardiography in the management of patients with left ventricular assist devices: recommendations from the American Society of Echocardiography. *J Am Soc Echocardiogr.* 2015;28(8):853-909.

**5. Correct Answer: B**

**Rationale:**

Cardiac ultrasound provides an opportunity to estimate cardiac output in a noninvasive manner. This can be a useful tool in the assessment of undifferentiated shock and correlates very well with thermodilution cardiac output measurements by PA catheter. The technique involves obtaining the velocity time integral (VTI) at the LVOT. When pulsed-wave Doppler is applied to a specific area of blood flow, a tracing is produced that has velocity of blood flow on the y-axis and time on the x-axis, as shown in the image below. This is the blood flow velocity versus time at that specific location, in this case the LVOT. When the integral (area under the curve) of that tracing is obtained for a single systolic period, the result is a specific distance. This is the distance that a disc that has the cross sectional area of the LVOT travels in systole. Thus, we end up with a 2D area of the LVOT and a height, allowing us to calculate the LV SV. The LVOT area is calculated by measuring the diameter in the parasternal long axis (transthoracic echocardiogram) or mid esophageal long axis (TEE). Assuming there is no aortic regurgitation, the SV calculated here multiplied by the heart rate provides us the cardiac output.

$$\text{LVOT Area} = (\text{LVOT diameter}/2)^2 \times 3.14$$

$$\text{SV} = \text{LVOT VTI} \times \text{LVOT Area}$$

$$\text{CO} = \text{HR} \times \text{SV}$$

To accurately measure the LVOT VTI, we must align the probe with the direction of blood flow. In typical hearts, this is best done in the apical 5-chamber view (transthoracic echocardiogram) and the deep transgastric 5-chamber view (TEE), making B the correct answer here. In the other answer choices, the Doppler beam will not align with the direction of blood flow and therefore the VTI will be underestimated.

### Reference

1. Mercado P, Maizel J, Beyls C, et al. Transthoracic echocardiography: an accurate and precise method for estimating cardiac output in the critically ill patient. *Critical Care.* 2017;21:136.

**6. Correct Answer: D**

**Rationale:**

This ultrasound image shows a dilated RV and an interventricular septum that is shifted toward the left ventricle. Acute RV failure from pressure overload is associated with a dilated and septal shifting toward the LV. In a short-axis view, this results in the LV forming a "D" shape.

In this patient with cardiogenic shock, a history of mitral valve replacement, and a dilated, hypokinetic RV, the two most likely differential diagnoses are pulmonary embolism and mitral stenosis. The PE was ruled out by the CT chest already. To investigate the gradient across the mitral valve, continuous-wave Doppler should be placed across the valve, making D the correct answer. In mitral stenosis, the pressure gradient across the stenotic valve will result in high velocity flow through the valve. In severe mitral stenosis, the elevated left atrial pressures result in postcapillary pulmonary hypertension that can result in right-sided heart failure.

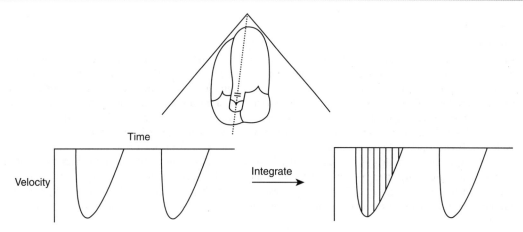

Demonstration of lower-extremity venous thrombus would not be useful after a PE has already been ruled out. Color Doppler of the main PA would likely not show any abnormality, even if a PE were present. The IVC will likely be plethoric, but again will not tell us the specific diagnosis.

**Reference**

1. Zoghbi WA, Chambers JB, Dumesnil JG, et al. Recommendations for evaluation of prosthetic valves with echocardiography and doppler ultrasound. *J Am Soc Echocardiogr.* 2009;22(9):975-1014.

---

**7.** Correct Answer: B

**Rationale:**

Cardiac ultrasound is extremely sensitive for the detection of pericardial effusions. It is also useful for determining the hemodynamic significance of pericardial effusions. In the setting of a pericardial effusion, signs of cardiac tamponade include IVC dilation, RA and RV diastolic collapse, elevated respiratory variation in trans-mitral and trans-tricuspid inflow, and septal "bounce." Of these, RA collapse in greater than one-third of the cardiac cycle is the most sensitive and specific for cardiac tamponade, making it the correct answer in this case.

Collapse of a cardiac chamber in tamponade occurs when the pericardial pressure exceeds the pressure in that chamber. As pericardial pressure increases, the right atrium will collapse first in early diastole. The longer the chamber remains collapsed, the longer the pericardial pressure exceeds the atrial pressure and the worse the tamponade.

The IVC will generally be plethoric in tamponade, but this can also be seen in other cardiac pathologies and is not specific to tamponade. The same applies to inspiratory variation in AV valve inflow. The size of the pericardial effusion correlates poorly with hemodynamic significance. A large pericardial effusion does not necessarily indicate tamponade.

**Reference**

1. Klein AL, Abbara S, Agler DA, et al. American Society of Echocardiography clinical recommendations for multimodality cardiovascular imaging of patients with pericardial disease: endorsed by the Society for Cardiovascular Magnetic Resonance and Society of Cardiovascular Computed Tomography. *J Am Soc Echocardiogr.* 2013;26(9):965-1012.e15.

---

**8.** Correct Answer: B

**Rationale:**

The image above shows a focal pericardial fluid collection adjacent to the left atrium. The fluid collection clearly distorts the left atrial anatomy and is responsible for the hypotension in this case. This is a good example of focal tamponade that can occur after cardiac surgery. That patient population tends not to have the classic hypoechoic and free-flowing pericardial effusion seen in classic tamponade, instead showing localized areas of semi-thrombosed blood products that impinge on specific cardiac chambers. Note the swirling echogenicity within the fluid collection here that is typical of static blood products.

The most common cause of pericardial bleeding after TAVR is RV perforation. However, aortic root rupture or LA/LV bleeding is possible and should be considered in surgical planning for this case.

The correct management here is surgical evacuation of the fluid collection. The posterior and lateral location of the fluid collection precludes percutaneous drainage. Because the fluid is pericardial and not pleural, chest tube placement would not be appropriate.

**Reference**

1. Fassa A, Himbert D, Vahanian A. Mechanisms and management of TAVR-related complications. *Nat Rev Cardiol.* 2013;10:685.

**9.** Correct Answer: A

**Rationale:**

Thoracic ultrasound provides a tool for the rapid assessment of patients with acute dyspnea. Lichtenstein and colleagues proposed an algorithmic diagnostic approach to respiratory failure. The first step is to look for lung sliding bilaterally. If present, lung sliding essentially rules out a pneumothorax. Then, evidence of interstitial or alveolar edema in the form of B lines is sought. If there is no evidence of pneumothorax, pulmonary edema, consolidation, or pleural effusion on lung ultrasound, the next differential to consider is pulmonary embolism. The next step in this case would be to look for venous thrombosis. If venous thrombus is demonstrated, then pulmonary embolism is very likely. An absence of DVT, however, does not rule out pulmonary embolism and further studies must be pursued.

Mitral regurgitation, which would be seen on color Doppler assessment, would result in pulmonary edema and B lines on imaging, which were absent on the examination. Abdominal fluid would not explain her acute dyspnea in the absence of other symptoms. Tissue Doppler assessment of diaphragmatic contraction velocity has been preliminarily investigated to predict ventilator weaning failure but has not been validated in the assessment of acute dyspnea.

### References

1. Lichtenstein DA, Mezière GA. Relevance of lung ultrasound in the diagnosis of acute respiratory failure. *Chest.* 2008;134(1):117-125.
2. Lichtenstein D. Novel approaches to ultrasonography of the lung and pleural space: where are we now? *Breathe.* 2017;13(2):100-111.

**10.** Correct Answer: D

**Rationale:**

Cross-sectional CT imaging of the noncardiogenic pulmonary edema seen in ARDS tends to show ground-glass opacities in the anterior (nondependent) lung fields and consolidation in the posterior (dependent) fields. On ultrasound examination, this presents as B lines in the areas containing interstitial edema and the appearance of consolidated lung in the dependent fields.

Consolidated lung on ultrasound will have a variable appearance depending on the pathophysiology. The first principle to remember is that normal lung is never ultrasonically visible. If lung can be "imaged" on ultrasound, then the alveoli are no longer gas filled. In the dense atelectasis that accompanies pleural effusions, the lung has a fine-textured uniform hypoechoic appearance similar to that of liver and spleen. The fluid-filled alveoli in pneumonia and ARDS create a different appearance on ultrasound. A hallmark of ARDS is the significant heterogeneity in consolidation density and aeration between lung units. This leads to areas of hypoechoic lung immediately adjacent to areas of better-aerated lung or bronchus, which will appear hyperechoic. The borders between these areas tend to be irregular and jagged, so the presence of a jagged interface between consolidated and aerated lung is known as the "shred sign."

Of the answer choices above, diffuse B lines without evidence of consolidation is more compatible with cardiogenic pulmonary edema. Large hypoechoic spaces subpleurally is consistent with pleural effusions. Answer choice C describes "lung point," which is a specific finding in pneumothorax. This is the ultrasound appearance of lung sliding (due to apposed visceral and parietal pleura) moving into and out of the imaged area of pneumothorax (lack of lung sliding) through the respiratory cycle.

### References

1. Copetti R, Soldati G, Copetti P. Chest sonography: a useful tool to differentiate acute cardiogenic pulmonary edema from acute respiratory distress syndrome. *Cardiovascular Ultrasound.* 2008;6(1):16.
2. Sekiguchi H, Schenck LA, Horie R, et al. Critical care ultrasonography differentiates ARDS, pulmonary edema, and other causes in the early course of acute hypoxemic respiratory failure. *Chest.* 2015;148(4):912-918.
3. Volpicelli G. Sonographic diagnosis of pneumothorax. *Intensive Care Med.* 2011;37(2):224-232.

# 29

# MANAGEMENT STRATEGIES (COAGULATION, VASOACTIVE MEDICATIONS)

Christoph G. S. Nabzdyk and Yvonne Lai

1. A 67-year-old male patient had a non-ST elevation myocardial infarction and is currently on a heparin drip and requires coronary artery bypass grafting. His baseline activated coagulation time (ACT) is 189 seconds. He is 78 kg and received a total of 28 000 units of heparin (350 Units/kg). Three minutes later, a second ACT is drawn and repeat ACT is 286 seconds. Another 10 000 units of heparin is administered, and targeted ACT is still not achieved. You suspect heparin resistance. What is NOT a predictor for heparin resistance?

   A. Antithrombin activity level
   B. Disseminated intravascular coagulation
   C. Prior heparin therapy
   D. Sepsis
   E. Factor IIa level

2. A 58-year-old female with diverticulitis developed free air and required intensive care unit admission. In the intensive care unit, she went into persistent atrial fibrillation and the team decided to start her on a heparin drip for stroke prevention. Her preoperative platelet count was 343 000/μL, and on hospital day 5, her platelet count is 86 000/μL. You suspect heparin-induced thrombocytopenia (HIT) but still need to provide anticoagulation. What is NOT an appropriate drug to administer?

   A. Argatroban
   B. Bivalirudin
   C. Enoxaparin
   D. Desirudin
   E. Hirudin

3. A 29-year-old male is hypotensive in the emergency department after a motor vehicle accident 2 hours ago despite fluid resuscitation. You suspect intra-abdominal hemorrhage and have heard that tranexamic acid may reduce mortality and death from hemorrhage. You decide to administer tranexamic acid knowing the possible complications from it. How is tranexamic acid metabolized?

   A. Renal
   B. Liver
   C. Lungs
   D. Plasma esterases
   E. CYP 450

4. A 68-year-old female in the intensive care unit on total parenteral nutrition due to ileus from recent abdominal surgery now has an ST-elevation myocardial infarction and was emergently taken to the cardiac catheterization laboratory. The cardiology team performs percutaneous coronary intervention in one of her coronary arteries and recommends continuation of antiplatelet agents. Because she cannot tolerate oral aspirin currently, which other medication can be used?

   A. Prasugrel
   B. Ticagrelor
   C. Cangrelor
   D. Clopidogrel
   E. Argatroban

5. You have decided to place a patient with a history of HIT on a bivalirudin infusion for anticoagulation. Which laboratory value shown below should you be able to monitor?

   A. Activated partial thromboplastin time (PTT)
   B. Prothrombin time (PT)
   C. Fibrinogen
   D. Anti-Xa
   E. Platelets

6. A 52-year-old male with a history of hypertrophic cardiomyopathy is nil per oral for right heart catheterization procedure. The patient is lightly sedated and the cardiology team obtains these numbers:

| | |
|---|---|
| Blood pressure | 80/42/55 mm Hg |
| Pulmonary capillary wedge pressure | 10 mm Hg |
| Pulmonary artery pressure | 28/10 mm Hg |
| Central venous pressure | 6 mm Hg |
| Cardiac output | 5.5 L/min |

   Based on the systemic vascular resistance and the rest of his numbers, what would be the best choice of vasopressor for this patient?

   A. Epinephrine
   B. Norepinephrine
   C. Phenylephrine
   D. Dobutamine
   E. Dopamine

7. A 43-year-old female presenting with urosepsis has persistent hypotension despite fluid resuscitation. You do a bedside echocardiogram on the patient showing normal biventricular function and measure an inferior vena cava size of 2.1 cm with minimal respiratory variation. Her blood pressure is 92/43 mm Hg on norepinephrine 30 µg/min, and you decide to add vasopressin 0.04 Units/min. What is the receptor that you are targeting by adding vasopressin?

   A. V1
   B. V2
   C. V3
   D. Alpha-1
   E. D2

8. A 56-year-old male with liver cirrhosis and hypertension (on angiotensin-converting enzyme inhibitors) presents to the intensive care unit postoperatively after a Whipple for pancreatic cancer. You note that he is on norepinephrine 30 µg/min, vasopressin 0.04 Units/min, and epinephrine 2 µg/min to maintain a mean arterial pressure of 58 mm Hg and heart rate 99 beats/min. His arterial line shows no pulse pressure variation. You do a bedside echocardiogram which shows hyperdynamic left ventricular function and measures inferior vena cava of 1.9 cm with <50% collapse. You want to add another agent to support his blood pressure to avoid kidney injury. Which among the following is the best medication to add?

   A. Milrinone
   B. Methylene blue
   C. Dopamine
   D. Isoproterenol
   E. Dobutamine

9. A 72-year-old female who is postoperative day 3 from a small bowel resection and is unable to take oral medications yet because of high nasogastric tube output. She is hypertensive, controlled on a nitroglycerin drip for a day now. What is the LEAST likely side effect of long-term nitroglycerin exposure?

   A. Headaches
   B. Tachycardia
   C. Cyanide toxicity
   D. Platelet aggregation
   E. Methemoglobinemia

10. A 69-year-old male is admitted to intensive care unit after four-vessel coronary artery bypass grafting for hemodynamic management. Upon awakening, he is hypertensive, has a central venous pressure of 12 mm Hg, and you start him on a nitroglycerin drip to maintain normotension. He then suddenly coughs and you notice 200 mL of blood in one of the chest tubes. He becomes hypotensive, and you stop the nitroglycerin drip. As this episode continues to develop, you see his central venous pressure is now 23 mm Hg and you need to start norepinephrine for hypotension. You suspect tamponade and perform a bedside echocardiogram. Which of the following is a specific sign for tamponade?

   A. Right atrial collapse
   B. Inferior vena cava plethora
   C. Pulsus paradoxus
   D. Diastolic collapse of right ventricle
   E. Tachycardia

# Chapter 29 ▪ Answers

1. Correct Answer: E

   **Rationale:**
   Heparin resistance is observed when large doses of heparin are required to achieve therapeutic prothrombin time (or ACT) despite an adequate heparin concentration. Some studies have shown that the incidence of heparin resistance before coronary revascularization is anywhere from 21% to 26%. Some of the predictors of heparin resistance include antithrombin activity level, platelet count, age, and prior heparin therapy. Many other clinical conditions are also associated with heparin resistance including sepsis, disseminated intravascular coagulation, liver disease, and elevated fibrinogen levels. On many occasions, a larger dose of heparin is sufficient to achieve adequate anticoagulation. If not, heparin resistance can be overcome by administering antithrombin 3, either by giving fresh frozen plasma or recombinant antithrombin 3.

   Reference
   1. *Kaplan's Cardiac Anesthesia.* 7th ed. Elsevier; 2016.

**2.** Correct Answer: C

**Rationale:**

HIT is a condition that develops after exposure to heparin (both unfractionated or low molecular weight heparin such as enoxaparin) and occurs in 5% to 28% of patients receiving heparin. Type 1 HIT is characterized by a mild decrease in platelet count that occurs within 2 days of exposure and is due to the platelet aggregation which is not clinically significant and not associated with thrombosis. Type 2 HIT usually occurs after more than 5 days of heparin administration (average time onset is 9 days). It is immune mediated, and antibodies bind to the heparin and platelet factor 4 complex to cause endothelial injury and complement activation. These antibody complexes can cause thrombosis and thrombocytopenia; the incidence of thrombotic complications can be 20% with a mortality rate as high as 40%. Diagnosis of HIT can be confirmed through a heparin-induced serotonin release assay or a heparin-induced platelet activation assay.

References

1. *Kaplan's Cardiac Anesthesia.* 7th ed. Elsevier; 2016.
2. Arepally GM. Heparin-induced thrombocytopenia. *Blood.* 2017;129:2864.

**3.** Correct Answer: A

**Rationale:**

Antifibrinolytics (aminocaproic acid, tranexamic acid, and aprotinin) inhibit fibrinolysis by binding to the plasminogen and inhibiting the formation of plasmin and displacing plasmin from fibrin. The CRASH-2 trial demonstrated that the tranexamic acid group had lower mortality and death from hemorrhage, with no differences in vascular occlusion complications. Tranexamic acid was further evaluated in the ATACAS trial in cardiac surgery which showed no difference in rate of thrombotic complications (myocardial infarction, stroke, pulmonary embolism, renal failure, or bowel infarction). Tranexamic acid is metabolized by the kidneys, and there is concern for a higher risk of seizures among patients with renal failure receiving tranexamic acid.

References

1. Levy JH, Koster A, Quinones QJ, Milling TJ, Key NS. Antifibrinolytic therapy and perioperative considerations. *Anesthesiology.* 2018;128(3):657-670
2. CRASH-2 trial collaborators; Shakur H, Roberts I, Bautista R, et al. Effects of tranexamic acid on death, vascular occlusive events, and blood transfusion in trauma patients with significant haemorrhage (CRASH-2): a randomised, placebo-controlled trial. *Lancet.* 2010;376:23.
3. Myles PS, Smith JA, Forbes A, et al. Tranexamic acid in patients undergoing coronary-artery surgery. *N Engl J Med.* 2017;376:136.

**4.** Correct Answer: C

**Rationale:**

The pathway for clot formation after percutaneous coronary intervention is primarily platelet mediated. Aspirin works by blocking platelet activation through irreversible acetylation of cyclooxygenase. The thienopyridines (ticlopidine, clopidogrel, and prasugrel), which are all oral drugs, bind to adenosine diphosphate (ADP) receptors. The GPIIb/IIIa receptor inhibitors are available in intravenous formulary (abciximab, eptifibatide, tirofiban, and cangrelor) making it useful when oral route of administration is not possible.

**Antiplatelet Therapy**

| DRUG TYPE | COMPOSITION | MECHANISM | INDICATIONS | ROUTE | HALF-LIFE | METABOLISM |
|---|---|---|---|---|---|---|
| Aspirin | Acetylsalicylic acid | Irreversible COX inhibition | CAD, AMI, PVD, PCI, ACS | Oral | 10 d | Liver, kidney |
| NSAIDs | Multiple | Reversible COX inhibition | Pain | Oral | 2 d | Liver, kidney |
| Adhesion inhibitors (e.g., dipyridamole) | Multiple | Block adhesion to vessels | VHD, PVD | Oral | 12 hr | Liver |
| ADP receptor antagonists (e.g., clopidogrel) | Thienopyridines | Irreversible inhibition of ADP binding | AMI, CVA, PVD, ACS, PCI | Oral | 5 d | Liver |

| DRUG TYPE | COMPOSITION | MECHANISM | INDICATIONS | ROUTE | HALF-LIFE | METABOLISM |
|---|---|---|---|---|---|---|
| GPIIb/IIIa receptor inhibitors; | | | | | | |
| Abciximab (ReoPro) | Monoclonal antibody | Nonspecific—binds to other receptors | PCI, ACS | IV | 12–18 hr | Plasma proteinase |
| Eptifibatide (Integrilin) | Peptide | Reversible—specific to GPIIb/IIIa | PCI, ACS | IV | 2–4 hr | Kidney |
| Tirofiban (Aggrastat) | Nonpeptide tyrosine derivative | Reversible—specific to GPIIb/IIIa | PCI, ACS | IV | 2–4 hr | Kidney |

ACS, acute coronary syndrome; AMI, acute myocardial infarction; CAD, coronary artery disease; COX, cyclooxygenase; CVA, cerebrovascular disease; IV, intravenous; NSAID, nonsteroidal anti-inflammatory drug; PCI, percutaneous coronary intervention; PVD, peripheral vascular disease; VHD, valvular heart disease.
Table from Kaplan's Cardiac Anesthesia. 7th ed. Elsevier; 2016.

### Reference

1. *Kaplan's Cardiac Anesthesia.* 7th ed. Elsevier; 2016.

---

**5.** Correct Answer: A

**Rationale:**

Direct thrombin inhibitors act by inhibiting factor IIa (thrombin) independently of antithrombin 3 or cofactors. These anticoagulant drugs are useful in patients with HIT, but the lack of an antidote and a prolonged duration of action are barriers to the drugs being more widely used. Intravenous direct thrombin inhibitors include bivalrudin, desirudin, hirudin, and argatroban. Dabigatran is an oral direct thrombin inhibitor. Activated PTT is the laboratory method of choice for monitoring, which measures both intrinsic and common coagulation pathways. Of note, the presence of antiphospholipid antibodies can prolong aPTT.

### References

1. Di Nisio M, Middeldorp S, Büller HR. Direct thrombin inhibitors. *N Engl J Med.* 2005;353:1028.
2. Warkentin TE, Greinacher A, Koster A. Bivalirudin. *Thromb Haemost.* 2008;99:830.
3. *Kaplan's Cardiac Anesthesia.* 7th ed. Elsevier; 2016.

---

**6.** Correct Answer: C

**Rationale:**
Systemic vascular resistance (SVR) is calculated by

$$SVR = MAP - CVP CO \times \wr$$

Normal value of 800 to 1200 dynes/sec/cm$^5$. Since this patient's calculated SVR is 740 dynes/sec/cm$^5$ in addition to his history of hypertrophic cardiomyopathy, the best vasopressor to use is phenylephrine (pure alpha agonist), which would increase SVR and reflexively decrease heart rate (beneficial for someone with hypertrophic cardiomyopathy).

### Reference

1. Gregory JS, Bonfiglio MF, Dasta JF, et al. Experience with phenylephrine as a component of the pharmacologic support of septic shock. *Crit Care Med.* 1991;19:1395.

---

**7.** Correct Answer: A

**Rationale:**
Vasopressin is formed in the hypothalamus and released from the pituitary. The primary function of vasopressin is to regulate extracellular fluid volume, but it is also a potent vasoconstrictor. There are three different types of vasopressin receptors. V1 is a receptor located in vascular smooth muscles that couples to a G protein to cause vasoconstriction. V2 receptor is located in the renal collecting duct to increase water reabsorption in the kidneys and forming a more concentrated urine through adenylyl cyclase. V3 receptor is located in the anterior pituitary gland that also couples to a G protein to release adrenocorticotropic hormone. It has been demonstrated that vasopressin has systemic vasoconstriction effects with minimal effect on pulmonary vascular resistance and thus does not increase right ventricular afterload.

References

1. Currigan DA, Hughes RJ, Wright CE, et al. Vasoconstrictor responses to vasopressor agents in human pulmonary and radial arteries: an in vitro study. *Anesthesiology*. 2014;121(5):930-936. doi:10.1097/ALN.0000000000000430.

2. Gordon AC, Mason AJ, Thirunavukkarasu N, et al. Effect of early vasopressin vs norepinephrine on kidney failure in patients with septic shock: the VANISH randomized clinical trial. *JAMA*. 2016;316:509.

## 8. Correct Answer: B

**Rationale:**

Methylene blue can be used as a rescue treatment for profound vasodilatory shock in the setting of normal cardiac function. It inhibits guanylate cyclase and the production of cyclic guanosine monophosphate, which reduces a vessel's response to nitric oxide and thus decreases smooth muscle relaxation. Methylene blue causes discoloration of urine and may interfere with pulse oximetry measurements. In this scenario, the patient has both liver dysfunction and use of an angiotensin-converting enzyme inhibitor that predisposes him to vasodilatory shock. Given his adequate cardiac function, he needs another agent to improve his systemic vascular resistance and methylene blue is a good choice. Milrinone, dobutamine, and isoproterenol decrease systemic vascular resistance and may cause hypotension. Dopamine may worsen tachycardia and thus not preferred.

References

1. Hosseinian L, Weiner M, Levin MA, Fischer GW. Methylene blue: magic bullet for vasoplegia? *Anesth Analg*. 2016;122(1):194-201. doi:10.1213/ANE.0000000000001045.

2. Booth AT, Melmer PD, Tribble B, Mehaffey JH, Tribble C. Methylene blue for vasoplegic syndrome. *Heart Surg Forum*. 2017;20(5):E234-E238. doi:10.1532/hsf.1806.

## 9. Correct Answer: C

**Rationale:**

Nitroglycerin is a parenteral nitrovasodilator drug that provides nitric oxide to induce vasodilation via the cyclic GMP pathway. Nitroglycerin provides relatively higher venodilation than arteriolar dilation as opposed to nitroprusside, which provides more arteriolar dilation. Headaches are a common side effect because of direct vasodilation; tachycardia usually results from reflex sympathetic activation. Nitroglycerin is metabolized by liver nitrate reductase, which produces a nitrite that oxidizes the ferrous iron of hemoglobin to methemoglobin. Nitroglycerin can also affect platelet aggregation by reducing the ability of platelets to adhere to damaged intima. Nitroprusside can cause cyanide toxicity, not nitroglycerin.

References

1. Kaplan K, Davison R. Nitroglycerin and methemoglobinemia. *Am J Cardiol*. 1986;57(11):1004.

2. Stamler JS, Loscalzo J. The antiplatelet effects of organic nitrates and related nitroso compounds in vitro and in vivo and their relevance to cardiovascular disorders. *J Am Coll Cardiol*. 1991;18:1529.

3. *Kaplan's Cardiac Anesthesia*. 7th ed. Elsevier; 2016.

## 10. Correct Answer: D

**Rationale:**

Specific signs of tamponade include electrical alternans, diastolic collapse of right ventricle, and left atrial collapse. Sensitive signs for tamponade include right atrial collapse, inferior vena cava plethora, and pulsus paradoxus. Right atrial collapse can occur in either tamponade or severe hypovolemia. Right atrial collapse for more than one-third of cardiac cycle is highly sensitive and specific for tamponade. Right ventricular diastolic collapse may not occur if right ventricle is hypertrophied (such as in pulmonary hypertension) or if diastolic pressure is greatly elevated.

References

1. Leimgruber PP, Klopfenstein HS, Wann LS, Brooks HL. The hemodynamic derangement associated with right ventricular diastolic collapse in cardiac tamponade: an experimental echocardiographic study. *Circulation*. 1983;68(3):612.

2. Kerber RE, Gascho JA, Litchfield R, Wolfson P, Ott D, Pandian NG. Hemodynamic effects of volume expansion and nitroprusside compared with pericardiocentesis in patients with acute cardiac tamponade. *N Engl J Med*. 1982;307(15):929.

# PULMONARY
# DISORDERS

# 30

# RESPIRATORY FAILURE

Jeffrey Gotts

1. A 40-year-old previously healthy 90-kg man (ideal body weight of 80 kg) walks into the Emergency Department (ED) complaining of 5 days of myalgias, fevers, rhinorrhea, and dry cough. Over the last day, he has become short of breath walking across the room. In the ED, he is febrile, hypotensive requiring vasopressors, with a respiratory rate of 30 and $SpO_2$ 88% on a non-rebreather face mask. He receives 30 mL/kg crystalloid and develops worsening work of breathing requiring endotracheal intubation 2 hours after arrival in ED. Endotracheal tube placement is confirmed by end-tidal $CO_2$ and bilateral breath sounds. His $SpO_2$ nadir is 75% but despite 5 minutes of bagging his $SpO_2$ remains in the mid-80s. His chest X-ray is shown below.

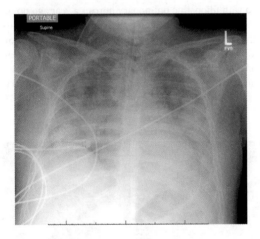

Which of the following statements is true?

A. Following ARDSnet ventilation at 6 mL/kg, if his Plateau airway pressure is 35 cm $H_2O$ on PEEP of 14, his goal tidal volume should be 480 mL
B. Given hypotension and severe respiratory failure, a PA catheter should be placed to optimize cardiac filling pressures and improve his chances of survival
C. A strategy of doing a recruitment maneuver followed by lowering PEEP until lung compliance is maximal will improve his chances of survival
D. Inhaled nitric oxide is likely to improve his $PaO_2$/$FiO_2$ ratio
E. Proning this early in ARDS has not been shown to favorably affect survival

**2.** A 52-year-old woman with a history of DVT on warfarin and active smoker develops several days of epigastric pain and melena and presents to the ED with a hemoglobin of 5.5 and tachycardia without hypotension, INR of 3.9, and a platelet count of 215,000/ μL. Following transfusion of 2 units PRBCs and 2 units FFP, she develops rapidly progressive acute hypoxemic respiratory failure and increased work of breathing requiring intubation, with CXR new confirming bilateral infiltrates. Which of the following statements is true of the most likely etiology for her respiratory decompensation?

   **A.** Risk factors include smoking and chronic alcohol use
   **B.** PRBCs, FFP, and platelets all confer equal risk of this process
   **C.** The incidence of this process has decreased dramatically in the last decade
   **D.** Neutrophils are not thought to play an important role in this process
   **E.** A diagnosis of transfusion-related acute lung injury (TRALI) can be made in patients with multiple risk factors for ARDS (eg, aspiration, shock, pneumonia)

**3.** A 53-year-old man with a history of mild asthma and alcoholic cirrhosis complicated by ascites (controlled with diuretics) presents to the ED with shoulder pain after a mechanical fall. Musculoskeletal examination and plain films yield a diagnosis of an acute acromioclavicular joint injury. Vitals obtained in the ED are notable for SpO$_2$ of 91% on RA. He uses albuterol MDI about once a week, denies dyspnea, and has no new pulmonary symptom. His lung examination is notable for subtle prolongation of the expiratory phase without wheezes and chest X-ray is clear. Which is true of the likely etiology for hypoxemia?

   **A.** Spider nevi are infrequently seen
   **B.** SpO$_2$ tends to drop further in the supine position
   **C.** Contrast echocardiography is the test of choice
   **D.** Asthma is a major contributor
   **E.** It is never an indication for liver transplantation

**4.** A 65-year-old man diagnosed with idiopathic pulmonary fibrosis a year ago not on supplemental oxygen therapy presents to the ED with a week and a half of worsening exercise tolerance, increased dry cough, myalgias, and subjective fevers. Over the last day he has been unable to walk across the room without resting. Physical examination is remarkable for SpO$_2$ of 85% on 6 L NC with tachypnea and increased work of breathing, bibasilar crackles. Laboratory test results reveal WBC 10,000/ μL (slightly increased absolute neutrophil count), normal metabolic panel and liver function tests, troponin of 0.1 ng/mL, and BNP of 120 pg/mL. Rapid flu is negative, and PCR panel is pending. CXR shows worsening bilateral opacities, and results of CT scan are shown in the figure that follows.

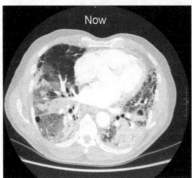 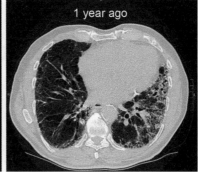

The patient is admitted to the ICU and placed on high flow nasal cannula at 40 LPM flow. Overnight FiO$_2$ has ranged between 0.7 and 0.9 to maintain SpO$_2$ in the low 90s, and he was unable to sleep because of dyspnea. On examination he appears to be tiring.

Which of the following statements is true?

   **A.** Intubation and mechanical ventilation in this setting are associated with in-hospital mortality approaching 90%
   **B.** The use of corticosteroids is supported by moderate- to high-quality trial data
   **C.** If metapneumovirus nucleic acid is detected in respiratory secretions, then it is not appropriate to diagnose "Acute exacerbation of IPF" (AE-IPF)
   **D.** Risk factors for AE-IPF include low BMI
   **E.** Lung biopsy would be most likely to show organizing pneumonia

**5.** A 60-year-old thin female smoker presents to the ED with several days of worsening dyspnea, productive cough, and high fevers. She remains hypotensive despite fluid resuscitation and develops worsening hypoxemia/ARDS requiring intubation and mechanical ventilation. A central line is placed in the right internal jugular vein for vasopressor administration, and she is admitted to the ICU and placed on low tidal volume ventilation protocol using the high PEEP/FiO$_2$ grid studied in the ALVEOLI trial. Twenty-four hours later admission blood cultures are positive for *Streptococcus pneumonia* and her respiratory status has continued to deteriorate, now on 6 mL/kg IBW with FIO$_2$ of 0.8 and PEEP of 20 cm H$_2$O with plateau pressure of 29 cm H$_2$O. ScVO2 is 75% while on moderate dose of norepinephrine and ABG is 7.32/40/65. Using volumetric capnography you measure dead space to be 75%. Several hours later she desaturates, and the FiO$_2$ is raised to 1.0 with PEEP 24 cm H$_2$O. Because making the ventilator change she has worsening hypotension and SpO$_2$ remains in the low 90s. SCVO2 is remeasured at 55% and repeat ABG is 7.24/48/59 with no change in minute ventilation from the prior ABG. In another 10 minutes, SpO$_2$ drops to the low 80s and you are adding a second vasopressor.

Which of the following should you do next?

**A.** Increase the PEEP
**B.** Start inhaled nitric oxide
**C.** Order urgent echocardiogram
**D.** PE protocol chest CT
**E.** Transiently disconnect the patient from the ventilator

**6.** Which of the following is not true of mortality in ARDS?

**A.** It has declined significantly over the last 15 years
**B.** It is associated with very low PaO$_2$/FiO$_2$
**C.** It is associated with high dead space (Vd/Vt)
**D.** It is higher in patients under age 60
**E.** It is higher in patients with kidney or liver dysfunction

**7.** A 45-year-old man with morbid obesity (BMI 55) presents to the ED at 6 AM with right leg pain, and cellulitis that has kept him awake all night. He is admitted to the ward and his fevers and skin examination are improved with antibiotics during the first 16 hours of hospitalization. At 2 AM you are called to evaluate the patient for ICU admission because of somnolence and hypoxemia (SpO$_2$ falling to high 70s on 2LNC). The rapid response team had difficulty waking the patient and ABG was performed before your arrival in the patient's room: 7.29/74/52. Following arterial puncture, the patient woke up and by your arrival he is able to converse but remains sleepy with eyes closed, denying dyspnea, with SpO$_2$ now 92% on 2LNC, and normal work of breathing. Medication history was reviewed and no opiates have been administered. The ward team is requesting ICU transfer because of acute hypercarbic respiratory failure and initiation of BiPAP. You review recent laboratory test results and note that serum bicarbonate has been 38 to 40 over the last 6 months.

Which of the following statements is true:

**A.** Obstructive sleep apnea (OSA) must be present
**B.** In this patient the PaCO$_2$ of 74 is likely to be a major cause of somnolence
**C.** Acetazolamide should be administered to increase his drive to breathe
**D.** The prevalence of Obesity Hypoventilation Syndrome (OHS) in patients with BMI >50 is as high as 50%
**E.** Narcan should be administered

**8.** A 24-year-old man with a history of severe asthma with multiple intubations presents to the ED with several days of worsening dyspnea despite the frequent use of albuterol nebs. The same morning, he visited a friend who has a cat and his dyspnea rapidly worsened. CXR shows hyperinflation and the ED physician gives solumedrol, continuous albuterol nebs, and initiates critical care consultation because of persistent accessory muscle use after an hour of care in the ED. Which of the following statements about severe asthma exacerbations is correct?

**A.** Peak expiratory flow (PEF) is predictive of arterial oxygen saturation
**B.** Intravenous magnesium is not recommended
**C.** The use of heliox (helium-oxygen mixtures) is well supported in the literature
**D.** Following intubation, the respiratory rate should be set 14 to 20 breaths/min
**E.** Increasing extrinsic PEEP may help improve breath triggering during the resolution phase

9. A 60-year-old man with very severe emphysema who is noncompliant with prescribed home oxygen therapy presents to the ED with a bleeding traumatic laceration on his foot. Triage vitals reveal T 36 C, HR 90, BP 120/50, RR 18, $SpO_2$ 71% RA. On further questioning he complains of chronic dyspnea on exertion but does not feel any worse than normal. Laboratory test results are notable for a hematocrit of 60%. Supplemental oxygen with a non-rebreathing mask is administered with $O_2$ sat quickly rising to 100%. Given the high acuity and census in the ED he is placed in the hallway to await physician evaluation and suturing. Thirty minutes later the patient is noted by the nurse to be unarousable, ABG 7.05/130/140 with bicarb 45. Which of the following statements is true?

   A. The mechanism of somnolence in acute hypercapnia is decreased cerebral blood flow
   B. Narcan is likely to be effective in restoring consciousness
   C. The Haldane effect is partially to blame
   D. Acetazolamide should be prescribed at discharge
   E. The acute increase in $PaCO_2$ is due almost entirely to reduced minute ventilation

10. The patient described in the preceding question is intubated, quickly regains his baseline level of alertness, and is extubated 4 hours later. He is alarmed by his need for mechanical ventilation and before discharge he asks you about his life expectancy. Which of the following measures is the best predictor of survival in COPD?

   A. FEV1
   B. BODE index
   C. Success in smoking cessation
   D. Age
   E. Presence of Diabetes Mellitus

# Chapter 30 ▪ Answers

**1.** Correct Answer: D

**Rationale:**

The ARMA trial randomly assigned 861 patients with ARDS to low tidal volume ventilation (6 mL/kg predicted body weight) or 12 mL/kg PBW. The 6 mL/kg group had a lower risk of 28-day mortality (RR 0.74, CI 0.61-0.88). A subsequent meta-analysis found similar results. Importantly, the ARMA protocol targeted both a tidal volume of 6 mL/kg and plateau pressure <30 cm $H_2O$. Because this patient had a plateau pressure of 35 cm $H_2O$ on 6 mL/kg PBW, the protocol would advise further reductions in tidal volume to a minimum of 4 mL/kg PBW.

The fluid and catheter treatment trial randomized 1,000 patients with acute lung injury to management with a central venous catheter or PA catheter, finding no difference in 60-day survival. Furthermore, there was no evident benefit of the PAC in the duration of shock, ventilator-free days, fluid balance, or measures of lung or kidney function. The PAC group had significantly more catheter-related complications, mostly arrhythmias (and some cases of conduction block).

Lungs afflicted with diffuse injury are edematous and have poor compliance. The multicenter ART trial randomized 1,010 patients with moderate to severe ARDS to low tidal volume ventilation using a low-PEEP $FIO_2$/PEEP grid (as in ARMA) or a recruitment maneuver/decremental PEEP strategy: following neuromuscular blockade and using pressure control ventilation, PEEP raised from 25 to 35 and then 45 cm $H_2O$ for 2 minutes, and then dropped to 23 cm $H_2O$ and reduced 3 cm $H_2O$ at a time down to a minimum of 11 cm $H_2O$ with static compliance measured at each step, settling on 2 cm $H_2O$ above the PEEP yielding the highest compliance. The recruitment maneuver group suffered a higher 28-day mortality (HR 1.20, CI 1.01-1.42), reduced ventilator-free days, and increased risk of barotrauma including pneumothorax-requiring drainage.

Inhaled nitric oxide has long-been known to improve oxygenation by selectively improving blood flow to aerated regions of lungs, improving ventilation-perfusion matching, which is frequently impaired during critical illness. Indeed, in a meta-analysis of 12 randomized trials, iNO was found to increase the $PaO_2$/$FiO_2$ ratio. However, this same meta-analysis showed that patients receiving iNO had a trend toward higher mortality (RR 1.10, CI 0.94-1.30) and significantly increased renal dysfunction (RR 1.50, CI 1.11-2.02).

The PROSEVA study randomized 455 patients with severe ARDS and intubated <36 hours to undergo prone-positioning of at least 16 hours daily or be left in the supine position. Prone positioning was associated with a dramatic improvement in 28-day mortality (HR 0.39, CI 0.25-0.63). Notably, prone positioning is occasionally utilized during the management of refractory hypoxemia in patients who have been intubated for many days. The PROSEVA study, by contrast, proned patients *early* in the course of their illness. The mechanism of benefit is not known with certainty, but speculated to be related to a reduction in ventilator injury owing to more even distribution of strain (because the proned ARDS lung has more uniform mechanical characteristics than the supine ARDS lung.)

### References

1. The Acute Respiratory Distress Syndrome Network. Ventilation with lower tidal volumes as compared with traditional tidal volumes for acute lung injury and the acute respiratory distress syndrome. *N Engl J Med.* 2000;342:1301-1308.
2. Petrucci N, De Feo C. Lung protective ventilation strategy for the acute respiratory distress syndrome. *Cochrane Database Syst Rev.* 2013;(2):CD003844. doi:10.1002/14651858.CD003844.pub4.
3. National Heart, Lung, and Blood Institute Acute Respiratory Distress Syndrome (ARDS) Clinical Trials Network, Wheeler AP, Bernard GR, Thompson BT, et al. Pulmonary-Artery versus central venous catheter to guide treatment of acute lung injury. *N Engl J Med.* 2006;354:2213-2224.
4. Writing Group for the Alveolar Recruitment for Acute Respiratory Distress Syndrome Trial (ART) Investigators, Cavalcanti AB, Suzumura ÉA, Laranjeira LN, et al. Effect of Lung Recruitment and Titrated Positive End-Expiratory Pressure (PEEP) vs Low PEEP on mortality in patients with acute respiratory distress syndrome: a randomized clinical trial. *JAMA.* 2017;318:1335-1345.
5. Adhikari NK, Burns KE, Friedrich JO, et al. Effect of nitric oxide on oxygenation and mortality in acute lung injury: systematic review and meta-analysis. *BMJ.* 2007;334:779.
6. Guérin C, Reignier J, Richard JC, et al. Prone positioning in severe acute respiratory distress syndrome. *N Engl J Med.* 2013;368:2159-2168.
7. Gattinoni L. Taccone P. Carlesso E. Marini JJ. Prone position in acute respiratory distress syndrome. Rationale, indications, and limits. *Am J Respir Crit Care Med.* 2013;188:1286-1293.

**2.** Correct Answer: C

**Rationale:**

TRALI is defined as new ARDS occurring within 6 hours of blood product administration, and in the absence of other risk factors for ARDS (such as aspiration, trauma, pneumonia). The incidence of TRALI declined dramatically in the last decade following a reduction in the use of plasma from multiparous female donors (which includes anti-HLA antibodies proportional to the number of pregnancies). Recipient risk factors include alcohol abuse, shock, and smoking. Although TRALI can occur after the transfusion of any blood product, high plasma components such as plasma, apheresis platelets, and whole blood have the highest risk per transfusion. TRALI most often occurs when passively transferred HLA and human neutrophil antigen antibodies activate neutrophils that have been sequestered in the lung microvasculature.

### References

1. Toy P, Popovsky MA, Abraham E, et al. Transfusion-related acute lung injury: definition and review. *Crit Care Med.* 2005;33:721-726.
2. Toy P, Gajic O, Bacchetti P, et al. Transfusion-related acute lung injury: incidence and risk factors. *Blood.* 2012;119:1757-1767.
3. Dunbar NM. Current options for transfusion-related acute lung injury risk mitigation in platelet transfusions. *Curr Opin Hematol.* 2015;22:554-558.

**3.** Correct Answer: C

**Rationale:**

This patient has a history of mild asthma and no active wheezing—hypoxemia is typically seen only in very severe life-threatening asthma attacks or with superimposed respiratory disease such as pneumonia. This patient likely has hepatopulmonary syndrome, defined as arterial hypoxemia in the setting of intrapulmonary vascular dilatations associated with liver disease and portal hypertension. Hepatopulmonary syndrome tends to be progressive, and when very severe can be an indication for liver transplantation. Diagnosis involves confirming arterial hypoxemia with an ABG and venous contrast-enhanced transthoracic echocardiography ("bubble study"), which visualizes contrast in the left side of the heart within 3 to 8 heart beats (more rapidly than normal, but less rapidly than with intracardiac shunting). Spider nevi are predictive of higher A-a oxygen gradients in patients with cirrhosis. Orthodeoxia (a decrease in $PaO_2$ or $SpO_2$ when the patient moves from supine to upright) is common in hepatopulmonary syndrome and is due to the redistribution of blood flow to lung zones with more intrapulmonary vascular dilatations.

### References

1. Rodriguez-Roisin R, Roca J, Agusti AG, et al. Gas exchange and pulmonary vascular reactivity in patients with liver cirrhosis. *Am Rev Respir Dis.* 1987;135:1085-1092.
2. Gómez FP, Martínez-Pallí G, Barberà JA, et al. Gas exchange mechanism of orthodeoxia in hepatopulmonary syndrome. *Hepatology.* 2004;40:660-666.

**4.** Correct Answer: A

**Rationale:**

This patient is experiencing an acute exacerbation of IPF (AE-IPF). In 2016, an International Working Group Report defined AE-IPF as "an acute, clinically significant respiratory deterioration characterized by evidence of new widespread alveolar abnormality" with the following diagnostic criteria:

- Previous or concurrent diagnosis of IPF
- Acute worsening or development of dyspnea typically <1-month duration

- CT with new bilateral ground-glass opacity and/or consolidation superimposed on a background pattern consistent with usual interstitial pneumonia pattern
- Deterioration not fully explained by cardiac failure or fluid overload

This report recommended that AE-IPF be subcategorized as "Triggered Acute Exacerbation" and "Idiopathic Acute Exacerbation." Thus the detection of a respiratory pathogen does not exclude the diagnosis but rather clarifies it as triggered. International guidelines make a weak recommendation against mechanical ventilation to treat acute respiratory failure in IPF because of estimated in-hospital mortality of nearly 90%. Although corticosteroids are commonly given during AE-IPF, no high-quality trial data support this practice, which is driven by anecdotal reports of benefit. Risk factors for AE-IPF include higher BMI. In autopsy series of patients with AE-IPF, the most common acute pathologic finding is diffuse alveolar damage.

### References

1. Collard HR, Ryerson CJ, Corte TJ, et al. Acute exacerbation of idiopathic pulmonary fibrosis. An International Working Group Report. *Am J Respir Crit Care Med*. 2016;194:265-275.
2. Raghu G, Collard HR, Egan JJ, et al. An official ATS/ERS/JRS/ALAT statement: idiopathic pulmonary fibrosis: evidence-based guidelines for diagnosis and management. *Am J Respir Crit Care Med*. 2011;183:788-824.
3. Oda K, Ishimoto H, Yamada S, et al. Autopsy analyses in acute exacerbation of idiopathic pulmonary fibrosis. *Respir Res*. 2014;15:109.

---

**5.**   Correct Answer: E

**Rationale:**

High levels of PEEP can lead to increased Zone 1 conditions in the lung while simultaneously reducing cardiac output (by reducing venous return into the heart and increasing pulmonary vascular resistance). This can be life threatening if presence of this positive feedback loop is not quickly recognized.

- Dead space increases and results in worsening hypercarbia despite increase in minute ventilation, causing pH to drop (which will tend to worsen ventilator dyssynchrony and hypotension). In patients with obstructive lung disease, dyssynchrony and tachypnea may further predispose to auto-PEEP, which will tend to exaggerate this problem.
- Lower cardiac output leads to lower central venous oxygen content. Given that the lungs are injured, they will be less effective in fully oxygenating the blood, which will result in a lower arterial oxygen content.
- The clinician or respiratory care practitioner may respond by increasing the PEEP further causing further hypoxemia.

The only option that is absolutely incorrect in this setting is (A). The intensivist should recognize this scenario and that the deteriorating hemodynamics is likely to produce cardiovascular collapse if quick action is not taken. Thus (C) and (D) would be wasting precious time. Nitric oxide may marginally improve V/Q matching and oxygenation but will not help with the hemodynamics, if the primary problem is reduced venous return. The intensivist must maintain a high index of suspicion for presence of this feedback loop and recognize that sometimes decreasing the PEEP will improve systemic oxygenation in addition to improving dead space and cardiac output. Intravascular volume expansion may also improve the above physiology but may not be necessary if hemodynamics rapidly improve with reduced airway pressure. Transient disconnection from ventilator and resuming ventilation at a lower PEEP would be the most appropriate intervention.

### Reference

1. Luecke T. Pelosi P. Clinical review: positive end-expiratory pressure and cardiac output. *Crit Care*. 2005;9(6):607-621.

---

**6.**   Correct Answer: D

**Rationale:**

Mortality in ARDS has declined substantially over the last 20 years, likely in large part due to improved supportive care, including the use of lung protective ventilation, and improved approaches to fluid management, transfusions, and sedation. In a study of 179 patients with ARDS, low $PaO_2/FIO_2$ ratio, low static respiratory compliance, oxygenation index, use of vasopressors, and dead space were all associated with increased mortality. Older patients are at an increased risk of death.

### Reference

1. Nuckton TJ, Alonso JA, Kallet RH, et al. Pulmonary dead-space fraction as a risk factor for death in the acute respiratory distress syndrome. N Engl J Med. 2002;346:1281-1286.

---

**7.**   Correct Answer: D

**Rationale:**

OHS is defined as alveolar hypoventilation in the awake state in a patient with BMI of 30 or higher without other cause. It likely results from the effects of obesity on multiple physiologic pathways including sleep-disordered breathing such as OSA, restrictive pulmonary mechanics, and altered ventilatory control. During sleep all patients experience reduced ventilatory responses to hypoxemia and hypercapnia, and this appears to be true to a greater extent in patients with OHS. In this patient, it is important to distinguish chronic versus acute pathology. The higher serum bicarbonate reflects a renal compensation to chronic hypercapnia, which is likely from OHS, especially in the absence of neuromuscular weakness or obstructive lung disease. In a patient with OHS in a deep sleep, an arterial pH of 7.29 with $PaCO_2$ of 74 is likely to be near the patient's baseline physiology.

OSA is common but not universal among patients with OHS. Acute hypercapnia may cause somnolence in eucapnic patients once $PaCO_2$ rises to greater than 75 mm Hg. However, patients with chronically elevated $PaCO_2$ are typically resistant to $CO_2$ narcosis until $PaCO_2$ rises to 90 to 100 mm Hg. Acetazolamide will cause the kidney to waste bicarbonate and may increase alveolar ventilation. However, in doing so it reduces the buffer against acute increases in $PaCO_2$ and may result in electrolyte abnormalities and other side effects and is not recommended as first line therapy for this disorder. OHS rises in prevalence with BMI and is present in up to 50% of patients with BMI >50. Narcan could be tried in this scenario but is very unlikely to be effective and may precipitate nausea. First line therapy for patients with OHS is CPAP, given that up to 90% of patients with OHS have coexisting OSA, though Bi-PAP may be used in patients who fail CPAP. Many hospitals have policies regarding new initiation of CPAP that would govern the decision on ICU admission. However, a strong argument could be made in this case that if the patient is otherwise ready for discharge the next day, an expedited outpatient sleep study might serve him better than a night in the ICU.

### Reference

1. Chau EH. Lam D. Wong J. Mokhlesi B. Chung F. Obesity hypoventilation syndrome: a review of epidemiology, pathophysiology, and perioperative considerations. *Anesthesiology.* 2012;117(1):188-205.

---

**8.** Correct Answer: E

**Rationale:**

Severe hypoxemia is unusual in asthma and suggests the presence of pneumonia or extensive mucous plugging. Reduced PEF generally predicts hypercapnia rather than hypoxemia. PEF below 50% of baseline suggests a severe exacerbation, but notably hypercapnia is rare until PEF falls to less than 25% of baseline. Asthmatic patients in exacerbation have high respiratory drive, and the presence of elevated $PaCO_2$ is a concerning sign that often heralds the imminent need for intubation and mechanical ventilation. Magnesium sulfate is generally recommended for asthma exacerbation when severe airflow limitation persists despite initial therapy with bronchodilators. Heliox has a lower density than air and thus reduces resistance to airflow. However, clinical trials have yielded conflicting results and its use limits the maximum $FiO_2$ to approximately 0.8 and requires the use of correction factors for ventilator gas flow. Survival in patients requiring mechanical ventilation for asthma exacerbations improved markedly following implementation of permissive hypercapnia ventilatory strategies. Dynamic hyperinflation creates intrinsic PEEP (air trapping), which can reduce venous return, place strain on the right ventricle, and may precipitate cardiovascular collapse. Ventilator adjustments that may be helpful include reducing the tidal volume (shorter inspiratory time and less volume to exhale), decreasing the rate, and optimizing triggering. Intrinsic PEEP can be measured during an expiratory pause although neuromuscular blockade may be necessary to obtain reliable measurements. Setting the extrinsic (applied) PEEP to up to 80% of the intrinsic PEEP can reduce the inspiratory effort required to trigger the ventilator without substantially increasing the risk of barotrauma. Notably patients with the most severe exacerbations may require paralysis that would obviate any benefit to improved triggering, and so this strategy is most useful during the ventilator weaning phase.

### References

1. Darioli R. Perret C. Mechanical controlled hypoventilation in status asthmaticus. *Am Rev Respir Dis.* 1984;129:385-387.
2. Oddo M. Feihl F. Schaller MD. Perret C. Management of mechanical ventilation in acute severe asthma: practical aspects. *Intensive Care Med.* 2006;32:501-510.

---

**9.** Correct Answer: C

**Rationale:**

This patient suffers from chronic hypercarbic hypoxemic respiratory failure (with secondary polycythemia) as a result of very advanced emphysema. Hypercapnia results from an increase in $CO_2$ production and/or a decrease in alveolar ventilation (which may be due to either decreased minute ventilation or increased dead space fraction). Acutely, increased $PaCO_2$ leads to increased brain blood flow and ICP but decreased level of consciousness. The mechanism of reduced LOC is not well established but probably involves global increases in inhibitory neurotransmitters. Narcan may be tried but can be expected to have minimal effect.

Patients with emphysema have major disruptions in v/q matching and increased dead space. They breathe with a lower tidal volume and higher respiratory rate to compensate, typically reaching a minute ventilation that is higher than normal. They variably develop chronic hypercapnia with compensatory metabolic alkalosis via renal compensation (increased serum bicarbonate). When severe hypoxemia accompanies advanced lung disease, compensatory polycythemia allows some improvement in oxygen delivery.

Most patients with COPD and chronic hypercapnia have at most a mild increase in $PaCO_2$ with oxygen therapy. However, excessive supplemental oxygen administration in a very small subset of patients with advanced chronic hypercarbic hypoxemic respiratory failure can lead to a vicious cycle of increased $PaCO_2$ and somnolence. The mechanisms by which this occurs remain somewhat controversial. The best study on this phenomenon dates to the early 1980s, in which Aubier and colleagues studied 22 patients with advanced COPD with mean age of 65 years, mean $PaO_2$ of 38, and mean $PaCO_2$ of 65. They were studied first on room air and then asked to breathe pure oxygen for 15 minutes. The mean increase in $PaCO_2$ in these patients at the end of the test period was 23 mm Hg, and although minute ventilation declined initially, by the end of the 15-minute period it had risen back to 93% of baseline. Furthermore, there was no correlation between the change in minute ventilation and the increase in $PaCO_2$ across the 22 patients. Subsequent analysis revealed that the majority of the increase in $PaCO_2$ was due to a combination of the Haldane effect (rightward displacement of the $CO_2$-Hb dissociation curve, causing the considerable red cell mass to liberate $CO_2$ in the presence of an acute increase in oxyhemoglobin) and an increase in dead space fraction, likely due to worsening V/Q mismatch in the setting of impaired hypoxic pulmonary vasoconstriction. Patients at highest risk for this phenomenon are those with advanced lung disease and a very low initial $PaO_2$ who have high levels of supplemental oxygen applied abruptly.

Acetazolamide may increase respiratory drive somewhat but can be dangerous by reducing the buffer against acute increases in $PaCO_2$. Nocturnal noninvasive ventilation may be considered but is best initiated in a sleep laboratory in patients who are likely to be compliant with close follow-up.

### Reference

1. Aubier M, Murciano D, Milic-Emili J, et al. Effects of the administration of O2 on ventilation and blood gases in patients with chronic obstructive pulmonary disease during acute respiratory failure. *Am Rev Respir Dis*. 1980;122:747-754.

---

**10.** Correct Answer: B

**Rationale:**

Postbronchodilator FEV1 (percent predicted) does have some predictive power for survival but is limited by high variability across patients. More recently the BODE index was developed: **B**MI, **O**bstruction (FEV1), **D**yspnea, and **E**xercise capacity (6-minute walk distance). Initially described in 2004, the BODE index is superior to FEV1 in predicting survival in patients with COPD.

### References

1. Traver GA. Cline MG. Burrows B. Predictors of mortality in chronic obstructive pulmonary disease. A 15-year follow-up study. *Am Rev Respir Dis*. 1979;119:895-902.
2. Celli BR, Cote CG, Marin JM, et al. The body-mass index, airflow obstruction, dyspnea, and exercise capacity index in chronic obstructive pulmonary disease. *N Engl J Med*. 2004;350:1005-1012.

# 31

# HYPOXEMIA AND OXYGEN DELIVERY

Christine Choi and Jeanine P. Wiener-Kronish

1. A 56-year-old male with advanced idiopathic pulmonary fibrosis presents to the ICU in respiratory distress. He is put on high flow nasal cannula with 50 L flow, 80% $FiO_2$. ABG obtained has a pH significant for 7.32, $PaO_2$ of 80 mm Hg, $PaCO_2$ of 20 mm Hg, $HCO_3$ of 30. Given his underlying disease, what is the primary physiological aberration leading to the patient's hypoxemia?

   A. Hypoventilation
   B. Reduced inspired oxygen tension
   C. Right to left shunt
   D. Diffusion limitation

2. A 72-year-old male with past medical history significant for pulmonary hypertension and congestive heart failure presents to the ICU in cardiogenic shock with hypotension. Despite initiation of vasopressor therapy, the patient remains hemodynamically unstable and develops worsening hypoxemia. Bedside transthoracic echocardiography shows bowing of the intra-atrial septum toward the left atrium with positive Doppler color flow across the intra-atrial septum and a hypokinetic right ventricle. What is the most likely cause of the patient's hypoxemia?

   A. V/Q mismatch
   B. Right to left shunt
   C. Left to right shunt
   D. Hypoxic pulmonary vasoconstriction

3. A 38-year-old, 155 cm, 50 kg, previously health female presents to the ICU with altered mental status, tachycardia, hypotension, and high fever. She is intubated for airway protection. Her laboratory test results reveal a markedly elevated T3 and T4 level with a decrease in thyroid-stimulating hormone level consistent with thyroid storm. Her arterial blood gas shows a pH of 7.24, $PaO_2$ of 80, $PaCO_2$ of 52, and $HCO_3$ of 22. Her ventilator settings are volume control, tidal volume of 350 mL, respiratory rate of 14, positive end expiratory pressure (PEEP) of 5, $FiO_2$ of 50%. Which of the following is the next appropriate step in management?

   A. Increase tidal volume to 500 mL
   B. Change from volume control mode to pressure support mode of ventilation
   C. Increase the PEEP from 5 to 8 mm Hg
   D. Increase the respiratory rate from 14 to 18
   E. Increase the $FiO_2$ to 70%

4. A 63-year-old male presents to the hospital in acute respiratory distress, with high fevers and cough with purulent sputum. The patient has a history of adenocarcinoma of the lung and has underwent a right upper lobectomy 10 days ago. His vitals are heart rate 120 bpm, blood pressure 152/91 mm Hg, $SpO_2$ 91% on 5 L nasal cannula. Chest X-ray reveals a 3 cm pneumothorax in the right chest. What is the next appropriate treatment option for this patient?

   A. Initiate noninvasive positive pressure ventilation (NIPPV)
   B. Apply high flow nasal cannula
   C. Insert a chest tube
   D. Draw blood cultures and start broad spectrum antibiotics
   E. Perform a diagnostic bronchoscopy

5. A 68-year-old male with past medical history significant for COPD, HTN, and heart failure with preserved ejection fraction with newly discovered left upper lobe speculated mass presents from a nursing home facility with complaints of acute onset shortness of breath and chest pain. The patient had undergone an uneventful left upper lobe wedge resection 10 days ago. Chest X-ray obtained in unremarkable except for bibasilar atelectasis. The patient's vital signs are heart rate of 101 bpm, blood pressure of 98/72 mm Hg, oxygen saturation of 90% on 50% $FiO_2$, on 50 L flow through high flow nasal cannula. Bedside point of care transthoracic ultrasound is showing normal function in the left ventricle, moderate tricuspid regurgitation, flattening of the intraventricular septum, and moderately depressed right ventricular function. Which physiologic factor is **not** involved in this patient's respiratory distress?

   A. Increase in shunt fraction
   B. Increase in dead space
   C. Limitation in diffusion
   D. Decreased cardiac output
   E. Ventilation/perfusion mismatch

6. Which among the following represent the changes in pulmonary respiratory parameters with aging?

| | FUNCTIONAL RESIDUAL CAPACITY | CLOSING CAPACITY |
|---|---|---|
| A | Increase | Increase |
| B | Increase | No change |
| C | Decrease | Increase |
| D | Decrease | No change |
| E | No change | Increase |

7. A 62-year-old male with past medical history significant for diabetes, hypertension, hyperlipidemia, and 60 pack year smoking history comes in with complaints of respiratory distress and flu-like symptoms for the past week. Vitals are HR 105 bpm, BP 170/91 mm Hg, $SpO_2$ 87% on 5 liters per minute of oxygen via nasal cannula. He is intermittently confused but is arousable and redirectable. His arterial blood gas shows pH of 7.26, $PaO_2$ of 97 mm Hg, $PaCO_2$ of 61 mm Hg and $HCO_3$ of 30. Which is the appropriate next step in intervention?

   A. Obtain sputum culture, start broad spectrum antibiotics, and high-dose steroids
   B. Emergently intubate the patient
   C. Initiate high flow nasal cannula at 50 L flow, 50% $FiO_2$
   D. Initiate Bi level Positive Pressure Ventilation
   E. Initiate heliox

8. A 81-year-old female with history of atrial fibrillation on Coumadin, hypertension, and recent hip fracture from a fall s/p trochanteric fixation of the femoral head who has been recovering in a skilled nursing facility is brought into the emergency department (ED) with complaints of altered mental status, high fevers, and productive cough. The patient is emergently intubated because of lethargy and is transferred to the ICU. On arrival to the ICU, the patient's vitals are HR 110 bpm, BP 90/65 mm Hg, $SpO_2$ 91% on 60% $FiO_2$ on the ventilator. ABG is showing pH of 7.38, $PaO_2$ of 88 mm Hg, $PaCO_2$ of 39 mm Hg, and $HCO_3$ of 22. Despite an increase of the $FiO_2$ on the ventilator, increase of PEEP, and repositioning of the ETT, the patient's oxygenation does not improve. A decision to obtain a CXR is made and the imaging obtained follows.

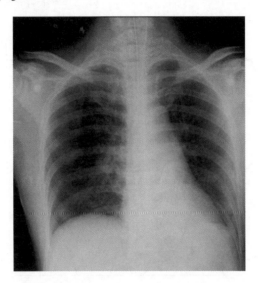

What is the next appropriate intervention given these clinical findings?

A. Perform needle decompression of the chest
B. Advance the endotracheal tube by 3 cm
C. Change the patient position from supine to prone
D. Perform a bronchoscopy
E. Insert chest tube on the left side of the chest

9. A 92-year-old female with mild dementia, atrial fibrillation on warfarin, and hypertension presents to the ED after suffering a mechanical fall after tripping over a rug at her nursing home. Chest X-ray reveals mildly displaced right-sided rib fractures from ribs 4 through 10. Her vital signs are heart rate 92, blood pressure 107/71, $SpO_2$ 89% on 8 L face mask. Arterial blood gas obtained shows pH 7.41, $PaO_2$ 72, $PaCO_2$ 37, $HCO_3$ 23. The patient is mildly confused and is only oriented toward self and place. The patient is complaining of shortness of breath and rib pain with every breath and continues to take rapid shallow breaths. She is also complaining of discomfort with the face mask and attempts to remove the face mask despite redirection. Given this clinical scenario, what would be the next appropriate clinical intervention to improve the patient's oxygenation?

A. Apply non-rebreather face mask at 10 L flow
B. Apply NIPPV with face mask (CPAP)
C. Apply Venturi mask
D. Intubate the patient
E. Apply heated and humidified high flow nasal oxygen (HFNC)

**10.** A 62-year-old male with past medical history significant for end stage liver disease secondary to alcohol abuse, portopulmonary syndrome, GI bleed, COPD, and type 2 diabetes presents to the ED with hematemesis. The patient is intubated for airway protection and is transferred up to the ICU for close monitoring. Gastroenterology specialists plan to perform an upper GI endoscopy to determine the etiology of the upper GI bleed. The patient is sedated on 30 mg/kg/min of propofol. The patient's vital signs are HR 102, BP 92/61, SPO$_2$ 100%. Ventilator settings are pressure control, tidal volume 700 mL, RR 14, FiO$_2$ 100%, PEEP 3 mm H$_2$O. You walk into the patient's room and notice these waveforms on the ventilator (see figure that follows). There are no ventilator or monitor alarms going off in the patient's room.

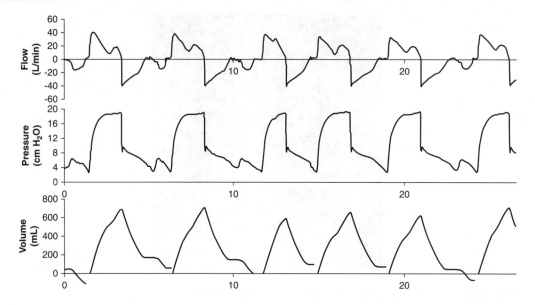

Given these findings, what is the next appropriate step in ventilator management?

**A.** Lower tidal volume
**B.** Lower trigger threshold
**C.** Decrease I:E ratio
**D.** Decrease inspiratory flow
**E.** Increase flow rate threshold
**F.** Keep the ventilator settings unchanged

# Chapter 31 ▪ Answers

**1.** Correct Answer: D

**Rationale:**
The patient may have several physiologic derangements, but given his diagnosis of fibrosis, diffusion limitation may be the primary physiologic aberration leading to hypoxemia.

There are several different mechanisms of hypoxemia: hypoventilation, V/Q mismatch, right to left shunt, diffusion limitation, and reduced inspired oxygen tension. Hypoventilation and reduced inspired oxygen tension will lead to reduced PAO$_2$, which results in hypoxemia. In the case of hypoventilation, a concurrent rise in PaCO$_2$ will also be noticed. Increasing ventilation and FiO$_2$ will improve oxygenation in these cases.

V/Q mismatch refers to an imbalance between alveolar ventilation and alveolar perfusion. A certain degree of V/Q mismatch exists in normal lungs with V/Q being higher in the apex of the lungs compared to the bases. In pulmonary disease states, the degree of V/Q mismatch will worsen resulting in hypoxemia. In cases of V/Q mismatch, worsening of A-a gradient will be noticed. Right to left shunt results from poorly oxygenated blood passing from the right to left side of the heart without being oxygenated, leading to hypoxemia. Two kinds of right to left shunt exist: anatomic and physiologic. Anatomic shunt refers to when the alveoli are bypassed as in cases of intracardiac shunt or AV malformations. Physiologic shunt refers to when nonventilated alveoli are perfused as in cases of atelectasis.

Diffusion limitation exists when there is a destruction of lung parenchymal tissue, which impairs the movement of oxygen from alveoli to pulmonary capillary. Often times in cases of lung parenchymal disease, V/Q mismatch and diffusion limitation coexists and the exact cause of hypoxemia can be difficult to distinguish.

References
1. Rodríguez-Roisin R, Roca J. Mechanisms of hypoxemia. *Intensive Care Med*. 2005;31:1017.
2. Williams AJ. ABC of oxygen: assessing and interpreting arterial blood gases and acid-base balance. *BMJ*. 1998;317:1213.

**2.** Correct Answer: B

**Rationale:**

In this scenario, based on the patient's echocardiography results, the patient is showing signs of right-sided heart failure with increase in right atrial pressure leading to right to left shunt through an atrial septal defect.

In patients with pulmonary hypertension, it is crucial to avoid hypoxemia, hypercarbia, and acidosis as this can increase pulmonary vascular resistance and if severe enough lead to right heart failure. When the right-sided heart fails to eject blood against the high pulmonary vascular resistance, significant tricuspid regurgitation can develop and rise in right atrial pressure higher than the left atrial pressure can result. Bowing of the intra-atrial septum toward the left atrium indicates increased right atrial pressure, which in presence of an atrial septal defect (seen as color Doppler flow across the septum) causes flow of unoxygenated blood from the right side of the heart to mix with oxygenated blood in the left atrium causing systemic hypoxemia. The resulting hypoxemia can further worsen the patient's pulmonary hypertension and lead to cardiopulmonary decompensation. Measures to decrease pulmonary hypertension may reduce the right to left shunting.

Reference
1. Rodríguez-Roisin R, Roca J. Mechanisms of hypoxemia. *Intensive Care Med*. 2005;31:1017.

**3.** Correct Answer: D

**Rationale:**

Increasing the patient's respiratory rate to increase minute ventilation is the next appropriate step in management of this patient.

The patient's ABG is shows primary respiratory acidosis with elevation in $PaCO_2$ levels. $PaCO_2$ is a measure of the patient's ventilation, whereas $PaO_2$ is a measure of oxygenation. Elevation in $PaCO_2$ indicates inadequate ventilation, which can be improved by increasing minute ventilation: either by increasing tidal volume or respiratory rate. Increasing the patient's tidal volumes to 500 mL would not be recommended as this is inconsistent with lung protective ventilation strategy. So, the appropriate course of action here would be to increase respiratory rate, which in turn will decrease $PaCO_2$ levels.

$PaO_2$ measures the patient's oxygenation and can be adjusted by altering the level of PEEP or fraction of inspired oxygen. Because the $PaO_2$ is within normal range, a change in this parameter is not warranted. Similarly, a change in mode of ventilation is also not indicated.

Reference
1. Slutsky AS. Mechanical ventilation. American College of Chest Physicians' Consensus Conference. *Chest*. 1993;104:1833.

**4.** Correct Answer: C

**Rationale:**

The first step in managing a bronchopleural fistula (BPF) is to insert a chest tube to allow drainage of air and fluid from the pleural space.

BPF is a known complication after lung resection surgery and carries a high mortality and morbidity. BPF should be suspected in patients with a recent history of lung surgery presenting with dyspnea, chest pain, and hemodynamic instability. Once BPF is suspected, imaging (chest X-ray or CT) should be obtained to look for evidence of pneumothorax, or pneumomediastinum. Although supportive therapy such as high flow nasal cannula, initiation of broad-spectrum antibiotics, and diagnostic bronchoscopy are all warranted, the first step in managing BPF is chest tube insertion to drain air and fluid. This prevents worsening of the patient's pneumothorax. Initiation of NIPPV should be deferred until a chest tube is inserted as it could also potentially worsen the pneumothorax.

A cardiothoracic surgery consult should then be obtained to determine if the patient is a candidate for surgical closure of the BPF. For those who are not a surgical candidate, placement of stents, angiographic coils, or other occlusive material can be considered as a treatment option.

References
1. Farkas EA, Detterbeck FC. Airway complications after pulmonary resection. *Thorac Surg Clin*. 2006;16:243.
2. Liberman M, Cassivi SD. Bronchial stump dehiscence: update on prevention and management. *Semin Thorac Cardiovasc Surg*. 2007;19:366.
3. Lois M, Noppen M. Bronchopleural fistulas: an overview of the problem with special focus on endoscopic management. *Chest*. 2005;128:3955.

**5.** Correct Answer: C

**Rationale:**

Based on the patient's clinical presentation (and presence of right heart strain), he is most likely suffering from an acute pulmonary embolism.

There are four main mechanisms behind hypoxemia: V/Q mismatch, right to left shunt, impaired diffusion, and hypoventilation. Shunt refers to areas of lung in which there is a complete cessation of ventilation but continued perfusion. Lung consolidation as seen in pneumonia, pleural effusions, or atelectasis represents shunt. In cases of shunt, increasing FiO$_2$ in the alveoli will have minimal improvement on hypoxemia. Technically, pulmonary emboli, a clot in the circulation, should only cause an increase in deadspace. But it also causes shunt and V/Q mismatch by causing edema around the clot. This patient had atelectasis on his chest X-ray, which increases shunt and added to his hypoxemia. Hypoventilation is usually accompanied by hypercapnia along with hypoxemia and can be treated by increasing minute ventilation in most cases (although in cases of severe hypermetabolism, hypoventilation may still exist despite having high minute ventilation).

Right- and left-sided heart failure can lead to a decrease in forward blood flow, leading to more desaturated blood returning to the pulmonary circulation and thus making it even more difficult to have the lungs oxygenate the blood in a normal fashion. Impaired diffusion is likely caused by destruction of lung parenchymal tissue as seen in interstitial lung disease, and hypoxemia is caused by inefficient exchange of gases in this case. This is not seen in pulmonary embolism.

Reference

1. Rodríguez-Roisin R, Roca J. Mechanisms of hypoxemia. *Intensive Care Med.* 2005;31:1017.

**6.** Correct Answer: A

**Rationale:**

The following diagram depicts various lung volumes and capacities.

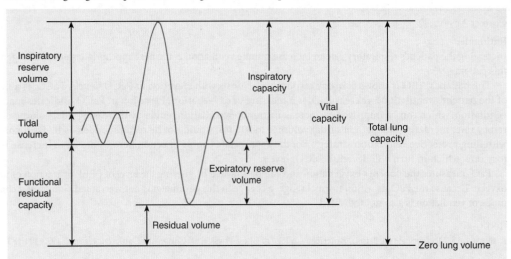

Functional residual capacity (FRC) is the volume of the lungs at the end of passive expiration. It is a sum of residual volume and expiratory reserve volume. FRC is determined by a balance between the inward "elastic recoil" force of the lung parenchymal tissue and the outward "passive recoil" force from the ribs, joints, and chest wall muscle. The FRC slightly increases with age and height. FRC is decreased with supine position, obesity, and the female sex.

Closing capacity is the point in which small airways start to close during expiration. With age, airway closing happens at a larger lung volume therefore closing capacity increases (approaches FRC). Closing of the small airways can happen at or above FRC around the age of 65 to 70 years, and this is partially what contributes to decreased oxygenation with aging. Closing capacity is independent of position.

Reference

1. Crapo RO. Pulmonary-function testing. *N Engl J Med.* 1994;331:25.

**7.** Correct Answer: D

**Rationale:**

The patient is experiencing COPD exacerbation likely brought on by recent flu. The patient's ABG is showing respiratory acidosis, and it would be most beneficial to start noninvasive bilevel positive pressure ventilation in this case.

NIPPV refers to a mode of ventilation in which positive pressure is delivered to the patient through a noninvasive mask interface (face mask, nasal pillow) compared to an invasive mode of ventilation (endotracheal tube, laryngeal mask, tracheostomy). Randomized controlled trials and meta-analysis have shown that NIPPV improves important clinical outcomes (mortality, rate of intubation, hospital length of stay) in patients having an acute exacerbation of COPD complicated by hypercapnic acidosis. Specific indications for NIPPV include COPD exacerbation with respiratory acidosis, cardiogenic pulmonary edema, and acute hypoxemic respiratory failure. Contraindications to NIPPV include cardiac or respiratory arrest, altered mental status, inability to clear airway secretions or protect airway, facial trauma, recent esophageal surgery, and high aspiration risk.

Although high flow nasal cannula has shown to provide patients with some degree of PEEP and improve oxygenation, the patient's primary problem in this case is hypercapnic respiratory failure, and HFNC is less efficacious in improving hypercapnia compared to NIPPV. Heliox can improve the patient's respiratory distress by delivering less-dense oxygen hence reducing resistance to airway flow. Although this may reduce the work of breathing for the patient, it would not improve the patient's hypercapnis brought on by COPD exacerbation. Intubation of the patient is not indicated at this point because the patient is hemodynamically stable and mentation is grossly intact.

Although steroids and antibiotics may be indicated in certain situations (severe COPD exacerbation with active sputum production, increased dyspnea), attempts to improve the patient's respiratory acidosis should be the primary focus at this point.

### References

1. Brochard L, Mancebo J, Wysocki M, et al. Noninvasive ventilation for acute exacerbations of chronic obstructive pulmonary disease. *N Engl J Med.* 1995;333:817.
2. Ferrer M, Esquinas A, Leon M, et al. Noninvasive ventilation in severe hypoxemic respiratory failure: a randomized clinical trial. *Am J Respir Crit Care Med.* 2003;168:1438.
3. Wysocki M, Tric L, Wolff MA, et al. Noninvasive pressure support ventilation in patients with acute respiratory failure. A randomized comparison with conventional therapy. *Chest.* 1995;107:761.
4. Kramer N, Meyer TJ, Meharg J, et al. Randomized, prospective trial of noninvasive positive pressure ventilation in acute respiratory failure. *Am J Respir Crit Care Med.* 1995;151:1799.

---

**8.** Correct Answer: D

**Rationale:**

Based on the chest X-ray obtained, the patient's hypoxemia is due to left lower lobe collapse. Given the patient's history of productive cough and purulent sputum, left lower lobe collapse is likely from mucous plugging, and bronchoscopy to clear the mucous plug is advised.

Left lower lobe collapse can be difficult to identify at times because of the cardiac shadow. The features to observe when left lower lobe is suspected is a triangular opacity in the posterior medial aspect of the left lung, a "double cardiac contour," loss of normal hemidiaphragmatic silhouette, or loss of the outline of the descending aorta. These features are also similar to how atelectasis would look on chest X-ray, so clinical correlation is necessary to distinguish between differential diagnosis of hypoxemia. In cases of lobe collapse due to mucous plugging, therapeutic bronchoscopy would be necessary to suction out the mucous plug. Although suctioning the endotracheal tube can partially alleviate symptoms of hypoxemia and mucous plugging, the suction catheter is limited in terms of the depth and specific location it can reach.

In case of a tension pneumothorax, contralateral shift of the mediastinum, increase in ipsilateral pleural space, and depression of the hemidiaphragm may be observed. If the tension pneumothorax is significant enough then it can also cause hemodynamic compromise. If a tension pneumothorax is suspected then a chest tube should be immediately inserted to the affected side to relieve the pneumothorax. If a chest tube is not readily available or if one is not familiar with insertion of a chest tube, then needle decompression should be immediately performed while help is called for. Needle decompression is typically performed with a large bore catheter needle, and it is inserted into the second intercostal space of the affected side along the mid-clavicular line.

Changing the patient's position from supine to prone is a technique that can be adopted to improve patient's oxygenation and V/Q mismatch. It is often employed as an adjunctive measure in patients with severe ARDS.

Movement of the endotracheal is not uncommon in the ICU setting. Especially with prolonged intubation, the endotracheal tube becomes warm and can be easily kinked or deformed. Movement of the ETT further into the trachea can cause right main stem intubation and can lead to hypoxemia and atelectasis of the contralateral lung, whereas movement of the ETT away from the carina can lead to air leaks and delivery of inadequate tidal volumes. Placement of ETT can be verified by listening to bilateral breath sounds, chest X-ray, or bronchoscopy.

### References

1. Du Rand IA, Blaikley J, Booton R, et al. Summary of the British Thoracic Society guideline for diagnostic flexible bronchoscopy in adults. *Thorax.* 2013;68:786.
2. Feinsilver SH, Fein AM, Niederman MS, et al. Utility of fiberoptic bronchoscopy in nonresolving pneumonia. *Chest.* 1990;98:1322.

---

**9.** Correct Answer: E

**Rationale:**

Given the patient's hypoxemia and mild confusion with complaints of discomfort of a face mask, applying a heated and humidified HFNC cannula would be the most appropriate treatment for this patient.

There are two main mechanisms to deliver oxygen: low-flow system versus high-flow system. Low-flow systems include nasal cannula and conventional oxygen face mask. High-flow system includes non-rebreather face mask, Venturi mask, and heated/humidified HFNC.

HFNC delivers heated and humidified oxygen at extremely high flow rates to minimize entrainment of room air. Patients who are in respiratory distress often times generate high inspiratory flow rates that exceed the oxygen flow rates of conventional oxygen delivery systems leading to entrainment of room air and reduction in the $FiO_2$ of oxygen delivered to the patient, contributing to hypoxemia. HFNC overcomes this issue by generating oxygen flow rates that are higher than the patient's inspiratory flow rate resulting in reliable and titratable $FiO_2$ delivery. HFNC is heated and humidified, which can promote clearance of secretions/mucous, decrease damage to the epithelial cells of the airway, and decrease work of breathing compared to the Venturi mask or a non-rebreather mask. The heat and the humidity along with the nasal prongs improves comfort for the patient. HFNC also has the added benefit of CPAP (for every 10 L/min flow increase, 0.7 cm $H_2O$ of PEEP is added) and wash out of nasopharyngeal deadspace. Given the patient's mild confusion with complaints of discomfort with the face mask, HFNC would be the best option for the patient to improve her oxygenation.

Venturi mask and non-rebreather masks are also considered high oxygen flow systems, but compared to HFNC, heating and humidification of oxygen is less effective hence leading to more discomfort for the patient. The wash out effect of the nasopharynx is also less leading to less fractional area available for effective gas exchange. Also both systems utilize a face mask that can add discomfort to patients who feel claustrophobic with a tight fitting mask.

BiPAP has similar benefits of HFNC and can deliver high amounts of positive pressure for respiratory support. BiPAP can also be utilized to improve hypercapnia, whereas HFNC is less effective in improving ventilation. Although BiPAP is not an unreasonable option for this patient, given the patient's complaint of discomfort with the face mask and no significant issues with the patient's ventilation status at this time, a trial of HFNC would be more reasonable at this time over BIPAP. If the patient's respiratory status continues to decline, then escalation to BIPAP would be reasonable.

### References
1. Rochwerg B, Brochard L, Elliott MW, et al. Official ERS/ATS clinical practice guidelines: noninvasive ventilation for acute respiratory failure. *Eur Respir J.* 2017;50.
2. Dysart K, Miller TL, Wolfson MR, Shaffer TH. Research in high flow therapy: mechanisms of action. *Respir Med.* 2009;103:1400.
3. Roca O, Riera J, Torres F, Masclans JR. High-flow oxygen therapy in acute respiratory failure. *Respir Care.* 2010;55:408.

**10.** Correct Answer: A

**Rationale:**
Based on the diagram presented above, the patient is ineffectively trigging the ventilator because of auto-PEEP. Given the answer choices, lowering tidal volumes would be the next appropriate step to improve the patient's ventilator dysynchrony.

Accurate assessment of patient-ventilator interactions and work of breathing is important in improving the patient comfort on the ventilator and to optimizing ventilator settings to achieve swift liberation from mechanical ventilator. The modern ventilator has many different modes of ventilation and many parameters that the physician can input to optimize ventilator support. Modern ventilators are also capable of displaying many real-time information including pressure-time graphs, flow-time graphs, and volume-time graphs. Using these types of various information, a physician's goal is to achieve patient-ventilator synchrony where the ventilator-assisted breathing coincides well with the patient's intrinsic breathing efforts. When the patient's inspiratory effort does not match with the ventilator triggered support, it is said that ventilator asynchrony has occurred. There are three main types of ventilator asynchrony: trigger-asynchrony, flow-asynchrony, and cycling-asynchrony.

Trigger asynchrony include ineffective triggering, double triggering, or auto-triggering. Ineffective triggering occurs when the patient attempts to initiate a breath, but the trigger threshold is not reached and the ventilator fails to trigger an effective breath. Ineffectively triggered breaths are not accounted for by the ventilator as respiratory rate and typically do not cause the ventilator to alarm. In the graph displayed in the question, two different respiratory wave forms can be observed. The effectively triggered breaths generate the set tidal volume of 700 mL. On the other hand, ineffectively triggered breaths produce a deflection in the pressure-time and flow-time graphs, but the set tidal volume is not achieved, leading to a trigger asynchrony. Also by observing the volume-time graph, one can conclude that the patient's inspiratory efforts (shown by deflection in the flow and pressure loops) are triggered before complete exhalation (volume loop does not return to baseline level of 0 before the deflection of pressure and flow loops) resulting in auto-PEEP. Air trapping due to insufficient exhalation time leading to auto-PEEP is a common cause of ventilator asynchrony in patients with a history of COPD. The ways to prevent auto-PEEP, therefore improve patient-ventilator synchrony, is to prolong expiratory time by adjusting the I:E ratio or by reducing tidal volume to allow complete exhalation.

Double-triggering occurs when a patient's inspiratory effort continues throughout the preset ventilator inspiratory time and remains present after ventilator inspiratory time has finished.

Auto-triggering occurs when the ventilator delivers an assisted breath that was not initiated by the patient.

Flow asynchrony may be due to ventilator flow being either too fast or too slow for the patient and may occur with either flow-targeted breaths or with pressure-targeted breaths.

Cycling refers to termination of ventilator-assisted inspiration. A patient's inspiratory effort may still be present at the time of termination of assisted inspiration. This termination of assisted breathing despite the patient's continued effort is referred to as premature cycling (the reference point is the patient and not the ventilator).

### References

1. MacIntyre NR. Branson RD. *Mechanical Ventilation*. 2nd ed. St Louis: Saunders Elsevier; 2009.
2. Hess D. Kacmarek RM. *Essentials of Mechanical Ventilation*. New York: McGraw-Hill (Health Professions Division); 1996.
3. Chao DC. Scheinhorn DJ. Stearn-Hassenpflug M. Patient-ventilator trigger asynchrony in prolonged mechanical ventilation. *Chest*. 1997;112(6):1592-1599.
4. Hill LL, Pearl RG. Flow triggering, pressure triggering, and autotriggering during mechanical ventilation. *Crit Care Med*. 2000;28:579.

# 32

# MECHANICAL VENTILATION

Jason H. Maley and Kathryn A. Hibbert

1. A 45-year-old previously healthy woman presents to the emergency department with 3 days of fevers and progressive dyspnea and is admitted to the intensive care unit (ICU) for influenza infection complicated by severe hypoxemia. She is intubated, and chest radiograph following intubation demonstrates an appropriately placed endotracheal tube with bilateral patchy opacities and interstitial markings throughout all lung fields, without effusions. Her bedside echocardiogram reveals a left ventricular ejection fraction of 0.75 with otherwise normal findings. Her ventilator settings are volume control, tidal volume (VT) 500 mL, respiratory rate (RR) 14 breaths per minute, $FiO_2$ 1.0, and positive end-expiratory pressure (PEEP) 5 cm $H_2O$. An initial arterial blood gas (ABG) is pH 7.30 $PCO_2$ 45 mm Hg and $PO_2$ 80 mm Hg. Which of the following therapies has been best shown to improve the survival of patients such as this woman?

   A. Diuresis to maintain a negative fluid balance
   B. Ventilation at a TV of 6 mL/kg of ideal body weight (IBW)
   C. Initiation of inhaled pulmonary vasodilator for severe hypoxemia
   D. Bronchoscopy to rule out additional infections
   E. Titration of PEEP with recruitment maneuver to optimize lung compliance

2. A 32-year-old man with severe asthma is admitted to the ICU with an acute asthma exacerbation. He is intubated, paralyzed, and mechanically ventilated. His ventilator settings are assist control/volume control, TV 400 mL, respiratory rate 20 breaths per minute, $FiO_2$ 0.5, and PEEP 5 cm $H_2O$. His ABG on these settings is pH 7.30 $PCO_2$ 55 mm Hg and $PO_2$ 150 mm Hg. On day 2 of his ICU stay, an end-expiratory hold maneuver is performed and his airway pressure is measured at 15 cm $H_2O$. Several hours later, he is noted to have progressive tachycardia, and his blood pressure has decreased from 120/90 to 75/55 mm Hg. A chest radiograph demonstrates similar findings to the prior day, without evidence of new infiltrate or pneumothorax. What is the best next step in management?

   A. Briefly disconnect the mechanical ventilator from the endotracheal tube
   B. Perform a needle decompression at the second intercostal space
   C. Perform an emergent bronchoscopy
   D. Increase the respiratory rate on the ventilator
   E. Decrease the set PEEP on the ventilator

3. A 68-year-old man with community-acquired pneumonia is intubated in the ICU with respiratory failure. Following induction of anesthesia, while paralyzed, his ventilator is set on volume assist-control, TV 450 mL, respiratory rate 14 breaths per minute, $FiO_2$ 0.8, and PEEP 5 cm $H_2O$. An inspiratory hold maneuver is performed and his peak inspiratory pressure is 25 cm $H_2O$ and plateau pressure is 15 cm $H_2O$. Which of the following is true regarding this patient's respiratory mechanics?

   A. The patient's lung compliance is 45 mL/cm $H_2O$.
   B. The patient's chest wall compliance is 30 mL/cm $H_2O$.
   C. The patient's lung compliance is 10 mL/cm $H_2O$.
   D. The patient's respiratory system compliance is 45 mL/cm $H_2O$.

4. A 70-year-old woman is intubated in the ICU for respiratory failure following an episode of aspiration with resulting pneumonitis. Which of the following practices is most likely to decrease her duration of mechanical ventilation?

   A. Spontaneous breathing trial performed when supervised by the attending physician
   B. Paired daily spontaneous breathing trial and spontaneous awakening trial
   C. Decremental pressure support wean as directed by respiratory therapist
   D. Early tracheostomy
   E. Spontaneous breathing trial performed when directed by the bedside nurse

5. A 68-year-old woman is admitted to the hospital with an acute exacerbation of chronic obstructive lung disease. She is intubated for worsening hypercarbia and transferred to the medical ICU. On day 8 of her ICU stay, she is felt to be clinically improving and close to extubation readiness when she develops intermittent desaturation and increased tracheal secretions. A portable chest radiograph demonstrates a new right lower lobe infiltrate. A tracheal aspiration is obtained for culture. Which of the following would be appropriate intravenous antibiotic regimen?

   A. Metronidazole
   B. Ceftriaxone and azithromycin
   C. Vancomycin and cefepime
   D. Cefepime and metronidazole
   E. Ceftriaxone and metronidazole

6. A 54-year-old man with ischemic cardiomyopathy is admitted to ICU for respiratory failure due to decompensated heart failure and cardiogenic pulmonary edema. On the day of admission, he requires intubation and mechanical ventilation, and aggressive diuresis is initiated. On day 3 of his ICU stay, his ventilator is set on pressure support, with a driving pressure of 5 cm $H_2O$, PEEP of 10 cm $H_2O$, and $FiO_2$ of 0.3. He is fully awake and breathing comfortably. He is placed on a spontaneous breathing trial with pressure support settings of driving pressure of 5 cm $H_2O$, PEEP of 0 cm $H_2O$, and $FiO_2$ of 0.3. Within minutes, he experiences oxygen desaturation, tachypnea, and respiratory distress. Which among the following in the MOST LIKELY cause for failure of his spontaneous breathing trial?

   A. Atelectrauma from collapse of alveoli with tidal breathing
   B. Mucous plugging from lower airway pressure
   C. Increased preload and decreased afterload
   D. Decreased preload and increased afterload
   E. Increased preload and increased afterload

7. A 75-year-old woman has been intubated for 7 days for community-acquired pneumonia. She is placed on a spontaneous breathing trial on ventilator settings of pressure support of 5 cm $H_2O$, PEEP of 0 cm $H_2O$, and $FiO2$ of 0.3. What is the most accurate explanation of how breaths are cycled (initiated or terminated) on this ventilator mode?

   A. Breaths are initiated based on a set respiratory rate and inspiratory:expiratory ratio.
   B. Breaths are terminated when inspiratory flow decreases to a set percentage of peak inspiratory flow.
   C. Breaths are terminated when a target volume is reached.
   D. Breathes are initiated based on diaphragmatic inspiratory effort.
   E. Breaths are terminated when a peak inspiratory flow is reached.

8. A 68-year-old woman with HIV is admitted to the ICU with respiratory failure secondary to pneumocystis pneumonia, requiring intubation and mechanical ventilation. A chest CT scan was performed before intubation and demonstrated cystic changes throughout the lungs, thought to be a sequela of past pneumocystis infection, with superimposed diffuse ground glass opacities. Her ventilator is set on volume assist-control, TV 6 mL/kg, respiratory rate 16 breaths per minute, $FiO2$ 0.8, and PEEP of 10 cm $H_2O$. On day 2 of her critical illness, her ventilator suddenly alarms for elevated peak pressures. She is observed to be deeply sedated and breathing passively on the ventilator. The peak pressure has risen from 25 cm $H_2O$ several hours before 50 cm $H_2O$. The patient has simultaneously experienced oxygen desaturation from 95% to 90%. She is otherwise hemodynamically stable. A chest radiograph is ordered. An inspiratory hold maneuver is performed and her plateau pressure is 20 cm $H_2O$. Which of the following is the MOST LIKELY explanation for this acute event?

   A. Rupture of a cyst leading to pneumothorax and acute decrease in lung compliance
   B. Mucous in the endotracheal tube leading to acute increase in airway resistance
   C. Mainstem intubation from migration of the endotracheal tube
   D. Biting on the endotracheal tube leading to acute increase in airway resistance
   E. Mucous plugging leading to lobar collapse and acute decrease in lung compliance

**9.** A 68-year-old man with chronic obstructive pulmonary disease ($FEV_1$ 30% predicted, on 3 L home $O_2$) presents to the emergency department with increased dyspnea for the past 3 days requiring a frequent albuterol-ipratropium nebulizer use at home. He is found to have labored breathing and his initial ABG shows pH 7.27 with a $PCO_2$ 90 mm Hg. His chest radiograph demonstrates no infiltrate but some increased interstitial markings consistent with volume overload. He is diagnosed with an acute exacerbation of chronic obstructive pulmonary disease and possible cardiogenic pulmonary edema and started on bronchodilators and given a dose of furosemide. On reevaluation, he is somnolent but arousable to sternal rub and is placed on bilevel positive airway pressure ventilation (BiPAP). Which of the following is most true regarding use of BiPAP in this patient?

   **A.** Treatment of patients like this with BiPAP is associated with increased mortality because it delays intubation.
   **B.** Treatment with BiPAP is associated with longer hospital length of stay.
   **C.** Coincident acute cardiogenic pulmonary edema is a relative contraindication to BiPAP.
   **D.** BiPAP is more likely to improve outcomes in patients with asthma than in this patient.
   **E.** His altered mental status is a relative contraindication to treatment with BiPAP.

**10.** A 48-year-old man with no prior medical history is admitted with community-acquired pneumonia and severe acute respiratory distress syndrome (ARDS). On day 1 of his illness, he is admitted to your ICU on volume control-assist control ventilation with a VT of 4 mL/kg IBW, respiratory rate 32 breaths per minute, PEEP 14 cm $H_2O$, and $FiO_2$ 1.0. On those settings, he is found to be hypoxemic with a $SaO_2$ of 86% with an ABG that demonstrates pH 7.28 $PCO_2$ 65 mm Hg and $PaO_2$ 55 mm Hg. Which of the following interventions is most likely to improve his survival?

   **A.** Prone positioning for at least 16 hours a day until oxygenation improves
   **B.** Initiation of extracorporeal membrane support (ECMO)
   **C.** PEEP titration using esophageal balloon pressures
   **D.** Initiation of high-frequency oscillatory ventilation
   **E.** Inhaled pulmonary vasodilator therapy

**11.** A 56-year-old woman with a history of recently diagnosed acute myeloid leukemia is admitted to the ICU after undergoing induction chemotherapy. She is febrile with temperature of 39°C and has a respiratory rate of 36 breaths per minute with $SaO_2$ 84% on 10L per minute oxygen by face mask. Her labs are otherwise notable for an absolute neutrophil count of 125. Which of the following is the most accurate statement regarding her management?

   **A.** Use on noninvasive ventilation instead of invasive ventilation is associated with increased mortality.
   **B.** Airway pressure release ventilation (APRV) is the preferred lung protective ventilator mode.
   **C.** Sedation with benzodiazepines is associated with longer ICU length of stay.
   **D.** Diuresis to a goal body balance of about even over the first 7 days is associated with decreased mortality.

**12.** A 22-year-old woman with a history of asthma (previously intubated twice) presents to the emergency department with worsening dyspnea over the past week and is found to have influenza. Her chest radiograph demonstrates bilateral patchy opacities and she is intubated for hypoxemic respiratory failure and receives empiric antibiotics, bronchodilators, and steroids. Ventilator settings are pressure control-assist control with an inspiratory pressure ($P_{Insp}$) of 25 cm $H_2O$, a PEEP of 5 cm $H_2O$, and a respiratory rate of 24 breaths per minute. On arrival to the ICU, she remains paralyzed after rapid sequence intubation, and on the above settings she is getting a TV of 200 mL (4 mL/kg IBW). Which of the following statements is MOST accurate regarding her ventilator settings and physiology?

   **A.** While she is paralyzed, her compliance can reliably be calculated from her inspiratory pressure and delivered volume.
   **B.** While she is paralyzed, you need to measure a pleural pressure to reliably calculate her pulmonary resistance.
   **C.** When her paralytics wear off, you would need to measure pleural pressure to reliably calculate her pulmonary compliance.
   **D.** Her pulmonary resistance is best assessed by looking at the difference between her peak inspiratory pressure and a pressure during an end-inspiratory pause.

**13.** An 84-year-old man with severe chronic obstructive pulmonary disease ($FEV_1$ 20% predicted, on 4 L/min home $O_2$) is admitted with severe hypoxemic respiratory failure due to a *Streptococcus pneumoniae* infection. He is intubated and placed on volume control-assist control ventilation with a set TV of 400 mL (6.5 mL/kg IBW), PEEP of 8 cm $H_2O$ and a respiratory rate of 30 breaths per minute. When the paralytic used for intubation wears off, the patient is noted to be triggering additional spontaneous breaths with a total respiratory rate of 36 breaths per minute, and his exhaled TVs vary from 100 to 800 mL. During an end-expiratory pause, his airway pressure is 18 cm $H_2O$. Which of the following is the MOST accurate statement regarding his ventilator settings?

**A.** Because the patient is on volume control, he is receiving lung-protective TVs.
**B.** The patient's intrinsic PEEP is likely overestimated by the measured end-expiratory airway pressure.
**C.** Changing the patient to pressure control will improve the patient's intrinsic PEEP.
**D.** The patient's intrinsic PEEP is likely making it more difficult for him to trigger spontaneous breaths.
**E.** Changing the patient to pressure control will provide more lung-protective TVs.

# Chapter 32 ▪ Answers

**1.** Correct Answer: B

**Rationale:**
This patient is presenting with severe ARDS, as defined by the Berlin criteria: onset within 1 week or presentation, bilateral opacities on imaging, edema not fully explained by cardiogenic etiology, and $PaO_2$:$FiO_2$ ratio of <100. The ARDSnet trial demonstrated a significant mortality benefit with lung protective, low-TV ventilation (6 mL/kg IBW) (answer B is correct). Diuresis to an even fluid balance increases ventilator-free days in patients with ARDS but has not been found to have a mortality benefit (answer A is incorrect). Similarly, while inhaled nitric oxide and PEEP titration may improve oxygenation, neither intervention has been demonstrated to improve survival (answers C and E are incorrect). Invasive respiratory cultures are not recommended in patients with severe community acquired pneumonia (answer D is incorrect).

References
1. Ranieri VM, Rubenfeld GD, Thompson BT, et al. Acute respiratory distress syndrome: the Berlin definition. *JAMA*. 2012;307(23):2526-2533.
2. The Acute Respiratory Distress Syndrome Network. Ventilation with lower tidal volumes as compared with traditional tidal volumes for acute lung injury and the acute respiratory disress syndrome. *N Engl J Med*. 2000;342:1301-1308.
3. Gebistorf F, Karam O, Wetterslev J, Afshari A. Inhaled nitric oxide for acute respiratory distress syndrome (ARDS) in children and adults. *Cochrane Database Syst Rev*. 2016;(6):CD002787.
4. Writing Group for the Alveolar Recruitment for Acute Respiratory Distress Syndrome Trial (ART) Investigators. Effect of lung recruitment effect of lung recruitment and titrated positive end-expiratory pressure (PEEP) vs low peep on mortality in patients with acute respiratory distress syndrome. *JAMA*. 2017;318(14):1335-1345.

**2.** Correct Answer: A

**Rationale:**
The patient has developed hemodynamic instability as a result of intrinsic PEEP, or dynamic hyperinflation, which increases intrathoracic pressure and decreases venous return. This is a life-threatening complication that requires immediate release of trapped gas from the lungs; this is best accomplished by disconnecting the ventilator circuit for a brief period of time (answer A is correct). Intrinsic PEEP can be very common in patients with obstructive lung disease on the ventilator.

Without evidence of pneumothorax on radiograph, ultrasound, or other high suspicion, a needle decompression is not warranted (answer B is incorrect). Bronchoscopy is occasionally utilized to clear mucous plugging in patient with severe asthma, however this would not explain the patient's hemodynamic instability (answer C is incorrect). An increase in the respiratory rate will decrease the patient's expiratory time and lead to worsening gas trapping (answer D is incorrect). A decrease in the extrinsic PEEP set on the ventilator will not decrease intrinsic PEEP and will not improve this patient's hemodynamics (answer E is incorrect).

Reference
1. MacIntyre NR, Cheng KC, McConnell R. Applied PEEP during pressure support reduces the inspiratory threshold load of intrinsic PEEP. *Chest*. 1997;111(1):188.

**3.** Correct Answer: D

**Rationale:**

The respiratory system compliance is equal to the change in volume divided by the change in pressure. In this case, the change in volume is the TV (450 mL) and the change in pressure is the plateau pressure minus the PEEP (15 cm $H_2O$ – 5 cm $H_2O$ = 10 cm $H_2O$) (answer D is correct). Without a measure of a pleural pressure, it is not possible to separately calculate lung and chest wall compliance (answers A, B and C are incorrect).

**4.** Correct Answer: B

**Rationale:**

Routine, protocolized implementation of a spontaneous breathing trial, paired with a spontaneous awakening trial, or interruption of sedation, results in a decreased duration of mechanical ventilation when compared with spontaneous breathing trial alone. Spontaneous breathing trials should be performed as a routine practice based on protocol, rather than when directed only by a medical provider (answers A and E are incorrect). Studies examining early tracheostomy have not demonstrated a decreased time on the ventilator, though this approach may be appropriate in select cases when reversal of the underlying process is not expected within several weeks (answer D is incorrect). In comparison with a decremental pressure support-based ventilator liberation strategy, spontaneous breathing trial is superior in ability to decrease the duration of mechanical ventilation (answer C is incorrect).

References

1. Girard TD, Kress JP, Fuchs BD, et al. Efficacy and safety of a paired sedation and ventilator weaning protocol for mechanically ventilated patients in intensive care (Awakening and Breathing Controlled trial): a randomised controlled trial. *Lancet.* 2008;371(9607):126-134.
2. Andriolo BNG, Andriolo RB, Saconato H, Atallah ÁN, Valente O. Early versus late tracheostomy for critically ill patients (Review). *Cochrane Database Syst Rev.* 2015;(1):CD007271.
3. Esteban A, Frutos F, Tobin MJ, et al. A comparison of four methods of weaning patients from mechanical ventilation. Spanish Lung Failure Collaborative Group. *N Engl J Med.* 1995;332(6):345-350.

**5.** Correct Answer: C

**Rationale:**

The patient has developed a ventilator-associated pneumonia (VAP), as defined by new worsening respiratory status, worsening volume and quality of sputum, and new radiographic infiltrate. VAPs frequently occur because of aspiration of secretions around the cuff of an endotracheal tube. Nosocomial pathogens, including *P. aeruginosa* and methicillin-resistant *S. aureus,* are common causes of VAP. Empiric coverage for these pathogens with an antipseudomonal beta-lactam and vancomycin is therefore recommended while awaiting culture results; choice of an antipseudomonal agent may depend on local resistance patterns (answer C is correct; answer D is incorrect). Treatment with ceftriaxone is inadequate as is does not provide coverage of *Pseudomonas* or methicillin-resistant *S. aureus.* Azithromycin is important when considering treatment of atypical organisms, particularly *Legionella* in community-acquired pneumonia, but would not be necessary for empiric VAP coverage (answer B and E are incorrect). Metronidazole adds additional anerobic coverage, which is not considered necessary in the treatment of VAP (answer A is incorrect).

Reference

1. Kalil AC, Metersky ML, Klompas M, et al. Management of adults with hospital-acquired and ventilator-associated pneumonia: 2016 clinical practice guidelines by the infectious diseases Society of America and the American Thoracic Society. *Clin Infect Dis.* 2016;63(5):e61-e111.

**6.** Correct Answer: E

**Rationale:**

The application of PEEP in both noninvasive and invasive positive pressure ventilation serves to decrease cardiac preload, through decreased venous return and decrease cardiac afterload as a result of decreased ventricular volume (and therefore radius) and transmural cardiac wall tension. In patients with baseline cardiac dysfunction, weaning-induced cardiac dysfunction may be observed when the absence of PEEP leads to an acute increase in cardiac preload and afterload (answer E is correct; answers C and D are incorrect).

Atelectrauma is a form of lung injury most common in ARDS, in which loss of surfactant and alveolar flooding result in alveolar instability and cyclic opening and closing of lung units with ventilation. Although atelectrauma can occur in other types of respiratory failure, it is less likely to result in such a rapid decompensation (answer A is incorrect). Mucous plugging can occur on any PEEP and is less likely to explain this increased respiratory distress associated with the reduction in positive pressure (answer B is incorrect).

Reference

1. Cherpanath TG, Lagrand WK, Schultz MJ, Groeneveld AB. Cardiopulmonary interactions during mechanical ventilation in critically ill patients. *Neth Heart J.* 2013;21(4):166-172.

**7.** Correct Answer: B

**Rationale:**

Pressure support breaths are cycled from inspiratory to expiratory when the patient's inspiratory flow reaches a set percentage of the peak inspiratory flow, often 25% of peak inspiratory flow by default (answer B is correct). Pressure assist-control, a form of continuous mandatory ventilation, cycles based on a set inspiratory time (answer A is incorrect). Volume assist-control, a form of continuous mandatory ventilation, cycles when a breath reaches a target TV, the time for which is dictated by an inspiratory flow rate (answer C is incorrect). Neurally assisted ventilation coordinates inspiratory support with diaphragmatic muscular effort (answer D is incorrect). There are no modes that are terminated by reaching a peak inspiratory flow (answer E is incorrect).

Reference

1. Gentile MA. Cycling of the mechanical ventilator breath. *Respir Care.* 2011;56(1):52-60.

**8.** Correct Answer: B

**Rationale:**

The ventilator mechanics reported here describe an acute increase in peak airway pressure with a normal plateau pressure. This indicates that the peak airway pressure is reflective of an acute increase in resistance within the respiratory system or endotracheal tube. Potential causes of this include biting or other kinking of the endotracheal tube, mucous within the endotracheal tube or airway without complete obstruction, bronchospasm, or airway edema/inflammation (answer B is correct). An increase in peak airway pressure, with a corresponding increase in plateau pressure, represents decrease in respiratory system compliance. This may be secondary to lobar collapse, mainstem intubation, pulmonary edema, pneumonia, ARDS, pleural effusion, pneumothorax, elevated intraabdominal pressure, or elevated chest wall pressure (answers A, C and E are incorrect). Given that the patient is deeply sedated, biting on the endotracheal tube is not a likely explanation for the increase in airway resistance (answer D is incorrect).

**9.** Correct Answer: E

**Rationale:**

Noninvasive positive pressure ventilation may reduce the rates of intubation, reduce the time to clinical improvement, and reduce mortality in patients with an acute exacerbation of chronic obstructive pulmonary disease with hypercarbia (answers A and B are incorrect). In patients with acute cardiogenic pulmonary edema, noninvasive positive pressure ventilation is associated with a decreased rate of intubation and decreased time to improvement in symptoms (answer C is incorrect).

Relative contraindications to BiPAP include significant secretions, altered mental status, and a patient's inability to protect their airway (answer E is correct). The data for use of BiPAP in patients with asthma are inconclusive and much less robust than data supporting use in chronic obstructive pulmonary disease (answer D is incorrect).

References

1. Osadnik CR, Tee VS, Carson-Chahhoud KV, et al. Non-invasive ventilation for the management of acute hypercapnic respiratory failure due to exacerbation of chronic obstructive pulmonary disease (Review). *Cochrane Database Syst Rev.* 2017;(7):CD00410.
2. Gray A, Goodacre S, Newby DE, et al. Noninvasive ventilation in acute cardiogenic pulmonary edema. *N Engl J Med.* 2008;359(2):142-151.

**10.** Correct Answer: A

**Rationale:**

Although prior data were conflicting, a recent large, multicenter randomized controlled study of prone positioning in patients with ARDS within the first 48 hours demonstrated a significant reduction in mortality in the prone position group (answer A is correct). Although ECMO is increasingly employed as a rescue therapy in patients with severe ARDS and refractory hypoxemia, there have been no trials that demonstrate a significant mortality benefit (answer B is incorrect). PEEP titration using an esophageal balloon improves oxygenation and pulmonary mechanics in patients with ARDS but does not improve mortality. High-frequency oscillatory ventilation has been shown to potentially harm patients with ARDS (answer D is incorrect). Although inhaled pulmonary vasodilators improve oxygenation in patients with ARDS, there are not data that they improve survival (answer E is incorrect).

References

1. Guerin C, Reignier J, Richards JC, et al. Prone positioning in severe acute respiratory distress syndrome. *N Engl J Med.* 2013;368:2159-2168.
2. Combes A, Hajage D, Capellier G, et al. Extracorporeal membrane oxygenation for severe acute respiratory distress syndrome. *N Engl J Med.* 2018;378:1965-1975.

3. Beitler JR, Sarge T, Banner-Godspeed VM, et al. Effect of titrating positive end-expiratory pressure (PEEP) With an Esophageal pressure–guided strategy vs an empirical high PEEP-Fio$_2$ strategy on death and days free from mechanical ventilation among patients with acute respiratory distress syndrome. *JAMA*. 2019;321:846-857.
4. Gebistorf F, Karam O, Wetterslev J, Afshari A. Inhaled nitric oxide for acute respiratory distress syndrome (ARDS) in children and adults. *Cochrane Database Syst Rev*. 2016;(6):CD002787.

## 11. Correct Answer: C

### Rationale:

Immunocompromised patients with ARDS are a unique population with both different epidemiology of infections and different data for management. Specifically, in patients with single-organ failure, the use of noninvasive ventilation has been associated with improved mortality compared with invasive ventilation (answer A is incorrect). Although APRV can increase mean airway pressure and therefore can improve oxygenation, there is no benefit to APRV compared with standard volume control-assist control ventilation and depending on the settings may not represent a volume-controlled mode (ie may be more injurious) (answer B is incorrect). Although diuresis to a goal body balance even over 7 days is associated with more ventilator-free days, it is not associated with decreased mortality (answer D is incorrect). Sedation with benzodiazepines, as compared with sedation with propofol or dexmedetomidine, is associated with longer length of stay and duration of mechanical ventilation (answer C is correct). Some studies also suggest an association between benzodiazepines and worse cognitive outcomes as well as increased short-term mortality. Sedation with nonbenzodiazepine-containing regimens is therefore preferred.

### References

1. Hilbert G, Gurson D, Vargas F, et al. Noninvasive ventilation in immunosuppressed patients with pulmonary infiltrates, fever, and acute respiratory failure. *N Engl J Med*. 2001;344(7):481-487.
2. ARDS Clinical Trials Network. Comparison of two fluid-management strategies in acute lung injury. *N Engl J Med*. 2006;354:2564-2575.
3. Fraser GL, Devlin JW, Worby CP, et al. Benzodiazepine versus nonbenzodiazepine-based sedation for mechanically ventilated, critically ill aduts: a systematic review and meta-analysis of randomized trials. *Crit Care Med*. 2013;41:S30-S38.

## 12. Correct Answer: C

### Rationale:

Unlike assist control-volume control, in a pressure-control mode of ventilation, the airway opening pressures are the target variables (ie the variable set on the ventilator). This means that her peak inspiratory pressure will be the same as the pressure that the ventilator has set during an inspiratory pause (in this case, 25 cm H$_2$O) and resistance cannot be calculated from these numbers (answer D is incorrect). Compliance can *sometimes* be calculated from the set change in pressure at the airway opening and the resulting volume delivered but there are important caveats. If flow does not reach zero at the end of inhalation (for example, in a patient with elevated airways resistance such as this patient or with very short inspiratory times) then you cannot reliably calculate a resistance from the set pressure and the delivered volume (answer A is incorrect). In addition, if the patient is making spontaneous effort in sync with the ventilator then the transpulmonary pressure (the distending pressure of the lung parenchyma) can only be calculated with a measurement of her pleural pressure with an esophageal balloon (answer C is correct). The pleural pressure is not necessary to calculate resistance (answer B is incorrect).

## 13. Correct Answer: D

### Rationale:

This patient is on a volume-control mode of ventilation but is asynchronous with variable exhaled TVs, which indicates "breath stacking," a type of cycle asynchrony in which patients do not fully exhale before taking their next breath. In this situation, the patient is no longer receiving the lung-protective TV that has been set despite being on a volume control mode (answer A is incorrect). If the ventilator setting were changed to pressure control, his TVs would vary with respiratory effort and therefore he would not be guaranteed to have more lung-protective TVs (answer E is incorrect).

The patient has evidence of intrinsic PEEP with an end-expiratory pressure that is greater than the set PEEP. In order to trigger breaths on the ventilator, or breath spontaneously, a patient needs to decrease their airway opening pressure and (depending on a ventilator trigger mode) create inspiratory flow. When a patient has intrinsic PEEP, they must overcome this PEEP to decrease their airway opening pressure or initiate inspiratory flow; this is the inspiratory threshold load and it increases the work of breathing both in spontaneously breathing and patients who are mechanically breathing and triggering breaths (answer D is correct). Changing the ventilator mode to pressure control will not necessarily decrease intrinsic PEEP (answer C is incorrect). The measurement of end-expiratory airway pressure often underestimates intrinsic PEEP because lung units that are slow emptying may not equilibrate with the airway opening and therefore the sickest lung units with the highest intrinsic PEEP are not fully represented by bedside measurements (answer B is incorrect).

### Reference

1. Nilsestuen JO, Hargett KD. Using ventilator graphics to identify patient-ventilator asynchrony. *Respir Care*. 2005;50(2):202-234.

# 33

# ACUTE RESPIRATORY DISTRESS SYNDROME

Rachel Steinhorn and Jeanine P. Wiener-Kronish

1. A 65-year-old woman with history of COPD, congestive heart failure with ejection fraction of 35%, Hepatitis C cirrhosis without ascites, and body mass index of 35 is intubated for hypoxemic respiratory failure after an aspiration event and transferred to the ICU for further management. A chest radiograph demonstrates bilateral patchy infiltrates, and initial $PaO_2$ is 145 on $FiO_2$ 100%. The patient remains hypoxemic on standard ventilation with tidal volumes 6 mL/kg and PEEP titrated to 12 cm $H_2O$ on $FiO_2$ 100%. Which clinical factor suggests this patient may benefit from esophageal pressure measurements to titrate ventilation parameters?

   A. COPD
   B. CHF with reduced EF
   C. HCV cirrhosis
   D. BMI 35

2. A 36-year-old man is admitted to the ICU intubated status post polytrauma, with trauma burden including multiple lacerations over the ventral chest wall and an uncleared c-spine. He develops progressive hypoxemia over the first 12 hours of admission, with $PaO_2$:$FiO_2$ ratios decreasing to <150 on $FiO_2$ 100%. Mechanical ventilation with tidal volumes 6 mL/kg and PEEP titrated to 12 cm $H_2O$ is initiated; however, arterial blood gas persistently shows pH 7.25 with $PaCO_2$ 68 and $PaO_2$ 67 on $FiO_2$ 100% over the subsequent 6 hours. The patient is adequately sedated, paralyzed, and demonstrates no ventilator asynchrony. What is the next best step?

   A. Use esophageal pressure measurements to titrate PEEP
   B. Initiate venovenous ECMO
   C. Prone the patient
   D. Initiate inhaled nitric oxide

3. A 29-year-old woman is admitted to the floor with a productive cough and fevers; her influenza swab is positive, and chest radiograph demonstrates bilateral patchy pulmonary opacities. She develops progressive hypoxemic respiratory failure requiring intubation on the first day of admission. On transfer to the ICU, her initial arterial blood gas shows a pH 7.35, $PaO_2$ 86, $PaCO_2$ 33 on $FiO_2$ 100%. What is the next best step?

   A. Ventilation with tidal volumes 4 to 6 mL/kg and PEEP >5
   B. Initiate venovenous ECMO
   C. Obtain a chest CT
   D. Blood cultures and broad spectrum antibiotics

**4.** A 66-year-old woman with *Haemophilus influenzae* pneumonia is intubated on the floor for hypoxemic respiratory failure and transferred to the ICU. Chest radiograph demonstrates bilateral patchy infiltrates; ABG is pH 7.34, $PaCO_2$ 47, $PaO_2$ 105 on $FiO_2$ 100%. Mechanical ventilation is titrated to tidal volumes 6 mL/kg with PEEP 8 cm $H_2O$, and plateau pressures remain <30 cm $H_2O$. The patient is paralyzed and sedated with no ventilator asynchrony noted. What is the next best step?

   **A.** Initiate venovenous ECMO
   **B.** Prone the patient
   **C.** Initiate inhaled nitric oxide
   **D.** Esophageal pressure monitoring to titrate PEEP

**5.** A 54-year-old man with a history of moderate COPD is transferred from the floor to the ICU one day after a witnessed aspiration event for increased work of breathing. On examination, pulmonary auscultation reveals bilateral rhonchi but no wheezing, and chest radiograph shows new bilateral, patchy pulmonary opacities. Respiratory rate is 36, and the patient communicates in one to three word sentences between breaths. Initial arterial blood gas analysis shows pH 7.34, $PaCO_2$ 65, $PaO_2$ 135 on 15L non-rebreather face mask. What is the next best step?

   **A.** Trial of noninvasive ventilation (NIV)
   **B.** Ipratropium/albuterol nebulizer
   **C.** Intubation and mechanical ventilation
   **D.** Furosemide IV bolus

**6.** A 65-year-old woman with a history of severe COPD and coronary artery disease is intubated for severe acute respiratory distress syndrome (ARDS) in the setting of pneumonia. Despite ventilation with 6 mL/kg tidal volumes and neuromuscular blockade, $PaO_2$:$FiO_2$ remains 85 on $FiO_2$ 100%. PEEP is increased from 5 to 10 cm $H_2O$, and mean arterial pressure subsequently decreases from 65 to 45. In what setting is increased PEEP *least* likely to improve oxygenation and hemodynamics?

   **A.** Right ventricular dysfunction
   **B.** Left ventricular (LV) dysfunction
   **C.** Severe ARDS
   **D.** Obesity

**7.** A 67-year-old woman was intubated for ARDS in the setting of pneumonia with septic shock and received muscular paralysis with cisatracurium to improve ventilator synchrony over the first 24 hours of mechanical ventilation. Her mean arterial pressure remains >65 on norepinephrine 35 µg/min. Cisatracurium was discontinued 12 hours prior, and the ventilator has been weaned to pressure support mode. She receives a spontaneous breathing trial (SBT) for 30 minutes on CPAP 5 cm $H_2O$ and $FiO_2$ 0.4. At this setting she has an $SpO_2$ 92%, generates a tidal volume of 4 mL/kg, and respiratory rate 28 breaths/min, with no signs of respiratory distress. What is the contraindication to extubation in the patient?

   **A.** There are no contraindications to extubation
   **B.** SBT <120 minutes
   **C.** SBT on CPAP 5 cm $H_2O$ instead of 0 cm $H_2O$
   **D.** Ongoing vasopressor support

**8.** Two 24-year-old males are admitted to the ICU intubated after polytrauma status post motor vehicle collision. Over the first 24 hours of admission, Patient 1 develops hypoxemia with bilateral pulmonary opacities on chest radiograph and $PaO_2$:$FiO_2$ 110. Patient 2 remains intubated for persistent altered mental status, and then on hospital day 4, develops bilateral pulmonary infiltrates with $PaO_2$:$FiO_2$ 220. Compared to Patient 2, Patient 1's clinical course likely includes:

   **A.** Lower thoracic trauma burden
   **B.** Higher mortality risk
   **C.** More severe hypotension on admission
   **D.** Increased likelihood of acute renal failure

# Chapter 33 ■ Answers

**1.** Correct Answer: D

**Rationale:**
The pressure in the lower third of the esophagus closely parallels the pressure in the adjoining pleura. The measurement is accurate when taken in the upright lung, without the pressure of the mediastinum compressing the esophagus. The esophageal pressure balloon can therefore be used to estimate the transpulmonary pressure ($P_{transpulmonary} = P_{airway\ opening} - P_{pleura}$). Referring to the transpulmonary pressure equation, elevated pleural pressure can result in negative end-expiratory transpulmonary pressure, which is clinically manifested as alveolar collapse. Esophageal pressure measurement as a proxy for pleural pressure allows for titration of PEEP to maintain positive transpulmonary pressure at end expiration, maintaining functional residual capacity and preventing airway collapse. Patients ventilated to achieve transpulmonary pressure 0 to 10 cm $H_2O$ had significantly improved oxygenation and lung compliance.

Esophageal pressure is most likely to be useful in patients with elevated pleural pressure due to a decrease in extrapulmonary compliance. Direct pulmonary causes of ARDS, such as aspiration or pneumonia, are associated with decreased lung compliance but often have normal chest wall compliance. They are characterized by alveolar consolidation, which is not typically responsive to changes in PEEP. By contrast, extrapulmonary decreases in compliance, caused by factors such as obesity, ascites, bowel edema, pancreatitis, peritonitis, or other intra-abdominal pathologies, manifest as atelectasis and have a greater potential for alveolar recruitment. COPD, congestive heart failure, and cirrhosis without ascites do not particularly decrease extrapulmonary compliance and thus are not likely to specifically benefit from esophageal pressure measurements.

## References

1. Akoumianaki E, Maggiore S, Valenza F, et al. The application of esophageal pressure measurement in patients with respiratory failure. *Am J Respir Crit Care Med*. 2014;189(5):520-531.
2. Talmor D, Sarge T, O'Donnell CR, et al. Esophageal and transpulmonary pressures in acute respiratory failure. *Crit Care Med*. 2006;34(5):1389-1394. doi:10.1097/01.CCM.0000215515.49001.A2.
3. Talmor D, Sarge T, Malhotra A, et al. Mechanical ventilation guided by esophageal pressure in acute lung injury. *N Engl J Med*. 2008;359(20):2095-2104. doi:10.1056/NEJMoa0708638.

**2.** Correct Answer: B

**Rationale:**
Mechanical ventilation can perpetuate lung injury in ARDS by overdistending ventilated alveoli and causing atelectrauma be repeated alveolar opening and collapse if PEEP is insufficient to maintain patency at end expiration. Venovenous ECMO can be used to bypass the pulmonary circuit in severe ARDS, performing gas exchange and minimizing further lung injury. It is typically a salvage therapy utilized when other rescue strategies such as prone positioning or neuromuscular blockade have failed or are contraindicated. Criteria for ECMO initiation include acute, reversible lung injury when conventional therapy is insufficient to sustain life in the setting of severe hypoxemia ($PaO_2:FiO_2$ <80) or uncompensated respiratory acidosis (pH <7.20). Contraindications include irreversible lung disease with no indication for lung transplant and intracranial bleeding.

In this stem, the patient has already shown no improvement after paralysis to ensure ventilator synchrony. An unstable vertebral fracture is an absolute contraindication to proning, whereas significant lacerations or burns over the ventral chest or abdomen are a relative contraindication. Inhaled nitric oxide results in transient improvement in oxygenation in patients with ARDS while therapy is continued but has shown no benefit on mortality and is associated with acute kidney injury. Esophageal pressure measurement can be used to individualize PEEP titration for improved alveolar recruitment, particularly in patients with decreased extrapulmonary compliance, such as those with ascites or obesity. However, it is unlikely to salvage the degree of refractory hypoxemia and respiratory acidosis seen in this patient. Thus, venovenous ECMO seems to be the next best strategy in this patient.

## References

1. Peek GJ, Clemens F, Elbourne D, et al. CESAR: conventional ventilatory support vs extracorporeal membrane oxygenation for severe adult respiratory failure. *BMC Health Serv Res*. 2006;6:163. doi:10.1186/1472-6963-6-163.
2. Combes A, Hajage D, Capellier G, et al. Extracorporeal membrane oxygenation for severe acute respiratory distress syndrome. *N Engl J Med*. 2018;378:1965-1975.
3. Aokage T, Palmer K, Ichiba S, Takeda S. Extracorporeal membrane oxygenation for acute respiratory distress syndrome. *J Intensive Care*. 2015;3(1):17.
4. Akmal AH, Hasan M. Role of nitric oxide in management of acute respiratory distress syndrome. *Ann Thorac Med*. 2008;3(3):100-103. doi:10.4103/1817-1737.41914.

**3.** Correct Answer: A

**Rationale:**

ARDS impacts as many as 10% of patients admitted to the ICU and 23% of mechanically ventilated patients, with a mortality of 46% in patients with severe ARDS. This patient clearly meets the diagnosis of severe ARDS by the Berlin criteria, which include:

| TIMING | WITHIN 1 WK OF KNOWN CLINICAL INSULT OR NEW/WORSENING RESPIRATORY SYMPTOMS |
|---|---|
| Chest imaging | Bilateral opacities not fully explained by effusions, lobar/lung collapse, or nodules |
| Origin of edema | Respiratory failure not fully explained by cardiac failure or fluid overload |
| Oxygenation | Measurement performed with PEEP or CPAP >5 cm $H_2O$ |
| Mild | 200 mm Hg < $PaO_2$:$FiO_2$ <300 mm Hg |
| Moderate | 100 mm Hg < $PaO_2$:$FiO_2$ <200 mm Hg |
| Severe | $PaO_2$:$FiO_2$ <100 mm Hg |

For all patients with ARDS, NHBI ARDS Network guidelines strongly suggest ventilation with low tidal volumes (goal 4-6 mL/kg predicted body weight) with plateau pressures <30 cm $H_2O$ and a minimum of PEEP 5 cm $H_2O$. In addition, patients should receive conservative fluid management, which has been shown to shorten the duration of assisted ventilation.

Venovenous ECMO can be used to support patients with severe ARDS when conventional therapy is insufficient to correct severe hypoxemia ($PaO_2$:$FiO_2$ <80) or hypercapnia (pH <7.20.) An increasing number of centers use ECMO in ARDS, particularly after 2009 H1N1 influenza A epidemic, where the patient population was typically young and otherwise healthy. Initial study of ECMO use for ARDS in patients with H1N1 found a mortality of 21%, leading to speculation that early initiation of ECMO may improve mortality. The EOLIA trial published in 2018, however, showed no mortality benefit with early initiation of ECMO as compared to ARDS Network mechanical ventilation with conventional rescue strategies that included ECMO.

A chest CT can be useful to confirm ARDS when chest radiographs fail to demonstrate opacities consistent with the diagnosis, given the heterogeneity of radiographic presentation, but it is not the next best step in this hypoxic patient. Likewise, although she will need blood cultures to rule out a superimposed bacterial pneumonia on viral influenza, improving oxygenation takes priority.

### References

1. Thompson BT, Chambers RC, Liu KD. Acute respiratory distress syndrome. *N Engl J Med.* 2017;377:562-572.
2. The Acute Respiratory Distress Syndrome Network. Ventilation with lower tidal volumes as compared with traditional tidal volumes for acute lung injury and the acute respiratory distress syndrome. *N Engl J Med.* 2000;342(18):1301-1308.
3. Thompson BT, Bernard GR. ARDS network (NHLBI) studies – successes and challenges in ARDS clinical research. *Crit Care Clin.* 2011;27(3):459-468. doi:10.1016/j.ccc.2011.05.011.
4. Davies A, Jones D, Bailey M, et al. Extracorporeal membrane oxygenation for 2009 influenza A(H1N1) acute respiratory distress syndrome. *JAMA.* 2009;302:1888-1895.
5. Combes A, Hajage D, Capellier G, et al. Extracorporeal membrane oxygenation for severe acute respiratory distress syndrome. *N Engl J Med.* 2018;378:1965-1975.

**4.** Correct Answer: B

**Rationale:**

In patients with severe ARDS (defined as $PaO_2$:$FiO_2$ <150 with an $FiO_2$ of >60%, PEEP >5 cm $H_2O$, and tidal volumes 6 mL/kg), changing from supine to the prone position is associated with decreased mortality. Best outcomes have been shown when performed early in the course (<48 hour), and in conjunction with neuromuscular blockade and tidal volume <6 mL/kg. It improves oxygenation and reduces the risk of ventilator-associated lung injury by homogenizing ventilation in the dependent and nondependent portions of lung, reducing ventral overdistension, and improving dorsal alveolar recruitment.

Contraindications to prone ventilation include patients with facial/neck trauma or spinal instability, patients with elevated ICP, recent sternotomy, large burns or lacerations over the ventral body area, massive hemoptysis, hemodynamic instability, or patients at high risk for needing CPR/defibrillation. Factors such as chest tubes, multiple lines, and large body habitus can require extensive coordination with the care team during turning but are not contraindications. Potential complications of the prone position include kinking or misplacement of the ETT, kinking of vascular access, temporary increase in oral or tracheal secretions that can occlude the ETT, facial pressure ulcers, facial edema, brachial plexus injury, and elevated intra-abdominal pressure, which can complicate enteral feeding.

Venovenous ECMO can be used in patients with ARDS or other causes of reversible pulmonary failure who experience refractory severe hypoxemia ($PaO_2:FiO_2$ <80) or hypercapnia (pH <7.20.) Early initiation has not been shown to have a mortality benefit in ARDS as compared to conventional low tidal volume ventilation strategies with standard supplementary maneuvers such as neuromuscular blockade, proning, and rescue ECMO. Inhaled nitric oxide transiently improves oxygenation in ARDS patients while therapy is maintained but has not been shown to improve mortality and is associated with acute renal injury. Esophageal pressure measurements can be used as a proxy for pleural pressure in patients with ARDS to titrate PEEP to maintain positive end-expiratory transpulmonary pressure, minimizing atelectotrauma and volutrauma, but has not been shown to have a mortality benefit.

### References

1. Guérin C, Reignier J, Richard JC, et al. Prone positioning in severe acute respiratory distress syndrome. *N Engl J Med.* 2013;368:2159-2168.
2. Koulouras V, Papathanakos G, Papathanasiou A, Nakos G. Efficacy of prone position in acute respiratory distress syndrome patients: a pathophysiology-based review. *World J Crit Care Med.* 2016;5(2):121-136.
3. Scholten E, Beitler J, Prisk G, Malhotra A. Treatment of ARDS with prone positioning. *Chest.* 2017;151(1):215-224.

**5.** Correct Answer: C

**Rationale:**

The patient meets criteria for ARDS, although severity stratification based on the Berlin criteria requires PEEP >5 cm $H_2O$.

**The Berlin Criteria for Acute Respiratory Distress Syndrome**

| TIMING | WITHIN 1 WK OF KNOWN CLINICAL INSULT OR NEW/WORSENING RESPIRATORY SYMPTOMS |
| --- | --- |
| Chest imaging | Bilateral opacities not fully explained by effusions, lobar/lung collapse, or nodules |
| Origin of edema | Respiratory failure not fully explained by cardiac failure or fluid overload |
| Oxygenation | Measurement performed with PEEP or CPAP >5 cm $H_2O$ |
| Mild | 200 mm Hg < $PaO_2:FiO_2$ <300 mm Hg |
| Moderate | 100 mm Hg < $PaO_2:FiO_2$ <200 mm Hg |
| Severe | $PaO_2:FiO_2$ <100 mm Hg |

Given the signs of increased work of breathing, with difficulty managing full sentences on face mask, an ABG demonstrating an uncompensated acute-on-chronic respiratory acidosis indicating progressive $CO_2$ retention, and persistent hypoxemia on non-rebreather, the patient should be intubated and receive mechanical ventilation with low tidal volumes (4-6 mL/kg), plateau pressure <30 cm $H_2O$, and PEEP >5 cm $H_2O$.

NIV can be used as an initial ventilatory support in patients with acute respiratory failure to spare the risks associated with sedation, muscular paralysis, and ventilator-associated complications. Several concerns remain regarding its use in the ARDS population, and the subgroups of ARDS most likely to benefit from it remain unclear. In particular, the use of prolonged NIV in the absence of respiratory function improvement may delay intubation and mechanical ventilation in patients who would benefit from conventional ARDS ventilation strategies. Recent data suggest that increased ARDS severity based on $PaO_2:FiO_2$ was associated with NIV failure, and that NIV used was associated with increased ICU (although not hospital) mortality. In particular, NIV use was associated with higher ICU mortality in patients with $PaO_2:FiO_2$ <150 mm Hg. NIV use may best be reserved for patients with mild ARDS ($PaO_2:FiO_2$ 201-300 mm Hg.) Other contraindications to NIV use include inability to cooperate because of altered mental status, inability to protect the airway or clear secretions, recent facial surgery or trauma, and recent esophageal anastomosis.

This patient with COPD may benefit from an ipratropium/albuterol nebulizer, but given adequate air excursion and the absence of wheezing, bronchospasm is likely not the central pathophysiology driving his clinical decompensation. Similarly, furosemide bolus is unlikely to significantly improve his ventilation in the absence of signs of volume overload.

### References

1. Bellani G, Laffey J, Pham T, et al. Noninvasive ventilation of patients with acute respiratory distress syndrome. Insights from the LUNG SAFE Study. *Am J Respir Crit Care Med.* 2017;195(1):67-77.
2. Rana S, Jenad H, Gay PC, Buck CF, Hubmayr RD, Gajic O. Failure of non-invasive ventilation in patients with acute lung injury: observational cohort study. *Crit Care.* 2006;10:R79.

3. Chawla R, Mansuriya J, Modi N, Pandey A, Juneja D, Chawla A, Kansal S. Acute respiratory distress syndrome: predictors of noninvasive ventilation failure and intensive care unit mortality in clinical practice. *J Crit Care.* 2016;31:26-30.
4. Ranieri VM, Rubenfeld GD, Thompson BT, et al; ARDS Definition Task Force. Acute respiratory distress syndrome: the Berlin definition. *JAMA.* 2012;307:2526-2533.

**6.** Correct Answer: A

**Rationale:**

Recruitment maneuvers and higher levels of PEEP are thought to protect against atelectrauma caused by repeated opening and closing of alveolar units in patients with ARDS. Higher PEEP has been shown to improve oxygenation and is not associated with worsened barotrauma or new organ failure. Its benefits are most established in patients with moderate to severe ARDS, and one meta-analysis found there may be a mortality benefit to higher PEEP in patients with severe ARDS.

Increased PEEP can also be beneficial for congestive heart failure with reduced LV ejection fraction. It reduces preload to the right-sided heart and increases right-sided heart afterload by increasing pulmonary vascular resistance, therefore, decreasing LV preload and placing an overfilled heart on a more favorable portion of the Frank–Starling curve to maximize contractility. It also decreases LV afterload (and thereby LV work) by reducing transmural pressure, and thus improves cardiac output in patients with poor LV function. On the other hand, cardiac output can decrease in patients with at risk for right-sided heart failure, as in this patient. COPD can lead to pulmonary hypertension, which in turn can lead to reduction in RV function and cor pulmonale. The decrease in RV preload and increase in RV afterload caused by PEEP can exacerbate preexisting RV dysfunction. The permissive hypercapnia seen in standard ARDS ventilation can likewise worsen RV dysfunction.

**References**

1. Brower RG, Lanken PN, MacIntyre N, et al. Higher versus lower positive end-expiratory pressures in patients with the acute respiratory distress syndrome. *N Engl J Med.* 2004;351:327-336.
2. Meade MO, Cook DJ, Guyatt GH, et al. Ventilation strategy using low tidal volumes, recruitment maneuvers, and high positive end-expiratory pressure for acute lung injury and acute respiratory distress syndrome: a randomized controlled trial. *JAMA.* 2008;299:637-645.
3. Mercat A, Richard JC, Vielle B, et al. Positive end-expiratory pressure setting in adults with acute lung injury and acute respiratory distress syndrome: a randomized controlled trial. *JAMA.* 2008;299:646-655.
4. Briel M, Meade M, Mercat A, et al. Higher vs lower positive end-expiratory pressure in patients with acute lung injury and acute respiratory distress syndrome: systematic review and meta-analysis. *JAMA.* 2010;303:865-873.
5. Pirrone M, Fisher D, Chipman D, et al. Recruitment maneuvers and positive end-expiratory pressure titration in morbidly obese ICU patients. *Crit Care Med.* 2016;44(2):300-307.
6. Luecke T, Pelosi P. Clinical review: positive end-expiratory pressure and cardiac output. *Crit Care.* 2005;9(6):607-621. doi:10.1186/cc3877.

**7.** Correct Answer: D

**Rationale:**

Extubation is contraindicated in hemodynamically unstable patients, including those requiring ongoing significant vasopressor support to maintain normotension. The NHLBI ARDS Network protocol recommends conducting a daily SBT for patients with ARDS when:

- $FiO_2 <0.4$ and PEEP $<8$ cm $H_2O$, or $FIO_2 <0.5$ and PEEP $<5$ cm $H_2O$
- PEEP and $FiO_2 <$ values of the previous day
- The patient has acceptable spontaneous breathing efforts
- Systolic BP $>90$ mm Hg without vasopressor support
- No neuromuscular blocking agents or blockade

If these criteria are met, an SBT can be conducted on a T-piece of trach collar with $FiO_2 <0.5$ and PEEP $<5$ cm $H_2O$. The patient can be assessed for tolerance of SBT for up to 120 minutes. Evidence of tolerance includes:

- $SpO_2 >90\%$ and/or $PaO_2 >60$
- Spontaneous tidal volumes $>4$ mL/kg
- Respiratory rate $<35$ breaths/min
- pH $>7.3$
- No signs of respiratory distress
  - HR $>120\%$ of baseline
  - Marked accessory muscle use
  - Abdominal paradox
  - Diaphoresis
  - Marked dyspnea

If the patient tolerates the SBT for 30 minutes, extubation should be considered. A 30 minute SBT is noninferior to a 120 minute trial, with no significant difference in percentage of patients extubated, percentage who remained extubated at 48 hours, reintubation rates, ICU mortality, and hospital mortality. For patients at high risk of extubation failure, extubation to noninvasive ventilation can significantly reduce ICU length of stay and mortality.

This patient satisfied the criteria to be extubated based on SBT. However, presence of high vasopressor support is considered a contraindication to SBT and extubation.

References
1. NHLBI ARDS Clinical Network. *Mechanical Ventilation Protocol Summary*; 2008:1-2. Accessed September 16, 2018. http://www.ardsnet.org/files/ventilator_protocol_2008-07.pdf.
2. Conti G, Mantz J, Longrois D, Tonner P. Sedation and weaning from mechanical ventilation: time for "best practice" to catch up with new realities? *Multidiscip Respir Med*. 2014;9(1):45. doi:10.1186/2049-6958-9-45.
3. Ouellette DR, Patel S, Girard TD, et al. Liberation from mechanical ventilation: an official American College of Chest Physicians/American Thoracic Society clinical practice guideline: inspiratory pressure augmentation during spontaneous breathing trials, protocols minimizing sedation, and non-invasive ventilation immediately after extubation. *Chest*. 2017;151(1):166-180.
4. Esteban A, Alia I, Tobin M, et al. Effects of spontaneous breathing trial duration on outcome of attempts to discontinue mechanical ventilation. Spanish Lung Failure Collaborative Group. *Am J Respir Crit Care*. 1999;159(2):512-518.

**8.** Correct Answer: C

**Rationale:**

ARDS is a clinical syndrome with a plethora of etiologies; the heterogeneity of its causes and their pathophysiology is being increasingly recognized and studied. Patients who develop ARDS after trauma can be separated into two temporal phenotypes: (1) early, defined as onset of ARDS within the first 48 hours of presentation, and (2) late, defined as ARDS diagnosis after 48 hours. Early-onset ARDS in trauma is associated with increased severity of thoracic trauma, more severe early hypotension, and increased red blood cell transfusion during initial resuscitation, as compared to the late-onset phenotype. Inflammatory biomarkers associated with endothelial injury and regulation of alveolar-capillary barrier integrity are more elevated in the early-onset group. This suggests that the early onset phenotype is characterized by a higher degree of hemorrhagic shock, with increased early vascular injury and disruption of the alveolar-capillary barrier. The late-onset phenotype, by contrast, is associated with progressive multiorgan system dysfunction and complications of prolonged mechanical ventilation, such as pneumonia. No significant difference in mortality has been found between the early- and late-onset phenotypes, however.

References
1. Reilly JP, Bellamy S, Shashaty MGS, et al. Heterogeneous phenotypes of acute respiratory distress syndrome after major trauma. *Ann Am Thorac Soc*. 2014;11(5):728-736. doi:10.1513/AnnalsATS.201308-280OC.
2. Calfee CS, Delucchi K, Parsons PE, et al. Latent class analysis of ARDS subphenotypes: analysis of data from two randomized controlled trials. *Lancet Respir Med*. 2014;2(8):611-620. doi:10.1016/S2213-2600(14)70097-9.

# 34

# OTHER PARENCHYMAL DISEASE AND PULMONARY EDEMA

Raffaele Di Fenza, Riccardo Pinciroli, and Lorenzo Berra

1. A 79-year-old male with a history of hypertension, dyslipidemia, and type-2 diabetes mellitus presents to the emergency department complaining of increasing shortness of breath, over the past 4 hours. Arterial blood gas (ABG) analysis at room air shows: $PaO_2$ 54 mm Hg, $PaCO_2$ 28 mm Hg, pH 7.48, $HCO_3-$ 22 mEq/L. Upon admission, the patient is administered oxygen via a face mask with oxygen reservoir at 15 L/min. The $SpO_2$ raises from 87% to 99%. Thirty minutes later, the patient is still dyspneic (respiratory rate: 32 breaths/min). Noninvasive blood pressure is 180/85 mm Hg, heart rate is 100 bpm. ABG now shows: $PaO_2$ 249 mm Hg, $PaCO_2$ 27 mm Hg. Chest auscultation reveals mild bilateral crackles at the bases of the lungs and mild wheezing. Body temperature is 36.2°C, WBC 6500/mL, creatinine 1.8 mg/dL, lactate 1.4 mmol/L. What is the **MOST** likely diagnosis?

   A. Pulmonary embolism
   B. Acute pulmonary edema
   C. Bilateral pneumonia
   D. Exacerbation of COPD

2. A 70-year-old male patient with a history of pulmonary hypertension and smoking has been admitted to the neurocritical care unit because of a Hunt and Hess Grade 4 subarachnoid hemorrhage (SAH) caused by a ruptured aneurysm of the anterior communicating artery (ACA). Successful endovascular clot retrieval was performed on day 1. On day 4, his hypoxemia worsened, reaching a ratio of $PaO_2$ to inspired oxygen ($FiO_2$) of less than 200 mm Hg at a $FiO_2$ of 0.6. The chest x-ray shows bilateral diffuse infiltrates suggestive of pulmonary edema. Which among the following is the best test to identify the cause of pulmonary edema?

   A. Transpulmonary thermodilution
   B. CT scan
   C. Lung ultrasound
   D. Serum catecholamine concentration

3. A 20-year-old male patient with no medical history is admitted in the operating room for emergent decompressive craniotomy after a motorbike accident causing a posterior cranial fossa epidural hematoma (diagnosed on CT scan). The neurosurgeon accesses the posterior fossa and relieves an opening pressure of 40 cm $H_2O$. Very quickly, the patient develops severe hypotension with a blood pressure of 50/30 mm Hg, for which high-dose norepinephrine is started. He also develops hypoxemia with an alveolar-arterial gradient of more than 100 mm Hg. In addition, the end-tidal $CO_2$ concentration drops by 10 mm Hg. With a high-dose noradrenaline infusion, the BP returns to normal, but hypoxia remains.

   Which among the following is most likely to be present in this patient?

   A. Ischemic changes in electrocardiogram
   B. Pink frothy sputum on tracheal aspiration
   C. Low cardiac index on pulse contour analysis
   D. Persistent reduction in end-tidal $CO_2$ concentration

4. A 31-year-old primiparous female gave birth 10 hours ago after preterm labor. The delivery was vaginal and proceeded without complications under epidural analgesia. The baby is a 25-week gestational age female and weighs 1780 g. Terbutaline administration failed in delaying the delivery. The mother has a history of anaphylaxis triggered by NSAIDs, past history of deep venous thrombosis, hypertension, and hypothyroidism. She has had a dry cough with mild fever and malaise for the past 10 days treated with amoxicillin. The patient now develops acute onset dyspnea and cannot speak in full sentences. She denies pain. Vitals are: respiratory rate is 32/min on non-rebreather face mask, blood pressure of 145/90 mm Hg, and a heart rate of 128/min. Bilateral rales and wheezing at the left base is heard on auscultation, cardiac sounds are normal, no jugular distension is observed, the skin is warm and well perfused. Blood gas analysis: pH 7.40, $pO_2$ 52 mm Hg, $pCO_2$ 30 mm Hg, lactate 2.2 mmol/L. What is the **MOST** likely cause of the patient's respiratory failure?

   **A.** Pulmonary embolism
   **B.** Pneumonia
   **C.** Tocolytic pulmonary edema
   **D.** Cardiac failure

5. A 5-year-old female patient has fallen from the balcony of her apartment located on a third floor. Impact on various branches of a tree before hitting the soil has dampened the velocity of the impact. Trauma burden includes two broken ribs on the right hemithorax, lung contusion, and a suspicion of spinal cord injury at the level of T1. She has to be sedated for a magnetic resonance imaging session. Which strategy could **BETTER** diminish the incidence of postprocedure atelectasis?

   **A.** Intubation, sedation with sevoflurane, PEEP of 5 cm $H_2O$, a tidal volume of 10 mL/kg, and a $FiO_2$ of 1.0
   **B.** Spontaneous breathing, sedation with propofol, and 15 L/min of oxygen on a non-rebreathing $O_2$ mask
   **C.** Noninvasive ventilation, sedation with midazolam, and a $FiO_2$ of 1.0
   **D.** Any strategy with the lowest possible $FiO_2$

6. A 74-year-old male patient weighing 80 kg with a history of essential hypertension and known subglottic laryngeal cancer is scheduled for elective surgery. He presents with dyspnea (respiratory rate of 45 breaths/min), hypoxemia ($SpO_2$ 80% in ambient air), and a high-pitched stridor that can be easily localized to the neck. Respiratory sounds are barely heard bilaterally on lung auscultation. A fiberoptic examination shows no space for nasotracheal or orotracheal intubation, so an emergency percutaneous tracheostomy is performed. Invasive mechanical ventilation initiated with assist control volume control ventilation (tidal volume of 600 mL and a PEEP of 8 cm $H_2O$). However, the patient remains hypoxemic with a $PO_2$ of 69 mm Hg despite an $FiO_2$ of 80%. An x-ray shows bilateral infiltrates.

   What would be the **MOST** appropriate first intervention on this patient?

   **A.** Switch to protective ventilation
   **B.** Administer diuretics
   **C.** Fiberoptic bronchoscopy of the bronchial tree
   **D.** CT scan of chest

7. Which among the following medications is indicated for treatment of high-altitude pulmonary edema, in absence of oxygen while awaiting for descent?

   **A.** Dexamethasone
   **B.** Salmeterol
   **C.** Nifedipine
   **D.** Sildenafil

8. A 28-year-old female patient was brought to the emergency room with a complaint of dyspnea. She is awake, breathing 34 times per minute with a $SpO_2$ of 93% in ambient air. She has a body temperature of 37.5°C and bilateral diffuse crackles on auscultation. The patient is a PhD student working in the same hospital where she is admitted, with symptoms starting just before leaving the lab to go back home. She regularly spends time in the animal facility as part of her PhD program. She denies allergies and admits to smoking 5 cigarettes per day. The chest x-ray is unremarkable.

   What would be the next **MOST** appropriate next test for this patient?

   **A.** Spirometry
   **B.** RAST test
   **C.** High resolution CT scan
   **D.** ImmunoCAP assay

**9.** A 55-year-old female patient is intubated for severe respiratory failure. A CT scan is then performed which shows diffuse bilateral ground glass opacities. On arrival in the intensive care unit, the patient desaturates due to abundant hemorrhagic secretions in the endotracheal tube. A fiberoptic bronchoscopy with deep bronchoalveolar lavages is then performed, yielding a very high percentage (>50%) of hemosiderin-laden macrophages in all samples.

Which among the following components in this patient's medical history supports the diagnosis?

     A. Acetylsalicylic acid prophylaxis for carotid artery disease
     B. Three spontaneous abortions all happened during the first trimester
     C. Polyarteritis nodosa treated with prednisone 60 mg daily
     D. Chronic hepatitis B with persistence of circulating HBV DNA

**10.** A female 50-year-old patient is undergoing induction of general anesthesia for gastric bypass surgery. Which of the following intraoperative measures would have the **MOST** impact on preventing the development of postoperative pulmonary atelectasis?

     A. Preoxygenation with a PEEP of 8 cm $H_2O$
     B. Induction and intubation using a $FiO_2$ of less than 0.6
     C. Setting an intraoperative PEEP of 10 cm $H_2O$
     D. Keeping the lowest possible $FiO_2$ before extubation

# Chapter 34 ▪ Answers

**1.** Correct Answer: B

**Rationale:**
Cardiogenic pulmonary edema triggers dyspnea through various mechanisms. In this scenario, acidosis and hypercapnia are absent. Here, the correction of hypoxia does not reduce the respiratory drive. No major alteration in respiratory mechanics is seen, except the increased respiratory rate. These observations indicate interstitial congestion as a potential trigger for the respiratory failure. The patient's past medical history of various cardiovascular risk factors pointing to congestive heart failure as a potential etiology. Nonetheless, no options can be safely excluded without the execution of primary diagnostic tests (ECG and chest x-ray). Bilateral wheezing is a sign of bronchial constriction. It may be caused by the irritation due to an underlying infectious disease (pneumonia), particularly in a context of chronic self-triggering inflammation, like that associated with a chronic obstructive pulmonary disease (COPD). Bronchospasm may be associated to pulmonary vascular congestion as well. The absence of a raised white blood cell count makes pneumonia and COPD exacerbation unlikely. The absence of signs of impaired respiratory mechanics such as the use of abdominal wall muscles to counteract outflow obstruction does not support this hypothesis either. Pulmonary embolism fits with the described scenario in which minute ventilation cannot be reduced without sedating the patient. Wheezing, however, is uncommon and a depressed $PO_2/FiO_2$ of less than 210 mm Hg in the setting of pulmonary embolism indicates a significant shunt and is usually accompanied by right heart failure and some degree of hemodynamic instability.

## References
1. Soldati G, Copetti R, Sher S. Sonographic interstitial syndrome: the sound of lung water. *J Ultrasound Med.* 2009;28(2):163-174.
2. Dyspnea. Mechanisms, assessment, and management: a consensus statement. American Thoracic Society. *Am J Respir Crit Care Med.* 1999;159(1):321-340.

**2.** Correct Answer: A

**Rationale:**
Neurogenic pulmonary edema typically occurs within 72 hours after the onset of neurologic injury, but can occur later as well. It results in a combination of cardiogenic and noncardiogenic pulmonary edema and occurs as a result of a large sympathetic stimulus causing hydrostatic as well as permeability pulmonary edema. In this patient, identifying the degree of contribution to lung edema from hydrostatic versus permeability will help guide therapy. Transpulmonary thermodilution technique allows the calculation cardiac index, extravascular lung water index (ELWI), and pulmonary vascular permeability index, which will help differentiate between purely hydrostatic (cardiogenic) pulmonary edema from that occurring due to increased capillary pulmonary permeability.

     Although, CT scan might give information on type of lung pathology, it would not differentiate between cardiogenic and noncardiogenic pulmonary edema. Similarly, lung ultrasound will not differentiate between types of pulmonary edema but is most effective in monitoring effect of treatment on pulmonary interstitial fluid. Measuring circulating levels of catecholamines is reasonable as well, but it only allows to identify a specific subset of patients who may benefit of alfa-adrenergic blockade.

### Reference

1. Busl KM, Bleck TP. Neurogenic pulmonary edema. *Crit Care Med.* 2015;43(8):1710-1715.

## 3. Correct Answer: B

**Rationale:**

The fulminant form of neurogenic pulmonary edema (NPE) develops between 30 and 60 minutes following neurologic injury and has been characterized by hypoxemia with an alveolar-arterial gradient of more than 100 mm Hg, a chest x-ray showing extensive pulmonary edema, the presence of a preserved cardiac output, and the absence of ischemic sign on the electrocardiogram. Typically, these patients have pink frothy fluid on tracheal aspiration or sputum if endotracheal intubation has not been performed yet. Cardiogenic pulmonary edema (CPE) is the main differential diagnosis and may be present at the same time as NPE. In this scenario, though, hypotension occurs specifically at posterior fossa decompression, which can be explained by waning of the Cushing reflex causing a drop in adrenal release of catecholamines. A persisting low end-tidal $CO_2$ concentration would indicate air embolism which typically occurs as a result of air entering a cerebral vein, especially when the patient is in a sitting position. In this case, the pressure of the posterior cranic fossa is positive making this unlikely.

### Reference

1. Busl KM, Bleck TP. Neurogenic pulmonary edema. *Crit Care Med.* 2015;43(8):1710-1715.

## 4. Correct Answer: C

**Rationale:**

Although infrequent, tocolytic pulmonary edema is triggered by drugs such as beta-agonists and calcium antagonists, with symptoms occurring within 12 hours after delivery. It is a purely hydrostatic edema occurring in the presence of normal cardiac function and results in a marked increase in the arterial-alveolar gradient and a hypoxic-nonhypercapnic respiratory failure. Pulmonary embolism (PE) is an important differential, especially with high alveolar-arterial gradient and history of deep venous thrombosis. However, PE with this degree of shunt would typically be accompanied by some degree of right heart failure. This patient does not have clinical signs of right cardiac failure (no gallop, jugular distension, or hypotension). The acuity of presentation makes pneumonia a less likely diagnosis. Peripartum cardiomyopathy and heart failure is another important differential. Although the respiratory signs and symptoms are compatible with cardiac failure, stable hemodynamics and adequate peripheral perfusion poorly fit with that clinical scenario.

### References

1. Biswas BK, Singh SN, Agarwal B, Sah BP, Chaturvedi A, Banerjee B. Respiratory failure after lumbar epidural anesthesia in a patient with uncontrolled hyperthyroidism. *Anesth Analg.* 2006;103(4):1061-1062.
2. O'Dwyer SL, Gupta M, Anthony J. Pulmonary edema in pregnancy and the puerperium: a cohort study of 53 cases. *J Perinat Med.* 2015;43(6):675-681.
3. Pisani RJ, Rosenow EC III. Pulmonary edema associated with tocolytic therapy. *Annals Intern Med.* 1989;110(9):714-718.

## 5. Correct Answer: D

**Rationale:**

Breathing an unnecessarily high $FiO_2$ leads to alveolar collapse (hyperoxic atelectasis) and, in addition, increases alveolar permeability, decreases surfactant production, and induces inflammatory mediators (thereby ventilation-induced lung injury). There is not an easy predictable PEEP value that protects all patients from atelectasis, although any value has been shown to be more protective than a PEEP of 0 cm $H_2O$. It has been shown that patients who are sedated and spontaneously breathing without invasive ventilation or PEEP have a lower risk for atelectasis when compared to those who were sedated and mechanically ventilated. Available physiological evidence suggests that breathing a lower $FiO_2$ was protective against atelectasis.

### References

1. Tusman G, Bohm SH, Warner DO, Sprung J. Atelectasis and perioperative pulmonary complications in high-risk patients. *Curr Opin Anaesthesiol.* 2012;25(1):1-10.
2. Duggan M, Kavanagh BP. Pulmonary atelectasis: a pathogenic perioperative entity. *Anesthesiology.* 2005;102(4):838-854.
3. Lutterbey G, Wattjes MP, Doerr D, Fischer NJ, Gieseke J Jr, Schild HH. Atelectasis in children undergoing either propofol infusion or positive pressure ventilation anesthesia for magnetic resonance imaging. *Pediatr Anesth.* 2007;17(2):121-125.
4. Kallet RH, Branson RD. Should oxygen therapy be tightly regulated to minimize hyperoxia in critically ill patients? *Respir Care.* 2016;61(6):801-817.

**6.** Correct Answer: A

**Rationale:**

The respiratory failure developing during severe upper airway obstruction typically originates from a negative-pressure pulmonary edema caused by the repeated negative airway pressure that the patient develops in order to overcome the resistance. This causes trans-vascular fluid extravasation and thereby interstitial and alveolar edema. This condition is purely hydrostatic and is generally relieved in 24 to 48 hours if positive pressure ventilation is ensured, and airway resistance is eliminated. The rate of alveolar fluid clearance in this condition is between 14% and 17% per hour, approaching physiological values, while in the presence of lung injury it may be as low as 0% to 3%/h. For this reason, the main intervention to take in this situation is to limit and prevent lung injury by guaranteeing a protective ventilation strategy (6 mL/kg of tidal volume with plateau pressure below 30 cm $H_2O$). Diuretics can accelerate the rate of fluid uptake, but their efficacy is limited in the presence of lung injury. Fiberoptic bronchoscopy may only reveal the presence of pink frothy transudate which may also present by simply performing a tracheal aspiration. The immediate execution of a CT scan is not indicated until the effects of positive pressure ventilation, PEEP, and alveolar clearance clarify the actual damage accumulated by the lung tissue, if any exists.

Reference

1. Bhattacharya M, Kallet RH, Ware LB, Matthay MA. Negative-pressure pulmonary edema. *Chest*. 2016;150(4):927-933.

**7.** Correct Answer: C

**Rationale:**

Sustained release oral nifedipine is the drug of choice in high-altitude pulmonary edema (HAPE) (Grade 1C). Other drugs reduce pulmonary vasoconstriction and thus might be useful in treatment of HAPE. However, their clinical efficacy has not been proven. While phosphodiesterase inhibitors have a strong biological rationale, data from prospective studies are missing. Use of inhaled beta-agonist is reported in literature, but there is not enough data to support these drugs. Dexamethasone has been proved to reduce the incidence of HAPE in a placebo-controlled trial, yet its role in treating the established acute disease has not been validated.

References

1. Bartsch P, Swenson ER. Clinical practice: acute high-altitude illnesses. *N Engl J Med*. 2013;368(24):2294-2302.
2. Pennardt A. High-altitude pulmonary edema: diagnosis, prevention, and treatment. *Curr Sports Med Rep*. 2013;12(2):115-119.

**8.** Correct Answer: C

**Rationale:**

Presence of a mild fever and potential occupational exposure to an antigen (triggering respiratory distress) in the absence of wheezing and a negative chest x-ray should point toward hypersensitivity pneumonitis (HP) as an important differential diagnosis. High-resolution CT (HRCT) scan is increasingly used in the initial evaluation of patients suspected with HP. Independently of the disease stage (acute vs subacute vs chronic HP), classic radiologic findings together with a history of appropriate exposure are adequate for establishing diagnosis, and a biopsy can be avoided. CT scan should not be delayed because the classic findings (ground glass opacification in the upper lobes with decreased attenuation of secondary lobules due to air trapping) are best seen during acute presentation and may disappear quickly while symptoms subside. Spirometry may show either a restrictive or an obstructive pattern or both, while diffusion lung carbon monoxide may be impaired in subacute patients and is always impaired in chronic patients. However, these tests are not diagnostic and should not be preferred over a potentially diagnostic HRCT scan. RAST test is useful in determining an IgE-mediated sensitization, which is less likely in this patient especially in the absence of wheezing. ImmunoCAP assay and other techniques to determine IgG-mediated sensitization are useful but may be inconclusive because they lack sensitivity and specificity. Positive findings are not diagnostic for HP and negative findings cannot exclude it. Furthermore, the patient is a smoker, which could yield false positives.

References

1. Lacasse Y, Selman M, Costabel U, et al. Clinical diagnosis of hypersensitivity pneumonitis. *Am J Resp Crit Care Med*. 2003;168(8): 952-958.
2. Vasakova M, Morell F, Walsh S, Leslie K, Raghu G. Hypersensitivity pneumonitis: perspectives in diagnosis and management. *Am J Resp Crit Care Med*. 2017;196(6):680-689.

**9.** Correct Answer: B

**Rationale:**

This patient has diffuse alveolar hemorrhage (DAH) based on the bronchoscopic findings. It is fundamental to quickly understand the underlying pathogenetic disorder in order to promptly prescribe the correct treatment regimen, which may include pulse-dose steroids, immune suppression, and plasmapheresis. The patient described in this scenario may have an undiagnosed primary or secondary (due to systemic lupus erythematosus) antiphospholipid syndrome, which, especially if untreated, is a frequent cause of DAH. In this setting a reasonable first line of treatment could be a combination of glucocorticoids and cyclophosphamide. Antiplatelet agents have been associated with the development of DAH, but this is true only when glycoprotein IIb/IIIa inhibitors, such as abciximab, are administered. Anticoagulant therapy is instead more frequently associated with DAH. Various autoimmune diseases may be involved in determining DAH, yet a link between polyarteritis nodosa and DAH is not described. To date, there is only one report in literature describing a patient with active hepatitis B and polyarteritis nodosa developing DAH, although this patient had multiple comorbidities which are strongly associated with DAH, such as cocaine abuse by inhalation. Chronic hepatitis C, especially in patients who develop cryoglobulinemia, is associated with DAH.

### References

1. Franks TJ, Koss MN. Pulmonary capillaritis. *Curr Opin Pulm Med*. 2000;6(5):430-435.
2. Jaffar R, Mohanty SK, Khan A, Fischer AH. Hemosiderin laden macrophages and hemosiderin within follicular cells distinguish benign follicular lesions from follicular neoplasms. *CytoJournal*. 2009;6:3.
3. Martínez-Martínez MU, Oostdam DAH, Abud-Mendoza C. Diffuse alveolar hemorrhage in autoimmune diseases. *Curr Rheumatol Rep*. 2017;19(5):27.
4. Miyakis S, Lockshin MD, Atsumi T, et al. International consensus statement on an update of the classification criteria for definite antiphospholipid syndrome (APS). *J Thromb Haemost*. 2006;4(2):295-306.
5. Guo X, Gopalan R, Ugbarugba S, et al. Hepatitis B-related polyarteritis nodosa complicated by pulmonary hemorrhage. *Chest*. 2001;119(5):1608-1610.

**10.** Correct Answer: D

**Rationale:**

Perioperative hypoxemia is a risk factor for perioperative mortality and for several perioperative complications including cardiac ischemia and delirium leading to increased postoperative length of stay. Perioperative atelectasis is one of the main causes of hypoxemia in surgical patients, with their prevention being mandatory and requiring a multistep approach in all phases of the perioperative period. After surgery, optimal pain control without residual anesthesia together with CPAP and postural changes are all fundamental to pursue this target.

A fundamental mechanism leading to postoperative atelectasis is hyperoxic reabsorption of gases from the alveolar space into circulation. Extubation with a $FiO_2$ of 1.0 has been shown to potentially jeopardize all previous intraoperative efforts to prevent and/or reduce atelectasis, even if a recruitment maneuver is performed prior to extubation. Keeping the lowest $FiO_2$ compatible with the patient's oxygenation requirements, not only before extubation but throughout the surgery, prevents atelectasis. Clinical studies evaluating fixed-ruled PEEP strategies have shown contradictory results, and thus there is no specific recommendation on the amount of PEEP. High PEEP has theoretical advantages in terms of protection from atelectasis. Studies comparing preset values of low versus high PEEP for intraoperative ventilation yield contradictory results. Preoxygenation with PEEP has a demonstrated role in reducing the incidence of postoperative atelectasis, yet it is not the most impactful strategy among those listed. Using an $FiO_2$ of less than 60% during preoxygenation, induction, and intubation has a dramatic effect leading in many cases to the absence of intraoperative atelectasis. However, this strategy cannot be implemented for safety reasons, especially since this will decrease the duration of safe apnea period.

### References

1. Tusman G, Bohm SH, Warner DO, Sprung J. Atelectasis and perioperative pulmonary complications in high-risk patients. *Curr Opin Anaesthesiol*. 2012;25(1):1-10.
2. Duggan M, Kavanagh BP. Pulmonary atelectasis: a pathogenic perioperative entity. *Anesthesiology*. 2005;102(4):838-854.
3. Levin MA, McCormick PJ, Lin HM, Hosseinian L, Fischer GW. Low intraoperative tidal volume ventilation with minimal PEEP is associated with increased mortality. *Br J Anaesth*. 2014;113(1):97-108.
4. Hemmes SN, Gama de Abreu M, Pelosi P, Schultz MJ. High versus low positive end-expiratory pressure during general anesthesia for open abdominal surgery (PROVHILO trial): a multicentre randomised controlled trial. *Lancet*. 2014;384(9942):495-503.

# 35

# AIRWAY DISEASES

Jenna McNeill and Charles Corey Hardin

1. A 70-year-old female with a history of diabetes, coronary artery disease, and hypothyroidism was admitted to the intensive care unit (ICU) for pneumonia complicated by acute respiratory distress syndrome (ARDS). She was intubated on the day of admission. Her ICU course was complicated by shock, delirium, and recurrent aspiration. She was successfully extubated on ICU day 14. Following extubation, she was noted to have significant coughing that seemed worse with the consumption of liquids. A barium swallow demonstrated a spillage of contrast from the esophagus into the trachea. Which of the following is a risk factor for this complication?

   A. Delirium
   B. Hypothryoidism
   C. ARDS
   D. Hypotension
   E. Advanced age

2. A 30-year-old female with a past medical history of moderate persistent asthma, substance abuse disorder, and allergic rhinitis was brought to the emergency department (ED) by paramedics after being found down in a subway station surrounded by empty medication bottles and was noted to have needle tracks on her arms. In the ED, she was intubated for airway protection with a 7.0 endotracheal tube. She was then admitted to the ICU where her toxicology panel was positive for cocaine, oxycodone, and methadone. Her mental status improved over the next 72 hours, and she was converted from volume control ventilation to pressure support. She was able to tolerate pressure support 5/5 with an $FiO_2$ of 0.30, a respiratory rate of 18, and tidal volume of 600 mL. Given her clinical improvement, the team contemplated extubation. Prior to extubation, her endotracheal cuff is deflated. The discrepancy between her inspiratory and expiratory volumes is less than 110 mL, but no audible cuff leak is appreciated. What is the next most appropriate step?

   A. Extubate the patient as she was intubated for less than 72 hours
   B. Extubate the patient as cuff leaks are not predictive of extubation success
   C. Retest for a cuff leak and, if absent, give 60 mg IV methylprednisolone and extubate tomorrow
   D. Retest for a cuff leak and, if absent, give 60 mg IV methylprednisolone and extubate in 6 hours.

3. A 60-year-old male with a history of type 2 diabetes and prior alcohol use presents to the emergency room with complaints of shortness of breath and mouth pain. His initial temperature is 102°F; he has a heart rate of 110, a blood pressure of 120/60, and a respiratory rate of 30. He states he recently had dental work performed. On examination, he appears uncomfortable with increased work of breathing. He is noted to have a swollen submandibular gland with surrounding erythema at the base of his face extending onto the proximal portion of his neck. His oropharyngeal examination is notable for poor dentition and one tooth with increased erythema along the gum line. There is a high-pitch wheeze with inspiration. The rest of his pulmonary examination is clear. His cardiac examination is notable for sinus tachycardia without murmurs. His labs were notable for an elevated white cell count of 16 000 and an elevated ESR and CRP. What is the next best step in management?

A. Nasotracheal intubation
B. CT neck and chest
C. Endotracheal intubation
D. Antibiotics and close monitoring in the ICU

---

4. A 70-year-old male with a history of chronic obstructive pulmonary disease (COPD), requiring prior intubation, and active tobacco use presents to the emergency department with shortness of breath. He states that over the last 24 hours, he has had increasing difficulty breathing. He denies fevers or chills at home and is not aware of any sick contacts. His initial vitals are temperature of 99.4 F, hear rate 90/min, blood pressure 130/80 mm Hg, respiratory rate 22/min, and $SpO_2$ 95%. On examination, he appears to have a mild increase in work of breathing. He is noted to have scattered wheezing throughout both lung fields. He is started on albuterol nebulizers and IV steroids. Three hours into his emergency room stay you are called to the bedside as the patient appears to be in more distress. His vitals demonstrate temperature of 99.8, HR 125, BP 120/70 with an RR of 35 and $SpO_2$ 90%. On examination, the patient is using accessory muscles, and his lung examination is notable for poor air movement with no wheezing. An arterial blood gas is performed pH 7.28, $PCO_2$ 50, and $PaO_2$ 65. A chest x-ray is performed and demonstrates hyperinflation of both lung fields with no infiltrate. He is intubated for hypoxemic respiratory failure and is subsequently paralyzed with a neuromuscular blocker secondary to ventilator dyssynchrony. He arrives to the ICU ventilated, with an $FiO_2$ of 0.8, PEEP 10, RR 30, and TV 420 mL/kg (the patient weighs 70 kg). His arterial blood gas demonstrates a pH 7.29/$PCO_2$ 50/$PaO_2$ 200. His blood pressure upon arrival to the ICU is 80/50 mm Hg.

His flow/time wave form is noted in the following figure:

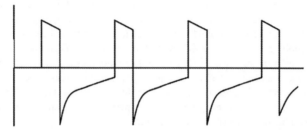

From Ward N, Dushay K. Clinical concise review: mechanical ventilation of patients with chronic obstructive pulmonary disease. *Crit Care Med.* 2008;36(5):1614-1619.

What would be the next step in management?

A. Increase his tidal volumes
B. Increase his PEEP from 10 to 15
C. Decrease the respiratory rate
D. Increase the inspiratory time

---

5. A 65-year-old male with a history of COPD and active tobacco use with no prior intubations presented to the emergency department with increased work of breathing and increased wheezing. In the emergency department, he was given stacked nebulizers and IV steroids and initiated on BIPAP. His initial blood gas demonstrated pH 7.2/ $pCO_2$ 75/ $pO_2$ 65. Following intubation, he was placed on volume control ventilation. His initial peak pressure (peak inspiratory pressure [PIP]) was 45 cm $H_2O$, and his plateau pressure (Pplat) was 35 cm $H_2O$. He was placed on a respiratory rate of 30, PEEP 15, $FiO_2$ 0.40 and his $SpO_2$ was 90%. Two hours after arrival to the ICU, his ventilator starts to alarm for high pressures. His peak pressures have increased to 65 cm $H_2O$, and his plateau pressure has increased to 55 cm $H_2O$. His heart rate increases from 80 beats per minutes to 110, and his blood pressure drops from 110/70 to 80/50 mm Hg. His $SpO_2$ drops to 75%. His examination is notable for continual wheezing and slight deviation of the trachea toward the left.

What is the most likely cause for this acute change?

A. Worsening bronchoconstriction
B. Unilateral pneumothorax
C. Biting down on the tube
D. Abdominal distention

6. A 50-year-old female with a history of atopic dermatitis and coronary artery disease on beta blockade presents to the emergency department with shortness of breath and hives. She is on vacation and was staying at a horse farm. Along with her shortness of breath, she reports an itchy feeling in the back of her throat, sneezing, and swelling around her lips and eyes. On physical examination, she is noted to have a blood pressure of 90/55 mm Hg, an RR of 32, and a heart rate of 110 and is afebrile. Her oropharyngeal examination is notable for tongue and lip swelling and some pooling of secretions at the back of her mouth. Her cardiac examination is notable for sinus tachycardia, and her pulmonary examination is notable for bilateral wheezes. IM epinephrine is given on the mid-outer thigh. After 5 minutes, the patient demonstrates no improvement in her symptoms and she is intubated for airway protection. Repeat IM epinephrine is given. Her repeat vitals demonstrate a blood pressure of 80/50 mm Hg and a heart rate of 115. Normal saline is hung and started via a peripheral IV. What next step could assist with the patient's hypotension?

   A. Administer diphendyramine 25 mg IV
   B. Administer methylprednisolone 125 mg IV
   C. Administer albuterol nebulizers via the endotracheal tube
   D. Administer glucagon 5 mg IV

7. A 35-year-old male with a history of moderate persistent asthma presents to the emergency department with complaints of shortness of breath and increased wheezing. His initial vitals were notable for a temperature of 100.4°F, blood pressure of 130/80 mm Hg, heart rate of 105, respiratory rate of 25, and oxygen saturation of 88%. On examination, the patient was noted to be in moderate distress with increased respiratory muscle use. He did not have evidence of stridor; his pulmonary examination was notable for bilaterally wheezing and cardiac examinmation notable for sinus tachycardia. His chest x-ray demonstrated hyperinflation with flattening of the diaphragms bilaterally with no clear infiltrate. In the emergency department, he was started on IV steroids and continuous albuterol nebulizers and placed on 3 L/min of oxygen via nasal cannula. His initial basic metabolic panel was unremarkable with an anion gap of 10. An arterial blood gas showed a pH 7.41, pCO$_2$ 34 mm Hg, and PaO$_2$ 90 mm Hg on supplemental oxygen. On arrival to the ICU, he continues to be in respiratory distress with accessory muscle use. A repeat basic metabolic panel is performed with labs notable for a creatinine of 0.80 and an anion gap of 24; lactate level was 8. A repeat arterial gas was performed and showed a pH 7.26, PCO$_2$ 46 mm Hg, and PaO$_2$ 80. What would be the next step in management?

   A. Stop the albuterol nebulizers
   B. Administer high-dose magnesium
   C. Intubate the patient given persistent work of breathing
   D. Provide patient with IV fluid bolus

8. A 50-year-old male with a history of obesity (BMI 35), type 2 diabetes, and GERD, who is status post right knee replacement 1 year prior, presented to the emergency room with complaints of right knee pain. His initial vitals are notable for a temperature of 101.1°F, heart rate of 110, and blood pressure of 90/50 mm Hg (baseline BP 140/80 mm Hg). His labs were notable for an elevated white blood cell count of 16 000 and a lactate of 3.0. He had a chest x-ray with no cardiopulmonary process noted. On examination, his right knee was noted to be erythematous and he was unable to flex is knee or extend his knee and was taken to the OR for concern for joint infection. Upon LMA removal at the end of the case, he was noted to be in distress with a respiratory rate of 35 with accompanying loud upper airway sounds concerning for stridor. His oxygenation saturations decreased to 83%, and given his hypoxemia and increased respiratory effort, the decision was made to reintubate the patient. A chest x-ray was performed demonstrating bilateral perihilar infiltrates. What was the most likely cause for the patient's respiratory distress status post extubation?

   A. Aspiration pneumonitis
   B. Acute cardiogenic pulmonary edema
   C. Anaphylaxis
   D. Negative pressure pulmonary edema

9. A 40-year-old female presents to the ED via EMS after being rescued from a house fire. Upon presentation, the patient has a temperature of 99.4, blood pressure of 120/80 mm Hg, heart rate of 95, oxygen saturation of 97% on room air, and respiratory rate of 22. The patient complains of a headache, pain on her face secondary to burn, and a hoarse voice. Her labs are notable for a carboxyhemoglobin level of 15%. On physical examination, she has a deep partial-thickness burn on the right side of her face extending from below her zygomatic arch to her jawline. She has soot in her nostrils bilaterally. She was placed on 100% oxygen. What would be the next step in management?

    **A.** Observe for 24 hours

    **B.** Fiberoptic bronchoscopy to assess the upper airway

    **C.** IV steroids

    **D.** Hyperbarbic oxygen chamber

**10.** A 40-year-old male with history of obesity (BMI 40) and substance abuse disorder was brought into the ED status post cardiac arrest from opioid overdose. Return of spontaneous circulation was achieved after 3 rounds of CPR and epinephrine prior to arrival to the ED. He was intubated and transferred to the ICU for further management. One week into his ICU admission, his neurologic status remained poor, and after discussion with family, the decision was made to pursue tracheostomy and PEG tube placement. He was taken to the OR for the placement of a Shiley 8 tracheostomy tube and was sedated for the procedure. Twelve hours following the tracheostomy placement, he was switched from volume control ventilation to spontaneous ventilation with an inspiratory pressure of 8 and PEEP of 10. He was noted to have increased tachypnea, and his heart rate increased to 120. The ventilator started to alert high pressures with PIPs of 40 cm $H_2O$ with each respiratory effort. What step could prevent the high pressures?

    **A.** Suctioning within the tracheostomy tube

    **B.** Decreasing the PEEP from 10 to 8

    **C.** Replacing the tracheostomy tube with a Shiley XLT 8

    **D.** Replacing the Shiley 8 tube with a T-piece

# Chapter 35 ■ Answers

**1.** Correct Answer: D

**Rationale:**

This patient has developed an acquired tracheoesophageal fistula (TEF). TEF is a rare but serious complication of prolonged mechanical ventilation. The most common etiology for acquired TEFs is malignancy, with esophageal malignancy as the most frequent cancer leading to TEF. Following malignancy, the most common cause of TEFs is endotracheal intubation. Endotracheal tube–related TEFs can occur in up to 3% of ventilated patients. Risk factors include prolonged intubation, diabetes, overinflation of the endotracheal cuff, hypotension leading to necrosis of the tracheal wall, and recurrent airway infections. In ventilated patients, TEFs can present with weight loss, recurrent infections or inability to liberate from the ventilator. In nonventilated patients, coughing is a common sign with a classic sign of coughing after consuming liquids (Ono's sign), particularly carbonated liquids. TEFs can be diagnosed via barium swallow, endoscopy, or bronchoscopy. Treatment is typically surgical; however, for nonoperable, malignant cases, stenting is an option. Extubation following correction of the TEF is key as positive pressure ventilation has been associated with poor anastomotic breakdown and stenosis.

Reference

1. Diddee R, Shaw IH. Acquired tracheo-oesophageal fistula in adults. *Contin Educ Anaesth Criti Care Pain*. 2006;6(3):105-108.

**2.** Correct Answer: D

**Rationale:**

The decision to test for an endotracheal cuff leak is controversial. Endotracheal intubation can lead to laryngeal edema and has been associated with an incidence of postextubation stridor that is 6% to 37%. The American Thoracic Society Guidelines indicate that a "cuff-leak" test to evaluate for laryngeal edema should only be performed in high-risk patients. High-risk patients are defined as those with traumatic intubation, intubation >6 days, large endotracheal tube, those who have been repeatedly reintubated and extubated, and women. This patient's largest risk factor is her gender. The guidelines then go on to recommend repeating a cuff-leak test if the initial testing demonstrated an absent leak. If no leak is present on the repeat testing, steroids are recommended. Lee et al. performed a randomized control trial of patients with less than 110 mL difference between inspiratory and expiratory volumes. Patients in the treatment arm received dexamethasone 5 mg q6h for 24 hours Cuff-leak volumes were checked every 6 hours, and the change in volumes in the steroid group demonstrated significant improvement within the first 6 hours with little additional benefit after.

References

1. Girard TD, Alhazzani W, Kress JP, et al. An Official American Thoracic Society/American College of Chest Physicians clinical practice guideline: liberation from mechanical ventilation in critically ill adults. Rehabilitation protocols, ventilator liberation protocols, and cuff leak tests. *Am J Respir Crit Care Med*. 2017;195(1):120-133. PubMed PMID:27762595.

2. Lee CH, Peng MJ, Wu CL. Dexamethasone to prevent postextubation airway obstruction in adults: a prospective, randomized, double-blind, placebo-controlled study. *Crit Care*. 2007;11(4):R72. PubMed PMID:17605780. Pubmed Central PMCID:2206529.

**3.** Correct Answer: A

**Rationale:**

Ludwig angina is characterized by cellulitis and edema of the floor of the mouth and soft tissues of the neck. Mortality is close to 8%. Risk factors for developing Ludwig angina include recent dental treatment, dental infections, diabetes, alcoholism, and immunosuppression. This patient is demonstrating evidence of airway compromise with increased respiratory rate, submandibular swelling, and stridor. The leading cause of death in Ludwig angina is airway compromise; therefore, the primary concern is securing the airway. Given that this patient appears to already have upper airway swelling, there is a high risk of failing with endotracheal intubation. If nasotracheal intubation is not an option or fails, then cricothyrotomy and tracheostomy should be performed. Once the airway has been secured, the focus should then switch to treating the underlying infection with antibiotics. *Streptococcus* and *Staphylococcus* are the most common bacteria that have been associated with Ludwig angina. A CT neck and chest would not be a good option for this patient given his tenuous airway.

References

1. Candamourty R, Venkatachalam S, Babu MR, Kumar GS. Ludwig's angina – an emergency: a case report with literature review. *J Nat Sci Biol Med*. 2012;3(2):206-208. PubMed PMID:23225990. Pubmed Central PMCID:3510922.
2. Crystal DK, Day SW, Wagner CL, Kranz J. Emergency treatment in Ludwig's angina. *Surg Gynecol Obstet*. 1969;129(4):755-757. PubMed PMID:5821231

**4.** Correct Answer: C

**Rationale:**

The figure above demonstrates air trapping or "auto-PEEP" as the exhalation wave form fails to reach zero before the next breath is taken. Auto-PEEP can cause decreased venous return which leads to a decrease in cardiac output and results in hypotension which was seen in this patient. To address air trapping, the key is to increase the expiratory time. Decreasing the respiratory rate is an affective way to achieve a longer exhalation period. Another way to enhance the expiratory time is to change the inspiration:expiratory ratio or the I:E time. This can be accomplished by increasing the inspiratory flow rate thus decreasing the inspiratory time. Increasing the patient's tidal volume could enhance the minute ventilation; however, it would not address the dynamic hyperinflation. Finally increasing PEEP can have variable effects on the intrathoracic pressure depending on the degree of expiratory flow limitation but is unlikely to decrease the auto-PEEP.

Reference

1. Ward N, Dushay K. Clinical concise review: mechanical ventilation of patients with chronic obstructive pulmonary disease. *Crit Care Med*. 2008;36(5):1614-1619.

**5.** Correct Answer: B

**Rationale:**

The incidence of overt barotrauma in mechanical ventilation ranges from 4% to 15% COPD is commonly associated with pneumothoraxes, as these patients may have underlying bullous disease and can require high airway pressures to overcome bronchial obstruction. In this case, the patient had a baseline elevated plateau pressure which placed him at higher risk for developing overdistention leading to a pneumothorax. Given that both parameters changed, the underlying issue does not deal solely with resistance. If resistance had suddenly increased, for example, with worsening bronchoconstriction, the peak airway pressures would likely have increased without an increase in the plateau pressures. Along with the increases in both pressures, there was also evidence of hemodynamic changes concerning for a tension pneumothorax. As the lung collapses, intrathoracic pressure causes a shift in mediastinal structures toward the noncollapsed lung which can cause tracheal deviation on examination. Biting on the endotracheal tube could result in an increase in airway pressures, but it is unlikely to have severe hemodynamic effects. Abdominal distention can also cause an increase in peak and plateau pressures and, in the setting of abdominal compartment syndrome, could cause hypotension; however, this would be less likely to occur so acutely and less likely to be associated with tracheal deviation.

Reference

1. Hsu CW, Sun SF. Iatrogenic pneumothorax related to mechanical ventilation. *World J Crit care Med*. 2014;3(1):8-14. PubMed PMID: 24834397. Pubmed Central PMCID:4021154.

**6.** Correct Answer: D

**Rationale:**

Epinephrine acts on both beta-1 receptors in the heart, beta-2 receptors within the smooth muscle, and alpha-1 receptors to increase peripheral vascular resistance. For patients who are on nonselective beta blockade, the effect of epinephrine could be diminished. Glucagon should be considered in patients on beta blockers who fail to respond to the initial doses of epinephrine. Glucagon has demonstrated a positive inotropic and chronotropic effect on the heart. Unlike epinephrine, glucagon does not work through the alpha or beta receptor pathway. Glucagon works via adenylyl cyclase stimulation and cyclic AMP-dependent phosphorylation of calcium channels which enhances inotropy. Glucagon is typically given in 1 to 5 mg IV doses over 5 minutes and followed by an infusion of 5 to 15 µg/min. The main side effect to be aware of with glucagon administration is vomiting. Histamines in the form of diphenhydramine have not been associated with the resolution of hypotension. Histamine medication is used to relieve the discomfort related to skin rash and can take up to 30 minutes to work. Similarly glucocorticoids are not associated with an increase in blood pressure. They can be used to prevent or lower the risk for a biphasic reaction in the setting of anaphylaxis as they can take numerous hours to have a full effect. Finally, bronchodilators help with airway resistance but do not improve the symptoms of shock related to anaphylaxis.

### References

1. Thomas M, Crawford I. Best evidence topic report. Glucagon infusion in refractory anaphylactic shock in patients on beta-blockers. *Emerg Med J*. 2005;22(4):272-273. PubMed PMID:15788828. Pubmed Central PMCID:1726748.
2. Mery PF, Brechler V, Pavoine C, Pecker F, Fischmeister R. Glucagon stimulates the cardiac $Ca^{2+}$ current by activation of adenylyl cyclase and inhibition of phosphodiesterase. *Nature*. 1990;345(6271):158-161. PubMed PMID:2159595.
3. Alqurashi W, Ellis AK. Do corticosteroids prevent biphasic anaphylaxis? *J Allergy Clin Immunol Pract*. 2017;5(5):1194-1205. PubMed PMID: 28888249.

---

**7.** Correct Answer: C

**Rationale:**

In asthmatic patients, two types of lactic acidosis can be present. Type A lactic acidosis can be seen in hypoxia as well as hypoperfusion. Type B lactic acidosis is typically seen in the setting of medication or errors of metabolism and is a result of increased lactate production or a decrease in lactate clearance. In asthmatic patients, type A lactic acidosis can be generated by multiple mechanisms. As the lung becomes hyperinflated, alveolar pressures can exceed pulmonary vascular pressures (increased West zone 1) leading to a situation where the alveolar pressure is increasingly the determinant of right-sided heart afterload. With greater afterload, there can be pressure overload of the RV and a reduction in cardiac output leading to impaired tissue perfusion. Elevated airway pressures at the end of expiration (intrinsic PEEP) also present an increased inspiratory load to the respiratory system. This requires large pleural pressure swings in order to initiate inspiration. The increase in muscle work can increase oxygen demands. The end result of either of these processes is type A lactic acidosis. Type B lactic acidosis has also been associated with asthma patients in the setting of albuterol use. Albuterol has been linked with an increase in glycolysis leading to enhanced pyruvate production which is converted to lactate. Albuterol has also been associated with increased lipolysis and production of free fatty acid. Fatty acid production inhibits pyruvate dehydrogenase which is the key cofactor needed for pyruvate to enter the Krebs cycle rather than be converted to lactate. While status asthmaticus patients can have two forms of lactate production, this patient had evidence of peak flows that were continuing to drop, evidence of pulsus paradoxus, and continued respiratory distress; therefore, type A lactic acidosis was the most likely driver. To combat the patient's high work of breathing, it would be recommended to intubate the patient to allow for rest and better control of the patient's ventilation. Magnesium can be used in asthmatic patients. Magnesium has been proposed to help enhance bronchial smooth muscle relaxation and enhance the receptor affinity for beta-2 agonists. It has not been demonstrated to reduce lactate production and, given the patient's compromised hemodynamics, should not be the next best step in management. Fluids can be helpful for hypotension secondary to low-flow states. The patient may benefit from the addition of IV fluids; however, without addressing the patient's respiratory distress, resolution of the lactate will be less likely.

### References

1. Dodda VR, Spiro P. Can albuterol be blamed for lactic acidosis? *Respir Care*. 2012;57(12):2115-2118. PubMed PMID:22613097.
2. Jardin F, Farcot JC, Boisante L, Prost JF, Gueret P, Bourdarias JP. Mechanism of paradoxic pulse in bronchial asthma. *Circulation*. 1982;66(4):887-894. PubMed PMID:7116605.
3. Song WJ, Chang YS. Magnesium sulfate for acute asthma in adults: a systematic literature review. *Asia Pac Allergy*. 2012;2(1):76-85. PubMed PMID:22348210. Pubmed Central PMCID:3269605.

---

**8.** Correct Answer: D

**Rationale:**

Negative pressure pulmonary edema (NPPE) occurs when significant negative intrathoracic pressures occur against a closed airway. In this case, the patient experiences laryngospasm after recent exposure to operative procedure. As the patient generates highly negative intrapleural and alveolar pressures in an attempt to overcome the upper airway obstruction, a pressure gradient is created and fluid moves out of the pulmonary capillaries and into the interstitial and alveolar spaces. The negative intrathoracic pressure also results in an increase in venous blood to the right side of the heart. This causes right-sided dilation and interventricular septum shift to the left. This reduces the stroke volume and cardiac output generated by the left ventricle. The increased venous return to the right side of the heart also increased the blood flow through the pulmonary vasculature. The increased blood increases hydrostatic forces within the pulmonary vasculature and creates a gradient in which fluid then leaks into the alveolar space. This phenomenon can be made worse as the patient becomes either more hypoxemic or acidic, as this will increase pulmonary vascular resistance which can further dilate the right side of the heart. This patient was at increased risk for laryngospasm, given he was a male and had GERD and an LMA was used which has higher rates of spasm in comparison to endotracheal tube intubation. Other risk factors for NPPE included upper airway infection, tumor, foreign body aspiration, or extended periods of time where a patient is biting down on the endotracheal tube.

NPPE can appear at times similar to cardiogenic pulmonary edema and can respond to similar treatment in the form of positive pressure and diuretics. NPPE distribution on imaging, however, can differ from cardiogenic pulmonary edema in the fact that it tends to form in the central and nondependent areas in the lungs. In these regions, a greater negative pressure is created when significant inspiratory effort is generated; therefore, these areas tend to form ground glass changes first. Cardiogenic pulmonary edema tends to favor dependent and peripheral regions.

Aspiration pneumonitis can cause acute respiratory distress; however, there is no clear history of an aspiration event. Anaphylaxis can present with bronchospasm and hypotension and can have pulmonary infiltrates. The patient did not have evidence of rash, urticaria, or swelling which can also be seen in anaphylaxis. The patient also had a clear distress that occurred after airway obstruction; therefore, the clinical picture is more aligned with NPPE. Finally, cardiogenic pulmonary edema is a very common cause of respiratory distress but does not typically follow laryngospasm.

### References

1. Bhaskar B, Fraser JF. Negative pressure pulmonary edema revisited: Pathophysiology and review of management. *Saudi J Anaesth*. 2011;5(3):308-313. PubMed PMID:21957413. Pubmed Central PMCID:3168351.
2. Guru PK, Agarwal A, Pimentel M, McLaughlin DC, Bansal V. Postoperative pulmonary edema conundrum: a case of negative pressure pulmonary edema. *Case Rep Crit Care*. 2018;2018:1584134. PubMed PMID:30345119. Pubmed Central PMCID:6174762.
3. Olsson GL, Hallen B. Laryngospasm during anesthesia. A computer-aided incidence study in 136,929 patients. *Acta Anaesthesiol Scand*. 1984;28(5):567-575. PubMed PMID:6496018.

**9.** Correct Answer: B

**Rationale:**
The patient presents with evidence of smoke inhalation injury secondary to a house fire. She has multiple risk factors for increased risk of inhalation injury which include history of inhalation in a closed space, facial burn, evidence of soot in her nasal cavity, and hoarseness. Approximately 10% to 20% of burns are associated with inhalation injury, and inhalation injury is an independent predictor of mortality. In patients with concern for inhalation injury, the greatest concern is for increasing swelling and inflammatory response which will lead to airway compromise. The mechanisms for inhalation injury include thermal injury to the upper airway, chemical irritation by combustion products which generate free radicals, damage to parenchymal tissue, and increased levels of carbon monoxide which displaces oxygen from hemoglobin and impairs mitochondrial function. Given that the patient presents with evidence of inhalation injury, after providing oxygen, a fiberoptic flexible bronchoscopy would be recommended to assess the degree of airway damage. An Abbreviated Injury Score has been created which grades the degree of injury seen on bronchoscopy by the amount of erythema, carbonaceous material, obstruction, and necrosis noted within the airway. The grading is on a 0 to 4 scale, with grades 2 to 4 on initial bronchoscopy demonstrating higher mortality in comparison to grade 0 to 1. In patients with higher grade injury seen on bronchoscopy, the decision may be made to electively intubate the patient as they are at higher risk for airway compromise.

This patient has multiple high-risk factors for airway compromise; therefore, the ideal situation would be to evaluate the airway with bronchoscopy rather than to solely observe the patient for 24 hours. If the patient were to have significant more swelling, an endotracheal tube may not be able to be passed in the coming hours and therefore an emergent tracheostomy may need to be performed. This patient also has evidence of elevated carboxyhemoglobin levels. The patient does not have a clear indication for hyperbaric chamber as her levels are less than 25; she has no evidence of ECG changes or end-organ dysfunction; and she did not have loss of consciousness. At this time, the initial therapy would be 100% oxygen. Finally, there has been no clear benefit demonstrated for steroids in inhalation injury. Steroids could potentially delay healing and increase infection risk.

### References

1. Tanizaki S. Assessing inhalation injury in the emergency room. *Open Access Emerg Med*. 2015;7:31-37. PubMed PMID:27147888. Pubmed Central PMCID:4806805.
2. Walker PF, Buehner MF, Wood LA, et al. Diagnosis and management of inhalation injury: an updated review. *Crit Care*. 2015;19:351. PubMed PMID:26507130. Pubmed Central PMCID:4624587.
3. Endorf FW, Gamelli RL. Inhalation injury, pulmonary perturbations, and fluid resuscitation. *J Burn Care Res*. 2007;28(1):80-83. PubMed PMID:17211205.
4. Bartley AC, Edgar DW, Wood FM. Pharmaco-management of inhalation injuries for burn survivors. *Drug Des Devel Ther*. 2009;2:9-16. PubMed PMID:19920889. Pubmed Central PMCID:2761179.

**10.** Correct Answer: C

**Rationale:**

The patient is demonstrating posterior trachea membrane occlusion status post tracheostomy placement. As the patient is transitioned to spontaneous mode of ventilation, he is able to generate his own inspiratory effort. In patients with a malpositioned or incorrectly sized tracheostomy tube, a significant inspiratory effort can cause the posterior membrane to collapse in on the distal end of the tracheostomy tube blocking air from entering. The occlusion will be seen on the ventilator in the form of high PIPs. The collapse of the posterior membrane can be diagnosed with bronchoscopy. Once the diagnosis is made, the tracheostomy tube can be replaced with a longer tube that may bypass the area of collapse, a tube with a different angle, or a tube that has a different shaft length. A T-piece tube would likely worsen the issue as there is no angle; therefore, the posterior membrane would directly be affected with each respiratory effort. If the tube cannot be exchanged quickly, the collapse of the posterior membrane may be reduced by increasing the PEEP rather than decreasing. Finally, suctioning is always recommended but is unlikely to correct the etiology for this patient's respiratory distress.

References

1. Hess DR, Altobelli NP. Tracheostomy tubes. *Respir Care*. 2014;59(6):956-971; discussion 71-3. PubMed PMID:24891201.
2. Singhal S, Kiran S, Das A. Posterior tracheal wall leading to life-threatening obstruction of tracheostomy tube. *Avicenna J Med*. 2013;3(2):48-49. PubMed PMID:23930242. Pubmed Central PMCID:3734631.

# 36

# DISEASES OF THE CHEST WALL

Charles Corey Hardin and Jenna McNeill

1. An 88-year-old male with a 55 pack-year smoking history and an additional past medical history of COPD, and stage IA non–small cell lung cancer was referred for bronchoscopy. Prior to the procedure the patient was alert and oriented, afebrile, with BP 130/70, RR 14, and $O_2$ saturation of 99% while breathing room air. The patient received a total of 100 µg IV fentanyl and 4 mg IV midazolam in divided doses during the bronchoscopy. Following the airway survey the diagnostic bronchoscope was removed and the patient received an additional 100 µg of fentanyl and 1 mg of midazolam prior to insertion of the scope for endobronchial ultrasound. Two minutes after insertion of the endobronchial ultrasound bronchoscope the patient developed a clenched hand and jaw and hypertension to 225/135 mm Hg. Respiratory motion was no longer evident upon examination of his chest wall. Oxygen saturation dropped to 81%. In addition to securing the airway the next most appropriate step would be:

   A. Rapidly obtain CT of the head
   B. Administer antihypertensives with a goal of lowering SBP 10% to 20% over an hour.
   C. Administer naloxone 0.2 mg IV
   D. Administer 2 mg benztropine

2. A 65-year-old female is scheduled for spinal surgery. Her pre-op CXR is shown below. She has a past medical history of CAD and HTN, atrial fibrillation. Which of the following is most helpful in predicting her risk of postoperative of respiratory failure?

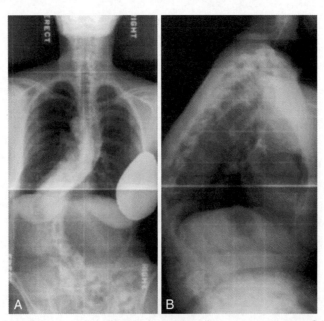

(From Taylor J, Gropper MA. Critical care challenges in orthopedic surgery patients. *Crit Care Med*. 2006;34(9 suppl):S191-S199.)

A. Vital capacity

B. History of atrial fibrillation

C. Nature of the surgery (orthopedic)

D. Age

3. A 49-year-old female is admitted to the hospital with community-acquired pneumonia. On presentation to the emergency department she is complaining of shortness of breath, temperature is 38.5, $O_2$ sat is 95% on 2 L NC, RR is 14, BP 120/80, and pulse is 98. CXR shows an RML lobar infiltrate. She is admitted to the general medical floor but that night complains of increased dyspnea that is worse when lying supine. She is noted to have a weak cough and difficulty clearing secretions. She is afebrile, with a pulse of 110 and BP 110/75. $O_2$ sat remains >95% on 2 to 4 L/min NC. Exam is notable for a regular cardiac rhythm, with no murmurs, rubs, or gallops. There are bronchial breath sounds noted over the right mid-lung zone. Peripheral pulses are intact, strength is normal in the b/l upper and lower extremities and there are normal deep tendon reflexes. CXR is unchanged from admission. Which will be most helpful in determining subsequent therapy and need for intubation?

A. Lumbar puncture and EMG

B. Measure vital capacity

C. Check BNP, obtain trans-throacic echocardiogram

D. Chest CT

4. A 77-year-old male presented to the emergency department after motor vehicle accident. On arrival, respirations were shallow and the right chest appeared to move inward with inspiration. $O_2$ saturation was 85% while breathing room air and pulse was 122. Chest x-ray and chest CT are shown in the figure that follows. What is the next most appropriate step in management?

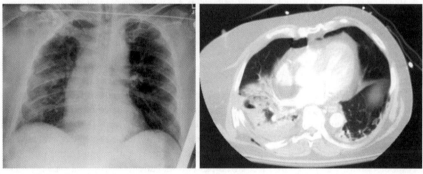

Figure from Kiraly L, Schreiber M. Management of the crushed chest. *Crit Care Med.* 2010;38(9 suppl):S469-S477.

A. Noninvasive positive pressure ventilation and IV morphine

B. Evaluation for surgical fixation of rib fracture

C. Intubation and adjustment of PEEP to improve oxygenation

D. Epidural catheter placement to decrease splinting

5. A 68-year-male is in the midst of a prolonged ICU stay for respiratory failure, ARDS, and gram-negative bacteremia. He initially presented with shock requiring high-dose vasopressors and stress-dose steroids as well as severe hypoxemia requiring mechanical ventilation and paralytics. By ICU day 10 he has repeatedly failed spontaneous breathing trials with low tidal volumes. His exam is notable for reduced strength in b/l upper and lower extremities without rigidity. Laboratory studies including creatine kinase are within normal limits. Head CT is normal and CSF studies are normal. Electrophysiologic testing is notable for significantly decreased sensory and motor nerve amplitudes in multiple nerves, prolonged compound muscle action potentials, and decreased motor amplitudes. Which of the following is an appropriate next step in management?

A. Dantrolene 2.5 mg/kg

B. Tracheostomy and physical therapy

C. Plasma exchange

D. IVIG

# Chapter 36 ▪ Answers

**1.** Correct Answer: C

**Rationale:**

This patient has likely experienced fentanyl-induced chest wall rigidity. Skeletal muscle rigidity following opiate administration, which may primarily affect the musculature of the chest and abdomen, was first described in 1953. While a rare complication of opioid analgesia, it is thought to be more commonly associated the lipophilic synthetic opioids such as fentanyl, remifentanil, and sufentanil. Risk factors include extremes of age, concurrent use of medications that alter dopamine levels, and higher doses or rapidity of injection. Skeletal muscle rigidity decreases the compliance of the chest wall and increases work of breathing or may even lead to the cessation of spontaneous breathing. Decreased chest wall compliance can also complicate efforts at mechanical ventilation. Treatment includes reversal of opioids with naloxone (answer C) or mechanical ventilation and neuromuscular blocking agents.

Head CT would be an appropriate diagnostic tool in cases of suspected stroke, but in this case the temporal association with fentanyl administration and the cessation of chest wall motion make rigidity the more likely diagnosis.

The patient developed acute hypertension along with atypical motion of the hand and arm which may suggest the possibility of hypertensive emergency. Acute therapy of hypertensive emergency is aimed at lowering of blood pressure by 10% to 20% but, in this case, the hypertension is secondary to respiratory distress.

Benztropine is indicated for therapy of dystonic reactions such as those associated with the administration of antipsychotic medications but is not the appropriate choice for the primary diagnosis here.

References

1. Hamilton WK, Culen SC. Effect of levallorphan tartrate upon opiate induced respiratory depression. *Anesthesiology*. 1953;14:550-554.
2. Coruth B, Tonelli M, Park D. Fentany-induced chest wall rigidity. *Chest*. 2013;143:1145-1146.
3. Ackerman WE, Phero JC, theodore GT. Ineffective ventilation during conscious sedation due to chest wall rigidity after intravenous midazolam and fentanyl. *Anesthe Prog*. 1990;37:46-48.

**2.** Correct Answer: A

**Rationale:**

As indicated by the CXR the patient suffers from severe kyphoscoliosis. Kyphosis refers to an excessive curvature of the thoracic spine. The prevalence of kyphosis increases with age due to the combined effects of vertebral fractures, muscle weakness, and degenerative disk disease. The increased curvature leads to a restrictive deficit on pulmonary function testing with decreased TLC and FVC. The restrictive deficit can be associated with atelectasis, intrapulmonary shunt, and arterial hypoxemia. It also places patients at greater risk of postoperative pulmonary complications including respiratory failure and need for mechanical ventilation. Patients with a vital capacity <35% of predicted are at increased risk and will frequently require postoperative ventilation. Atrial fibrillation has a small effect on risk of overall mortality but is not known to specifically increase risk of respiratory failure. In general, orthopedic surgery is associated with a lower complication rate than other procedures. Age >70 is associated with increased mortality in orthopedic patients but this patient is 65.

References

1. Schneider D, von Muhlen D, Barrett-Connor E, sartoris D. Kyphosis does not equal vertebral fractures: the Rancho Bernardo study. *J Rheumatol*. 2004;31:747-752.
2. Leech J, Dulberg C, Kellie S, Pattee L, Gay J. Relationship of lung function to severity of osteoporosis in women. *Am Rev Respir Dis*. 1990;141:68-71.
3. Taylor JM, Gropper MA. Critical care challenges in orthopedic surgery patients. *Crit Care Med*. 2006;34:S191-S199.

**3.** Correct Answer: B

**Rationale:**

This patient is presenting with signs and symptoms consistent with myasthenic crisis. Myasthenic crisis can be the first presentation of myasthenia gravis, an autoimmune disorder caused by development of autoantibodies which attack the neuromuscular junction. Common precipitants of crisis in patients with myasthenia include infection, with bacterial pneumonia being most common, and drugs including fluoroquinolones. Clinical features include bulbar weakness and dysphagia, dyspnea, respiratory muscle weakness (often manifested as worsening respiratory function when supine—a position in which the abdominal contents impede the motion of the diaphragm more so than in the upright position), and decreased vital capacity. Elective intubation should be considered when vital capacity declines below 15 to 20 mL/kg. Additional therapies for myasthenic crisis include plasma exchange and IVIG. Myasthenia can be associated with generalized weakness, but a proportion of patients will present with primarily respiratory weakness. Lumbar puncture and EMG can be helpful in the diagnosis of Guillain-Barre syndrome but weakness in the Guillain-Barre syndrome typically starts in the legs and is associated with a lack of deep tendon reflexes. Heart failure and subsequent pulmonary edema can lead to worsening dyspnea when lying flat. BNP and TTE can be helpful in making that diagnosis, but the normal cardiac exam and unchanged CXR make that diagnosis less likely here. Heart failure would also not explain the dysphagia. Chest CT could be helpful in establishing a diagnosis of aspiration, which occurs in the setting of bulbar weakness, but in this case the CXR is unchanged and there is minimal change in the degree of hypoxemia.

### References

1. Thomas CE, Mayer SA, Gungor Y, et al. Myasthenic crisis: clinical features, mortality, complications, and risk factors for prolonged intubation. *Neurology.* 1997;48:1253-1260.
2. Berrouschot J, Baumann I, Kalischewski P, Sterker M, Schneider D. Therapy of myasthenic crisis. *Crit Care Med.* 1997;25:1228-1235.
3. Willison HJ, Jacobs BC, van Doorn PA. Guillain-Barre syndrome. *Lancet.* 2016;388:717-727.

**4.** Correct Answer: C

**Rationale:**
The patient has suffered significant thoracic trauma as the result of a motor vehicle collision. He has multiple right-sided rib fractures on CXR and flail chest on exam. In addition, the chest CT scan reveals significant pulmonary contusion and atelectasis. Management of flail chest includes pain control, management of pulmonary injury, and, in selected patients, surgical fixation. Importantly, this patient presents in respiratory distress with evidence of pulmonary contusion on chest CT. There are small trials of noninvasive ventilation in chest injury, but in this patient with distress and established lung injury this would not be appropriate. In addition, IV analgesia carries the risk of respiratory depression. Locoregional (epidural, paravertebral) analgesia is often preferred. There is increasing interest in surgical fixation of flail chest, but in patients with underlying contusion there is no benefit over nonoperative management. Epidural catheter placement can be a key component of pain control in flail chest but does nothing to treat the pulmonary contusion which is likely a larger risk factor for mortality.

### References

1. Majercik S, Pieracci F. Chest wall trauma. *Thorac Surg Clin.* 2017;27:113-121.
2. Kiraly L, Schreiber M. Management of the crushed chest. *Crit Care Med.* 2010;38:S469-S477.

**5.** Correct Answer: B

**Rationale:**
This patient is likely suffering from critical illness polyneuropathy and myopathy (CIP/CIM). CIP/CIM is a form of generalized weakness that results from skeletal muscle dysfunction and peripheral neuropathy. Risk factors include prolonged ICU stay, sepsis, use of steroids and neuromuscular blocking agents, and hyperglycemia during ICU stay. The etiology of CIP/CIM is not entirely understood, but it is thought to result from some combination of nerve ischemia, decreased muscle protein synthesis, disordered inflammatory signaling. Typical clinical features include failure to wean from mechanical ventilation, peripheral limb weakness, and the described features on electrodiagnostic testing. Patients with CIP/CIM can experience prolonged weakness and resolution, if it occurs, typically occurs over weeks to months. Treatment is primarily supportive with aggressive physical therapy and potentially prolonged mechanical ventilation. The differential diagnosis of CIP/CIM includes rare neuromuscular disorders such as the Guillain-Barre syndrome (GBS), but GBS more typically presents with an elevated CSF protein (with normal CSF cell count). Plasma exchange and IVIG are used in GBS and myasthenic crisis associated with Myasthenia Gravis, but there is no role for either in CIP/CIM. Dantrolene has been used in neuroleptic malignant syndrome (NMS), but in this case there is no mention of the use of neuroleptics nor is there fever of rigidity on exam.

### References

1. Bercker S, Weber-Carstens S, Deja M, et al. Critical illness polyneuropathy and myopathy in patients with acute respiratory distress syndrome. *Crit Care Med.* 2005;33:711-715.
2. Callahan LA, Supinkski GS. Sepsis-induced myopathy. *Crit Care Med.* 2009;37:S354-S367.

# 37

# THROMBOEMBOLIC DISEASE AND HEMOPTYSIS

Maram Marouki, Joanna Brenneman, and Roshni Sreedharan

1. A 55-year-old female with a history of renal cell carcinoma with metastases to the spine is scheduled for a spinal separation procedure to facilitate radiation therapy. The surgical procedure was uneventful. Following skin closure, there was a sudden drop in oxygen saturation to 86% with an increase in heart rate to 124/min and blood pressure of 85/41 mm Hg. The peak airway pressure was 25 cm $H_2O$ and the ETCO$_2$ is 15 mm Hg. 100% oxygen was administered and the patient was started on an epinephrine infusion to support hemodynamics. Which of the following statements is **LEAST** likely to be true if you are considering a diagnosis of pulmonary embolism in this patient?

A. S1Q3T3 on ECG is seen in less than 20% of the patients
B. The VQ mismatch is due to an increase in dead space ventilation
C. Hemoptysis is an uncommon presenting symptom
D. Intravenous heparin infusion is the treatment of choice in this patient

2. Which of the following statements regarding monitoring modalities for venous air embolism (VAE) is **MOST** accurate?

A. Precordial Doppler is the most sensitive monitoring modality available for the detection of VAE
B. Changes in end tidal nitrogen occur earlier than changes in end tidal carbon dioxide
C. Pulmonary artery catheter is the most sensitive monitor for the detection of VAE
D. Mill-wheel murmur auscultated with an esophageal stethoscope is an early sign of VAE

3. A 40-year-old female is admitted to the intensive care unit with worsening shortness of breath. She states that she had a clot in her lung "a long time ago" for which she "took blood thinners for a few months." Her initial transthoracic echocardiogram reveals enlarged right-sided chambers with severe tricuspid regurgitation and a large thrombus in the pulmonary artery with severe pulmonary hypertension. This patient is **MOST** likely to belong to which of the groups of the World Health Organization clinical classification of pulmonary hypertension.

A. Group 1
B. Group 2
C. Group 3
D. Group 4
E. Group 5

4. A 56-year-old male with 30-pack year smoking history, CAD, and advanced liver disease due to alcoholic cirrhosis is being evaluated for a liver transplantation. He complains of worsening shortness of breath. His heart rate is 110/min, blood pressure is 97/64 mm Hg, respiratory rate is 32/min, and saturation 90% on 5 L/min nasal cannula. When asked to sit up in bed, the patient states that he "*usually breathes better*" when lying supine. Which of the following is the **MOST** likely pathophysiology behind the diagnosis?

A. Decreased FRC resulting in increasing closing capacity leading to atelectasis
B. Acute on chronic pulmonary thromboembolism
C. Increased production or decreased clearance of endogenous nitric oxide
D. Increased venous congestion leading to pulmonary edema

5. A 67-year-old female with a history of DVT/PE, hypertension, diabetes mellitus, and coronary artery disease undergoes a hemicolectomy with end ileostomy for colorectal carcinoma. On postoperative day 4, she aspirates following an episode of emesis. She is intubated and transferred to the ICU for further management. Ventilator settings are as follows:

Mode: Assist control—volume control
Tidal volume: 450 mL
Respiratory rate: 12/min
$FiO_2$: 100%
PEEP: 18 mm Hg
I:E ratio: 1:2

Her HR is 105 bpm; BP is 127/64 mm Hg, saturation 85%. Her most recent ABG reveals a pH 7.31, $paCO_2$ 48, $paO_2$ 59, Hgb 7.0. Which of the following interventions is **MOST** likely to improve the oxygen delivery in this patient?

   A. Change the mode of ventilation to pressure control
   B. Decrease the I:E ratio
   C. Transfuse 1 unit of PRBC
   D. Start norepinephrine infusion

6. A 24-year-old male with no major medical history has been receiving treatment for a lower respiratory tract disease for the past 5 days. He had a large bout of hemoptysis this evening, which prompted his visit to the emergency room. His BP is 120/70 mm Hg, HR 120/min, and RR is 30/min. Physical examination reveals bilateral rales and a diastolic murmur. Patients with which of the following valvular disorders are **MOST** likely to present with hemoptysis?

   A. Tricuspid stenosis
   B. Mitral stenosis
   C. Aortic stenosis
   D. Aortic regurgitation

7. Which of the following statements regarding the signs and symptoms of venous air embolism (VAE) is **INCORRECT**?

   A. Bradyarrhythmias are the most common arrhythmias that occur with VAE
   B. Substernal chest pain, right heart failure, and cardiovascular collapse commonly occur with entrained volumes over 2 mL/kg
   C. Increased end tidal nitrogen and decreased end tidal carbon dioxide can be seen with less than 0.5 mL/kg of air entrainment
   D. Paradoxical air embolism could occur across the lung vascular bed in patients with VAE

8. A 34-year-old male undergoing an emergent open reduction and internal fixation of his left femur suddenly develops tachycardia, hypotension and hypoxemia. Fat embolism syndrome (FES) is suspected. All of the following are considered a part of the major clinical criteria for the diagnosis of FES proposed by Gurd **EXCEPT**:

   A. Respiratory symptoms with radiographic changes
   B. Tachycardia
   C. Petechial rash
   D. Central nervous system signs unrelated to trauma or other alternative pathology

# Chapter 37 ▪ Answers

1. Correct Answer: D

   **Rationale:**
   Advancing age, immobilization, and a diagnosis of cancer confer an increased risk of deep vein thrombosis and pulmonary embolism (PE). Contrast-enhanced chest CT scan is the most commonly used modality to confirm the diagnosis of a PE. As PE represents a perfusion defect, there is an increase in dead space ventilation in these patients. In addition to initial stabilization, volume infusion, and vasopressor therapy, systemic anticoagulation is initiated

in most patients with a PE as long as there are no contraindications. Recent surgery, especially in closed spaces like brain/spinal cord, active bleeding, and malignant hypertension are considered contraindications for systemic anticoagulation. Thrombolytic therapy is reserved for patients with PE who present with hemodynamic instability. Although it could rapidly restore pulmonary circulation and improve right ventricular function, it confers a higher risk of bleeding. Catheter-directed thrombolysis can be considered in patients in whom the risk of bleeding with systemic therapy outweighs the benefits.

### References

1. Jimenez D, Yusen R, Hull R. Pulmonary embolism. In: Vincent JL, Abraham E, Moore FA, Kochanek PM, Fink MP, eds. *Chapter 71. Textbook of Critical Care*. 7th ed. 2016:442-455.
2. Wood K. Major pulmonary embolism. *Crit Care Clin*. 2011;27(4):885-906.

## 2. Correct Answer: B

### Rationale:

Transesophageal echocardiography (TEE) is the most sensitive monitoring modality to detect venous air embolism. TEE can detect as little as 0.02 mL/kg of air. Precordial Doppler is the most sensitive noninvasive monitoring modality with the ability to detect 0.05 mL/kg of air. Other available monitoring modalities for the detection of VAE include transcranial Doppler, esophageal stethoscope, pulmonary artery catheter, end tidal carbon dioxide and nitrogen. Changes in end tidal nitrogen are seen to occur 30 to 90 seconds prior to the changes in end tidal carbon dioxide. Although their sensitivities seem equivalent, for large volume entrainment, the sensitivity of end tidal nitrogen might exceed that of end tidal $CO_2$. Pulmonary artery catheters are fairly insensitive monitors for this purpose. The mill-wheel murmur auscultated with an esophageal stethoscope has a low sensitivity and is not an early sign (1.7 mL/kg/min).

### References

1. Mirski M, Lele A, Fitzsimmons L, Toung T. Diagnosis and treatment of vascular air embolism. *Anesthesiology*. 2007;106: 164-177.
2. Shaikh N, Ummunisa F. Acute management of vascular air embolism. *J Emerg Trauma Shock*. 2009;2(3):180-185.

## 3. Correct Answer: D

### Rationale:

The World Health Organization clinical classification of pulmonary hypertension categorizes this diagnosis into groups based on similarities in pathophysiology, clinical presentation, and therapeutic measures. The five broad groups are as follows:

*Pulmonary arterial hypertension* (Group 1)—Pulmonary hypertension that is idiopathic; drug-, toxin-, or infection-induced; and those that are associated with systemic diseases fall into this category.

*Pulmonary hypertension due to left heart disease* (Group 2)—Pulmonary hypertension arising from left heart disease, be it atrial, ventricular, or valvular falls under this category. This is probably the most common etiological class for pulmonary hypertension. Left-sided disease leading to elevated left atrial pressure results in back pressure into the pulmonary vasculature. Over time, increases in pulmonary vasomotor tone and pulmonary vascular remodeling result in worsening pulmonary arterial pressures.

*Pulmonary hypertension due to lung disease* (Group 3)—Pulmonary hypertension as a result of intrinsic lung disease and/or hypoxia falls under this category.

*Chronic thromboembolic pulmonary hypertension (CTEPH)* (Group 4)—Thromboemboli either forming in or traveling to the lung resulting in pulmonary hypertension fall under this group.

*Pulmonary hypertension with unclear or multifactorial mechanisms* (Group 5)—Disorders wherein the mechanism of pulmonary hypertension is poorly understood fall under this category. A few of these include sarcoidosis, Langerhans cell histiocytosis, and certain anemias.

Given the clinical presentation, this patient seems to have a large clot in the pulmonary artery with enlarged right-sided chambers and pulmonary hypertension. She most likely has CTEPH and belongs to group 4.

### References

1. Simonneau G, Robbins IM, Beghetti M, et al. Updated clinical classification of pulmonary hypertension. *J Am Coll Cardiol*. 2009; 54:S43-S54.
2. Simonneau G, Gatzhoulis M, Adatia I, et al. Updated clinical classification of pulmonary hypertension. *J Am Coll Cardiol*. 2013;62(25):D34-D41.

## 4. Correct Answer: C

### Rationale:

The development of intrapulmonary vascular dilatations (IVPD) in the presence of advanced liver disease and portal hypertension results in hepatopulmonary syndrome (HPS). Several mediators included nitric oxide, endothelin 1, TNF alfa, and vascular endothelial growth factor have been implicated in the development of these IVPDs. The dilation of these blood vessels results in shunting of blood, leading to V/Q mismatch, hypoxemia, and an increased alveolar arterial oxygen gradient. These IVPDs tend to occur predominantly in the base of the lungs, resulting in worsening of the shunt while upright. This manifests as platypnea-orthodeoxia. Contrast-enhanced echocardiography can aid with the diagnosis of HPS and microaggregated albumin (MAA) can help distinguish and quantify hypoxemia resulting from IVPD in patients with other lung parenchymal disorders. Liver transplantation is the definitive treatment. Although several experimental medical therapies have been tried, none of them have consistently shown to be of benefit in the treatment of HPS.

### References

1. Krowka MJ, Fallon MB, Kawut SM, et al. International Liver Transplant Society practice guidelines: diagnosis and management of hepatopulmonary syndrome and portopulmonary hypertension. *Transplantation*. 2016;100:1440.
2. Grace J, Angus P. Hepatopulmonary syndrome: update on recent advances in pathophysiology, investigation and treatment. *J Gastroenterol Hepatol*. 2013;28:213-219.

### 5. Correct Answer: C

**Rationale:**

Increase in dead space ventilation contributes to the V/Q mismatch in patients with pulmonary embolism. Oxygen attached to hemoglobin contributes a great extent to the overall oxygen content in the arterial system. The other factors that contribute to the arterial oxygen content include the oxygen saturation and partial pressure of oxygen in the blood or the dissolved oxygen. This is depicted by the equation, $CaO_2 = (1.34 \times Hgb \times SaO_2) + (0.0031 \times PaO_2)$. The role of the dissolved component of oxygen is negligible as it is multiplied by a factor of 0.0031. The saturation of oxygen has an upper limit of 100% which limits its ability to improve the content above a certain limit. Consequently, PRBC transfusion is most effective in increasing the oxygen content of arterial blood, especially in an anemic patient. Oxygen delivery is a product of oxygen content and cardiac output. Although inotropes could increase cardiac output, this patient has appropriate hemodynamics at this time which would not warrant inotropic support.

### References

1. Hess D, Kacmarek R. Blood gases. *Chapter 28. Essential of Mechanical Ventilation*. 4th ed. 2014.
2. Lumb A. Oxygen. *Nunn's Applied Respiratory Physiology, Chapter 10*. 8th ed. 2017:169-202, E3.

### 6. Correct Answer: B

**Rationale:**

Massive hemoptysis is most commonly defined as a volume over 500 mL in 24 hours or over 100 mL per hour. Hemoptysis could be the presenting symptom in a patient with mitral stenosis, although uncommon in patients with a known diagnosis. Several pathophysiological mechanisms have been postulated for this presentation. In patients with severe MS, shunts occur between the pulmonary and bronchial venous vasculature. Rupture of these vessels could result in hemoptysis which could occasionally be massive resulting in pulmonary apoplexy. Other causes of hemoptysis in patients with mitral stenosis include pulmonary edema and infarction.

### References

1. Thomas J, Bonow R. *Braunwald's Heart Disease: A Textbook of Cardiovascular Medicine, Chapter 69*. 11th ed. 1415-1444.
2. Wood P. An appreciation of mitral stenosis. *Br J Med*. 1954;1:1051, 1113.

### 7. Correct Answer: A

**Rationale:**

The clinical effects of VAE depend on the volume and rate of entrainment of air. Spontaneous respiration with negative intrathoracic pressure could facilitate further entrainment of air. Venous air embolism can present with arrhythmias. Tachyarrhythmias are common but bradyarrhythmias can occur, as well. Associated substernal chest pain could be a presenting symptom. Right heart failure and cardiovascular collapse are more often seen with large volumes of entrainment—around 2 mL/kg. Changes in levels of monitored gases like nitrogen and carbon dioxide can occur with smaller volumes of air entrainment. Fundoscopy is typically normal. Rarely, air bubbles can be seen within the retinal vessels. Paradoxical embolism could happen either through a patent foramen ovale or by overwhelming the capacity of the lungs to filter the air emboli.

### References

1. Mirski M, Lele A, Fitzsimmons L, Toung T. Diagnosis and treatment of vascular air embolism. *Anesthesiology*. 2007;106:164-177.
2. Muth C, Shank E. Gas embolism. *N Engl J Med*. 2000;342:476-482.

**8.** Correct Answer: B

**Rationale:**

Fat embolism syndrome (FES) is most often seen in orthopedic patients with long bone fractures. Although rare, liposuction, bone marrow harvest, and sickle cell crisis could also be complicated by FES. The clinical manifestations of FES are considered to occur as a result of the proinflammatory and prothrombotic effects of fat cells, resulting in either mechanical obstruction or biochemical injury. Gurd criteria are the most commonly used or cited diagnostic criteria for FES. Gurd criteria typically require the presence of one major and four minor criteria to make a clinical diagnosis of FES. The major criteria include respiratory insufficiency, cerebral involvement, and petechial rash. The minor criteria include tachycardia, fever, jaundice, retinal changes, and renal changes. The treatment of FES is largely supportive with some studies advocating the use of heparin and corticosteroids.

### References

1. Gurd AR. Fat embolism: an aid to diagnosis. *J Bone Joint Surg Br*. 1970;52:732-737.
2. Kosova E, Bergmark B, Piazza G. Fat embolism syndrome. *Circulation*. 2015;131:317-320.

# 38

# PLEURAL DISORDERS

Galen Royce-Nagel

1. A 64-year-old female presents with a 5-day history of exertional dyspnea and orthopnea. Her medical history is significant for SLE and diastolic heart failure. Chest X-ray reveals significant bilateral pleural effusions. The decision is made to perform a thoracentesis. Which laboratory value would indicate that the effusions are a result of her known diagnosis of SLE?

   A. Pleural fluid to serum protein ratio less than 0.5
   B. Pleural fluid LDH less than two-thirds the upper limit of normal serum LDH
   C. Pleural fluid to serum LDH ratio greater than 0.6
   D. Pleural fluid cholesterol less than 45 mg/dL

2. A 45-year-old male was admitted to the ICU after sustaining a gunshot wound to the chest. The resulting hemothorax was initially managed with a chest tube. On hospital day 4 he developed a fever, and leukocytosis and broad spectrum antibiotics were started. A CT of the chest revealed a multiloculated effusion that was concerning for empyema. The next **best** step in management is:

   A. Place a second chest tube
   B. Continue systemic antibiotics and monitor for resolution
   C. Flush the chest tube with 100 mL normal saline
   D. Consult thoracic surgery for washout and debridement

3. A 72-year-old male with congestive heart failure is undergoing thoracentesis for a right pleural effusion. Shortly after draining 1.5 L of fluid, the patient develops dyspnea and hypoxia. What measure, if taken, could reduce the risk of this complication?

   A. Limit end-expiratory pleural pressures to less than (−) 20 cm $H_2O$
   B. Limit total volume removed to less than 0.5 L
   C. Administer IV albumin in a 1:1 ratio for fluid removed
   D. Increase the volume removed to 2 L

4. The proper position for chest tube placement in a patient with a pneumothorax is:

   A. Second intercostal space mid-axillary line
   B. Fifth intercostal space posterior axillary line
   C. Third intercostal space mid-clavicular line
   D. Fourth intercostal space anterior axillary line

5. A 90-year-old female with a history of atrial fibrillation on Eliquis presents with right rib pain and dyspnea after a mechanical fall from standing. She is hemodynamically stable, but her chest CT reveals right rib fractures 3 to 5 with associated hemothorax. The next best step in management includes:

A. Placement of a large bore chest tube for hemothorax evacuation
B. Placement of an epidural for pain control and prevention of respiratory decompensation
C. Consult thoracic surgery for emergent VATS
D. Initation of broad spectrum antibiotics

# Chapter 38 ▪ Answers

**1.** Correct Answer: C

**Rationale:**
When evaluating pleural fluid obtained from a thoracentesis, Light's criteria can be used to differentiate a transudative effusion, which is due to an imbalance in hydrostatic and oncotic pressure, from an exudative effusion, which can be secondary to a myriad of alternative problems. A transudative effusion can be treated usually without undergoing the extent of investigation that is required if the effusion is exudative in origin. Transudative effusions tend to be seen in patients with known heart failure, nephrotic syndrome, and cirrhosis. Exudative effusions can be secondary to cancer, pneumonia, viral infections, TB, and pulmonary emboli. Exudative effusions result from a disruption in the capillary membrane, and the increased permeability leads to the leakage of cells, protein, and fluid into the pleural space. If one of the following is positive then the fluid is considered an exudate:

Pleural fluid protein to serum protein ratio >0.5
Pleural fluid LDH to serum LDH ratio >0.6
Pleural fluid LDH > two-thirds the upper limit of normal serum LDH

Alternative criteria include the two-test and three-test rules. Only one criteria need be met for the fluid to be considered an exudate.

**Two-test rule:**
Pleural fluid cholesterol >45 mg/dL
Pleural fluid LDH >0.45 times the upper limit of normal serum LDH

**Three-test rule:**
Includes the above two criteria plus pleural fluid protein >2.9 g/dL

Reference
1. Heffner JE, Brown LK, Barbieri CA. Diagnostic value of tests that discriminate between exudative and transudative pleural effusions. *Chest.* 1997;111(4):970.

**2.** Correct Answer: D

**Rationale:**
Retained hemothorax is a risk factor for subsequent development of empyema. The AATS consensus guidelines for empyema management class IIa recommendation is that VATS, chest washout should be the first line approach in all patients with stage II acute empyema (loculated effusions or positive culture/gram stain from pleural fluid). Unfortunately, when the hemothorax or empyema is loculated, another chest tube and antibiotics are not curative.

Reference
1. Shen KR, Bribriesco A, Crabtree T, et al. The American Association for Thoracic Surgery Consensus Guidelines for the Management of Empyema. *J Thorac Cardiovasc Surg.* 2017;153:e129-e146.

**3.** Correct Answer: A

**Rationale:**
This patient is likely suffering from re-expansion pulmonary edema (RPE). RPE is a potential complication from thoracentesis for pneumo- or hydrothoraces. The clinical presentation of RPE is characterized by a rapid onset of dyspnea and tachypnea with symptoms most often occurring within 1 hour of the re-expansion of the collapsed lung. Although the exact pathophysiology of RPE is not entirely clear, it is suspected that the mechanism includes the abrupt conclusion of hypoxic pulmonary vasoconstriction, as the alveoli are no longer hypoxic as blood flow returns. There is reperfusion of the lung, bringing in oxygen supply, and there then may be formation of reactive oxygen species. During reperfusion, there are increases in lipid and polypeptide mediators and immune complexes, which lead to damage of the endothelium, which is one way in which pulmonary edema may ensue.

Feller-Kopman et al found that volume of fluid removed was not correlated with development of RPE. Instead, an end-expiratory pleural pressure greater than (−)20 cm $H_2O$ was associated with this potential complication. Treatment consists of supportive therapy, with the application of mechanical ventilation and PEEP.

References

1. Feller-Kopman D, Berkowitz D, Boiselle P, Ernst A. Large-volume thoracentesis and the risk of reexpansion pulmonary edema. *Ann Thorac Surg*. 2007;84(5):1656.
2. Sivrikoz MC, Tuncozgur B, Cekmen M, et al. The role of tissue reperfusion in the reexpansion injury of the lungs. *Euro J Cardio-thorac Surg*. 2002;22:721-727.

**4.** Correct Answer: D

**Rationale:**

Chest tube insertion for evacuation of air is most appropriately placed in the fourth or fifth intercostal space at the mid to anterior axillary line. Placement more posterior runs the risk of liver or spleen injury depending on side. Placement more superiorly into the axilla runs the risk of nerve or vascular damage.

Reference

1. Dalbec DL, Krome RL. Thoracostomy. *Emerg Med Clin North Am*. 1986;4(3):441.

**5.** Correct Answer: A

**Rationale:**

Prompt drainage of a hemothorax addresses treatment before the development of clot. Retained hemothorax carries the risk of empyema. An epidural would not be appropriate at this time as the patient has been on anticoagulation. A consult to thoracic surgery may eventually be required if the initial output is greater than 1.5 L or the patient develops a retained hemothorax, but it is not emergently necessary in a hemodynamically stable patient. Prophylactic antibiotics are indicated in the first 24 hours after chest tube placement for a hemothorax; however, broad spectrum antibiotics would not be necessary at this time.

Reference

1. Boersma WG, Stigt JA, Smit HJM. Treatment of haemothorax. *Respir Med*. 2010;104(11):1583-1587.

# 39

# SLEEP APNEA

Dario Winterton, Riccardo Pinciroli, and Lorenzo Berra

1. You assess a 55-year-old male patient who is a candidate for bariatric surgery. He is 175 cm, 120 kg and has arterial hypertension for which he takes ramipril. His wife tells you the patient snores during the night. His blood pressure (BP) is 125/75 mm Hg and pulse oximetry is 89% on room air. What is the MOST appropriate management of this patient?

   A. Proceed to surgery without further testing
   B. Postpone surgery and proceed with a sleep study
   C. Perform an arterial blood gas analysis
   D. Recommend positive airway pressure (PAP) treatment at night and proceed to surgery

2. A 65-year-old male with a history of heart failure and central sleep apnea with Cheyne-Stokes (CSA-CSB) breathing presents to your clinic for evaluation. He had been started on continuous positive airway pressure (CPAP) therapy but did not tolerate it. His recent echocardiogram shows an ejection fraction (EF) of 40%. His medical therapy has already been optimized. What is the MOST appropriate management of this patient?

   A. Initiate adaptive servo-ventilation (ASV)
   B. Perform an in-laboratory polysomnography (PSG)
   C. Initiate supplemental nocturnal oxygen
   D. Initiate bilevel positive airway pressure in a spontaneous timed mode (BPAP-ST)

3. You evaluate a 49-year-old patient who has been referred to you because of excessive daytime sleepiness. His past medical history includes drug-controlled hypertension, obesity (body mass index [BMI] 36 kg/m²), and low back pain for which he has been taking daily nonsteroidal anti-inflammatory drugs (NSAIDs) and oxycodone for the past 5 years. Upon questioning his wife reports loud snoring during the night, to the point where she has sometimes had to sleep in another room. She does not think she has witnessed any apneic episodes but states she cannot be certain. What is the MOST appropriate next step in the management of this patient?

   A. Overnight PSG for further investigation of sleep apnea
   B. Overnight home sleep apnea testing (HSAT), for further investigation of sleep apnea
   C. Initiating PAP treatment, as the diagnosis of sleep apnea can be made based on the information provided
   D. Overnight pulse oximetry for further investigation of sleep apnea

4. You are asked to evaluate a 45-years-old female who is scheduled to undergo elective laparoscopic cholecystectomy. Her past medical history includes hypertension, which is controlled with an angiotensin-receptor blocker (ARB), and obesity (BMI 39 kg/m²). Upon questioning, she tells you she snores loudly during the night and often dozes off during the day. Investigating further, she reports she has been told she sometimes stops breathing during the night. Her vital signs during your examination are a BP of 135/75, heart rate (HR) 67, and $SpO_2$ 97% on room air. She presents you with a recent echocardiogram, which is unremarkable. You take an arterial blood gas, which shows pH 7.38, $pCO_2$ 42, $pO_2$ 87, and $HCO_3$– 25. What is the MOST appropriate management of this patient?

**A.** Advise the patient immediate further testing is necessary and postpone surgery

**B.** Make the patient aware she has a high probability of obstructive sleep apnea (OSA) and the implied risks and proceed to surgery without further immediate testing

**C.** Initiate PAP treatment and proceed to surgery

**D.** Perform a follow-up echocardiogram

5. A 43-year-old female is referred to your clinic by her primary care physician after undergoing a polysomnographic study, which supports a diagnosis of OSA (Apnea-Hypopnea Index [AHI] 25). Her BMI is 36 kg/m², her BP is 135/70, HR 82 bpm, and $SpO_2$ 88% on room air. She presents you with a recent arterial blood gas on room air (pH 7.35, $pCO_2$ 51 mm Hg, $pO_2$ 60 mm Hg, and $HCO_3-$ 31 mEq/L), chest x-ray (which is reported as normal), and spirometry (showing a restrictive picture). She denies ever smoking or taking recreational drugs and only takes simvastatin for her high serum cholesterol levels (now under control). What is the MOST likely diagnosis?

**A.** Chronic obstructive pulmonary disease (COPD)

**B.** OSA

**C.** Overlap syndrome

**D.** OSA and obesity hypoventilation syndrome (OHS)

# Chapter 39 ▪ Answers

**1.** Correct Answer: B

**Rationale:**
In the above case, the patient has a STOP-Bang (1) score of at least 5 (snoring, hypertension, male gender, BMI, and age; no information is given on daytime tiredness, observed apneas, or neck circumference), identifying him as a high-risk patient for OSA. He also has medically controlled hypertension and resting hypoxemia. The Society for Anesthesia and Sleep Medicine guidelines (2, 3) recommend additional evaluation for preoperative cardiopulmonary optimization in patients who have a high probability of having OSA where there is indication of an additional problem with ventilation or gas exchange, as is the case of this patient (option B).

Considering the increased risk of postoperative complications and the potential optimization of the patient, it is unwise to proceed to elective surgery without further testing (option A). An arterial blood gas analysis would provide further information on gas exchange; however there is already indication of a high-risk patient with impaired gas exchange, so an arterial blood gas analysis would not be the most appropriate (option C). Initiation of PAP treatment (option D) is a likely step in the management of this patient; however, it is only to be started after confirmation of underlying OSA and only a part of the workup and preoperative optimization of the patient.

References
1. Chung F, Yegneswaran B, Liao P, et al. STOP questionnaire: a tool to screen patients for obstructive sleep apnea. *Anesthesiology.* 2008;108(5):812-821.
2. Chung F, Memtsoudis SG, Ramachandran SK, et al. Society of anesthesia and sleep medicine guidelines on preoperative screening and assessment of adult patients with obstructive sleep apnea. *Anesth Analg.* 2016;123(2):452-473.
3. Madhusudan P, Wong J, Prasad A, et al. An update on preoperative assessment and preparation of surgical patients with obstructive sleep apnea. *Curr Opin Anaesthesiol.* 2018;31(1):89-95.

**2.** Correct Answer: C

**Rationale:**
The optimal treatment of CSA-CSB in patients with an EF ≤45% who do not tolerate CPAP is uncertain. Although ASV use was recommended by the 2012 American Academy of Sleep Medicine (AASM) guidelines (1), a distinction was made in the 2016 update (2) between its use in patients with EF ≤45% (in whom it is contraindicated, option A is therefore wrong) and in patients with EF >45% (in whom it may be considered). Currently, the guidelines suggest initiation of supplemental nocturnal oxygen (option C). In the presence of an established diagnosis of CSA-CSB, another in-laboratory PSG is not indicated (option B). Finally, use of BPAP-ST is only indicated by the guidelines if there is no response to an adequate trial of CPAP and oxygen therapies (therefore option D is incorrect).

References
1. Aurora RN, Chowdhuri S, Ramar K, et al. The treatment of central sleep apnea syndromes in adults: practice parameters with an evidence-based literature review and meta analyses. *Sleep.* 2012;35(1):17-40.
2. Aurora RN, Bista SR, Casey KR, et al. Updated adaptive servo-ventilation recommendations for the 2012 AASM guideline: "The treatment of central sleep apnea syndromes in adults: practice parameters with an evidence-based literature review and meta-analyses". *J Clin Sleep Med.* 2016;12(5):757-761.

**3. Correct Answer: A**

**Rationale:**

The patient in the presented case has an increased risk of moderate to severe OSA, as he presents with excessive daytime sleepiness, loud snoring, and diagnosed hypertension. The AASM guidelines on diagnostic testing for adult OSA (1) recommend that prediction algorithms, diagnostic tools, and questionnaires (such as the Berlin Questionnaire, the STOP-Bang questionnaire, the Epworth Sleepiness Scale, etc) should not be used to diagnose OSA in adults in the absence of PSG or HSAT (therefore answer C is wrong). An uncomplicated patient is defined by the absence of (A) conditions that place the patient at increased risk of nonobstructive sleep–disordered breathing (including chronic use of opioid medication); (B) concern for significant nonrespiratory sleep disorder(s) that require evaluation or interfere with the accuracy of HSAT; (C) environmental or personal factors that preclude the adequate acquisition and interpretation of data from HSAT. The guidelines recommend either PSG or HSAT in uncomplicated patients at an increased risk of moderate to severe risk of OSA, and in case of patients who do not fit this definition of uncomplicated, the guidelines recommend PSG rather than HSAT (answer A is therefore correct; answer B is wrong). Overnight pulse oximetry does not provide enough clinical or laboratory information to formulate a diagnosis of OSA (option D is incorrect)

**Reference**

1. Kapur VK, Auckley DH, Chowdhuri S, et al. Clinical practice guideline for diagnostic testing for adult obstructive sleep apnea: an American Academy of sleep medicine clinical practice guideline. *J Clin Sleep Med*. 2017;13(3):479-504.

**4. Correct Answer: B**

**Rationale:**

In the presented case, the patient has a STOP-Bang (1) score of at least 5 (snoring, tiredness, hypertension, observed apneas, and BMI; no information is given on neck circumference), identifying her as a high-risk patient for OSA. Her vital signs and arterial blood gas are normal (no sign of resting hypoxemia or hypoventilation), and her recent echocardiogram shows no signs of pulmonary hypertension. The Society for Anesthesia and Sleep Medicine guidelines (2, 3) recommend that all perioperative providers, and the patient, are made aware of the high likelihood of OSA and its potential impact on morbidity and recommend proceeding to surgery without further testing provided: (A) there is no indication of uncontrolled systemic condition or additional problems with ventilation or gas exchange (hypoventilation syndromes, pulmonary hypertension, or resting hypoxemia), as in this case and (B) strategies for mitigation of postoperative complications are implemented (option B).

Considering the nature of the surgery (not major) and the stable conditions of the patient, immediate further testing is not necessary and is not a reason to delay surgery (option A). Initiation of PAP treatment in the absence of a confirmed diagnosis of OSA is incorrect, albeit it is a likely therapy the patient will undergo after her diagnostic workup (option C). A further echocardiogram, in the presence of a recent normal one, is unlikely to add any clinical information (option D).

**References**

1. Chung F, Yegneswaran B, Liao P, et al. STOP questionnaire: a tool to screen patients for obstructive sleep apnea. *Anesthesiology*. 2008;108(5):812-821.
2. Chung F, Memtsoudis SG, Ramachandran SK, et al. Society of anesthesia and sleep medicine guidelines on preoperative screening and assessment of adult patients with obstructive sleep apnea. *Anesth Analg*. 2016;123(2):452-473.
3. Madhusudan P, Wong J, Prasad A, et al. An update on preoperative assessment and preparation of surgical patients with obstructive sleep apnea. *Curr Opin Anaesthesiol*. 2018;31(1):89-95.

**5. Correct Answer: D**

**Rationale:**

OHS is defined as a combination of obesity (BMI >30 Kg/m$^2$) and daytime hypercapnia (PaCO$_2$ >45 mm Hg) in the absence of other causes that could account for awake hypoventilation, such as lung or neuromuscular disease. The patient in the presented case meets diagnostic criteria for both OSA (positive PSG with AHI 25) and OHS (PaCO$_2$ 51) (1, 2) (option D).

The patient's spirometry showing a restrictive, rather than obstructive, picture and the absence of smoking history make the diagnosis of COPD unlikely (option A). Overlap syndrome is the combination of COPD and OSA and, for the same reason, is unlikely (option C). Finally, the patient has a clear laboratory diagnosis of OSA, as stated in the description, but option D is a more complete explanation of the clinical picture than option B.

**References**

1. Piper AJ, Grunstein RR. Obesity hypoventilation syndrome: mechanisms and management. *Am J Respir Crit Care Med*. 2011;183(3):292-298.
2. Raveedran R, Wong J, Singh M, et al. Obesity hypoventilation syndrome, sleep apnea, overlap syndrome: perioperative management to prevent complications. *Curr Opin Anaesthesiol*. 2017;30(1)146-155.

# 40

# PULMONARY INFECTIONS

Jason H. Maley and Kathryn A. Hibbert

1. A 68-year-old woman with a history of hypertension and poorly controlled diabetes mellitus presents to the emergency department (ED) with fevers and 5 days of progressive shortness of breath and cough. She presented to her primary care physician 3 days ago and was prescribed amoxicillin. Despite this treatment, her symptoms worsened; she has no other associated symptoms. On arrival to the ED, her vital signs are notable for T 38.4°C, blood pressure (BP) 118/75 mm Hg, heart rate (HR) 90 beats per minute, respiratory rate 14 breaths per minute, and $SpO_2$ 83% breathing ambient air. She is placed on high-flow nasal cannula at 60 L/min and $FiO_2$ 0.6 in the ED, and vancomycin and cefepime administered. She is subsequently admitted to the intensive care unit (ICU) for severe community-acquired pneumonia (CAP). Which of the following is the BEST next step in her management?

   A. Perform flexible bronchoscopy and bronchoalveolar lavage to obtain bacterial culture
   B. Add levofloxacin to her antibiotic regimen
   C. Send quantitative respiratory cultures and blood cultures
   D. Change her antibiotic regimen to ceftriaxone and azithromycin
   E. Change vancomycin to linezolid

2. A 45-year-old man was diagnosed 1 month ago with a squamous cell lung cancer involving his left hilum and has been receiving chemotherapy. He is now admitted to the ICU with hypoxemia and fever. He reports about 10 days of low-grade fevers and loss of appetite, which has progressed to worsening shortness of breath and a cough productive of foul-smelling, purulent sputum. His chest radiograph demonstrates dense consolidation of his left lower lobe with evidence of an abscess. A computed tomography (CT) scan is ordered and he is started on vancomycin, cefepime, and metronidazole. Sputum cultures are pending. Which of the following is the most accurate regarding his diagnosis?

   A. His current antibiotic regimen is appropriate.
   B. He should receive a standard 7 to 10 day course of antibiotics.
   C. His pneumonia is unlikely to recur if appropriately treated.
   D. If his sputum cultures do not show anaerobic species, then his coverage can be narrowed.

3. A 65-year-old man with congestive heart failure is intubated and mechanically ventilated in the ICU for acute decompensated heart failure complicated by pulmonary edema. His extubation is delayed by ongoing delirium. On day 5 of his ICU stay, he is noted to have a new fever, with a temperature of 38.5°C. He is on pressure support ventilation, with an inspiratory pressure of 5 cm $H_2O$, positive end-expiratory pressure (PEEP) of 5 cm $H_2O$, and $FiO_2$ 0.4. The remainder of his vital signs are BP 130/75 mm Hg, HR 75 beats per minute, respiratory rate 12 breath per minute, and $SpO_2$ 98%. His examination reveals clear lung fields with auscultation and no other notable findings. A diagnostic workup, including blood cultures, urinalysis, and chest radiograph, are performed. Chest radiograph reveals clear lung fields. His urinalysis and blood cultures are unrevealing. Over the next 48 hours, he has one additional fever, and the respiratory therapist notes increased thick secretions suctioned from his endotracheal tube that are sent for sputum culture. His vent settings, chest radiograph, and vital signs remain unchanged. Which of the following is the MOST appropriate management at this time?

A. Initiate treatment with vancomycin and cefepime
B. Perform flexible bronchoscopy with bronchoalveolar lavage
C. Initiate treatment with vancomycin, cefepime, and azithromycin
D. Close observation
E. Initiate treatment with cefepime

4. A 25-year-old man with a history of mild intermittent asthma is admitted to the ICU with rapidly progressive hypoxemic respiratory failure following 4 days of fevers, myalgias, and cough at home. He is intubated and mechanically ventilated on volume assist-control with a tidal volume of 6 mL/kg, respiratory rate 14 breaths per minute, $FiO_2$ 0.8, and PEEP of 10 cm $H_2O$. His arterial blood gas on these settings is pH 7.30, $PaCO_2$ 50, and $PaO_2$ 85. His chest radiograph demonstrates diffuse bilateral patchy opacities, and his rapid influenza testing is positive for influenza A. Which of the following statements is MOST accurate regarding diagnosis and treatment for this patient?

A. With his history of asthma, he should receive methylprednisolone at 1 mg/kg daily.
B. Antibacterial coverage can be discontinued as he is positive for influenza A.
C. Treatment with oseltamivir 75 mg twice daily is not indicated as he is 4 days into his illness.
D. If a sputum culture cannot be obtained, a diagnostic bronchoscopy with bronchioalveolar lavage is indicated.
E. This patient does not meet criteria for acute respiratory distress syndrome (ARDS) and does not need low tidal volume ventilation.

5. A 65-year-old man with acute myeloid leukemia is admitted to the ICU with worsening hypoxemia while receiving induction chemotherapy on the oncology ward. His chest radiograph reveals bibasilar opacities, and he is started on treatment with vancomycin and cefepime. His hypoxemia improves by day 3 of treatment, however his fevers continue. On day 5 of treatment, chest radiograph reveals opacification of the right lower lung fields with loss of visualization of the right hemidiaphragm and costophrenic angle. A thoracic ultrasound demonstrates a pleural effusion, and diagnostic thoracentesis is performed with removal of 60 mL of fluid. Pleural fluid analysis demonstrates cloudy tan fluid, pH 7.1, glucose 30 mg/dL, lactate dehydrogenase (LDH) 2000 U/L, cholesterol 85 mg/dL, and protein 4.5 g/dL. Gram stain and cultures are pending. What is the next best step in management?

A. Broaden antibiotic coverage and await results of gram stain and culture
B. Perform tube thoracostomy and continue antibiotic therapy
C. Continue antibiotic therapy with serial imaging, drainage if no response
D. Repeat thoracentesis to drain pleural space
E. Perform video-assisted thoracoscopic surgery to clear pleural space

6. A 38-year-old man with human immunodeficiency virus (HIV) and a CD4+ count of 100 cells/μL is admitted to the ICU with respiratory failure from the medical ward. He reports 1 week of progressive dyspnea on exertion and chills. He had been treated with vancomycin and meropenem since his arrival to the ED 1 day ago. He is intubated and mechanically ventilated on volume control-assist control, tidal volume 6 mL/kg ideal body weight, respiratory rate 18/min, $FiO_2$ 0.7, and PEEP 8 cm $H_2O$. His initial vital signs are T 38.5°C, BP 110/75 mm Hg, HR 85 beats per minute, and $SpO_2$ 94%. Initial laboratory data are remarkable for a (1,3)-beta-D-glucan >200 pg/mL and LDH 100 U/L. On day 1 of his ICU stay, a bronchoscopy with bronchoalveolar lavage is performed and the *Pneumocystis* examination is negative. Which of the following can result in an elevated 1-3 beta-D-glucan blood test in this patient?

A. Treatment with meropenem
B. *Cryptococcus neoformans*
C. *Blastomyces dermatitidis*
D. Treatment with vancomycin
E. Mucormycosis

7. A 58-year-old man with idiopathic pulmonary fibrosis is admitted to the ICU with an acute exacerbation of interstitial lung disease. He reports 4 days of worsening dyspnea and dry cough, without fevers, chills, night sweats, or other associated symptoms. His examination is notable for diffuse crackles throughout inspiration. He reports that he is originally from India and moved to the United States 20 years ago, where he has lived since. He is placed on high-flow nasal cannula with $FiO_2$ 0.5 and flow of 40 L/min. Methylprednisolone 50 mg daily is administered, along with vancomycin, ceftriaxone, and azithromycin. A chest CT reveals basilar predominant honeycombing with new superimposed multifocal ground glass opacities, along with new scattered right upper and middle lobe centrilobular nodules compared with CT scan 1 year prior. A sputum culture is obtained and sent for bacterial, fungal, and mycobacterial cultures along with acid-fast bacilli (AFB) stain. The sputum is found to have 2+ AFB. A nucleic acid amplification test (NAAT) for tuberculosis (TB) is negative. A repeat sputum sample is collected and again results with 2+ AFB and negative TB NAAT with no presence of NAAT inhibitors detected by the laboratory. What is the best next step and interpretation of this finding?

A. Obtain past records of Bacille Calmette-Guérin (BCG) vaccination as this may cause a false-negative TB PCR

B. Order an interferon gamma release assay test to confirm TB infection

C. Await cultures, findings indicate nontuberculous mycobacterial infection

D. Await cultures, findings indicate latent tuberculosis infection

E. Await cultures and start antimicrobial therapy for tuberculosis

8. A 75-year-old woman is admitted to the ICU after coronary artery bypass graft complicated by cardiogenic shock. She is improving on ICU day 4, and her ventilator settings are pressure support 10 cm $H_2O$, PEEP 8 cm $H_2O$, and $FiO_2$ 0.4. She is noted later that day to have increased frequency of thick secretions requiring suctioning through her endotracheal tube and develops a new fever at 39°C. Over the course of the evening, she experiences frequent oxygen desaturation, requiring an increase in her $FiO_2$ to 0.6. A chest radiograph reveals a new opacity in the right lower lung field, and she is started on vancomycin and levofloxacin. Sputum culture grows *Acinetobacter baumannii* after 48 hours without other organisms identified over the next 24 hours. What is the BEST next step in her management?

A. Continue levofloxacin, discontinue vancomycin

B. Discontinue vancomycin and levofloxacin, start meropenem

C. Discontinue vancomycin, add ceftriaxone to levofloxacin

D. Discontinue vancomycin and levofloxacin, start linezolid

E. Continue vancomycin and levofloxacin

9. A 75-year-old man with hypertension, mild Alzheimer disease marked by occasional short-term memory difficulties, and a past history of squamous cell carcinoma of the tongue with prior surgical resection and radiation to the neck presents from his assisted living facility with productive cough and shortness of breath. The assisted living facility staff reports that he is routinely noted to be coughing while eating meals, and his dyspnea and cough began while eating yesterday. His medications include hydrochlorothiazide and amlodipine. In the ED, his vital signs are T 37.8°C, BP 110/70 mm Hg, HR 90 beats per minute, respiratory rate 20/min, and $SpO_2$ 88% on ambient air. A CT scan of his chest reveals patchy bibasilar ground glass opacities and tree-in-bud opacities. Supplemental oxygen is provided via a venturi mask at $FiO_2$ 0.5 and admitted to the ICU. Which of the following is most accurate concerning this patient's pneumonia?

A. This patient has a healthcare-associated pneumonia (HCAP) and should receive appropriate broad spectrum antibiotics.

B. Placement of a gastrostomy tube for future nutrition will reduce his risk of recurrent pneumonia.

C. The patient's Alzheimer disease is a significant risk factor for future pneumonia.

D. Empiric antibiotics do not have to include anaerobic coverage.

10. A 54-year-old woman develops fevers and cough on the final day of her vacation on a cruise ship in the Caribbean. She returns to her home in Florida, and over the following 3 days, she has continued fevers, productive cough, and new dyspnea on exertion. She presents to the ED and her vitals at that time are T 39°C, BP 110/80 mm Hg, HR 95 beats per minute, respiratory rate 21 breaths per minute, and $SpO_2$ 85% breathing ambient air. Her chest radiograph demonstrates multifocal patchy opacities and increased interstitial markings throughout all lung fields. Ceftriaxone and azithromycin are administered, along with 2 L of lactated ringers solution intravenously and her urinary *Legionella* antigen subsequently returns positive. She is admitted to the ICU on high-flow nasal cannula at $FiO_2$ 0.7 and flow 50 L per minute. Which of the following statements is most accurate regarding *Legionella* pneumonia?

A. *Legionella pneumophila* urine antigen is highly sensitive for both serogroups 1 and 2.

B. Most recognized *Legionella* outbreaks occur in hotels, cruise ships, and healthcare facilities.

C. *Legionella* culture from sputum has a sensitivity of greater than 95%.

D. If *Legionella* does not grow from sputum culture quickly (<48 hours), it is unlikely to be the pathogen in question.

E. *Legionella* is less likely to cause severe pneumonia than other atypical pneumonia pathogens.

# Chapter 40 ▪ Answers

---

**1.** Correct Answer: B

**Rationale:**

The patient presents with severe CAP. Common pathogens explaining this presentation include *S. pneumoniae, H. influenzae, Legionella,* Enterobacteriaceae species, *S. aureus,* and *Pseudomonas.* The narrowest recommended antibiotic regimen for patients admitted to the ICU with CAP must include: (1) an antipneumococcal beta-lactam antibiotic and (2) **either** a macrolide (eg azithromycin) **or** a respiratory fluoroquinolone. For patients with risk factors for *S. aureus* and *Pseudomonas* infection (which include outpatient antibiotic failure, past healthcare exposure, structural lung disease, and recent IV antibiotic exposure), empiric coverage is recommended. Given this patient's recent antibiotic exposure and failure of outpatient antibiotic therapy, empiric treatment for methicillin-resistant *S. aureus* and *Pseudomonas* species is appropriate (answer D is incorrect). However, addition of a macrolide or fluoroquinolone is recommended to cover atypical pathogens including *Legionella*—at least 20% of severe pneumonia is thought to be because of atypical bacterial pathogens (answer B is correct). There are no data to support the use of bronchioalveolar lavage over routine respiratory gram stain and culture for CAP (answer A is incorrect). Additionally, although blood cultures are recommended for patients who are hospitalized with CAP, there is no additional value of quantitative respiratory cultures over routine respiratory gram stain and cultures. There is no indication for empiric treatment of vancomycin-resistant species such as *Enterococcus* (answer E is incorrect)

### Reference

1. Mandell LA, Wunderink RG, Anzueto A, et al. Infectious diseases Society of America/American Thoracic Society consensus guidelines on the management of community-acquired pneumonia in adults. *Clin Infect Dis.* 2007;44(suppl 2):S27-S72.

---

**2.** Correct Answer: A

**Rationale:**

The patient's presentation is concerning for postobstructive pneumonia and abscess in the setting of bronchial obstruction and immunosuppression. Given the severity of his illness and his recent chemotherapy, his antibiotic regimens should include empiric treatment of methicillin-resistant *S. aureus*, gram-negative organisms including *Pseudomonas* species, and anaerobic organisms (answer A is correct). Obligate anaerobic organisms will not grow in routine sputum microbiologic cultures but are considered important pathogens in postobstructive pneumonia and should be treated empirically (answer D is incorrect). Antibiotic regimens for anaerobic coverage may include beta-lactam/beta lactamase inhibitor combination, metronidazole, clindamycin, or carbapenem antibiotics. Lung abscesses often require prolonged treatment that is guided by repeat imaging (answer B is incorrect). Unfortunately, unless his cancer is successfully treated, he will be at ongoing risk for postobstructive pneumonia (answer C is incorrect).

### References

1. Rolston KVI, Nesher L. Post-obstructive pneumonia in patients with cancer: a review. *Infect Dis Ther.* 2018;7(1):29-38.
2. Mandell LA, Wunderink RG, Anzueto A, et al. Infectious diseases Society of America/American Thoracic Society consensus guidelines on the management of community-acquired pneumonia in adults. *Clin Infect Dis.* 2007;44(suppl 2):S27-S72.

---

**3.** Correct Answer: D

**Rationale:**

The patient is presenting with fevers and increased sputum production without evidence of infiltrate on examination, chest imaging, and with a stable and/or improved respiratory status. The clinical presentation suggests tracheobronchitis. Current guidelines recommend observation without empiric antibiotic treatment for tracheobronchitis, given lack of evidence suggesting a clinical benefit to treatment (answer D is correct). Vancomycin and cefepime may be an appropriate regimen for a ventilator-associated pneumonia (VAP) depending on local resistance patterns, but this patient does not have evidence of pneumonia (answer A is incorrect). Further workup for pneumonia including bronchoscopy is also not indicated (answer B is incorrect). Routine coverage for atypical organisms with a macrolide is not recommended for hospital-acquired or VAP or tracheobronchitis (answer C is incorrect). Monotherapy with cefepime is not indicated either for tracheobronchitis or VAP (answer E is incorrect).

### Reference

1. Kalil AC, Metersky ML, Klompas M, et al. Management of adults with hospital-acquired and ventilator-associated pneumonia: 2016 clinical practice guidelines by the infectious diseases Society of America and the American Thoracic Society. *Clin Infect Dis.* 2016;63(5):e61-e111.

**4.** Correct Answer: D

**Rationale:**

This patient is presenting with respiratory failure secondary to influenza A infection. He meets clinical criteria for ARDS, which include acute onset of bilateral infiltrates with associated hypoxemia in the absence of evidence of explanatory cardiogenic pulmonary edema (answer E is incorrect). Mainstays of treatment for severe influenza pneumonia include antiviral therapy with oseltamivir (answer C is incorrect) and empiric treatment of possible secondary bacterial infection (answer B is incorrect). Common bacterial pathogens that coinfect with influenza include *S. pneumoniae, Staphylococcus aureus,* and *Haemophilus influenzae,* and coverage should be targeted to these organisms. Treatment with steroids in patients with influenza infection is associated with an increased risk of mortality, and although these data are observational, the consensus is that steroids should be avoided if possible (answer A is incorrect).

References

1. ARDS Definition Task Force. Acute respiratory distress syndrome: the berlin definition. *JAMA.* 2012;307(23):2526-2533.
2. Mandell LA, Wunderink RG, Anzueto A, et al. Infectious diseases Society of America/American Thoracic Society consensus guidelines on the management of community-acquired pneumonia in adults. *Clin Infect Dis.* 2007;44(suppl 2):S27-S72.
3. Rodrigo C, Leonardi-Bee J, Nguyen-Van-Tam J, Lim WS. Corticosteroids as adjunctive therapy in the treatment of inluenza. *Cochrane Database Syst Rev.* 2016;3:CD010406.

**5.** Correct Answer: B

**Rationale:**

This patient presents with continued fevers while being treated of pneumonia and is found to have a pleural effusion with diagnostic tests highly suggestive of an empyema—these include frankly purulent pleural fluid, an LDH greater than 1000, low pH, and low glucose. The first step in management of empyema is the placement of the tube thoracostomy to completely drain the pleural space (answer B is correct). Delay in drainage may lead to increased morbidity and mortality (answer A and answer C are incorrect). Drainage with thoracentesis alone is not recommended because of the likelihood of fluid reaccumulating, making ongoing drainage necessary (answer D is incorrect). When drainage cannot be achieved through thoracostomy, thoracic surgical intervention may be necessary but is not usually the initial management strategy (answer E is incorrect).

References

1. Light RW. Parapneumonic effusions and empyema. *Proc Am Thorac Soc.* 2006;3(1):75-80.
2. Colice GL, Curtis A, Deslauriers J, et al. Medical and surgical treatment of parapneumonic effusions: an evidence-based guideline. *Chest.* 2000;118(4):1158.
3. Shen KR, Bribriesco A, Crabtree T, et al. The American Association for thoracic surgery consensus guidelines for the management of empyema. *J Thorac Cardiovasc Surg.* 2017;153(6):e129.

**6.** Correct Answer: A

**Rationale:**

The (1,3)-beta-D-glucan test is a common, commercially available assay that detects a polysaccharide element of fungal cell walls that is found in most fungi. Notable exceptions to this are cryptococci, zygomycetes (eg mucormycoses), and *Blastomyces dermatitidis*, which either completely lack this element or produce it at minimal levels (answer B, answer C, and answer E are incorrect). This test, therefore, cannot be used to rule out infection with these fungal organisms. Notably, beta-lactam antibiotics may react with this assay and produce false-positive results (answer A is correct; answer D is incorrect). The (1,3)-beta-D-glucan has been studied as a noninvasive diagnostic test for pneumocystis pneumonia and has good sensitivity in patients with HIV. However, bronchoalveolar lavage remains the gold standard of the diagnosis of pneumocystis pneumonia.

Reference

1. Karageorgopoulos DE, Qu JM, Korbila IP, Zhu YG, Vasileiou VA, Falagas ME. Accuracy of β-D-glucan for the diagnosis of Pneumocystis jirovecii pneumonia: a meta-analysis. *Clin Microbiol Infect.* 2013;19(1):39-49.

**7.** Correct Answer: C

**Rationale:**

This patient presents with worsening hypoxemia in the setting of structural lung disease and has new findings of ground glass opacities and centrilobular nodules. Sputum testing reveals AFB with a negative NAAT for tuberculosis on repeated specimens. Latent tuberculosis infection should not result in AFB smear positive sputum (answer D is incorrect). NAAT has high sensitivity and specificity for tuberculosis in AFB smear positive sputum samples. Less than 5% of NAAT testing is falsely negative on AFB smear positive samples because of the presence of nucleic acid amplification inhibitors. If the presence of these inhibitors is excluded, repeat AFB smear positive and NAAT negative samples suggest a nontuberculous mycobacterium (NTM) infection (answer C is correct; answer E is incorrect). NTM infection occurs most commonly in patients with structural lung disease and is a chronic, indolent infection. Prior BCG vaccination may cause a reaction to tuberculin skin testing resulting in a false-positive result; it does not affect the performance of TB PCR (answer A is incorrect). Interferon gamma release assays are testing modalities for latent tuberculosis infection and cannot rule in or out active tuberculosis disease (answer B is incorrect).

### Reference

1. Lewinsohn DM, Leonard MK, LoBue PA, et al. Official American Thoracic Society/Infectious Diseases Society of America/Centers for disease control and prevention clinical practice guidelines: diagnosis of tuberculosis in adults and children. *Clin Infect Dis.* 2017;64:e1.

---

**8.** Correct Answer: B

**Rationale:**

This patient is presenting with VAP, as indicated by the development of fevers, increased sputum production, radiographic infiltrate, and worsening respiratory status after 4 days of mechanical ventilation. Common organisms in VAP include methicillin-resistant *S. aureus*, *P. aeruginosa*, and other gram-negative bacilli including *Acinetobacter* species. Although empiric coverage for *Acinetobacter* is not necessary unless there is a high degree of suspicion based on past infections, the isolation of this organism in sputum culture warrants appropriate antibiotic coverage. The treatments of choice for *Acinetobacter* species are either a carbepenem or ampicillin/sulbactam, with further treatment guided by antimicrobial susceptibility testing and local antibiogram data (answer B is correct; answers A, C, and D are incorrect). Ongoing empiric coverage for other organisms is not necessary in VAP once cultures have resulted (answer E is incorrect)

### Reference

1. Kalil AC, Metersky ML, Klompas M, et al. Management of adults with hospital-acquired and ventilator-associated pneumonia: 2016 clinical practice guidelines by the infectious diseases Society of America and the American Thoracic Society. *Clin Infect Dis.* 2016;63(5):e61-e111.

---

**9.** Correct Answer: D

**Rationale:**

This patient presents with dyspnea, hypoxemia, and cough, with a reported history of coughing while eating, suggestive of aspiration. His chest imaging is notable for inflammatory changes in a gravity-dependent distribution, along with tree-in-bud opacities, all supportive of aspiration pneumonitis versus pneumonia. He also has a prior history of surgery and radiation to his tongue and neck, which likely resulted in oropharyngeal dysphagia. HCAP is no longer a distinct category of pneumonia, and he should therefore be treated as a CAP, given the absence of specific risk factors for resistant organisms (answer A is incorrect). Additionally, his presentation is not characteristic of an anaerobic pneumonia, which is often more indolent and occurs in patients with specific risk factors, and so he does not require anaerobic coverage as part of his initial empiric regimen (answer D is incorrect). Although advanced dementia may be a risk factor for aspiration, this patient has very mild symptoms of dementia (answer C is incorrect). Although feeding tubes allow for more effective nutrition in patients with dysphagia, they do not reduce the risk of aspiration pneumonia (answer B is incorrect).

### References

1. Mandell LA, Wunderink RG, Anzueto A, et al. Infectious diseases Society of America/American Thoracic Society consensus guidelines on the management of community-acquired pneumonia in adults. *Clin Infect Dis.* 2007;44(suppl 2):S27-S72.
2. Taylor JK, Fleming GB, Singanayagam A, Hill AT, Chalmers JD. Risk factors for aspiration in community-acquired pneumonia: analysis of a hospitalized UK cohort. *Am J Med.* 2013;126(11):995-1001.
3. Fox KA, Mularski RA, Sarfati MR, et al. Aspiration pneumonia following surgically placed feeding tubes. *Am J Surg.* 1995;170(6):564.

---

**10.** Correct Answer: B

**Rationale:**

*Legionella* infection of the lungs results from exposure to aerosolized *Legionella* species that reside in water sources. The most recognized sites of outbreaks have been cruise ships, hotels, resorts, and healthcare facilities where large water storage and heating systems are present. The most common causative agent is *Legionella pneumophila* serogroup 1, which is also the only species reliably detected by urinary antigen testing (answer A is incorrect). Serogroup 1 may account for nearly 85% of cases by some estimates, and urine-antigen testing is estimated to have a sensitivity of at least 70%. *Legionella* culture is technically challenging for a number of reasons: at least half of the patients with legionella have no sputum production, culture requires specific agar (buffered charcoal yeast extract), the bacteria can be slow growing (5+ days), and the sensitivity is highly dependent on the technical skill of the diagnostic laboratory. For this reason, *Legionella* culture is generally insensitive, with a sensitivity that is estimated to range from 20% to 80% (answers C and D are incorrect). The identification of *Legionella* on sputum culture is 100% specific for *Legionella* infection. *Legionella* is more prevalent among patients with severe CAP than in nonhospitalized patients with pneumonia and accounts for an even greater proportion of pneumonia in patients requiring ICU admission; no other atypical pathogen commonly causes severe CAP requiring ICU admission (answer E is incorrect).

## References

1. Mandell LA, Wunderink RG, Anzueto A, et al. Infectious diseases Society of America/American Thoracic Society consensus guidelines on the management of community-acquired pneumonia in adults. *Clin Infect Dis.* 2007;44(suppl 2):S27-S72.
2. Murdoch DR. Diagnosis of legionella infection. *Clin Infect Dis.* 2003;36(1):64-69.

# 41

# NEOPLASM

Jenna McNeill and Charles Corey Hardin

1. A 34-year-old male presented to the emergency department (ED) with a chief complaint of hemoptysis. His past medical history (PMH) was notable for recurrent pneumonias. Chest x-ray (CXR) demonstrated a right middle lobe infiltrate. Chest computed tomoghraphy (CT) revealed an endobronchial lesion at the level of the bronchus intermedius. Flexible bronchoscopy was notable for bloody secretions, and a broad-based lesion in the bronchus intermedius is shown in the figure that follows. What is the next most appropriate step in management?

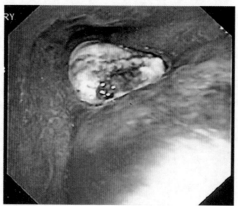

Figure from Boyd M, Sahebazamani M, Ie S, Rubio E. The safety of cryobiopsy in diagnosing carcinoid tumors. *J Bronchology Interv Pulmonol.* 2014;21(3):234-236.

A. Forceps biopsy
B. Rigid bronchoscopy
C. Interventional radiology (IR) embolization
D. Human immunodeficiency virus (HIV) testing

2. A 59-year-old female presents to her primary care doctor with a chief complaint of progressive shortness of breath and nonproductive cough. She denies chest pain, palpitations, or wheezing. Her PMH is notable only for right-sided inflammatory breast cancer, diagnosed 1 year prior to presentation and treated with doxorubicin/cyclophosphamide/paclitaxel followed by x-ray telescope (XRT) and mastectomy. At rest, her room air saturation is 95% and other vital signs are normal. Chest CT is negative for pulmonary embolus but notable for patchy consolidation and ground glass opacities in the right lung as well as traction bronchiectasis. Her WBC is normal and sputum gram stain shows no organisms. What is the most appropriate treatment?

A. Ceftriaxone and azithromycin
B. Cefepime and vancomycin
C. High-dose prednisone
D. Albuterol

3. A 46-year-old male with a remote history of resected stage IIA non–small-cell lung cancer presents to the emergency room with dyspnea and chest pain. He is tachycardic, tachypneic, and hypotensive. CXR shows mediastinal lymphadenopathy and bilateral pleural effusions. Bedside transthoracic echocardiogram (TTE) was performed and an image is shown below. What is the next most appropriate step in management?

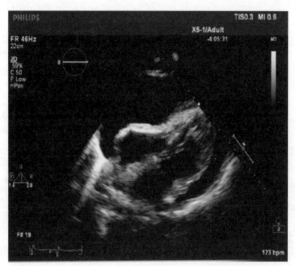

Figure from McCurdy MT, Shanholtz CB. Oncologic emergencies. *Crit Care Med.* 2012;40(7):2212-2222.

    **A.** Heparin
    **B.** Cardiac surgical consult
    **C.** Aspirin, clopidogrel, and heparin
    **D.** Fluid resuscitation

4. A 47-year-old male with a PMH of lung cancer presents with confusion and lethargy. He has postural hypotension and low central venous pressure on examination. There is no fever, cough, sputum, or rash. The remainder of the examination is notable only for tachycardia. CXR shows a right upper lobe mass similar to prior films and mediastinal lymphadenopathy and left lower lobe nodules. Serum creatinine is 2 mg/dL. Serum calcium is 18 mg/dL and electrocardiogram EKG is shown in the figure that follows.

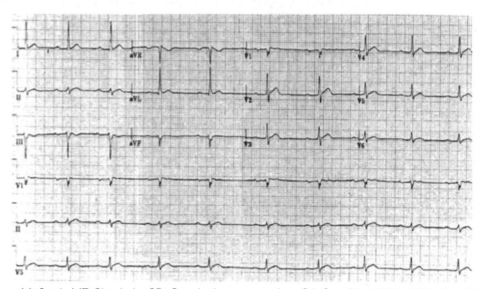

Figure from McCurdy MT, Shanholtz CB. Oncologic emergencies. *Crit Care Med.* 2012;40(7):2212-2222.

What is the most appropriate treatment?

A. Measurement of serum albumin
B. Saline and furosemide
C. Pamidronate
D. Head CT

5. A 60-year-old female was diagnosed with right-sided proximal bronchogenic carcinoma and underwent right-sided pneumonectomy 8 months ago. She presents to the ED with a 1-month history of progressive dyspnea, cough, stridor, and occasional low-grade fevers. A CT chest was performed and shown in the two figures that follow. What should be the next step in management?

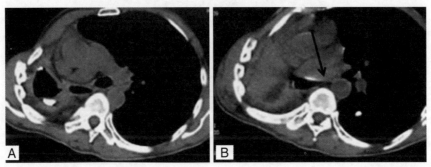

Figure from Chandrashekhara SH, Bhalla AS, Sharma R, Gupta AK, Kumar A, Arora R. Imaging in postpneumonectomy complications: a pictorial review. *J Cancer Res Ther.* 2011;7(1):3-10.

A. Insertion of a chest tube
B. Barium swallow study
C. IV steroids
D. Surgery

6. A 65-year-old female with 50 pack-year tobacco history presents to the ED after being involved in a motor vehicle accident. Her vitals on arrival were temperature of 98.6°F, heart rate 95, blood pressure 142/86 mm Hg, and $SpO_2$ of 91% on room air. She underwent a CT head, chest, abdomen, and pelvis. The CT chest demonstrated a 5 cm spiculated nodule in the right middle lobe. Thoracic surgery was consulted for possible lobectomy. Pulmonary function tests were performed which demonstrated a forced expiratory volume (FEV1) of 1.4 L (53% predicted), forced vital capacity (FVC) of 2.39 L (71% predicted), and a diffusing capacity of the lungs for carbon monoxide (DLCO) of 48% predicted. What would be the next step in management?

A. Stair climbing assessment
B. Calculate perioperative lung function
C. Cardiopulmonary exercise testing
D. Proceed with surgery as the patient is low risk
E. Arterial $PO_2$

7. A 75-year-old male with a history of tobacco use (50 pack year), chronic obstructive pulmonary disease (COPD), hypertension (HTN), and recent diagnosis of adenocarcinoma of the lung for which he has not started treatment presents to the ED with a 4-day history of increased dyspnea at rest and with exertion, productive cough, and subjective fevers at home. His initial vitals were notable for a temperature of 101°F, heart rate of 105, blood pressure 120/80 mm Hg, and saturation of 84% on room air with a respiratory rate of 26. He was placed initially on a nonrebreather and his saturations increased to 92%. He had a CXR performed which showed a dense consolidation in the right lower lobe. He was started on ceftriaxone and azithromycin for community-acquired pneumonia (CAP) and admitted to the ICU given his high oxygen requirements. Three days into his ICU course, his high flow requirements remained unchanged. He remained tachycardic in the low 100s and continued to have low-grade fevers. What would be the next step in management?

A. Add vancomycin for greater antibiotic coverage
B. Add steroids for COPD exacerbation in the setting of pneumonia
C. Perform a CT-PE (pulmonary embolism)
D. Continue with current management

# Chapter 41 ▪ Answers

**1.** Correct Answer: B

**Rationale:**

This patient likely has a bronchial carcinoid tumor. Carcinoid tumors of the lung are rare neuroendocrine tumors accounting for less than 1% of all lung tumors. The lung, however, is the second most common presenting site (after the gut) for carcinoid tumor. Typical presenting symptoms include cough, hemoptysis, and/or symptoms of bronchial obstruction. Carcinoid tumors are far more common in the larger airways. The tumors are highly vascular and grow intraluminally as well as extraluminally and are mostly covered by bronchial epithelium. Definitive treatment is with surgical resection, which typically carries an excellent prognosis. Historically there has been concern for massive hemorrhage following forceps biopsy secondary to the highly vascular nature of the tumor . While this complication is actually fairly rare, it is common to sample suspected carcinoid tumors via rigid bronchoscopy, so that any bleeding may be more effectively controlled. Cryobiopsy has also been reported to be preferable to forceps biopsy. IR embolization would not allow for the tissue sampling needed to make the diagnosis of carcinoid. Pulmonary Kaposi sarcoma is characterized by violaceous endobronchial lesions but is typically a late manifestation of HIV and more likely to present with other constitutional symptoms. In addition, the bronchoscopic appearance in this case is far more typical of carcinoid.

### References

1. Kaifi T, Kayser G, Passlick B. The diagnosis and treatment of bronchopulmonary carcinoid. *Dtsch Arztebl Int.* 2015;112:479-485.
2. Hurt R, Bates M. Carcinoid tumors of the bronchus: a 33 year experience. *Thorax.* 1984;39:617-623.
3. Ayache M, Donatelli C, Roncin K, et al. Massive hemorrhage after inspection bronchoscopy for carcinoid tumor. *Respir Med Case Rep.* 2018;24:125-128.
4. Boyd M, Sahebazamani M, Ie S, Rubio E. The safety of cryobiopsy in diagnosing carcinoid tumors. *J Bronchology Interv Pulmonol.* 2014;21:234.
5. Nwabudike M, Hemmings S, Paul Y, et al. Pulmonary Kaposi Sarcoma: an uncommon cause of respiratory failure in the era of highly active antiretroviral therapy- case report and review of the literature. *Case Rep Infect Dis.* 2016;2016:1-4.

**2.** Correct Answer: C

**Rationale:**

This patient with a PMH of inflammatory breast cancer and recent (<1 year) radiation to the chest is likely presenting with radiation-induced pneumonitis. Inflammatory breast cancer is a rare but aggressive form of breast cancer that classically presents with a finding of "peau d'orange"—warm, thickened, firm skin over the affected breast. Treatment, as in this case, is multimodal with neoadjuvant chemo, surgery, and radiation. Patients who undergo thoracic radiation are at risk for radiation pneumonitis, which can present weeks to months after therapy. Radiation pneumonitis is thought to result from radiation-induced injury to type II penumocytes and endothelial cells. It typically presents with shortness of breath and dry cough. Chest CT findings include patchy consolidation, fibrotic changes, and ground glass that does not respect lobar borders. Newer radiation techniques make the classic radiographic finding of a portal line marking the boundary of the radiation field less likely. The mainstay of treatment of high-dose prednisone. Ceftriaxone and azithromycin would be appropriate treatment for CAP but the subacute onset, negative gram stain, and lack of other infectious signs and symptoms make that diagnosis less likely here. Similarly, vancomycin and cefepime would not be the most appropriate therapy. Obstructive lung disease (asthma and COPD) can present with dyspnea and would be appropriately treated with bronchodilators such as albuterol, but there are no physical examination findings or history to support that diagnosis here.

### References

1. Van Uden DJ, van Laarhoven HW, Westenberg A, deWilt JH, Blanken-Peeters C. Inflammatory breast cancer: an overview. *Crit Rev Oncol Hematol.* 2015;93:116-126.
2. Ikezoe J, Takashima S, Morimoto S, et al. CT appearence of acute radiation-induced injury in the lung. *Am J Roentgenol.* 1988;150:765-770.
3. Bledsoe TJ, Nath SK, Decker RH. Radiation pneumitis. *Clin Chest Med.* 2017;38:201-208.

**3.** Correct Answer: B

**Rationale:**

The subcostal view image from the TTE demonstrates a large pericardial effusion and right ventricular compression. Given the history and findings on CXR, this is highly likely to be a malignant pericardial effusion. Malignant pericardial effusion has a high probability of recurrence often requiring pericardial window for definitive management. Drainage of the effusion and subsequent referral for definitive management is also a reasonable approach, but that option is not given here. Malignant pericardial effusion can be seen in numerous tumor types, with lung being the most common. In lung cancer, it is thought to occur via spread from local lymphatics rather than direct pericardial invasion. It is associated with a very poor prognosis, although long-term survival is occasionally seen in the current era of targeted therapeutics. Prognosis is most strongly related to treatability of the underlying malignancy rather than any details of the tamponade. Heparin would be appropriate therapy for pulmonary embolus, which can present with shortness of breath and chest pain, but that diagnosis would not explain the echo findings. Aspirin, clopidogrel, and heparin could be a reasonable step in management of an acute coronary syndrome, but that diagnosis is again not consistent with the echo. Fluid resuscitation is mainstay of therapy for hypotension, but, in this case, there is a readily reversible cause of low blood pressure and intervention should be carried out without delay.

### References

1. Wilkes JD, Fidias P, Vaickus L, Perez RP. Malignancy-realted pericardial effusion: 127 cases from the Roswell Park Cancer Institute. *Cancer*. 1995;76:1377-1387.
2. Li BT, Pearson A, Pavlakis N, et al. Malignant cardiac tamponade from non-small cell lung cancer: case series from the era of molecular targeted therapy. *J Clin Med*. 2015;4:75-84.
3. McCurdy MT, Shanholtz CB. Oncologic emergencies. *Crit Care Med*. 2012;40:2212-2222.

---

**4.** Correct Answer: B

**Rationale:**

This patient with advanced lung cancer (lymphadenopathy and contralateral nodules on CXR, in addition to the presumably primary lung mass) is presenting with severe hypercalcemia, which is a medical emergency. Hypercalcemia of malignancy is a late complication in a number of tumors and is associated with poor outcomes. Up to one-half of all patients diagnosed with malignancy-associated hypercalcemia will die within a month of diagnosis. Serum calcium levels are regulated by a balance between bone resorption, intestinal absorption, and renal excretion. Parathyroid hormone (PTH) modulates all of these processes by increasing bone resorption, decreasing renal calcium excretion, and increasing intestinal excretion by converting calcidiol to calcitriol. Hypercalcemia can occur in malignancy via direct osteolysis in the case of bony metastasis, ectopic PTH secretion, or the action of PTH-related proteins. Therapy for hypercalcemia includes aggressive volume repletion, loop diuretics to maintain high urine output, and bisphosphonates such as pamidronate to decrease bone resorption. While pamidronate should be initiated as soon as hypercalcemia is diagnosed, the peak effect is not achieved for 2 to 4 days making other supportive measures, such as fluid resuscitation, important. Serum calcium measurements can be affected by albumin, and there exist formulas for the correction of measured calcium for hypoalbuminemia. However, this patient has classic signs of hypercalcemia (including shortened QT interval of EKG, altered mental status, and hypovolemia) as well as very elevated uncorrected calcium. Head CT is an important part of the workup of altered mental status, but there is adequate evidence to support a diagnosis of hypercalcemia, and treatment should be initiated as soon as possible.

### References

1. McCurdy MT, Shanholtz CB. Oncologic emergencies. *Crit Care Med*. 2012;40:2212-2222.
2. Stewart AF. Hypercalcemia associated with cancer. *N Engl J Med*. 2005;352:373-379.

---

**5.** Correct Answer: D

**Rationale:**

The image demonstrates stretching of the left main bronchus between the pulmonary artery and vertebral body which can occur in postpneumonectomy syndrome. Postpneumonectomy syndrome is a rare complication that typically occurs 6 months or later after pneumonectomy. It is characterized by extreme shift of the mediastinum, and common symptoms include increasing dyspnea, cough, stridor, and recurrent pulmonary infections. The syndrome is more common after right-sided pneumonectomy as there is greater volume loss with removal of the right lung. Treatment for postpneumonectomy syndrome involves shifting the mediastinum closer to the midline to remove the compression on the airway and vessels. This procedure is typically performed by inserting saline-filled prostheses on the side of the pneumonectomy. A chest tube would be an appropriate next step for empyema formation, which can be a late complication of pneumonectomy. On imaging, this could be characterized by air fluid levels or a loculated pleural effusion on the side of the surgery which was not visualized in this patient. A barium swallow would be helpful in diagnosing an esophagopleural fistula. An esophagopleural fistula in the late stages is typically caused by residual tumor burden eroding into the esophagus. It will typically present with an empyema, and a barium swallow will demonstrate the spilling of contrast into the airway. Finally IV steroids can be used for pulmonary edema that can occur post pneumonectomy. This is typically an early complication within 72 hours of surgery, therefore would not fit with this patient's delayed time course.

### References

1. Chandrashekhara SH, Bhalla AS, Sharma R, Gupta AK, Kumar A, Arora R. Imaging in postpneumonectomy complications: a pictorial review. *J Cancer Res Ther*. 2011;7(1):3-10. PubMed PMID:21546734.
2. Sharifpour M, Bittner EA. Postpneumonectomy syndrome: a case of shifting priorities. *Anesthesiology*. 2014;121(6):1334. PubMed PMID:24047857.

**6. Correct Answer: B**

**Rationale:**

Prior to pneumonectomy or lobectomy, the American College of Chest Physicians (ACCP) and the British Thoracic Society (BTS) recommend starting with pulmonary function tests. A reduced FEV1 has been associated with increased respiratory mortality rates post surgery In the BTS guidelines, a preoperative FEV1 >2 L (or 80% predicted) generally suggests the patient would tolerate a pneumonectomy well and for lobectomy, the FEV1 cutoff is 1.5 L. In patients with a FEV1 <30%, the incidence of respiratory morbidity has been as high as 43% but drops to 12% in patients with a FEV1 >60%. DLCO is also recommended for all patients prior to lung resection surgery. Ferguson et al. demonstrated that DLCO <60% was associated with 25% mortality and 40% pulmonary morbidity. If patients do not fall into a low-risk category (FEV1 >80% and DLCO >80%), it is recommended that a postoperative (PPO) pulmonary function test be calculated. A PPO calculation involves using the preoperative FEV1 or DLCO and multiplying by 1—the fraction of total perfusion in the to-be-resected lung. This involves the use of a ventilation/perfusion scan. If the PPO FEV1 and PPO DLCO are >60% predicted, no additional testing is recommended. If the PPO FEV1 and PPO DLCO are <60% and greater than 30%, either a stair testing or shuttle testing is recommended. If the PPO FEV1 and PPO DLCO are <30%, a cardiopulmonary exercise test is recommended. An arterial $PO_2$ has not been shown to predict mortality prior to lung resection surgery. For this patient, given the FEV1 and DLCO do not clearly place the patient into a low-risk category, the next best step would be to calculate a PPO and then determine if stair climbing or a cardiopulmonary exercise test was necessary.

References

1. Brunelli A, Kim AW, Berger KI, Addrizzo-Harris DJ. Physiologic evaluation of the patient with lung cancer being considered for resectional surgery: Diagnosis and management of lung cancer, 3rd ed: American College of Chest Physicians evidence-based clinical practice guidelines. *Chest.* 2013;143:e166S-e190S.
2. British Thoracic Society; Society of Cardiothoracic Surgeons of Great Britain and Ireland Working Party. BTS guidelines: guidelines on the selection of patients with lung cancer for surgery. *Thorax.* 2001;56:89.
3. Ferguson MK, Little L, Rizzo L, et al. Diffusing capacity predicts morbidity and mortality after pulmonary resection. *J Thorac Cardiovasc Surg.* 1988;96:894-900.

**7. Correct Answer: C**

**Rationale:**

The patient continues to demonstrate tachycardia, hypoxemia, and low-grade fevers. However, he also displays clinical and subjective findings to suggest improvement in his pneumonia with reduced cough and rhonchi. Given the patient has an underlying diagnosis of non–small-cell lung cancer, he is at increased risk for the development of PE. In comparison to cancer-free controls, patients with lung cancer were six times more likely to develop a PE. He also has a recent diagnosis of malignancy, and the incidence of PE is greatest within the first 6 months of lung cancer diagnosis. The patient has been diagnosed with adenocarcinoma which independently is a risk factor for PE (OR 3.6). Given is lack of improvement and his associated risk factors, a CT-PE would be warranted to rule out a PE as the cause for his continual symptoms. Adding on vancomycin would not be appropriate, given the patient has low methicillin-resistant *Staphylococcus aureus* (MRSA) risk factors. Steroids would likely not be helpful as clinically the patient does not appear to have a COPD exacerbation and his sputum production is improving and he has no evidence of wheeze on examination. In patients, without significant risk factors for PE, it may be appropriate to wait for clinical improvement, given the patient did have an initial diagnosis of pneumonia, however, missing a PE in this patient could be life threatening.

References

1. Li Y, Shang Y, Wang W, Ning S, Chen H. Lung cancer and pulmonary embolism: what is the relationship? a review. *J Cancer.* 2018;9(17):3046-3057.
2. Ma L, Wen Z. Risk factors and prognosis of pulmonary embolism in patients with lung cancer. *Medicine (Baltimore).* 2017;96(16):e6638.

# 42

# LUNG TRANSPLANTATION, COMPLICATIONS, AND VV ECMO

Archit Sharma and Bharathram Vasudevan

1. A 45-year-old female with history of idiopathic pulmonary fibrosis is admitted to the intensive care unit (ICU) after compatible bilateral lung transplantation. The surgery required the use of intraoperative cardiopulmonary bypass (CPB). Postoperatively, she is on lung protective ventilation with low tidal volumes. She has progressive increase in oxygen requirements and is requiring an $FiO_2$ of 0.7 with a PEEP of 10 to maintain saturations of 92%. At 24 hours, her $PaO_2/FiO_2$ ratio is 175 and chest radiography reveals bilateral diffuse infiltrates. She has a HR of 90/min, BP of 105/76 mm Hg, and a CVP of 7 mm Hg. A bronchoscopy is performed which is unremarkable except for mild erythema in the bronchi. Which of the following is the MOST appropriate next step in managing this patient?

    A. Initiation of veno-venous (VV) ECMO
    B. Administration of inhaled nitric oxide
    C. Therapeutic plasma exchange
    D. Systemic anticoagulation

2. Which of the following patients on mechanical lung support in ICU is best suited for lung transplantation?

    A. A 40-year-old male on "awake" VV ECMO for worsening idiopathic pulmonary fibrosis
    B. A 25-year-old female on VV ECMO for ARDS due to sepsis and dialysis for AKI
    C. A 47-year-old morbidly obese female (BMI-42) with severe restrictive lung disease on mechanical ventilation
    D. A 76-year-old male with a recent history of bladder cancer resection on mechanical ventilation for acute exacerbation of end-stage COPD.

3. A 58-year-old male patient is admitted to the hospital 6 months after receiving bilateral lung transplantation. He complains of increasing shortness of breath with a "barking" cough and inability to clear secretions over the past 2 months. He mentions that he has been sleeping in his recliner chair due to dyspnea when lying flat. He is afebrile with a HR of 88/min, BP of 140/80 mm Hg, $SpO_2$ of 94% on room air, and a respiratory rate of 30/min. He is using his accessory neck muscles, and right-sided rhonchi are noted during the chest examination. Administration of bronchodilators fails to improve his symptoms. He is started on noninvasive positive pressure ventilation, which leads to a marked improvement. Which of the following is the gold standard test to diagnose his condition?

    A. Pulmonary function testing with spirometry
    B. Standard CT scan of the chest
    C. Flexible fiber-optic bronchoscopy
    D. Sputum for microbiological analysis

4. Three months after bilateral lung transplantation, a 50-year-old female patient is admitted to the ICU with complaints of worsening shortness of breath, low grade fever, and cough. She is compliant with her drug regimen consisting of prednisone, tacrolimus, azathioprine, valganciclovir, and trimethoprim-sulfamethoxazole. Examination reveals bilateral crackles and decreased breath sounds over the left lower chest wall. She has a temperature of 38°C, HR of 90/min, BP of 105/65 mm Hg, RR of 25/min, and $SpO_2$ of 91% on room air. She is started on oxygen therapy, and a chest CT is obtained, which reveals bilateral ground glass opacities with a left-sided pleural effusion. Laboratory testing is unremarkable except for slight eosinophilia. Bronchoalveolar lavage reveals lymphocytic predominance and transbronchial biopsy is significant for dense perivascular and bronchial mononuclear infiltrates with a negative C4d staining. Which of the following is the best next step in management?

   A. Intravenous methyl prednisone
   B. Intravenous ganciclovir and piperacillin-tazobactam
   C. Intravenous immunoglobulins (IvIg) and rituximab
   D. Therapeutic plasma exchange

5. A 62-year-old male patient with end-stage emphysema undergoes left-sided single-lung transplantation. He arrives at the ICU after his surgery and is mechanically ventilated on volume assist control mode. The initial ventilator settings are $FiO_2$ of 0.4, PEEP of 10 cm $H_2O$, tidal volume of 380 mL, and respiratory rate of 20 breaths/minute. A few hours later, arterial blood gas reveals hypoxia with hypercapnia. In response, his ventilator settings are changed to $FiO_2$ of 0.5, PEEP of 12 cm $H_2O$, and respiratory rate of 26 breaths/min. One hour later, he has a HR of 120/min, BP of 80/60 mm Hg and $SpO_2$ of 89%. Chest examination reveals bilateral air entry with coarse breath sounds on the left. Arterial blood gas shows worsening hypoxia and hypercapnia. He is started on norepinephrine, and FiO2 is further increased to 0.6. What is the next best step in management of this patient?

   A. Chest tube insertion on the right side
   B. Increase PEEP and respiratory rate
   C. Decrease PEEP and respiratory rate
   D. Obtain a CT scan of the thorax

6. A 35-year-old female patient is admitted to the hospital with pneumonia. She was recently diagnosed with end-stage renal disease and is on maintenance dialysis through a tunneled right subclavian dialysis catheter. Hospital course is complicated by respiratory failure and acute respiratory distress syndrome requiring mechanical ventilation. Due to progressive hypoxia, VV ECMO is instituted via bilateral femoral cannulas. Mechanical ventilation is reduced to resting ventilation with a low $FiO_2$, tidal volume, and respiratory rate. Twelve hours later the patient has a drop in arterial oxygen saturation from her baseline of 94% to 82%. The oxygen saturation of blood drawn from the femoral venous line, which is pre-oxygenator, has increased during the same time from 65% to 80%. What is the most appropriate next step in management?

   A. Increase pump speed
   B. Radiographic evaluation of the cannulas
   C. Change oxygenator
   D. Add an additional parallel ECMO circuit

7. A 22-year-old male is admitted to the ICU with acute respiratory distress syndrome secondary to pneumonia. The clinical course is complicated by progressive hypoxemia, which does not improve with prone ventilation. VV ECMO is instituted with a 31 Fr right internal jugular double-lumen cannula, and the pump flow is at 4.5 L/min. The patient has a HR of 90/min, BP of 110/70 mm Hg with a norepinephrine infusion at 0.05 μg/kg/min, and a $SpO_2$ of 90%. One hour later, the ECMO specialist mentions of "chugging" in the drainage circuit with low inlet pressures. The ECMO flow has reduced to 3 L/min. There is a drop in $SpO_2$ to 84%, and the norepinephrine requirement has increased to 0.1 μg/kg/min. An arterial blood sample sent to the critical care laboratory reveals a pH of 7.30, $PaCO_2$ of 35, $PaO_2$ of 49, $HCO_3$ of 19, hematocrit of 42%, and a lactate 4.2. The most appropriate next step in management is to:

   A. Start epinephrine to improve cardiac contractility
   B. Increase pump speed to increase ECMO flow
   C. Urgent blood transfusion
   D. Administer a 500 mL fluid bolus

**8.** A 42-year-old female is admitted to the ICU after a motor vehicle accident. She develops ARDS secondary to lung contusions and is initiated on VV ECMO. The clinical course is complicated by worsening acute kidney injury. The latest laboratory workup reveals acidosis with a pH of 7.18 and hyperkalemia of 6.5 mEq/L. Sodium bicarbonate, calcium gluconate, and insulin-dextrose are administered. Although adding on a continuous renal replacement therapy circuit to the ECMO circuit, the patient develops a short run of ventricular tachycardia, which quickly degenerates into asystole. What is the immediate next step in managing this patient?

**A.** Initiate chest compressions
**B.** Administer epinephrine only and avoid chest compressions
**C.** Urgent conversion to VA ECMO
**D.** Defibrillation with 200 J

# Chapter 42 ■ Answers

**1.** Correct Answer: B

**Rationale:**

The most probable diagnosis in this patient with worsening hypoxemia after lung transplantation is primary graft dysfunction (PGD), which is most likely to improve with inhaled nitric oxide. PGD is a common complication occurring in the first 72 hours and is a leading cause for early morbidity and mortality. It is considered a form of ischemia-reperfusion injury and is characterized by hypoxemia associated with diffuse alveolar infiltrates on chest radiography. Donor risk factors for PGD include aspiration, chest trauma or lung contusion, undersized donor, and heavy alcohol use. Significant recipient risk factors for PGD are female sex, African American race, obesity, prior pleurodesis and a pretransplant diagnosis of idiopathic pulmonary fibrosis, sarcoidosis, or idiopathic pulmonary arterial hypertension. Operative risk factors include the use of CPB, prolonged ischemia time, high reperfusion $FiO_2$, and large volume blood transfusion.

Given the similarities between PGD and ARDS, management strategies for ARDS have been extrapolated to PGD. The mainstay of management involves lung protective ventilation with fluid restriction. In patients with severe PGD, inhaled nitric oxide and inhaled prostacyclins have been tried to improve oxygenation. Nitric oxide (NO) availability is reduced in ischemia-reperfusion injury, and animal studies have shown improved allograft function with NO treatment (B). Posttransplant ECMO (A) is generally reserved for patients with severe hypoxemia ($PaO_2/FiO_2$ <100) who fail to improve with the above strategies. Patients who require ECMO for PGD have higher complication rates and poor outcomes when compared to those who improve with other supportive management. Hyperacute rejection is another rare complication and has to be ruled out by reviewing the results of pretransplant panel reactive antibody testing and the donor-recipient cross match. In the presence of donor-specific HLA antibodies, treatment of rejection includes therapeutic plasma exchange (C) and other immunosuppressive therapies. Systemic anticoagulation (D) is used in the treatment of pulmonary embolism and thrombosis of venous anastomosis.

References

1. Snell GI, Yusen RD, Weill D, et al. Report of the ISHLT Working Group on Primary Lung Graft Dysfunction, part I: definition and grading-A 2016 Consensus Group statement of the International Society for Heart and Lung Transplantation. *J Heart Lung Transplant.* 2017;36:1097-1103.
2. Diamond JM, Arcasoy S, Kennedy CC et al. Report of the International Society for Heart and Lung Transplantation Working Group on Primary Lung Graft Dysfunction, part II: epidemiology, risk factors, and outcomes-A 2016 Consensus Group statement of the International Society for Heart and Lung Transplantation. *J Heart Lung Transplant.* 2017;36:1104-1113.
3. Porteous MK, Lee JC. Primary graft dysfunction after lung transplantation. *Clin Chest Med.* 2017;38:641-654.

**2.** Correct Answer: A

**Rationale:**

Lung transplantation is considered for patients with end-stage lung disease who carry an expected 2-year mortality rate of greater than 50%. Expected likelihood of survival at 90 days and 5 years posttransplantation are also taken into consideration when selecting candidates for transplantation. Mechanical ventilation and/or extracorporeal life support (ECLS) are considered as "relative" contraindications for lung transplantation. At the same time, it is important to review and rule out other absolute and relative contraindications in a patient on mechanical support. There is a growing interest in using ECMO in awake, nonintubated patients as a bridging modality. "Awake" ECMO (A) offers the advantage of participation in physical therapy and rehabilitation before transplant. Successful transplantation with better outcomes has been reported with this strategy when compared to traditional mechanical support.

| ABSOLUTE CONTRAINDICATIONS | RELATIVE CONTRAINDICATIONS |
|---|---|
| • Significant major organ dysfunction (eg, liver, kidney, heart, brain) **(B)**<br>• Class II or III obesity (BMI>35 kg/m²) **(C)**<br>• Recent malignancy (5-y disease-free interval required for many malignancies) **(D)**<br>• Significant CAD not amenable to revascularization<br>• Acute medical condition (eg, sepsis, myocardial infarction)<br>• Poor baseline functional status<br>• Active substance abuse | • Age >65 with other relative contraindications<br>• Class I obesity<br>• Severe malnutrition<br>• Severe osteoporosis<br>• Prior extensive chest surgery with lung resection<br>• Chronic colonization or infection with resistant/virulent organisms<br>• Active medical conditions that have not been optimized—atherosclerosis, coronary heart disease, diabetes mellitus, hypertension |

### References

1. Weill D, Benden C, Corris PA, et al. A consensus document for the selection of lung transplant candidates: 2014–an update from the Pulmonary Transplantation Council of the International Society for Heart and Lung Transplantation. *J Heart Lung Transplant*. 2015;34:1-15.
2. Fuehner T, Kuehn C, Welte T, Gottlieb J. ICU care before and after lung transplantation. *Chest*. 2016;150:442-450.
3. Biscotti M, Gannon WD, Agerstrand C, et al. Awake extracorporeal membrane oxygenation as bridge to lung transplantation: a 9-year experience. *Ann Thorac Surg*. 2017;104:412-419.

**3.** Correct Answer: C

**Rationale:**

The patient described here has most likely developed tracheobronchomalacia with or without bronchial stenosis, which will require visualizing with a fiber-optic bronchoscope (C). Malacia is defined as greater than 50% reduction in the airway lumen during expiration. It can be localized to the anastomotic site or diffusely affect the donor airways. Clinical features include dyspnea that may be aggravated in the recumbent position, chronic "barking" cough, wheezing, inability to clear secretions, and recurrent infections. Spirometry (A) may show a reduction in FEV1 and forced expiratory flow at 25% to 75% but is not confirmatory. Variable obstructive pattern may be seen in flow-volume loops. A *dynamic* CT scan of the chest may show the respiratory change in airway lumen, but a standard CT scan will not be diagnostic (B). Bronchoscopy is the gold standard tool for diagnosing airway complications including tracheobronchomalacia. It allows for direct visualization of the dynamic luminal narrowing during expiration. It can be present alone or at a site of bronchial stenosis. A sputum culture (D) would help to diagnosis if this patient had pneumonia, but the chance of a pneumonia with the patient being afebrile and producing clear secretions is fairly low.

Management of tracheobronchomalacia can be challenging. Observation is recommended for asymptomatic disease. Medical management is initially considered for symptomatic disease and involves chest physiotherapy, mucolytics, and noninvasive positive pressure ventilation. More invasive options such as stenting and trachea-bronchoplasty may be considered for severe malacia that is localized to the central airways.

### References

1. Crespo MM, McCarthy DP, Hopkins PM, et al. ISHLT consensus statement on adult and pediatric airway complications after lung transplantation: definitions, grading system, and therapeutics. *J Heart Lung Transplant*. 2018;37:548-563.
2. Varela A, Hoyos L, Romero A, et al. Management of bronchial complications after lung transplantation and sequelae. *Thorac Surg Clin*. 2018;28:365-375.
3. Frye L, Machuzak M. Airway complications after lung transplantation. *Clin Chest Med*. 2017;38:693-706.

**4.** Correct Answer: A

**Rationale:**

Patient seems to be undergoing acute cellular rejection and will need to be treated with intravenous corticosteroids such as methylprednisone **(A)**. Spirometry typically shows a decrease in FEV1 in acute rejection. CT scan findings in acute rejection include ground-glass opacities, interlobular septal thickening, pleural effusions, and lung volume loss. The gold standard test to diagnose rejection is flexible bronchoscopy with bronchoscopic alveolar lavage and transbronchial biopsy. Two main histopathological components used for grading are the severities of lymphocytic bronchiolitis and perivascular mononuclear cell infiltrates. Intravenous high-dose corticosteroids are the mainstay of treatment for symptomatic or high-grade acute cellular rejection. Other treatment options that have been used for acute cellular rejection include antithymocyte globulin, extracorporeal photopheresis, and alternative immunosuppressive agents such as alemtuzumab and sirolimus or everolimus. Acute rejection episodes are important risk factors for the development of chronic lung allograft dysfunction. Therefore, prevention and treatment of acute rejection by appropriate immunosuppressive regimen is essential. CMV pneumonitis is unlikely in a patient who is already on valganciclovir prophylaxis. Therefore, intravenous ganciclovir in this patient is not warranted (B).

The main differential diagnoses of acute cellular rejection include humoral rejection and infections. Humoral rejection can be hyperacute rejection or acute antibody-mediated rejection. Hyperacute rejection presents in the first 24 hours following transplantation and is due to preformed donor-specific antibodies (DSA).

Acute antibody-mediated rejection presents later and is due to DSA that developed or increased in titers after transplantation. The diagnoses require demonstration of DSA along with ruling out other conditions. The histopathological hallmark of acute antibody-mediated rejection is subendothelial deposition of C4d demonstrated by immunohistochemistry but is not essential for diagnosis. Specific treatment options for humoral rejection include intravenous immunoglobulins (IvIg), therapeutic plasma exchange (D), rituximab (C), and bortezomib.

### References
1. Martinu T, Howell DN, Palmer SM. Acute cellular rejection and humoral sensitization in lung transplant recipients. *Semin Respir Crit Care Med.* 2010;31:179-188.
2. Hachem RR. Acute rejection and antibody-mediated rejection in lung transplantation. *Clin Chest Med.* 2017;38:667-675.
3. Stewart S, Fishbein MC, Snell GI, et al. Revision of the 1996 working formulation for the standardization of nomenclature in the diagnosis of lung rejection. *J Heart Lung Transplant.* 2007;26:1229-1242.

**5.** Correct Answer: C

**Rationale:**

The clinical picture in this patient is suggestive of clinically significant acute native lung hyperinflation. Recipients of single lung transplantation for emphysema are prone to develop native lung hyperinflation. The native lung is highly compliant when compared to the graft lung in patients with COPD. It has severe expiratory airflow limitation that can lead to dynamic hyperinflation and air trapping and hence will improve by decreasing the respiratory rate and PEEP (C). The patient has breath sounds bilaterally and hence does not need a chest tube (A). Increasing PEEP and respiratory rate (B) in this situation can worsen dynamic hyperinflation. Obtaining a CT scan will not help in the acute hemodynamic instability that this patient is in because it does not offer any additional information about his mechanical ventilation (D).

Acute hyperinflation with mediastinal shift to the opposite site can compromise hemodynamic and respiratory functions. The increase in intrathoracic pressure impairs venous return and causes hypotension, often requiring vasopressors. Marked compression of the graft lung results in atelectasis, hypoxia, and hypercapnia.

Positive pressure ventilation in such cases must be tailored to the characteristics of the native lung. The best approach to mechanical ventilation in these patients is to maximize the expiratory time by having a shorter inspiratory time and a lower respiratory rate with minimal PEEP. Acute symptomatic hyperinflation has also been treated by temporarily disconnecting the endotracheal tube from ventilator to allow deflation of the native lung. Ventilation can be very challenging if the graft lung develops edema or PGD. Severe respiratory or hemodynamic compromise in such patients can be treated with differential lung ventilation by placing a double-lumen tube. This allows for independent ventilation of the native and graft lungs with suitable ventilator settings.

### References
1. Diamond J, Kotloff RM. Lung transplantation for chronic obstructive pulmonary disease: special considerations. *Semin Respir Crit Care Med.* 2010;31:115-122.
2. Barnes L, Reed RM, Parekh KR, et al. Mechanical ventilation for the lung transplant recipient. *Curr Pulmonol Rep.* 2015;4:88-96.
3. Fuehner T, Kuehn C, Welte T, Gottlieb J. ICU care before and after lung transplantation. *Chest.* 2016;150:442-450.
4. Mitchell JB, Shaw AD, Donald S, Farrimond JG. Differential lung ventilation after single-lung transplantation for emphysema. *J Cardiothorac Vasc Anesth.* 2002;16:459-462.

**6.** Correct Answer: B

**Rationale:**

Increase in oxygen saturation of the pre-oxygenator venous blood with a decrease in arterial oxygen saturation raises the concern for clinically significant recirculation in this patient and hence requires radiographic evaluation of cannula position to verify that the two lumens are separate from each other (B). Recirculation is a phenomenon unique to VV ECMO wherein the oxygenated blood from the return cannula reenters the ECMO circuit through the drainage cannula before reaching the systemic circulation. The distance between the ports of drainage and return cannulas influence the amount of recirculation. Recirculation is also affected by the type of cannulation for VV ECMO. Femoro-femoral and femoral-internal jugular configurations carry higher risks of significant recirculation when compared to a dual-lumen configuration.

Increase in pump speed and ECMO flow rate have shown to be associated with a higher fraction of recirculation (A). Oxygenator failure is fairly unlikely to occur in just 12 hours after initiation of support but can be easily ruled out with a postoxygenator ABG (C). Adding another parallel circuit will not provide any additional benefit, if the cannulas are malpositioned (D). Other factors that may influence recirculation include changes in intrathoracic and intra-cardiac pressures and changes in patient positioning.

Clinically significant recirculation can lead to hypoxia and subsequent end-organ damage. Management of new-onset recirculation involves radiographic or ultrasound evaluation to check the positions of the drainage and return cannulas. Increasing the distance between the two cannulas by withdrawing the drainage cannula can reduce recirculation. Other strategies to reduce recirculation include addition of a new drainage cannula, use of a bicaval dual-lumen cannula, or manipulation of the reinfusion cannula to direct the return jet toward the tricuspid valve.

References

1. Abrams D, Bacchetta M, Brodie D. Recirculation in venovenous extracorporeal membrane oxygenation. *ASAIO J.* 2015;61:115-121.
2. Xie A, Yan TD, Forrest P. Recirculation in venovenous extracorporeal membrane oxygenation. *J Crit Care.* 2016;36:107-110.
3. Broman M, Frenckner B, Bjällmark A, Broomé M. Recirculation during veno-venous extra-corporeal membrane oxygenation–a simulation study. *Int J Artif Organs.* 2015;38:23-30.

---

**7.** Correct Answer: D

**Rationale:**

"Chugging" or "chattering" of the ECMO circuit refers to back and forth swinging of the drainage and return tubes. This occurs because of fluctuations in venous drainage pressures. Hypovolemia and high pump speeds are two common scenarios where chugging can occur. In both cases, increased negative pressure at the venous inflow port of the drainage cannula leads to a temporary venous collapse. This causes low flows through the ECMO circuit even at high pump speeds, and hence increasing ECMO pump flows will not help (B). The normal negative pressure in the drainage cannula is between -50 to -80 mm Hg. Pressures lower than -100 mm Hg are abnormal and are seen during chugging episodes. The hypovolemia can be treated by administering a fluid bolus (D).

In the presence of chugging, the patient should be evaluated for signs of low intravascular volume. Tachycardia and hypotension may be present requiring vasopressor initiation or up titration. There might be desaturation due to decreased ECMO flows. Management involves administration of fluid bolus or blood transfusion if hematocrit is low. Inotropes are not usually required if baseline cardiac function is normal (A). Because the hematocrit is normal, the patient does not need a blood transfusion (C). Point of care ultrasound can be utilized to guide hemodynamic management. The ECMO pump speed can be reduced temporarily to decrease the flows to avoid chugging and subsequent venous suck down.

Low ECMO flows despite high pump speeds can also be encountered when there is some obstruction in the circuit. Obstruction could be due to kinking of the tubes or due to the presence of blood clots in the oxygenator. Isolated postoxygenator tubing chugging can be due to high flows and unrelated to hypovolemia. It is also important to rule out malposition of the cannulas.

References

1. Sidebotham D. Troubleshooting adult ECMO. *J Extra Corpor Technol.* 2011;43:P27-P32.
2. Walter JM, Kurihara C, Corbridge TC, Bharat A. Chugging in patients on veno-venous extracorporeal membrane oxygenation: an under-recognized driver of intravenous fluid administration in patients with acute respiratory distress syndrome? *Heart Lung.* 2018;47:398-400.
3. Staudacher DL, Bode C, Wengenmayer T. Fluid therapy remains an important cornerstone in the prevention of progressive chugging in extracorporeal membrane oxygenation. *Heart Lung.* 2018;47:432.

---

**8.** Correct Answer: A

**Rationale:**

VV ECMO provides pulmonary support with little cardiac support. The patient on VV ECMO is completely dependent on his native cardiac function to maintain cardiac output and hemodynamics. Any decrease in cardiac or hemodynamic function in such patients should be supported in the same way as a patient who is not on ECMO. Therefore, in the event of a cardiac arrest, it is prudent to follow the advanced cardiac life support algorithm and initiate CPR (A). In this patient it would mean initiating high-quality chest compressions (B), as well as administering intravenous epinephrine. Because asystole is not a shockable rhythm, defibrillation is unlikely to help in this case (D).

During a cardiac arrest, there is no cardiac output, and this impairs the flows through VV ECMO. But with high-quality chest compressions, it is possible to run the pump at low flows, which may be adequate to maintain oxygenation. The $FiO_2$ on the ventilator can be turned up to 1.0 as a safety precaution to protect against hypoxia in the event of inadequate pump flows. Institution of VA ECMO is recommended in case of refractory cardiac arrest when there is a strong suspicion for a reversible cause of cardiac arrest. The survival rates and neurological outcomes after ECPR are influenced by the time to initiation of VA ECMO after cardiac arrest. It seems reasonable to consider ECPR after 10 minutes of high-quality conventional CPR in a patient with a potentially reversible cause of cardiac arrest. In this patient on VV ECMO, conversion to VA ECMO by arterial cannulation should be considered if initial CPR fails to achieve return of spontaneous circulation (C).

References

1. Link MS, Berkow LC, Kudenchuk PJ, et al. Part 7: adult advanced cardiovascular life support: 2015 American Heart Association guidelines update for cardiopulmonary resuscitation and emergency cardiovascular care. *Circulation.* 2015;132:S444-S464.
2. Makdisi G, Wang IW. Extra corporeal membrane oxygenation (ECMO) review of a lifesaving technology. *J Thorac Dis.* 2015;7:E166-E176.
3. King CS, Roy A, Ryan L, et al. Cardiac support: emphasis on venoarterial ECMO. *Crit Care Clin.* 2017;33:777-794.

# 43

# RESPIRATORY DIAGNOSTIC MODALITIES AND MONITORING

Phat Tan Dang, Christopher Dinh, Abdulaziz S. Almehlisi, and Ulrich Schmidt

1. A 22-year-old man with a history of severe reactive airway disease and polysubstance abuse is brought to the emergency department following a motor vehicle collision. Endotracheal intubation is performed and placement confirmed by continuous capnography. Peak inspiratory pressure on the ventilator is 45 cm $H_2O$. Which of the following describes the **MOST LIKELY** appearance of his capnogram?

   A. Box shaped with a flat phase III
   B. Biphasic with a rounded phase III
   C. Shark finned with up-sloped phase III
   D. Flat

2. A 72-year-old female (body mass index of 27 kg/m$^2$), admitted for exacerbation of chronic obstructive pulmonary disease (COPD), is started on noninvasive ventilation on the floor. She is claustrophobic, and the intern orders lorazepam for mask tolerance. Soon after, the patient is found to be obtunded and a code is called. During laryngoscopy, particulate gastric contents are noted in the posterior pharynx. Her postintubation vitals are temperature 100.3°F, blood pressure 98/62 mm Hg, heart rate 108 beats/min, SpO$_2$ 88% on 100% FiO$_2$, respiratory rate 14 breaths/min, and peak end expiratory pressure of 8 cm $H_2O$ with tidal volume of 8 mL/kg ideal body weight. Despite adjustment of ventilatory parameters and maximal bronchodilator therapy, airway inspiratory pressures remain high. Which of the following actions would be BEST next step in the management of this patient?

   A. Surface ultrasound of the heart and lungs
   B. Arterial blood gas
   C. Chest x-ray
   D. Bronchoscopy

3. A 68-year-old man in stable atrial fibrillation with rapid ventricular response undergoes transesophageal echocardiogram and successful synchronized cardioversion under conscious sedation in the medical intensive care unit (ICU). Topical 20% benzocaine spray is used for oropharyngeal anesthesia prior to transesophageal probe insertion. His starting SpO$_2$ is 99% on 6 L/min oxygen via nasal cannula. Within a few minutes, the patient appears blue-gray and SpO$_2$ decreases to 84%. His saturation fails to improve on 10 L/min oxygen via simple face mask. The rest of the vital signs remain stable. Which of the following findings would be **LEAST** consistent with the patient's clinical condition?

   A. Carboxy-Hgb 18%
   B. Normal SpO$_2$ waveform
   C. PaO$_2$ 265 mm Hg
   D. PaCO$_2$ 55 mm Hg

4. An 88-year-old woman with an acute GI bleed undergoes endoscopic evaluation and subsequently remains intubated in the ICU in anticipation of further intervention the following day. She is 5′6″ and has her ideal body weight of 60 kg throughout her life. Her arterial blood gas (ABG) shows pH 7.30, $PCO_2$ 58, $PaO_2$ 68, $HCO_3$ 25 on assist control-volume control ventilation with tidal volume 320 mL, respiratory rate 14/min, PEEP 7 cm $H_2O$, and 50% $FiO_2$. She is hemodynamically stable, and her airway pressures are low. Which of the following is the MOST appropriate next step in her management?

   A. Increase $FiO_2$
   B. Increase tidal volume
   C. Increase PEEP
   D. Decrease $FiO_2$

5. You are the sole intensivist at a rural hospital, and the overnight hospitalist asked you to evaluate a patient with a left-sided malignant pleural effusion who is experiencing dyspnea. You determine that the patient has a very large pleural effusion, and you decide that a thoracentesis will be needed. Under ultrasound guidance, you place a chest tube and begin to aspirate the pleural effusion. At what point should you stop your thoracentesis to maximize your drainage and minimize complication(s)?

   A. Stop after draining 1 L of pleural effusion
   B. Stop after patient complains of chest discomfort
   C. Stop after your pleural manometer goes below −20 cm $H_2O$
   D. Stop after patient coughs

6. A 45-year-old man with a history of idiopathic pulmonary fibrosis is admitted to the ICU intubated and sedated after single lung transplantation. On postoperative day 1, the patient's oxygen requirement increases. He remains afebrile, and his arterial blood gas shows $PaO_2$ 90 mm Hg on $FiO_2$ 50%. The respiratory therapist reports increased secretions from his endotracheal tube. The patient is on ceftazidime, vancomycin, voriconazole, inhaled amphotericin B, and valganciclovir. Which of the following is the BEST next step in management?

   A. Lighten the sedation and try to extubate him today
   B. Perform a bronchoscopy and send the bronchial lavage from the native lung for culture and expand antibiotic coverage meropenem
   C. Give the patient a pulse steroid therapy with methylprednisolone
   D. Increase his $FiO_2$ to 100%

7. A 52-year-old man with severe COPD underwent bilateral lung transplant 10 days ago. His postoperative course was unremarkable. He was extubated and transferred to the floor on postoperative day 5. Today, he starts to complain of shortness of breath. The physical examination is significant for chest wall subcutaneous emphysema. Images from a chest CT scan follow.

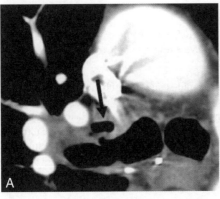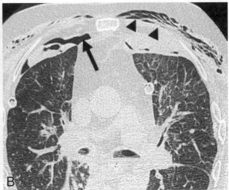

   What is the BEST next step in management?

   A. Pulse dose of methylprednisolone
   B. Flexible bronchoscopy
   C. Open surgical exploration and repair
   D. Observation and serial chest x-rays

8. A previously healthy 28-year-old man presents to the emergency department with severe respiratory distress, flu-like symptoms, and cough. The emergency physician intubates the patient for hypoxic respiratory failure. His postintubation chest x-ray shows diffuse, bilateral pulmonary infiltrations, and appropriate endotracheal tube position. The initial mechanical ventilation settings are $FiO_2$ 50%, PEEP 18 cm $H_2O$, and tidal volume (TV) 6 mL/kg ideal body weight (IBW). The patient is transferred to the ICU, and 6 hours later you are informed that the patient is hypoxic on $FiO_2$ 100%, PEEP 24 cm $H_2O$, and tidal volume (TV) 8 mL/kg ideal body weight (IBW). His plateau pressure is 42 cm $H_2O$, and his ABG shows $PaO_2$ of 54. You decided to place the patient on venovenous extracorporeal membrane oxygenation (V-V ECMO).

Which of the following mechanical ventilation settings are **BEST** after V-V ECMO initiation?

A. Pressure controlled 25 cm $H_2O$, rate 5, PEEP 15 cm $H_2O$, $FiO_2$ 50%
B. Pressure controlled 30 cm $H_2O$, rate 14, PEEP 10 cm $H_2O$, $FiO_2$ 50%
C. Volume controlled, TV 5 mL/kg IBW, rate 14 PEEP 10 cm $H_2O$, $FiO_2$ 50%
D. Volume controlled, TV 8 mL/kg IBW, rate 5, PEEP 10 cm $H_2O$, $FiO_2$ 50%

9. A 5'7" middle-aged man, with unknown medical history, has just arrived in the operating room for emergent exploratory laparotomy following intubation in the emergency department with appropriate hypnotic and 100 mg rocuronium. The initial ventilator settings are tidal volume 450 mL, rate 16 breaths/min, PEEP 5 cm $H_2O$ and $FiO_2$ 40%, and inspiratory:expiratory (I:E) ratio 1:2. The $EtCO_2$ waveform follows.

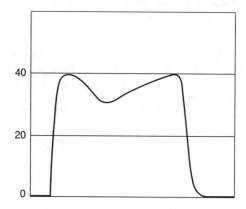

Based on the $EtCO_2$ waveform, what would be the **BEST** next course of action?

A. Give an additional dose of muscle relaxation
B. Increase minute ventilation to 600 mL
C. Continue current ventilator setting
D. Change the I:E ratio to 1:3

10. A 59-year-old male with history of COPD is admitted to the ICU for pneumonia and hypoxic respiratory failure. Four hours after admission, the patient continues to be in severe respiratory distress with $O_2$ saturation of 85% on BiPAP (10 cm $H_2O$ IPAP, 5 cm $H_2O$ EPAP, and $FiO_2$ 100%).

You decided to intubate the patient, and immediately after rapid-sequence intubation, the patient oxygen saturation decreases to 78% with blood pressure 110/65 mm Hg and heart rate 95 bpm. Ventilator settings were tidal volume 6 mL/kg, respiratory rate 14 breaths/min, $FiO_2$ 100%, and PEEP 5 cm $H_2O$. The ventilator is alarming for peak air pressure of 45 cm $H_2O$ with plateau pressure of 40 cm $H_2O$. You next perform a point-of-care ultrasound of the lungs, and it shows an absence of pleural sliding on the left lung with positive A-lines and positive pulse sign on the left lung. Which of the following is the **MOST** appropriate next step in management?

A. Perform left tube thoracostomy
B. Perform left needle thoracostomy
C. Start the patient on cisatracurium infusion
D. Adjust endotracheal tube

11. An 89-year-old bedridden man with a history of dementia, non–insulin-dependent diabetes, hip fracture (treated conservatively), diastolic heart failure, and chronic kidney disease was admitted to the medicine service for confusion and possible UTI. The patient had a one week hospital admission for UTI one month ago. While he was waiting for bed assignment, he starts to desaturate in the emergency department. His vital signs are heart rate 115 beats/min, blood pressure 100/60 mm Hg, respiratory rate 26 breaths/min, SpO$_2$ 86% on room air. Lung auscultation was unrevealing. You were consulted by the medicine team to evaluate the patient for possible ICU admission for hypoxic repository failure. Portable x-ray was negative for any acute process per radiology official read. Your bedside lung ultrasound images show the following:

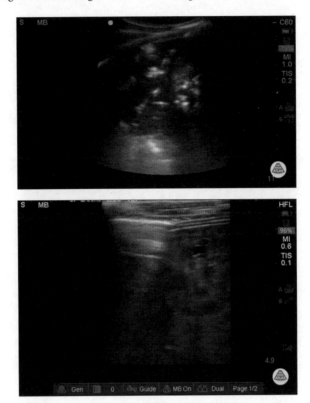

Besides placing the patient on oxygen, what would be the **BEST** next step in management?

A. Start the patient on antibiotics hospital acquire pneumonia
B. Order a STAT CT angiogram of the chest to rule out pulmonary embolism
C. Order furosemide to treat pulmonary edema
D. Place chest tube to treat pleural effusion

12. A 65-year-old female patient presents with acute respiratory failure to the ICU. She is intubated and placed on pressure support ventilation. The driving pressure is set at 10 cm H$_2$O. The PEEP is set at 10 cm H$_2$O. Esophageal balloon is placed, and a pressure of negative 12 cm H$_2$O is obtained at end inspiration.

Given these measurements please estimate transpulmonary pressure.

A. 22 cm H$_2$O
B. 8 cm H$_2$O
C. 32 cm H$_2$O
D. 20 cm H$_2$O

13. A 48-year-male patient with a BMI of 48 kg/m$^2$ is undergoing a spontaneous breathing trial in anticipation of extubation. What is the best position to optimize his respiratory mechanics?

A. Supine position
B. Trendelenburg
C. Beach chair position
D. Reversed Trendelenburg

**14.** A 47-year-old male patient (BMI 55 kg/m²) with methicillin-resistant *Staphylococcus aureus* pneumonia suffers an aspiration event. His oxygen saturation on a nonrebreather face mask is 72%. His previous endotracheal intubation was described as "straightforward." What is the best initial approach for airway management?

   **A.** Awake fiberoptic intubation
   **B.** Rapid-sequence induction followed by intubation via direct laryngoscopy
   **C.** Noninvasive ventilation
   **D.** Rapid-sequence induction followed by intubation via video laryngoscopy

**15.** A 67-year-old patient (BMI 40 kg/m²) is admitted to the ICU in acute respiratory failure. What is the best way to optimize the patient's end expiratory lung volume?

   **A.** PEEP setting guided by measurement of transpulmonary pressures
   **B.** Recruitment maneuver followed by PEEP optimization guided by measurements of transpulmonary pressures
   **C.** Zero PEEP
   **D.** PEEP set by clinician preference

# Chapter 43 ▪ Answers

**1.** Correct Answer: C
   **Rationale:**

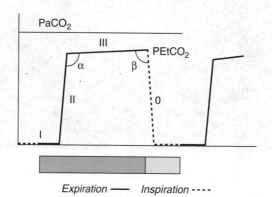

Normal capnogram.

A timed capnograph has 4 segments with phase 0 representing inspiration. In a mechanically ventilated patient, a "normal" capnograph takes a relatively box-shaped appearance with a relatively flat phase III (A, Normal Capnogram figure).

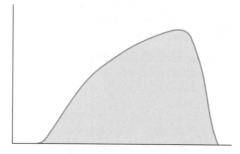

Obstructive lung disease.

The clinical scenario in the question suggests obstructive lung pathology which manifests as an up-sloped phase III which some have described as "shark-finned" appearance (C, Obstructive Lung Disease figure).

Any airway obstruction, including obstruction of the endotracheal tube, can result in this waveform. A biphasic capnograph has been previously described but is not specific for endobronchial intubation (B). Regardless, its presence should prompt further investigation.

Capnography has additional utility as a noninvasive cardiac output monitor. Current American Heart Association/Advanced Cardiac Life Support guidelines recommend the use of continuous capnography during cardiopulmonary resuscitation as an assessment for adequacy of cardiopulmonary resuscitation and a sensitive detector for return of spontaneous circulation. A flat capnograph should alert the physician to possible esophageal intubation or inadvertent extubation, as adequate ventilation should produce a waveform (D).

### References

1. Cook TM, Woodall N, Harper J, Benger J. on behalf of the Fourth National Audit Project. Major complications of airway management in the UK: results of the Fourth National Audit Project of the Royal College of Anaesthetists and the Difficult Airway Society. Part 2: intensive care and emergency departments. *BJA Br J Anesth.* 2011;106(5):632-642.
2. Bhavani Shankar Kodali. Capnography outside the operating rooms. *Anesthesiology.* 2013;118(1):192-201.
3. Link MS, Berkow LC, Kudenchuk PJ, et al. Part 7: adult advanced cardiovascular life support: 2015 American Heart Association Guidelines Update for Cardiopulmonary Resuscitation and Emergency Cardiovascular Care. *Circulation.* 2015;132(suppl 2):S444-S464.

**2.** Correct Answer: D

**Rationale:**

High-quality randomized control trials support the use of noninvasive ventilation as a first-line intervention for patients with acute hypercapnic respiratory failure due to exacerbation of COPD. It is associated with decreased mortality and a lower likelihood of invasive ventilation. However, vigilance is required, particularly as failure necessitates intubation. Furthermore, as this is a "nonsecure" ventilation modality, there is a potential risk for gastric aspiration.

For this patient, diagnostic studies such as surface ultrasonography, ABG, chest x-ray (answers A, B, and C) are all reasonable management steps that should be taken, as they can be helpful in narrowing the differential diagnosis. The presence of gastric contents in the pharynx on laryngoscopy does not guarantee aspiration but should raise suspicion. Most aspirated gastric content is liquid and quickly disperses, but in the event of particulate aspiration, bronchoscopy (answer D) could be both diagnostic and therapeutic and should be the next step in management.

### References

1. Osadnik CR, Tee VS, Carson-Chahhoud KV, Picot J, Wedzicha JA, Smith BJ. Non-invasive ventilation for the management of acute hypercapnic respiratory failure due to exacerbation of chronic obstructive pulmonary disease. *Cochrane Database Syst Rev.* 2017;(7):CD004104.
2. Kabadayi S, Bellamy MC. Bronchoscopy in critical care. *BJA Educ.* 2017;17(2):48-56.
3. Raghavendran K, Nemzek J, Napolitano LM, Knight PR. Aspiration-induced lung injury. *Crit Care Med.* 2011;39(4):818-826.

**3.** Correct Answer: A

**Rationale:**

Conventional pulse oximeter determines the ratio of light absorbance at two wavelengths (660 nm-red and 940 nm-infrared) and plots this against direct measurements (arterial oxygen saturation, $SaO_2$) to determine the peripheral oxygen saturation ($SpO_2$). $SpO_2$ generally correlates well with arterial $SaO_2$; however, this relationship can be inaccurate when local tissue perfusion is impaired.

The given clinical context of recent benzocaine use and presence of normal vital signs except $SpO_2$ suggest benzocaine-induced methemoglobinemia. This patient needs to be further evaluated by co-oximetry. In this case, $PaO_2$ will remain normal (answer C) since it measures the oxygen dissolved in blood and methemoglobin affects the oxygen carrying capacity of hemoglobin. However, if the $PaO_2$ were lower, causes for an elevated A-a gradient should be explored (ie, aspiration, bronchospasm, etc.). Mild hypercarbia due to hypoventilation is likely during procedural sedation (answer D). Since this patient's vital signs are stable (after cardioversion), it is reasonable to expect a normal $SpO_2$ waveform, as compared to the poor waveforms seen in low perfusion states (answer B).

### References

1. Jubran A. Pulse oximetry. *Crit Care.* 2015;19(1):272.
2. Hampson NB. Pulse oximetry in severe carbon monoxide poisoning. *Chest.* 1998;114(4):1036-1041.
3. Bozeman WP, Myers RA, Barish RA. Confirmation of the pulse oximetry gap in carbon monoxide poisoning. *Ann Emerg Med.* 1997;30(5):608-611.
4. Louw A, Cracco C, Cerf C, et al. Accuracy of pulse oximetry in the intensive care unit. *Intensive Care Med.* 2001;27:1606.

**4.** Correct Answer: B

**Rationale:**

This patient has a minute ventilation of ~4.5 L, which is inadequate, as the ABG indicates a respiratory acidosis. Since physiologic and anatomic dead space both increase with age, this is not entirely surprising.

The patient has an additional issue—her oxygenation is adequate but suboptimal. A $PaO_2$ of 68 on 50% $FiO_2$ indicates a large A-a gradient. The patient's relatively low Tv (5.3 mL/kg) should raise suspicion of atelectasis from hypoventilation. This could be combated with frequent recruitment maneuvers and increasing PEEP (answers C and D).

However, increasing the tidal volume would increase the minute ventilation and improve atelectasis and is a reasonable first step in management of this patient (answer B). For instance, increasing tidal volume to 400 mL (7 mL/kg ideal body weight) would still be well within the lung protective paradigm while increasing the patient's minute ventilation by 25%.

### References

1. Determann RM, Royakkers A, Wolthuis EK, et al. Ventilation with lower tidal volumes as compared with conventional tidal volumes for patients without acute lung injury: a preventive randomized controlled trial. *Crit Care*. 2010;14(1):R1. doi:10.1186/cc8230.
2. Wrigge H, Pelosi P. Tidal volume in patients with normal lungs during general anesthesia: lower the better? *Anesthesiology*. 2011;114(5):1011-1013.

---

**5. Correct Answer: B**

**Rationale:**

Re-expansion pulmonary edema (RPE) can be a life-threatening complication during thoracentesis for pleural effusion. Some evidence suggests that RPE occurs due to the sudden decrease in pleural pressure. It had been recommended to stop thoracentesis when pleural pressure dropped below −20 cm $H_2O$ (answer C) or when more than 1 L of fluid was removed (answer A). However, various studies have shown that large volume thoracentesis (more than 1 L) can be performed without adverse events, even if the final pleural pressure is below −20 cm $H_2O$. In addition, further investigation show that there is little change in pleural pressure when the patient coughs, so coughing should not be an end point for thoracentesis (answer D). However, chest discomfort is recommended as the point at which thoracentesis would be stopped, due to the potential of development of unsafe negative pressure (answer B).

### References

1. Grabczak EM, Krenke R, Zielinska-Krawczyk M, Light RW. Pleural manometry in patients with pleural diseases – the usefulness in clinical practice. *Respir Med*. 2018. pii:S0954-6111(18)30023-4. doi:10.1016/j.rmed.2018.01.014.
2. Feller-Kopman D, Walkey A, Berkowitz D, Ernst A. The relationship of pleural pressure to symptom development during therapeutic thoracentesis. *Chest*. 2006;129(6):1556-1560.

---

**6. Correct Answer: C**

**Rationale:**

Acute graft rejection after lung transplantation is one of the major causes of early graft loss. There are two mechanisms in which acute rejection could present: acute cellular rejection (ACR) and antibody-mediated rejection (AMR). ACR is the leading cause of acute graft rejection in lung transplant patients. AMR is uncommon due to the extensive cross-matching between the donor and recipient for patients undergoing lung transplantation.

ACR could present with a wide range of symptoms, from asymptomatic, cough, shortness of breath to acute respiratory failure. Pulse steroids are the treatment of choice of ACR (answer C). AMR, on the other hand, can be resistant to steroids, and plasmapheresis might be an effective option.

Primary graft dysfunction (PGD) is another major cause of early morbidity and mortality after lung transplantation. It can present as mild to severe lung injury, and chest x-ray can reveal diffuse allograft infiltrations. Donor risk factors such as smoking history, alcohol use, African American race, female gender, and age are associated with increased risk of PGD. Prevention and treatment of PGD are unclear due to lack of appropriately powered clinical studies. However, lung protective ventilation therapy is recommended. ECMO could be used as salvage therapy for patients that remains hypoxemic despite maximum ventilation support.

Lung transplant patient should remain intubated (answer A) if there is a suspicion of acute rejection, as this process is progressive and may lead to severe respiratory failure. Since this patient is afebrile and on appropriate antimicrobial prophylaxis, the addition of a carbapenem (answer B) would not add any benefit. Increasing $FiO_2$ does not add any clinical benefits to this patient, and may be harmful.

### References

1. Habre C, Soccal PM, Triponez F, et al. Radiological findings of complications after lung transplantation. *Insights Imaging*. 2018. doi:10.1007/s13244-018-0647-9.
2. Potestio C, Jordan D, Kachulis B. Acute postoperative management after lung transplantation. *Best Pract Res Clin Anaesthesiol*. 2017;31(2):273-284.
3. Morrison MI, Pither TL, Fisher AJ. Pathophysiology and classification of primary graft dysfunction after lung transplantation. *J Thorac Dis*. 2017;9(10):4084-4097.

---

**7. Correct Answer: B**

**Rationale:**

Bronchial dehiscence is a feared complication after lung transplantation. Its incidence ranges between 1% and 10% of all lung transplantation. Bronchial arterial circulation is usually not reconstructed during transplant which could lead to bronchial ischemia and dehiscence. Bronchial artery circulation typically reestablished within 4 weeks by collateral formation. Bronchial dehiscence is classified as a partial or complete, and it usually occurs within the first 5 weeks postoperatively. Patients typically present with dyspnea, pneumomediastinum, pneumothorax, persistent chest tube air leak, or subcutaneous emphysema.

Chest CT is highly sensitive and specific for diagnosing bronchial dehiscence. Radiological signs such as bronchial wall defects, bronchial wall irregularities, or extraluminal air around anastomosis area are suggestive for bronchial dehiscence. Although CT scan is an excellent diagnostic modality, flexible bronchoscopy remains essential for making the final diagnosis. CT scan is not reliable for detecting mucosal necrosis as bronchoscopy. Moreover, bronchoscopy is superior to CT scan in assessing the severity of dehiscence. Depending on the severity of bronchial dehiscence, management could include conservative treatment, bronchoscopic or open repair. Conservative treatment includes antibiotics and close monitoring. Bronchoscopic interventions include the use of stents, cyanoacrylate glue, growth factors, and autologous platelet-derived wound-healing factor. Open repair includes reanastomosis, flap bronchoplasty, pneumonectomy, or retransplantation.

Acute rejection (answer A) is in the differential diagnosis for any posttransplant lung transplant patients with shortness of breath; however, CT scan results and physical examination in this patient suggest airway complication rather than rejection. Confirmation of diagnosis and severity assessment should be done by flexible bronchoscopy to guide management (answer B). Serial chest x-ray has no role in confirming or evaluation of the severity of bronchial dehiscence (answer D).

References

1. Habre C, Soccal PM, Triponez F, et al. Radiological findings of complications after lung transplantation. *Insights Imaging.* 2018. doi:10.1007/s13244-018-0647-9.
2. Santacruz JF, Mehta AC. Airway complications and management after lung transplantation: ischemia, dehiscence, and stenosis. *Proc Am Thorac Soc.* 2009;6(1):79-93. doi:10.1513/pats.200808-094GO.
3. Mahajan AK, Folch E, Khandhar SJ, et al. The diagnosis and management of airway complications following lung transplantation. *Chest.* 2017;152:627-638.

---

**8.** Correct Answer: A

**Rationale:**

Venovenous ECMO can be used as salvage therapy in severe acute respiratory distress syndrome (ARDS). The ECMO circuit membrane lung (often called the oxygenator) can provide full gas exchange without relying on the patient lungs. It improves oxygenation by providing prepulmonary oxygen-rich blood and ventilation by removing $CO_2$ with the sweep gas in the membrane lung. When a patient is on full V-V ECMO support, mechanical ventilation strategy should focus on preventing ventilator-induced lung injuries. High PEEP during the early course of V-V ECMO (10-14 cm $H_2O$) is associated with decreased mortality in ARDS patients. The Extracorporeal Life Support Organization (ESLO) recommends placing the patient on pressure controlled ventilation at 25/15, I:E 2:1, rate 5, and $FiO_2$ 50% for the first 24 hours (answer A). After 24 to 48 hours, ELSO recommends reducing the pressure to 20/10, but keeping I:E ratio at 2:1, $FiO_2$ 20% to 40%, rate at 5 and allow for spontaneous breathing.

References

1. Schmidt M, Stewart C, Bailey M, et al. Mechanical ventilation management during extracorporeal membrane oxygenation for acute respiratory distress syndrome: a retrospective international multicenter study. *Crit Care Med.* 2015;43(3):654-664. doi:10.1097/CCM.0000000000000753.
2. Extracorporeal Life Support Organization. *ELSO Guidelines for Adult Respiratory Failure v1.4.* Available at https://www.elso.org/Portals/0/ELSO%20Guidelines%20For%20Adult%20Respiratory%20Failure%201_4.pdf. Accessed October 24, 2018.

---

**9.** Correct Answer: D

**Rationale:**

A biphasic $EtCO_2$ waveform suggests that the patient had undergone single lung transplantation, most likely from severe emphysema. The first peak shows $CO_2$ emptying of an allograft with normal compliance and airway resistance. The second peak reflects the obstruction of the native emphysematous lung. Since the emphysematous lung is more compliant than the donor lung, most of the tidal volume will preferably go to the native lung. As a result, the native lung, which has a severe expiratory obstruction, is prone to hyperinflation and auto-PEEP. Therefore, expiratory time should be allowed as long as possible to allow time to completely empty the native lung (answer D).

Answer A is incorrect because the waveform does not show recovery from muscle relaxation. When the patient recovers from muscle relaxation, a curare cleft will appear in the $EtCO_2$ tracing as shown below:

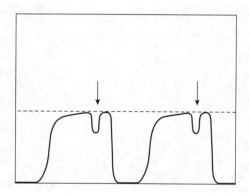

Answer B is incorrect because the patient predicted body weight given his height and gender is around 66 kg. A tidal volume of 600 mL then would be 9 mL/kg IBW. Since we want to use lung protective ventilation, especially in a patient with a history of lung transplant, this tidal volume would be too high.

### References
1. Figure 1. Single Lung Transplant. Available at https://aneskey.com/wp-content/uploads/2017/06/image01049.jpeg.
2. Figure 2. Capnography. Available at https://www.csems.org/wp-content/uploads/2018/04/Capnography.png.
3. Rai HS, Boehm JK, Stoller JK. Biphasic capnogram in a single-lung transplant recipient: a case report. *Respir Care*. 2014;59(8):E108-E109.
4. Barnes L, Reed RM, Parekh KR, et al. Mechanical ventilation for the lung transplant recipient. *Curr Pulmonol Rep*. 2015;4(2):88-96.

**10.** Correct Answer: D

**Rationale:**

Lung sliding sign is a created by the movement of visceral pleura on parietal pleura. The presence of lung sliding suggests that visceral and parietal pleurae are opposing, which excludes pneumothorax. The absence of lung sliding alone, however, does not diagnose pneumothorax. It has to be accompanied by the presence of lung point and absence of B-lines and lung pulse.

B-lines originate from visceral pleura, and their presence indicates that parietal and visceral pleurae are in contact and excludes pneumothorax. Lung pulse was described by Lichtenstein et al. as a sign of mainstem intubation. A completely atelectatic lung transmits the rhythmic movement of the heart to the pleura. An opposed parietal and visceral pleurae are required to transfer the heart pulses; hence, the presence of lung pulse excludes pneumothorax.

Neuromuscular blockade can help patient-ventilator synchrony. However, this is not the reason for this patient's acute hypoxemia.

### References
1. Lichtenstein DA, Lascols NPrin SMezière G. The "lung pulse": an early ultrasound sign of complete atelectasis. *Intensive Care Med*. 2003;29(12):2187-2192. doi:10.1007/s00134-003-1930-9.
2. Volpicelli G. Sonographic diagnosis of pneumothorax. *Intensive Care Med*. 2011;37(2):224-232.
3. Volpicelli G, Elbarbary M, Blaivas M, et al. International evidence-based recommendations for point-of-care lung ultrasound. *Intensive Care Med*. 2012;38:577-591.
4. Lichtenstein DA. BLUE-protocol and FALLS-protocol: two applications of lung ultrasound in the critically ill. *Chest*. 2015;147(6):1659-1670.

**11.** Correct Answer: A

**Rationale:**

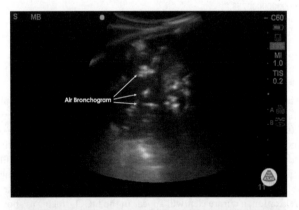

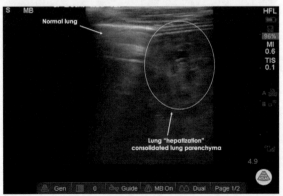

Based on the ultrasound images, this patient likely has pneumonia (answer A). The negative auscultation findings and negative chest x-ray cannot rule out pneumonia due to their low accuracy and negative predictive values. Moreover, chest x-ray diagnostic accuracy for pneumonia has been questioned. Bourcier et al. showed that chest x-ray has low sensitivity in diagnosing pneumonia when compared to lung ultrasound (95 vs. 60%).

Multiple sonographic signs were described in the literature to assist in the diagnosis of pneumonia. These signs include b-lines, air bronchograms, subpleural consolidations "hepatization," pleural line abnormalities, and pleural effusions. Air bronchograms and subpleural consolidations "hepatization" are the most specific sonographic signs. Air bronchograms are thought to be caused by air trapped in small airways within a consolidated lung. On ultrasound, it will look like hyperechoic dots and lines (air) within a hypoechoic (fluid) area (Figure 1). Subpleural consolidations, which also known as "hepatization," is a sonographic sign of consolidated lung. Typically, the lung parenchyma is not visible on ultrasound since air does not conduct sound waves, but when small airways and alveoli get filled by purulent fluid, sound waves will be able to go through the lung parenchyma. Sonographically, consolidated lungs will have the echotexture of the liver, hence the name hepatization of lungs.

Answers C and D are both incorrect because the patient does not have sonographic signs suggesting pleural edema or effusion. Pulmonary embolism can cause peripheral lung parenchyma infarction, which sonographically appears like consolidation. The presence of air bronchograms, on the other hand, is pathognomonic of pneumonia.

### References

1. Metlay JP, Kapoor WN, Fine MJ. Does this patient have community-acquired pneumonia? Diagnosing pneumonia by history and physical examination. *JAMA*. 1997;278:1440-1445.
2. Bourcier JE, Paquet J, Seinger M, et al. Performance comparison of lung ultrasound and chest x-ray for the diagnosis of pneumonia in the ED. *Am J Emerg Med*. 2014;32(2):115-118.
3. Ticinesi A, Lauretani F, Nouvenne A, et al. Lung ultrasound and chest x-ray for detecting pneumonia in an acute geriatric ward. *Medicine*. 2016;95:e4153.
4. Blaivas M. Lung ultrasound in evaluation of pneumonia. *J Ultrasound Med*. 2012;31(6):823-826.
5. Figure 1. The POCUS Atlas. Available at http://www.thepocusatlas.com/pulmonary-1/ohidf6dvg076d2jzmel6c733cs2y5w. Accessed November 1, 2018.
6. Figure 2. The POCUS Atlas. Available at http://www.thepocusatlas.com/pulmonary-1/7z96r1evhnr2eyjwagn2e8o8jacqbh. Accessed November 1, 2018.

---

**12.** Correct Answer: C

**Rationale:**

Transpulmonary pressure is defined as the difference between alveolar pressure and pleural pressure.

Alveolar pressure (at end inspiration) is the driving pressure plus PEEP (here, 10 cm $H_2O$ + 10 cm $H_2O$ = 20 cm $H_2O$).

The pressure measured by the esophageal balloon is a surrogate for the intrapleural pressure and is measured at −12 cm $H_2O$ for this patient. Therefore, the estimated transpulmonary pressure is 32 cm $H_2O$. Elevated transpulmonary pressures increase the strain on the lung and worsened lung injury. It is important for clinicians to consider the impact of the pleural pressure on the transpulmonary pressures to identify patients at risk for worsening lung injury and to institute better ventilation strategies.

### References

1. Schmidt UH, Hess DR. Does spontaneous breathing produce harm in patients with the acute respiratory distress syndrome? *Respir Care*. 2010;55(6):784-786.
2. Kassis EB, Loring SH, Talmor D. Mortality and pulmonary mechanics in relation to respiratory system and transpulmonary driving pressures in ARDS. *Intensive Care Med*. 2016;42(8):1206-1213.

---

**13.** Correct Answer: D

**Rationale:**

Morbid obese patients have a marked reduction in functional residual capacity mainly due to a reduction in expiratory reserve volume. The diaphragm is displaced upward decreasing lung and chest wall compliance. In contrast to supine position, both beach chair and reversed Trendelenburg positions increase functional residual capacity as well as spontaneous tidal volume. However, there is a larger increase seen in reversed Trendelenburg position. This is potentially because the lower leg position exerts less upward pressure on the abdomen and diaphragm. Hence, in morbidly obese individuals, it is recommended to perform spontaneous breathing trial, extubation, and preoxygenation in reverse Trendelenburg position.

### Reference

1. Couture EJ, Provencher S, Somma J, Lellouche F, Marceau S, Bussières JS. Effect of position and positive pressure ventilation on functional residual capacity in morbidly obese patients: a randomized trial. *Can J Anesth*. 2018;65(5):522-528.

**14.** Correct Answer: B

**Rationale:**

The patient is acutely hypoxic, and invasive mechanical ventilation seems to be the safest option. While noninvasive ventilation has a role in management of respiratory failure in the morbid obese population its use in acute hypoxic respiratory failure is limited. Given that the patient is already hypoxemic, an awake fiberoptic intubation would be not easily tolerated and likely result in further potentially dangerous hypoxemia. Morbid obese critically ill patients desaturate quickly during airway manipulation due to limited reserve. Rapid-sequence induction followed by intubation via direct laryngoscopy is the fastest way to secure the airway and hence the safest. In this patient, previous record of intubation without difficulty is further reassuring. However, fiberoptic intubation and video laryngoscopy are important backup options in this patient, if direct laryngoscopy fails.

Reference

1. Andersen LH, Rovsing L, Olsen KS. GlideScope videolaryngoscope versus Macintosh direct laryngoscope for intubation of morbidly obese patients: a randomized trial. Acta Anaesthesiol Scand. 2011;55:1090-1097.

**15.** Correct Answer: B

**Rationale:**

Generally, clinicians set a lower PEEP than what was used during a recruitment maneuver. This becomes more important in obese individuals where the transpulmonary pressure is higher. It has been shown that measurement of transpulmonary pressures by esophageal balloon following a recruitment maneuver lead to same PEEP settings as after a decremental PEEP trial. In obese patients, the latter strategies had no negative hemodynamic effects but improved lung mechanics as well as oxygenation significantly.

References

1. Pirrone M, Fisher D, Chipman D, et al. Recruitment maneuvers and positive end-expiratory pressure titration in morbidly obese ICU patients. Crit Care Med. 2016;44(2):300-307.
2. Goligher EC, Hodgson CL, Adhikari NK, et al. Lung recruitment maneuvers for adult patients with acute respiratory distress syndrome. A systematic review and meta-analysis. Ann Am Thorac Soc. 2017;14(suppl 4):S304-S311.

# RENAL, ELECTROLYTE AND ACID BASE DISORDERS

# 44

# ACUTE RENAL FAILURE

Qasim AlHassan, Madiha Syed, and Roshni Sreedharan

1. A 62-year-old male presents to the hospital complaining of nonradiating back pain for the past 2 days. He has a past medical history of hypertension, hyperlipidemia, and chronic back pain for which he takes ibuprofen, atorvastatin, and hydrochlorothiazide. He mentions that he tried to take a few extra doses of analgesics which did not seem to help, and it seems like his regular water pill is not working either. His vitals and laboratory work are as follows

   Heart rate (HR) 110 bpm, respiratory rate (RR) 18/min, blood pressure (BP) 95/54 mm Hg, SpO$_2$ 98%, and temp 37.3°C.
   WBC 5.08 k/μL, hemoglobin (Hb) 14 g/dL, hematocrit (Hct) 37%, and platelet (Plt) count 290 k/μL.
   Sodium (Na) 143 mmol/L, potassium (K) 4.3 mmol/L, CO 18 mmol/L, chloride (Cl) 109 mmol/L, BUN 30 mg/dL, and serum creatinine (Scr) 2.0 mg/dL. Anion gap is 16 mmol/L.

   Which of the following etiologies for acute renal injury (AKI) should **ALWAYS** be excluded first?

   **A.** Dehydration
   **B.** Nonsteroidal anti-inflammatory overdose
   **C.** Septic shock
   **D.** Chronic anemia

2. A 35-year-old obese female with a past medical history of type 2 diabetes, chronic kidney disease (CKD) stage 3, chronic obstructive pulmonary disease (COPD), and deep vein thrombosis (DVT) is brought to the emergency room with acute-onset shortness of breath. She is on home oxygen for the COPD, warfarin, and subcutaneous insulin therapy. Her chest x-ray reveals hyperinflated lung fields, and CT angiogram did NOT reveal pulmonary embolism (PE). She was admitted and treated for COPD exacerbation. Serum creatinine is noticed to have increased to 2.6/dL from a baseline of 1.3 mg/dL with concern for contrast-induced acute kidney injury (CI-AKI). Which of the following strategies is **MOST** likely to prevent CI-AKI?

   **A.** Use of isotonic saline infusion before and after CT angiogram
   **B.** Use of a lower-osmolality, lower-viscosity contrast agent
   **C.** Use of V/Q scan to rule out PE
   **D.** Use of N-acetyl cysteine (NAC) before and after the angiogram

3. A healthy 24-year-old male is admitted to the intensive care unit (ICU) for AKI and hyperkalemia. History is remarkable for a recent episode of sinusitis for which amoxicillin-clavulanate therapy was initiated. Physical examination is notable for a temperature of 37.6°C, skin rashes, and joint pain. Urine microscopy shows a few RBC's and eosinophils. Laboratory results are given below

   WBC 12.5 k/μL, Hb 14.3 g/dL, Hct 38%, Plt 256 k/μL, and eosinophilia.
   Na 137 mmol/L, K 5.7 mmol/L, Cl 106 mmol/L, CO 22 mmol/L, BUN 18 mg/dL, Scr 2.3 mg/dL, and glucose 176 mg/dL.

   What is the MOST appropriate next step in the management of this patient?

    A. Add amikacin
    B. Discontinue amoxicillin-clavulanate
    C. Add vancomycin
    D. Send patient for kidney biopsy

**4.** A 33-year-old muscular male is brought to emergency room after being rescued from under a collapsed concrete building. Physical examination reveals multiple lower extremity bone fractures and skin lacerations. CT scan is negative for traumatic brain injury. Vitals and laboratory parameters are as follows

HR 110 bpm, BP 100/65 mm Hg, RR 20/min, $SpO_2$ 96%, and temp 37.5°C.
Hb 10 g/dL, Na 143 meq/L, K 4.0 meq/L, Cl 109 meq/L, creatine kinase (CK) 15 000 units/L.
He has received a liter of lactated ringers so far. His urine output is dark brown and only 10 mL for the past hour.

Which of the following is the next **BEST** step in the management of this patient?

    A. Administer 40 mg of furosemide
    B. Administer 1 g/kg of mannitol
    C. Administer 1 L of normal saline (0.9% NS)
    D. Administer 50 meq of sodium bicarbonate

**5.** Which of the following statements is **MOST ACCURATE** regarding the pathophysiology behind bilateral *obstructive nephropathy*?

    A. Glomerular filtration rate (GFR) is increased by increasing renal blood flow and decrease in tubular hydrostatic pressure.
    B. Sodium excretion is partially stimulated after relief of obstruction due to upregulation of atrial natriuretic peptide.
    C. Arterial blood gas will demonstrate a hypokalemic, metabolic alkalosis.
    D. Renal ultrasound is NOT a useful screening tool for obstructive uropathy due to low specificity.

**6.** A 65-year-old male admitted to the ICU with septic shock and develops nonoliguric AKI. Urinary microscopy reveals muddy brown, granular, and epithelial cell casts. Serum creatinine does not improve with fluid resuscitation. Which of the following sets of laboratory parameters is **MOST** consistent with a diagnosis of acute tubular necrosis?

|   | $FE_{NA}$ (%) | URINE OSMOLALITY (MOSMOL/KG) | URINE NA (MEQ/L) | BUN/SCR RATIO (MG/DL) * |
|---|---|---|---|---|
| A | 1.2 | 500 | 30 | 15/1 |
| B | 0.8 | 600 | 10 | 20/1 |
| C | 0.9 | 300 | 15 | 20/1 |
| D | 2.4 | 350 | 60 | 15/1 |

$FE_{Na}$ *fractional excretion of sodium; Scr, serum creatinine.*

**7.** A 42-year-old female presents with acute oliguric renal failure 3 days after initiation of chemotherapy for newly diagnosed non-Hodgkin lymphoma. Urine sediment analysis demonstrates amber crystals shaped like hexagonal plates, barrels, and needles.

Which of the following therapies is **LEAST** likely to be beneficial in the prophylaxis and management of this nephropathy?

    A. Rasburicase
    B. Aggressive intravenous hydration
    C. Allopurinol
    D. Sodium bicarbonate

**8.** A 33-year-old male underwent a necrosectomy for necrotizing pancreatitis 4 days ago. For the past 2 days, he has been complaining of watery diarrhea. He has not noticed any blood in his stool. Laboratory parameters are as follows

Na 142 mmol/L, Cl 118 mmol/L, K 3.1 mmol/L, $CO_2$ 15 mmol, BUN 25 mg/dL, Scr 1.03 mg/dL, and glucose 130 mg/dL.

pH 7.25, $PCO_2$ 32 mm Hg, $PO_2$ 110 mm Hg, $HCO_3$ 15 mmol/L, and base excess—4.

Which of the following findings in this patient would be MOST consistent with metabolic acidosis attributed to diarrhea?

A. Hypokalemia and positive value of urine anion gap (UAG)
B. Hyperchloremia and negative value of UAG
C. Hyperchloremia and positive value of UAG
D. Hyperkalemia and negative value of UAG

9. A 38-year-old male with multiple enterocutaneous fistulae and chronic malnutrition on total parenteral nutrition (TPN) is admitted to the ICU with lethargy and hypotension. His medical history is significant for Crohn disease requiring multiple bowel surgeries. Soon after arrival in the ICU, he starts seizing and exhibits tetany.

Which of the following electrolyte abnormalities is MOST consistent with this presentation?

A. Hypophosphatemia
B. Hypomagnesemia
C. Hyperkalemia
D. Hyperphosphatemia

10. A 19-year-old female was on a hiking trip with her friends who brought her to the emergency room with lethargy. The only significant medical history she mentions is that she has diabetes and problems with her thyroid. Other than hypotension, the rest of her physical examination is unrevealing.

Which of the following clinical profiles is MOST consistent with a diagnosis of adrenal insufficiency in this patient?

A. Hypotension that is responsive to fluid resuscitation
B. Hypernatremia and excessive urine output
C. Refractory hyponatremia and hyperkalemia
D. Hypokalemia and hypocalcaemia

# Chapter 44 ▪ Answers

1. Correct Answer: A

**Rationale:**
Renal blood flow constitutes 20% of cardiac output. A large part of the renal perfusion (80%-90%) goes to renal cortex where glomerular filtration occurs. Prerenal azotemia as a consequence of reduction in renal perfusion, accounts for approximately 70% of the community-acquired and 40% of hospital-acquired cases of AKI. As this is a reversible process, most of the time, once the underlying inciting process is addressed, prerenal etiology (eg, vomiting, dehydration, and hemorrhage) should be excluded in all cases of AKI.

The renin-angiotensin-aldosterone system (RAAS) becomes activated secondary to a decrease in renal blood flow with subsequent increase in sodium reabsorption at the level of the proximal and distal tubule induced by angiotension II and aldosterone, respectively. As a result, the urine sodium concentration is less than 20 mmol/L and fractional excretion of sodium ($FE_{Na}$) is less than 1%. Medications like nonsteroidal anti-inflammatory drugs (NSAIDs) or RAAS inhibitors which interfere with the renal autoregulatory mechanisms could worsen prerenal azotemia, which seems likely in this patient.

Patients with NSAID overdose typically present with a wide spectrum of gastrointestinal symptoms, altered mental status, and arterial blood gas consistent with an anion gap metabolic acidosis. C and D are unlikely due to lack of neurological symptoms and patient not being in shock, respectively. *Prerenal etiology should be excluded in all cases of AKI due to its reversible nature in the majority of cases.*

Reference
1. Elhassan E, Schrier R. Acute kidney injury. In: Vincent JL, Abraham E, Moore FA, Kochanek PM, Fink MP, eds. *Chapter 109: Textbook of Critical Care.* 7th ed. 773-783.

**2.** Correct Answer: C

**Rationale:**

CI-AKI is the most common iatrogenic cause of AKI. The incidence is reported to be as high as 20% to 30% in patients with preexisting renal dysfunction. The most effective method of preventing CI-AKI is avoidance of iodinated contrast unless absolutely indicated, especially in patients with compromised kidney function.

Reduction in renal blood flow, tubular cell damage, and tubular obstruction are implicated in the pathogenesis of CI-AKI. Therefore, volume expansion with normal saline has been used extensively with the goal of improving medullary blood flow, diluting the contrast agent in the tubule, and increasing urinary flow. Low-osmolality contrast agents are less toxic to the kidneys as compared to high-osmolality agents.

Although NAC has antioxidant and anti-inflammatory properties and proposed to have a beneficial role in the prevention of CI-AKI, the largest trial on this subject did not confirm this. *The most effective method of preventing CI-AKI is avoiding studies requiring IV contrast administration.*

References

1. Akbari A, Hiremath S. Contrast-induced acute kidney injury. In: Vincent JL, Abraham E, Moore FA, Kochanek PM, Fink MP, eds. *Chapter 111: Textbook of Critical Care.* 7th ed. 790-793.
2. ACT investigators. Acetyl cysteine for prevention of renal outcomes in patients undergoing coronary and peripheral vascular angiography: main results from randomized acetyl cysteine for contrast-induced nephropathy trial (ACT). *Circulation.* 2011;124(11):1250-1259.

**3.** Correct Answer: B

**Rationale:**

Acute interstitial nephritis (AIN) is an important cause of AKI characterized by inflammation of the renal interstitium and tubules. AIN results from a hypersensitivity reaction, most commonly induced by medications, infections, and autoimmune disorders. Common offending agents are antibiotics (penicillins, cephalosporins, sulfonamides, ciprofloxacin, and rifampin), anticonvulsants (phenytoin, carbamazepine, phenobarbital, valproate), diuretics (thiazides, loop diuretics, triamterene), NSAIDs, and proton pump inhibitors. Medications account for over two-thirds of all the AIN cases. Patients with AIN could present with sterile pyuria, hematuria, eosinophilia, and fever. The majority of the patients have complete recovery of renal function.

It is important to differentiate AIN from acute tubular necrosis (ATN). The diagnosis of AIN is difficult as symptoms could mimic infection. Sterile pyuria and eosinophiluria could suggest the diagnosis.

Removal of the offending agent is the most important component of AIN treatment. Treatment is largely supportive with use of renal replacement therapy as needed. Corticosteroid therapy in these patients is controversial. *Discontinuation of the inciting agent is the cornerstone of treatment of acute interstitial nephritis.*

References

1. Burgardt S, Sanghani V, Falk R, Hladik G. Acute interstitial nephritis. In: Vincent JL, Abraham E, Moore FA, Kochanek PM, Fink MP, eds. *Chapter 113: Textbook of Critical Care.* 7th ed. 799-801.
2. Clarkson MR, Giblin L, O'Connell PF, et al. Acute interstitial nephritis: clinical features and response to corticosteroid therapy. *Nephrol Dial Transplant.* 2004;19:2778-2783. PMID:15340098.

**4.** Correct Answer: C

**Rationale:**

Patients with rhabdomyolysis-induced AKI present with an elevated CK and reddish brown urine with absent erythrocytes on microscopic examination. They could have associated electrolyte abnormalities including hyperkalemia, hyperphosphatemia, and hypocalcemia. Early aggressive intravascular volume expansion is the most important measure to prevent worsening AKI from rhabdomyolysis. The goal is to enhance renal perfusion and flush the renal tubules off obstructing casts.

Fluid repletion is continued until the plasma CK level is stable and maintained <5000 units/L. The Renal Disaster Relief Task Force (RDRTF) of the International Society of Nephrology (ISN) recommends use of isotonic solution due to its ready availability and equivalent efficacy at volume expansion compared to sodium bicarbonate. Despite the theoretical benefits of using sodium bicarbonate in severe rhabdomyolysis, there is no concrete evidence that suggests that alkaline diuresis is more effective than saline diuresis in preventing AKI.

References

1. Better OS, Stein JH. Early management of shock and prophylaxis of acute renal failure in traumatic rhabdomyolysis. *N engl J Med.* 1990;322(12):825. PMID:2407958.
2. Vanholder R, Sever M, Erek E, Lameire N. Rhabdomyolysis. *J Am Soc Nephrol.* 2000;11(8):1553-1561.
3. Sever MS, Vanholder R, Lameire N. Management of crush-related injuries after disasters. *N Engl J Med.* 2006;354(10):1052.
4. Huerta-Alardin AL, Varon J, Marik PE. Bench-to-bedside review: rhabdomyolysis-an overview for clinicians. *Crit Care.* 2005;9(2):158. Epub 2004 Oct 20.

**5.** Correct Answer: B

**Rationale:**

Often renal sodium excretion increases after relief of the obstruction. Two mechanisms that could potentially contribute to this include the downregulation of the apical membrane transporters and an upregulation of atrial natriuretic peptide. In patients with obstructive uropathy, reduction in GFR occurs due to an increase in tubular hydrostatic pressure, which alters the balance between the glomerular capillaries and the renal tubules. The hyperkalemia and metabolic acidosis in these patients are most likely a reflection of a reduced GFR and renal function. Ultrasound is utilized as a good screening tool for patients with new-onset or unexplained AKI to rule out urinary tract obstruction as a potential etiology.

References

1. Montford J, Teitelbaum I, Liebman S. Urinary tract obstruction. In: Vincent JL, Abraham E, Moore FA, Kochanek PM, Fink MP, eds. *Chapter 110: Textbook of Critical Care.* 7th ed. 790-793.
2. Mourmouris P, Chiras T. Obstructive uropathy: from etiopathology to therapy. *World J Nephrol Urol.* 2014;3(1):1-6.

**6.** Correct Answer: D

**Rationale:**

There are three major diagnostic approaches that are used to distinguish prerenal disease from ATN:

1. Urinalysis: Urinalysis with sediment examination is typically normal in prerenal disease. In patients with ATN, muddy brown, granular, and epithelial cell casts are seen. Although these findings are common in ATN, they do not always indicate the presence of ATN, and conversely, their absence does not exclude ATN.

2. Fractional excretion of sodium ($FE_{Na}$): Kidneys with intact tubular function tend to conserve the sodium resulting in a low urine sodium concentration (<20 mEq/L). This is seen with the prerenal etiologies. Tubular function is impaired in ATN leading to high urine sodium concentrations (>40-50 mEq/L) as a result of defective reabsorption. $FE_{Na}$ is not affected by urine volume and is valuable in the evaluation of AKI. $FE_{Na}$ is typically <1% in prerenal disease and greater than 2% in patients with ATN.

3. Response to fluid resuscitation: Response to fluid repletion is helpful to differentiate between prerenal from intrinsic renal disease. Return of the serum creatinine to previous baseline within 24 to 72 hours with fluid resuscitation most likely indicates prerenal disease, whereas persistence of AKI is most likely indicative of ATN.

References

1. Miller TR, Anderson RJ, Linas SL, et al. Urinary diagnostic indices in acute renal failure. *Ann Intern Med.* 1978;89(1):47. PMID:666184.
2. Espinel CH, Gregory AW. Differential diagnosis of acute renal failure. *Clin Nephrol.* 1980;13(2):73. PMID:7363517.
3. Perazella MA, Coca SG, Kanbay M, Brewster UC, Parikh CR. Diagnostic value of urine microscopy for differential diagnosis of acute kidney injury in hospitalized patients. *Clin J Am Soc Nephrol.* 2008;3(6):1615. Epub 2008 Sep 10. PMID:18784207.
4. Steiner RW. Interpreting the fractional excretion of sodium. *Am J Med.* 1984;77(4):699. PMID:6486145.

**7.** Correct Answer: D

**Rationale:**

This patient most likely has tumor lysis syndrome (TLS) and AKI as a consequence. Uric acid precipitation in the renal tubules results in AKI in patients with acute urate nephropathy. This could occur due to overproduction and excretion of the excess uric acid, particularly after chemotherapy or radiation in patients with lymphoma, leukemia, or other myeloproliferative diseases. That being said, patients with a large tumor burden could present with spontaneous TLS, without antecedent chemotherapy.

Uric acid nephrolithiasis may manifest with flank pain if there is renal pelvic or ureteral obstruction. The diagnosis should be suspected in presence of acute renal failure in patients at high risk for TLS (increased tumor burden, volume depletion, preexisting CKD, and hyperuricemia).

Uric acid nephropathy is associated with a marked hyperuricemia, with plasma urate levels >15 mg/dL. Urinalysis may show uric acid crystals.

Prophylaxis in patients at high risk for TLS involves the use of allopurinol or febuxostat (xanthine oxidase inhibitors) along with rasburicase (recombinant urase oxidase that catalyzes conversion of uric acid to allantoin). The cornerstone of treatment of TLS and urate nephropathy is aggressive intravenous hydration to ensure adequate renal blood flow and glomerular filtration. Volume expansion has shown to delay and reduce the need for renal replacement therapy in these patients.

Sodium bicarbonate infusion and alkalization of urine could reduce solubility and increase the risk of calcium phosphate precipitation. Further rise in serum pH with bicarbonate infusion could result in exacerbation in hypocalcemia. For these reasons, urinary alkalinization is not recommended in this setting.

References

1. Cosmai L, Porta C, Ronco C, Gallieni M. Acute kidney injury in oncology and tumor lysis syndrome. Chapter 41. *Crit Care Nephrol*:234-250.
2. Coiffier B, Altman A, Pui CH, Younes A, Cairo MS. Guidelines for the management of pediatric and adult tumor lysis syndrome: an evidence-based review. *J Clin Oncol.* 2008;26(16):2767. PMID:18509186.

**8.** Correct Answer: B

**Rationale:**

This patient has hyperchloremic, nonanion gap metabolic acidosis due to excessive GI bicarbonate loss consequent to diarrhea. The response of the kidneys in this case is to reabsorb the chloride instead of bicarbonate, yielding no net change in the serum anion gap (AG).

Measurement of serum anion gap helps deduce the etiology for metabolic acidosis. Serum AG represents the difference in the measured cations (mainly sodium) and anions (chloride and bicarbonate). Serum AG is usually around $12 \pm 4$ mEq/L but can vary depending on the laboratory.

Hyperchloremic metabolic acidosis could result from impaired renal acid excretion, bicarbonate loss, or administration of chloride-rich solutions during resuscitation.

UAG is the difference between measured urine cations and anions (UAG = Na + K − Cl) and helps differentiate renal causes of non–anion gap acidosis from the gastrointestinal causes.

Normally, the sum of the excreted urine sodium and urine potassium is greater than the amount of excreted urine chloride resulting in a positive UAG. With diarrhea and other nonrenal causes of hyperchloremic acidosis, the kidneys compensate by increasing the net acid excretion. The excretion of ammonium occurs in conjunction with chloride. In such situations, urine chloride exceeds the sum of urine sodium and potassium, resulting in a negative UAG. *Urine AG is a useful tool to differentiate renal from GI causes in hyperchloremic metabolic acidosis.*

References

1. Tolwani A, Saha M, Wille K. Metabolic acidosis and alkalosis. In: Vincent JL, Abraham E, Moore FA, Kochanek PM, Fink MP, eds. *Chapter 104: Textbook of Critical Care.* 7th ed. 726-742.
2. Gennari J, Weise W. Acid base disturbances in gastrointestinal disease. *Clin J Am Soc Nephrol.* 2008;3(6):1861-1868.

**9.** Correct Answer: B

**Rationale:**

Hypomagnesemia is a common in critically ill patients. Magnesium plays an important role in several vital biochemical and physiological functions of the body including neuromuscular and cardiac conduction, maintenance of cardiac contractility, and vascular tone.

Hypomagnesemia could result from either gastrointestinal (GI) or renal losses. GI causes include diarrhea, intestinal fistulae, and malabsorption syndromes. Renal causes include chronic parenteral fluid therapy, osmotic diuretics, and chronic alcohol consumption. It is important to note that several medications including diuretics, antibiotics, and immunosuppressants can lead to hypomagnesemia through renal mechanisms

Intracellular magnesium depletion has potential to cause atrial and ventricular arrhythmias, impaired cardiac contractility, and vasoconstriction. Nervous system manifestations include hyperactivity, tremors, and tetany with a positive chvostek sign. Severe hypomagnesemia could result in altered mental status and seizures. *Magnesium depletion can present with neuromuscular symptoms that are similar to those of calcium deficiency, including hyperactive reflexes, muscle tremors, and tetany.*

References

1. Hansen B, Bruserud O. Hypomagnesemia in critically ill patients. *J Intensive Care.* 2018;6:21.
2. Vincent JL, Abraham E, Moore FA, Kochanek PM, Fink MP. *Textbook of Critical Care.* 7th ed.

**10.** Correct Answer: C

**Rationale:**

Patients with type 2 polyendocrine syndrome could present with type 1 diabetes, thyroid autoimmunity, and adrenal insufficiency. Hyponatremia and hyperkalemia are commonly seen in patients with adrenal insufficiency due to diminished cortisol and aldosterone production.

Aldosterone enhances sodium reabsorption and increases urinary potassium secretion. The hyperkalemia that is seen in adrenal insufficiency is largely related to the aldosterone deficiency. Cortisol has a direct suppressive effect on antidiuretic hormone (ADH) secretion, and a deficiency of cortisol results in hyponatremia due to the effect of increased ADH.

Treatment of hyponatremia in adrenal insufficiency requires cortisol and volume repletion. The administration of saline alone is relatively ineffective as the water retention due to ADH persists if cortisol is not supplemented. Cortisol replacement with hydrocortisone helps with the potassium excretion through its mineralocorticoid activity. Hypoaldosteronism should be considered in patients with persistent hyperkalemia accompanied by hyponatremia.

References

1. Eisenbarth GS, Gottlieb PA. Autoimmune polyendocrine syndromes. *N Engl J Med.* 2004;350:2068.
2. Quinkler M, Oelkers W, Remde H, Allolio B. Mineralocorticoid substitution and monitoring in primary adrenal insufficiency. *Best Pract Res Clin Endocrinol Metab.* 2015;29:17.

# 45

# OLIGURIA AND POLYURIA

Abdulaziz S. Almehlisi, Phat Tan Dang, Ji Sun "Christina" Baek, Anushirvan Minokadeh, Alan S. Nova, Zeb McMillan, Kimberly S. Robbins, and Ulrich Schmidt

1. A previously healthy 18-year-old woman presents to the emergency department 4 hours ago with headache and photophobia. Her parents state that her symptoms began as a mild fever and headache, and today, she appears to be a bit confused and has been urinating a lot. On physical examination, she is alert and oriented but slow to answer questions. There are no focal neurological signs. Her labs reveal elevated leukocytosis and hypernatremia. Blood cultures were sent. What is the next **BEST** step in management?

   A. Start broad-spectrum antibiotics
   B. Obtain urine sodium, chloride, creatinine, and osmolality
   C. Obtain spinal fluid sample
   D. Obtain CT scan of head

2. A 45-year-old man is admitted for urgent laparoscopic cholecystectomy for severe cholecystitis. His medical history was significant for chronic kidney disease and moderate to severe pulmonary hypertension which is being treated with continuous epoprostenol infusion at home. Intraoperative transesophageal echocardiogram showed depressed right ventricular systolic function. Intraoperative course was complicated by blood loss, requiring 2 units of packed red blood cells and 500 mL of lactated ringer. Postoperatively, he remained sedated and intubated and transferred to the intensive care unit (ICU) for close monitoring. His home-dose IV epoprostenol was continued intraoperatively and in the ICU. During his first postoperative day, he made minimal urine. Oxygen saturation is 100%, and estimated pulmonary artery pressure is at baseline, however, central venous pressure has increased.

   Which of the following is the next **BEST** step in management?

   A. Repeat transesophageal echocardiogram to reassess the right ventricular function
   B. Obtain a nephrology consult to start continuous renal replacement therapy
   C. Switch intravenous epoprostenol to inhaled epoprostenol
   D. Administer a bolus of albumin in to improve the urine output

3. A 62-year-old woman with medical history of hypertension and smoking presents to the hospital after sudden onset of severe headache followed by collapse. In the emergency department, CT scan of the head showed diffuse subarachnoid hemorrhage and CT angiogram revealed a left middle cerebral artery aneurysm. An extraventricular drain is placed by neurosurgery team. On day 7 of hospitalization, the patient develops new aphasia. The urine output has been 1800 mL in the past 3 hours, while the serum sodium has decreased from 138 to 132 mmol/L.

   What is the best next step in management to address this high urine output?

   A. Start fluid restriction and continue to monitor the sodium every 6 hours
   B. Aggressively replace volume deficit by giving bolus of 2 L of 0.9% normal saline and recheck sodium after the bolus
   C. Start fludrocortisone and salt tablets
   D. Stop maintenance intravenous fluids and give 250 mL of 3% hypertonic saline, recheck sodium level after administration
   E. Continue administration of intravenous normal saline for maintenance and to replete urine output. Give a 250 mL bolus of 3% hypertonic saline

4. A 52-year-old man with history of bipolar disorder and headaches is admitted for elective pituitary macroadenoma resection in the early morning. Following the otherwise uncomplicated neurosurgical procedure, he is admitted to the ICU for postoperative observation. You receive a call near midnight reporting that urine output has increased to 1000 mL in the past 3 hours while serum sodium increased from 142 to 146 mmol/L.

What are the next steps you should take to prevent worsening of hypernatremia?

A. Start maintenance fluids with dextrose 5% in water until sodium level returns to baseline
B. Ask for the value of urine specific gravity and if <1.005, administer a dose of desmopressin while asking patient to drink to thirst
C. Increase rate of maintenance IV fluids with 0.9% normal saline
D. Institute fluid restriction to 1.5 L/d and recheck sodium in the morning before rounds
E. Call neurosurgery and ask if 3% hypertonic saline was given intraoperatively

5. A 75 kg, 70-year-old male with a history of hypertension, coronary artery disease, and benign prostatic hypertrophy gets admitted to the ICU after a partial colectomy and liver resection for colon cancer. Placement of indwelling urinary catheter placement was challenging due to his enlarged prostate causing some hematuria. The operative procedure was complicated by bleeding, requiring 4 units of packed red blood cell transfusion. Postoperative hemoglobin was 8.2 g/dL.

His vitals on admission at noon are heart rate 75 beats/min, blood pressure 120/68 mm Hg, respiratory rate 20 breaths/min, and $SpO_2$ 100% on 4 L oxygen via nasal cannula. Over the next 12 hours, his abdominal drain produced 700 mL of sanguineous output and his urine output decreases from 80 mL/h in immediate postoperative period to 20, 10, and 5 mL, respectively, in the last 3 consecutive hours. His vitals 12 hours after admission are now heart rate 105 beats/min, blood pressure 85/50 mm Hg, respiratory rate 20 breaths/min, and $SpO_2$ 100% on 2 L oxygen via nasal cannula. Which of the following would be **LEAST** likely in this patient?

A. A serum BUN:Cr ratio of 10:1
B. Fractional excretion of sodium ($FE_{Na}$) >3%
C. High urine specific gravity
D. RBC casts on urine microscopy

6. The patient continues to have persistent blood drainage from his abdominal drain overnight. He stops making urine for last 6 hours, which was not identified until morning. In the morning, his vitals are heart rate 110 beats/min, blood pressure 80/45 mm Hg, respiratory rate 25 breaths/min, and $SpO_2$ 100% on 2 L oxygen. He has the following lab values:

Hemoglobin 5.6 g/dL
Serum urea 24 mg/dL
Creatinine 1.8 mg/dL

You transfuse him 3 units of packed red blood cells and 1 unit of fresh frozen plasma and notify the surgeon of the bleeding. He is taken to the operating room where his surgical bleeding is identified and repaired. He receives 2 L of crystalloid, 2 unit fresh frozen plasma, and 2 units of platelets in the operating room, but his urine output does not improve. In the next 12 hours, his vitals are normalized but he remains anuric. Which of the following is most likely to prevent the need for dialysis?

A. Mannitol
B. Lasix to treat his oliguria
C. Dopamine at 3 μg/min
D. None of the above

# Chapter 45 ▪ Answers

1. Correct Answer: A

**Rationale:**
Central diabetes insipidus (DI) is a rare complication of bacterial meningitis. The presence of polyuria and hypernatremia is concerning for the development of DI in this patient. While it is important to obtain urine electrolytes and osmolality (Answer C) to confirm the diagnosis of DI, the most concerning issue here is the potential for bacterial meningitis in this patient. Therefore, prompt diagnosis and treatment are needed to prevent morbidity and mortality.

According to the 2004 Infectious Diseases Society of America guidelines, a CT scan of head is indicated when a patient is immunosuppressed, has new onset of seizure, a history of an intracranial mass lesion, altered mental status, or focal neurological deficit. However, this patient does not have any of these features, making choice D incorrect.

Obtaining a sample of spinal fluid is essential for diagnosis of meningitis. However, in this case, there was a delay in antibiotics initiation since the patient has been in the emergency department for 4 hours before consultation with no antibiotics initiated. Delay in antibiotic administration is associated with worse outcomes in patients with bacterial meningitis. Retrospective data suggest a 10% increase of in-hospital mortality and risk for unfavorable outcomes with each hour of delay. Thus, antibiotic administration takes precedence in this patient.

### References
1. Tunkel AR. *Clinical Features and Diagnosis of Acute Bacterial Meningitis in Adults.* Uptodate. 2018. https://www.uptodate.com/contents/clinical-features-and-diagnosis-of-acute-bacterial-meningitis-in-adults.
2. Bichet DG. *Evaluation of Patients with Polyuria.* Uptodate. 2019. https://phstwlp2.partners.org:2057/contents/evaluation-of-patients-with-polyuria.
3. Bodilsen J, Dalager-Pedersen M, Schonheyder HC, Nielsen H. Time to antibiotic therapy and outcome in bacterial meningitis: a Danish population-based cohort study. *BMC Infectious Diseases.* 2016;16:392. Epub 2016/08/11. doi:10.1186/s12879 to 016 to 1711-z.

### 2. Correct Answer: B

**Rationale:**

Acute right ventricular failure can occur in patients with moderate to severe pulmonary hypertension. Compared to the left ventricle, the right ventricle is more sensitive to increases in afterload. As a result, in this patient, who already has right ventricular dysfunction, efforts must be made to minimize right ventricular afterload. Factors such as hypoxemia, hypercapnia, hypothermia, high airway pressure, positive end-expiratory pressure, and acidosis can increase pulmonary vascular resistance.

Additional fluid challenge could be detrimental in this patient with depressed right ventricular function. It may increase the risk of right heart failure, especially since the increasing central venous pressure is an indicator of right heart volume overload (nswer D). Renal failure and associated metabolic acidosis will also be poorly tolerated by this patient, since acidosis will worsen pulmonary vascular resistance and right ventricular afterload. Hence, early intervention with renal replacement therapy to avoid renal acidosis is most beneficial. Moreover, renal replacement therapy will also help correct volume status, especially since he is anuric (Answer B).

The patient's pulmonary artery pressure and pulmonary vascular resistance remained stable which indicates that the intravenous epoprostenol has been effective. Inhaled and intravenous administration of epoprostenol is similarly effective and therefore no indication to change (Answer C). While transesophageal echocardiogram allows direct assessment of ventricular function, it requires equipment and the availability of an expert who can acquire and interpret the images. As a result, in the patient with impending sign of right ventricular failure, transesophageal echocardiogram should not be a priority (Answer A).

### References
1. Gordon C, Collard CD, Pan W. Intraoperative management of pulmonary hypertension and associated right heart failure. *Curr Opin Anaesthesiol.* 2010;23(1):49-56. doi:10.1097/ACO.0b013e3283346c51.
2. Subramaniam K, Yared JP. Management of pulmonary hypertension in the operating room. *Semin Cardiothorac Vasc Anesth.* 2007;11(2):119-136
3. Cioccari L, Baur HR, Berger D, et al. Hemodynamic assessment of critically ill patients using a miniaturized transesophageal echocardiography probe. *Crit Care.* 2013;17(3):R121. doi:10.1186/cc12793.

### 3. Correct Answer: E

**Rationale:**

In the setting of acute intracranial injury, both syndrome of inappropriate secretion of antidiuretic hormone (SIADH) and cerebral salt wasting (CSW) are potential causes of hyponatremia. The main difference between the two is the patient's volume status which can be difficult to determine using clinical criteria.

In SIADH, the patient is typically in an euvolemic or hypervolemic state, while in CSW, the patient is hypovolemic. Consistent with the above description, CSW is associated with large urine output volumes, whereas SIADH is associated with low to normal amounts of urine output volumes. Evaluation for CSW begins with a basic metabolic panel to identify the hyponatremia (serum sodium less than 135 mEq/L). Urine studies are commonly checked for urine sodium and osmolality. Urine sodium is typically elevated above 40 mEq/L. Urine osmolality is elevated above 100 mosmol/kg. The patient must also have signs or symptoms of hypovolemia such as hypotension, decreased central venous pressure, lack of skin turgor, or elevated hematocrit. Laboratory parameters common between SIADH and CSW are hyponatremia and increased urine sodium. However, with SIADH, the patient is euvolemic to hypervolemic from the retained free water, compared to the hypovolemic picture of CSW.

High urine output with reduction in serum sodium, in a patient with subarachnoid hemorrhage, likely suggests CSW syndrome. The treatment for CSW involves repletion of fluid and salt to prevent volume contraction (Answer E).

Additionally, in subarachnoid hemorrhage, the risk of vasospasm is increased with hypovolemia. Answer A is incorrect because this case scenario does not describe SIADH. Answer B does not address the decrease in sodium. Answer C may be a step in management of neurogenic hyponatremia seen in SAH patients but is not typically done until later in the course. Further, this answer choice does not immediately address the volume or sodium deficit. Answer D does not address the fluid deficit.

### Reference

1. Torbey MT. Cerebral salt wasting syndrome. In: Kruse JA ed. *Neurocritical Care.* 1st ed. New York, NY: Cambridge University Press; 2009:405-406.

---

## 4. Correct Answer: B

**Rationale:**

Low urine specific gravity in the context of polyuria and a rise in serum sodium are sufficient to make the diagnosis of DI. This postoperative neurosurgical patient is most likely experiencing central DI. Here, there is a decrease in antidiuretic hormone (ADH) which leads to polyuria (urine output >30 mL/kg body weight or >200 mL/h for 2 hours), a hallmark of DI. Additional tests that help confirm the diagnosis are measurement of urine specific gravity and serum sodium. In DI, urine will be dilute, evidenced by low urine specific gravity <1.005. With loss of dilute urine, serum sodium is expected to rise. A patient with adequate mental status may demonstrate polydipsia due to significant thirst.

Desmopressin (DDAVP) is a synthetic vasopressin analog, which acts specifically on the V2 receptor. Administration of desmopressin in central DI to replace the lack of ADH reverses the effects of central DI and thereby prevents rise in serum sodium (Answer B).

Answer A is incorrect because the relative hyponatremia is not causing clinical signs or symptoms, at this time. It is also preferable to avoid hypotonic fluids such as D5W in immediate postoperative neurosurgical or other patients with potential for cerebral edema. Answer C is not correct because increasing the rate of maintenance IV fluids (normal saline) with hypotonic fluid loss in urine (seen in DI) may further increase serum sodium. Fluid restriction (Answer D) would cause hypovolemia and may raise serum sodium.

### Reference

1. Schreckinger M, Szerlip N, Mittal S. Diabetes Insipidus following resection of pituitary tumors. *Clin Neurol Neurosurg.* 2013;115(2):121-126. doi:10.1016/j.clineuro.2012.08.009.

---

## 5. Correct Answer: D

**Rationale:**

Important causes for low urine output may be classified into prerenal, intrarenal, and postrenal causes. Based on presentation sanguineous output from abdominal drain, hypotension, and tachycardia are consistent with a prerenal etiology. A common cause of prerenal disease is volume depletion, which may occur from hypovolemia caused by hemorrhage, dehydration, diuretics, or gastrointestinal fluid losses (vomiting/diarrhea). Prerenal physiology and renal hypoperfusion may also occur due to heart failure causing poor cardiac output, or cirrhosis causing splanchnic venous pooling and systemic vasodilation. Prerenal physiology is often characterized by azotemia, caused by increased sodium and urea absorption in the proximal tubule in an attempt to increase circulating blood volume. In such patients, the BUN is often increased to a greater proportion than the creatinine such that the serum BUN:Cr ratio is greater than 20:1 (Answer A). In prerenal disease, the $FE_{Na}$ is typically less than 1% due to decreased urinary sodium excretion (due to reabsorption of sodium) in an attempt to retain water and circulating blood volume (Answer B). Urine with a high specific gravity (Answer C) indicates very concentrated urine, which occurs when the kidney is trying to retain additional free water. RBC casts in the urine (Answer D) are virtually diagnostic of some form of glomerulonephritis or vasculitis and indicate microscopic bleeding in the kidney. They are not associated with trauma to an enlarge prostate on insertion of a foley catheter and are not associated with prerenal or acute tubular necrosis. Acute tubular necrosis typically results in "muddy brown casts" consisting of renal tubular epithelial cells.

### Reference

1. Sladen RN. Oliguria in the ICU. Systematic approach to diagnosis and treatment. *Anesthesiol Clin North Am.* 2000;18(4):739-752, viii.

---

## 6. Correct Answer: D

**Rationale:**

Based on the information provided, this patient's acute kidney injury has likely progressed to acute tubular necrosis (ATN). Treatment of ATN is generally supportive and involves establishing and maintaining adequate renal blood flow and mean arterial pressure to prevent further ischemia and injury while the kidney recovers. Dialysis can be used to address complications of renal failure such as fluid overload, hyperkalemia, signs of uremia, or severe metabolic acidosis. Diuretics (Answers A and B) are often used to manage volume overload in patients with nonoliguric

ATN and hypervolemia who are responsive to diuretics. It has not been shown to promote renal recovery but can be useful in volume management. When infused in low doses, (0.5-3 µg/kg/min), dopamine dilates the interlobular arteries and both the afferent and efferent arterioles. The net effect is a relatively large increase in renal blood flow with a lesser or no elevation in glomerular filtration rate. Despite this effect on renal vasculature, dopamine at "renal doses" has not been shown to improve mortality, prevent the progression of prerenal disease to ATN, or prevent the need for dialysis (Answer C).

## References

1. Lassnigg A, Donner E, Grubhoefer G, Presterl E, Druml W, Hiesmayer M. Lack of renoprotective effects of dopamine and furosemide during cardiac surgery. *J Am Soc Nephrol*. 2000;11(1):97

2. Friedrich JO, Adhikari N, Herridge MS, Beyene J. Meta-analysis: low-dose dopamine increases urine output but does not prevent renal dysfunction or death. *Ann Intern Med*. 2005;142(7):510.

3. Bellomo R, Chapman M, Finfer S, Hickling K, Myburgh J. Low-dose dopamine in patients with early renal dysfunction: a placebo-controlled randomised trial. Australian and New Zealand Intensive Care Society (ANZICS) Clinical Trials Group. *Lancet*. 2000;356(9248):2139.

# 46

# RENAL REPLACEMENT THERAPY

Riaz M. Karukappadath, Faith Natalie Factora, and Roshni Sreedharan

1. Which of the following statements is **MOST** likely to be true of continuous renal replacement therapy (CRRT) in comparison to intermittent hemodialysis (IHD):

   A. CRRT is more likely to induce dialysis-associated increase in intracranial pressure.
   B. CRRT is associated with less hemodynamic changes during treatment.
   C. CRRT allows for earlier mobilization of patients.
   D. CRRT is less efficient in removing solutes and fluid.

2. A 44-year-old male with a long-standing history of insulin-dependent diabetes mellitus is admitted to the intensive care unit (ICU) with diabetic ketoacidosis. He has acute kidney injury (AKI) and is being started on hemodialysis in the ICU. Which of the following is the **LEAST** preferred route for vascular access insertion for renal replacement therapy (RRT)?

   A. Right internal jugular vein
   B. Left internal jugular vein
   C. Femoral vein
   D. Subclavian vein

3. Which of the following techniques does hemodialysis employ for solute clearance?

   A. Diffusion
   B. Convection
   C. Osmosis
   D. Both diffusion and convection

4. A 63-year-old female has been admitted to the ICU from another hospital with ongoing acute upper gastrointestinal bleeding, necessitating multiple blood transfusions. She has a history of a previous coronary artery bypass grafting and end-stage renal disease (ESRD) on dialysis. The records from the other hospital indicate that she was recently diagnosed with heparin-induced thrombocytopenia (HIT). She is due to get her dialysis today and feels short of breath after the blood transfusions. Which of the following is the MOST ideal anticoagulation strategy for hemodialysis in this patient?

   A. Low–molecular weight heparin can be safely used in the circuit
   B. Regional citrate anticoagulation
   C. Dabigatran can be used
   D. Dialysis cannot be safely performed at this time and needs to be deferred

5. In which of the following clinical scenarios is RRT **LEAST** likely to be urgently initiated?

   A. 30-year-old female with postoperative acute renal insufficiency with serum magnesium >8 mEq/L with anuria and absent deep tendon reflexes
   B. 50-year-old male with ESRD, on scheduled MWF dialysis, with serum potassium of 6 mEq/L
   C. 45-year-old male with septic shock and anuric AKI on pressors with a PH of 7.0 and bicarbonate of 12 mEq/L
   D. 60-year-old female with acute oliguric renal failure not responding to diuretic therapy with hypoxia and shortness of breath

6. A 64-year-old female with ESRD and nonischemic cardiomyopathy with a left ventricular ejection fraction of 20% underwent IHD the day before. She developed flash pulmonary edema and is currently on epinephrine infusion for hemodynamic support. Which of the following modalities would be **MOST** effective for fluid removal in this patient?

   A. IHD
   B. Slow continuous ultrafiltration (SCUF)
   C. Intravenous furosemide
   D. Continuous venovenous hemodialysis

7. A 55-year-old male with history of diabetes mellitus, hypertension, and ESRD has been admitted to the ICU following a polytrauma. He suffered a mild concussion of his brain and multiple orthopedic injuries including a fractured pelvis and pelvic bleeding which required coiling in the interventional radiology suite. He is protecting his airway and has been hemodynamically stable for the past 24 hours. He is being started on IHD, as his blood urea nitrogen (BUN) is 180 mg/dL and creatinine is 8 mg/dL. Following IHD, he develops nausea, vomiting, and altered mental status concerning for dialysis disequilibrium syndrome. Which of the following interventions if used is MOST likely to prevent the occurrence of this syndrome?

   A. Use of CRRT with slow removal of fluids and solutes
   B. Intubation prior to institution of dialysis
   C. Avoiding anticoagulation during dialysis
   D. Infusion of mannitol during dialysis

8. A 55-year-old female with a history of chronic obstructive pulmonary disease and chronic kidney disease on peritoneal dialysis (PD), presents to the emergency department with fever, dry cough, and wheezing. She does not complain of any abdominal pain. An upper respiratory tract infection is suspected. On admission, her hemoglobin is 9.8 mg/dL, white blood cell count is 11.2 K/μL, and lactate 3.8 mmol/L. Her vital signs are BP 100/70 mm Hg, HR 88 bpm, and oxygen saturation 95% on room air. She has been afebrile since admission. What is the **MOST** appropriate next step in the management of this patient?

   A. Abdominal computerized tomography scan to confirm diagnosis of bowel ischemia
   B. Admit to the ICU as she is likely to develop peritonitis and septic shock
   C. Observation and treatment of symptoms
   D. Start on empiric antibiotic therapy

9. What is the recommended delivered dose of the effluent in CRRT?

   A. 10 to 20 mL/kg/h
   B. 20 to 25 mL/kg/h
   C. 30 to 40 mL/kg/h
   D. 50 to 60 mL/kg/h

10. A 34-year-old female with a history of hypertension and diabetes is admitted to the ICU after an exploratory laparotomy following a motor vehicle accident. Her vital signs include HR 110 bpm and BP 90/66 mm Hg. She is currently intubated and mechanically ventilated and has developed AKI requires RRT. It is anticipated that she would need several trips to the operating room in the next few days for debridement and subsequent closure of the abdomen. Which of the following would be the **MOST** efficient modality of RRT in this patient?

    A. Continuous renal replacement therapy (CRRT)
    B. Prolonged intermittent renal replacement therapy (PIRRT)
    C. Slow continuous ultrafiltration (SCUF)
    D. Intermittent hemodialysis (IHD)

# Chapter 46 ▪ Answers

---

**1.** Correct Answer: B

**Rationale:**

IHD is an efficient dialysis technique, which is performed over 3 to 4 hours. CRRT is less efficient, as it is continuous over an entire 24-hour period. IHD allows for early mobilization of patients compared to CRRT but is not tolerated well in hemodynamically unstable patients. Hence the most recent KDIGO guidelines recommend CRRT in hemo-dynamically unstable patients. Dialysis-induced increase in intracranial pressure is more likely to occur in patients undergoing IHD. This is postulated to occur due to the rapid removal of solutes and consequent fluid shifts. The slower fluid and solute removal with CRRT minimizes its occurrence.

References

1. KDIGO clinical practice guidelines for acute kidney injury. *Kidney Int Suppl.* 2012;2(1). Section 5, Chapter 5.6.
2. Gemmell L, Docking R, Black E. Renal replacement therapy in critical care. *BJA Educ.* 2017;17(3):88-93.

---

**2.** Correct Answer: D

**Rationale:**

The site and length of vascular access catheters play an important role in the provision of optimal RRT. The subcla-vian vein is the least preferred route for vascular access insertion intended for RRT. Contact of the catheter with the vessel wall and subsequent thrombosis could result in vessel stenosis, jeopardizing the possibility for an arteriove-nous fistula in case the patient remains dialysis-dependent.

Right internal jugular vein is the preferred vein for hemodialysis access as the vein takes a straight path into the superior vena cava (SVC). Access through the left internal jugular vein requires the catheter makes two right angles prior to reaching the SVC resulting in a higher incidence of catheter dysfunction. The length of the catheter is equally important with optimal flows occurring when the catheter tip is positioned in the right atrium SVC junction for internal jugular access and in the inferior vena cava for femoral access. Appropriate lengths of catheters need to be chosen for this purpose. The right internal jugular, femoral, left internal jugular, and subclavian are recommended in order as options for vascular access in patients requiring RRT. The right internal jugular vein should be the first consideration for hemodialysis access.

References

1. KDIGO clinical practice guidelines for acute kidney injury. *Kidney Int Suppl.* 2012;2(1). Section 5, Chapter 5.4.
2. Gemmell L, Docking R, Black E. Renal replacement therapy in critical care. *BJA Educ.* 2017;17(3):88-93.
3. Clinical practice guidelines for hemodialysis adequacy, update 2006. *Am J Kidney Dis.* 2006;48(Suppl 1):S2-S90.
4. Hernández D, Díaz F, Rufino M, Lorenzo V, Pérez T, Rodríguez A, et al. Subclavian vascular access stenosis in dialysis patients: natural history and risk factors. *J Am Soc Nephrol.* 1998;9(8):1507-1510.

---

**3.** Correct Answer: A

**Rationale:**

The goals of RRT could be one or a combination of the following—solute and fluid clearance, normalization of elec-trolytes, and acid-base status. This could be achieved through diffusion or convection, depending on the modality of RRT.

In diffusion, which is employed in hemodialysis, blood and the dialysate fluid flow in a countercurrent fashion on either side of the semipermeable membrane of the hemofilter. The driving force that moves solutes across the semi-permeable membrane is the solute concentration gradient. Diffusion is effective in removing small molecules, such as potassium, ammonium, and creatinine (<20 kDa). It is less efficient in removing larger solutes and water.

In hemofiltration, a convective process is utilized wherein solutes and water are transported across the membrane by a pressure differential. Pressure forces water and consequently "drags" solutes with it from the blood compartment to the so-called effluent compartment. The permeability coefficient of the membrane and the difference in pressure between both sides of the membrane determine the amount of fluid and solutes transported across the membrane. With a large amount of fluid removed, crystalloid replacement is given back to the patient to restore circulating volume.

References

1. Pannu N, Gibney RN. Renal replacement therapy in the intensive care unit. *Ther Clin Risk Manag.* 2005;1(2):141-150.
2. KDIGO clinical practice guidelines for acute kidney injury. *Kidney Int Suppl.* 2012;2(1).
3. Gemmell L, Docking R, Black E. Renal replacement therapy in critical care. *BJA Educ.* 2017;17(3):88-93.

**4.** Correct Answer: B

**Rationale:**

All forms of heparin should be avoided in a patient with recent history of HIT. Anticoagulation strategies in patients with HIT requiring hemodialysis include regional anticoagulation with citrate or use of direct thrombin inhibitors. Parenteral direct thrombin inhibitors—argatroban, danaparoid, and lepirudin—have been used for this purpose. Dabigatran, an oral direct thrombin inhibitor is contraindicated in patients with ESRD and hence cannot be used in this patient. Dialysis without anticoagulation can be used in an acutely bleeding patient, requiring hemodialysis, but filter clogging can lead to acute drop in hematocrit from blood lost in the dialysis circuit and is not usually preferred. Regional citrate anticoagulation is an option in patients with HIT, requiring dialysis.

References

1. Mariano F, Bergamo D, Gangemi E, Hollo Z. Citrate anticoagulation for continuous renal replacement therapy in critically ill patients: success and limits. *Int J Nephrol.* 2011;2011:748320.
2. KDIGO clinical practice guidelines for acute kidney injury. *Kidney Int Suppl.* 2012;2(1). Chapter 5.3.

**5.** Correct Answer: B

**Rationale:**

While hyperkalemia >6 mEq/L with ECG abnormalities is an absolute indication for RRT, asymptomatic hyperkalemia >6 mEq/L is only a relative indication, especially in a patient with ESRD. In the setting of AKI, metabolic acidosis with a pH <7.15, diuretic resistant fluid overload, and hypermagnesemia >8 mEq/L with anuria and absent deep tendon reflexes are absolute indications for RRT. In patients with AKI, refractory metabolic acidosis, diuretic resistant fluid overload, and hypermagnesemia >8 mEq/L with anuria are absolute indications for initiation of RRT.

References

1. KDIGO clinical practice guidelines for acute kidney injury. *Kidney Int Suppl.* 2012;2(1). Chapter 5.1.
2. Gibney N, Hoste E, Burdmann EA, et al. Timing of initiation and discontinuation of renal replacement therapy in AKI: unanswered key questions. *Clin J Am Soc Nephrol.* 2008;3:876-880.

**6.** Correct Answer: B

**Rationale:**

SCUF is used exclusively to remove fluids and therefore a useful modality to treat isolated fluid overload. SCUF is not useful in patients who are uremic or hyperkalemic, because solute removal is minimal. SCUF can safely remove up to 8 L of fluid per day. The slow rate of fluid removal is beneficial in patients who have a tenuous hemodynamic status.

References

1. Granado R, Macedo E, Mehta R. Indications for continuous renal replacement therapy: renal replacement versus renal support. *Critical Care Nephrology.* 2019:987-993.e2:chap 163.
2. Ronco C, Ricci Z, Brendolan A, Bellomo R, Bedogni F. Ultrafiltration in patients with hypervolemia and congestive heart failure. *Blood Purif.* 2004;22(1):150-163.

**7.** Correct Answer: A

**Rationale:**

Dialysis disequilibrium syndrome can occur when using aggressive/rapid RRT in a severely uremic patient. The shift of water into brain tissue due to the abrupt lowering of plasma tonicity during IHD may lead to an acute increase in intracranial pressure and cerebral hypoperfusion. Caution should be exercised in patients who are at risk of cerebral edema prior to initiation of RRT. To avoid brain edema caused by large variations in osmolality, several preventative measures can be employed. They include targeting a reduction in the plasma urea nitrogen of 40% at the most, reducing blood and dialysate flow, using a small dialyzer, and limiting the length of treatment. The use of a sodium-enriched dialysate may further reduce the risk. Dialysis disequilibrium syndrome is a significant risk with rapid clearance in severe azotemia when instituting RRT.

Reference

1. Patel N, Dalal P, Panesar M. Dialysis disequilibrium syndrome: a narrative review. *Semin Dial.* 2008;21:493-498.

**8.** Correct Answer: C

**Rationale:**

Lactate is the most commonly used buffer in PD solutions. An abnormal lactate value is often seen in PD patients presenting to the ED. It does not necessarily indicate tissue hypoperfusion or gut ischemia. This patient with acute respiratory symptoms needs to be treated and observed for any further worsening. Hyperlactatemia could be a coincidental occurrence in patients who undergo PD.

References
1. Trinh E, Saiprasertkit N, Bargman JM. Increased serum lactate in peritoneal dialysis patients presenting with intercurrent illness. *Perit Dial Int.* 2018;38(5):363-365.
2. Anderson YS, Curtis NJ, Hobbs JA, et al. High serum D-lactate inpatients on continuous ambulatory peritoneal dialysis. *Nephrol Dial Transplant.* 1997;12(5):981-983.

**9.** Correct Answer: B

**Rationale:**

Two large randomized controlled trials found no significant difference in mortality with effluent doses above 20 to 25 mL/kg/h. There were no significant differences in the secondary outcomes such as renal recovery and nonrenal organ failure as well. Of note, there were a few serious adverse events in the higher-intensity group. The KDIGO clinical practice guidelines recommend delivering an effluent dose of 20 to 25 mL/kg/h for CRRT in patients with AKI. Higher effluent rates confer no mortality benefit compared to a rate 20 to 25 mL/kg/h.

References
1. Palevsky PM, Zhang JH, O'Connor TZ, Chertow GM, Crowley ST, Choudhury D, et al. Intensity of renal support in critically ill patients with acute kidney injury. *N Engl J Med.* 2008;359:7-20.
2. Investigators, The RENAL replacement therapy study. Intensity of continuous renal-replacement therapy in critically ill patients. *N Engl J Med.* 2009;361:1627-1638.

**10.** Correct Answer: B

**Rationale:**

PIRRT is a renal replacement modality wherein treatment sessions last over 8 to 12 hours but are intermittent (about three times a week). It is a hybrid treatment wherein the hemodynamic stability achieved with CRRT is combined with the intermittent nature of IHD. Diffusion, convection, or a combination of the two techniques could be used with this modality. It is especially useful in patients who are not hemodynamically stable enough to initiate IHD but require several interruptions in therapy (potentially due to required procedures) which would make provision for CRRT challenging. To be effective, CRRT needs to be performed over 24 hours with minimal interruptions. As PIRRT has scheduled time off of dialysis and anticoagulation, procedures could be strategically scheduled over those times. PIRRT is sometimes referred to as sustained low-efficiency (daily) dialysis (SLEDD), sustained low-efficiency (daily) diafiltration (SLEDD-f), extended daily dialysis (EDD), or slow continuous dialysis (SCD). SCUF exclusively removes fluid and would be ineffective in patients requiring solute clearance as well. PIRRT is an effective hybrid renal replacement modality in hemodynamically unstable patients who are anticipated to have interruptions in CRRT.

References
1. Bellomo R, Baldwin I, Fealy N. Prolonged intermittent renal replacement therapy in the intensive care unit. *Crit Care Resusc* 2002;4:281.
2. Naka T, Baldwin I, Bellomo R, Fealy N, Wan L. Prolonged daily intermittent renal replacement therapy in ICU patients by ICU nurses and ICU physicians. *Int J Artif Organs.* 2004;27(5):380-387.

# 47

# DRUG DOSING IN RENAL FAILURE

Abdulaziz S. Almehlisi, Phat Tan Dang, Ji Sun "Christina" Baek, and Ulrich Schmidt

1. A 67-year-old man with a history of syringomyelia, benign prostatic hypertrophy, and chronic pain with an intrathecal pump with morphine and baclofen presents with altered mental status. His vitals are temperature 37.2°C, blood pressure (BP) 116/70 mm Hg, heart rate (HR) 90 beats/ min, respiratory rate 4/min, and SpO$_2$ 92%. His basic laboratory data are potassium 5.0 mEq/L, sodium 142 mEq/L, creatinine 2.9 mg/dL, and glomerular filtration rate 22 mL/min/1.73 m². On examination, the patient appears somnolent, and his neurological examination is significant for constricted pupils. On further questioning, the patient's wife states that he has had his intrathecal pump for 12 years with no issues and denies any recent change in the dose of intrathecal medications. You suspect that impaired renal excretion of his intrathecal medications has caused the patient's altered mental status. Which of the following is the MOST LIKELY cause for this patient's clinical presentation?

   A. Morphine-6-glucuronide (M6G)
   B. Morphine-3-glucuronide (M3G)
   C. Normorphine
   D. Baclofen

2. Which of the following statements is **correct** with regards to drug dosing in chronic kidney disease (CKD)?

   A. The loading dose of vancomycin needs to be decreased in patients with chronic renal failure.
   B. The induction dose of propofol for intubation in CKD patients must be significantly reduced.
   C. The dose of tobramycin needs to be reduced in patients with CKD.
   D. The duration of action of cisatracurium is not prolonged in renal failure because of its Hoffman elimination.

3. You are called to evaluate a 70-year-old man who underwent cystoscopy and ureteral stent placement under general anesthesia for potential intensive care unit (ICU) admission. The post anesthesia care unit nurse tells you that the patient was shivering in the immediate postoperative period, but now he is exhibiting more pronounced jerky movements of his extremities. He has a past medical history of hypertension, diabetes, CKD, and mild dementia. Laboratory data are hematocrit 40%, platelets 182 000/μL, potassium 5.1 mEq/L, creatinine 2.7 mg/dL, and glomerular filtration rate 48 mL/min/1.73 m². You are told that he has received some medications for his pain and shivering. Suddenly, the patient begins to seize. Which of the therapies administered to the patient MOST LIKELY explains this outcome?

   A. Fentanyl
   B. Meperidine
   C. Acetaminophen
   D. Ondansetron

4. A 71-year-old man with a history of diabetes, hypertension, and CKD is in the ICU for septic shock secondary to a urinary tract infection. The patient has a complicated psychiatric and social history that includes posttraumatic stress disorder, depression, and generalized anxiety disorder in the setting of homelessness. He currently complains of severe anxiety to the point that he has not been able to get any rest since being admitted. He says that he takes some medication for his anxiety and sees a psychiatrist for it sporadically. You order a one-time dose of alprazolam 0.5 mg PO. One hour later, the nurse pages you and states that the patient has become overly sedated. What is the most likely pharmacokinetic explanation for why this medication produced an exaggerated clinical effect in this patient with CKD?

**A.** With lowered protein binding in CKD, there is an increase in the free fraction of alprazolam, potentiating its clinical effect.

**B.** Secondary to impaired renal excretion, there is a rapid accumulation of the metabolite of alprazolam, causing oversedation.

**C.** Owing to the decrease in volume of distribution found in CKD patients, there is a higher concentration of alprazolam in the plasma, leading to greater clinical effect.

**D.** The metabolism of alprazolam is heavily dependent on the kidneys. In CKD, the decreased metabolism of benzodiazepines can often lead to an overdose of the medication.

5. A 42-year-old male with history of positive human immunodeficiency virus status with poor compliance to antiretroviral therapy presents to the ICU with altered mental status and severe hypotension, requiring aggressive intravenous fluid resuscitation, vasopressor therapy, and endotracheal intubation with sedation. He has recently been in a skilled nursing facility and was lost to follow-up on discharge. Cultures are drawn, and he is placed on broad-spectrum antimicrobial therapy as further workup is being performed. His basic labs show that he has acute kidney injury with creatinine 2.3 mg/dL with estimated glomerular filtration rate (eGFR) 38 mL/min/1.73 m². Which of the following is **FALSE** regarding antibiotic treatment in this patient?

**A.** Checking a trough level for vancomycin is a useful tool to help determine an appropriate dose for the individual patient.

**B.** As many antimicrobial medications are renally excreted, a dose reduction should be considered based on the eGFR to avoid overdose.

**C.** When patients are placed on continuous renal replacement therapy (CRRP), antimicrobials tend to reach supratherapeutic levels because of further decrease in the clearance of these medications.

**D.** There are two main ways to adjust the total dosage of antimicrobials given to the patient—changing the dosing interval and the dose of medication given each time.

6. A 70-year-old male with mild dementia and history of intravenous drug abuse, currently on methadone, was admitted to the ICU with obstructive nephropathy. Based on the initial workup, it is likely secondary to advanced prostate cancer with metastatic disease to the bones. He has postobstructive renal acute kidney injury and has been admitted for further care. He was placed on his home dose of methadone. Which of the following is **TRUE** regarding methadone?

**A.** Methadone undergoes extensive hepatic metabolism by the cytochrome P450 family.

**B.** Methadone has two main active metabolites.

**C.** The primary elimination of methadone is through the liver.

**D.** In addition to its action on the mu receptors, methadone also acts as an agonist to N-methyl-D-aspartate (NMDA) receptors.

7. Which of the following antibiotics requires dose adjustment in stage 5 CKD patient?

**A.** Linezolid
**B.** Moxifloxacin
**C.** Ceftriaxone
**D.** Cefazolin
**E.** Clindamycin

8. A patient with chronic renal failure and 60 % (body surface area) burns is undergoing a 20-minute dressing change in the ICU. Which of the following opioids has the most favorable profile?

**A.** Morphine
**B.** Remifentanil
**C.** Hydromorphone
**D.** Meperidine

# Chapter 47 ▪ Answers

1. Correct Answer: A

**Rationale:**
Morphine is a prototypical opioid medication that provides pain relief through its actions on the mu-opioid receptors in the central nervous system. It is primarily metabolized by the liver via glucuronidation into two

major water-soluble metabolites, M6G and M3G. M6G is an active metabolite that acts on mu-opioid receptors, producing potent analgesic and sedative effects. M3G, on the other hand, is inactive and has no effects on mu-opioid receptors. Normorphine is another metabolite that is produced by demethylation. Normorphine is a minor metabolite with little opioid activity. This patient is presenting with altered mental status, respiratory depression, and miosis, which are consistent with opioid toxidrome. The most likely explanation for the above clinical presentation is the accumulation of the active morphine metabolite M6G secondary to decreased renal function. Morphine is primarily eliminated by the kidneys although some of the morphine glucuronide metabolites undergo excretion in the bile.

Baclofen is a muscle relaxant that acts as a gamma-aminobutyric acid B (GABAB) agonist. The majority of baclofen (~80%) is eliminated in its unchanged form by the kidneys. The remainder is metabolized by the liver via deamination. Baclofen toxicity can cause respiratory and central nervous system depression as well, but typically does not cause miosis.

### References

1. Barash PG. *Clinical Anesthesia*. 7th ed. Philadelphia, PA: Wolters Kluwer Health/Lippincott Williams & Wilkins; 2013:1412.
2. Leung NY, Whyte IM, Isbister GK. Baclofen overdose: defining the spectrum of toxicity. *Emerg Med Australas*. 2006;18(1):77-82.
3. Janicki PK. Pharmacology of morphine metabolites. *Curr Pain Headache Rep*. 1997;1:264-270.

---

**2.** Correct Answer: D

**Rationale:**

Vancomycin is nephrotoxic, especially in patients with chronic renal failure. The loading dose is not affected as it is imperative to reach the target concentration as soon as possible. However, reduction in maintenance dose or longer dosing intervals may be necessary in patients in renal insufficiency.

With an initial intravenous bolus of propofol, the termination of central nervous system effects depends primarily on the redistribution of the drug from the central compartment to the peripheral compartments. Therefore, the induction dose of propofol is unchanged in CKD patients. Cisatracurium undergoes degradation by Hoffman elimination and ester hydrolysis, both independent of renal function. Therefore, its dose does not need to be adjusted in renal failure.

### References

1. Barash PG. *Clinical Anesthesia*. 7th ed. Philadelphia, PA: Wolters Kluwer Health/Lippincott Williams & Wilkins; 2013:1410-1411.
2. Salem MM. "Pathophysiology of hypertension in renal failure." *Semin Nephrol*. 2002;22(1):17-26.
3. Thomas R, Kanso A, Sedor JR. "Chronic kidney disease and its complications." *Primary care*. 2008;35(2):329, vii.

---

**3.** Correct Answer: B

**Rationale:**

Patient likely received meperidine for post-op shivering. In the setting of kidney injury, the renal excretion of the meperidine metabolite is compromised. The accumulation of normeperidine, the active metabolite of meperidine, can cause significant neurotoxic side effects, such as tremors, myoclonus, and seizures.

### References

1. Barash PG. *Clinical Anesthesia*. 7th ed. Philadelphia, PA: Wolters Kluwer Health/Lippincott Williams & Wilkins; 2013:1412.
2. Hellums JS, Ross EL. *Long-Acting Opioids. In Pain Medicine*. Cham: Springer; 2017:153-155.

---

**4.** Correct Answer: A

**Rationale:**

Benzodiazepines are GABAA agonists that can be used for anxiolysis. They are primarily metabolized by the liver-hepatic oxidation and reduction (by cytochrome P450) and glucuronide conjugation. Subsequently they undergo renal elimination.

In patients with CKD, there is usually an increase in volume of distribution and lowered protein binding. Benzodiazepines are highly protein bound molecules. With less protein binding, there is an increased free fraction of the benzodiazepine available to exert clinical effects. This likely explains why alprazolam has been shown to have more sedative effects in CKD patients compared with those without renal disease. If one were to administer an infusion of a benzodiazepine, however, the accumulation of metabolites due to compromised renal clearance would be another way in which CKD patients may experience a more dramatic clinical effect from benzodiazepines.

### References

1. Barash PG. *Clinical Anesthesia*. 7th ed. Philadelphia, PA: Wolters Kluwer Health/Lippincott Williams & Wilkins; 2013.
2. http://paindr.com/wp-content/uploads/2015/10/Revised-BZD_-9-30.pdf.
3. Fissell W. Antimicrobial dosing in acute renal replacement. *Adv Chronic Kidney Dis*. 2013;20(1):85-93. doi:10.1053/j.ackd.2012.10.004. https://www.ackdjournal.org/article/S1548-5595(12)00194-2/pdf.

**5.** Correct Answer: C

**Rationale:**

Renal dysfunction is a commonly associated with sepsis, especially in the setting of septic shock with hemodynamic instability. As many antimicrobial medications are renally excreted, dose reductions may be warranted. Vancomycin is one of the few drugs for which trough level is available to help guide dose adjustments. Appropriate antimicrobial dosing is critical to treat the underlying infection in sepsis while avoiding the negative side effects from suprathera-peutic levels. For example, an excessive dose of imipenem/cilastatin may cause seizures.

When patients are placed on CRRT, drugs are also removed as well. As a result, patients placed on CRRT may have subtherapeutic levels of their antimicrobial therapy. Therefore, it would be important to consider increasing the dosing of antimicrobials that are more readily cleared by CRRT.

References

1. http://med.stanford.edu/bugsanddrugs/guidebook/_jcr_content/main/panel_builder_1454513702/panel_0/download_1586531681/file.res/Sepsis%20ABX%202017-05-25.pdf.
2. https://www.nebraskamed.com/sites/default/files/documents/for-providers/asp/Renal-Dose-Adjustment-Guidelines-for-Antimicrobial.pdf.
3. Heintz BH, Matzke GR, Dager WE. Antimicrobial dosing concepts and recommendations for critically ill adult patients receiving continuous renal replacement therapy or intermittent hemodialysis. *Pharmacotherapy*. 2009;29(5):562-577.

**6.** Correct Answer: A

**Rationale:**

Methadone is a unique opioid medication with a long duration of action that can be useful in the treatment of opioid addiction. It is also used for cancer-related pain and chronic pain conditions. Methadone is a mu-receptor agonist and an NMDA receptor antagonist. Similar to other opioids, it undergoes hepatic metabolism by the cytochrome P450 family via N-methylation. It has no active metabolites. Fecal elimination is the primary process through which methadone is excreted. There is a minimal amount of renal elimination. Therefore, there is no need for a dose adjustment for those with renal dysfunction.

References

1. https://pdfs.semanticscholar.org/17b3/8e679ae89e851b66dc301d85b443255e5dc7.pdf.
2. https://www.drugbank.ca/drugs/DB00333.
3. Kharasch ED, Regina KJ, Blood J, Friedel C. Methadone pharmacogenetics CYP2B6 polymorphisms determine plasma concentrations, clearance, and metabolism. *Anesthesiology*. 2015;123(5):1142-1153.

**7.** Correct Answer: D

**Rationale:**

There are multiple antibiotics that have significant nonrenal excretion routes. Antibiotics such as azithromycin, ceftriaxone, clindamycin, doxycycline, linezolid, metronidazole, moxifloxacin, nafcillin, oxacillin, rifampin, and tigecycline do not require dose adjustment in patients with severe renal disease. Cefazolin, on the other hand, requires dose adjustment based on creatinine clearance.

References

1. Letourneau A, Hooper D, Bloom A. *Penicillin, Antistaphylococcal Penicillins, and Broad-Spectrum Penicillins*. https://www.uptodate.com/contents/penicillin-antistaphylococcal-penicillins-and-broad-spectrum-penicillins.
2. Lexi–Drug, Lexi–Comp® [Internet database]. Hudson, OH: Lexi–Comp, Inc. Available at http://www.crlonline.com. Accessed October 2018.
3. Stanford Hospital & Clinics Antimicrobial Dosing Reference Guide 2014. Available at http://med.stanford.edu/content/dam/sm/bugsanddrugs/documents/dosingprotocols/2014%20SHC%20ABX%20Dosing%20Guide.pdf. Accessed October 2018.

**8.** Correct Answer: B

**Rationale:**

All of the opioids listed undergo significant renal elimination except for remifentanil. Remifentanil undergoes rapid metabolism in the blood by plasma esterases. Although its metabolite remifentanil acid requires renal elimination, it has not been shown to be clinically significant.

References

1. Barash PG. *Clinical Anesthesia*. 7th ed. Philadelphia, PA: Wolters Kluwer Health/Lippincott Williams & Wilkins; 2013:1412.
2. Dean M. Opioids in renal failure and dialysis patients. *J Pain Symptom Manage*. 2004;28:497-504.

# 48

# RENAL TRANSPLANTATION

Hassan Farhan

1. Which of the following is the MOST appropriate initial treatment for acute rejection of a renal allograft?

   A. 3.375 g piperacillin/tazobactam
   B. Plasmapheresis
   C. 500 mg IV methylprednisolone
   D. Rabbit antithymocyte globulin

2. A 54-year-old man is 18 months post kidney transplant. He presents with headaches and oliguria. Serum creatinine is 2.5 mg/dL from a baseline of 1.32 post transplant. His blood pressure is 190/101 mm Hg. He has no focal neurological signs. On reviewing his operative note from the kidney transplant, you note that the renal allograft was deemed a "difficult procurement," and his postoperative course was complicated by delayed graft function (DGF). Biopsy is not consistent with rejection. Which of the following is the next best step in workup of this patient?

   A. CT abdomen
   B. Renal ultrasound
   C. 24 hour urine catecholamines
   D. Renal arteriography

3. A 63-year-old woman is 5 hours post live donor renal transplant and is complaining of abdominal pain. The nurse looking after the patient notices that the urinary catheter has not drained any urine in the last 90 minutes despite 1:1 replacement of fluids (1 mL of crystalloid infusion for every 1 mL of urine output during the previous hour). Obstruction of the catheter is ruled out. Which of the following is the most likely cause?

   A. Postoperative hemorrhage
   B. Hyperacute rejection
   C. Renal artery thrombosis
   D. Bladder rupture

4. Delayed graft function (DGF) after renal transplant is most commonly defined as:

   A. Dialysis requirement within 7 days of transplantation
   B. Failure of decrease in serum creatinine after transplantation
   C. Proteinuria >1 g/d
   D. Urine output <0.5 mL/kg for 1 week

# Chapter 48 ■ Answers

**1.** Correct Answer: C

**Rationale:**

Acute rejection typically presents in the first 6 months after renal transplantation and is cell mediated. The incidence of acute rejection has declined with current practices in induction and maintenance of immunosuppression. There are two histological forms of acute rejection, Acute T cell–mediated rejection and acute antibody-mediated rejection. Risk factors include human leukocyte antigen (HLA) mismatches, blood group incompatibility, prolonged cold ischemia time, DGF, and patients with previous episodes of rejection. Most patients are asymptomatic; the first sign is usually a rise in serum creatinine. Worsening hypertension and proteinuria >1 g/d are other signs of acute rejection. Diagnosis is confirmed with allograft biopsy. Treatment is with pulse methylprednisolone in most centers, with the dose and duration of pulse therapy depending on the grade of rejection. Maintenance immunosuppression therapy may also be intensified (eg, aim for higher tacrolimus levels). Antithymocyte globulin is typically used as a second-line agent and is coadministered with glucocorticoid therapy in higher grade rejection or rejection refractory to glucocorticoid pulse therapy. The expected reversal rate for a first episode of acute rejection is 60% to 70% with this regimen. Plasmapharesis can be effective in antibody-mediated rejection, but it is not first-line therapy. Therapy success is indicated by increases in urine output and a decrease in serum creatinine within 5 days of initiating treatment.

## References

1. Lamarche C, Côté JM, Sénécal L, Cardinal H. Efficacy of acute cellular rejection treatment according to banff score in kidney transplant recipients: a systematic review. *Transplant Direct.* 2016;2:e115.
2. Vineyard GC, Fadem SZ, Dmochowski J, et al. Evaluation of corticosteroid therapy for acute renal allograft rejection. *Surg Gynecol Obstet.* 1974;138:225.
3. Burton SA, Amir N, Asbury A, et al. Treatment of antibody-mediated rejection in renal transplant patients: a clinical practice survey. *Clin Transplant.* 2015;29:118.

**2.** Correct Answer: D

**Rationale:**

Transplant renal artery stenosis (TRAS) usually occurs between 3 months and 2 years after renal transplantation, but it can present at any time. It is a potentially curable cause of posttransplant hypertension, allograft dysfunction, and graft loss. Renal artery stenosis usually occurs close to the allograft renal artery surgical anastomosis. Risk factors include difficulties in procurement and surgical technique, atherosclerotic disease, cytomegalovirus infection, and DGF. It presents in most cases as refractory hypertension and allograft dysfunction. Although noninvasive imaging modalities such as Doppler ultrasonography, spiral computed tomography, and magnetic resonance angiography are useful in screening for TRAS, arteriography is the definitive diagnostic and treatment modality when TRAS is suspected based on noninvasive tests or clinical presentation. Once identified by arteriography, the stenosis can be corrected directly with angioplasty and stenting. It is important to rule out rejection before arteriography to optimize chances of graft function recovery.

## References

1. Bruno S, Remuzzi G, Ruggenenti P. Transplant renal artery stenosis. *J Am Soc Nephrol.* 2004;15:134.
2. Audard V, Matignon M, Hemery F, et al. Risk factors and long-term outcome of transplant renal artery stenosis in adult recipients after treatment by percutaneous transluminal angioplasty. *Am J Transplant.* 2006;6:95.

**3.** Correct Answer: C

**Rationale:**

Renal artery thrombosis is a devastating posttransplant complication that usually results in graft loss. Fortunately, it is an uncommon complication occurring in less than 1% of patients. Early identification and intervention is most important. It usually presents with sudden cessation of urine output and a tender, swollen graft. Risk factors include hypotension, hypercoagulable state, and multiple renal arteries. Diagnosis is usually made with color flow Doppler studies. Once the diagnosis is made, urgent surgical exploration and thrombectomy is indicated. Outcomes are unfavorable as the transplanted kidney does not have collateral vessels, and its tolerance of warm ischemia is poor.

## References

1. Humar A, Matas AJ. Surgical complications after kidney transplantation. *Semin Dial.* 2005;18:505.
2. Bakir N, Sluiter WJ, Ploeg RJ, et al. Primary renal graft thrombosis. *Nephrol Dial Transplant.* 1996;11:140.

**4.** Correct Answer: A

**Rationale:**

Although there are over 10 definitions of DGF in the literature, it is most commonly defined as the need for dialysis within 7 days of transplantation (69% of studies reviewed between 1984 and 2007 use this criteria for their definition). This definition offers a standard by which centers can report outcomes and define a clinical entity that can be studied to help improve graft and patient survival. It occurs in 20% to 50% of patients receiving a first cadaveric graft. It is characterized by acute tubular necrosis following renal transplantation. DGF occurs more commonly among recipients of deceased donor transplants compared with live donor transplants. DGF has significant effects on graft and patient survival as it can be associated with both acute and chronic allograft nephropathy and increased risk of graft failure. Risk factors include deceased donor and prolonged allograft ischemia times. Studies are currently ongoing to look at pretransplant, intraoperative, and posttransplant interventions that may reduce the risk of DGF and subsequent graft failure. These treatments focus on immunosuppression, ischemic preconditioning, and vasodilatory agents.

References
1. Perico N, Cattaneo D, Sayegh MH, Remuzzi G. Delayed graft function in kidney transplantation. *Lancet*. 2004;364:1814-1827.
2. Siedlecki A, Irish W, Brennan DC. Delayed graft function in the kidney transplant. *Am J Transplant*. 2011;11(11):2279-2296.

# 49

# DIAGNOSIS AND MONITORING IN RENAL FAILURE

Abdulaziz S. Almehlisi, Phat Tan Dang, Ji Sun "Christina" Baek, Anushirvan Minokadeh, Alan S. Nova, Zeb McMillan, Kimberly S. Robbins, and Ulrich Schmidt

1. You are asked to consult on a previously healthy 68-year-old woman who presented with malaise and one episode of hematuria. She visited her primary care doctor 5 days ago for a "bladder infection" and was prescribed trimethoprim-sulfamethoxazole, which she has been taking. She is alert and oriented, and her physical examination is within normal limits. Her vital signs are normal. Her laboratory data are unremarkable except for elevated eosinophils, creatinine of 3 mg/dL, and urea 41 mg/dL.

   What would you expect to see in urine analysis?

   A. Muddy brown cast
   B. Red blood cell cast
   C. White blood cell cast
   D. Envelopelike crystals

2. What management should you pursue next?

   A. Administer fomepizole
   B. Discontinue trimethoprim-sulfamethoxazole
   C. Administer 500 mL bolus of normal saline
   D. Obtain a computed tomography (CT) abdomen/pelvis with intravenous (IV) contrast

3. Which of the electrolyte abnormalities is **associated** with advanced chronic kidney disease?

   A. Hyponatremia
   B. Hypophosphatemia
   C. Hypomagnesemia
   D. Hypokalemia

4. You are working as an intensivist in a rural hospital where the emergency physician calls you to evaluate a patient for intensive care unit (ICU) admission. When you come to the emergency department (ED), you see a disheveled, cachectic, old gentleman who was brought in by his neighbor for altered mental status. His neighbor reports that the patient has been complaining about back pain, and he was taking some "over-the-counter" (OTC) pain medication. You cannot elicit any history from the patient, and his physical examination is unremarkable. His laboratory data show elevated creatinine of 2.1 mg/dL, sodium 147 mEq/L, potassium 5.8 mEq/L, chloride 113 mEq/L, bicarbonate 22 mEq/L, albumin 2 mg/dL, and glucose 98 mg/dL. His arterial blood gas shows pH 7.39 and $pCO_2$ 38.

   What is the next test that you would order?

   A. Obtain an acetaminophen level
   B. Obtain a salicylate level
   C. Obtain an alcohol level
   D. Obtain a ketone level

5. What is the **BEST** next step of management?

   A. Administer N-acetylcysteine
   B. Start an insulin drip
   C. Start emergent hemodialysis
   D. Proceed with urine alkalization

6. A 42-year-old man with a history of insulin-dependent diabetes mellitus, hypertension, and end-stage renal disease on hemodialysis is admitted to the surgical ICU after a motor vehicle collision resulting in femur fracture and subdural hematoma. The patient is alert and oriented. His vital signs are blood pressure (BP) 185/100 mm Hg, heart rate (HR) 110 beats per minute, respiratory rate 12/min, and SpO$_2$ 95% on room air. His blood work is significant for creatinine 4 mg/dL, urea 80 mg/dL, and potassium 5.8 mEq/L. The patient states that he missed a dialysis session two days ago and that he was on his way to the dialysis center when he had the car accident.

   Which of the following dialysis modalities is **INAPPROPRIATE** for this patient?

   A. Intermittent hemodialysis (iHD)
   B. Continues renal replacement therapy (CRRT)
   C. Sustained low efficiency dialysis (SLED)
   D. Extended daily dialysis (EDD)

7. A 64-year-old male with a history of cirrhosis secondary to hepatitis C is being evaluated for abdominal pain. The patient reports worsening generalized abdominal pain and fever for the past 4 days. He denies hematemesis or melena. His BP was 110/60 mm Hg, and HR was 95 beats per minute. His physical examination is significant for icterus, ascites, and generalized abdominal tenderness. Laboratory analysis is notable for white blood cell count of 18 000/μL, creatinine 1.1 mmol/L (baseline 0.8 mmol/L), blood urea nitrogen 36 mg/dL, and total bilirubin is >4.3 mg/dL. The patient received broad-spectrum antibiotics.

   Which of the following drugs is **MOST** appropriate to administer to reduce risk for renal failure in this patient?

   A. Terlipressin 1 mg IV bolus now and then every 6 hours plus 1 g/kg of albumin
   B. Albumin 1.5 g per kg now and 1.0 g/kg on day 3
   C. Midodrine 7.5 mg orally now and then every 8 hours plus 1 g/kg of albumin
   D. Octreotide subcutaneous injection 100 μg now and then every 8 hours plus 1 g/kg of albumin

8. A 22-year-old man presented to the ED with vomiting, altered mental status, and fever. The patient's roommate states that the patient has not been feeling well for 2 days, yesterday was complaining of fever and headache. This morning the patient had a new-onset seizure and altered mental status. The patient's roommate is not aware of any history of drug abuse other than marijuana. In the ED, a CT scan was done and did not show any acute intracranial pathology. Urine toxicology screen was positive for cannabis. A lumbar puncture was done in the ED and resulted cell count consistent with viral meningitis/encephalitis. Cerebrospinal fluid herpes simplex virus (HSV) PCR and bacterial cultures were ordered, and results are pending. The patient was started on empirical vancomycin, ceftriaxone, and acyclovir. The patient was admitted to the ICU for monitoring. The next day, the patient's mental status improved and the patient was transferred out of the ICU to the medical floor. The following day (48 hours after admission), the patient starts to have nausea, oliguria, abdominal, and flank pain. Repeated blood works were significant for creatinine 3.2 mg/dL, urea 56 mg/dL, potassium 5.3 mEq/L, and sodium 142 mEq/L. Urine analysis shows white blood cells 5 cells/HPF, red blood cells 5 cells/HPF, protein 100 mg/dL, and crystals.

   Which of the following is the **MOST LIKELY** cause of acute kidney injury (AKI)/failure in this patient?

   A. Vancomycin
   B. Synthetic marijuana
   C. Acyclovir
   D. Ceftriaxone

9. A 75-year-old male is in postoperative day 3 in the ICU status post liver resection. He was aggressively resuscitated with IV fluids in the perioperative period. Currently, he is mechanically ventilated and hemodynamically stable; however over the last 24 hours, his urine output has decreased significantly to 5 mL/h. What is the best test to assess his AKI?

   A. Serum urea/creatinine
   B. Urine sodium
   C. Renal ultrasound with Doppler
   D. Abdominal CT scan

# Chapter 49 ▪ Answers

**1.** Correct Answer: C

**Rationale:**

Acute interstitial nephritis (AIN) is a rare cause of AKI. Most patients present with nonspecific signs and symptoms of acute kidney failure. The classical triad of fever, rash, and eosinophilia occurs only in 10% of the population. Moreover, patients can be oliguric or nonoliguric, and hematuria can occur in 5% of them. The most common cause of AIN is drug-associated, such as trimethoprim-sulfamethoxazole that the patient has been taking. Other causes include infection, idiopathic, or associated with systemic autoimmune diseases. Laboratory results usually show an increase in creatinine level, eosinophilia or eosinophiluria, white blood cells or white blood cell casts in urine (question 1—choice C), and a variable degree of proteinuria.

Muddy brown cast is usually seen in acute tubular necrosis (ATN), which is associated with prolonged prerenal insult or nephrotoxin induced. Red blood cell cast is associated with acute glomerulonephritis, in which immunological mechanisms cause glomerular inflammation. These mechanisms could be infection-related, cancer, or exposure to drugs of toxins. Enveloplike, calcium oxalate crystals are seen in patients with ethylene glycol poisoning. As the patient is healthy and does not have any risk factors, and her examination is normal, ATN, acute glomerulonephritis, or ethylene glycol poisoning are very unlikely.

## Reference

1. Moledina DG, Perazella MA. Drug-induced acute interstitial nephritis. *Clin J Am Soc Nephrol*. 2017;12:2046-2049.

**2.** Correct Answer: B

**Rationale:**

Treatment of AIN includes discontinuing the offending agent (question 2—choice B) or treating the underlying disease. In severe cases of biopsy-confirmed AIN, steroids can be administered. Answer A is incorrect because fomepizole is the treatment for ethylene glycol poisoning, not AIN. Her urea/creatinine ratio is less than 20, making prerenal cause unlikely, so fluid bolus would not be needed here. Also, CT scan with IV contrast would not be the best choice as there is no indication for this study, and IV contrast should be avoided in patients with AKI (answer D).

## References

1. Praga M, Appel GB. *Clinical Manifestations and Diagnosis of Acute Interstitial Nephritis*. Retrieved from Uptodate. https://www.uptodate.com/contents/clinical-manifestations-and-diagnosis-of-acute-interstitial-nephritis.
2. Roberts PR, Todd SR. *Acute and chronic renal failure and management (including hemodialysis and continuous renal replacement. therapies)*. In: *Comprehensive Critical Care: Adult*. 2nd ed. USA: Society of Critcal Care Medicine; 2017:365-376:Chap 33.
3. Kshirsagar AV, Falk RJ. *Treatment of Acute Interstitial Nephritis*. Retrieved from Uptodate. https://www.uptodate.com/contents/treatment-of-acute-interstitial-nephritis.
4. Ronco P. *Mechanisms of Immune Injury of the Glomerulus*. Retrieved from Uptodate. https://www.uptodate.com/contents/mechanisms-of-immune-injury-of-the-glomerulus.
5. Sivilotti MLA. *Methanol and Ethylene Glycol Poisoning*. Retrieved from Uptodate. https://www.uptodate.com/contents/methanol-and-ethylene-glycol-poisoning.

**3.** Correct Answer: A

**Rationale:**

Kidneys play an essential role in the body to maintain normal acid-base status and electrolyte levels. In addition, kidneys excrete acids in the form of ammonium chloride. As kidney disease progresses, patients lose the ability to effectively neutralize and excrete acids, leading to metabolic acidosis.

As the glomerular filtration decreases, renal failure patients lose the ability to concentrate urine, which can lead to hyponatremia. Studies suggest that a decreased clearance of vasopressin also contributes to the development of dysnatremia. It is not uncommon for hyperkalemia, hyperphosphatemia, and hypermagnesemia to occur as the kidneys lose their ability to excrete these electrolytes.

## References

1. Barash PG. *Clinical Anesthesia*. 7th ed. Philadelphia, PA: Wolters Kluwer Health/Lippincott Williams & Wilkins; 2013:1410.
2. Cadnapaphornchai MA, Schrier RW. "Pathogenesis and management of hyponatremia." *Am J Med*. 2000;109(8):688-692.
3. Dhondup T, Qian Q. "Electrolyte and acid-base disorders in chronic kidney disease and end-stage kidney failure." *Blood Purif*. 2017;43(1–3):179-188. doi:10.1159/000452725. Epub 2017 January 24.

**4.** Correct Answer: B

**Rationale:**

Because we cannot obtain any useful history from the patient, we need to look for clues from his physical examination and laboratory results. His anion gap (corrected for serum albumin) is $147 - 113 - 22 + 2.5(4 - 2) = 17$, indicating a high-gap metabolic acidosis. Based on the Winter's formula, his expected $pCO_2$ should be $1.5 \times 22 + 8 = 41$ mm Hg. However, as his $pCO_2$ is 38, he also has a respiratory alkalosis.

In the presence of a high-gap metabolic acidosis, we need to identify if there is a third process. The patient's $\Delta$ gap = $17 - 12 = 5$, and $\Delta$ bicarbonate = $24 - 22 = 2$. As $\Delta$ gap > $\Delta$ bicarbonate, he also has a metabolic alkalosis.

The history of taking OTC medications and the combination of metabolic acidosis and respiratory alkalosis make aspirin toxicity high on the differential diagnosis. Aspirin could also cause altered mental status, confusion, and possible seizure at a toxic dose. Moreover, aspirin could cause GI upset, which could explain his metabolic alkalosis.

Although euglycemic diabetes ketoacidosis has been described in the literature, a normal glucose level makes diabetic ketoacidosis very unlikely. Similarly, alcohol intoxication is less likely to cause respiratory alkalosis, which makes it lower in the differential diagnosis.

Because of its availability OTC and the potential combination with aspirin in some formulary, acetaminophen level should be checked; however, it would not be the best choice as it does not typically cause mixed metabolic acidosis and respiratory alkalosis. Moreover, acetaminophen overdose typically presents with gastrointestinal signs and symptoms.

**Reference**

1. O'Malley GF. Emergency department management of the salicylate-poisoned patient. *Emerg Med Clin North Am.* 2007;25:333-346.

**5.** Correct Answer: C

**Rationale:**

In a patient with salicylate toxicity, the presence of altered mental status is an indication for emergent dialysis. Other indications for emergent dialysis are pulmonary edema, seizure, decreased renal function impairing salicylate elimination (consider when creatinine >2 mg/dL or 1.5 mg/dL for elderly or glomerular filtration rate <45 mL/min per 1.73 m²), severe volume overload, severe acidemia, and serum salicylate level >90 mg/dL. Urine alkalization is indicated in salicylate poisoning to enhance its elimination; however, the presence of altered mental status and AKI makes dialysis the best choice for this patient.

**References**

1. Boyer EW, Weibrecht KW. *Salicylate (Aspirin) Poisoning in Adults.* Retrieved from Uptodate. https://www.uptodate.com/contents/salicylate-aspirin-poisoning-in-adults.

2. Heard K, Dart R. *Acetaminophen (Paracetamol) Poisoning in Adults: Treatment.* Retrieved from Uptodate. https://www.uptodate.com/contents/acetaminophen-paracetamol-poisoning-in-adults-treatments.

**6.** Correct Answer: A

**Rationale:**

Intermittent hemodialysis (iHD) is associated with an increased risk of causing dialysis disequilibrium syndrome (DDS). DDS is characterized by different neurological symptoms of varying severity. Its symptoms range from nausea, headache, dizziness to seizure, coma, and death. DDS is primarily caused by fluid shifts that result in brain edema. Removal of urea across the blood-brain barrier occurs at a much slower rate than urea removal from plasma. This cause the brain cells to be "relatively" hyperosmolar to plasm and promotes water movement to brain cells.

Moreover, patients with end-stage renal disease are in a chronic hyperosmolar state; this leads to the development of "idiogenic osmoles," which add to the "relative" hyperosmolarity of the brain following dialysis. It has been reported that brain volume increases by an average of 3% after hemodialysis, which makes iHD inappropriate for patients with head trauma, intracranial bleeding, stroke, or any intracranial pathology that leads to increased intracranial pressure.

The use of dialysis modality that removes solute and fluid at lower rates do not cause significant elevation of intracranial pressure and lower the risk for DDS. CRRT, SLED, and EDD can be used for patients at risk for DDS, and they all have similar effects on intracranial pressure and hemodynamics.

**References**

1. Davenport A. Practical guidance for dialyzing a hemodialysis patient following acute brain injury. *Hemodial Int.* 2008;12(3):307-312. doi:10.1111/j.1542-4758.2008.00271.x.

2. Kumar A, Cage A, Dhar R. Dialysis-induced worsening of cerebral edema in intracranial hemorrhage: a case series and clinical perspective. *Neurocrit Care.* 2015;22:283-287.

3. Wu VC, Huang TM, Shiao CC, et al. The hemodynamic effects during sustained low-efficiency dialysis versus continuous veno-venous hemofiltration for uremic patients with brain hemorrhage: a crossover study. *J Neurosurg.* 2013;119:1288-1295. doi:10.3171/2013.4.JNS122102.

4. Khwaja A. KDIGO clinical practice guidelines for acute kidney injury. *Nephron Clin Pract.* 2012;120(4):c179-c184.

**7. Correct Answer: B**

**Rationale:**

The patient in the vignette is presenting with signs and symptoms concerning for spontaneous bacterial peritonitis (SBP). Cirrhosis patients with SBP are at high risk of developing renal failure secondary to hepatorenal syndrome. The risk can be reduced (from 30% to 10%) with IV albumin infusion. Albumin appears to be most effective in patients with serum creatinine >1 mg/dL and total bilirubin >4 mg/dL, but its effect is unclear in patients who had lower creatinine and bilirubin levels. The European Association for the Study of the Liver guidelines recommend starting albumin infusion in all patients with SBP. The recommended dose is 1.5 g per kg at the time of diagnosis and 1.0 g/kg body weight on day 3. Terlipressin, midodrine, and octreotide used as treatment options for hepatorenal syndrome but not for prevention.

### References

1. European Association for the Study of the Liver. EASL clinical practice guidelines on the management of ascites, spontaneous bacterial peritonitis, and hepatorenal syndrome in cirrhosis. *J Hepatol.* 2010;53(3):397-417. doi:10.1016/j.jhep.2010.05.004. https://www.ncbi.nlm.nih.gov/pubmed/20633946.
2. Sort P, Navasa M, Arroyo V, et al. Effect of intravenous albumin on renal impairment and mortality in patients with cirrhosis and spontaneous bacterial peritonitis. *N Engl J Med.* 1999;341:403-409. https://www.ncbi.nlm.nih.gov/pubmed/10432325.

**8. Correct Answer: C**

**Rationale:**

This patient presented to the ED with possible HSV encephalitis/meningitis. The patient was started on empirical antimicrobial, including acyclovir. After appropriate treatment with acyclovir, the patient mental status improved but developed AKI. Acyclovir and vancomycin, both are nephrotoxic. Acyclovir can cause AKI by forming crystals that precipitate in renal tubules. Vancomycin, on the other hand, does not cause crystal-induced nephropathy. Acyclovir crystal–induced nephropathy can be asymptomatic or present with nausea, abdominal pain, flank pain, asterixis, multifocal myoclonus, seizures, hallucination, and altered mental status. Symptoms typically within 24 to 48 hours after therapy. Crystal-induced nephropathy can be avoided by appropriate volume repletion before starting acyclovir infusion, slow IV acyclovir infusion over 1 to 2 hours, and dose adjustment for patients with renal impairment. Treatment of acyclovir crystal–induced nephropathy range from IV hydration and loop diuretics to hemodialysis depending on the severity of symptoms.

There are case reports for AKI associated with synthetic marijuana. There are reports of calcium oxalate crystal on kidney biopsy of patients who had renal impairment associated with synthetic marijuana abuse. As the patient does not have a history of synthetic marijuana abuse, it is less likely to be the cause of his renal impairment. Conventional urine drug screen does not test for synthetic marijuana.

### References

1. Gentry JL III, Peterson C. Death delusions and myoclonus: acyclovir toxicity. *Am J Med.* 2015;128:692-694. doi:10.1016/j.amjmed.2015.03.001.
2. Perazella M, Palevsky P, Forman J. *Crystal-Induced Acute Kidney Injury.* Uptodate. www.uptodate.com/contents/crystal-induced-acute-kidney-injury. Accessed 11/1/2018.
3. Perazella MA, Crystal-induced acute renal failure. *Am J Med.* 1999;106(4):459.
4. Kazory A, Aiyer R. Synthetic marijuana and acute kidney injury: an unforeseen association. *Clin Kidney J.* 2013;6:330-333. doi:10.1093/ckj/sft047.

**9. Correct Answer: C**

**Rationale:**

Renal ultrasound with Doppler can easily detect obstruction and can be performed at the bedside. In addition, Doppler measurements allow for assessment of renal perfusion. The renal resistive index (RI) is defined as peak systolic velocity—end diastolic velocity/peak systolic velocity and is measured at the renal arcuate or interlobar arteries. It has a specificity and sensitivity of about 90% to discern between states of no AKI, kidney injury, and persistent AKI. It can also guide therapy to optimize renal perfusion. Normal RI is approximately 0.58 ± 0.10 and values >0.70 are considered to be abnormal and a high renal RI on ICU admission may be predictive for developing AKI. RI is unaffected by changes in sodium or creatinine in urine or serum after diuretics or hemodialysis.

Serum urea and creatinine are late markers of renal failure and are not predictive of permanent renal failure. These laboratory parameters in conjunction with urine sodium might potentially help to predict whether the patient is in a prerenal or renal state, however this information is often unreliable in critically ill patients. Abdominal CT scan will show renal pathology, however this necessitates transport of the patient. Additionally, contrast is often required for best images and this might further decrease renal function.

References

1. Lerolle N, Guerot E, Faisy C, Bornstain C, Diehl JL, Fagon JY. Renal failure in septic shock: predictive value of Doppler-based renal arterial resistive index. *Intensive Care Med.* 2006;32:1553.

2. Darmon M, Schortgen F, Vargas F, et al. Diagnostic accuracy of Doppler renal resistive index for reversibility of acute kidney injury in critically ill patients. *Intensive Care Med.* 2011;37:68-76.

3. Deruddre S, Cheisson G, Mazoit JX, Vicaut E, Benhamou D, Duranteau J. Renal arterial resistance in septic shock: effects of increasing mean arterial pressure with norepinephrine on the renal resistive index assessed with Doppler ultrasonography. *Intensive Care Med.* 2007;33:1557.

4. Bellomo R, Bagshaw S, Langenberg C, Ronco C. Pre-renal azotemia: a flawed paradigm in critically ill septic patients? *Contrib Nephrol.* 2007;156:1.

# 50

# SODIUM

Jaya Prakash Sugunaraj and Ngoc-Tram Ha

1. A 78-year-old man is brought to the hospital after being found down by his daughter at his home this morning. He was functional at baseline and last seen normal yesterday. He is a life-time smoker with chronic obstructive pulmonary disease (COPD) and was recently diagnosed with lung cancer. On physical examination, he is lethargic, has unsteady gait, and is confused. His temperature is 37.4°C, blood pressure is 127/94 mm Hg, pulse rate is 74 beats/min, and respiratory rate is 11 breaths/min. On examination, he has a normal jugular venous pressure, but he has decreased air entry at the lung bases. A CT head obtained shows age-related atrophic changes. Laboratory studies obtained are as follows:

Sodium 120 mEq/L (mmol/L)
BUN 9 mg/dL
Bicarbonate 30 mmol/L
Creatinine 1.0 mg/dL
Urine osmolality 275 mOsm/kg $H_2O$
Urine sodium 45 mEq/L (mmol/L)
Serum osmolality 264 mOsm/kg $H_2O$
Glucose 84 mg/dL (4.6 mmol/L)

Which of the following is the MOST appropriate next step in management of this patient?

A. Fluid restriction to 800 mL
B. Desmopressin
C. Isotonic saline infusion
D. Tolvaptan
E. Hypertonic saline infusion

2. A 17-year-old college student is admitted to the hospital after sustaining a traumatic hit to the head during football practice, resulting in subdural hemorrhage. Upon arrival, his Glasgow Coma Scale is 4. He is started on hypertonic saline and undergoes emergent neurosurgical intervention. His exam remains unchanged overnight, but during morning rounds, the nurse reports that his urine output increased to over 300 mL/h.

Laboratory studies obtained show serum sodium 167 mEq/L, specific gravity 1.013, random urine sodium 55 mEq/L (mmol/L), random urine creatinine 51 mg/dL, urine osmolality 199 mOsm/kg $H_2O$, and serum osmolality 338 mOsm/kg $H_2O$.

Which is the MOST likely cause of his increased urine output?

A. Syndrome of inappropriate antidiuretic hormone secretion (SIADH)
B. Central diabetes insipidus (DI)
C. Cerebral salt wasting (CSW) syndrome
D. Nephrogenic diabetes insipidus (NDI)
E. Osmotic diuresis

**3.** A 68-year-old man presents to his primary care physician complaining of frequent urination at night. He reports a strong urinary stream without any feeling of incomplete emptying. His medications include aspirin, pravastatin, lithium, and amlodipine. On physical examination, he is afebrile, his blood pressure 138/75 mm Hg, pulse rate 74 beats/min, and respiratory rate 18 breaths/min. Which of the following laboratory studies are MOST consistent with the patient's clinical presentation?

| | PLASMA SODIUM | URINE OSMOLALITY | PLASMA OSMOLALITY |
|---|---|---|---|
| A. | 133 mg/dL | 281 mOsm/kg $H_2O$ | 210 mOsm/kg $H_2O$ |
| B. | 149 mg/dL | 370 mOsm/kg $H_2O$ | 280 mOsm/kg $H_2O$ |
| C. | 144 mg/dL | 262 mOsm/kg $H_2O$ | 310 mOsm/kg $H_2O$ |
| D. | 134 mg/dL | 239 mOsm/kg $H_2O$ | 234 mOsm/kg $H_2O$ |

**4.** A 58-year-old woman with past medical history of alcohol abuse and bipolar schizophrenia presents to the hospital after a fall complicated by numerous rib fractures seen on chest x-ray. She is currently not taking any medications. On physical examination, her temperature is 37.1°C, blood pressure is 138/88 mm Hg, pulse rate is 99 beats/min, and respiratory rate is 14 breaths/min, oxygen saturation is 95% on room air. Her neurological, cardiovascular, and abdominal examinations are normal. She exhibits tenderness to palpation over the left chest wall with decreased bibasilar breath sounds. Her chemistry panel is as follows:

Sodium 122 mEq/L (mmol/L)
Potassium 2.8 mEq/L (mmol/L)
BUN 5 mg/dL
Creatinine 0.7 mg/dL
Urine osmolality 117 mOsm/kg
Urine sodium 18 mEq/L (mmol/L)
Serum osmolality 266 mOsm/kg
Glucose 105 mg/dL
Thyroid stimulating hormone 2.20 mIU/L
Morning cortisol 16 µg/dL
Total cholesterol 140 mg/dL
HDL cholesterol 55 mg/dL
LDL cholesterol 124 mg/dL
Triglycerides 162 mg/dL

What is the MOST appropriate management of her hyponatremia?

**A.** Conivaptan
**B.** Desmopressin
**C.** Normal saline infusion
**D.** Fluid restriction
**E.** Observation with repeat laboratory testing in 4 to 6 hours

**5.** A 62-year-old woman is brought to the hospital with sudden onset headache followed by nausea and vomiting. Upon arrival to the emergency room, she is lethargic with a Glasgow Coma Scale of 5. Significant vital signs include a blood pressure of 220/130 mm Hg. She is emergently intubated. CT scan of the head reveals subarachnoid hemorrhage in the basilar cisterns. She undergoes placement of a right frontal extraventricular device and coiling with improvement of her neurological examination. Over the following days, she is weaned off propofol. However, on the seventh day, her urine output increases to 4 L/d and she becomes hypotensive with blood pressure of 89/60 mm Hg and pulse rate of 118 beats/min. Laboratory data show hyponatremia with a sodium level of 130 mEq/L, potassium of 3.3 mEq/L, plasma osmolality of 269 mOsm/kg, urine sodium concentration of 71 mEq/L, urine osmolality of 93 mmol/L, glucose 172 mg/dL, TSH 3.1 mIU/L, and triglyceride of 118 mg/dL.

What is the MOST likely cause for the patient's acute changes?

**A.** CSW syndrome
**B.** Central DI
**C.** Osmotic diuresis
**D.** SIADH
**E.** Pseudohyponatremia

6. A 68-year-old male with long-standing smoking and alcohol use history presents to his primary care physician. His wife noticed progressively worsening jaundice and poor appetite with an associated weight loss of 35 lbs over the past 2 months. He also reports early satiety and vague abdominal pain.

His temperature is 37.5°C, blood pressure is 110/75 mm Hg, pulse rate is 84 beats/min, and respiratory rate is 12 breaths/min. An ultrasound of his abdomen confirms a mass in the head of the pancreas. He is admitted for surgical intervention, and laboratory data obtained show the following:

Sodium 131 mEq/L (mmol/L)
Potassium 3.8 mEq/L (mmol/L)
BUN 7 mg/dL
Creatinine 1.0 mg/dL
Total bilirubin 8.7 mg/dL
Amylase 90 U/L
Lipase 67 U/L
Total cholestrol 485 mg/dL
LDL cholesterol 157 mg/dL
HDL cholesterol 42 mg/dL
Triglycerides 349 mg/dL
Plasma osmolality 295 mOsm/kg
Urine osmolality 420 mOsm/kg
TSH 2.1 mIU/L
Glucose 93 mg/dL

What is the MOST likely cause for the patient's hyponatremia?

A. Beer potomania
B. Psychogenic polydipsia
C. SIADH
D. Adrenal insufficiency
E. Pseudohyponatremia

7. A 24-year-old woman is brought to the emergency department by her boyfriend for worsening lethargy. He reports that she has no known medical history and was doing well until 2 days ago after they returned home from a hiking trip on the Appalachian trail. She started experiencing diarrhea after drinking from the fresh springs. Vital signs are as follows: temperature is 37.8°C, blood pressure is 97/64 mm Hg, pulse rate is 112 beats/min, and respiratory rate is 14 breaths/min. On physical examination, abdominal examination reveals tenderness in the left lower quadrant and weak radial pulses.

Sodium 144 mEq/L (mmol/L)
Potassium 3.9 mEq/L (mmol/L)
Chloride 110 (mmol/L)
Bicarbonate 18 (mmol/L)
BUN 42 mg/dL
Creatinine 1.2 mg/dL
Glucose 123 mg/dL
Urine sodium 24 mEq/L

What is the next BEST step in management of this patient's condition?

A. Normal saline with 20 KCl mEq/L
B. Ringer lactate
C. ½ normal saline
D. ½ normal saline with D5W
E. Normal saline with D5W

8. A 38-year-old male is brought to the hospital after a witnessed seizure. The patient's medical history is only significant for bipolar disease. His sister also reports that he recently started a new diet regimen using herbal supplements that he purchased online. On physical examination, his vital signs are unremarkable. He appears unkempt, and there is a small laceration noted over his tongue. His serum sodium is 128 mEq/L (mmol/L). Other laboratory findings before and after water deprivation test (WDT) are shown below:

|  | BEFORE WDT | AFTER WDT |
| --- | --- | --- |
| Serum osmolality | 268 mOsm/kg | 305 mOsm/kg |
| Urine osmolality | 137 mOsm/kg | 780 mOsm/kg |
| Specific gravity | 1.009 | 1.023 |

What is the MOST likely diagnosis in this patient?

A. Nephrogenic DI
B. Pseudohyponatremia
C. Psychogenic polydipsia
D. SIADH
E. Central DI

9. A 19-year-old woman with past medical history of type I diabetes mellitus and seizures on oxcarbazepine is admitted for fever, chills, and myalgia. She works as a nurse assistant in the local skilled nursing facility where a few patients recently have been diagnosed with the flu. Her appetite has been poor since her symptoms started, and she also reports bouts of diarrhea. On physical examination, she is febrile with a temperature of 38.7°C, blood pressure is 102/76 mm Hg, pulse rate is 120 beats/min, and respiratory rate is 12 breaths/min. Laboratory values show the following:

Sodium 130 mEq/L (mmol/L)
Potassium 4.1 mEq/L (mmol/L)
Chloride 95 (mmol/L)
Bicarbonate 9 (mmol/L)
BUN 9 mg/dL
Creatinine 0.7 mg/dL
Glucose 623 mg/dL

What is the MOST likely underlying cause for her hyponatremia?

A. Poor solute intake
B. SIADH
C. Medication related
D. Hyperglycemia
E. Diarrhea

10. A 56-year-old man with a past medical history of hypertension, hyperlipidemia, and type II diabetes mellitus presents to his primary care physician for a follow-up visit. He started working as a welder 6 months ago and was recently diagnosed with hypersensitivity pneumonitis after complaining of worsening shortness of breath at the time. He was prescribed a medication whose name he is unable to recall but stopped taking them abruptly after 2 months because of his busy schedule. His other medications include amlodipine, atorvastatin, and hydrochlorothiazide though he admits being noncompliant with those, too.

Today, he reports fatigue, unintentional weight loss of 7 lbs in 2 weeks, nausea, and lightheadedness.

Pertinent vital signs include a temperature of 37.6°C, blood pressure of 117/58 mm Hg, pulse rate of 92 beats/min, and respiratory rate of 12 breaths/min.

What are the MOST likely laboratory findings in this patient?

|   | SERUM SODIUM | SERUM POTASSIUM | SERUM OSMOLALITY | URINE SODIUM |
|---|---|---|---|---|
| A. | 130 mg/dL | 4.7 mg/dL | 295 mOsm/kg | 32 mEq/L |
| B. | 128 mg/dL | 5.4 mg/dL | 260 mOsm/kg | 45 mEq/L |
| C. | 145 mg/dL | 3.8 mg/dL | 265 mOsm/kg | 48 mEq/L |
| D. | 149 mg/dL | 4.0 mg/dL | 285 mOsm/kg | 53 mEq/L |
| E. | 132 mg/dL | 5.2 mg/dL | 280 mOsm/kg | 25 mEq/L |

# Chapter 50 ▪ Answers

**1.** Correct Answer: E

**Rationale:**
The patient's history and laboratory studies are consistent with hypotonic euvolemic hyponatremia. The important differentials are SIADH, adrenocortical insufficiency, polydipsia, physiological stimulus antidiuretic hormone (ADH) release (nausea, pain, anxiety), and hypothyroidism. Based on presentation, the most likely etiology of hyponatremia in this patient is SIADH. Patients with lung cancer, particularly small cell lung cancer, have a reported incidence of up 18.9%. SIADH is caused by the secretion of ADH from the posterior pituitary gland or unregulated ectopic production by tumor cells. Elevated levels of ADH lead to hyponatremia and hypoosmolality by decreasing the renal excretion of free water. While not all cases of hyponatremia require correction with hypertonic saline, this patient has acute onset, severe hyponatremia and has moderate symptoms. Symptoms of hyponatremia include headache, nausea, vomiting, confusion, disorientation, and seizures. Though his sodium needs correction with hypertonic saline, the sodium should not be corrected by more than 9 mEq/L in 24 hours to avoid osmotic demyelination syndrome (ODS). It is important to note that neurological effects related to ODS can take up to 1 week to manifest, including dysarthria and dysphagia.

References
1. Fiordoliva I, Meletani T, Baleani MG, et al. Managing hyponatremia in lung cancer: latest evidence and clinical implications. *Ther Adv Med Oncol.* 2017;9:711-719.
2. Hoorn EJ, Zietse R. Diagnosis and treatment of hyponatremia: compilation of the guidelines. *J Am Soc Nephrol.* 2017;28:1340-1349.

**2.** Correct Answer: B

**Rationale:**
Central DI occurs in the setting of inadequate production of ADH. Normally, ADH is secreted by the posterior pituitary gland. However, in patients who sustained traumatic brain injury, a decrease or cessation of ADH production can occur, thereby decreasing reabsorption of water leading to hypernatremia. In otherwise healthy patients, the lack of ADH will cause increased thirst and lead to polydipsia. These symptoms might not be apparent in a critically ill patient.

Water deprivation test and administration of desmopressin, as depicted in the flowchart below, may be used to confirm the diagnosis. However, the test is relatively contraindicated in hypovolemic and hypernatremic patients due to risk of exacerbating these. Further testing is not needed in our patient, since the clinical presentation and laboratory studies are consistent with central DI. Diagnostic evaluation for suspected DI includes serum sodium, serum, and urine osmolality, which are expected to show hypernatremia with decreased urine osmolality <600 mOsm/kg and serum osmolality of >295 mOsm/kg. In patients with central DI, the urine osmolality is expected to increase by >100% after administration of desmopressin.

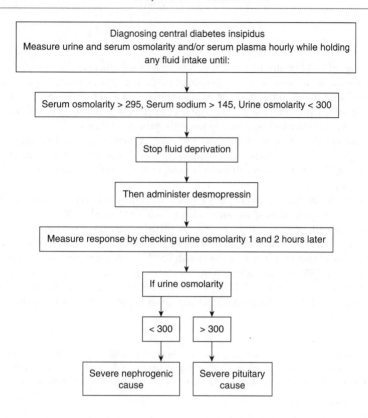

References
1. Robertson GL. Diabetes insipidus. *Endocrinol Metab Clin North Am.* 1995;24(3):549-572.
2. Makaryus AN, McFarlane AI. Diabetes insipidus: diagnosis and treatment of a complex disease. *Clev Clin J Med.* 2006;73(1):65-71.

### 3. Correct Answer: C

**Rationale:**

The patient's history and presentation is consistent with lithium-induced NDI. In NDI, the kidney's ability to concentrate the urine is decreased despite the presence of sufficient ADH, due to insufficient water reabsorption in the collecting duct. Vasopressin is responsible for regulating the water permeability in the collecting duct and water reabsorption based on the tonicity of the medullary interstitium. Lithium causes NDI by entering the principal cells in the collecting tubules and interfering with aquaporin function, thereby decreasing the ability to concentrate urine.

Other causes for NDI include hypercalcemia, hypercalciuria, and obstructive uropathy. In the setting of a positive water deprivation test, the administration of desmopressin can further differentiate primary polydipsia from central and nephrogenic DI. Patients with NDI will not respond to the administration of desmopressin, whereas patients with central DI will have an increased urine osmolality.

In NDI, the urine osmolarity is typically lower than serum osmolarity (option C). Since water intake is maintained by compensatory polydipsia, patients do not typically develop overt hypernatremia.

References
1. Bockenhauer D, Bichet D. Pathophysiology, diagnosis and management of nephrogenic diabetes insipidus. *Nat Rev Nephrol.* 2015;11:576-588.
2. Sands JM, Bichet DG. Nephrogenic diabetes insipidus. *Ann Intern Med.* 2006;144:186-194.

### 4. Correct Answer: D

**Rationale:**

This patient's hyponatremia is due to low solute intake associated with increased consumption of beer which is also known as beer potomania. Beer is low in solutes and electrolytes. Excessive consumption with an otherwise nutritionally poor diet leads to impaired water clearance and therefore dilutional hyponatremia. Typical laboratory findings include low urine sodium, low urine osmolality, and low ADH levels. However, it should be noted, that the concomitant use of diuretics can make the diagnosis of beer potomania more difficult as diuretics will cause increased sodium excretion in urine and thus result in higher than expected urine sodium and osmolality concentrations.

References
1. Joshi R, Chou S. Beer potomania: a view on the dynamic process of developing hyponatremia. *Cureus.* 2018;10:3024.
2. Rafei H, Yunus R, Khurana P. Beer potomania: a challenging case of hyponatremia. *J Endocrinol Metab.* 2016;6:123-126.

**5.** Correct Answer: A

**Rationale:**

The pathophysiology of CSW syndrome remains poorly understood. There are two proposed mechanisms that lead to CSW. One of the mechanisms involves the disruption of the sympathetic neural input which normally promotes the reabsorption of sodium. The other mechanism is natriuresis induced by natriuretic peptides that are released in patients with brain injury. Both of these mechanisms lead to decreased activation of the renin-angiotensin-aldosterone system, leading to decreased sodium absorption at the proximal tubules.

CSW syndrome and SIADH both have similar laboratory values, including low serum osmolality, high urine osmolality, and high urine sodium levels. The most important distinguishing feature is the extracellular fluid volume status. Patients with CSW will have low extracellular fluid, reflected by their hypotension, whereas SIADH patients are generally euvolemic.

Evaluation of 24 hour uric acid excretion may also aid in the diagnosis as patients with SIADH. Uric acid is normally resorbed in the proximal tubule along with sodium. Both SIADH and CSW results in loss of uric acid via urine. However, an important differentiating feature is that in patients with SIADH, serum uric acid level and fractional excretion of uric acid normalize after correction of the serum sodium level, whereas the uric acid level remains low and uric acid excretion remains elevated in patients with CSW, despite correction of hyponatremia.

Common causes for CSW include subarachnoid hemorrhage, intracranial tumors and infections. Overall, the prevalence of CSW is less common than SIADH, but it is important to exclude as the treatment for CSW and SIADH vary vastly. The treatment for CSW includes administration of fluids and mineralocorticoids. In contrast, SIADH is treated with water restriction.

**References**

1. Maesaka JK, Imbriano L, Mattana J, Gallagher D, Bade N, Sharif S. Differentiating SIAD from cerebral/renal salt wasting: failure of the volume approach and need for a new approach to hyponatremia. *J Clin Med.* 2014;3:1373-1385.
2. Momi J, Tang CM, Abcar A, Kujubu DA, Sim JJ. Hyponatremia – What is cerebral salt wasting? *Perm J.* 2010;12(2):62-65.

**6.** Correct Answer: E

**Rationale:**

While the patient's calculated plasma osmolality is 270 mOsm/kg $H_2O$, his measured plasma osmolality is normal at 295 mOsm/kg $H_2O$, making the diagnosis of pseudohyponatremia most likely.

Plasma osmolality (mOsm/kg $H_2O$) = 2 × serum sodium (mEq/L) + plasma glucose (mg/dL)/18 + blood urea nitrogen (mg/dL)/2.8.

Plasma consists of 93% water and 7% lipids and proteins. However, in the presence of other substances, such as elevated lipids or paraproteins, the aqueous fraction of plasma will be diluted and thereby falsely lower the serum sodium concentration while the actual serum sodium concentration remains normal. Pseudohyponatremia is due to a laboratory error in the measurement of the serum sodium that leads to low reported sodium with normal plasma osmolality in the presence of total serum cholesterol and lipoprotein X as in patients with obstructive jaundice. Other causes for pseudohyponatremia include severe hypertriglyceridemia, diabetic ketoacidosis, plasma cell dyscrasia, such as in patients with multiple myeloma, and obstructive jaundice as in this patient.

**References**

1. Hussain I, Ahmad Z, Garg A. Extreme hypercholesterolemia presenting with pseudohyponatremia – a case report and review of the literature. *J Clin Lipidol.* 2015;9(2):260-264.
2. Vo I, Gosmanov AR, Garcia-Rosell M, Wall BM. Pseudohyponatremia in acute liver disease. *Am J Med Sci.* 2013;345(1):62-64.

**7.** Correct Answer: B

**Rationale:**

In patients who cannot tolerate oral rehydration therapy (ORT), the usage of isotonic fluids such as lactated Ringers (LR) is the most appropriate. The lactate found in LR is converted to bicarbonate in the liver and replaces the bicarbonate that is lost with diarrhea (which contains high level of sodium, bicarbonate and potassium). Thus, persistent diarrhea will lead to a hypokalemic, hyperchloremic metabolic acidosis in most patients which should be replaced by isotonic fluids, such as LR. However, close monitoring of potassium should be performed as the correction of the metabolic acidosis will lead to an intracellular shift of potassium leading to hypokalemia.

**Reference**

1. Pandya S. *Practical Guidelines on Fluid Therapy.* 2nd ed. Bhalani Medical Book House; 2012.

**8.** Correct Answer: C

**Rationale:**

The cause for his hyponatremia is due to increased free water intake which may manifest in patients with underlying psychiatric disorders, such as schizophrenia, depression, and bipolar disorder in particular. When patients present with polyuria, WDT can help differentiate between psychogenic polydipsia and DI. It is believed that patients with psychogenic polydipsia have a dysregulated thirst mechanism with a reduced osmotic threshold for thirst compared to the ADH threshold, causing them to drink more than needed. It rarely occurs as the amount of free water intake needed to cause hyponatremia is greater than 7 L/d. In patients with polydipsia, an increase in serum osmolarity from water deprivation leads to a marked increase in urine osmolality. On the other hand, urine osmolality will remain low in a patient with DI. Other important differentiating feature is that DI causes hypernatremia while patients with polydipsia are either eunatremic or mildly hyponatremic. Desmopressin has no effect since endogenous release is intact. SIADH and pseudohyponatremia do not cause polyuria.

References

1. Goldman MB. The influence of polydipsia on water excretion in hyponatremic, polydipsic, schizophrenic patients. *Endocrinol Metab.* 1996;81(4):1465-1470.
2. Hariprasad MK, Eisinger RP, Nadler IM. Hyponatremia in psychogenic polydipsia. *Arch Intern Med.* 1980;140(12):1639-1642.
3. Trimpou P, Olsson DS, Ehn O, Ragnarsson O. Diagnostic value of the water deprivation test in the polyuria-polydipsia syndrome. *Hormones (Athens).* 2017;16(4):414-422.

**9.** Correct Answer: D

**Rationale:**

Glucose is an osmotically active solute. In the presence of hyperglycemia, the serum osmolality increases which leads to water movement out of the cells. This leads to a dilutional hyponatremia. Generally, for any glucose level greater that 100 mg/dL, an additional 1.6 mEq/L should be added to the measured serum sodium level. In this case, the patient's corrected sodium level is approximately 138 mEq/L.

Reference

1. Liamis G, Liberopoulos E, Barkas F, Elisaf M. Diabetes mellitus and electrolyte disorders. *World J Clin Cases.* 2014;2(10):488-496.

**10.** Correct Answer: B

**Rationale:**

Sudden withdrawal of prolonged steroid therapy can lead to low adrenocorticotropic hormone (ACTH) levels due to suppression of the hypothalamic-pituitary-adrenal axis, leading to mineralocorticoid and glucocorticoid deficiency. The patient likely developed adrenal insufficiency after abrupt cessation of his prednisone that he was prescribed for treatment for hypersensitivity pneumonitis. The symptoms vary based on the severity of adrenal insufficiency; however, they most commonly manifest with fatigue, weight loss, and GI symptoms, such as nausea and vomiting. Mineralocorticoid deficiency results in excessive sodium loss and insufficient potassium excretion in the urine. Significant laboratory findings include hyponatremia, hyperkalemia, and anemia which are all due to the mineralocorticoid and glucocorticoid deficiency due to suppressed hypothalamic-pituitary dysfunction.

Reference

1. Broersen LHA, Pereira AM, Jørgensen JO, Dekkers OM. Adrenal insufficiency in corticosteroids use: systematic review and meta-analysis. J Clin Endocrinol Metab. 2015;100(6):2171-2180.

# 51

# POTASSIUM

Jaya Prakash Sugunaraj and Debdoot Saha

1. A 78-year-old lady was found at her home after a fall earlier in the day by her daughter. Medication history is significant for aspirin, statin, glipizide, and acetaminophen use for chronic low back pain. She recently visited her primary care physician with significant weight loss and failure to thrive. She is currently admitted in the intensive care unit (ICU) for multiple rib fractures and flail chest. Her urine analysis and labs are as follows:

| | |
|---|---|
| pH—7.26 | $pCO_2$—16 |
| $pO_2$—101 | $HCO_3$—10 |
| Na—136 mEq/L | K—5.7 mEq/L |
| Cl—101 mEq/L | Glucose—234 mg/dL |
| Ketones—absent | Lactate—0.9 |

What is the most likely cause for her acid-base abnormality and hyperkalemia?

A. Ketones from starvation ketosis
B. 5-Oxoproline
C. Isopropyl alcohol
D. Lactic acidosis

2. A 55-year-old male with a long-standing diabetes, heart failure with reduced ejection fraction, and open-angle glaucoma presents to the emergency room. He reports loose stools for last few days. His list of medications includes metoprolol, acetazolamide, atorvastatin, aspirin, and metformin.

Serum:

1. pH—7.30
2. $pCO_2$—40 mm Hg
3. Na—145 mEq/L
4. K—3.0 mEq/L
5. $HCO_3$—10 mEq/L
6. Cl—125 mEq/L
7. Albumin—4 g/dL

Urine:

1. Na—56 mEq/L
2. K—10 mEq/L
3. Cl—76 mEq/L

The most likely cause of this patient's acidosis is:

A. Diarrhea
B. Renal tubular acidosis
C. Spironolactone use
D. Acetazolamide use

3. A 59-year-old female with a history of hypertension and gout is admitted in the ICU for observation status post thrombolysis for ischemic stroke. Her outpatient medications include metoprolol, colchicine, aspirin, metformin, and meloxicam. Vitals are normal except for sinus tachycardia with a heart rate (HR) of 108 beats per minute. Low bicarbonate is noted on labs prompting an arterial blood gas (ABG), and patient is found to be mildly acidotic. Lab values are given below:

| pH | 7.32 | $PaCO_2$ | 38 mm Hg |
|---|---|---|---|
| Na | 140 mEq/L | K | 5.9 mEq/L |
| Cl | 110 mEq/L | Bicarb | 18 mEq/L |
| BUN | 18 mg/dL | Cr | 1.1 mg/dL |
| Glucose | 76 mg/dL | Lactic acid | 1.0 |
| Albumin | 4 g/dL | | |

Urine electrolytes:

1. Na—56 mEq/L
2. K—10 mEq/L
3. Cl—56 mEq/L

Which of the following can most likely be expected to be the cause of this?

A. Chronic diarrhea
B. Type 1 renal tubular acidosis
C. Type 4 renal tubular acidosis
D. Bartter syndrome

4. A 55-year-old female presents with headaches and generalized weakness. Her mental status is intact. Her vital signs are blood pressure (BP) 170/80 mm Hg, HR 120/min, respiratory rate (RR) 18/min, and temperature 36.8°C.

Lab values:

| pH | 7.48 | $PaCO_2$ | 46 mm Hg |
|---|---|---|---|
| Na | 152 mEq/L | K | 3.1 mEq/L |
| Cl | 100 mEq/L | Bicarb | 34 mEq/L |

What is the next best test to determine the cause of this acid-base abnormality?

A. Serum cortisol
B. Urine electrolytes
C. Serum ionized calcium
D. Liver function test

5. A 30-year-old male with history of alcohol abuse presents with nausea and vomiting. He is jaundiced, agitated, and endorsing visual hallucinations. Vital signs are as follows:

| BP | 105/100 mm Hg | RR | 22/min |
|---|---|---|---|
| HR | 110/min | Temperature | 38°C |

Labs and ABG values are shown below:

| pH | 7.48 | PaCO$_2$ | 28 mm Hg |
|---|---|---|---|
| Na | 138 mEq/L | K | 3.0 mEq/L |
| Cl | 80 mEq/L | Bicarb | 22 mEq/L |
| PaO$_2$ | 100 mm Hg | Albumin | 4 g/dL |

Which of the following best describes the acid-base disorder?

**A.** Metabolic acidosis/respiratory alkalosis
**B.** Respiratory alkalosis
**C.** Combined respiratory alkalosis, metabolic acidosis, and metabolic alkalosis
**D.** Metabolic alkalosis and respiratory alkalosis

# Chapter 51 ▪ Answers

**1.** Correct Answer: B

**Rationale:**
This patient has high anion gap metabolic acidosis with resultant acidosis-induced hyperkalemia. One of the overlooked causes of metabolic acidosis is elevation of serum oxoproline levels, seen more commonly in undernourished patients taking acetaminophen regularly. The patient has no lactate or ketones in their lab workup. Isopropyl alcohol toxicity causes an osmolar gap only and no anion gap (choices A, C, and D are incorrect).

Causes of high anion gap metabolic acidosis can be remembered with the mnemonic—GOLDMARK
Glycols
Oxoproline
L-Lactate
D-Lactate
Methanol
Aspirin
Renal failure
Ketoacidosis

When a source of high anion gap metabolic acidosis is not obvious, elevated 5-oxoproline level (also called pyroglutamic acid) should be considered, especially if there is a history of acetaminophen use.

References
1. Mehta A, Emmett JB, Emmett M. GOLD MARK: an anion gap mnemonic for the 21st century. *Lancet*. 2008;372(9642):892.
2. Aronson PS, Giebisch G. Effects of pH on potassium: new explanations for old observations. *J Am Soc Nephrol*. 2011; 22:1981.

**2.** Correct Answer: A

**Rationale:**
The pH suggests acidosis. The anion gap is 10, which is appropriate for an albumin of 4. There is no respiratory-driven acidosis as denoted by the normal pCO$_2$ of 40. Therefore, this patient has normal anion gap metabolic acidosis (NAGMA). The next step is to determine the etiology using a calculation of the urine anion gap (UAG)

$$Na + K - Cl = 56 + 10 - 76 = -10$$

A positive numerical value on UAG in NAGMA can be seen with renal tubular acidosis, spironolactone, and acetazolamide use. Diarrhea typically results in numerically negative UAG. Typically acidosis is associated with hyperkalemia unlike in this scenario, which can be explained by GI loss of potassium, resulting in hypokalemia in spite of academia.

Reference
1. Goldstein MB, Bear R, Richardson RMA, et al. The urine anion gap: a clinically useful index of ammonium excretion. *Am J Med Sci*. 1986;292(4):198-202.

**3.** Correct Answer: C

**Rationale:**

The blood gas suggests a metabolic acidosis. The anion gap is 12, which is appropriate for an albumin of 4. There is no respiratory-driven acidosis component as denoted by normal $pCO_2$ of 38 mm Hg. This patient has NAGMA. The next step is to calculate the UAG

$$U.Na + U.K - U.Cl = 56 + 10 - 56 = 10.$$

A positive numerical value on UAG in NAGMA can be seen in renal tubular acidosis (type 1 and type 4), spironolactone, and acetazolamide use. This patient has serum chemistry consistent with renal tubular acidosis type 4 with hyperkalemia not explained by any other etiology. Types of renal tubular acidosis with their respective differentiating features are depicted in the table below.

| | TYPE 1 DISTAL | TYPE 2 PROXIMAL | TYPE 4 |
|---|---|---|---|
| **Defect** | Impaired H+ excretion in distal tubule | Impaired $HCO_3$—reabsorption in the proximal tubule | Impaired cation exchange in distal tubule |
| **Urine pH** | Usually >5.5 | Usually <5.5 | Usually <5.5 |
| **Serum $HCO_3$** | <15 | >15 | >15 |
| **Serum K** | low-normal | low-normal | High |
| **Renal stones** | Yes | No | No |
| **Urine anion gap** | Positive | Negative | Positive |

References

1. Goldstein MB, Bear R, Richardson RMA, Marsden PA, Marsden ML, Haleperin ML. The urine anion gap: a clinically useful index of ammonium excretion. *Am J Med Sci.* 1986;292(4):198-202.
2. Soriano JG. Renal tubular acidosis: the clinical entity. *J Am Soc Nephrol.* 2002;13:2160-2170.

**4.** Correct Answer: B

**Rationale:**

The patient has a pH of 7.48, with a bicarbonate level of 34 mEq/L, suggesting metabolic alkalosis as the acid-base disorder. Hypokalemia is also noted with potassium of 3.1 mEq/L consistent with metabolic alkalosis. In differentiating the cause of metabolic alkalosis, urine chloride levels can be utilized. Urine chloride level less than 10 mmol/L suggests volume responsive or contraction alkalosis that can be corrected with saline replacement. Urine chloride greater than 20 mmol/L is associated with alkalosis that is resistant to volume expansion such as excess aldosterone, severe potassium deficiency, diuretic therapy, or Bartter syndrome. Metabolic alkalosis can be a feature of Cushing syndrome, but ordering a serum cortisol level would not be the first-line investigation (choice A). Liver function tests and serum ionized calcium are not typically useful for the investigation of metabolic acidosis (choices C and D).

References

1. Galla JH. Metabolic alkalosis. *J Am Soc Nephrol.* 2000;11:369.
2. Palmer BF, Alpern RJ. Metabolic alkalosis. *J Am Soc Nephrol.* 1997;8(9):1462.
3. Khanna A, Kurtzman NA. Metabolic alkalosis. *J Nephrol.* 2006;19(9):86.
4. Luke RG, Galla JH. It is chloride depletion alkalosis, not contraction alkalosis. *J Am Soc Nephrol.* 2012;23:204.

**5.** Correct Answer: C

**Rationale:**

The patient has a significant anion gap of 36 [138−(22 + 80) = 36], which makes high anion gap metabolic acidosis as one of the acid-base derangements even though the pH is alkalotic. Using Winters formula, the patient's $CO_2$ to compensate for the acidosis should be

$$\left(1.5 \times 22\right) + 8 \pm 2 = 41 \pm 2$$

This value is more than the $pCO_2$ of the patient which is 28, suggesting more $CO_2$ washout, thus adding respiratory alkalosis as a component of the acid-base disorder. Additionally, the patient's albumin is 4, making the normal anion gap for this patient as 12; the difference between the normal anion gap and patient's anion gap is 36 − 12 = 24. This means the acid-base disorder has caused the original bicarbonate level to decrease by 24. So, by adding 24 to the patient's current bicarbonate level of 22, we can get the original bicarbonate level this patient started out with, which would be 22 + 24 = 46, thus making the patient's original acid-base problem as metabolic alkalosis. The patient has a combined respiratory alkalosis, metabolic acidosis, and metabolic alkalosis.

### Reference

1. Berend K, De Vries APJ, Gans ROB. Physiological approach to assessment of acid–base disturbances. *N Engl J Med.* 2014;371:1434-1445.

# 52

# CALCIUM, PHOSPHATE, AND MAGNESIUM

Jaya Prakash Sugunaraj and Debdoot Saha

1.  A 32-year-old G2P1 female at 34 weeks gestation and a history of chronic kidney disease develops hypertension and altered mental status followed by seizures. She is started on intravenous magnesium with seizure resolution. She becomes somnolent 3 hours later, and physical examination reveals hyporeflexia. What is the immediate management for this symptom?

    A. Hypotonic IV fluids
    B. Calcium gluconate infusion
    C. Hemodialysis
    D. Furosemide

2.  A 66-year-old homeless man presents to the emergency department with severe weakness for last few weeks. His vitals are as follows:

    Temperature 36.9°C, HR 70 beats/min, RR 22 breaths/min, oxygen saturation 94% on room air.
    He is alert and oriented to time and person. The patient denies any specific complaints besides back pain for several days. Routine chest radiograph and ECG are performed:

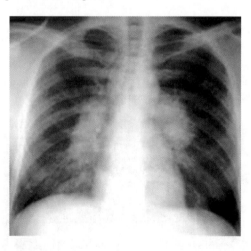

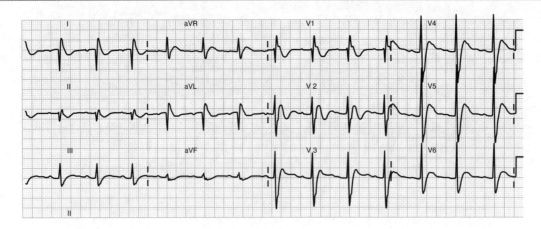

These ECG changes are most likely explained by

**A.** Cold exposure
**B.** Hyperthyroidism
**C.** Hypercalcemia
**D.** Acute coronary syndrome

3. A 65-year-old male nursing home resident with a history of quadriplegia is admitted to the ICU for respiratory failure. He is intubated and sedated. Tube feeds are initiated. Electrolyte levels are as follows.

Serum calcium—7.0 mg/dL
Serum phosphorus—0.9 mg/dL
Serum magnesium—1.6 mg/dL
Serum potassium—3.6 mg/dL
Serum sodium—138 mg/dL
What replacement strategy should be initiated for this patient?

**A.** IV Calcium followed IV Phosphorus
**B.** IV phosphorus followed by IV calcium
**C.** IV calcium followed by oral phosphorus replacement
**D.** Oral phosphorus replacement only

4. A 65-year-old male with a history of end-stage renal disease on hemodialysis presents to the emergency room with history of fever for the last few days. Vitals are as follows:

Bp 130/70 mm Hg, RR 20 breaths/min, Temp 36.6°C, HR 78 beats/min
Lap values are notable for parathyroid hormone (PTH) 350 pg/mL and calcium 12 mg/dL.
Physical examination reveals the following skin lesions:

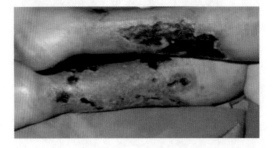

Which of the following is the most appropriate first-line pharmacological therapy for this patient?

**A.** Antibiotics
**B.** Sodium thiosulphate infusion
**C.** Sodium thiosulphate infusion and cinacalcet
**D.** Treat with analgesics till surgical parathyroidectomy

5. A 67-year-old male is admitted to the trauma ICU for management of anaphylaxis. He is intubated for airway swelling. 3 hours from the onset of symptoms the patient is hemodynamically stable without a pressor requirement. Routine labs ordered show the following:

Calcium: 8.0 mEq/L
Ionized calcium: 1.03 mEq/L
Sodium: 136 mg/dL
Potassium: 4.0 mEq/L
Which of the following electrolytes require repletion?

A. Potassium, magnesium, and IV calcium
B. Potassium only
C. Neither potassium or IV calcium
D. Potassium and magnesium

6. A 54-year-old male presents to the emergency department with agitation. The ED physician orders haloperidol for agitation before learning that patient is taking high-dose methadone for back pain and has a history of substance abuse and dependence. Labs are awaited. His ECG strip on telemetry is shown in the figure that follows. He converts to normal sinus rhythm after receiving 2 g of magnesium. 10 minutes later the arrhythmia shown below recurs. He is alert and talking comfortably.

BP: 110/68
Vitals: 110/60
SpO$_2$: 94% on 2 L/min oxygen via nasal cannula

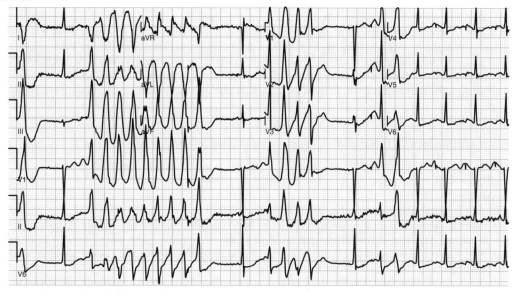

What should be the next immediate step?

A. Give more magnesium
B. Synchronized cardioversion
C. IV isoproterenol to increase heart rate
D. Overdrive pacing to increase heart rate

7. A 45-year-old male with past medical history of COPD is admitted for acute hypoxemic respiratory failure secondary to influenza H1N1. He is intubated for 7 days. On hospital day 7, his P/F ratio has improved to 220 and the patient's chest x-ray looks improved. He fails spontaneous breathing trial for two consecutive days secondary to low tidal volumes. He has poor cough reflex and was given 5 days of steroids for his acute illness.

Which electrolyte is most likely to be deficient in this patient?

A. Serum phosphorus
B. Serum free cortisol
C. Serum calcium
D. Serum potassium

8. A 65-year-old male nursing home resident with a history of quadriplegia is admitted to the ICU for respiratory failure. He was intubated and placed on mechanical ventilation, and tube feeds were initiated on hospital day 2. Electrolyte levels are as follows on day 3.

Serum calcium: 7.0 mg/dL
Serum phosphorus: 0.9 mg/dL
Serum magnesium: 1.6 mg/dL
Serum potassium: 3.6 mg/dL
Serum sodium: 138 mg/dL
Besides electrolyte repletion, what should be the strategy with regard to his nutrition?

**A.** Stop tube feeds
**B.** Decrease rate of tube feeds
**C.** Continue same rate of tube feeds with phosphorus supplementation in feeds
**D.** Make no change to tube feeds rate/type.

# Chapter 52 ▪ Answers

**1.** Correct Answer: B

**Rationale:**
The signs and symptoms elicited by this patient are consistent with hypermagnesemia. This patient is predisposed to higher levels of serum magnesium due to underlying renal impairment. Although hemodialysis will be the most definitive management for removing magnesium from the system in this patient with chronic kidney disease, immediate and first-line management of central nervous system and cardiac side effects should be by administration of IV calcium which acts as a magnesium antagonist. Unless the patient is anuric, medical management with intravenous fluids and loop diuretics should also be initiated (choice D) after giving calcium, especially in severe or symptomatic cases.

Reference
1. Mordes JP, Wacker WE. Excess magnesium. *Pharmacol Rev.* 1977;29(4):273-300.

**2.** Correct Answer: C

**Rationale:**
The chest radiograph shows hilar enlargement consistent with sarcoidosis. The ECG shows Osborn waves and, given the presentation above, is most consistent with severe hypercalcemia. Sarcoidosis is known to cause high levels of serum calcium due to the uncontrolled synthesis of 1,25-dihydroxyvitamin D3 by macrophages. 1,25-dihydroxyvitamin D3 leads to an increased absorption of calcium in the intestine and to an increased resorption of calcium in the bone.

Severe cold exposure and acute coronary syndrome can both cause similar ST changes (Osborn waves), but the patient's temperature on presentation is normal. These ECG changes are not typical of hyperthyroidism.

Reference
1. Otero J, Lenihan DJ. The "normothermic" Osborn wave induced by severe hypercalcemia. *Tex Heart Inst J.* 2000;27(3):316-317.

**3.** Correct Answer: A

**Rationale:**
This patient has hypophosphatemia from refeeding syndrome. This patient has concomitant low serum calcium levels. Early replacement of phosphorus is warranted in refeeding syndrome; however, hypocalcemia can worsen with phosphorus replacement; therefore, calcium should be replaced before phosphorus correction.

It is recommended to replace phosphorus with IV supplementation instead of oral due to absorption issues often encountered in this patient group (choice C).

Reference
1. Mehanna HM, Moledina J, Travis J. Refeeding syndrome: what it is, and how to prevent and treat it. *BMJ.* 2008;336:1495.

**4.** Correct Answer: C

**Rationale:**

This patient has calciphylaxis. Sodium thiosulfate is an agent with antioxidant and vasodilatory properties that also inhibits adipocyte calcification and blocks the ability of adipocytes to induce calcification of vascular smooth muscle cells. Two studies have shown effectiveness of sodium thiosulphate in treatment of calciphylaxis. Also, in addition to sodium thiosulphate, patients who have elevated serum PTH levels (>300 pg/mL) are treated with cinacalcet. Several case reports have suggested cinacalcet can be effective in the management of this condition.

References
1. Nigwekar SU, Thadhani R, Brandenburg VM. Calciphylaxis. *N Engl J Med.* 2018;378:1704-1714.
2. Nigwekar SU, Brunelli SM, Meade D, et al. Sodium thiosulfate therapy for calcific uremic arteriolopathy. *Clin J Am Soc Nephrol.* 2013;8:1162-1170.
3. Zitt E, König M, Vychytil A, et al. Use of sodium thiosulphate in a multi-interventional setting for the treatment of calciphylaxis in dialysis patients. *Nephrol Dial Transplant.* 2013;28:1232-1240.
4. Velasco N, MacGregor MS, Innes A, et al. Successful treatment of calciphylaxis with cinacalcet-an alternative to parathyroidectomy? *Nephrol Dial Transplant.* 2006;21:1999.
5. Robinson MR, Augustine JJ, Korman NJ. Cinacalcet for the treatment of calciphylaxis. *Arch Dermatol.* 2007;143:152.
6. Sharma A, Burkitt-Wright E, Rustom R. Cinacalcet as an adjunct in the successful treatment of calciphylaxis. *Br J Dermatol.* 2006;155:1295.

**5.** Correct Answer: C

**Rationale:**

IV calcium replacement is recommended only when severe effects of hypocalcemia like neurological symptoms (tetany and seizures), hypotension, prolonged QT interval, or in asymptomatic patients with an acute decrease in serum corrected calcium to ≤7.5 mg/dL. This patient does not meet criteria for treatment.

Reference
1. Kraft MD, Btaiche IF, Sacks GS, Kudsk KA. Treatment of electrolyte disorders in adult patients in the intensive care unit. *Am J Health Syst Pharm.* 2005;62:1663-1682.

**6.** Correct Answer: A

**Rationale:**

The management of Torsades de Pointes begins with assessing if the patient is hemodynamically stable. Most episodes of torsades are self-limiting. However, the danger lies in those patients who go on to develop ventricular fibrillation. Synchronized cardioversion should be performed on a hemodynamically unstable patient in torsades who has a pulse (100 J monophasic, 50 J Biphasic). Pulseless torsades should be defibrillated.

This patient is hemodynamically stable. Studies have shown that levels of magnesium drop precipitously a short time after a bolus infusion. It is recommended to start an infusion soon after the bolus dose of magnesium or supplement with intermittent magnesium pushes and follow labs for magnesium levels and monitor patient for magnesium overdose effects.

References
1. Biesenbach P, Mårtensson J, Lucchetta L, et al. Pharmacokinetics of magnesium bolus therapy in cardiothoracic surgery. *J Cardiothorac Vasc Anesth.* 2018;32(3):1289-1294.
2. Tzivoni D, Banai S, Schuger C, et al. Treatment of torsade de pointes with magnesium sulfate. *Circulation.* 1988;77(2):392-397.

**7.** Correct Answer: A

**Rationale:**

Low serum phosphorus has been strongly associated with diaphragmatic weakness. Since the duration of steroid therapy was short, the probability of steroid induced myopathy is low.

Reference
1. Aubier M, Murciano D, Lecocguic Y, et al. Effect of hypophosphatemia on diaphragmatic contractility in patients with acute respiratory failure. *N Engl J Med.* 1985;313(7):420-424.

**8.** Correct Answer: B

**Rationale:**

The patient has refeeding syndrome. Studies suggest significant benefit in decreasing the rate of tube feed in patients who develop refeeding syndrome after initiation of tube feeds, correcting electrolyte disturbances and only then increasing back to a target rate after electrolytes have stabilized.

Reference
1. Doig GS, Simpson F, Heighes P, et al. Restricted versus continued standard caloric intake during the management of refeeding syndrome in critically ill adults: a randomised, parallel-group, multicentre, single-blind controlled trial. *Lancet Respir Med.* 2015;3(12):943-952.

# 53

# ACID BASE DISORDERS

Jaya Prakash Sugunaraj and Ngoc-Tram Ha

1. A 33-year-old woman presents to the primary care physician for a month-long history of palpations and diarrhea. She has no known medical history. She denies taking any prescribed medication and has not traveled anywhere recently; however, she reports being exposed to "lots of sick people" as part of her job as a nurse. On physical examination, she appears anxious, but the rest of her examination results, including vital signs, are within normal limits. Her BMI is 21 kg/m². Laboratory studies are as follows:

Sodium 139 mEq/L (mmol/L)
Potassium 3.6 mEq/L (mmol/L)
Chloride 117 mEq/L (mmol/L)
Bicarbonate 16 mEq/L (mmol/L)
Glucose 135 mg/dL
BUN 12 mg/dL
Creatinine 0.7 mg/dL
Albumin 4.2 g/dL

Which of the following is the MOST likely cause for her laboratory abnormalities?

**A.** Laxative abuse
**B.** Bulimia nervosa
**C.** Factious disorder
**D.** Exogenous insulin use
**E.** Diuretic use

2. A 43-year-old man is brought by the police to the emergency department after being found unresponsive on the street. He appears unkempt and disheveled. On physical examination, his temperature is 36.0°C, blood pressure is 146/92 mm Hg, pulse rate is 84 beats/min, and respiratory rate is 10 breaths/min. He is not oriented to time and place. Laboratory data show the following:

Sodium 144 mEq/L (mmol/L)
Potassium 4.3 mEq/L (mmol/L)
Chloride 108 mEq/L (mmol/L)
Bicarbonate 8 mEq/L (mmol/L)
Glucose 135 mg/dL
BUN 18 mg/dL
Creatinine 1.1 mg/dL
Albumin 4.0 g/L
Lactate 0.8 mmol/L
TSH 3.60 mIU/L
An arterial blood gas is also obtained which shows a pH 7.28, $pCO_2$ 18 mm Hg, and plasma osmolality 278 mOsm/kg $H_2O$.

Which of the following is the MOST likely diagnosis in this patient?

A. Ethylene glycol poisoning
B. Starvation ketoacidosis
C. Lactic acidosis
D. Isopropyl ingestion
E. Propylene glycol toxicity

3. An 87-year-old lady is being evaluated in the nursing home after being found to be more lethargic. She had been complaining of decreased appetite due to abdominal pain and ongoing diarrhea for the last 3 days. Her past medical history is significant for hypertension, type II diabetes mellitus, chronic back pain, and diverticulosis. Her medications include metformin, insulin, lisinopril, and naproxen. On physical examination, her temperature is 37.8°C, blood pressure is 118/82 mm Hg, pulse rate is 104 beats/min, and respiratory rate is 10 breaths/min.

Laboratories obtained show the following:

Sodium 140 mEq/L (mmol/L)
Potassium 3.4 mEq/L (mmol/L)
Chloride 99 mEq/L (mmol/L)
Bicarbonate 20 mEq/L (mmol/L)
Glucose 243 mg/dL
BUN 22 mg/dL
Creatinine 1.6 mg/dL (baseline 1.1)
Albumin 3.7 g/L
Lactate 1.0 mmol/L
ABG
pH 7.52
$pCO_2$ 20 mm Hg

Which of the following is the MOST likely diagnosis in this patient?

A. Metabolic acidosis with compensation
B. Respiratory acidosis with metabolic alkalosis
C. Respiratory alkalosis with increased anion gap metabolic acidosis
D. Respiratory alkalosis with acute compensation
E. Mixed disorder

4. A 32-year-old male is referred to the nephrologist for abnormal laboratory values. He was recently seen by his primary care physician for his annual physical examination. During his visit, he was told that his "urine was abnormal." The patient does not have any known medical history except for a 26-year pack-year smoking history. He is normothermic with a blood pressure of 128/90 mm Hg, pulse rate of 58 beats/min, and respiratory rate of 12 breaths/min. The rest of his physical examination is unremarkable. His family history is only significant for arthritis and "thyroid disease." Further laboratory studies obtained show the following:

Sodium 142 mEq/L (mmol/L)
Potassium 3.3 mEq/L (mmol/L)
Chloride 117 mEq/L (mmol/L)
Bicarbonate 10 mEq/L (mmol/L)
Glucose 243 mg/dL
BUN 22 mg/dL
Creatinine 1.3 mg/dL (baseline is 1.1)
Albumin 4.2 g/L
Urine pH 5.6
Urine sodium 62 mEq/L
Urine potassium 85mEq/L
Urine chloride 126 mEq/L
Urine calcium 378 mg/dL

What is the MOST likely diagnosis in this patient?

A. Gitelman syndrome
B. Renal tubular acidosis (RTA) type 1
C. RTA type 2
D. Bartter syndrome
E. Salicylate toxicity

5. A 64-year-old woman is being treated in the local intensive care unit (ICU) for septic shock due to *Streptococcus pneumoniae*. She weighs 120 kg. She is started on empiric antibiotics and resuscitated with 30 mL/kg of normal saline without significant improvement. She is therefore temporarily started on vasopressor support. She improves after 4 days and is weaned off all vasopressors. She extubated to noninvasive ventilation. However, her voice remains hoarse, and she fails her swallow evaluation. She remains on intravenous fluids for hydration for 3-day history of diarrhea.

Laboratory data obtained on admission:

|  | ON ADMISSION | ON THE SIXTH DAY OF ADMISSION |
|---|---|---|
| Sodium | 141 mEq/L (mmol/L) | 148 mEq/L (mmol/L) |
| Potassium | 4.3 mEq/L (mmol/L) | 3.8 mEq/L (mmol/L) |
| Chloride s | 102 mEq/L (mmol/L) | 120 mEq/L (mmol/L) |
| Bicarbonate | 24 mEq/L (mmol/L) | 19 mEq/L (mmol/L) |
| BUN | 32 mg/dL | 23 mg/dL |
| Creatinine | 1.2 mg/dL | 1.4 mg/dL |
| Albumin | 3.7 g/L | 2.8 g/L |
| Lactate | 5.2 mg/dL | 2.0 mg/dL |
| pH | 7.29 | 7.31 |
| $pCO_2$ | 30 mm Hg | 24 mm Hg |

What is the MOST likely cause for her laboratory abnormalities?

A. Contraction alkalosis
B. Diuresis
C. Fluid administration
D. RTA
E. Hypoalbuminemia

6. A 62-year-old man with past medical history of benign prostate hyperplasia, congestive heart failure, and hyperlipidemia presents to his primary care physician for a routine follow-up visit. Today, he complains of progressively worsening fatigue and back pain for the past 4 weeks. He states that there are days that he feels so tired that he does not leave the house. He no longer enjoys playing golf or fishing on the weekends. On physical examination, his temperature is 37.2°C, blood pressure is 134/72 mm Hg, pulse rate is 74 beats/min, and respiratory rate is 12 breaths/min. Pallor conjunctiva and point tenderness are noted over his lumbar spine. The rest of the physical examination is unremarkable. His medications include pravastatin, furosemide, and tamsulosin. He also has been taking aspirin daily for his back pain. Laboratory data show the following:

Sodium 133 mEq/L (mmol/L)
Potassium 3.4 mEq/L (mmol/L)
Chloride 104 mEq/L (mmol/L)
Bicarbonate 16 mEq/L (mmol/L)
Glucose 243 mg/dL
BUN 28 mg/dL
Creatinine 1.7 mg/dL
Albumin 2.9 g/L
Calcium 11.3 mg/dL
Phosphorous 3.0 mg/dL
Total protein 6.2 g/dL
WBC 8200/μL
Hemoglobin 8.9 g/dL
Hematocrit 27.3 g/dL
Platelets 250,000/μL
ABG
pH 7.42
$pCO_2$ 38 mm Hg

What is the MOST likely cause for the patient's acid-base disturbance?

A. Starvation ketoacidosis
B. D-lactic acidosis
C. Normal anion gap metabolic acidosis
D. High anion gap metabolic acidosis
E. Dehydration

7. A 54-year-old male was brought to the emergency department with nausea and vomiting. He has a long-standing history of alcohol abuse and cardiomyopathy. He complains of severe abdominal pain. On physical examination, his temperature is 37.6°C, blood pressure is 94/67 mm Hg, pulse rate is 122 beats/min, and respiratory rate is 20 breaths/min. His BMI is 17. He is tender to palpation over the epigastrium, and guarding is noted. He is kept NPO and treated with aggressive fluid resuscitation. Given his poor respiratory status, he is intubated and admitted to the ICU. After 8 days, he is clinically improving but remains unable to tolerate enteral feeds for which he is started on total parenteral nutrition (TPN) for 5 days.

Laboratory data obtained:

|  | ON ADMISSION | ON THE 13TH DAY OF ADMISSION |
| --- | --- | --- |
| Sodium | 137 mEq/L (mmol/L) | 142 mEq/L (mmol/L) |
| Potassium | 3.1 mEq/L (mmol/L) | 4.4 mEq/L (mmol/L) |
| Chloride | 110 mEq/L (mmol/L) | 97 mEq/L (mmol/L) |
| Bicarbonate | 22 mEq/L (mmol/L) | 34 mEq/L (mmol/L) |
| BUN | 32 mg/dL | 15 mg/dL |
| Creatinine | 1.2 mg/dL | 0.9 mg/dL |
| Albumin | 2.8 g/L | 3.1 g/L |
| Hemoglobin | 17.1 mg/dL | 13.2 mg/dL |
| Hematocrit | 54.8% | 48.0% |
| Lipase | 620 U/L | 120 U/L |
| Magnesium | 2.7 mg/dL | 1.9 mg/dL |
| Phosphorus | 3.2 mg/dL | 2.2 mg/dL |
| pH | 7.36 | 7.48 |
| $pCO_2$ | 38 mm Hg | 42 mm Hg |

Based on the information provided, what is the BEST explanation for his acid-base abnormalities?

A. Excessive vomiting
B. Administration of normal saline
C. Malnutrition
D. TPN
E. Acute respiratory distress syndrome

8. A 72-year-old woman with a past medical history of hypertension, hyperlipidemia, and congestive heart failure (most recent echocardiogram 3 months ago showed an ejection fraction of 45%) is intubated in the ICU for septic shock in the setting of *Escherichia coli* bacteremia. She received 9 L total of IV fluids, and on examination, she is awake and cooperative, though she has anasarca. She is unable to be weaned off the ventilator due to high respiratory rate, and a chest x-ray obtained shows bilateral vascular congestion. She is given furosemide over the next few days and started on enteral feedings.

After 3 days, repeat laboratory data show the following:

Sodium 146 mEq/L (mmol/L)
Potassium 3.2 mEq/L (mmol/L)
Chloride 110 mEq/L (mmol/L)
Bicarbonate 16 mEq/L (mmol/L)
Glucose 143 mg/dL
BUN 27 mg/dL
Creatinine 1.2 mg/dL
Albumin 4.1 g/L
Calcium 9.8 mg/dL
ABG
pH 7.48
pCO$_2$ 45 mm Hg

Which of the following is MOST likely the cause of her acid-base disturbances?

A. Bartter syndrome
B. Diuretic usage
C. Primary respiratory acidosis
D. Milk-Alkali syndrome
E. RTA type 2

9. An 89-year-old man with a past medical history of chronic kidney disease stage III, diabetes mellitus type II, and hypertension who is 4 days status post small bowel resection for a small bowel obstruction. He has a persistent ileus with nasogastric decompression. On the fifth day, he develops palpitations and lethargy. An ECG and laboratory parameters are shown below:

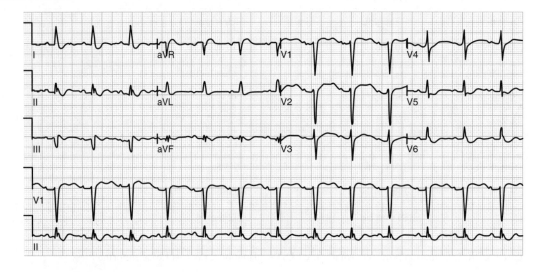

Sodium 146 mEq/L (mmol/L)
Potassium 3.0 mEq/L (mmol/L)
Chloride 90 mEq/L (mmol/L)
Bicarbonate 18 mEq/L (mmol/L)
Glucose 243 mg/dL
BUN 22 mg/dL
Creatinine 1.8 mg/dL
Albumin 3.7 g/L
Lactate 1.0 mmol/L

ABG
pH 7.28
pCO$_2$ 28
HCO$_3$ 33
PO$_2$ 98%

Based on this, what do you expect his urine pH value to be?

A. 4.1
B. 8.9
C. 6.0
D. 7.4
E. 3.1

10. A 23-year-old man is brought to the hospital by his girlfriend. She states that he has not been feeling well, complaining of nausea and abdominal pain for the past 2 days. His younger sister was recently treated for rotavirus, though she denies that anyone else had any other symptoms. Given his lethargy, he has not taken any of his medications. She also admits that he "binge drinks" on occasion but has not consumed any alcohol over 2 months.

On physical examination, his temperature is 36.8°C, blood pressure is 92/60 mm Hg, pulse rate is 124 beats/min, and respiratory rate is 10 breaths/min. His oral mucosa is dry, and his pulse is palpable though thready.

Sodium 132 mEq/L (mmol/L)
Potassium 4.2 mEq/L (mmol/L)
Chloride 102 mEq/L (mmol/L)
Bicarbonate 10 mEq/L (mmol/L)
Glucose 656 mg/dL
BUN 42 mg/dL
Creatinine 1.4 mg/dL
Albumin 4.1 g/L
Calcium 9.8 mg/dL
ABG
pH 7.48
$pCO_2$ 45 mm Hg

| Urine ketones | Positive | Urine nitrite | Negative |
|---|---|---|---|
| Urine glucose | Positive | Urine leukocyte esterase | Negative |
| Urine protein | Negative | Urine clarity | Clear |
| Specific gravity | 1.029 | Urine color | Yellow |
| Urine pH | 7.0 | Urine urobilinogen | 0.5 |
| Urine blood | Negative | Urine bilirubin | Negative |

Which of the following is MOST likely the cause of his acid-base disturbances?

A. Starvation ketoacidosis
B. Acute kidney injury
C. Alcoholic ketoacidosis
D. D-Lactic acidosis
E. Diabetic ketoacidosis (DKA)

11. A 74-year-old man presents to his primary care physician for worsening lower extremity edema. He has advanced chronic obstructive pulmonary disease and benign prostatic hyperplasia and is a former alcoholic. He is prescribed a diuretic and returns to the office 1 week after. His swelling has improved, but he is complaining about worsening shortness of breath. Given that, an ABG on room air is obtained and shows the following.

ABG
pH 7.47
$PaO_2$ 82 mm Hg
$PCO_2$ 53 mm Hg
$HCO_3$ 38 mEq/L

What is the MOST likely acid-base disturbance?

A. Chronic respiratory alkalosis
B. Acute respiratory alkalosis with metabolic compensation
C. Acute metabolic alkalosis with respiratory compensation
D. Mixed acid-base disorder
E. Chronic metabolic alkalosis

**12.** A previously healthy 23-year-old woman is taken to the hospital by her boyfriend for weakness since 2 weeks. They recently returned from a trip to Caribbean after which she developed an upper respiratory infection. She was given Levofloxacin by the urgent care provider. While her cough improved, she noticed weakness in her feet that subsequently traveled up to her arms. On physical examination, vital signs are unremarkable except for a respiratory rate of 8 breaths/min. Deep tendon reflexes are diminished bilaterally.

Sodium 137 mEq/L (mmol/L)
Potassium 3.9 mEq/L (mmol/L)
Chloride 109 mEq/L (mmol/L)
Bicarbonate 32 mEq/L (mmol/L)
Glucose 121 mg/dL
BUN 16 mg/dL
Creatinine 0.8 mg/dL
Arterial blood gas
pH 7.26
$PCO_2$ 72 mm Hg

What is the MOST likely acid-base disturbance in this patient?

**A.** Acute on chronic respiratory acidosis
**B.** Respiratory alkalosis with increased anion gap metabolic acidosis
**C.** Mixed disorder
**D.** Respiratory acidosis with metabolic alkalosis
**E.** Uncompensated acute respiratory acidosis

**13.** A 78-year-old man presents from his skilled nursing facility for generalized weakness and a "funny feeling in his ears." He recently sustained a fall complicated by a left femur fracture. He underwent open reduction and internal fixation a week ago and has been undergoing physical rehabilitation. He has medical history of hypertension, coronary artery disease, and chronic obstructive pulmonary disease (COPD).

On physical examination, his blood pressure is 152/86 mm Hg, pulse rate is 64 beats/min, and respiratory rate is 22 breaths/min. He is confused to time and place. Laboratory data show the following:

Sodium 140 mEq/L (mmol/L)
Potassium 3.8 mEq/L (mmol/L)
Chloride 111 mEq/L (mmol/L)
Bicarbonate 10 mEq/L (mmol/L)
Glucose 95 mg/dL
BUN 22 mg/dL
Creatinine 1.4 mg/dL (baseline 1.0 mg/dL)
Albumin 3.7 g/L
Lactate 1.0 mmol/L
An arterial blood gas (ABG) is also obtained which shows a pH 7.21, $pCO_2$ 38 mm Hg, and plasma osmolality 288 mOsm/kg $H_2O$.

What is the MOST likely acid-base disturbance in this patient?

**A.** Anion gap metabolic acidosis and metabolic alkalosis
**B.** Anion gap metabolic acidosis and respiratory acidosis
**C.** Respiratory acidosis and metabolic alkalosis
**D.** Normal anion gap metabolic acidosis
**E.** Respiratory acidosis

**14.** A 67-year-old man is brought to the local hospital for severe onset of acute abdominal pain. He has chronic obstructive pulmonary disease and hypertension and is an active smoker. On physical examination, his vital signs are unremarkable except for a blood pressure of 188/94 mm Hg and pulse rate of 118 beats/min. He is tender to abdominal palpation and unable to lie still due to pain. A CT angiogram reveals an aortic dissection for which he is taken to the operating room emergently. He receives a total of 12 units of packed red blood cells during the case. He remains intubated postoperatively, and laboratory data obtained after surgery reveal the following:

Sodium 147 mEq/L (mmol/L)
Potassium 3.2 mEq/L (mmol/L)
Chloride 100 mEq/L (mmol/L)
Bicarbonate 37 mEq/L (mmol/L)
BUN 18 mg/dL
Creatinine 1.2 mg/dL
Calcium 7.8 mg/dL
Urine pH 5.8
ABG
pH 7.52
$pCO_2$ 48 mm Hg

What is the MOST appropriate treatment for his acid-base disturbance?

**A.** Furosemide
**B.** Bicarbonate infusion
**C.** Lactated Ringer
**D.** Normal saline
**E.** Acetazolamide

**15.** A 43-year-old woman is brought to the emergency department by her neighbor by ambulance after being found unresponsive. She has a known past medical history of bipolar disease, seizures, and previous suicide attempts. Her medications include lithium and levetiracetam. She was in her usual state of health prior to this; however, he recalls she was recently treated with "some antibiotic" for acute bronchitis. On physical examination, her temperature is 37.2°C, blood pressure is 110/72 mm Hg, pulse rate is 98 beats/min, and respiratory rate is 8 breaths/min. She is lethargic and unable to follow commands or answer questions. A tongue bite mark and a soiled underwear are also noted. Laboratory data obtained after 6 days are shown below:

Sodium 134 mEq/L (mmol/L)
Potassium 4.2 mEq/L (mmol/L)
Chloride 102 mEq/L (mmol/L)
Bicarbonate 12 mEq/L (mmol/L)
Glucose 99 mg/dL
BUN 24 mg/dL
Creatinine 1.6 mg/dL
Lactate 4.4 mmol/L
Plasma osmolality 289 mOsm/kg $H_2O$
ABG
pH 7.48
$pCO_2$ 45 mm Hg

| Urine ketones | Negative | Urine nitrite | Trace |
|---|---|---|---|
| Urine glucose | Negative | Urine leukocyte esterase | Negative |
| Urine protein | Negative | Urine clarity | Cloudy |
| Specific gravity | 1.010 | Urine color | Dark yellow |
| Urine pH | 6.5 | Urine urobilinogen | 0.7 |
| Urine blood | Negative | Urine bilirubin | Negative |
| Urine RBC | Positive | | |

What is the MOST likely cause of her acid-base disturbance?

**A.** Methanol overdose
**B.** Acute kidney injury
**C.** Rhabdomyolysis
**D.** Aspirin-induced
**E.** Isopropyl poisoning

# Chapter 53 ▪ Answers

**1.** Correct Answer: A

**Rationale:**

This patient has a normal anion gap metabolic acidosis which can be seen in patients abusing laxatives. Stool contains a significant amount of bicarbonate along with potassium and sodium. With increased amounts of diarrhea, bicarbonate is lost, leading to a metabolic acidosis. Other causes of normal anion gap metabolic acidosis include renal causes, such as RTA, which emphasizes the importance of measurement of the urine anion gap ($U_{Na} + U_K - U_{Cl}$). The urine anion will aid in estimating the kidneys' ability to excrete acid. A positive urine anion gap is suggestive of renal causes of a normal anion gap metabolic acidosis, whereas a negative urine anion gap points toward a gastrointestinal source, such as diarrhea.

The first step with this kind of presentation is to determine the type of acid-base and electrolyte disturbance. Once it is determined that it is a normal anion gap metabolic acidosis, the second step is to differentiate between renal causes versus extrarenal causes by calculating the urine anion gap; a positive urine anion gap points toward renal causes whereas a negative urine anion gap is mostly of gastrointestinal etiology.

**Reference**

1. Goldstein MB, Bear R, Richardson RMA, Marsden PA, Marsden ML, Haleperin ML. The urine anion gap: a clinically useful index of ammonium excretion. *Am J Med Sci.* 1986;292(4):198-202.

**2.** Correct Answer: A

**Rationale:**

The patient presents with an increased anion gap metabolic acidosis of 26—calculated anion gap = $Na - (HCO_3 + Cl)$. In addition, his serum bicarbonate level is reduced to 8 mEq/L with a plasma osmolal gap of 12 mOsm/kg $H_2O$. Altogether, this points to ethylene intoxication.

The osmolal gap is defined as the difference between the measured and the calculated plasma osmolality using the formula below:

Calculated plasma osmolality = (2 × plasma sodium) + glucose/18 + BUN/2.8

Ethylene glycol is commonly found in automotive coolants and cleaners, and ingestion of ethylene glycol will cause an increased anion gap metabolic acidosis with increased plasma osmolal gap of >10 mOsm/kg $H_2O$. Of note, methanol poisoning will also lead to similar findings. Isopropyl poisoning will also have an increased osmolal gap of >10 mOsm/L, but it does not usually cause an anion gap metabolic acidosis.

**Reference**

1. Jacobsen D, Bredesen JE, Eide I, Østborg J. Anion and osmolal gaps in the diagnosis of methanol and ethylene glycol poisoning. *J Intern Med.* 1982;212(1):17-20.

**3.** Correct Answer: E

**Rationale:**

The patient has a mixed acid-base disorder. Her pH is alkalotic. Upon closer look, it appears that she has a respiratory alkalosis (pCO$_2$ 20 mm Hg). To determine whether this is an acute or chronic respiratory alkalosis, the following formula can be used: *1-2-4-5 rule.*

METABOLIC COMPENSATION IN RESPIRATORY ACIDOSIS/ALKALOSIS

| EVERY 10 mm Hg CHANGE IN PaCO$_2$ | HCO$_3$– mmol/L | |
| --- | --- | --- |
| | ACUTE | CHRONIC |
| PaCO$_2$ (Increases) | 1 | 4 |
| PaCO$_2$ (Decreases) | 2 | 5 |

In acute respiratory alkalosis, for every decrease in $PaCO_2$ by 10, the $HCO_3^-$ decreases by 2.

In chronic respiratory alkalosis, for every decrease in $PaCO_2$ by 10, the $HCO_3^-$ decreases by 5.

Based on that, her expected $HCO_3^-$ is approximately 14 mEq/L. However, in this case, it is 21 mEq/L which is higher than expected. This suggests that there is concurrent metabolic alkalosis present. This is also confirmed by calculating the Δ-Δ ratio—(calculated AG – expected AG)/24 – measured $HCO_3^-$—which aids in determining the presence of any other normal AG metabolic acidosis or if this is a pure high AG metabolic acidosis.

In this case, the Δ-Δ ratio is >1, indicating that there is in fact a metabolic alkalosis present. A Δ-Δ ratio < 1 suggests a normal AG metabolic acidosis.

### Reference

1. Berend K, De Vries APJ, Gans ROB. Physiological approach to assessment of acid–base disturbances. *N Engl J Med.* 2014;371:1434-1445.

---

**4.** Correct Answer: B

**Rationale:**

This patient likely has RTA type 1. In patients with RTA type 1, there is impairment of acidification in the distal part of the nephrons. Because the kidney is unable to excrete hydrogen ions, this defect leads to the secretion of $NH^{4+}$. Patients with RTA type 1 usually have non–anion gap acidosis (which is also found in patients with RTA type 2 and 4). However, the main difference between the types of RTA is that type 1 will also have very low levels of $HCO_3^-$, high urine pH of >5.5 (as the kidney is unable to maximally acidify the urine), and positive urine anion gap. In this case, the patient's urine anion gap is 19 based on the formula, Urine anion gap = $U_{Na} + U_K - U_{Cl}$.

Main causes of RTA type I include autoimmune diseases, such as rheumatoid arthritis and Sjögren syndrome, obstructive nephropathy, and nephrotoxins, including toluene and amphotericin B. There is a hereditary cause for RTA type 1 which is usually diagnosed in infants or childhood. Though the clear mechanism of acquired RTA type I is unclear, it has been suggested that this due to defective $H^+$-$K^+$ ATPase function at the apical surface of the α-type intercalated cells of the collecting duct.

In children, this can manifest with polyuria, stunted growth, recurrent nephrocalcinosis, and hypercalciuria. In adults, RTA type 1 will also lead to nephrocalcinosis. Treatment consists of managing the underlying disorders but can sometimes include usage of thiazide diuretics and/or $NaHCO_3$ and $K^+$ supplementation.

While all types of RTA lead to hyperchloremic non–anion gap metabolic acidosis, the main differences between types of RTA are laid out in the table that follows.

| | TYPE 1 DISTAL | TYPE 2 PROXIMAL | TYPE 4 |
|---|---|---|---|
| **Defect** | Impaired $H^+$ excretion in distal tubule | Impaired $HCO_3^-$ reabsorption in the proximal tubule | Impaired cation exchange in distal tubule |
| **Urine pH** | Usually >5.5 | Usually <5.5 | Usually <5.5 |
| **Serum $HCO_3$** | <15 | >15 | >15 |
| **Serum K** | Low-normal | Low-normal | High |
| **Renal stones** | Yes | No | No |
| **Urine anion gap** | Positive | Negative | Positive |

### Reference

1. Soriano JG. Renal tubular acidosis: the clinical entity. *J Am Soc Nephrol.* 2002;13:2160-2170.

---

**5.** Correct Answer: C

**Rationale:**

Iatrogenic causes of non–anion gap metabolic acidosis are common in the setting of critical ill patients, who require aggressive fluid administration, particularly when chloride-rich solutions such as 0.9% saline are used. When large amounts of sodium chloride–containing solutions are administered, the chloride concentration in the serum will rise more than that of sodium as the serum chloride levels are normally lower than serum sodium. Therefore, the strong ion difference (SID) decreases and leads to a reduction of the positive plasma charge. To compensate for this, the chloride reacts with bicarbonate to produce protons and buffer the pH. This leads to depletion of bicarbonate stores and subsequently an acidosis.

### Reference

1. Kraut J, Kurtz I. Treatment of acute non-anion gap metabolic acidosis. *Clin Kidney J.* 2015;8(1):93-99.

**6.** Correct Answer: D

**Rationale:**

Based on the patient's symptoms of fatigue and back pain, along with laboratory studies, including anemia and hypoalbuminemia, the patient most likely has multiple myeloma (MM). Patients with MM also commonly have hypoalbuminemia for which a correction factor needs to be applied. For any 1 g/L decrease of albumin, the anion gap increases by 2.5. So, while the anion gap without albumin is normal at 11, after correction factor for albumin, the anion gap is >12.

Corrected anion gap (AG) = AG + 2.5 × (4.5 − measured albumin [g/dL])

When calculating the anion gap, attention should be paid to patients with hypoalbuminemia and hypophosphatemia as this will increase the anion gap further.

### References

1. Zampieri FG, Park M, Ranzani OT, et al. Anion gap corrected for albumin, phosphate, and lactate is a good predictor of strong ion gap in critically ill patients: a nested cohort study. *Rev Bras Ter Intensiva*. 2013;25(3):205-211.
2. Lee S, Kang KP, Kang SK. Clinical usefulness of the serum anion gap. *Electrolyte Blood Press*. 2006;4:44-46.

**7.** Correct Answer: D

**Rationale:**

In patients who receive parental nutrition, close monitoring of electrolytes and acid-base status is required as complications such as refeeding syndrome and other metabolic disturbances can occur. Parenteral nutrition consists of various cations, such as sodium, potassium, and calcium along with other anions such as chloride. However, in lieu of chloride, acetate is a solution commonly used in parenteral nutrition as a substitute for chloride (as a buffer) as it reduces the incidence of metabolic acidosis and hyperchloremia.

In this case, the patient has developed a metabolic alkalosis after TPN was started. In TPN, if the acetate content is too high, this can lead a metabolic alkalosis because acetate is metabolized to bicarbonate. Similarly, low chloride in TPN solutions will also lead to a metabolic alkalosis. Therefore, to correct this, the chloride content should be increased whereas the amino acid levels should be reduced to aid in reducing the acetate concentration in the TPN.

### References

1. Peters O, Ryan S, Matthew L, Cheng K, Lunn J. Randomized controlled trial of acetate in preterm neonates receiving parenteral nutrition. *Arch Dis Child*. 1997;77:12-15.
2. Johnson P. Review of micronutrients in parenteral nutrition for the NICU population. *Neonatal Netw*. 2014;33(3):155-161.

**8.** Correct Answer: B

**Rationale:**

The patient has primary metabolic alkalosis which is most likely due to diuretic usage. Diuretics such as furosemide increase sodium and water delivery to the distal nephron, which subsequently increases the urinary hydrogen and potassium secretion, thereby leading to metabolic alkalosis and hypokalemia. Furthermore, the contraction of extracellular fluid (ECF) leads to renin and aldosterone secretion, which slows the sodium loss but in turn increases the secretion of potassium and hydrogen ions. This is also known as "contraction alkalosis" which is due to the loss of low bicarbonate–containing extracellular fluid.

Patients with Bartter syndrome will have similar findings, but with the recent usage of diuretics and lack of previous history, this is less likely the cause here. Treatment consists of replacement of potassium chloride.

### References

1. Greenberg A. Diuretic complications. *Am J Med Sci*. 2000;319(1):10-24.
2. Sica DA, Carter B, Cushman W, Hamm L. Thiazide and loop diuretics. *J Clin Hypertens*. 2011;13(9):639-643.

**9.** Correct Answer: A

**Rationale:**

The patient has a hypokalemic hypochloremic metabolic alkalosis caused by excessive gastrointestinal losses. This can be caused with prolonged nasogastric suctioning, vomiting, and high ileostomy ostomy output. Of note, despite the low serum chloride, the patients develop a paradoxical aciduria which is due the sodium exchange for hydrogen ion in the kidney.

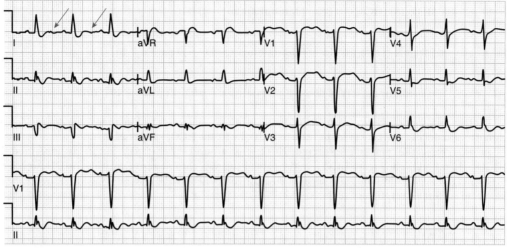

The above arrows point to "U wave" which can be seen on ECGs in the presence of hypokalemia.

References

1. Galla JH. Metabolic alkalosis. *J Am Soc Nephrol.* 2000;11(2):369-375.
2. Aspelund G, Langer JC. Current management of hypertrophic pyloric stenosis. *Semin Pediatr Surg.* 2007;16(1):27-33.

**10.** Correct Answer: E

**Rationale:**

Both diabetic and alcoholic ketoacidosis can lead to increased anion gap metabolic acidosis. However, given the patient's elevated blood glucose and ketones in the urine, this is more suggestive of DKA. Patients with DKA generally present with nausea, vomiting, and abdominal pain. Patients with diabetes can develop DKA due to a reduction in effective insulin leading to increased conversion of free fatty acids into ketones, including β-hydroxybutyrate and acetoacetic acid, thereby leading to ketoacidosis. In this case, the patient's elevated β-hydroxybutyrate also points toward DKA, though it may not be present in all cases. Treatment includes insulin and fluid administration as most of the patients are volume depleted.

References

1. Dunger DB, Sperling MA, Acerini CL, et al. ESPE/LWPES consensus statement on diabetic ketoacidosis in children and adolescents. *Arch Dis Child.* 2004;89:188-194.
2. Viallon A, Zeni F, Lafond P, et al. Does bicarbonate therapy improve the management of severe diabetic ketoacidosis? *Crit Care Med.* 1999;27(12):2690-2693.

**11.** Correct Answer: C

**Rationale:**

This patient has metabolic alkalosis with respiratory compensation due to his recent diuretic use. Diuretics such as thiazide and loop diuretics will lead to a net loss of chloride with free water without affecting the bicarbonate excretion. This therefore leads to a so-called "contraction alkalosis." As a compensatory mechanism, the elevated pH will depress the respiratory centers, thereby leading to an increase of $PaCO_2$ to correct the pH. The formula below can be used to assess for the expected respiratory compensation:

$$PCO_2 = 0.7 \times \Delta \left[ HCO_3^- \right]$$

In other words, for every 1 mEq/L rise in $HCO_3^-$, there will be a 0.7 mm Hg increase in $PCO_2$.

References

1. Palmer BF, Naderi ASA. Metabolic complications associated with use of thiazide diuretics. *J Am Soc Hypertens.* 2007;1(6):381-392.
2. Sood P, Paul G, Puri S. Interpretation of arterial blood gas. *Indian J Crit Care Med.* 2010;14(2):57-64.

**12.** Correct Answer: A

**Rationale:**

The patient has a respiratory acidosis due to Guillain-Barre syndrome. Her pH is acidic and her inappropriately elevated $pCO_2$ points toward a primary respiratory etiology. To determine whether there is any compensation, the following formula can be used.

$$\text{Expected}\left[HCO_3\right] = 24 + \left[\left(\text{Measured pCO}_2 - 40\right)/10\right]$$

$$\text{Acute respiratory acidosis} - \text{Decrease in pH} = 0.08 \times \left[\left(\text{paCO}_2 - 40\right)/10\right]$$

$$\text{Chronic respiratory acidosis} - \text{Decrease in pH} = 0.03 \times \left[\left(\text{pCO}_2 - 40\right)/10\right]$$

In other words, for every increase in $PaCO_2$ by 10, the $HCO_3-$ increases by 1 in acute respiratory acidosis and in chronic respiratory acidosis, for every increase in $PaCO_2$ by 10, the $HCO_3-$ increases by 4.

In this case, the patient's expected $HCO_3-$ is around 27 mEq/L, but it is measured higher ($HCO_3-$ 32 mEq/L). The higher $HCO_3-$ in the patient suggests chronic respiratory acidosis. However, the low pH points towards an additional uncompensated acute component to the respiratory acidosis. hence the patient has acute on chronic respiratory acidosis.

### Reference

1. Rose B, Post T. *Clinical Physiology of Acid-Base and Electrolyte Disorders*. 5th ed. USA: McGraw-Hill; 2001.

---

**13. Correct Answer: B**

**Rationale:**

Based on the patient's pH, there is acidosis which is likely metabolic given his low $HCO_3-$. The next step is to calculate the anion gap (AG).

$$\text{Calculated anion gap} = Na - \left(HCO_3 + Cl\right)$$

In this case, the patient has an AG of 19. The next step is to see whether there is any respiratory compensation via Winter's formula as follows:

$$\text{Expected PaCO}_2 = \left(HCO_3^- \times 1.5\right) + 8 +/-2$$

When using Winter's formula, the expected $PaCO_2$ is 21 to 25. However, in this patient, the $PaCO_2$ is higher than that, suggesting that there is respiratory acidosis present in addition to the anion gap metabolic acidosis. In this case, patient has aspirin overdose which explains the tinnitus and metabolic acidosis along with COPD leading to a respiratory acidosis.

### Reference

1. Kellum JA. Disorders of acid-base balance. *Crit Care Med.* 2007;35(11):2630-2636.

---

**14. Correct Answer: E**

**Rationale:**

The patient has a metabolic alkalosis that is caused by citrate from numerous blood transfusions. Citrate is used as an anticoagulant in blood bags as a preservative and is converted from citrate to form three moles of sodium bicarbonate via the liver. Another mechanism that leads to metabolic alkalosis includes the depletion of chloride due to the reduced chloride concentration content of the donor's blood. Both mechanisms lead to hypochloremic metabolic alkalosis. This is best treated with acetazolamide as it is carbonic anhydrase inhibitor and cause $NaHCO_3-$ diuresis by inhibiting the reabsorption of bicarbonate ions from renal tubules. Other complications from massive blood transfusions include hypocalcemia due calcium chelation and hypomagnesemia.

### References

1. Calladine M, Gairdner D, Naidoo BT, Orrell DH. Acid-base changes following exchange transfusion with citrated blood. *Arch Dis Child.* 1965;40:626-631.
2. Li K, Xu Y. Citrate metabolism in blood transfusions and its relationship due to metabolic alkalosis and respiratory acidosis. *Int J Clin Exp Med.* 2015;8(4):6578-6584.

---

**15. Correct Answer: C**

**Rationale:**

The patient has increased anion gap metabolic acidosis of 20—calculated anion gap = $Na - (HCO_3 + Cl)$. However, her osmolal gap is <10 mOsm/kg $H_2O$ which rules out ethylene or isopropyl intoxication. Furthermore, she has acute kidney injury with positive urine RBC indicative of myoglobin release in the absence blood in the urine. Altogether, this points toward rhabdomyolysis in the setting of seizures. In patients with severe rhabdomyolysis, this can lead to the release of lactic acid caused by muscle breakdown leading to metabolic acidosis and acute renal failure.

The osmolal gap is defined as the difference between the measured and the calculated plasma osmolality using the formula below:

Calculated plasma osmolal = (2 × plasma sodium) + glucose/18 + BUN/2.8. The patient's calculated plasma osmolality is 282 mOsm/kg $H_2O$ which is close to the measured plasma osmolality.

References
1. Hunter JD, Gregg K, Damani Z. Rhabdomyolysis. *Contin Edu Anaesth Crit Care Pain.* 2006;6(1):141-143.
2. Chatzizisis YS, Misirli G, Hatzitolios AI, Giannoglou GD. The syndrome of rhabdomyolysis: complications and treatment. *Eur J Intern Med.* 2008;19(8):568-574.

# ENDOCRINE DISORDERS

# 54

# DIABETES MELLITUS

Jean Kwo

1. A 75-year-old male with a history of hypertension, chronic renal insufficiency, and type 2 diabetes mellitus is admitted to the intensive care unit (ICU) with shock secondary to bowel perforation. His blood glucose is 304 mg/dL on presentation and 275 mg/dL on recheck an hour later. Which of the following is the MOST appropriate for management of hyperglycemia?

   A. Start insulin glargine 0.2 mg/kg/d and correction insulin with a sliding scale of regular insulin every 6 hours with a goal glucose target between 80 and 110 mg/dL
   B. Start insulin glargine 0.2 mg/kg/d and correction insulin with a sliding scale of regular insulin every 6 hours with a goal glucose target between 140 and 180 mg/dL
   C. Start an insulin infusion targeting a blood glucose of 80 to 110 mg/dL
   D. Start an insulin infusion targeting blood glucose of 140 to 180 mg/dL

2. Which of the following statements is FALSE regarding intensive glucose control (target blood glucose between 81 and 108 mg/dL) compared to conventional glucose control (target blood glucose <180 mg/dL) in critically ill patients.

   A. Patients receiving intensive glucose control are 15 times more likely to develop hypoglycemia when compared to patients receiving conventional glucose control
   B. Intensive glucose control is not associated with decreased mortality in surgical patients
   C. Deaths from cardiovascular causes were more common in the intensive glucose control group than in the conventional glucose control group
   D. Patients in the conventional glucose control group were more likely to have blood cultures positive for pathogenic organisms

3. Which of the following statements regarding agents used to treat Type 2 diabetes mellitus is FALSE?

   A. Metformin is contraindicated in patients with an eGFR of less than 60 mL/min/1.73 m$^2$
   B. Sodium-glucose co-transporter 2 (SGLT2) inhibitors can cause hypovolemia and acute kidney injury
   C. Sulfonylureas reduce both microvascular and macrovascular complications of diabetes
   D. Both glucagon-like peptide-1 (GLP-1) receptor agonists and dipeptidyl peptidase-4 (DPP-4) inhibitors are associated with acute pancreatitis

4. All of the following contribute to the development of diabetic ketoacidosis (DKA) EXCEPT:

   A. Insulin deficiency
   B. Increased secretion of catecholamines, cortisol, and growth hormone
   C. Glucagon deficiency
   D. Increased lipolysis

341

5. A 27-year-old man with a history of obesity and substance abuse is found obtunded. His laboratory findings are:

| | VALUE |
|---|---|
| **Chemistry** | |
| Sodium | 135 mmol/L |
| Potassium | 3.0 mmol/L |
| Chloride | 105 mmol/L |
| $CO_2$ | 10 mmol/L |
| Blood Urea Nitrogen | 42 mg/dL |
| Creatinine | 2.1 mg/dL |
| Glucose | 570 mg/dL |
| **Arterial Blood Gas** | |
| pH | 7.21 |
| $PaCO_2$ | 24 |
| $PaO_2$ | 95 |
| Serum ketones | positive |

Initial treatment for him should include all of the following EXCEPT:

A. Normal saline at 500 to 1,000 mL/h during the first 1 to 2 hours
B. Replete potassium by administering potassium chloride
C. Intravenous insulin infusion to correct serum glucose
D. Identify and treat precipitating event

6. An 85-year-old male is admitted to the ICU with urosepsis. His blood sugar is 720 mg/dL. Which of the following is TRUE about hyperglycemic hyperosmolar state (HHS)?

A. Positive urine ketones means that this cannot be a HHS
B. Mortality in HHS is similar to mortality in DKA
C. His free water deficit is likely higher than a patient with DKA
D. Acidemia rules out a diagnosis of HHS

7. You calculate the Δ anion gap/Δ bicarbonate ratio in your patient with DKA and find that it is greater than 1. Explanations include all of the following EXCEPT:

A. Impaired renal function
B. A coexisting nonanion gap metabolic acidosis
C. A coexisting metabolic alkalosis
D. It may be normal for your patient

8. A 68-year-old female with a history of type 2 diabetes mellitus is admitted to the ICU with pancreatitis. Her ICU course is notable for vasodilatory shock requiring vasopressors, respiratory failure requiring mechanical ventilation, renal failure requiring renal replacement therapy, and multiple episodes of hypoglycemia (blood glucose <80 mg/dL). TRUE statements include:

A. Hypoglycemia is a cause of mortality in critically ill patients
B. ICU length of stay is not associated with the incidence of hypoglycemia
C. Patients with hypoglycemia have an increased risk for death from vasodilatory shock
D. A history of well-controlled diabetes (preadmission Hgb A1c level <6.5) is associated with increased risk of hypoglycemia

# Chapter 54 ▪ Answers

**1.** Correct Answer: D

**Rationale:**

A single center trial published in 2001 involving approximately 1,500 surgical ICU patients showed significantly decreased ICU mortality in patients who were managed with intensive glucose control (target blood glucose of 80-110 mg/dL) when compared to patients with conventional glucose control (target blood glucose of 180-200 mg/dL). Most of the patients in this trial had undergone cardiac surgery and the mortality benefit was in patients who were in the ICU for 5 days or longer. This mortality benefit was not seen in 1,100 critically ill medical patients from the same center.

The subsequent Normoglycemia in Intensive Care Evaluation — Survival Using Glucose Algorithm Regulation (NICE-SUGAR) trial was a larger (approximately 6,000 patients), multicenter trial that showed that intensive glucose control (target blood glucose 81-108 mg/dL) was associated with higher mortality and increased risk of hypoglycemia when compared to conventional glucose control (target blood glucose <180 mg/dL). Furthermore, a post hoc analysis of the NICE-SUGAR database showed that hypoglycemia was associated with increased mortality. Based on these findings, the Surviving Sepsis guideline recommend a protocolized approach to glucose control targeting a blood glucose <180 mg/dL. Other experts recommend a target glucose between 140 and 180 mg/dL from the NICE-SUGAR trial (patients in the conventional glucose management group had a mean time-weighted glucose level of 144 ± 23 mg/dL).

Although a basal/bolus insulin regimen is recommended for management of hyperglycemia in non-ICU patients, absorption of subcutaneously delivered medications can be variable because of shock or edema. Continuous intravenous insulin infusions are recommended for glucose management in ICU patients. The half-life of iv insulin is short (<15 minutes) and can be titrated to bring a patient's blood glucose levels to targeted range more rapidly than subcutaneous insulin. Insulin infusions can also be adjusted quickly based on changes in the patient's clinical status.

References
1. Finfer S, Chittock DR, Blair D, et al. Intensive versus conventional glucose control in critically ill patients. *N Engl J Med.* 2009;360:1283-1297.
2. Rhodes A, Evans LE, Alhazzani W, et al. Surviving sepsis campaign: international guidelines for the management of sepsis and septic shock: 2016. *Crit Care Med.* 2017;45:486-552.
3. Van den Berghe G, Wouters P, Weekers F, et al. Intensive insulin therapy in critically ill patients. *N Engl J Med.* 2001;345:1359-1367.
4. Van den Berghe G, Wilmer A, Hermans G, et al. Intensive insulin therapy in the medical ICU. *N Engl J Med.* 2006;354:449-461.

**2.** Correct Answer: D

**Rationale:**

The NICE-SUGAR study was an international, multicenter trial involving 6,104 patients designed to test the hypothesis that intensive glucose control reduces mortality at 90 days. It found that intensive glucose control (target blood glucose between 81-108 mg/dL) was associated with a 2.6% increase in mortality at 90 days when compared to conventional glucose control (target blood glucose of <180 mg/dL). There were more hypoglycemic events in the intensive glucose control group. There was no difference between the two groups in overall length of stay, ICU length of stay, time on mechanical ventilation, time on renal replacement therapy, incidence of new organ failure, positive blood cultures, or red blood cell transfusions.

Although a previous trial showed intensive glucose control improved survival among surgical ICU patients, there was no difference in 90-day mortality in surgical and nonsurgical patients in the NICE-SUGAR trial.

References
1. Finfer S, Chittock DR, Blair D, et al. Intensive versus conventional glucose control in critically ill patients. *N Engl J Med.* 2009;360:1283-1297.
2. Van den Berghe G, Wouters P, Weekers F, et al. Intensive insulin therapy in critically ill patients. *N Engl J Med.* 2001;345:1359-1367.

**3.** Correct Answer: A

**Rationale:**

Metformin is the first drug recommended when starting treatment for type 2 diabetes. It reduces hemoglobin A1c by 1% to 1.5% and is associated with decreases in both the microvascular and macrovascular complications of diabetes. Recommendations against the use of metformin in patients with mild to moderate chronic kidney disease were removed by the FDA, as recent studies did not show an increased risk of lactic acidosis in these patients. However, metformin is contraindicated in patients with an eGFR <30 mL/min/1.73 m².

Sulfonylureas also decrease hemoglobin A1c by 1% to 1.5% and have been shown to reduce long-term macrovascular and microvascular events. Adverse effects include weight gain and hypoglycemia.

GLP-1 receptor agonists also lower hemoglobin A1c by 1% to 1.5% and are associated with weight loss. They are associated with a reduced risk of cardiovascular mortality. Adverse effects include nausea, vomiting, diarrhea, acute renal failure due to volume depletion from vomiting and diarrhea, and acute pancreatitis.

DPP-4 inhibitors produce a small reduction in hemoglobin A1c (0.5%-1%). It has been associated with acute pancreatitis as well as hypersensitivity reactions.

SGLT2 inhibitors also produce a small reduction in hemoglobin A1c (0.5%-1%) and are also associated with a small decrease in systolic blood pressure and weight loss. Because SGLT2 inhibitors also increase sodium excretion, acute renal injury due to hypovolemia can occur.

### References

1.  Drugs for type 2 diabetes. *Med Lett Drugs Ther*. 2017;59(1512):9-18.
2.  Qaseem A, Barry MJ, Humphrey LL, et al. Oral pharmacologic treatment of type 2 diabetes mellitus: a clinical practice guideline update from the American College of Physicians. *Ann Intern Med*. 2017;166(4):279-290.

---

**4.** Correct Answer: C

**Rationale:**

DKA results from insulin deficiency and increased levels of glucagon. In addition, there is increased secretion of catecholamines, cortisol, and growth hormone, which counteract the action of any residual insulin. Absolute insulin deficiency results in increased lipolysis resulting in increased free fatty acids that are oxidized to ketone bodies in the liver. Increased levels of catecholamines, cortisol, and growth hormone result in increased gluconeogenesis and glycogenolysis, and hyperglycemia.

### References

1.  Hirsch IB, Emmett M. Diabetic ketoacidosis and hyperosmolar hyperglycemic state in adults: epidemiology and pathogenesis. In: Nathan DM, Wolfsdorf JI, eds. *UpToDate*. Waltham, MA: UpToDate, Inc. http://www.uptodate.com. Accessed August 28, 2018.
2.  Umpierrez G, Korykowski M. Diabetic emergencies – ketoacidosis, hyperglycemic hyperosmolar state, and hypoglycemia. *Nat Rev Endocrinol*. 2016;12:222-232.

---

**5.** Correct Answer: B

**Rationale:**

Diagnostic criteria for DKA consist of the triad of hyperglycemia (serum glucose >250 mg/dL), acidemia (pH <7.3), and ketonemia. The osmotic diuresis associated with glycosuria results in total body water, sodium, potassium, and phosphate deficits. Initial treatment consists of administration of normal saline to restore intravascular volume and renal perfusion. If the serum potassium is less that 3.3 mmol/L, potassium should be repleted before starting insulin as correction of volume depletion and acidosis, and insulin can all worsen hypokalemia. Once the serum sodium is greater than 3.3 mmol/L, insulin should be started. The recommended dose for regular intravenous insulin is a bolus of 0.1 U/kg followed by a continuous infusion at 0.1 U/kg/h. In patients with mild to moderate DKA, subcutaneous rapid-acting insulin analogues can also be considered.

A search for a precipitating event should be initiated. The most common associated events are infection and inadequate insulin therapy. Other precipitating factors include medications that affect carbohydrate metabolism (glucocorticoids, thiazide diuretics, sympathomimetic agents), SGLT2 inhibitors, cocaine use, and malfunction of continuous subcutaneous infusion devices.

### References

1.  Kitabchi AE, Umpierrez GE, Murphy MB, et al. Hyperglycemic crises in adult patient with diabetes: a consensus statement from the American Diabetes Association. *Diabetes Care*. 2006;29(12):2739-2748.
2.  Umpierrez G, Korykowski M. Diabetic emergencies – ketoacidosis, hyperglycemic hyperosmolar state, and hypoglycemia. *Nat Rev Endocrinol*. 2016;12:222-232.

---

**6.** Correct Answer: C

**Rationale:**

Though HHS is usually associated with type 2 diabetes mellitus and older age, the pathophysiology is similar to that of DKA. However, unlike DKA, patients with HHS usually have enough insulin to prevent ketosis. It should be noted that there is a subpopulation of patients with type 2 diabetes that can present with ketosis.

Given its slower onset (over several days to several weeks), patients with HHS usually have greater free water and electrolyte deficits than patients with DKA due to more prolonged glycosuria and lack of hydration due to concomitant illness. This results in a hyperosmolar state with a serum osmolarity of >320 mmol/kg.

ADA guidelines for diagnosis of HHS include a glucose level of >600 mg/dL, pH >7.3, and bicarbonate level >20 mEq/L. Although HHS is usually not associated with a metabolic acidosis, acidosis may occur due to dehydration and lactate acidosis, concomitant illness (sepsis), or renal failure.

Mortality in HHS ranges from 5% to 16%, which is 10 times higher than mortality in DKA. The higher mortality may reflect the precipitating factor and not hyperglycemia and concomitant metabolic disarray.

## References

1. Kitabchi AE, Umpierrez GE, Murphy MB, et al. Hyperglycemic crises in adult patient with diabetes: a consensus statement from the American Diabetes Association. *Diabetes Care.* 2006;29(12):2739-2748.
2. Milanesi A, Weinreb J. Hyperglycemichyperosmolar state. In: DeGroot LJ, Chrousous G, Dungan K, et al. eds. *Endotext.* South Darmouth, MA: MDText.com, Inc. www.endotext.org. Accessed December 20, 2018.

## 7. Correct Answer: B

**Rationale:**

The "delta ratio" or the (change in anion gap)/(change in bicarbonate) is used to determine whether a mixed acid base disorder is present in the setting of a high anion gap metabolic acidosis. A delta ratio of 1 is indicative of an uncomplicated high anion gap metabolic acidosis.

Conditions that increase the serum bicarbonate concentration (metabolic alkalosis or chronic respiratory acidosis) cause a smaller change in bicarbonate and an increased delta ratio (typically >2).

Young patients with diabetes have relatively normal renal function and can excrete large quantities of ketoacids in the urine and thus, have a delta ratio of 1 or less. However, if renal function is abnormal (eg due to diabetic nephropathy or volume depletion), less ketoacid anions are excreted resulting in an increased change in anion gap as compared to the change in bicarbonate.

A nonanion gap metabolic acidosis results from an increased chloride and decreased bicarbonate. A delta ratio of <1 is indicative of a combined anion gap metabolic acidosis and nonanion gap metabolic acidosis.

Calculation of the delta ratio is to diagnose mixed acid base disorders in patients with anion gap metabolic acidosis is controversial. Sources of error include the assumption that all buffering of acid occur in the extracellular space, acid anions are buffered solely by bicarbonate, and the distribution and clearance of acid anions and H$^+$ are the same. Furthermore, the calculation of anion gap is derived from the measurement of three or four electrolytes (sodium, potassium, chloride, and bicarbonate) each with its own measurement error. As well, there is the assumption that the normal anion gap is 12 and the normal serum bicarbonate is 24. Thus, the delta ratio should not be used as the sole method to diagnose mixed acid base disturbances in the patient with anion gap metabolic acidosis.

## References

1. Rastegar A. Use of the $\Delta$AG/$\Delta$HCO$_3$– ratio in the diagnosis of mixed acid-base disorders. *JASN.* 2007;18(9):2429-2431.
2. Emmett M, Palmer BF. The delta anion gap/delta HCO3 ratio in patients with a high anion gap metabolic acidosis. In: Forman JP, ed. *UpToDate.* Waltham, MA: UpToDate, Inc. http://www.uptodate.com. Accessed August 14, 2018.
3. Umpierrez G, Korykowski M. Diabetic emergencies – ketoacidosis, hyperglycemic hyperosmolar state, and hypoglycemia. *Nat Rev Endocrinol.* 2016;12:222-232.

## 8. Correct Answer: C

**Rationale:**

The NICE-SUGAR trial showed that patients receiving intensive glucose control (target blood glucose 81-108 mg/dL) had more episodes of severe hypoglycemia (blood glucose ≤40 mg/dL) than patients in the conventional glucose control (blood glucose <180 mg/dL) group. A subsequent study using data from the NICE-SUGAR database examined the relationship between hypoglycemia and mortality. This study found an increased mortality in patients with hypoglycemia. Furthermore, patients with severe hypoglycemia (blood glucose <40 mg/dL) had a higher risk of death when compared to normoglycemic patients than patients with moderate hypoglycemia (blood glucose between 40 and 79). Patients with more than 1 day of hypoglycemia were also more likely to die than those with 1 day of hypoglycemia. Although hypoglycemia occurred more frequently in patients in the intensive glucose control group, the association between hypoglycemia and death was similar in the two groups.

Patients who had an ICU stay of 7 days or longer were more likely to have moderate/severe hypoglycemia than those whose ICU length of stay was shorter. Patients with moderate and severe hypoglycemia also had an increased risk of death from vasodilatory shock when compared with patients who did not have hypoglycemia.

This study did not show a difference between risk of death with moderate and severe hypoglycemia in patients with and without diabetes. However, another study showed that poorly controlled diabetic patients (as reflected by Hgb A1c level within a 3-month period preceding ICU admission) were more likely to have moderate/severe hypoglycemia and higher risk of death.

Although these studies show an association between hypoglycemia and death, they do not prove causality. The current consensus for blood sugar management in critically ill patients is to target a blood sugar between 140 to 180 mg/dL. Patients with poorly controlled diabetes may benefit from closer blood sugar monitoring as they are more likely to become hypoglycemic and have poorer outcomes.

## References

1. Egi M, Bellomo R, Stachowski E, et al. Hypoglycemia and outcome in critically ill patients. *Mayo Clin Proc.* 2010;85:217-224.
2. Egi M, Krinsley JS, Maurer P, et al. Pre-morbid glycemic control modifies the interaction between acute hypoglycemia and mortality. *Int Care Med.* 2016:42:562-571.
3. NICE-SUGAR Investigators. Hypoglycemia and risk of death in critically ill patients. *N Engl J Med.* 2012;367:1108-1118.

# 55

# THYROID

Kenneth Potter and Kunal Karamchandani

1. A 27-year-old man with primary sclerosing cholangitis and ulcerative colitis presents with high ileostomy output and abdominal pain for last few weeks associated with a 9-kg weight loss. He has no other medical history. Despite fluid resuscitation and pharmacologic therapy, his symptoms persist. He develops fever to 39.7°C and is transferred to the ICU with concerns for sepsis. On admission to the ICU, he is somnolent and lethargic, heart rate is 160 beats/min, blood pressure is 156/80 mm Hg, respiratory rate is 25/min, and his pulse oximeter reads 98% on room air. His sepsis workup is negative, but his laboratory work is remarkable for a low TSH level. What is the diagnosis?

   A. Serotonin syndrome
   B. Hyperthyroidism
   C. Thyroid storm
   D. Malignant hyperthermia
   E. Malignant neurolept syndrome

2. What is the best **initial** treatment?

   A. High-dose Iodine
   B. Propanolol
   C. Diltiazem
   D. Hydrocortisone
   E. Cholestyramine

3. A 79-year-old female is admitted to the ICU after repair of a pathologic femur fracture with an estimated blood loss of 1.2 L. She is oxygenating well on room air, is hemodynamically stable, and is appropriately alert and oriented. Physical examination is remarkable for incision site tenderness and signs of malnutrition. Laboratory studies reveal normal electrolytes, normal liver function tests, normal TSH and T4, and decreased levels of T3. What would be the most appropriate management of her deranged thyroid function test?

   A. Supportive care with appropriate nutrition
   B. Supplementation with T4
   C. Supplementation with T3
   D. Hydrocortisone

4. A 78 year-old female is admitted to the ICU with a 6 month history of generalized fatigue and muscle cramps, which are worsened with exercise. Her symptoms have been progressively worsening and now she is unable to ambulate. On physical examination, pressure stimulus on the muscles of the arm leads to formation of a palpable, painless ridge around the site of the stimulus, which subsides gradually returning the muscle contour to normal in a few seconds. She is also noted to have delayed deep tendon reflexes and anasarca. Her laboratory studies are within normal limits, except for an elevated TSH level. Which of the following is most likely the cause of her symptoms?

   A. Recent influenza vaccine
   B. Recent CVA
   C. Multiple sclerosis
   D. Muscular dystrophy
   E. Chronic hypothyroidism

5. An 81-year-old female is admitted to the ICU with altered mental status. She is lethargic and does not provide a good history. On physical examination, her skin is dry and pale, and her temperature is 35°C. She is noted to have decreased deep tendon reflexes. Which of the following clinical/physiologic derangements is most likely to be present in the patient?

   A. Decreased systemic vascular resistance
   B. Decreased cardiac contractility
   C. Respiratory Alkalosis
   D. Diarrhea
   E. Hyperglycemia

# Chapter 55 ▪ Answers

1. Correct Answer: C

2. Correct Answer: B

**Rationale:**
Thyroid storm is a rare, life-threatening condition characterized by severe clinical manifestations of thyrotoxicosis. The incidence ranges between 0.02% and 1.3% and is associated with significant mortality. It may be precipitated by an acute event such as thyroid or nonthyroidal surgery, trauma, and infection. In addition to specific therapy directed against the thyroid, supportive therapy in an intensive care unit (ICU) and recognition and treatment of any precipitating factors is essential to prevent morbidity and mortality.

The diagnosis of thyroid storm is based on the presence of severe and life-threatening symptoms such as hyperpyrexia, cardiovascular dysfunction, and/or altered mentation along with biochemical evidence of hyperthyroidism (elevation of free T4 and/or T3 and suppression of TSH). A scoring system was devised in 1993 by Burch and Wartofsky using clinical criteria for the identification of thyroid storm (Table 55.1). A score of 45 or more is highly suggestive of thyroid storm, whereas a score below 25 makes thyroid storm unlikely. A score of 25 to 44 is suggestive of impending storm. Although this scoring system is likely sensitive, it is not very specific.

The patient was not exposed to any drugs that could trigger malignant hyperthermia (anesthetic agents or succinylcholine), malignant neurolept syndrome (neuroleptic medications), or serotonin syndrome (serotonergic medications).

Treatment includes controlling the symptoms and signs induced by increased adrenergic tone, blocking the peripheral conversion of T4 to T3, decreasing the production of thyroid hormones, and decreasing enterohepatic recycling of thyroid hormones. Decreased production and secretion of thyroid hormones can be achieved with thionamide medications, such as propylthiouracil and methimazole. High-dose iodine can also reduce production; however, it is only effective after initial blockade with other agents. Glucocorticoids, such as hydrocortisone, are useful to block the peripheral conversion of T4 to T3, but take time. Medications such as propanolol block the sympathetic surge present during thyroid storm and avoid life-threatening complications.

Calcium channel blockers, such as diltiazem, can be used to decrease sympathetic surge if beta blockers are contraindicated. Cholestyramine and hydrocortisone are not the initial agents as they take time to act.

**349**

**TABLE 55.1 The Burch-Wartofsky Point Scale for diagnosis of thyroid storm**

| CRITERIA | POINTS |
| --- | --- |
| **Thermoregulatory dysfunction** | |
| Temperature (°C) | |
| 37.2-37.7 | 5 |
| 37.8-38.3 | 10 |
| 38.4-38.8 | 15 |
| 38.9-39.3 | 20 |
| 39.4-39.9 | 25 |
| ≥40.0 | 30 |
| **Cardiovascular** | |
| Tachycardia (beats per minute) | |
| 90-109 | 5 |
| 110-119 | 10 |
| 120-129 | 15 |
| 130-139 | 20 |
| ≥140 | 25 |
| Atrial fibrillation | |
| Absent | 0 |
| Present | 10 |
| **Congestive heart failure** | |
| Absent | 0 |
| Mild | 5 |
| Moderate | 10 |
| Severe | 15 |
| **Gastrointestinal-hepatic dysfunction** | |
| Manifestation | |
| Absent | 0 |
| Moderate (diarrhea, abdominal pain, nausea/vomiting) | 10 |
| Severe (jaundice) | 20 |
| **Central nervous system disturbance** | |
| Manifestation | |
| Absent | 0 |
| Mild (agitation) | 10 |
| Moderate (delirium, psychosis, extreme lethargy) | 20 |
| Severe (seizure, coma) | 30 |

| CRITERIA | POINTS |
|---|---|
| **Precipitating event** | |
| Status | |
| Absent | 0 |
| Present | 10 |

(Adapted from Burch HB, Wartofsky L. Life-threatening thyrotoxicosis. Thyroid storm. *Endocrinol Metab Clin North Am.* 1993;22(2):263-277.)

### References

1. Akamizu T, Satoh T, Isozaki O, et al. Diagnostic criteria, clinical features, and incidence of thyroid storm based on nationwide surveys. *Thyroid.* 2012;22(7):661.
2. Sarlis NJ, Gourgiotis L. Thyroid emergencies. *Rev Endocr Metab Disord.* 2003;4(2):129-136.
3. Satoh T, Isozaki O, Suzuki A, et al. 2016 Guidelines for the management of thyroid storm from The Japan Thyroid Association and Japan Endocrine Society (First edition). *Endocr J.* 2016;63(12):1025-1064.
4. Burch HB, Wartofsky L. Life-threatening thyrotoxicosis. Thyroid storm. *Endocrinol Metab Clin North Am.* 1993;22(2):263-277.
5. Nayuk B, Burman K. Thyrotoxicosis and thyroid storm. *Endocrinol Metab Clin N Am.* 2006:663-686.

3. **Correct Answer: A**

**Rationale:**

Euthyroid sick syndrome (ESS), also known as nonthyroidal illness syndrome, is often seen in patients with severe critical illness, deprivation of calories, and following major surgeries. Common causes include infection, trauma, cardiopulmonary bypass, and malignancy. Although the exact mechanism is not known, one possible hypothesis is that the presence of thyroid binding hormone inhibitor in serum and body tissues inhibits the binding of thyroid hormone to thyroid-binding protein. Cytokines such as interleukin 1, interleukin 6, tumor necrosis factor alpha, and interferon-beta may affect the hypothalamus and pituitary, thus inhibiting TSH, thyroid-releasing hormone, thyroglobulin, T3, and thyroid-binding globulins production have also been implicated. ESS has been classified as (1) low T4 syndrome, (2) low T3-low T4 syndrome, (3) high T4 syndrome, and (4) other abnormalities. Low serum total T3 is the most common abnormality in ESS, and it is seen in about 70% of hospitalized patients. Both low T3 and the T4 syndromes are observed in critically ill patients admitted to intensive care units. Low-serum total T4 correlates with a bad prognosis; the probability of death correlates with the level of serum total T4. When total T4 levels drop below 4 μg/dL, the probability of death is approximately 50%, and when serum T4 levels are below 2 μg/dL, the probability of death reaches 80%.

Thyroid hormone replacement is not needed in patients with ESS (Choices B and C), and there is no role of steroids in the management of ESS (Choice D). Treatment and management of underlying medical illness is sufficient (Choice A).

### References

1. Ganesan K, Wadud K. *Thyroid, euthyroid sick syndrome.* In: *StatPearls* [Internet]. Treasure Island, FL: StatPearls Publishing; January 2018. Updated 2018 January 3, 2018. Available from https://www.ncbi.nlm.nih.gov/books/NBK482219/.
2. Gutch M, Kumar S, Gupta KK. Prognostic value of thyroid profile in critical care condition. *Indian J Endocrinol Metab.* 2018;22(3):387-391.

4. **Correct Answer: E**

**Rationale:**

Hypothyroid myopathy is a complication of untreated or uncontrolled hypothyroidism. Although most cases are not clinically significant, severe cases can lead to muscle disease and functional limitations. The exact mechanism is not understood; however, it is believed to be related to intracellular changes secondary to decreased T4 levels. T4 deficiency leads to reduced mitochondrial oxidative capacity, abnormal glycogenolysis, and an insulin-resistant state of the cell causing selective atrophy of type 2 muscle fibers (fast-twitching type), which leads to slowing of muscle contraction seen clinically in patients with hypothyroidism.

"Myoedema" is characteristic of hypothyroid myopathy. It is demonstrated by percussion or a pressure stimulus on the muscles of the arm, which causes the muscle to form a palpable, painless ridge around the site of the stimulus. The swelling subsides gradually returning the muscle contour to normal in a few seconds. This is believed to be caused by prolonged muscle contraction due to delay in calcium reuptake by the sarcoplasmic reticulum after the stimulus causes local calcium release. This sign if elicited can help differentiate hypothyroid myopathy from other types of myopathies.

Four main types of myopathies are associated with hypothyroidism: Myasthenic syndrome, Atrophic form, Kocher-Debre-Semelaigne, and Hoffman syndrome. Hoffmann syndrome is usually seen in adults and characterized by pseudohypertrophy, painful spasms, proximal muscle weakness, and stiffness. Management of hypothyroidism is the mainstay of treating hypothyroid myopathy. It is reversible with timely diagnosis and prompt treatment.

References

1. Fariduddin MM, Bansal N. *Thyroid, hypothyroid myopathy*. In: *StatPearls* [Internet]. Treasure Island, FL: StatPearls Publishing; January 2018. Updated August 15, 2018. Available from https://www.ncbi.nlm.nih.gov/books/NBK519513/.
2. Bloise FF. Oliveira TS, Cordeiro A, Ortiga-Carvalho TM. Thyroid hormones play role in sarcopenia and myopathies. *Front Physiol*. 2018;9:560.

**5.** Correct Answer: B

**Rationale:**

Based on the presentation, this patient likely has severe hypothyroidism causing myxedema coma. Myxedema coma is a severe manifestation of hypothyroidism that can carry up to 50% mortality. Patients experience decreased metabolic rate and decreased oxygen consumption. Systemic vascular resistance is increased (choice A) secondary to decreased beta adrenergic activity. Myocardial depression (choice B) results in profound hypotension. Hypothermia is common, occurring in up to 88% of patients. Central respiratory depression occurs, resulting in respiratory acidosis (choice C). Decreases in gastrointestinal motility typically manifests with constipation (choice D).

References

1. Sarlis NJ, Gourgiotis L. Thyroid emergencies. *Rev Endocr Metab Disord*. 2003;4:129-136.
2. Wartofsky L. Myxedema coma. *J Intensive Care Med*. 2007;35:687-698.
3. Sanders V. Neurologic manifestations of myxedema coma. *N Eng J Med*. 1962;266:547-551.

# 56

# PARATHYROID AND CALCIUM

Nathan M. Lee

1. A 58-year-old female with history of end-stage renal disease and hyperthyroidism is admitted to the intensive care unit after a complicated total thyroidectomy with reimplantation of parathyroid glands. Intravenous calcium supplementation is initiated. However, the patient continues to fail her spontaneous breathing trials with inadequate tidal volumes and negative inspiratory force (NIF) of −20 mm Hg. Labs on postoperative day 4 showed continued hypocalcemia despite supplementation and normal parathyroid hormone (PTH) levels. Which of the following statement regarding her condition is **NOT** correct?

   **A.** The syndrome most often occurs in patients with chronic increase in bone resorption induced by high levels of PTH.
   **B.** Patients often present with hypocalcemia, hypophosphatemia, hypomagnesemia, and hypokalemia.
   **C.** Sudden withdrawal of PTH causes an imbalance between osteoblast-mediated bone formation and osteoclast-mediated bone resorption.
   **D.** It can occur despite normal or even elevated levels of PTH.

2. Which of the following is **NOT** a symptom of acute hypoparathyroidism?

   **A.** Focal seizure
   **B.** Laryngospasm
   **C.** PR interval prolongation
   **D.** Anxiety

3. Which of the following medications may mimic hyperparathyroidism?

   **A.** Lithium
   **B.** Haloperidol
   **C.** Clozapine
   **D.** Spironolactone

4. A previously healthy 62-year-old female is admitted to the intensive care unit for airway watch after sustaining numerous rib fractures in a motor vehicle accident. On additional workup, she is noted to have mild hypercalcemia of 11.5 mg/dL (normal 8.9-10.1 mg/dL) and mildly elevated PTH of 124 pg/mL (normal 10-65 pg/mL). Review of her CT scans demonstrates mild-moderate osteoporosis and bilateral nephrocalcinosis. Which of the following is the recommended management for this patient's hyperparathyroidism?

   **A.** Alendronate
   **B.** Vitamin D supplementation
   **C.** Cinacalcet
   **D.** Parathyroidectomy

5. A 55-year-old male patient arrives to the emergency department complaining of worsening fatigue, vomiting, and weight loss over the last 2 weeks. A basic metabolic panel demonstrates the following: Sodium 148 mEq/L, potassium 3.1 mEq/L, chloride 112 mEq/L, bicarbonate 18 mEq/L, BUN 38 mg/dL, creatinine 1.8 mEq/L, glucose 98 mg/dL, and calcium 14 mg/dL. What is the best next step in management?

   **A.** Aggressive fluid bolus of 0.9% NaCl
   **B.** Administration of calcitonin
   **C.** Initiation of furosemide infusion
   **D.** Hemodialysis

# Chapter 56 ▪ Answers

**1.** Correct Answer: B

**Rationale:**
Hypocalcemia is a common problem after parathyroidectomy or thyroidectomy. The acute withdrawal of PTH causes an increase in osteoblast-mediated bone formation and a decrease in osteoclast-mediated bone resorption. Hypocalcemia after surgery is usually transient, as the degree of bone disease is typically mild and normal parathyroid tissue recovers function within a few days. Severe or prolonged hypocalcemia is called the hungry bone syndrome, and most often occurs in patients with chronic increase in bone resorption induced by high levels of PTH or in patients with high bone turnover induced by excess thyroid hormone. Hungry bone syndrome can occur despite normal or even elevated levels of PTH.

   Patients with hungry bone syndrome often present with concurrent hypophosphatemia, hypomagnesemia, and hyperkalemia. These imbalances reflect increased bone influx and efflux. Treatment consists of aggressive electrolyte supplementation and may necessitate a continuous infusion of calcium. Severe cases can be managed with dialysis with high-calcium bath.

References
1. Ho LY, Wong PN, Sin HK, et al. Risk factors and clinical course of hungry bone syndrome after total parathyroidectomy in dialysis patients with secondary hyperparathyroidism. *BMC Nephrol.* 2017;18:12.
2. Brasier AR, Nussbaum SR. Hungry bone syndrome: clinical and biochemical predictors of its occurrence after parathyroid surgery. *Am J Med.* 1988;84:654.
3. Tohme JF, Bilezikian JP. Diagnosis and treatment of hypocalcemic emergencies. *Endocrinologist.* 1996;6:10.

**2.** Correct Answer: C

**Rationale:**
Acute hypoparathyroidism is often the result of postsurgical or autoimmune damage to the parathyroid glands. Its clinical manifestations are due to acute hypocalcemia, of which the hallmark is tetany. Calcium normally blocks sodium channels and inhibits nerve depolarization; reduced calcium levels lower the threshold for depolarization. This is the reason for Trousseau sign (carpal spasm elicited by inflating the blood pressure cuff) and Chvostek sign (facial spasm elicited by tapping of the cheekbone), as well as hyperactive tendon reflexes.

   Laryngospasm, bronchospasm, and diaphragmatic weakness secondary to hypocalcemia can contribute to respiratory failure requiring intubation. Cardiac arrhythmias can occur, and QT prolongation can place the patient at high risk for torsades de pointes. However, PR interval prolongation is not reported. Hypocalcemia itself causes both a negative chronotropic and inotropic effect on the heart and can lead to acute heart failure and cardiogenic shock.

   Neurological complications can include focal or generalized seizures, as well as less specific symptoms such as fatigue, hyperirritability, anxiety, and depression.

References
1. Tohme JF, Bilezikian JP. Hypocalcemic emergencies. *Endocrinol Metab Clin North Am.* 1993;22:363.
2. Levine SN, Rheams CN. Hypocalcemic heart failure. *Am J Med.* 1985;78:1033.

**3.** Correct Answer: A

**Rationale:**
Lithium, primarily used as a psychiatric medication, can decrease parathyroid gland sensitivity to calcium, increasing serum levels of both calcium and PTH. It may also reduce urinary calcium excretion, further compounding its effect. Approximately 10% to 20% of patients taking lithium will develop hypercalcemia and hypocalciuria. Serum calcium concentration often returns to normal after discontinuation of lithium.

   Other serious side effects of lithium include hypothyroidism, diabetes insipidus, and lithium toxicity.

### References

1. Lehmann SW, Lee J. Lithium-associated hypercalcemia and hyperparathyroidism in the elderly: what do we know? *J Affect Disord.* 2013;146:151.
2. Meehan AD, Udumyan R, Kardell M, et al. Lithium-associated hypercalcemia: pathophysiology, prevalence, management. *World J Surg.* 2018;42:415.

---

**4.** Correct Answer: D

**Rationale:**

This patient has primary hyperparathyroidism but was previously asymptomatic. Studies have shown that most asymptomatic patients do not have progression of the disease, evidenced by worsening hypercalcemia, hypercalciuria, bone disease, and/or nephrolithiasis. However, the Fourth International Workshop on Asymptomatic Primary Hyperparathyroidism guidelines suggest that patients who meet at least one of the following criteria are at an increased risk for developing end-organ effects of primary hyperparathyroidism and thus should have surgical intervention:

- Serum calcium concentration of 1.0 mg/dL or more above the upper limit of normal
- Bone density score less than −2.5
- Previous asymptomatic vertebral fracture
- eGFR <60 mL/min
- 24-hour urinary calcium > 400 mg/d
- Nephrolithiasis or nephrocalcinosis on imaging
- Age less than 50 years

This patient above meets criteria based on serum calcium and nephrocalcinosis. Thus, parathyroidectomy is indicated.

Calcimimetic agents such as cinacalcet are recommended for patients who meet the above criteria but are not surgical candidates. Cinacalcet activates the calcium-sensing receptor in the parathyroid gland and inhibits PTH secretion. Patients who do not meet the above criteria should be treated with bisphosphonates. Bisphosphonates are potent inhibitors of bone resorption and can improve low bone mass in patients with untreated primary hyperparathyroidism. 25-hydroxyvitamin D levels should also be checked and supplemented if low.

### Reference

1. Bilezikian JP, Brandi ML, Eastell R, et al. Guidelines for the management of asymptomatic primary hyperparathyroidism: summary statement from the Fourth International Workshop. J Clin Endocrinol Metab. 2014;99:3561.

---

**5.** Correct Answer: A

**Rationale:**

Hypercalcemic crisis, or severe hypercalcemia, is a life-threatening emergency often in the setting of malignancy, primary hyperparathyroidism, or medication use. Patients may exhibit a variety of symptoms including neurologic, gastrointestinal, and renal manifestations of hypercalcemia, particularly dehydration. Immediate attention and management is crucial. The first step should be aggressive intravenous rehydration with normal saline at 200 to 300 mL/h, then adjusted to maintain urine output at 100 to 150 mL/h.

Once resuscitation is initiated, management should be focused on promoting urinary excretion of calcium and to identify the underlying cause of hypercalcemia. Calcitonin (4 IU/kg), pamidronate (60-90 mg over 2 hours), or zoledronic acid (4 mg over 15 minutes) can further prevent bone resorption and stabilize serum calcium levels. These medications may take some time to exert their effect (calcitonin 12-48 hours, bisphosphonates 24-96 hours) and should be administered quickly. Furosemide increases urinary calcium excretion and should be administered only when the patient is in a euvolemic state. For hypercalcemia unresponsive to other measures, mithramycin should be administered. Hemodialysis should be reserved for severely symptomatic patients or those who do not demonstrate a reduction in calcium levels after the above treatments have been initiated.

### References

1. Zeigler R. Hypercalcemic crisis. *J Am Soc Nephr.* 2001;12(suppl 1):S3-S9.
2. Trabulus S, Oruc M, Ozgun E, et al. The use of low-calcium hemodialysis in the treatment of hypercalcemic crisis. *Nephron.* 2018;139:319-331.

# 57

# PITUTARY

Nathan M. Lee

1. A 42-year-old man is brought to the emergency department by his family after suffering a generalized seizure that lasted for 10 seconds. His past medical history includes depression, schizophrenia, 20 pack-year smoking history, heavy alcohol use, but no documented cirrhosis. His pulse is 94 beats/min, blood pressure 108/62 mm Hg, respiration rate 14 breaths/min, and is afebrile. Physical examination demonstrates normal skin turgor, clear lungs, normal cardiac examination, trace edema, and nonfocal neurologic examination. Head computed tomography (CT) is negative and chest X-ray shows a possible hilar/perihilar mass with mediastinal widening. His labs are sodium 118 mEq/L, potassium 4.2 mEq/L, chloride 87 mEq/L, bicarbonate 23 mEq/L, urea nitrogen 12 mg/dL, creatinine 1.2 mg/dL, and glucose 118 mg/dL. Measured serum osmolality is 265 mOsm/kg. Urine sodium is 36 mEq/L and urine osmolality is 355 mOsm/kg. Alcohol level is 0 and toxicology screen is negative. What is the most likely etiology of this patient's symptoms?

   A. Syndrome of inappropriate antidiuretic hormone (ADH)
   B. Psychogenic polydipsia
   C. Cerebral salt wasting
   D. Early cirrhosis

2. A 22-year-old previously healthy female is brought to the emergency department from a rave party with a chief complaint of "dizziness." Per her friends, the patient had taken a tablet of "ecstasy." There was no report of other drug use or excessive water intake. Her blood pressure is 108/62 mm Hg, pulse 115 beats/min, respiration rate 18 breaths/min, pulse oximetry 98% on room air, and afebrile. Physical examination demonstrates normal skin turgor, normal cardiac examination, clear lungs, no edema, and nonfocal neurologic examination. Head CT and chest X-ray are negative. Her labs are sodium 128 mEq/L, potassium 3.7 mEq/L, chloride 87 mEq/L, bicarbonate 19 mEq/L, urea nitrogen 6 mg/dL, creatinine 0.7 mg/dL, and glucose 118 mg/dL. Measured serum osmolality is 250 mOsm/kg. Urine sodium is 105 mEq/L and urine osmolality is 352 mOsm/L. Alcohol level is 0 and toxicology screen is negative. What is the next best step in management?

   A. Neurosurgical consult
   B. Administration of hypertonic saline
   C. Demeclocycline
   D. Fluid restriction

3. A 49-year-old man who presented with chief complaint of "severe headache" was diagnosed with a subarachnoid hemorrhage (SAH) without hydrocephalus and significant neurological defects. After successful intravascular coiling of a right posterior communicating artery aneurysm, he is admitted to the intensive care unit (ICU). On postoperative day 1, patient complains of feeling weak, then becomes progressively more confused. Labs drawn prior to his seizure demonstrate the following: sodium 122 mEq/L, potassium 3.4 mEq/L, chloride 91 mEq/L, bicarbonate 26 mEq/L, urea 12 mg/dL, and creatinine 0.6 mEq/L. Fingerstick glucose is 89 mg/dL. Additional studies are ordered which demonstrate urine sodium of 40 mmol/L, urine osmolality of 452 mOsm/kg, and serum osmolality of 265 mOsm/kg. The patient then suffers a grand mal seizure which is terminated with intravenous levetiracetam. Which is the most appropriate next step in management?

    **A.** Immediate reimaging and neurosurgical consult
    **B.** Administration of hypertonic saline
    **C.** Demeclocycline
    **D.** Fluid restriction

4. Which of the following is **NOT** associated with nephrogenic diabetes insipidus (DI)?

    **A.** Amphotericin B
    **B.** Lithium
    **C.** Hyperkalemia
    **D.** Hypercalcemia

5. A 26-year-old, previously healthy, G1P0 female at 36 weeks gestational age comes to the emergency department due to polyuria, nocturia, and polydipsia. Her pulse is 78 beats/min, blood pressure 102/63 mm Hg, and weight 53 kg (BMI 22.6 kg/m$^2$). Physical examination is normal except for decreased skin turgor and dry mucous membranes. Laboratory data reveal low urine osmolality 89 mOsmol/kg (normal 350-1000), serum osmolality 308 mOsmol/kg (normal 278-295), serum sodium 144 mEq/L, potassium 4.1 mEq/L, chloride 109 mEq/L, blood urea nitrogen 10 mg/dL, creatinine 0.7 mg/dL, glucose 110 mg/dL, and HbA1c 5.3%. Serum ADH is 0.5 pg/mL (normal 1-5 pg/mL). MRI of her brain demonstrates no acute findings. Which of the following statements best explains her symptoms?

    **A.** Kidney disease affecting renal sensitivity to ADH
    **B.** Ischemic insult decreasing release of ADH
    **C.** Placental trophoblasts producing excessive vasopressinase
    **D.** Autoimmune destruction of the pituitary

6. A 70-year-old male with past medical history of hypertension and headaches presents to the emergency department with a severe headache, double vision, nausea, and vomiting. Initial evaluation demonstrated hyponatremia, hyperkalemia, and intravascular volume depletion. Given concern for an intracranial process, an MRI was performed which demonstrated a hemorrhagic pituitary macroadenoma. You would like to initiate corticosteroid therapy. Which of the following choices has the correct order of steroids from least to most potent?

    **A.** Hydrocortisone < cortisone < prednisone < dexamethasone
    **B.** Cortisone < hydrocortisone < dexamethasone < prednisone
    **C.** Cortisone < hydrocortisone < prednisone < dexamethasone
    **D.** Cortisone < dexamethasone < hydrocortisone < prednisone

7. A 28-year-old with history of severe postpartum hemorrhage 1 month ago is sent to the ED from primary care clinic for hypotension and worsening weakness and fatigue over the last few days. On review of systems, she notes that she has been having trouble with her memory, cold intolerance, low appetite, and has been unable to breastfeed since her previous discharge from the hospital. Vitals are pulse 110, blood pressure 81/49, respiratory rate 16, and oxygen saturation of 98% on room air. Basic metabolic panel shows sodium of 128 mEq/L, potassium of 5.8 mEq/L, chloride of 98 mEq/L, bicarbonate 26 mEq/L, urea 36 mg/dL, and creatinine 1.6 mg/dL. Complete blood count demonstrates hemoglobin 10.2 g/dL, hematocrit 33%, WBC 4.0 × 10$^3$/μL, and platelets 120 × 10$^3$/μL. Thyroid-stimulating hormone (TSH) is 0.1 mIU/L (normal 0.5-4 mIU/L). Injection of 500 μg of thyrotropin-releasing hormone elicits no increase in serum TSH or prolactin. Which of the following hormones is most likely to have normal levels?

    **A.** Aldosterone
    **B.** Cortisol
    **C.** Follicle-stimulating hormone
    **D.** Gonadotropin-releasing hormone

8. A 72-year-old female with history of hypertension, chronic kidney disease stage IV, and worsening headaches over the last few weeks is brought to the ICU for airway watch after falling in her bathroom and suffering multiple rib fractures and mild respiratory distress. CT head without contrast demonstrates no signs of acute cranial bleed but notes "an enlarged pituitary with concern for sellar mass." What is the best imaging procedure to further investigate?

    **A.** Computed tomography
    **B.** Magnetic resonance imaging
    **C.** Magnetic resonance imaging with gadolinium
    **D.** Positron emission tomography

# Chapter 57 ▪ Answers

**1.** Correct Answer: A

**Rationale:**

Hyponatremia, defined as serum sodium <135 mEq/L, is the most common electrolyte abnormality in hospitalized patients and presents in 12% to 17% patients admitted to the ICU. Most patients fall in the mild range of 130 to 135 mEq/L, some are moderate 125 to 129 mEq/L, and few are severe <125 mEq/L, as in this patient. Symptoms of hyponatremia include lethargy, dysarthria, disorientation, and seizures. This patient is presenting with severe symptomatic hypotonic hyponatremia, likely due to subsequently diagnosed small-cell lung cancer as suggested by findings on the chest imaging.

This patient has hypotonic hyponatremia. The next step is to assess the patient's volume status. This patient has euvolemic hypotonic hyponatremia as suggested by normal skin turgor and lack of significant edema. If the patient was hypovolemic (with decreased skin turgor), this patient's process would be more consistent with cerebral salt wasting. On the other hand, cirrhosis causes hypervolemic hypotonic hyponatremia.

In a patient with euvolemic hypotonic hyponatremia, the next step is to assess the urine osmolality. If urinary osmolality is low (<100 mOsm/kg), it suggests primary psychogenic polydipsia such as in schizophrenia or other psychoses. Other causes include low solute intake from beer potomania syndrome. The high urine osmolality seen in this patient indicates an abnormal concentrating effect, also indicated by urinary sodium >20 mEq/L. Syndrome of inappropriate antidiuretic hormone (SIADH) is the most likely cause of hyponatremia in this patient with hypotonic hyponatremia, euvolemia, natriuresis, and inappropriately concentrated urine. SIADH is a diagnosis of exclusion made in the correct clinical context. SIADH can be caused by small-cell lung cancer, pneumonia, lung abscess, cystic fibrosis, SAH, stroke, brain tumors, meningitis, or brain abscess, and common medications, such as nonsteroidal agents, tricyclic antidepressants, selective serotonin reuptake inhibitors, chemotherapy agents, opiates, and haloperidol.

References

1. Decaux G, Musch W. Clinical laboratory evaluation of the syndrome of inappropriate secretion of antidiuretic hormone. *Clin J Am Soc Nephr*. 2008;3(4):1175-1184.
2. Ellison DH, Berl T. Clinical practice. The syndrome of inappropriate antidiuresis. *N Engl J Med*. 2007;356:2064.
3. Feldman BJ, Rosenthal SM, Vargas GA, et al. Nephrogenic syndrome of inappropriate antidiuresis. *N Engl J Med*. 2005;352:1884.

**2.** Correct Answer: D

**Rationale:**

This patient presents with mildly symptomatic hyponatremia in the setting of ingestion of the drug 3,4-methylenedioxymethamphetamine (MDMA, the active ingredient in ecstasy). Her physical examination demonstrated no signs of hypovolemia, which would suggest either fluid/electrolyte loss with hypotonic repletion, or hypervolemia, which would suggest a complex neuroendocrine response from cirrhosis or congestive heart failure. Instead, her euvolemic status makes SIADH the most likely etiology of this patient's condition. MDMA is a serotonin agonist, and there is sufficient data that not only is ADH release mediated by serotonin, but ADH levels increases with MDMA administration. This is also consistent with the association of selective serotonin reuptake inhibitors with SIADH.

Treatment of any patient should begin with assessment of airway, breathing, and circulation. This patient has no serious symptoms, with dizziness her main complaint. Given her mild symptoms, this patient should be treated with fluid restriction of less than 800 mL/d, which is the mainstay of treatment for most patients with SIADH. If fluid restriction does not improve serum sodium >130 mEq/L, oral salt tablets can be given. Loop diuretics are used when the urine osmolality is more than twice that of the plasma. Other therapies, such as tolvaptan, demeclocycline, or lithium, are not recommended for the patient with mild symptoms. Hypertonic saline is reserved for more serious symptoms such as confusion, lethargy, and seizures.

References

1. Cooke CR, Turin MD, Walker WG. The syndrome of inappropriate antidiuretic hormone secretion (SIADH): pathophysiologic mechanisms in solute and volume regulation. *Medicine (Baltimore)*. 1979;58:240.
2. Ellison DH, Berl T. Clinical practice. The syndrome of inappropriate antidiuresis. *N Engl J Med*. 2007;356:2064.
3. Verbalis JG, Greenberg A, Burst V, et al. Diagnosing and treating the syndrome of inappropriate antidiuretic hormone secretion. *Am J Med*. 2016;129:537.e9.

**3.** Correct Answer: B

**Rationale:**

The patient is severely hyponatremic and symptomatic, with evidence that he has SIADH. With his underlying intracranial disease, the serum sodium must be raised quickly to prevent further cerebral edema and prevent irreversible neurologic injury. To raise the serum sodium concentration, electrolyte concentration of the fluid given must be greater than the electrolyte concentration of the urine. Thus, the administration of hypertonic saline is the only rapid way to raise the serum sodium and improve neurologic symptoms in patients with symptomatic severe hyponatremia. Fluid restriction should not be done in patients with SAH, as it may promote cerebral vasospasm.

Although there is no set protocol of hypertonic saline therapy, various studies recommend 100 mL of 3% saline given as an intravenous bolus, which should raise serum sodium approximately 1.5 mEq/L in men and 2 mEq/L in women. If neurologic symptoms persist, a 100 mL bolus of 3% saline can be repeated up to two more times at 10-minute intervals.

Of note, the serum sodium should not be raised greater than 8 to 12 mEq/L in a 24-hour period. Overly rapid correction of sodium increases risk of central pontine myelinolysis.

### References
1. Woo CH, Rao VA, Sheridan W, et al. Performance characteristics of a sliding-scale hypertonic saline infusion protocol for the treatment of acute neurologic hyponatremia. *Neurocrit Care.* 2009;11:228.
2. Sterns RH, Nigwekar SU, Hix JK. The treatment of hyponatremia. *Semin Nephrol.* 2009;29:282.

### 4. Correct Answer: C

**Rationale:**

Nephrogenic DI is caused by an improper response of the kidney to ADH, leading to a decrease in the ability of the kidney to concentrate the urine by removing free water. This differs from central DI, which is caused by insufficient levels of ADH, usually due to decreased secretion from the posterior pituitary.

Common causes of nephrogenic DI include hereditary mutations, chronic lithium ingestion, hypercalcemia, and hypokalemia. Hereditary mutations include the x-linked vasopressin V2 receptor gene mutation and the aquaporin-2 gene mutation that has both autosomal dominant and recessive modes of inheritance. Lithium exerts its effect by disrupting the aquaporin-2 water channel. Hypercalcemia and hypokalemia decrease collecting tubule responsiveness to ADH, as well as decrease sodium chloride reabsorption in the thick ascending limb.

Other causes of nephrogenic DI include a variety of renal disease (sickle cell disease or trait, polycystic kidney disease, renal amyloidosis, and Sjogren syndrome), drugs (cidofovir, foscarnet, amphotericin B, ofloxacin, orlistat, and didanosine), pregnancy, and craniopharyngioma surgery.

### References
1. Garofeanu CG, Weir M, Rosas-Arellano MP, et al. Causes of reversible nephrogenic diabetes insipidus: a systematic review. *Am J Kidney Dis.* 2005;45:626.
2. Bockenhauer D, Bichet DG. Pathophysiology, diagnosis and management of nephrogenic diabetes insipidus. *Nat Rev Nephrol.* 2015;11:576.

### 5. Correct Answer: C

**Rationale:**

Gestational DI is a rare complication of pregnancy, occurring in about 1 in 30,000 pregnancies. It usually develops at the end of the second or third trimester of pregnancy and will resolve spontaneously 4 to 6 weeks after delivery. The pathophysiology of gestational DI is different from both central and nephrogenic DI; rather than a deficiency in ADH secretion or decreased ADH receptor sensitivity, gestational DI involves excessive vasopressinase activity. Vasopressinase is an enzyme expressed by placental trophoblasts during pregnancy, and it metabolizes ADH. The level of activity is proportional to the placental weight, explaining its higher activity in the third trimester or in multiple pregnancies. Vasopressinase is metabolized by the liver, and thus pregnant women with liver dysfunction, such as hemolysis, elevated liver enzymes, low platelet count (HELLP) syndrome, acute fatty liver of pregnancy, hepatitis, and cirrhosis, have higher concentrations.

Patients with gestational DI should be treated with desmopressin, which is not metabolized by vasopressinase. Fluid restriction is not recommended in gestational DI as it can lead to significant dehydration and complications such as oligohydramnios and intrauterine growth restriction.

### References
1. Marques P, Gunawardana K, Grossman A. Transient diabetes insipidus in pregnancy. *Endocrinol Diabetes Metab Case Rep.* 2015;2015:150078.
2. Rodrigo N, Hocking S. Transient diabetes insipidus in a post-partum woman with pre-eclampsia associated with residual placental vasopressinase activity. *Endocrinol Diabetes Metab Case Rep.* 2018;2018:18-52.

### 6. Correct Answer: C

**Rationale:**

This patient has pituitary apoplexy secondary to his hemorrhagic pituitary adenoma. As pressure inside the sella turcica rises, surrounding structures such as the optic nerve and contents of the cavernous sinus are compressed. This further decreases the blood supply to the pituitary, leading to tissue death and hypopituitarism.

Treatment involves stabilization of the circulatory system, as acute adrenal insufficiency can cause hypotension. Administration of a glucocorticoid replacement is required; for patients without a prior diagnosis of adrenal insufficiency, dexamethasone 4 mg IV bolus is preferred as it is not measured in serum cortisol assays. For patients with a known diagnosis of adrenal insufficiency who present with adrenal crisis, hydrocortisone 100 mg IV bolus or dexamethasone is recommended.

In order of potency: cortisone < hydrocortisone < prednisone < dexamethasone.

The decision to surgically decompress the pituitary gland is mainly dependent on the severity of visual loss and defects. Surgery is most likely to improve vision if there was some remaining vision prior to surgery and if the surgery is performed within a week of onset of symptoms.

### References

1. Nawar RN, AbdelMannan D, Selman WR, et al. Pituitary tumor apoplexy: a review. *J Intens Care Med.* 2008;23(2):75-90.
2. Murad-Kejbou S, Eggenberger E. Pituitary apoplexy: evaluation, management, and prognosis. *Curr Opin Ophthalmol.* 2009;2(6):456-461.
3. Van Aken MO, Lamberts SW. Diagnosis and treatment of hypopituitarism: an update. *Pituitary.* 2005;8(3-4):183-191.

---

**7.** Correct Answer: A

**Rationale:**

This patient has symptoms of new adrenal insufficiency and hypothyroidism that is unresponsive to an injection of thyrotropin-releasing hormone. This is indicative of destruction of pituitary tissue responsible for adrenocorticotropic hormone and TSH production. Her history of severe postpartum hemorrhage, along with agalactorrhea, strongly suggests Sheehan syndrome as the etiology of her symptoms.

Sheehan syndrome is hypopituitarism caused by ischemic damage from excessive hemorrhage. The pituitary is enlarged and more metabolically active during pregnancy and, thus, more prone to hypoxemia and infarction from hypovolemic shock. The blood vessels are also more susceptible to vasospasm due to elevated estrogen levels.

Damage to the pituitary can be variable; some or all hormones produced by the pituitary may be affected, as well as those downstream. These include ACTH, TSH, luteinizing hormone, follicle-stimulating hormone, prolactin, growth hormone, and melanocyte-stimulating hormone. Of note, ACTH stimulates adrenal glands to produce cortisol and other hormones, but aldosterone production is regulated by angiotensin II and serum potassium levels. Thus, aldosterone levels should be unaffected in Sheehan syndrome.

### References

1. Kovacs K. Sheehan syndrome. *Lancet.* 2003;361(9356):520-522.
2. Shivaprasad C. Sheehan's syndrome: newer advances. *Indian J Endocrinol Metab.* 2011;15(3):S203-S207.

---

**8.** Correct Answer: B

**Rationale:**

Magnetic resonance imaging (MRI) is the diagnostic modality of choice for most sellar masses. Compared to CT, MRI provides greater soft-tissue contrast, which allows clear visualization of pituitary morphology and neighboring structures, including the optic chiasm, optic nerves, cavernous sinuses, and carotid arteries. The one exception is that calcifications in a craniopharyngioma or meningioma are seen better by CT scan. Regardless, the initial study of a suspected sellar mass should be a MRI scan.

Gadolinium is used as an intravenous contrast agent to enhance and improve the quality of MRI imaging. Normal pituitary tissue takes up gadolinium more than surrounding tissue and will exhibit a higher intensity signal. Micro- and macroadenomas, craniopharyngiomas, and meningiomas take up gadolinium to a less degree than normal pituitary tissue but more than surrounding tissue; this characteristic can help identify a sellar mass. Gadolinium should not be used in patients with moderate to advanced renal failure (eGFR <30 mL/min), as it has been associated with nephrogenic systemic fibrosis. Patients should be well informed of the risks associated with gadolinium administration if its use is warranted.

### References

1. Gsponer J, De Tribolet N, Déruaz JP, et al. Diagnosis, treatment, and outcome of pituitary tumors and other abnormal intrasellar masses. Retrospective analysis of 353 patients. *Medicine (Baltimore).* 1999;78:236.
2. Connor SE, Penney CC. MRI in the differential diagnosis of a sellar mass. *Clin Radiol.* 2003;58(1):20-31.
3. FitzPatrick MF, Tartaglino LM, Hollander MD, et al. Imaging of sellar and parasellar pathology. *Radiol Clin North Am.* 1999;37(1):101-121.

# 58

# ENDOCRINE TUMORS

Nathan M. Lee

1. Pheochromocytomas are associated with all of the following familial disorders **EXCEPT?**

    A. von Hippel-Lindau (VHL) syndrome
    B. Multiple endocrine neoplasia type 2 (MEN2)
    C. Hereditary nonpolyposis colorectal cancer (HPNCC)
    D. Neurofibromatosis type 1 (NF1)

2. A 48-year-old female with family history of pheochromocytoma is undergoing laparoscopic nephrectomy for newly diagnosed renal cell carcinoma. The surgeons note an adrenal mass not previously seen on imaging, and manipulation of the kidney causes severe hypertension up to 225/135 mm Hg. The case is aborted, with the patient transferred to the intensive care unit for blood pressure management. In this scenario, which of the following biochemical testing is most recommended?

    A. 24-hour urine catecholamines
    B. Plasma catecholamines
    C. 24-hour urine-fractionated metanephrines
    D. Plasma-fractionated metanephrines

3. Which of the following is the appropriate management strategy of pheochromocytoma-associated hypertension?

    A. α-adrenergic blockade only
    B. β-adrenergic blockade only
    C. α-adrenergic blockade first, then β-adrenergic blockade
    D. β-adrenergic blockade first, then α-adrenergic blockade

4. Which of the following statements regarding neuroendocrine tumors is **FALSE?**

    A. Tumor production of histamine and bradykinin causes vasodilation and flushing.
    B. Carcinoid syndrome only occurs in the presence of liver metastases.
    C. Carcinoid tumors may arise in lung, liver, and anywhere in the gastrointestinal tract.
    D. Serotonin can stimulate fibroblast and fibrogenesis causing valvular lesions.

5. Which of the following diagnostic tests is most appropriate for suspected carcinoid tumor?

    A. 24-hour urinary excretion of 5-hydroxyindoleacetic acid (5-HIAA)
    B. 24-hour urinary excretion of serotonin
    C. Plasma chromogranin A
    D. Plasma serotonin

# Chapter 58 ▪ Answers

**1.** Correct Answer: C

**Rationale:**
Pheochromocytomas are rare catecholamine-secreting neuroendocrine tumors that originate from chromaffin cells of the adrenal medulla. While the majority are sporadic neoplasms, up to 40% have the disease as part of a familial disorder. These familial disorders all exhibit autosomal dominant inheritance and include MEN2 (mutations in *RET* proto-oncogene), VHL syndrome (mutations in the *VHL* tumor suppressor gene), and NF1 (mutation sin the *NF1* gene). HNPCC is a genetic condition that demonstrates autosomal dominant inheritance; however, it is not associated with pheochromocytomas.

Approximately 50% of patients with MEN2, 20% of patients with VHL, and 1% of patients with NF1 will have a pheochromocytoma. When compared with each other, MEN2 patients are often more symptomatic with higher incidences of hypertension and higher plasma metanephrine (epinephrine metabolite) concentrations. VHL patients have higher plasma normetanephrine (norepinephrine) concentrations than MEN2 patients. When pheochromocytomas are diagnosed in the setting of no known familial disorder, clinicians should monitor closely for findings such as retinal angiomas in VHL syndrome, a thyroid mass in MEN2, café au lait spots, and neurofibromas in NF1. Any of these findings or a family history of pheochromocytoma should warrant genetic testing for early diagnosis and management.

### References
1. Erlic Z, Neumann HP. Familial pheochromocytoma. *Hormones (Athens)*. 2009;8(1):29-38.
2. Pawlu C, Bausch B, Reisch N, Neumann HP. Genetic testing for pheochromocytoma-associated syndromes. *Ann Endocrinol (Paris)*. 2005;66:178.
3. Eisenhofer G, Walther MM, Huynh TT, et al. Pheochromocytomas in von Hippel-Lindau syndrome and multiple endocrine neoplasia type 2 display distinct biochemical and clinical phenotypes. *J Clin Endocrinol Metab*. 2001;86:1999.

**2.** Correct Answer: D

**Rationale:**
Measuring plasma-fractionated metanephrines is the recommended first-line test when there is a high index of suspicion for pheochromocytoma. It has the highest sensitivity (96%-100%) and moderate specificity (85%-91%) among all biochemical testing for pheochromocytoma, with the highest area under the receiver operating characteristic curve. The nearly maximal negative predictive value of plasma free metanephrines suggests that pheochromocytoma can be ruled out when the test result is within the normal range. However, the false-positive rate is high when the blood is not drawn per recommendation (i.e., supine with an indwelling cannula over 30 minutes). Since plasma-fractionated metanephrines is associated with a high–false-positive rate, it should only be used when there is a high index of suspicion. The following scenarios warrant a high index of suspicion: family history of pheochromocytoma, genetic syndrome that is associated with pheochromocytoma (MEN2, VHL, NF1), prior resection of pheochromocytoma, or adrenal mass consistent with pheochromocytoma. The patient above had a family history of pheochromocytoma and an incidentally found adrenal mass, which qualify for a high index of suspicion and thus further confirmation with plasma-fractionated metanephrines.

24-hour urine-fractionated metanephrines is the recommended test for patients with low index of suspicion. It has a sensitivity of 92% to 98% and a specificity of 94% to 98% and thus less sensitive than plasma metanephrines but more specific. Measurement of plasma or urinary catecholamines is less sensitive than the aforementioned tests, likely due to the sporadic secretion of parent catecholamines compared to the continuous diffusion of intratumorally produced metanephrines into the circulation.

### References
1. Lenders JW, Pacak K, Walther MM, et al. Biochemical diagnosis of pheochromocytoma: which test is best? *JAMA*. 2002;287(11):1427.
2. Lenders JW, Eisenhofer G. Update on modern management of pheochromocytoma and paraganglioma. *Endocrinol Metab (Seoul)*. 2017;32(2):152-161.

**3.** Correct Answer: C

**Rationale:**
Blood pressure management is critical in the preoperative management of pheochromocytoma prior to definitive treatment via surgical resection. α-adrenergic receptor blockade (particularly α1-mediated vasoconstriction) should be established prior to β-adrenoreceptor blockade, as unopposed α-adrenergic receptor stimulation can cause a hypertensive crisis and place a patient at high risk for heart attack, stroke, and death.

Phenoxybenzamine is a long-acting, nonselective, noncompetitive α-antagonist (α1 > α2) often used to control blood pressure prior to surgery. Phentolamine is an intravenous, rapid-acting, nonselective α-antagonist (α1 = α2) often used to control blood pressure perioperatively. While selective α1-blockers such as prazosin, terazosin, and doxazosin may offer a more favorable adverse effect profile, they are not used to prepare patients for surgery due to their incomplete α-blockade.

Once α-blockade is established, β-blockade should be initiated to treat or prevent tachycardia. Both noncardioselective β-blockers, such as propranolol, and cardioselective β-blockers, such as metoprolol, have been used for heart rate control prior to surgery. Esmolol is an intravenous, rapid, short-acting, β1-selective blocker often to control heart rate perioperatively.

Metyrosine is an oral medication which inhibits tyrosine hydroxylase, the rate-limiting step in catecholamine synthesis. It is often used for patients with malignant pheochromocytoma or in whom surgery is contraindicated. Of note, it can also be prescribed for patients with a pheochromocytoma who do not respond to phenoxybenzamine or phentolamine therapy, or as an adjunct to therapy.

### References

1. Waguespack SG, Rich T, Grubbs E, et al. A current review of the etiology, diagnosis, and treatment of pediatric pheochromocytoma and paraganglioma. *J Clin Endocrinol Metab*. 2010;95(5):2023-2037.
2. Därr R, Lenders JWM, Hofbauer LC, et al. Pheochromocytoma: update on disease management. *Ther Adv Endo Metab*. 2012;3(1):11-26.

## 4. Correct Answer: B

**Rationale:**

Carcinoid syndrome is a paraneoplastic syndrome that occurs in approximately 5% of carcinoid tumors. It is caused by endogenous secretion of serotonin, histamine, prostaglandins, and kallikrein, an enzyme that catalyzes conversion of kininogen to bradykinin. These bioactive molecules cause a wide variety of symptoms, but the most notable are diarrhea (from serotonin), flushing (from histamine and bradykinin), wheezing (from histamine and bradykinin), and cardiac lesions (from serotonin-stimulated fibrogenesis). The liver inactivates many of these bioactive molecules, and thus, it is commonly thought that carcinoid syndrome only occurs with liver dysfunction or metastasis. This is not true, as several case reports describe carcinoid syndrome in the absence of liver metastases. Carcinoid tumors were found in the lungs, ovaries, and testis, and it is thought that carcinoid syndrome may arise in these situations because of the tumors draining directly into the systemic circulation, bypassing portal circulation and subsequent inactivation. Thus, one should consider the possibility of carcinoid syndrome in the absence of liver metastases.

### References

1. Datta S, Williams N, Suortamo S, et al. Carcinoid syndrome from small bowel endocrine carcinoma in the absence of hepatic metastasis. *Age Ageing*. 2011;40:760.
2. Haq AU, Yook CR, Hiremath V, et al. Carcinoid syndrome in the absence of liver metastasis: a case report and review of literature. *Med Pediatr Oncol*. 1992;20:221.
3. Feldman JM. Carcinoid tumors and syndrome. *Semin Oncol*. 1987;14:237.

## 5. Correct Answer: A

**Rationale:**

24-hour urinary excretion of 5-HIAA is the recommended test for suspected carcinoid tumor. 5-HIAA is the main metabolite of serotonin, and normal urinary excretion ranges from 2 to 8 mg/d, greater than 25 mg/d is diagnostic of a carcinoid tumor.

The test has high sensitivity (>90%) and high specificity (>90%) and is most useful in patients with primary midgut (jejunoileal, appendiceal, ascending colon) tumors which produce the highest levels of serotonin. Foregut (gastroduodenal, bronchus) and hindgut (transverse, descending, sigmoid, rectum, genitourinary) tumors rarely secrete serotonin and thus, 5-HIAA levels may not be elevated in the urine. False-positive results can occur with intake of acetaminophen, guaifenesin, ephedrine, methamphetamine, nicotine, caffeine, and tryptophan-/serotonin-rich foods such as spinach, eggplant, wine, and cheese. False negatives can occur with intake of ethanol, levodopa, methyldopa, monoamine oxidase inhibitors, aspirin, heparin, isoniazid, and fluoxetine.

24-hour urinary excretion of serotonin, plasma serotonin, and chromogranin assays is of interest but have not been validated in large clinical series. The sensitivities and specificities of these tests are not well established and inferior to the 24-hour urinary excretion of 5-HIAA and thus offer little diagnostic value and are not recommended.

### References

1. O'Toole D, Grossman A, Gross D, et al. ENETS consensus guidelines for the standards of care in neuroendocrine tumors: biochemical markers. *Neuroendocrinology*. 2009;90(2):194-202.
2. Feldman JM. Urinary serotonin in the diagnosis of carcinoid tumors. *Clin Chem*. 1986;32:840.

# 59

# RENIN-ANGIOTENSIN-ALDOSTERONE SYSTEM

Nathan M. Lee

1. An 18-year-old male with a history of headaches presents to the emergency department with complaints of severe headache. His vitals are HR of 112 beats/min, BP 215/125 mm Hg, respiratory rate 14 breaths/min, and temperature 36.9°C. CT scan of the brain showed diffuse cerebral edema but no acute intracranial bleed. ECG demonstrates sinus tachycardia but is otherwise normal. Despite multiple administrations of antihypertensives, his blood pressure is still 194/110, and he is admitted for hypertensive crisis. Workup demonstrates mild hypokalemia. Hormonal studies were significant for elevated plasma renin and aldosterone levels, but normal renin/aldosterone ratio. Plasma metanephrines, thyroid-stimulating hormone, T3, T4, and free T4 are normal. Imaging shows a juxtaglomerular mass on the right kidney and no evidence of renal artery stenosis. Which of the following regarding his diagnosis is **correct**?

   A. Patients often present with concurrent metabolic acidosis.
   B. Renal ultrasound is the diagnostic modality of choice.
   C. The patient should undergo alpha-blockade prior to beta-blockade.
   D. Blood pressure is often difficult to control before resection.

2. A 68-year-old male with a history of coronary artery disease/myocardial infarction treated with a drug-eluting stent and controlled hypertension develops microscopic hematuria and is scheduled for cystoscopy. His medication list includes metoprolol XL 100 mg daily, losartan 50 mg daily, atorvastatin 80 mg daily, and aspirin 81 mg. His preoperative examination is unremarkable, and patient reports exercise capacity >4 METs. Per his instructions from his surgeon, he has continued taking all his medications except for holding his lisinopril and metformin the night before. After an uneventful induction and intubation, the patient's blood pressure drops from 132/68 to 70/42 mm Hg, with pulse continuing at 66 beats/min. The patient's five-lead electrocardiogram demonstrates sinus rhythm but with new 1 mm ST depressions in his precordial leads. End-tidal $CO_2$ and pulse oximetry are unchanged. The blood pressure does not improve with repeated boluses of phenylephrine and ephedrine, or with a fluid bolus of 500 mL, necessitating vasopressin and epinephrine boluses. Bedside transthoracic echocardiogram demonstrates a hyperdynamic and collapsed LV, no wall motion abnormalities, no valvular lesions, and no pericardial effusion. Decision is made to postpone the patient's elective surgery and awaken him. Upon emergence, the patient's blood pressure recovers to 124/62 mm Hg and pulse 60 beats/min. The patient is extubated successfully with no neurological sequelae. Which of the following is the most likely etiology of the patient's hypotension?

   A. Hypovolemia
   B. Medication effect
   C. Acute myocardial infarction
   D. Pulmonary embolism

3. An 18-year-old male with multiple stab wounds to his abdomen is brought by ambulance to the trauma bay. He is bleeding profusely, with HR 128 beats/min, BP 72/41 mm Hg, $SpO_2$ 92% on 15 L oxygen via nonrebreathing face mask. Of the following statements regarding this patient's renin-angiotensin-aldosterone system (RAAS), which is **FALSE**?

**A.** Decreased oxygenation in the macula densa activates the RAAS.

**B.** Increased conversion of angiotensin I to II via renin results in angiotensin (AT1)-receptor–mediated vasoconstriction of arteriolar smooth muscle.

**C.** Angiotensin II has a greater effect on efferent glomerular arterioles than afferent, preserving glomerular pressure.

**D.** Aldosterone release promotes sodium and water retention in the kidneys leading to greater volume retention.

4. Which of the following lab results is most consistent with isolated hypoaldosteronism?

|   | SERUM PH | SERUM NA⁺ | SERUM K⁺ | SERUM CL⁻ | SERUM $HCO_3^-$ |
|---|---|---|---|---|---|
| A | 7.30 | 140 | 6.0 | 105 | 22 |
| B | 7.30 | 130 | 5.5 | 115 | 20 |
| C | 7.35 | 140 | 5.5 | 115 | 22 |
| D | 7.35 | 130 | 6.0 | 101 | 20 |

# Chapter 59 ▪ Answers

**1.** Correct Answer: D

**Rationale:**

The patient presents with hypertensive crisis, hypokalemia, high plasma aldosterone, and high plasma renin, but normal renin/aldosterone ratio which suggests secondary hyperaldosteronism from excess renin. Normal plasma metanephrines rules out pheochromocytoma or paraganglioma. The presence of a juxtaglomerular mass further suggests that this patient's symptoms are likely due to a juxtaglomerular cell tumor secreting renin, or reninoma.

Renin is normally secreted from the juxtaglomerular kidney cells in response to: (1) a decrease in renal perfusion pressure detected via stretch receptors in the vascular walls of the juxtaglomerular cells and (2) signaling from the macula densa when sodium delivery to the distal tubule decreases. It hydrolyzes angiotensinogen into angiotensin I, which is further cleaved in the lungs by endothelial-bound angiotensin-converting enzyme (ACE) into angiotensin II, a potent vasoconstrictor peptide. Angiotensin II also acts on the adrenal glands to release aldosterone, which stimulates the epithelial cells in the distal tubule and collecting ducts of the kidney to increase reabsorption of sodium and water and excretion of potassium and hydrogen ions. This results in an increase in intravascular volume, hypertension, hypokalemia, and metabolic alkalosis.

While abdominal ultrasonography is noninvasive and easily performed, it may miss small lesions. Contrast-enhanced computed tomography or magnetic resonance imaging is recommended as the diagnostic modality of choice. Medical management consists of antihypertensives, particularly ACE inhibitors, angiotensin receptor blockers (ARBs), and aldosterone antagonists. Definitive treatment is by surgical resection with most patients becoming and remaining normotensive.

References

1. Martin SA, Mynderse LA, Lager DJ, et al. Juxtaglomerular cell tumour: a clinicopathologic study of four cases and review of the literature. *Am J Clin Pathol*. 2001;116:854-863.
2. Venkateswaran R, Hamide A, Dorairajan LN, et al. Reninoma: a rare cause of curable hypertension. *BMJ Case Rep*. 2013;2013:bcr2012008367.

**2.** Correct Answer: B

**Rationale:**

Losartan is a highly selective angiotensin (AT1) receptor blocker (ARB), and like other ARBs and ACE inhibitors, is used for treatment of hypertension, heart failure, and prevention of cardiac remodeling after myocardial infarction. By displacing angiotensin II from the AT1 receptor, ARBs antagonize AT1-receptor–induced vasoconstriction, aldosterone, catecholamine and arginine-vasopressin release, water intake, and hypertrophic responses. During general anesthesia, maintenance of blood pressure is dependent on the RAAS and AT1 activation. By blocking AT1, losartan may precipitate severe hypotension under general anesthesia. Chronic AT1-blockade can also reduce the vasoconstrictor response to alpha1 receptors activated by norepinephrine, causing resistance to direct and indirect pharmacologic intervention, as seen in this patient. Clinical studies have shown that vasopressin can restore the sympathetic response and is useful in cases of refractory hypotension in patients with chronic RAAS inhibition undergoing general anesthesia. Norepinephrine, with much more potent alpha1 activation than phenylephrine, is also recommended as it may have a more favorable effect on splanchnic perfusion and oxygen.

While the patient's NPO status may result in hypovolemia, the lack of response to a fluid bolus makes hypovolemia alone a less likely cause of this patient's hypotension during general anesthesia. The patient reported great exercise capacity, no symptoms of heart failure, no signs of acute infarction on ECG, and return to normal blood pressure after discontinuation of general anesthesia, making an acute myocardial infarction or pulmonary embolism unlikely.

### References

1. Brabant SM, Eyraud D, Bertrand M, et al. Refractory hypotension after induction of anesthesia in a patient chronically treated with angiotensin receptor antagonists. *Anesth Analg.* 1999;89(4):887-888.
2. Ryckwaert F, Colson P, Andre E, et al. Haemodynamic effects of an angiotensin-converting enzyme inhibitor and angiotensin receptor antagonist during hypovolaemia in the anaesthetized pig. *Br J Anaesth.* 2002;89(4):599-604.
3. Colson P, Ryckwaert F, Coriat P. Renin angiotensin system antagonists and anesthesia. *Anesth Analg.* 1999;89(5):1143-1145.

**3.** Correct Answer: A

**Rationale:**

There are many compensatory biological and neuroendocrine mechanisms in response to acute hypovolemic shock. In the juxtaglomerular apparatus, renin is released in response to three stimuli: (1) low arterial blood pressure, which activates the baroreceptors in the afferent arterioles; (2) decreases in chloride ion concentration in the distal tubules, secondary to decreased renal perfusion and glomerular filtration rate; and (3) β1-adrenergic receptor activation via catecholamines and sympathetic nervous system activity.

Renin hydrolyzes angiotensinogen into angiotensin I, which is further cleaved in the lungs by endothelial-bound ACE into angiotensin II, a potent vasoconstrictor which acts directly on the AT1-receptor on arteriolar smooth muscles to maintain systemic perfusion. Angiotensin II also acts on glomerular arterioles, with greater vasoconstrictive effect on efferent arterioles than afferent. This preserves glomerular pressure and the glomerular filtration rate in shock states.

Angiotensin II also stimulates the adrenal glands to release aldosterone, which triggers the epithelial cells in the distal tubule and collecting ducts of the kidney to increase reabsorption of sodium and water and excretion of potassium and hydrogen ions.

### References

1. Bock HA, Hermle M, Brunner FP, et al. Pressure dependent modulation of renin release in isolated perfused glomeruli. *Kidney Int.* 1992;41:275.
2. Lorenz JN, Weihprecht H, Schnermann J, et al. Renin release from isolated juxtaglomerular apparatus depends on macula densa chloride transport. *Am J Physiol.* 1991;260:F486.
3. Heyeraas KJ, Aukland K. Interlobular arterial resistance: influence of renal arterial pressure and angiotensin II. *Kidney Int.* 1987;31:1291.

**4.** Correct Answer: C

**Rationale:**

Aldosterone is the main mineralcorticoid hormone produced by the zona glomerulosa of the adrenal cortex. It promotes sodium retention and potassium excretion by: (1) upregulating and activating the basolateral Na⁺/K⁺ pump in the distal tubule and collecting ducts; (2) upregulating epithelial sodium channels in the collecting duct and colon; (3) stimulating Na⁺ and water reabsorption from the gut, and salivary and sweat glands in exchange for K⁺; and (4) stimulating secretion of K⁺ into the tubular lumen.

Hypoaldosteronism presents with hyperkalemia and an associated mild (normal anion gap) metabolic acidosis. Although aldosterone plays a key role in sodium homeostasis, isolated hypoaldosteronism is not typically associated with sodium wasting as the kidney compensates via angiotensin II. Hyponatremia is also uncommon, as ADH is not released in a patient who is otherwise euvolemic. The presence of hyponatremia should warrant workup for primary adrenal insufficiency and other causes. Option C demonstrates eunatremia, mild non-gap metabolic acidosis and hyperkalemia, making it the right answer.

The potassium imbalance in hypoaldosteronism can also impair urinary excretion of ammonium, a condition called type 4 renal tubular acidosis.

The most common causes of acquired hypoaldosteronism are hyporeninemic hypoaldosteronism, pharmacologic inhibition of angiotensin II or aldosterone, heparin therapy, and critical illness. Hyporeninemic hypoaldosteronism is common in patients with mild to moderate renal insufficiency due to diabetic nephropathy or chronic interstitial nephritis but can also occur in acute glomerulonephritis and in patients taking nonsteroidal anti-inflammatory drugs or calcineurin inhibitors. Pharmacologic inhibition of angiotensin II with medications such as ACE inhibitors, angiotensin II receptor blocks, and aldosterone receptor blockers are often initiated to improve survival in patients with heart failure and to prevent cardiac remodeling. Heparin has a direct toxic effect on the production of aldosterone in the adrenal cortex. Decreased adrenal production can occur in severely ill patient, whereas stress-induced production of cortisol may divert substrates away from aldosterone production.

Treatment is with replacement therapy with mineralocorticoid effect, such as fludrocortisone.

### References

1. DeFronzo RA. Hyperkalemia and hyporeninemic hypoaldosteronism. *Kidney Int.* 1980;17:118.
2. Rodríguez Soriano J. Renal tubular acidosis: the clinical entity. *J Am Soc Nephrol.* 2002;13:2160.
3. White PC. Disorders of aldosterone biosynthesis and action. *N Engl J Med.* 1994;331:250.

# 60

# HYPOTHALAMIC-PITUITARY-ADRENAL AXIS

Ilan Mizrahi

1. A 35-year-old man presents to the emergency department with fever, nausea, vomiting, and diarrhea for the last 2 days. His vital signs are temperature 100.6°F, HR 115 bpm, BP 70/50 mm Hg, and RR 25/min. His abdominal examination is soft and nontender. His only past medical history is unexplained orthostasis. Despite administration of 6 L of normal saline over 3 hours, he remains hypotensive and is started on a norepinephrine infusion. Point of care ultrasound reveals normal cardiac function. Which of the following laboratory tests would be most immediately helpful to establishing a diagnosis and to guide treatment?

   A. Cortisol
   B. ACTH stimulation
   C. Insulin
   D. Aldosterone

2. A 76-year-old man with COPD, and prior head and neck radiation for a pituitary tumor, and worsening dementia presents with hypotension after running out of his medications last week. He is admitted to the ICU for management of hypotension. Which of the following electrolyte values are most likely present?

   A. Na 129 mEq/L; K 5.4 mEq/L; $HCO_3$ 18 mEq/L; BUN 30 mg/dL; Glucose 84 mg/dL
   B. Na 129 mEq/L; K 3.9 mEq/L; $HCO_3$ 20 mEq/L; BUN 12 mg/dL; Glucose 84 mg/dL
   C. Na 140 mEq/L; K 2.7 mEq/L; $HCO_3$ 28 mEq/L; BUN 30 mg/dL; Glucose 180 mg/dL
   D. Na 145 mEq/L; K 4.3 mEq/L; $HCO_3$ 24 mEq/L; BUN 12 mg/dL; Glucose 140 mg/dL

3. A 56-year-old woman with hypertension, rheumatoid arthritis, and gastroesophageal reflux disease presents with perforated diverticulitis. Her home medications include lisinopril 10 mg, prednisone 15 mg, and omeprazole 40 mg. After emergent small bowel resection she was admitted to the ICU with low-dose norepinephrine. She is initially treated with piperacillin-tazobactam, and her home prednisone is continued. She remains vasopressor-dependent despite 30 mL/kg of normal saline and the addition of vasopressin. Which of the following treatment regimens is most appropriate at this time?

   A. Change antibiotics to cefepime and metronidazole
   B. Start intravenous corticosteroids
   C. Give additional bolus of 2 L of albumin
   D. Start an epinephrine infusion

4. A 26-year-old woman with a history of seizures controlled on phenytoin has been undergoing chemotherapy for treatment of acute myelogenous leukemia. She is admitted to the ICU with fungal pneumonia. She is intubated with etomidate and rocuronium, started on ketoconazole, and given 30 mL/kg of normal saline. Thirty-six hours later she becomes increasingly hypotensive despite escalating vasopressor doses. She is subsequently treated with hydrocortisone with good response. Which of the following medications likely contributed to her clinical decompensation?

   A. Phenytoin
   B. Etomidate
   C. Ketoconazole
   D. All of the above

5. A 56-year-old woman is admitted to the ICU with septic shock from community-acquired pneumonia. She is intubated with etomidate and rocuronium, fluid resuscitated with 30 mL/kg of normal saline and treated with cefepime and levofloxacin. Despite treatment she becomes increasingly hypotensive requiring escalating vasopressor doses. A random cortisol level is sent to test for adrenal insufficiency. Which of the following levels would be the lowest indicating an ADEQUATE adrenal response?

   A. 4 μg/dL
   B. 13 μg/dL
   C. 25 μg/dL
   D. 50 μg/dL

6. A 48-year-old man with a history of asthma treated with intermittent steroids, and a history of kidney stones, is admitted to the ICU with urosepsis. He is intubated, started on antibiotics, and fluid resuscitated with 30 mL/kg of normal saline. Despite this therapy he becomes increasingly hypotensive requiring escalating vasopressor doses. An ACTH stimulation test is performed revealing a baseline cortisol of 10 μg/dL and a 30-minute peak of 16 μg/dL.

   Which of the following interventions is most appropriate given the ACTH test results?

   A. Administer corticosteroids, she is adrenally insufficient
   B. A second test is needed to rule out daily variation
   C. Do not administer corticosteroids, she has adequate adrenal function
   D. Do not administer corticosteroids, the ACTH stimulation test is unreliable in sepsis

7. A 75-year-old man is admitted to the ICU with septic shock. Broad spectrum antibiotics are initiated, and he undergoes fluid resuscitation. Despite receiving 5 L of lactated ringers, he remains hypotensive requiring high-dose norepinephrine and vasopressin infusions. Cardiac ultrasound reveals hyperdynamic ventricular function without other abnormalities. Which of the following statements regarding administration of systemic corticosteroids is most appropriate for this patient?

   A. Perform an ACTH stimulation test and give methylprednisolone if adrenally insufficient
   B. Perform an ACTH stimulation test and give hydrocortisone if adrenally insufficient
   C. Give hydrocortisone, there is no need for ACTH stimulation testing
   D. Do not start corticosteroids in this patient

8. A 56-year-old woman with hypertension, rheumatoid arthritis, and gastroesophageal reflux disease is admitted to the ICU after undergoing a bowel resection for perforated diverticulitis. Her home medications include lisinopril 10 mg, prednisone 15 mg, and omeprazole 40 mg. She is treated with piperacillin-tazobactam and receives adequate fluid resuscitation over the next 24 hours but continues to require vasopressors for hypotension. Given a concern for adrenal insufficiency, which of the following steroids is most appropriate to administer to this patient?

   A. Prednisone
   B. Dexamethasone
   C. Fludrocortisone
   D. Hydrocortisone

# Chapter 60 ▪ Answers

1. Correct Answer: A

   **Rationale:**
   This patient's presentation is consistent with adrenal insufficiency, and he is suffering from adrenal crisis. Primary adrenal insufficiency is the inability of the adrenal gland to produce steroid hormones even when the stimulus by the pituitary gland via corticotropin is adequate or increased. Chronic primary adrenal insufficiency (Addison disease) results from the destruction of the adrenal cortex. The most common causes are autoimmune destruction (70%-80%), tuberculosis (~20%), and adrenal metastases. In primary disorders, both glucocorticoid (cortisol) and mineralocorticoid (aldosterone) secretion are affected. Typical features of primary adrenal insufficiency fatigue, orthostasis, hyperpigmentation, and scant axillary and pubic hair. About 25% of patients with adrenal insufficiency present with adrenocortical crisis. The symptoms are nonspecific and include sudden dizziness, weakness, dehydration, hypotension, and shock. In many cases, the clinical picture may be indistinguishable from shock because of loss

of intravascular fluid volume. Glucocorticoid (cortisol) deficiency decreases vascular responsiveness to angiotensin II, and norepinephrine reduces the synthesis of renin and increases the production and effects of prostacyclin and other vasodilatory hormones. In acute cases, mineralocorticoid deficiency leads to hypotension.

The diagnosis of adrenal crisis in this patient would be best supported by a low serum cortisol level. Serum cortisol and aldosterone levels would be low in patients with primary adrenal insufficiency. However, patients with secondary adrenal insufficiency have normal aldosterone levels and can also present in the refractory shock due to adrenal crisis. Thus, measurement of just the aldosterone level is not sufficient. Though serum ACTH level is expected to be high in primary insufficiency, it could be elevated in other conditions too. Lastly although the cortisol response to ACTH stimulation is the standard way to interrogate the function of the hypothalamic-pituitary-adrenal axis, the results may be impacted by critical illness and might lead to misdiagnosis. It also takes two repeated measurement to generate results. Thus, for patients in the ICU it remains extremely difficult to recognize acute, absolute adrenal insufficiency based on clinical symptoms. Because a missed diagnosis is often fatal, patients with sudden deterioration and unexplained catecholamine resistant should be initially screened with a cortisol level for adrenal insufficiency. The insulin-induced hypoglycemia test is used to evaluate integrity of the full hypothalamic-pituitary-adrenal axis as hypoglycemia acts centrally to stimulate hypothalamic corticotropin-releasing hormone release and, therefore, ACTH release. In this test, blood is drawn to measure the blood glucose and cortisol levels, followed by an injection of fast-acting insulin. Blood glucose and cortisol levels are measured again at 30, 45, and 90 minutes after the insulin injection. The normal response is for blood glucose levels to fall and cortisol levels to rise. In most settings the ACTH stimulation test provides nearly the same information, is less difficult to perform, and is without risk to the patient.

### References

1. Shenker Y, Skatrud JB. Adrenal insufficiency in critically ill patients. *Am J Respir Crit Care Med.* 2001;163:1520-1523.
2. Vincent JL, Abraham E, Moore FA, et al, eds. *Textbook of Critical Care.* 7th ed. Philadelphia, PA: Elsevier; 2017.

---

**2.** Correct Answer: B

**Rationale:**

This patient likely has secondary adrenal insufficiency from radiation affecting the pituitary gland, resulting in a deficit in ACTH production. Other potential causes of secondary insufficiency include pituitary tumors or craniopharyngiomas, postpartum hypopituitarism ("Sheehan's syndrome"), and pituitary infiltrative diseased (hemochromatosis, sarcoidosis). There may be clinical manifestations of a pituitary or hypothalamic tumor, such as symptoms and signs of deficiency of other anterior pituitary hormones, headache, or visual field defects. This patient has developed adrenal crisis because he has been unable to take his daily replacement steroids. When differentiating primary from secondary adrenal insufficiency, it is important to remember that mineralocorticoid production is affected in primary but unchanged in secondary adrenal insufficiency (ACTH does not play a major role in regulation of aldosterone). Thus, hyperkalemia is usually present in primary insufficiency but absent in secondary. Hyponatremia is a feature of both, but in primary insufficiency it is associated with volume contraction resulting in an elevated blood urea nitrogen (BUN) and creatinine; whereas in secondary adrenal insufficiency, hyponatremia is dilutional because of decreased ability to excrete water and increased vasopressin levels. Hypoglycemia is present in both primary and secondary because of cortisol deficiency. Hyperaldosteronism is characterized by a normal sodium, hypokalemia, alkalemia, and hyperglycemia.
Thus

- Na 129 mEq/L; K 5.4 mEq/L; $HCO_3$ 18 mEq/L; BUN 30 mg/dL; Glucose 84 mg/dL—Primary adrenal insufficiency
- Na 129 mEq/L; K 3.9 mEq/L; $HCO_3$ 20 mEq/L; BUN 12 mg/dL; Glucose 84 mg/dL—Secondary adrenal insufficiency
- Na 140 mEq/L; K 2.7 mEq/L; $HCO_3$ 28 mEq/L; BUN 30 mg/dL; Glucose 180 mg/dL—Hyperaldosteronism
- Na 145 mEq/L; K 4.3 mEq/L; $HCO_3$ 24 mEq/L; BUN 12 mg/dL; Glucose 140 mg/dL—Normal

### Reference

1. Vincent JL, Abraham E, Moore FA, et al, eds. *Textbook of Critical Care.* 7th ed. Philadelphia, PA: Elsevier; 2017.

---

**3.** Correct Answer: B

**Rationale:**

This patient likely has a suppressed hypothalamic-pituitary-adrenal axis due to long-term exogenous glucocorticoid intake. These patients do well with normal activities but may be unable to mount an adequate steroid response to the stress of surgery or critical illness. Typical patients are those with chronic autoimmune or inflammatory diseases (asthma, ulcerative colitis, rheumatoid arthritis), or those with underlying primary or secondary adrenal insufficiency who take chronic steroid supplementation. Although past recommendations have indicated that all patients on chronic steroids require "stress dose," it is now generally accepted to be necessary only for patients taking 5 mg or greater of prednisone, per day, for more than 3 weeks. In addition to their typical daily maintenance dose, patients should receive additional steroids commensurate with the anticipated stress. A reasonable approach is to use 50 mg of hydrocortisone followed by 25 mg every 8 hours for surgeries with minor (eg hernioplasty, colonoscopy) or moderate surgical stress (eg total joint replacement, cholecystectomy). A higher initial dose of 100 mg followed by 50 mg every 8 hours is recommended for surgeries with major surgical stress such as cardiac surgery. A higher dose may be needed for critical illness–related corticosteroid insufficiency. In contrast to nonendocrine diseases, patients with organic primary or secondary adrenal insufficiency are not capable of augmenting their serum cortisol levels at all, and these patients should always receive supplemental glucocorticoids.

There is no indication that the current antibiotic regimen is insufficient as it adequately covers for abdominal sepsis, and cultures have not shown any resistant organisms. She has received adequate fluid resuscitation for septic shock, and there is no clinical reason to bolus further. Although epinephrine may be added to support her blood pressure, it will not treat the underlying cause of adrenal insufficiency.

### References

1. Annane D, Pastores SM, Rochwerg B, et al. Guidelines for the Diagnosis and Management of Critical Illness-Related Corticosteroid Insufficiency (CIRCI) in Critically Ill Patients (Part I): Society of Critical Care Medicine (SCCM) and European Society of Intensive Care Medicine (ESICM) 2017. *Crit Care Med.* 2017;45(12):2078-2088.
2. Liu MM, Reidy AB, Saatee S, Collard CD. Perioperative steroid management: approaches based on current evidence. *Anesthesiology.* 2017;127(1):166-172.
3. Bancos I, Hahner S, Tomlinson J, Arlt W. Diagnosis and management of adrenal insufficiency. *Lancet Diabetes Endocrinol.* 2015;3(3):216-26.

**4. Correct Answer: D**

**Rationale:**

Critical illness-related corticosteroid insufficiency (CIRCI), formerly known as relative adrenal insufficiency, results from inadequate cellular corticosteroid activity for the severity of a patient's illness. Most individuals will mount a strong corticosteroid response to critical illness, but a certain subset fail to do so. Although relative adrenal insufficiency relies on measurement of deficiency cortisol concentrations, CIRCI is a clinical diagnosis. The clinical presentation of this patient, like other adrenal insufficiency, is catecholamine-dependent vasoplegic shock that responds to steroids. Morphologic and structural changes in the adrenal gland in these cases are generally minor, with some adrenal cortical hyperplasia. There is also peripheral glucocorticoid resistance mediated by systemic inflammation, although absolute cortisol levels might be normal. In septic shock specifically, insufficiency may be due to impaired pituitary corticotropin release, attenuated adrenal response to corticotropin, and reduced cortisol synthesis. Various medications used in critical care may interfere with the hypothalamic-pituitary-adrenal axis: either by increased metabolism of cortisol (phenytoin, rifampin) or impairing steroid synthesis (etomidate, ketoconazole).

### References

1. Shenker Y, Skatrud JB. Adrenal insufficiency in critically ill patients. *Am J Respir Crit Care Med.* 2001;163:1520-1523.
2. Annane D, Pastores SM, Rochwerg B, et al. Guidelines for the Diagnosis and Management of Critical Illness-Related Corticosteroid Insufficiency (CIRCI) in Critically Ill Patients (Part I): Society of Critical Care Medicine (SCCM) and European Society of Intensive Care Medicine (ESICM) 2017. *Crit Care Med.* 2017;45(12):2078-2088.

**5. Correct Answer: C**

**Rationale:**

Cortisol secretion normally exhibits a diurnal variation, with peak concentrations in the morning (around 8:00 AM) correlating with waking and accelerating activity after sleeping. For outpatient testing, early morning "peak" measurements are typically used for diagnosing adrenal insufficiency. However, the timing of such testing is not always appropriate in the critical care setting. Providers can measure "random" cortisol levels as a gross test of hypothalamic-pituitary-adrenal axis integrity. Values below an established threshold indicate adrenal insufficiency that would respond to steroid administration. For critically ill patients, a lower bound of 20 to 25 µg/dL (depending on desired diagnostic sensitivity) is considered an adequate random cortisol. A level less than 5 µg/dL constitutes adrenal insufficiency with 100% specificity. In unstressed individuals (ie outpatients) a random cortisol >15 µg/dL is sufficient to rule out adrenal insufficiency. A level of 50 µg/dL would be considered adequate response in a critically ill patient.

### References

1. Annane D, Pastores SM, Rochwerg B, et al. Guidelines for the Diagnosis and Management of Critical Illness-Related Corticosteroid Insufficiency (CIRCI) in Critically Ill Patients (Part I): Society of Critical Care Medicine (SCCM) and European Society of Intensive Care Medicine (ESICM) 2017. *Crit Care Med.* 2017;45(12):2078-2088.
2. Bancos I, Hahner S, Tomlinson J, Arlt W.Diagnosis and management of adrenal insufficiency. *Lancet Diabetes Endocrinol.* 2015;3(3):216-226.

**6. Correct Answer: A**

**Rationale:**

Administering ACTH (cosyntropin) is a way of interrogating the hypothalamic-pituitary-adrenal axis to determine its function in response to systemic stress. The ACTH stimulation test involves measuring a baseline (random) cortisol level, administering 250 µg of ACTH, and measuring the rise in serum cortisol after 30 to 60 minutes. A peak cortisol of 18 to 20 µg/dL is considered a normal response to ACTH stimulation and excludes primary and nearly all cases of secondary adrenal insufficiency. In critical illness an incremental increase of less than 9 µg/dL is the most sensitive and specific cutoff of identify nonresponders. Thus, in this patient a peak level of 16 µg/dL and rise of only 6 µg/dL indicate adrenal insufficiency, and she would likely benefit from corticosteroids. There is no indication that repeat testing is necessary as long as the peak levels are drawn at the appropriate time. The 250 µg cosyntropin stimulation tests raised the ACTH concentration to 60,000 pg/mL, which dwarfs the physiologic 100 pg/mL of ACTH needed to maximally stimulate the adrenal cortex. However, it is possible that patients who respond to these supra-maximal doses may still be adrenally insufficient when this stimulus is removed. Corticosteroid administration has been shown to be useful in shock reversal in patients with critical illness–related corticosteroid insufficiency.

### References

1. Annane D, Pastores SM, Rochwerg B, et al. Guidelines for the Diagnosis and Management of Critical Illness-Related Corticosteroid Insufficiency (CIRCI) in Critically Ill Patients (Part I): Society of Critical Care Medicine (SCCM) and European Society of Intensive Care Medicine (ESICM) 2017. *Crit Care Med*. 2017;45(12):2078-2088.
2. Bancos I, Hahner S, Tomlinson J, Arlt W.Diagnosis and management of adrenal insufficiency. *Lancet Diabetes Endocrinol*. 2015;3(3):216-226.

---

**7.** Correct Answer: C

**Rationale:**

The surviving sepsis guidelines recommend low-dose steroids in patients who are fluid-resuscitated in vasopressor-dependent shock who are unable to reach their target MAP goal. It is not necessary to perform an ACTH stimulation test. Steroid use is associated with improved MAP and shorter duration of vasopressor use. This is a low-strength recommendation, but steroids may be warranted in this decompensating patient.

Early research using high-dose methylprednisolone (supra-physiologic) did not show improved survival and possible harm. Subsequent trials using physiologic doses arrived at conflicting results. The study by Annane and colleagues (2002) and the APROCCHSS trial (2018) showed that patients with septic shock had faster reversal of shock and decreased mortality after receiving low-dose hydrocortisone and fludrocortisone. On the other hand, the CORTICUS trial in 2008 and the ADRENAL trial in 2018 found a faster resolution of shock, but no difference in 28-day mortality with hydrocortisone administration. Thus, evidence is mixed against recommending routine use in patients who are adrenally insufficient. Guidelines do not recommend routine ACTH testing as it may be unreliable in critical illness and may be affected by numerous medications.

### References

1. Annane D, Pastores SM, Rochwerg B, et al. Guidelines for the Diagnosis and Management of Critical Illness-Related Corticosteroid Insufficiency (CIRCI) in Critically Ill Patients (Part I): Society of Critical Care Medicine (SCCM) and European Society of Intensive Care Medicine (ESICM) 2017. *Crit Care Med*. 2017;45(12):2078-2088.
2. Annane D, Cariou A, Maxime V, et al. Corticosteroid treatment and intensive insulin therapy for septic shock in adults: a randomized controlled trial. *JAMA*. 2010;303:341-348.
3. Rhodes A, Evans LE, Alhazzani W, et al. Surviving sepsis campaign: international guidelines for management of sepsis and septic shock: 2016. *Intens Care Med*. 2017;43:304-377.
4. Venkatesh B, Finfer S, Cohen J, et al. Adjunctive glucocorticoid therapy in patients with septic shock. *N Engl J Med*. 2018;378:797-808.

---

**8.** Correct Answer: D

**Rationale:**

This patient has vasopressor-resistant septic shock despite adequate IV fluid resuscitation which may be due to adrenal insufficiency. Current guidelines on critical illness–related corticosteroid insufficiency recommend IV hydrocortisone <400 mg/d for ≥3 days in patients with septic shock that is not responsive to fluid resuscitation and requires moderate- to high-dose vasopressor therapy. Hydrocortisone is the synthetic equivalent to the physiologic final active compound, cortisol, so treatment with hydrocortisone directly replaces cortisol independently from metabolic transformation. In these large doses it provides both glucocorticoid and mineralocorticoid coverage. A potential disadvantage of hydrocortisone administration is that diagnostic testing of adrenal function cannot be performed while receiving the medication.

Dexamethasone does not have any intrinsic mineralocorticoid activity and therefore would not provide full repletion. Fludrocortisone would not be an adequate choice as it is pure mineralocorticoid and does not have any glucocorticoid activity. Additional mineralocorticoid replacement is not needed as long as the dose of cortisol exceeds 50 mg daily. If a patient is completely adrenally insufficient, then fludrocortisone should also be administered. Prednisone and cortisone are typically avoided in critically ill patients because they require hydroxylation to create the active compound (prednisone to prednisolone and cortisone to cortisol). In addition, these are only available for oral administration, and their use is limited in critical care where enteral absorption may be compromised.

### References

1. Annane D, Pastores SM, Rochwerg B, et al. Guidelines for the Diagnosis and Management of Critical Illness-Related Corticosteroid Insufficiency (CIRCI) in Critically Ill Patients (Part I): Society of Critical Care Medicine (SCCM) and European Society of Intensive Care Medicine (ESICM) 2017. *Crit Care Med*. 2017;45(12):2078-2088.
2. Vincent JL, Abraham E, Moore FA, et al, eds. *Textbook of Critical Care*. 7th ed. Philadelphia, PA: Elsevier; 2017.

# 61

# MANAGEMENT DURING CRITICAL ILLNESS

Ilan Mizrahi

1. A 48-year-old woman presents with severe headache. She has a history of refractory hypertension, intermittent headaches, and palpitations. Her vital signs are notable for blood pressure of 242/100 mm Hg and oxygen saturation of 85% on room air. Chest X-ray shows diffuse pulmonary edema, and oxygenation improves with high flow nasal cannula. She is admitted to the ICU for blood pressure management and respiratory support. Collection of 24-hour urinary vanillylmandelic acid and metanephrines are started. Until these results return, which of the following medications would be most appropriate to start to manage her hypertension?

   A. Labetalol
   B. Esmolol
   C. Phentolamine
   D. Phenoxybenzamine

2. A 72-year-old woman is admitted to the ICU with hypoxemic respiratory failure and sepsis. Her medical history is notable for hypertension, COPD, and CKD (Cr 1.9). Her vital signs are temperature is 38.5°C, heart rate 107 bpm, blood pressure 87/55, $O_2$ saturation 89% on 60% $FiO_2$. She is intubated, undergoes fluid resuscitation and vasopressor support, and receives broad spectrum antimicrobials and is started on a norepinephrine infusion. In addition to routine laboratory studies a thyroid function panel is sent, which is notable for a T3 of 60 ng/dL (normal 80-180) and a TSH 8 µg/dL (normal 0.5-5). Based on these laboratory studies, which of the following interventions is most appropriate?

   A. No further treatment necessary
   B. Send free T4, reverse T3
   C. Start IV levothyroxine
   D. Start iodine supplementation

3. A 48-year-old woman with a history of Grave's disease undergoes an urgent appendectomy. Four hours after surgery she is found to be confused and diaphoretic. Her vital signs are T 102.7, HR 130/min, and BP 184/106 mm Hg and $O_2$ saturation of 93% on RA. On physical examination there is no evidence of rigidity. An arterial blood gas ABG shows pH 7.51, $pCO_2$ 30, $pO_2$ 98. Thyroid function tests are sent. Although awaiting the results, which of the following medications would be most appropriate to give?

   A. Aspirin
   B. Propranolol
   C. Bromocriptine
   D. Dantrolene

4. A 48-year-old woman with a history of Grave's disease undergoes an urgent appendectomy. Fours hours after surgery she is found to have altered mental status and diaphoresis. Her vital signs are T 102.7, HR 130/min, and BP 184/106 mm Hg. On physical examination there is no evidence of rigidity. ABG shows pH 7.51, $pCO_2$ 30, $pO_2$ 98. TSH is <0.01 µg U/mL. Two liters of normal saline and intravenous propranolol are administered. Which of the following medications is NOT indicated for immediate treatment in this patient?

A. Iodine
B. Propylthiouracil
C. Methimazole
D. Corticosteroids

5. A 65-year-old woman is admitted to the ICU after being found down at home. Her only medical history is a remote history of Grave's disease and thyroid ablation. Vital signs are T 89°F, HR 50 bpm, BP 105/61 mm Hg. On physical examination she obtunded, and brittle hair, macroglossia, and periorbital edema are noted. An ABG shows pH 7.30, $PaCO_2$ 55, $PaO_2$ 65. She is intubated for airway protection ventilatory support. Urine, sputum, and blood cultures are sent, and she is treated with broad spectrum antibiotics. Thyroid function tests are sent and she is started on IV levothyroxine. Which of the following additional therapies is most appropriate at this time?

A. Hydrocortisone
B. Insulin
C. Iodine
D. Active rewarming

6. A 68-year-old woman presents to the emergency department after being found at home with confusion and lethargy. Her medical history includes GERD, obesity, non–insulin dependent type 2 diabetes, and depression with prior suicide attempts. Empty bottles of omeprazole, glyburide, and sertraline were found in her home. She is intubated for airway protection. Her admission laboratory test results are notable for a blood glucose of 33 mg/dL, and she is treated with an IV bolus of dextrose 50. Repeat laboratory tests an hour later show blood glucose 52 mg/dL. Which of the following is most appropriate to treat her hypoglycemia?

A. Glucagon IM
B. D50 bolus and octreotide
C. D50 bolus followed by glucose infusion
D. D50 bolus and recheck glucose in 1 hour

7. A 22-year-old man with type 1 diabetes since age 11 presents with fever, drowsiness, and abdominal pain. These symptoms started 2 days ago, and he has been unable to tolerate food or water. Vital signs are T 38.2 HR 122 and BP 105/70 mm Hg. Laboratory tests are notable for glucose 480 mg/dL, Sodium 154 mEq/L, Potassium 5.5 mEq/L, Chloride 114 mEq/L. An ABG shows pH 7.2, $PaCO_2$ 28 mm Hg, $PaO_2$ 95 mm Hg, $HCO_3$ 9 mEq/L. Serum and urine ketones are positive. He undergoes fluid resuscitation with normal saline and receives an IV insulin bolus followed by a continuous insulin infusion. After 3 hours of treatment, his blood glucose is 250 mg/dL. What is the most appropriate IV fluid management at this time?

A. Continue normal saline infusion and add glucose and potassium
B. Continue normal saline infusion and add glucose
C. Start half-normal saline with glucose and potassium
D. Start half-normal saline with glucose

8. A 58-year-old man is admitted to the ICU with pneumonia and sepsis. His medical history is notable for coronary artery disease and COPD. He is intubated and receiving a norepinephrine infusion to support blood pressure. On his serum, glucose has ranged from 191 to 283 mg/dL over the last 12 hours. What is the most appropriate treatment at this time for his blood glucose?

A. No treatment is necessary
B. Start insulin infusion with target blood glucose <150 mg/dL
C. Start Lantus insulin
D. Start sliding scale insulin and target blood glucose <180 mg/dL

9. A 60-year-old man with bipolar disorder on chronic lithium therapy undergoes an uncomplicated appendectomy. In the PACU he becomes delirious and agitated. His vital signs are within normal limits. He weighs 75 kg. Laboratory values are notable for sodium 148 mEq/L. He is maintained overnight on dextrose in half-normal saline at 125 mL/h. Urine output is approximately 300 mL/h overnight. In the morning serum sodium has increased to 155 mEq/L. His urine osmolality is 120 mOsm/kg, and urine sodium is 22 mEq/L. Arginine vasopressin is administered without a change in urine output. What is the most appropriate change in IV fluids for treatment of his hypernatremia?

    **A.** Increase the infusion rate to 400 mL/h
    **B.** Change to D5 water at 200 mL/h
    **C.** Change to D5 water at 400 mL/h
    **D.** Change to D5 water at 300 mL/h and add desmopressin

**10.** A 22-year-old, 70-kg man sustained unrecoverable traumatic brain injury and is undergoing evaluation for donation of his heart, liver, and lungs. During transplant evaluation and preparation, he becomes progressively hypotensive, with increased urine output, and laboratory evaluation is notable for a sodium of 148 mEq/L (from initial of 139 mEq/L). Administration of which of the following medications is most appropriate to increase the chances of successful organ recovery?

    **A.** Vasopressin infusion 0.04 U/min and desmopressin 1 µg every 6 hours
    **B.** Methylprednisolone 1000 mg IV
    **C.** Levothyroxine IV 20 µg followed by infusion
    **D.** All of the above

# Chapter 61 ▪ Answers

**1.** Correct Answer: C

**Rationale:**
This patient presents in hypertensive emergency secondary to pheochromocytoma. The triad of refractory hypertension, headaches, and palpitations is classic for pheochromocytoma. The diagnosis is confirmed with elevated urinary VMA and metanephrine levels. The essential tenet of pheochromocytoma management is alpha-adrenergic blockade and correction of intravascular volume depletion. The typical agents for alpha blockade are phentolamine and phenoxybenzamine. Phentolamine is available as an intravenous agent and has an onset of action of 1 to 2 minutes, lasting 3 to 10 minutes. Phenoxybenzamine is only available orally and would be inappropriate for immediate blood pressure lowering in this symptomatic patient. Beta-blockade should not be administered initially as the impairment of beta-mediated vasodilation can result in unopposed alpha-mediated vasoconstriction and may lead to circulatory collapse. Thus, labetalol and esmolol are not appropriate first line agents.

**Reference**

1. Vincent JL, Abraham E, Moore FA, et al, eds. *Textbook of Critical Care*. 7th ed. Philadelphia, PA: Elsevier; 2017.

**2.** Correct Answer: A

**Rationale:**
This patient presenting with hypoxemic respiratory failure and sepsis has a nonthyroidal illness syndrome (NTIS), which had previously been called the euthyroid sick syndrome. NTIS, which was previously called the euthyroid sick syndrome, is characterized by low T3, usually elevated reverse T3, normal or low TSH, and if prolonged, low T4 levels in clinically euthyroid patients experiencing critical illness (trauma, sepsis, DKA, CKD, malnutrition). A variety of mechanisms have been proposed to explain these thyroid hormone abnormalities, including decreased conversion of T4 to T3, decreased binding to thyroid-binding globulin, and the effect of circulating cytokines and oxidative stress.

    Diagnosis of primary hypothyroidism can be difficult in patients who are severely ill and not known to have hypothyroidism before admission to the ICU because serum thyroid hormones, especially $T_3$, are decreased in most patients in the ICU because of NTIS. In patients clinically suspected to have severe hypothyroidism, the most useful test for diagnosis is measurement of plasma TSH, because a normal plasma TSH excludes primary hypothyroidism. In patients with a combination of primary hypothyroidism and NTIS, serum TSH concentration is still high and responsive to levothyroxine treatment. However, of note is that in patients who have hypothyroidism the high serum TSH concentration might decrease during the acute phase of illness especially if dopamine or high doses of glucocorticoids are given. Thus, high serum TSH in combination with low serum $T_4$ is indicative of hypothyroidism

**References**

1. Fliers E, Bianco AC, Langouche L, Boelen A. Thyroid function in critically ill patients. *Lancet Diabetes Endocrinol*. 2015;3:816-825.
2. Van den Berghe G. Non-thyroidal illness in the ICU: a syndrome with different faces. *Thyroid*. 2014;24:1456-1465.
3. Vincent JL, Abraham E, Moore FA, et al, eds. *Textbook of Critical Care*. 7th ed. Philadelphia, PA: Elsevier; 2017.

**3. Correct Answer: B**

**Rationale:**

This patient has thyrotoxicosis (thyroid storm), an acute, life-threatening hypermetabolic state resulting from excessive thyroid hormone. It clinically manifests as altered mental status, fever, tachycardia, and hypertension, which can lead to cardiomyopathy, congestive heart failure, and cardiovascular collapse. In patients with underlying hyperthyroidism it may be precipitated by illness, surgery, or other severe stress. Management is generally supportive with cooling and administration of fluids, as well as measures to inhibit the effects of the excessive thyroid hormones, reduce thyroid hormone synthesis, and prevent further release. The underlying cause of the thyroid storm should also be treated.

Propranolol is effective at blocking the hyperadrenergic manifestations of thyrotoxicosis. Propranolol is a nonselective beta blocker that crosses the blood-brain barrier and is known to decrease the conversion of T4 to T3. Although antipyretic agents should also be administered, aspirin is generally avoided as it may displace thyroid hormone from thyroid binding globulin and exacerbate symptoms. Bromocriptine is a dopamine agonist that is used in treatment of neuroleptic malignant syndrome. Dantrolene expresses excitation-contraction coupling in skeletal muscle by acting as a receptor antagonist to the ryanodine receptor and is the treatment for malignant hyperthermia. Neuroleptic malignant syndrome and malignant hyperthermia are hypermetabolic states that can present similarly to thyrotoxicosis (tachycardia, hyperthermia, altered mental status) but also more commonly result in muscle rigidity, metabolic acidosis, and hypercarbia.

References

1. Chiha M, Samarasinghe S, Kabaker AS. Thyroid storm: an updated review. *J Intensive Care Med*. 2015;30:131-140.
2. Vincent JL, Abraham E, Moore FA, et al, eds. *Textbook of Critical Care*. 7th ed. Philadelphia, PA: Elsevier; 2017.

**4. Correct Answer: A**

**Rationale:**

This patient has thyrotoxicosis (thyroid storm), an acute, life-threatening hypermetabolic state of excessive thyroid hormone. Management is supportive and aimed at blocking further hormone synthesis, release, and peripheral conversion. This thyroid hormone blockade has been referred to as the four 'Bs': **B**eta-blockade; **B**lock synthesis (ie antithyroid drugs); **B**lock release (ie iodine); **B**lock conversion of T4 into T3 (propranolol, corticosteroids).

Thyroid hormone synthesis can be inhibited by either the drugs propylthiouracil (PTU) or methimazole, which prevent the enzyme thyroid peroxidase from iodination of tyrosine residues on thyroglobulin. PTU also inhibits the peripheral conversion of T4 to T3. Even if synthesis is blocked, the thyroid gland still contains stores of thyroid hormone and will continue to release it for days to weeks. To suppress thyroid hormone release, large doses of iodine can be administered. Either potassium iodine or sodium iodine can be used. However, if iodine is administered before blocking thyroid hormone synthesis with an antithyroid agent, it will merely be incorporated into further thyroid hormone production. Therefore, iodine should not be administered for at least 1 hour after PTU or methimazole. Corticosteroids (hydrocortisone) inhibit peripheral conversion of T4 into T3. Moreover, many patients in thyroid storm also have suppression of the HPA axis and are adrenally insufficient.

References

1. Chiha M, Samarasinghe S, Kabaker AS. Thyroid storm: an updated review. *J Intensive Care Med*. 2015;30:131-140.
2. Vincent JL, Abraham E, Moore FA, et al, eds. *Textbook of Critical Care*. 7th ed. Philadelphia, PA: Elsevier; 2017.

**5. Correct Answer: A**

**Rationale:**

This patient is in myxedema coma. It is often the result of prolonged noncompliance with thyroid supplementation in the face of absent thyroid function, such as following thyroid ablation. Triggers of myxedema coma include physiologic stresses such as MI and sepsis. Certain drugs that can cause hypothyroidism include amiodarone, propylthiouracil, lithium, and sulfonamides. The hallmark of myxedema is altered mental status and hypothermia, with associated bradycardia and hypotension. On physical examination these patients may have brittle hair, macroglossia, and generalized edema. Laboratory studies of patients with myxedema coma patients may reveal a low $PaO_2$, high $PaCO_2$ (from blunted respiratory responses), hyponatremia (from impaired free water excretion), hypoglycemia (from hypothyroidism alone or from concomitant adrenal insufficiency), and elevated CPK levels. TSH will also be significantly elevated.

The treatment of myxedema coma should begin based on clinical suspicion and should not await laboratory confirmation. The primary treatment is IV thyroxine, with a loading dose followed by daily administration. Unsuspected adrenal insufficiency is frequently coexisting, and all patients with myxedema coma should also empirically receive hydrocortisone. Insulin administration is not indicated as these patients are commonly hypoglycemic and require supplemental glucose. There is no role for iodine in this patient who has undergone complete thyroid ablation and is receiving IV levothyroxine. Moreover, patients with some intrinsic thyroid function generally do not develop myxedema coma, and the giving high-dose iodine can inhibit thyroid hormone release. Although these patients are profoundly hypothermic, active rewarming is avoided as it can cause peripheral vasodilation and may lead to worsening hypotension and potentially cardiovascular collapse. Passive rewarming is preferred.

### References
1. Kwaku MP, Burman K. Myxedema coma. *J Intensive Care Med.* 2007;22:224-231.
2. Vincent JL, Abraham E, Moore FA, et al, eds. *Textbook of Critical Care.* 7th ed. Philadelphia, PA: Elsevier; 2017.
3. Klubo-Gwiezdzinska J, Wartofsky L. Thyroid emergencies. *Med Clin North Am.* 2012;96:385-403.

**6.** Correct Answer: B

**Rationale:**
Critically ill patients can be hypoglycemic for numerous reasons, including the effects of medications, ethanol, sepsis, hepatic failure, renal failure, and the cessation of TPN. This patient's hypoglycemia most likely results from an overdose of glyburide, a sulfonylurea oral hypoglycemic medication. Sulfonylureas act by increasing insulin release from pancreatic beta cells. The initial treatment for all hypoglycemic episodes should be a bolus of glucose, typically 0.5 to 1 g/kg of D50W. If a patient does not have intravenous access for emergent D50 administration, then IM glucagon is an effective alternative—raising blood glucose by promoting glycogenolysis and gluconeogenesis. After administering an initial glucose bolus, a dextrose infusion is typically required until the underlying cause of hypoglycemia has resolved. However, after sulfonylurea overdose a continuous glucose infusion can stimulate endogenous insulin production, leading to further hypoglycemia. If not recognized this can lead to a cycle of repeated glucose boluses and hypoglycemia episodes. Thus, after sulfonylurea overdose and an initial glucose bolus, octreotide is the preferred treatment. Octreotide is a long-acting somatostatin analog that binds to pancreatic beta cells and blocks insulin secretion. Octreotide can be administered either as an intravenous bolus followed by infusion, or subcutaneously. This patient failed to maintain normoglycemia after an initial D50 bolus, and starting a glucose infusion would likely contribute to further insulin release and repeated hypoglycemia. This patient has a functioning IV and does not require glucagon IM.

### References
1. Klein-Schwartz W, Stassinos GL, Isbister GK. Treatment of Sulfonylurea and insulin overdose. *Br J Clin Pharmacol.* 2015;81:496-504.
2. Vincent JL, Abraham E, Moore FA, et al, eds. *Textbook of Critical Care.* 7th ed. Philadelphia, PA: Elsevier; 2017.

**7.** Correct Answer: C

**Rationale:**
This patient presents in diabetic ketoacidosis. The immediate treatment is fluid resuscitation with normal saline to restore intravascular volume and an insulin IV bolus of 0.1 to 0.2 U/kg, followed by a continuous IV infusion at 0.10 U/kg/h. Serum glucose should be assessed hourly with the goal of lowering it by 50 mg/dL/h. The insulin infusion should be titrated downward as glucose levels are reduced. Serum electrolytes should be assessed every 2 to 4 hours. When the serum glucose is in the 200 range, glucose is added to the intravenous fluids. Starting glucose avoids hypoglycemia, while allowing continued administration of IV insulin to reverse ketogenesis. Once intravascular volume is restored, intravenous fluids should be changed to hypotonic saline to treat the ongoing free-water deficit and avoid hyperchloremic acidosis that can result from administration of large volumes of normal saline. Despite initial presence of hyperkalemia, with the administration of insulin and correction of acidosis hypokalemia will develop and should be treated with IV potassium.

### References
1. Boord JB, Graber AL, Chistman JW, Powers AC. Practical management of diabetes in critically ill patients. *Am J Respir Crit Care Med.* 2001;164:1763-1767.
2. Kohler K, Levy N. Management of diabetic ketoacidosis: a summary of the 2013 joint british diabetes societies guidelines. 2014;15(3).
3. Vincent JL, Abraham E, Moore FA, et al, eds. *Textbook of Critical Care.* 7th ed. Philadelphia, PA: Elsevier; 2017.

**8.** Correct Answer: D

**Rationale:**
This patient is critically ill with sustained hyperglycemia, blood glucose >180 mg/dL. Sustained hyperglycemia has been associated with increased morbidity and mortality across various patient population. Thus, although hyperglycemia should be avoided, there may additional morbidity associated with hypoglycemia resulting from targeting lower blood glucose levels. Although single center studies showed an apparent benefit to such "intensive insulin therapy," large randomized multicenter trials have shown the opposite—that intensive insulin therapy (blood glucose 81-108 mg/dL) is associated with a higher morbidity and mortality than a conventional regimen (blood glucose <180 mg/dL).

Given the repeated blood glucose measurements >180 mg/dL, this patient should be started on insulin therapy. As explained above there is no role for a lower target of 150 mg/dL instead of 180 mg/dL as attempts at tighter control are associated with worse outcomes. Administering long acting insulin to a critically ill patient with blood glucose variability may increase the risk of hypoglycemia. Starting sliding scale insulin that can be adjusted to the specific glucose level is an appropriate starting point for this patient.

### References

1. Finfer S, Chittock DR, Su SY, et al. Intensive versus conventional glucose control in critically ill patients. *N Engl J Med.* 2009;360:1283-1297.
2. Fahy BG, Sheehy AM, Coursin DB. Glucose control in the intensive care unit. *Crit Care Med.* 2009;37(5):1769-1776.
3. Clain J, Ramar K, Surani SR. Glucose control in critical care. *World J Diabetes.* 2015;6(9):1082-1091.
4. Vincent JL, Abraham E, Moore FA, et al, eds. *Textbook of Critical Care.* 7th ed. Philadelphia, PA: Elsevier; 2017.

**9.** Correct Answer: C

### Rationale:

Based on the medical history and laboratory results this patient likely has nephrogenic diabetes insipidus (DI) from long-term lithium therapy. Nephrogenic DI can be caused by several drugs, including lithium, demeclocycline, amphotericin B, and antiretroviral drugs such as tenofovir and indinavir. He developed severe hypernatremia from ongoing free water loss when he was unable to maintain oral intake. The goal of treatment is to correct his free water deficit by half over the 24 hours and then fully correct the sodium level within 3 days.

To determine the appropriate amount of fluid to administer, we must calculate the free water deficit. Assuming a total body water (TBW) of 60% lean body mass (this may be an overestimation in women or the elderly), this patient's normal TBW is approximately 45 L (0.6 × 75 kg). Assuming normal sodium of 140 mEq/L, his current TBW = normal TBW × (normal sodium/current sodium) = 45 × (140/155) = 45 × 0.9 = 40.5 L. Thus, his free water deficit = 45 − 40 = 5 L. We would aim to replace half of this in 24 hours, or about 2.5 L. We also must account for urinary free water loss resulting from the elevated urine output 300 mL/h × 24 h = 7.2 L. Thus the total free water repletion for 24 hour should be 2.5 + 7.2 = 9.7 L. Averaged per hour, this is approximately 400 mL/h.

Thus, changing to D5 Water at 400 mL/h should appropriately correct his free water deficit. D5 half-normal saline at 300 mL/h would provide approximately one-fourth of the needed free water. And D5W at 200 mL/h is only half that required. Administering D5W at 300 mL/h would only provide three quarters of the needed free water. In addition he did not respond to arginine vasopressin, so response to the synthetic vasopressin analogue desmopressin would be unlikely.

### References

1. Adler SM, Verbalis JG. Disorders of body water homeostasis in critical illness. *Endrocinol Metab Clin North Am.* 2006;35:873-894.
2. Makaryus AN, McFarlane SI. Diabetes insipidus: diagnosis and treatment of a complex disease. *Cleve Clin J Med.* 2006;73:65-71.
3. Vincent JL, Abraham E, Moore FA, et al, eds. *Textbook of Critical Care.* 7th ed. Philadelphia, PA: Elsevier; 2017.

**10.** Correct Answer: D

### Rationale:

Patients with severe brain injury and subsequent brain death before organ donation often develop multiple endocrine abnormalities. The HPA axis is particularly susceptible to ischemic injury from elevated intracranial pressure. Up to 80% of patients with brain death develop DI from reduced antidiuretic hormone (vasopressin). Hypothyroidism and hypocortisolism are also reported, albeit at lower rates. Numerous animal and clinical studies suggest that hormone replacement promotes hemodynamic stability, improves organ function, and increases the number or organs retrieved.

Several studies show that together, thyroid hormone, vasopressin, and methylprednisolone significantly increase successful organ recovery and may be associated with better cardiac recipient survival.

If DI develops and there is significant polyuria (>3 mL/kg/h), hypernatremia (sodium >145-150) and desmopressin may be administered (1-4 μg initially) and then titrated every 6 hours to urine output and osmolality, and serum sodium. If there is associated hypotension, vasopressin infusion 0.01 to 0.04 U/min may adequately treat the hypotension as well as the treat DI. Both a vasopressin infusion and desmopressin may also be administered together if one is not sufficient.

High-dose corticosteroids (methylprednisolone 1000 mg IV) reduce the inflammatory effects of brain death on organ function and may improve graft function after transplantation.

There is some controversy regarding the benefit of thyroid hormone supplementation, as not all studies have shown benefit. It seems to have the most benefit in hemodynamically unstable donors under consideration for cardiac donation. In this patient it would be warranted given his hypotension and potential cardiac donation, with little potential for harm.

### References

1. Kotloff RM, Blosser S, Fulda GJ. Management of the potential organ donor in the ICU: SCCM/ACCP/AOPO consensus statement. *Crit Care Med.* 2015;43:1291-1325.
2. Vincent JL, Abraham E, Moore FA, et al, eds. *Textbook of Critical Care.* 7th ed. Philadelphia, PA: Elsevier; 2017.

# INFECTIONS AND IMMUNOLOGIC DISEASE

# 62

# SYSTEMIC INFECTIONS

Lisa M. Bebell

1. A 26-year-old man presents to the emergency room with fevers and headache for the last 2 days. His temperature is 39.1°C, heart rate 123 beats/min, blood pressure 88/54 mm Hg, and respiratory rate 28 breaths/min. He appears diaphoretic and pale on examination but has no rash and no other abnormal physical findings. His white blood cell count is $3.9 \times 10^9$/L, hemoglobin 5.6 g/dL, platelet count 112,000/µL, and creatinine 2.7 mg/dL. He is oliguric. He is a medical student and returned from Uganda 6 days ago, where he has been conducting research for the last year. He reports no sexual contacts within the last six months. Which of the following is the **MOST** likely cause of his acute illness?

   A. Strongyloides hyperinfection syndrome
   B. Zika virus infection
   C. *Plasmodium falciparum* malaria
   D. Brucellosis

2. Which of the following statements are **TRUE** about empiric antibiotic selection for patients in septic shock?

   A. Selection should account for recently received antibiotics, prior organisms, and susceptibility patterns for each patient, and local antimicrobial resistance patterns
   B. The broadest-spectrum antibiotic combination available should be used until microbiologic testing results return
   C. Two antipseudomonal antibiotics of the same class should be used when there is concern for *Pseudomonas aeruginosa* bacteremia
   D. A and C

3. A 19-year-old woman is admitted to the intensive care unit for massive hemoptysis. Computed tomography (CT) of the chest reveals a large, cavitated lesion in the right middle lobe. The patient has no known past medical history, lives with her family, and recently immigrated from China. What is the **MOST** appropriate management strategy?

   A. Place the patient in a negative-pressure isolation room, and continue negative-pressure isolation until three sputum samples are negative for acid-fast bacteria and an alternative diagnosis has been established
   B. Place the patient in a negative-pressure isolation room, and continue negative-pressure isolation until three sputum samples are negative for acid-fast bacteria
   C. Place the patient in a positive-pressure isolation room, and continue positive-pressure isolation until two sputum samples are negative for acid-fast bacteria and an alternative diagnosis has been established
   D. Place the patient in a positive-pressure isolation room, and continue positive-pressure isolation until three sputum samples are negative for acid-fast bacteria

4. You admit a 61-year-old man to the intensive care unit after a witnessed generalized tonic-clonic seizure at home. He has a history of sarcoidosis and has been treated with prednisone 10 to 60 mg for the last year. Before admission, he had no cough or sputum production and had felt well. CT of the head, chest, abdomen, and pelvis reveals a 2.5 cm pulmonary nodule in the right upper lobe and 3 cm parenchymal brain lesion. What is the MOST likely diagnosis?

A. *Pneumocystis jirovecii* (formerly *carinii*) infection
B. Sarcoidosis
C. Tuberculosis
D. Nocardiosis

5. A 71-year-old man with diabetes, obesity, hypertension, and benign prostatic hypertrophy is admitted to the intensive care unit with abrupt-onset groin pain, fever, and a rapidly spreading erythematous groin and lower abdominal rash with ill-defined margins. The rash is exquisitely tender and firm to palpation. He develops hypotension with mean arterial pressure measured at 52 mm Hg, refractory to intravenous fluid resuscitation. What is the **MOST** appropriate sequence of events to manage his disease?

A. Insert a central venous catheter, start vasopressors, obtain two sets of blood cultures, and start antibiotic therapy with vancomycin, meropenem, and clindamycin
B. Start antibiotic therapy with vancomycin, meropenem, and clindamycin; obtain two sets of blood cultures, surgical consult for emergent debridement, and start vasopressors
C. Start vasopressors, obtain two sets of blood cultures, start antibiotic therapy with vancomycin, piperacillin-tazobactam, and clindamycin; surgical consult for emergent debridement
D. Start vasopressors, obtain two sets of blood cultures, start antibiotic therapy with vancomycin, piperacillin-tazobactam, and clindamycin; obtain CT or magnetic resonance image (MRI) of pelvis, surgical consult for emergent debridement

6. A 77-year-old woman with chronic obstructive pulmonary disease is brought from her skilled nursing facility to the emergency room with fever and mixed hypoxemic-hypercarbic respiratory failure. She was last hospitalized 4 months ago for a hip fracture and last received antibiotics during that hospitalization. She has no known history of multidrug resistant infections, and no risk factors for methicillin-resistant *Staphylococcus aureus* infection. Chest X-ray demonstrates a right middle lobe infiltrate, and she is admitted to the intensive care unit for hypoxemia. What is the **MOST** appropriate antibiotic choice and duration for her pneumonia?

A. Piperacillin-tazobactam for 5 to 7 days
B. Cefepime for 7 to 8 days
C. Levofloxacin for 7 to 8 days
D. Cefepime plus levofloxacin for 5 to 10 days

7. A 66-year-old man is admitted to the intensive care unit in respiratory distress. He was attending a conference in a local hotel when he developed fevers and shortness of breath, followed by mild confusion. He also has end-stage renal disease managed with thrice-weekly hemodialysis and is anuric. Chest X-ray demonstrates a patchy infiltrate in the left upper lobe. As you admit him to the intensive care unit, you are called by the emergency department for a second admission—this time for a 52-year-old woman with chronic obstructive pulmonary disease who also attended the same conference. In addition to fever and tachypnea, the second patient has a serum sodium of 119 mEq/L, diarrhea, and vomiting. Her chest X-ray demonstrates diffuse bilateral patchy infiltrates. What is the **MOST** sensitive test to diagnose the organism causing these patients' symptoms?

A. Urinary antigen
B. Polymerase chain reaction (PCR) performed on a lower respiratory tract specimen
C. Microbiologic culture of a lower respiratory tract specimen
D. Gram stain

8. You admit a 28-year-old man to the intensive care unit in July for a generalized tonic-clinic seizure in the setting of 2 days of fevers, headache, and myalgias. The patient's girlfriend tells you that they were backpacking in Tennessee's Great Smoky Mountains National Park the week before the patient became ill, and 3 weeks before he became ill they went for a hike in the woods on Massachusetts' Cape Cod. Chest X-ray is clear, and his white blood cell count is normal. Platelet count on presentation is 139,000/μL, and hemoglobin and hematocrit are normal. Two days after admission, he develops worsening thrombocytopenia and a rash. What is the **MOST** likely diagnosis?

A. Babesiosis
B. Rocky Mountain Spotted Fever (RMSF)
C. Mumps
D. Lyme disease

9. Which of the following patients should receive antiviral medication for seasonal influenza infection?

   A. A breastfeeding 32-year-old woman who is 6 weeks postpartum
   B. A 25-year-old man receiving a TNF-α antagonist for inflammatory bowel disease
   C. A 56-year-old man with cirrhosis from alcohol use
   D. Both B and C

10. A 47-year-old woman with poorly controlled insulin-dependent diabetes mellitus presents to the emergency room with diabetic ketoacidosis. She reports severe pain in her paranasal sinuses with purulent discharge from the bilateral nares for 1 day. On examination, you notice swelling of the paranasal soft tissues and a dark eschar over the left nasal mucosa. What is the **BEST** management strategy?

    A. Emergent surgical debridement and liposomal amphotericin B
    B. Emergent surgical debridement and voriconazole
    C. Blood cultures followed by vancomycin, meropenem, and clindamycin
    D. Insulin infusion plus liposomal amphotercin B plus voriconazole

# Chapter 62 ▪ Answers

**1.** Correct Answer: C

**Rationale:**

Malaria is the most common infection among returned travelers, and *P. falciparum* is the malaria species causing the vast majority of malaria infections in travelers to sub-Saharan Africa. Diagnosis is traditionally made using thick and thin peripheral blood smears but requires an experienced microscopist. Rapid diagnostic tests using immunochromatography to detect malaria antigens are also commonly used for diagnosis. Because malaria is the most common infection among returned travelers, this is the most likely cause of this patient's illness. The illness described is less likely to be Strongyloides hyperinfection syndrome (Answer A), which usually presents in an immune-suppressed patient, often with a high white blood cell count and signs of meningitis. Zika virus infection (Answer B) is often mild or asymptomatic and does not fit well with the scenario of extremis presented here. Brucellosis (Answer D) is usually an indolent infection presenting as fever of unknown origin with malaise and mylagias.

References

1. Freedman DO, Weld LH, Kozarsky PE, et al. Spectrum of disease and relation to place of exposure among ill returned travelers. *N Engl J Med*. 2006;354:119-130.
2. Wilson ME, Weld LH, Boggild A, et al. Fever in returned travelers: results from the GeoSentinel Surveillance Network. *Clin Infect Dis*. 2007;44:1560-1568.

**2.** Correct Answer: A

**Rationale:**

Empiric antibiotic selection for sepsis and septic shock should be tailored to the individual. Clinicians should take into account each patient's medical history and comorbidities, immune deficits, prior microbiologic history including known antimicrobial-resistant infections, recent hospitalization or facility contact, suspected site of infection, presence of invasive or indwelling devices, and local infection prevalence and antimicrobial resistance patterns. Most patients with septic shock should receive at least two antibiotics from two different classes (combination therapy), especially if a gram-negative pathogen is suspected. If severe *P. aeruginosa* infection is suspected, one or two antibiotics can be used empirically, but if two antibiotics are used, they should be from different classes. The broadest-spectrum antibiotic combination available is not always appropriate, as broad-spectrum antimicrobial use has the potential to drive antimicrobial resistance, confer additional toxicities, and may not benefit the patient.

References

1. De Waele JJ, Akova M, Antonelli M, et al. Antimicrobial resistance and antibiotic stewardship programs in the ICU: insistence and persistence in the fight against resistance. A position statement from ESICM/ESCMID/WAAAR round table on multi-drug resistance. *Intensive Care Med*. 2018;44:189-196.
2. Johnson MT, Reichley R, Hoppe-Bauer J, Dunne WM, Micek S, Kollef M. Impact of previous antibiotic therapy on outcome of Gram-negative severe sepsis. *Crit Care Med*. 2011;39:1859-1865.

**3.** Correct Answer: A

**Rationale:**

*Mycobacterium tuberculosis* infection can present as primary disease or reactivation of latent disease. Hemoptysis in a patient with epidemiologic risk factors for tuberculosis should raise the specter of active pulmonary tuberculosis, which is a public health concern. Management principles include admission to a negative-pressure isolation (airborne infection isolation) room. Positive-pressure or "reverse" isolation rooms are used to protect patients with systemic immune defects against airborne infections and are not used for management of tuberculosis. Healthcare workers caring for patients with suspected tuberculosis should wear N95 respirator masks or powered air-purifying respirators when entering the patient's room. Empiric tuberculosis therapy would be reasonable in this patient with signs, symptoms, and epidemiologic risk factors compatible with active pulmonary tuberculosis. Discontinuation of negative-pressure isolation in patients suspected of tuberculosis requires a determination that (1) infectious tuberculosis is unlikely, and one or more of the following: (2a) an alternative diagnosis has been established, (2b) three or more consecutive sputum samples are smear-negative for acid-fast bacteria, or (2c) two or more sputum samples are negative for *M. tuberculosis* DNA using the Xpert MTB/RIF assay. Note that these are not the same requirements for discontinuing negative-pressure isolation in patients diagnosed with active tuberculosis.

### References

1. Cowan JF, Chandler AS, Kracen E, et al. Clinical impact and cost-effectiveness of Xpert MTB/RIF testing in hospitalized patients with presumptive pulmonary tuberculosis in the United States. *Clin Infect Dis.* 2017;64:482-489.
2. Jensen PA, Lambert LA, Iademarco MF, Ridzon R. Guidelines for preventing the transmission of Mycobacterium tuberculosis in health-care settings, 2005. *MMWR Recomm Rep.* 2005;54:1-141.

**4.** Correct Answer: D

**Rationale:**

This case presentation is most consistent with nocardiosis, a classic "brain and lung" infectious syndrome (Answer D). Although nocardiosis typically presents in immune-compromised patients, up to one-third are immunocompetent. Infections caused by aerobic actinomycetes in the genus *Nocardia* are characterized by their ability to spread to any organ (especially the central nervous system) and a tendency to relapse or progress despite appropriate therapy. Glucocorticoids depress the phagocytic function of alveolar macrophages and neutrophils and alter antigen presentation and lymphocyte activation, increasing risk of bacterial and fungal infections. Virtually every chronic illness that requires prolonged glucocorticoid therapy has been associated with nocardiosis. *P. jirovecii* (formerly *carinii*) (Answer A) and sarcoidosis (Answer B) are not associated with parenchymal mass–like brain lesions. Although tuberculosis (Answer C) can present with masslike lesions in the brain parenchyma (tuberculomas), it is very uncommon to have simultaneously pulmonary and central nervous system tuberculomas/nodules. Furthermore, most patients with pulmonary tuberculosis present with cough.

### References

1. Brouwer MC, Tunkel AR, McKhann GMII, van de Beek D. Brain abscess. *N Engl J Med.* 2014;371:447-456.
2. Brook I. Microbiology and treatment of brain abscess. *J Clin Neurosci.* 2017;38:8-12.

**5.** Correct Answer: C

**Rationale:**

This scenario describes the clinical presentation of necrotizing fasciitis, specifically Fournier gangrene, a necrotizing soft tissue infection of the perineum. The microbiology of this disease comprises facultative organisms (*Escherichia coli*, *Enterococcus* spp.) and anaerobes (anaerobic or microaerophilic streptococci, *Bacteroides*, *Clostridium*, *Fusobacterium*). Thus, antimicrobial therapy should target this spectrum of bacterial pathogens and should also include clindamycin, for its antitoxin properties against toxin-producing streptococci and staphylococci. Meropenem or piperacillin-tazobactam is an appropriate component of first-line regimens, which should also include clindamycin. Patients with risk factors for methicillin-resistant *S. aureus* should also be given vancomycin or daptomycin. Hemodynamic instability is common with necrotizing soft tissue infections and requires aggressive supportive care with intravenous fluids and vasopressors. Vasopressor therapy should not be delayed until a central line can be placed, and hypotensive shock should be addressed before or simultaneously as blood cultures are drawn and antibiotics are started, and not delayed. Surgical consult should not be delayed by obtaining CT, MRI, or other imaging looking for soft tissue gas collections to support a diagnosis of necrotizing soft tissue infection. Surgical exploration is the only way to truly establish the diagnosis and obtain source control. Early surgical debridement has also been shown to improve outcomes.

### References

1. Stevens DL, Bryant AE. Necrotizing soft-tissue infections. *N Engl J Med.* 2017;377:2253-2265.
2. Sorensen MD, Krieger JN. Fournier's gangrene: epidemiology and outcomes in the general US population. *Urol Int.* 2016;97:249-259.

**6.** Correct Answer: D

**Rationale:**

In 2016, the category of healthcare-associated pneumonia was eliminated from the American Thoracic Society and Infectious Diseases Society of America guidelines, as it was thought to be overly sensitive and lead to increased, inappropriately broad, antibiotic use. The 2016 guidelines include the categories of community-acquired pneumonia (CAP), hospital-acquired pneumonia (HAP), and ventilator-associated pneumonia. The HAP category is reserved for patients who develop pneumonia at least 48 hours into hospitalization. Antibiotic choices for answers A, B, and C above are appropriate selections for HAP, although the recommended duration is generally 7 to 8 days, if the patient demonstrates sufficient clinical improvement on therapy. The patient in this scenario does not meet criteria for HAP and should be treated in a similar fashion to a patient with CAP admitted to the intensive care unit, accounting for additional risk factors. Residing in a skilled nursing facility is a risk factor for *Pseudomonas* pneumonia, and two antipseudomonal antibiotics are recommended as initial therapy. The duration of therapy can be tailored to clinical course, but no less than 5 days' and no more than 10 days' therapy is generally recommended.

References

1. Mandell LA, Wunderink RG, Anzueto A, et al. Infectious Diseases Society of America/American Thoracic Society consensus guidelines on the management of community-acquired pneumonia in adults. *Clin Infect Dis*. 2007;44(suppl 2):S27-S72.
2. Kalil AC, Metersky ML, Klompas M, et al. Management of adults with hospital-acquired and ventilator-associated pneumonia: 2016 clinical practice guidelines by the Infectious Diseases Society of America and the American Thoracic Society. *Clin Infect Dis*. 2016;63:e61-e111.

**7.** Correct Answer: B

**Rationale:**

These two patients present with Legionnaire's disease, pneumonia due to the intracellular pathogen *Legionella pneumophilia*. The scenario portrayed here likely represents an outbreak because both patients were attending the same conference. Although certain features such as gastrointestinal symptoms and hyponatremia increase suspicion of *Legionella* pneumonia, the presentation can also closely mimic other types of CAP. PCR testing of lower respiratory tract specimens is the most sensitive diagnostic assay, although exact sensitivity and specificity are difficult to determine owing to lack of a perfect reference standard. Urinary antigen testing appears to be 70% to 80% sensitive and nearly 100% specific for *Legionella* disease, and it is a reasonable alternative when PCR is not available or a lower respiratory tract specimen cannot be obtained. Culture performed on lower respiratory tract specimens is nearly 100% specific for *Legionella*, but sensitivity varies widely from <10% up to 80% and is thought to be significantly lower than PCR. Because *Legionella* is an intracellular pathogen, Gram stain plays no role in diagnosis of Legionnaire disease.

References

1. Bellew S, Grijalva CG, Williams DJ, et al. Pneumococcal and legionella urinary antigen tests in community-acquired pneumonia: prospective evaluation of indications for testing. *Clin Infect Dis*. 2018.
2. Viasus D, Di Yacovo S, Garcia-Vidal C, et al. Community-acquired Legionella pneumophila pneumonia: a single-center experience with 214 hospitalized sporadic cases over 15 years. *Medicine*. 2013;92:51-60.

**8.** Correct Answer: B

**Rationale:**

RMSF (Answer B) is the most common tick-borne illness in the United States, with a broad distribution across most of the lower 48 states. Symptoms on presentation are often nonspecific. The classic rash (which often eventually involves palms and soles) is rarely present when the patient becomes ill and commonly develops 3 to 5 days into the course of illness. RMSF has an incubation period of 2 to 14 days after being bitten by an infected tick, and many patients do not recall any tick bite. Although Lyme disease (Answer D) can cause thrombocytopenia, confusion and seizures are not common with central nervous system Lyme disease; nor is late presentation of rash. Mumps (Answer C) often begins as a nonspecific illness of fever and malaise, but rarely presents with fever or seizures, and usually involved salivary gland swelling within 2 days of developing symptoms. Babesiosis (Answer A) is also a tick-borne disease that can be contracted on Massachusetts' Cape Cod, but usually presents with anemia and does not cause seizures. Coinfections should always be considered when evaluating a patient with suspected tick-borne illness, as it is not uncommon for a single tick bite to transmit multiple infectious pathogens.

References

1. Helmick CG, Bernard KW, D'Angelo LJ. Rocky Mountain spotted fever: clinical, laboratory, and epidemiological features of 262 cases. *J Infect Dis*. 1984;150:480-488.
2. Hardstone Yoshimizu M, Billeter SA. Suspected and confirmed vector-borne Rickettsioses of North America Associated with human diseases. *Trop Med Infect Dis*. 2018;3.

**9.** Correct Answer: D

**Rationale:**

People at risk of severe seasonal influenza disease and poor outcomes include pregnant women and women up to 2 weeks postpartum; immunosuppressed patients and immunodeficient patients including people living with HIV and a CD4 T-cell count <200 cells/mL, adults over the age of 65 years, people with active malignancy, chronic liver, kidney, lung, or cardiovascular disease (except isolated hypertension), among others. When seasonal influenza is suspected or confirmed in any of these groups, prompt initiation of antiviral therapy is recommended.

References

1. Centers for Disease Control and Prevention. *Influenza Antiviral Medications: Summary for Clinicians.* https://www.cdc.gov/flu/professionals/antivirals/summary-clinicians.htm. Accessed November 21, 2018.
2. Fiore AE, Fry A, Shay D, Gubareva L, Bresee JS, Uyeki TM. Antiviral agents for the treatment and chemoprophylaxis of influenza -- recommendations of the Advisory Committee on Immunization Practices (ACIP). *MMWR Recomm Rep.* 2011;60:1-24.

**10.** Correct Answer: A

**Rationale:**

This patient has rhino-orbital mucormycosis, which is best managed with a combination of surgical debridement and broad-spectrum antifungal therapy. Voriconazole are not effective against the *Mucorales* species causing mucormycosis, nor are antibacterial agents. Treating diabetic ketoacidosis, metabolic acidosis, and reducing immune suppression are helpful adjunctive therapies, when possible. Almost all patients presenting with this disease have an underlying predisposing comorbidity, including diabetes mellitus (often with diabetic ketoacidosis), hematologic malignancy, hematopoetic stem cell transplantation, trauma, glucocorticoid treatment, solid organ transplant, AIDS, or malnutrition.

References

1. Roden MM, Zaoutis TE, Buchanan WL, et al. Epidemiology and outcome of zygomycosis: a review of 929 reported cases. *Clin Infect Dis.* 2005;41:634-653.
2. Jeong W, Keighley C, Wolfe R, et al. The epidemiology and clinical manifestations of mucormycosis: a systematic review and meta-analysis of case reports. *Clin Microbiol Infect.* 2018.

# 63

# CNS INFECTIONS

Nitin Das Kunnathu Puthanveedu and Fatima I. Adhi

1. A 55-year-old man with a history of well-controlled diabetes and hypertension presents to the emergency department (ED) with a 5-day history of worsening headache and fever. He requests that the light in his room to be turned off as it worsens his headache. Review of systems is otherwise significant only for cough productive of clear phlegm for the last 1 week and intermittent dizziness for 24 hours before presentation. His vital signs are T 102.4°F, heart rate (HR) 118 bpm, respiratory rate (RR) 24 bpm, and blood pressure (BP) 106/60 mm Hg. He is alert and oriented to time, place, and person. Systemic examination, including a detailed neurological examination, is normal except for a 2/6 ejection systolic murmur in the aortic region and mild nuchal rigidity. Kernig signs are positive. Diagnostic lumbar puncture (LP) is planned. Which of the following sequences of diagnostic and therapeutic steps is MOST appropriate for the care of this patient?

   A. Blood culture, empiric antibiotics, LP, transfer to intensive care unit (ICU), computed tomography (CT) head with contrast
   B. Blood cultures, CT head without contrast, steroids, empiric antibiotics, LP
   C. Blood cultures, LP, steroids, empiric antibiotic therapy
   D. CT head without contrast, blood cultures, LP, empiric antibiotics, steroids
   E. Blood cultures, LP, empiric antibiotic therapy, steroids, magnetic resonance imaging (MRI) of brain with gadolinium

2. A 66-year-old woman is brought to the ED after being found down in her home by her maid; no family member is reachable. On arrival, she has a BP of 80/40 mm Hg, HR 128, RR 20, temperature 102°F, and is saturating 94% on room air (RA). Her mental status is altered with a Glasgow Coma Scale (GCS) of 8, but her physical examination is otherwise normal including a nonfocal neurological examination. Soon after presentation, she has multiple emetic episodes and is intubated for airway protection. A head CT shows no signs of an acute intracranial process. A urine toxicology screen is negative. Empiric antimicrobial therapy with vancomycin and ceftriaxone is initiated after blood cultures are obtained, and she is transferred to the ICU for further care. Contact is finally established with her husband who reports that she had been having severe headaches, body aches, and fever for the past few days. He also reports that she has a history of osteoarthritis and well-controlled diabetes and was in a motor vehicle accident several years ago requiring emergent splenectomy. Her vaccination status is not known. An LP is performed approximately 13 hours after initial antibiotics administration, which shows cerebrospinal fluid (CSF) glucose 52 mg/dL, total protein 180 mg/dL, white blood cells (WBCs) 2000 cells/µL (90% neutrophils, 10% other forms), red blood cells (RBCs) 2 cells/µL. CSF gram stain is negative, and cultures have no growth at 48 hours. Multiplex polymerase chain reaction (PCR) on CSF is positive for *Neisseria meningitidis*. Which of the following interpretations of the CSF findings is MOST correct?

   A. Prior antibiotics do not affect CSF glucose or CSF protein and do not alter the yield of CSF cultures.
   B. Prior antibiotics do not affect CSF glucose or CSF protein but do alter the yield of CSF cultures.
   C. Prior antibiotics decrease both CSF glucose and CSF protein and decrease the yield of CSF cultures within a few hours of initiation.
   D. Prior antibiotics alter both CSF glucose and protein and decrease the yield of CSF cultures within a few hours of initiation.

**3.** A 42-year-old woman is admitted to the neurological ICU after presenting with worsening mentation and the finding of a new intracranial mass on MRI. She is intubated for airway protection and has a external ventricular drain (EVD) placed for management of obstructive hydrocephalus. On ICU day 1, she is afebrile and hemodynamically stable. Over the next 3 days, she has a low-grade fever (99.5-100°F), and on ICU day 5, she has a fever of 100.8°F. CSF drawn from the EVD on day 4 to day 6 shows the following results:

| PARAMETER | DAY 4 | DAY 5 | DAY 6 |
| --- | --- | --- | --- |
| CSF/serum glucose ratio | 0.7 | 0.6 | 0.5 |
| Protein | 34 mg/dL | 72 mg/dL | 108 mg/dL |
| WBC count | 48 cells/µL | 114 cells/µL | 146 cells/µL |
| Gram stain/culture | Negative | Negative | Negative |

Based on the CSF results, what is the most appropriate next step in management?

**A.** Repeat the MRI to inform further management of the intracranial disease process
**B.** Defer any intervention unless CSF cultures show any growth
**C.** Start empiric intraventricular vancomycin and cefepime
**D.** Start empiric intravenous (IV) vancomycin and cefepime

**4.** A 42-year old woman is brought to the ED from home after she was difficult to arouse from sleep in the morning. She has no significant past medical history but had been complaining of malaise for 1 week as well as new onset headache and fever for 2 days before presentation. She has not had other symptoms except for cold sores, which she gets this time every year. She had also been taking care of her 7-year-old grandson who had fevers and a severe nonproductive cough. In the ED, her vital signs are T 103°F, BP 110/70 mm Hg, HR 110, RR 22, and saturating 94% on RA. On examination, she is only responsive to noxious stimuli with eye opening and withdrawal of all four extremities. Her pupils are reactive to light bilaterally; there is no nuchal rigidity. Skin examination is normal with no visible rash. Heart, lung, and abdominal examination are unremarkable. During the examination, she has a generalized tonic-clonic seizure and is intubated for airway protection. A head CT is performed, which does not show any acute abnormality. An LP is performed, and results are pending. She is started on vancomycin, ceftriaxone, and dexamethasone for concern of bacterial meningitis. After that, a brain MRI is also performed, which shows altered signal in the left orbitofrontal cortex with enhancement on postgadolinium images. What further diagnostic and therapeutic interventions are MOST appropriate at this time?

**A.** Await results of the LP for further intervention
**B.** Add *Herpes simplex* virus (HSV) IgG to the CSF laboratory testing and begin empiric IV acyclovir
**C.** Add *Varicella zoster* virus (VZV) IgG to the CSF laboratory testing and begin empiric IV acyclovir
**D.** Add HSV PCR to the CSF laboratory testing and begin empiric IV acyclovir

**5.** A 66-year-old man is brought to the ED with a 3-week history of generalized malaise and worsening right-sided headaches not responding to acetaminophen or ibuprofen. He has a past medical history significant for hypertension, hyperlipidemia, moderate obesity, and recurrent otitis media and had an episode of pneumonia about 4 years ago. He is awake, alert, and well-oriented. Vital signs are within normal limits. Heart and lung sounds are normal, abdomen is soft and nontender, and neurological examination including cranial nerves is normal and symmetrical. Complete blood count and metabolic panel are within normal limits except for a mild leukocytosis and mild hyponatremia. Erythrocyte sedimentation rate (ESR) is 62 mm/h and a nasal swab for methicillin-resistant *Staphylococcus aureus* is negative by PCR. A CT of the head without contrast shows a single 2 cm lesion in the right temporal lobe with mild surrounding edema, which the radiologist reports as concerning for an abscess. Also seen are some microvascular ischemic changes and opacification of right mastoid air cells. The patient is started on vancomycin and piperacillin/tazobactam and transferred to the neurological ICU for further management. Which of the following changes to the antibiotic regimen is MOST appropriate for this patient

**A.** Continue vancomycin and piperacillin/tazobactam. Start voriconazole
**B.** Continue vancomycin. Stop Piperacillin/Tazobactam. Start Cefriaxone and Metronidazole
**C.** Continue Vancomycin. Stop piperacillin/tazobactam. Start ceftriaxone, metronidazole, and amphotericin B
**D.** Stop vancomycin and piperacillin/tazobactam. Start ceftriaxone and metronidazole

**6.** A previously healthy 42-year-old man is brought to the ED by his wife who noticed that he was stumbling and almost fell down on two occasions over the past few hours. He had been having nausea and vomiting for the last few days followed by global headaches and subjective fevers. This morning he woke up complaining of double vision, and his wife noticed that he was limping when he got up from his bed. In the ED, his vital signs are BP 120/80 mm Hg, HR 120, RR 20, T 102.5°F, and $O_2$ saturation 92% on RA. On examination, he was alert and oriented. Cardiovascular, respiratory, and abdominal examination were normal. He did not have nuchal rigidity, but lateral gaze of the right eye was restricted; he had mild left-sided hemiparesis and decreased sensation on the left side of the body. Laboratory data included a hemoglobin of 12.3 g/dL, WBC count 16 000/dL (90% neutrophils), platelets 235 000/dL, sodium 126 mmol/L, creatinine 1.5 mg/dL (no prior data available), aspartate aminotransferase 37 U/L, alanine aminotransferase 26 U/L, and total bilirubin 1.0 mg/dL. A CT head without contrast was obtained, which did not show any acute abnormality. He was empirically started on vancomycin and ceftriaxone for community-acquired bacterial meningitis and transferred to the floor. Overnight, his level of consciousness decreased and respiratory status deteriorated resulting in the need for intubation before being transferred to the medical ICU. Bedside electroencephalography did not show any seizure activity. He continued to spike high-grade fevers and eventually underwent an LP, which showed mild neutrophilic pleocytosis and mildly elevated protein, suggestive of aseptic meningitis but was otherwise normal. A brain MRI with contrast was planned; however, before this could happen, the patient's neurological status worsened with loss of cranial nerve reflexes and the family decided to withdraw care. Blood cultures from admission showed growth of gram-positive bacteria in two of two bottles at 48 hours, about 24 hours after the patient's death. Final pathology from autopsy reported severe inflammation of the brainstem, which led to herniation. Which of the following is true regarding the management of this patient?

**A.** Empiric therapy with acyclovir should have been started pending diagnostic workup.
**B.** Empiric therapy with ampicillin would have decreased his risk of mortality
**C.** The brain stem inflammation was an autoimmune manifestation of an occult malignancy.
**D.** Early initiation of dexamethasone may have prevented this poor outcome.

**7.** A 76-year-old male with rheumatoid arthritis managed with rituximab infusions is brought in to the ED with altered mental status. Four days before presentation, he developed fevers up to 103°F and headaches about a week after he returned from a camping trip in rural Wyoming. He was seen in his primary care physician's office 2 days ago for these symptoms and was noted to have a nonblanchable maculopapular rash over the left side of his trunk. He was managed symptomatically with antipyretics, but his headaches worsened and he was found to be confused this morning. On examination, he has limited ability to move his left lower extremity, which appears floppy. The rest of his examination is unremarkable, and no rash is seen. His complete blood profile and chemistry is normal. He has no risk factors for human immunodeficiency virus (HIV). Diagnostic workup is started for stroke, and he is empirically started on IV vancomycin, ceftriaxone, ampicillin, and acyclovir for possible meningoencephalitis. A CT head without contrast does not show an acute abnormality. An LP is performed, which reveals mildly elevated protein, normal glucose, no RBCs, and WBCs 1000 cells/μL (80% neutrophils). Gram stain is negative, and culture is pending. Brain MRI with gadolinium shows nonspecific enhancement of left basal ganglia. PCR for HSV on CSF is negative. Over the next 24 hours, his fevers persist, level of consciousness worsens, and he requires intubation for airway protection. Which of the following laboratory tests is MOST likely to reveal the etiology of his presentation?

**A.** Echovirus PCR of CSF
**B.** Echovirus PCR of serum
**C.** West Nile virus PCR of CSF
**D.** West Nile virus IgG of serum

**8.** A 38-year-old male is brought to the ED when family noticed that he was confused. Per report, he was well until about 3 weeks ago when he developed generalized malaise and a dry cough followed by daily fevers of 100.6°F to 100.8°F. Over the last week, he had been feeling increasingly short of breath. His past medical history is significant for HIV for which he is receiving highly active antiretroviral therapy (HAART), untreated hepatitis C infection complicated by cirrhosis, and smoking-related chronic obstructive pulmonary disease (COPD) for which he has been receiving prednisone 40 mg daily for the last 2 weeks. His CD4 count 1 month ago was 640 cells/mL with an undetectable HIV viral load. He has no history of opportunistic infections. On physical examination, he has normal heart sounds, coarse crackles on the right lung base, his abdomen is soft and nontender without evidence of ascites, and his neurological examination is unremarkable except that he is not oriented to time, place, or person. In the ED, laboratory data are significant for a WBC count 14 000 cells/dL, platelets 165 000/dL, creatinine 1.1 mg/dL, aspartate aminotransferase 56 U/L, alanine aminotransferase 48 U/L, alkaline phosphatase 110 U/L, and total bilirubin 0.9 mg/dL. Chest x-ray shows a right lower lobar consolidation. Two sets of blood cultures are drawn, and he is started on vancomycin and piperacillin/tazobactam. Over the next 72 hours, his oxygen requirements increase to requiring 6 L via nasal cannula and he continues to spike fevers. His increasing confusion is attributed to delirium, and he is started on lactulose for possible hepatic encephalopathy. On day 5 of admission, he is transferred to the ICU with worsening hypoxia requiring intubation. He undergoes bronchoscopy for diagnostic bronchoalveolar lavage (BAL). The initial stain shows yeast with thick capsules, and the following day cultures show growth of pigmented colonies. What is the next best step in management for this patient?

A. Check bacterial multiplex PCR on BAL fluid for identification of the causative organism
B. Check cytomegalovirus (CMV) PCR on BAL fluid and if positive, start ganciclovir
C. Start micafungin for Candida pneumonia
D. Perform an LP and if positive, start liposomal amphotericin B and flucytosine

# Chapter 63 ▪ Answers

**1.** Correct Answer: C

**Rationale:**

There are multiple factors that determine the optimal sequence of events in cases of suspected community-acquired meningitis. In an ideal scenario without any absolute indication for head imaging, a patient with suspected bacterial meningitis has blood cultures drawn, LP performed, and consideration for steroid therapy in quick succession before timely initiation of appropriate empiric antimicrobial therapy.

Appropriate empiric antimicrobial therapy should be initiated as soon as possible. A delay in the administration of appropriate antimicrobials for bacterial meningitis by 6 to 8 hours has been associated with an increased fatality risk from <5% to 45% and up to 75% for delay of 8 to 10 hours. If interventions are likely to substantially delay antimicrobial administration, the benefits of such interventions should be carefully weighed against the potential of increased mortality risk associated with delayed antimicrobial administration—if a significant delay is anticipated, antimicrobials should take precedence.

Blood cultures should always be obtained before administration of antimicrobials for any infection where microbiological diagnosis has not been achieved.

A CT head is sometimes obtained before LP to look for signs of increased intracranial pressure that can place a patient at risk of brain herniation from the sudden CSF loss during LP. However, in the absence of an absolute indication, this can inadvertently lead to increased door-to-antibiotic time, which in turn affects mortality. Therefore, screening of patients for clinical signs of raised intracranial pressure and factors that are known to predispose to complications of LP is strongly encouraged. The Infectious Diseases Society of America (IDSA) recommends a CT head before performance of LP only in the following circumstances:

- Immunocompromised state—HIV infection, non-HIV immunosuppressed conditions, or on immunosuppressive therapy
- Known central nervous system (CNS) disease such as mass lesion, recent stroke, or focal infection such as abscess
- New-onset seizures within 1 week of presentation
- Papilledema
- Abnormal level of consciousness (altered sensorium, stupor, coma)
- Focal neurological deficit

When taken together, these criteria have a negative predictive value of 97% and a negative likelihood ratio of 0.1 for an abnormal CT head. Therefore, in the absence of any of the above findings, it is deemed safe to proceed with LP without head imaging.

The administration of steroids *before or with* empiric antimicrobial therapy in patients with suspected pneumococcal meningitis has been associated with a trend toward lower mortality as well as fewer neurological sequelae, a benefit that is lost if steroids are given *after* initiation of antimicrobials. If suspicion of pneumococcal meningitis is confirmed by LP, steroid therapy should be continued for 4 days.

## References

1. Proulx N, Fréchette D, Toye B, Chan J, Kravcik S. Delays in the administration of antibiotics are associated with mortality from adult acute bacterial meningitis. *QJM*. 2005;98:291-298.
2. Young N, Thomas M. Meningitis in adults: diagnosis and management. *Intern Med J*. 2018;48:1294-1307.
3. April MD, Long B, Koyfman A. Emergency medicine myths: computed tomography of the head prior to lumbar puncture in adults with suspected bacterial meningitis – due diligence or antiquated practice? *J Emerg Med*. 2017;53:313-321.
4. Brouwer MC, McIntyre P, Prasad K, van de Beek D. Corticosteroids for acute bacterial meningitis. *Cochrane Database Syst Rev*. 2015;(9):CD004405.

**2.** Correct Answer: D

**Rationale:**

In suspected bacterial meningitis, LP should ideally precede empiric antibiotic therapy. However, multiple factors including overreliance on CT imaging before LP have increasingly led to delay in LP until after initiation of antimicrobials. Antimicrobials can affect measurements of CSF glucose, protein, and potentially other indices as well, and decrease the yield of CSF cultures making accurate diagnosis more challenging. The data on postantimicrobial CSF analysis is very limited, is largely retrospective, and mostly extrapolated to the adult population from pediatric literature. CSF culture has a reported sensitivity of 88% for microbiological diagnosis, which decreases to 70% with any prior antibiotic use and sensitivity declines further as the duration of time receiving antibiotics increases. As duration of antimicrobial therapy increases, CSF glucose levels increase and CSF protein levels decrease as compared with preantimicrobial measurements, which is likely a reflection of pathogen clearance from the CSF. Complete clearance of meningococcus from the CSF occurs within 2 hours of antimicrobial therapy initiation, and pneumococcus clearance begins around 4 hours into therapy. Other pathogens seem to be more persistent. However, it is important to note that CSF pleocytosis and neutrophilic count are not as readily affected by antibiotics, and the counts are relatively preserved even after 24 hours of antimicrobial therapy.

The following parameters predict bacterial infection with high accuracy and should therefore inform differential diagnosis even in the absence of microbiological data and regardless of administration of antimicrobial therapy:

- CSF glucose level <34 mg/dL
- CSF to blood glucose ratio <0.23
- CSF protein level >220 mg/dL
- CSF leukocytes >2000 cells/uL
- CSF absolute neutrophil count >1180 cells/$\mu$L

### References

1. Kanegaye JT, Soliemanzadeh P, Bradley JS, Lumbar puncture in pediatric bacterial meningitis: defining the time interval for recovery of cerebrospinal fluid pathogens after parenteral antibiotic pretreatment. *Pediatrics.* 2001;108:1169-1174.
2. Nigrovic LE, Malley R, Macias CG, et al. Effect of antibiotic pretreatment on cerebrospinal fluid profiles of children with bacterial meningitis. *Pediatrics.* 2008;122:726-730.
3. Venkatesh B, Scott P, Ziegenfuss M. Cerebrospinal fluid in critical illness. *Crit Care Resusc.* 2000;2:42-54.

---

**3.** Correct Answer: D

**Rationale:**

The patient has evidence of a ventriculostomy-related infection and should be treated with broad-spectrum empiric IV antimicrobial therapy.

Healthcare-associated ventriculitis and meningitis (HAVM) accounts for a significant proportion of CNS infections seen in institutions with neurosurgical facilities. However, diagnosis of HAVM based on CSF findings can be challenging especially in the setting of a known neurological disease process or recent neurosurgical intervention. The microbiology of healthcare-associated meningitis differs fundamentally from community-acquired meningitis. The most common pathogens in the healthcare setting are *Staphylococcus aureus, Staphylococcus epidermidis, Propionibacterium acnes,* and *Enterobacteriaceae* (including *Serratia* in the postoperative setting).

CSF drain–related ventriculitis has an incidence of 8% to 9% per patient or per EVD placement. However, the diagnosis is often difficult to establish in critically ill patients where clinical examination and symptomatic assessment are limited. Clinical symptoms which should raise suspicion for HAVM include CSF pleocytosis, hypoglychorrachia, increasing CSF protein and/or cell counts, and positive CSF gram stain or cultures. In general, an isolated positive CSF gram stain and/or culture is not considered diagnostic for HAVM, and contamination or colonization is more likely. Given the indolent nature of some pathogens common in this setting (eg *Staphylococcus epidermidis, Propionibacterium acnes*), CSF cultures may take several days to show growth, which may mislead clinicians and delay the diagnosis of HAVM. Lozier's classification is often used to support treatment decisions for HAVM:

**Lozier's Classification of CSF Infections in Patients With Ventriculostomy**

| CLASS | FEATURES |
| --- | --- |
| Contamination | Single positive CSF gram stain or culture with normal CSF basic chemistries and cell counts |
| Colonization | Multiple positive CSF gram stains or cultures with *same* organism with normal CSF basic chemistries and cell counts |
| Suspected ventriculostomy-related infection | CSF basic chemistries and cell counts suggestive of a developing infection, ie dropping glucose levels, increasing protein, and cell counts but with negative CSF gram stain and culture |
| Ventriculostomy-related infection | CSF chemistries as well as cell counts suggestive of infection (as with suspected infection) with one or more positive CSF gram stains or cultures in the absence of clinical symptoms other than fever |
| Ventriculitis | CSF chemistries and cell counts suggestive of infection with one or more positive CSF gram stains or cultures with clinical symptoms of meningitis other than just fever |

Empiric therapy for HAVM is directed at the common pathogens and often consists of IV vancomycin and a third or fourth generation cephalosporin to provide Pseudomonas coverage. Intrathecal therapy is usually reserved for poor response to IV therapy or when pathogens are known to have high minimum inhibitory concentrations (MICs), which are not likely to be attainable via the IV route. In a penicillin- or cephalosporin-allergic patient, aztreonam may be used instead of a cephalosporin.

### References

1. Lozier AP, Sciacca RR, Romagnoli MF, Connolly ES. Ventriculostomy-related infections: a critical review of the literature. *Neurosurgery*. 2008;62(suppl 2):688-700.
2. Tunkel AR, Hasbun R, Bhimraj A, et al. 2017 Infectious diseases Society of America's clinical practice guidelines for healthcare-associated ventriculitis and meningitis. *Clin Infect Dis*. 2017. doi:10.1093/cid/ciw861.
3. O'Horo JC, Sampathkumar P. Infections in neurocritical care. *Neurocrit Care*. 2017;27:458-467.

### 4. Correct Answer: D

**Rationale:**

The patient's presentation and imaging findings are classic for HSV encephalitis. Empiric therapy should include high-dose IV acyclovir while awaiting HSV PCR on CSF, which is the test of choice for definitive diagnosis.

Encephalitis or encephalomyelitis should be considered in the differential diagnosis for any patient presenting with behavioral changes, altered mental status, and/or depressed level of consciousness. In the absence of nuchal rigidity and peripheral symptoms, this should be high on the differential. The presence of parenchymal involvement on brain imaging is virtually diagnostic of encephalitis. Microbiological diagnosis is usually made by serological tests or PCR on CSF.

HSV is the most common cause of encephalitis (including both infectious and noninfectious causes) in adults. 90% of the cases are caused by HSV-1 during primary infection (more common in young adults) or recurrence (more common in older adults) from latent virus reactivation either as peripheral infection spreading to the CNS or de novo reactivation within the CNS. Temporal lobe involvement is pathognomic but less commonly the temporal lobe may be spared with involvement of other areas such as the orbitofrontal cortex, cingulate gyrus, or insula. This patient's presentation of an episode of orolabial herpes followed by fever, headaches, and altered consciousness is classic for HSV encephalitis. High-dose acyclovir 10 mg/kg/dose IV every 8 hours should be started empirically if HSV encephalitis is a consideration even before diagnostics are performed as mortality is high with delay in therapy. The diagnostic test of choice is HSV DNA PCR performed on CSF. This test is highly sensitive and specific but may be falsely negative very early in the course of the disease. If the clinical suspicion for HSV encephalitis is high, especially if supported by imaging findings, then acyclovir should be continued despite an initial negative PCR and an LP should be repeated with HSV PCR retesting in 3 to 7 days. Serologies are not helpful in the diagnosis of HSV encephalitis either in the serum or on CSF.

VZV is a neurotropic virus that establishes latency in ganglionic cells of the nervous system during primary infection and dermatomal reactivation can occur in times of immunocompromise (old age, immunosuppression, HIV/AIDS). CNS manifestations of infection range from strokes and subarachnoid hemorrhages to arterial ectasias, but encephalitis is also a common presentation. Unlike HSV, VZV IgG detection in CSF is more sensitive than VZV PCR for diagnosis. Treatment is with high-dose IV acyclovir as well.

### References

1. Rabinstein AA. Herpes virus encephalitis in adults: current knowledge and old myths. *Neurol Clin*. 2017;35:695-705.
2. Gaieski DF, O'Brien NF, Hernandez R. Emergency neurologic life support: meningitis and encephalitis. *Neurocrit Care*. 2017;27:124-133.
3. Gilden D, Cohrs RJ, Mahalingam R, Nagel MA. Varicella zoster virus vasculopathies: diverse clinical manifestations, laboratory features, pathogenesis, and treatment. *Lancet Neurol*. 2009;8:731-740.

### 5. Correct Answer: D

**Rationale:**

This patient has a temporal lobe abscess associated with recurrent otitis media infection and mastoiditis. He does not have a history of transplantation or immunocompromise, and MRSA PCR is negative. Consequently there is no need of antimicrobial coverage for methicillin-resistant *Staphylococcus aureus* (MRSA), atypical bacteria, fungi, or parasites. He should be empirically treated with a third-generation cephalosporin and metronidazole.

Although cryptogenic brain abscesses do occur, most focal brain parenchymal infections are associated with either a contiguous focus of infection (dental infection, otitis media, mastoiditis, sinusitis, meningitis), introduced directly by disruption of physical barriers in the area (recent dental or neurological procedure, head trauma), or via hematogenous spread from distant source (endocarditis, lung infection). When the source is adjacent, there is usually only a solitary abscess, whereas multiple abscesses are commonly seen with hematogenous spread from more distant sources. The location of the abscess also can provide some clues to the etiology. The causative organisms in these cases are typically the ones causing the primary infection. However, underlying host characteristics can predispose to brain abscesses by unusual or atypical bacteria, parasites, and/or fungi, for example in patients with HIV, solid organ transplant (SOT), hematopoietic stem cell transplant (HSCT), neutropenia, other forms of immunosuppression, or in those with diabetes and cyanotic heart disease (see table). The source of infection and the predisposing factors should therefore be taken into consideration while designing an empiric antimicrobial regimen.

**Brain—common culprit organisms and location where abscesses are commonly seen**

| HOST CHARACTERISTIC | ORGANISMS | LOCATION OF ABSCESS |
|---|---|---|
| **HIV infection** | Toxoplasma, Cryptococcus, Nocardia and Mycobacterium | Middle cerebral artery (MCA) distribution |
| **Neutropenia** | Aerobic gram negative bacilli, Fungal organisms such as Aspergillus, Mucorales, Candida | Middle cerebral artery distribution |
| **Transplantation** | Fungal organisms such as Aspergillus, Candida, Mucorales. Toxoplasma, Mycobacterium, Nocardia | Middle cerebral artery distribution |
| **Cyanotic heart disease** | Streptococcus and Hemophilus | Middle cerebral artery distribution |

**Common culprit organisms for brain abscess based on route of entry**

| ROUTE OF ENTRY | ORGANISMS | LOCATION OF ABSCESS |
|---|---|---|
| **Neurosurgery or penetrating trauma** | Staphylococcus aureus, Staphylococcus epidermidis, Streptococcus, Enterobacteriaceae | Depends on site of neurosurgery |
| **Otitis media or mastoiditis** | Streptococcus, Bacteroides, Enterobacteriaceae | Inferior temporal lobe and cerebellum |
| **Paranasal sinusitis** | Streptococcus, Bacteroides, Enterobacteriaceae | Frontal lobe (especially frontal/ethmoid sinus infection) and temporal lobe |
| **Dental infection** | Polymicrobial infection—Fusobacterium, Prevotella, Actinomyces, Streptococcus | Frontal lobe |
| **Hematogenous spread** Lung abscess, empyema Endocarditis | Nocardia, anaerobes such as Fusobacterium or Bacteroides. Staphylococcus aureus, Streptococcus | Multiple brain abscesses at gray-white junction usually in the middle cerebral artery distribution |

Based on the principles discussed above, the empiric antibiotic therapy for suspected brain abscess can be summarized as:

- Empiric coverage in an immunocompetent patient with a suspected or confirmed contiguous route of entry of infection such as otitis media/mastoiditis or paranasal sinusitis is a combination of third-generation cephalosporin (eg ceftriaxone) plus metronidazole for anaerobic coverage.
- In cryptogenic cases where there is no identifiable source and MRSA is a potential pathogen, vancomycin should be added to the basic empiric regimen of third-generation cephalosporin plus metronidazole.
- In the setting of prior neurosurgical intervention or in trauma, an antipseudomonal cephalosporin (eg cefepime or ceftazidime) should be used in combinmation with vancomycin to cover for healthcare associated MRSA.
- In HIV-infected patients, empiric coverage for toxoplasmosis, Cryptococcus, and Nocardia should be considered depending on the clinical scenario. Therapy for tuberculosis is reserved for confirmed cases or in whom other diagnoses have been reasonably excluded and, in general, should not be started as part of an empiric regimen.
- For SOT and HSCT recipients, empiric coverage for toxoplasmosis and Nocardia should be considered as well as empiric fungal coverage for Candida and/or Aspergillus.

References

1. Brouwer MC, Coutinho JM, van de Beek D, Clinical characteristics and outcome of brain abscess: systematic review and meta-analysis. *Neurology.* 2014;82:806-813.
2. Brouwer MC, Tunkel AR, McKhann GM II, van de Beek D. Brain abscess. *N Engl Med.* 2014;371:447-456.
3. Brook I. Microbiology and treatment of brain abscess. *J Clin Neurosci.* 2017;38:8-12.

**6.** Correct Answer: B

**Rationale:**

*Listeria monocytogenes* can cause invasive CNS disease in otherwise healthy individuals requiring a very high level of suspicion for diagnosis. Early administration of ampicillin, which is the treatment of choice, significantly alters morbidity and mortality.

Inflammation of the brainstem, also known as rhomboencephalitis, is a well-described syndrome that can result from a variety of infectious and noninfectious insults. In immunocompromised individuals such as those with HIV and slowly progressing infections such as *Cryptococcus* and tuberculosis are seen more commonly, but HSV-1 and *Listeria monocytogenes* can affect immunocompetent individuals as well. In contrast to its other manifestations, *Listeria monocytogenes* rhomboencephalitis typically occurs in young healthy individuals. This syndrome is distinct from the more commonly seen *Listeria* meningitis in neonates, in the immunosuppressed and elderly. It classically presents as a biphasic illness with 72 to 96 hours of prodromal symptoms consisting most commonly of fevers, headaches, nausea, and vomiting, which are followed by rather rapid progression of focal neurological deficits involving the brainstem. Meningeal signs may be completely absent in these patients, and CSF analysis may or may not be suggestive of meningoencephalitis. Blood cultures are positive in up to half of these cases, and CSF PCR for *Listeria monocytogenes* (as part of multiplex panels) may aid in diagnosis. The treatment of choice is ampicillin, with trimethoprim-sulfamethoxazole as an alternative in the setting of penicillin allergy. Mortality without early initiation of adequate therapy is up to 50%. Even with treatment, high mortality and morbidity from persistent neurological deficits have been reported. As this syndrome occurs in young, otherwise healthy individuals in whom *Listeria* is not usually considered a causative organism of meningitis and for whom *Listeria* coverage is not usually included in empiric antimicrobial regimen for CNS infections, the diagnosis requires high index of suspicion and early initiation of empiric treatment while awaiting diagnostic studies.

Consideration should also be given to noninfectious etiologies of rhomboencephalitis including multiple sclerosis and autoimmune or paraneoplastic syndromes; however, antimicrobial therapy should be started early while workup is in process for other noninfectious etiologies. Although HSV can cause rhomboencephalitis, the presence of bacteremia with *Listeria* argues against this being the etiological agent. The addition of dexamethasone during treatment of invasive Listeriosis was associated with a trend toward worsened outcomes in a large French study and is therefore discouraged.

References

1. Charlier C, Perrodeau É, Leclercq A, et al. Clinical features and prognostic factors of listeriosis: the MONALISA national prospective cohort study. *Lancet Infect Dis.* 2017;17:510–519.
2. Miranda González G, Orellana PP, Dellien ZH, Switt RM. Listeria monocytogenes rhomboencephalitis. Report of three cases. *Rev Med Chil.* 2009;137:1602-1606.
3. Abbs A, Nandakumar T, Bose P, Mooraby D. Listeria rhomboencephalitis. *Pract Neurol.* 2012;12:131-132.

**7.** Correct Answer: C

**Rationale:**

The patient has a classical presentation for West Nile virus meningoencephalitis. The diagnostic test of choice is measurement of West Nile IgM in the CSF unless there is concern for impaired antibody production in which case PCR on CSF can be helpful.

West Nile is the most common mosquito-borne illness in the United States. It was first reported in an outbreak in New York City in 1999, but the disease has spread rapidly across the continent and has now been reported from almost all continental states in the United States. Culex mosquitoes are primary vectors of transmission, which occurs seasonally in summer and fall. Transmission has also been reported via blood transfusion, organ transplantation, breastfeeding, and even transplacentally. Eighty percent of infections are asymptomatic and if present, symptoms are usually limited to a brief flulike illness with or without a nonspecific maculopapular rash, which is present for hours to days. Neuroinvasive disease is seen in less than 1% of cases and has three distinct presentations–acute flaccid paralysis, encephalitis, and meningitis (very rare in isolation)–although a combination of these presentation may also be seen. Meningismus is often absent, and LP usually reveals a mild aseptic meningitis picture without any predilection for lymphocyte or neutrophil predominance. When history is suggestive, diagnosis is usually made by West Nile virus IgM in the CSF. Serum IgM can also be supportive. Serologies may be negative early on in the disease, and a convalescent titer should be checked if suspicion remains high. IgM is not an option in the answers for this question; IgG in CSF or serum is insensitive in the acute phase. The next best diagnostic option is West Nile virus PCR in CSF. West Nile virus is notable in that unlike most other viruses, PCR is less sensitive and becomes negative very early on in the disease process. In patients who have known impairment of antibody production—either from an underlying disease such as chronic lymphocytic leukemia or iatrogenic (as in this case) from rituximab, antibody testing is not reliable and therefore PCR is very useful. It should be noted that West Nile virus is *not* included in most commercially available viral PCR panels and West Nile virus–specific PCR needs to be specifically sent to a reference laboratory. Most state labs and the Centers for Disease Control and Prevention (CDC) offer West Nile virus testing.

The above presentation of encephalitis with aseptic meningitis and flaccid paralysis following a prodrome of fevers, headaches, and transient maculopapular rash after a camping trip is not consistent with Echovirus or Coxsackie virus infection—these viruses typically cause self-limited aseptic meningitis.

### References

1. Kramer LD, Li J, Shi PY. West Nile virus. *Lancet Neurol.* 2007;6:171-181.
2. Montgomery RR, Murray KO. Risk factors for West Nile virus infection and disease in populations and individuals. *Expert Rev Anti Infect Ther.* 2015;13:317-325.
3. Curren EJ, Lehman J, Kolsin J. et al. West Nile virus and other nationally notifiable arboviral diseases – United States, 2017. *MMWR Morb Mortal Wkly Rep.* 2018;67:1137-1142.

**8.** Correct Answer: D

**Rationale:**

This scenario is concerning for disseminated cryptococcosis involving the lungs and meninges. LP should therefore be performed to measure opening pressure and to establish whether CNS involvement is present as this would directly affect management.

*Cryptococcus neoformans* is one of the most common causes of meningitis in HIV positive individuals and usually occurs when CD4 counts fall below 100 cells/mL. *Cryptococcus* is being increasingly recognized as causative of lung, CNS, and disseminated disease in other immocompromised populations including organ or stem cell transplantation, receiving other forms of immunosuppression, and in patients with diabetes. Cirrhosis, which leads to impaired humoral as well as cell-mediated immunity, is also considered to be a risk factor for cryptococcosis. Even in the absence of any of these risks, immunocompetent individuals can also occasionally be affected. The primary mode of transmission is inhalation of the fungus with dissemination from the lung through hematogenous spread. Invasive cryptococcal disease classically presents as a meningoencephalitis, but lung involvement in the form of lobar pneumonia, nodules, or even cavitary lesions is common in HIV-negative individuals either alone or concomitant with CNS infection. Skin involvement may occur with a variable presentation ranging from papular rash to cellulitis and even ulceration. cryptococcal meningitis is usually an indolent and subacute process presenting with a few weeks of headache, malaise, fever, and/or altered mental status. It is uncommon to have rapid progression of disease with significant neurological impairment although that can occur. Signs of meningeal irritation may or may not be present.

Whenever a diagnosis of extraneural cryptococcosis is made, including that of isolated Cryptococcemia, an LP is indicated to establish CNS involvement. CNS cryptococcosis is treated with amphotericin ideally in combination with flucytosine, whereas fluconazole alone may otherwise be sufficient for isolated lung, skin, or other organ disease. Additionally, intracranial pressures may be very high in cryptococcal meningitis in which case repeat LPs for therapeutic drainage or drain/shunt placement may be indicated. Other than high opening pressures, the CSF analysis is usually of limited utility with low to normal glucose, mildly elevated protein, and mild, if any, pleocytosis. Culture of CSF remains the gold standard for diagnosis. The identification of cryptococcal antigen in the CSF has very high sensitivity and specificity and is also useful for monitoring the effect of treatment. Serum cryptococcal antigen is also highly sensitive for meningoencephalitis (not for other organs) and if positive, is sufficient to rule in CNS involvement in patients with an absolute contraindication to LP.

Although the patient's HIV is well controlled, his steroid use and cirrhosis place him at risk for cryptococcosis. The presence of non-Candida yeast in the BAL, which grows with pigmented colonies (due to melanin production) on culture is characteristic of *Cryptococcus neoformans*. Candida, CMV, typical bacterial pneumonia, or nontuberculous mycobacterial disease would not fit this clinical picture.

### References

1. Abassi M, Boulware DR, Rhein J. Cryptococcal meningitis: diagnosis and management update. *Curr Trop Med Rep.* 2015;2:90-99.
2. Asawavichienjinda T, Sitthi-Amorn C, Tanyanont V, Serum cyrptococcal antigen: diagnostic value in the diagnosis of AIDS-related cryptococcal meningitis. *J Med Assoc Thai.* 1999;82:65-71.
3. Chuang YM, Ho YC, Chang HT, et al. Disseminated cryptococcosis in HIV-uninfected patients. *Eur J Clin Microbiol Infect Dis.* 2008;27:307-310.

# 64

# HEAD AND NECK, UPPER AIRWAY INFECTIONS

Ilan Mizrahi

1. A 19-year-old woman presents with 5 days of progressive swelling around her right eye. She reports a week of prior nasal pain. On examination, her right eyelid is swollen, the globe is proptotic, and eye movement is limited by pain. Visual acuity is intact. Vital signs are temperature 38°C, HR 94 beats/min, BP 128/76 mm Hg. A CT scan demonstrates inflammation of extraocular muscles, fat stranding, and anterior displacement of the globe, with frontal sinusitis. There is no evidence on CT of intracranial inflammation, nor any vascular compromise. While awaiting the results of blood cultures, which of the following antibiotic regimens is MOST appropriate to administer at this time?

   A. Levofloxacin
   B. Vancomycin and metronidazole
   C. Vancomycin and ceftriaxone
   D. Piperacillin-tazobactam

2. A 55-year-old male with no medical history presents with headache which has lasted for the last 8 days. Approximately 2 weeks ago, he had a furuncle adjacent to the right nares drained. This morning he developed fever, diplopia, and right eye ptosis. On examination, he is febrile to 38.4°C, somnolent but arousable, and hemodynamically stable. He has ptosis and proptosis of the right eye, with a dilated pupil. Neurologic examination shows right third and fourth nerve palsy and decreased sensation on the right side of his face. A high-resolution CT scan with contrast shows regions of decreased enhancement, thickening of the lateral walls, and bulging of the cavernous sinus. Which is the MOST likely causative organism of the infection?

   A. *Rhizopus*
   B. *Staphylococcus aureus*
   C. *Streptococcus pneumoniae*
   D. *Fusobacterium*

3. A 28-year-old woman presents with increasing pain and progressive swelling of her neck over the last day. She recently underwent a dental extraction for an abscess but did not complete her course of antibiotics. She denies any respiratory difficulty or distress. On examination, her neck is inflamed, erythematous, with areas of fluctuance and crepitus on palpation. She is to be taken emergently for surgical debridement. After cultures are obtained in the operating room, what is the MOST appropriate antibiotic regimen to administer?

   A. Vancomycin and clindamycin
   B. Meropenem
   C. Piperacillin-tazobactam and vancomycin
   D. Meropenem and vancomycin and clindamycin

4. A 55-year-old male with acute respiratory distress syndrome (ARDS) and ventilator-associated pneumonia (VAP) due to a pansensitive *Klebsiella* continues to have fevers and a persistently elevated white blood cell count. Blood, sputum, and urine cultures remain negative. His medical history includes prior chest radiation, atrial fibrillation currently managed with a heparin gtt, and a prior cholecystectomy. He is tolerating tube feeding via a nasogastric tube and has solid formed stool. Which of the following diagnostic tests is MOST likely helpful?

A. CT head
B. Right-upper-quadrant ultrasound
C. Difficile toxin testing
D. Lower extremity duplex ultrasound

5. A 43-year-old man presented to the emergency department with complaints of dysphagia and fever. He has felt ill and unable to eat for 2 days. He has a history of type 2 diabetes and reports frequent alcohol use. On examination, he is noted to have poor dentition and is drooling. The floor of the mouth is firm, and the submandibular glands are enlarged and tender. Laboratory testing reveals a leukocytosis to 20,000. He is treated with ampicillin-sulbactam and clindamycin and admitted to the ICU. Over the next 4 hours, he complains of increasing tongue swelling and shortness of breath. Which of the following is the more appropriate next step in management?

A. Proceed to the OR for intubation or tracheostomy
B. Proceed with intubation in the ICU
C. Administer bronchodilators
D. Drain the submandibular gland

# Chapter 64 ▪ Answers

**1.** Correct Answer: C

**Rationale:**
This patient's clinical presentation and CT findings are characteristic of orbital cellulitis, an infection involving the contents of the orbit. Orbital cellulitis may cause loss of vision and even loss of life. It is distinguished from preseptal cellulitis (a less severe infection of the anterior portion of the eyelid) by ophthalmoplegia, pain with eye movements, proptosis, and characteristic findings of infection on CT including inflammation of extraocular muscles, fat stranding, and anterior displacement of the globe. CT or MR venography should also be performed to rule out cavernous sinus thrombosis. Most patients with uncomplicated orbital cellulitis can be treated with antibiotics alone. A broad-spectrum regimen should be administered to target *Staphylococcus aureus* (including methicillin-resistant *Staphylococcus aureus* [MRSA]), *Streptococcus pneumoniae,* and other streptococci, as well as gram-negative bacilli. When intracranial extension is suspected, the regimen should also include coverage for anaerobes. Of the options provided for this patient, vancomycin and ceftriaxone would be the most appropriate coverage regimen. Levofloxacin or piperacillin-tazobactam alone or the combination of vancomycin and metronidazole would not be broad enough to cover likely pathogens. Moreover, since there is minimal concern for intracranial involvement, the anaerobic coverage of metronidazole is not needed.

References
1. Seltz LB, Smith J, Durairaj VD, et al. Microbiology and antibiotic management of orbital cellulitis. *Pediatrics.* 2011;127:e566.
2. Amin N, Syed I, Osborne S. Assessment and management of orbital cellulitis. *Br J Hosp Med (Lond).* 2016;77:216-220.

**2.** Correct Answer: B

**Rationale:**
This patient presents with concern for septic cavernous sinus and thrombosis. The multiple trabecula of the cavernous sinus acts as sieves to trap bacteria and consequently makes it the most frequent dural sinus to become thrombosed. Infections of the face including the orbit (orbital cellulitis), around the nose, and soft palate can spread to the cavernous sinus from the facial veins and the pterygoid plexus. In this patient, bacterial spread likely resulted from the drained furuncle. Cranial nerves III, IV, ophthalmic ($V_1$) and maxillary($V_2$) branches of the trigeminal nerve, and VI all travel through the cavernous sinus. Headache and cranial nerve deficits should alert the clinician to the possibility of this condition. CT or MR venography can readily identify septic cavernous sinus thrombosis characteristically demonstrating regions of decreased or irregular enhancement, thickening of the lateral walls, and bulging of the sinus.

The causative organism reflects the primary site of infection. *Staphylococcus aureus* accounts for 70% of all infections, and community-acquired MRSA is increasingly reported. Less commonly streptococci (*Streptococcus pneumoniae*) are found. Anaerobes (*Fusobacterium, Bacteroides*) most often occur with dental or tonsillar infections. Fungal pathogens (*Rhizopus*) have been reported but are quite rare. High-dose intravenous antibiotics against the most probable organisms should be instituted promptly and continued for a prolonged period (at least 3 weeks) to ensure sterilization.

References
1. Ferro JM, Canhao P, Bousser MG, et al. Cerebral vein and dural sinus thrombosis in elderly patients. *Stroke.* 2005;36:1927.
2. Fam D, Saposnik G. Critical care management of cerebral venous thrombosis. *Curr Opin Crit Care.* 2016;22:113.

**3. Correct Answer: D**

**Rationale:**

The finding of severe pain, fluctuance, and crepitus in the setting of recent infection is typical of a necrotizing soft-tissue infection. Necrotizing soft-tissue infection is a surgical emergency that requires immediate debridement. Necrotizing soft-tissue infections of the head and neck infection can rapidly spread leading to mediastinitis and possibly death from associated complications. These infections can result from a disruption in the oropharyngeal mucus membrane such as following surgery for a dental infection. The infection is usually polymicrobial caused by mouth anaerobes (fusobacteria, anaerobic streptococci, *Bacteroides*). Monomicrobial infections due to group A *Streptococcus* can also occur. Empiric treatment of a necrotizing infection is three-pronged and should include: (1) coverage for gram-positive, gram-negative, and anaerobic organisms with a carbapenem (meropenem) or beta-lactam-beta-lactamase inhibitor (piperacillin-tazobactam, or ampicillin-sulbactam); (2) coverage for methicillin-resistant *Staphylococcus aureus* (vancomycin); (3) clindamycin for its antitoxin effects against streptococci and staphylococci.

**References**

1. Reynolds SC, Chow AW. Severe soft tissue infections of the head and neck. *Lung*. 2009;187:271.
2. Vincent JL, Abraham E, Moore FA., et al, eds. *Textbook of Critical Care*. 7th ed. Philadelphia, PA: Elsevier; 2017.

**4. Correct Answer: A**

**Rationale:**

This patient has evidence of infection despite treatment for VAP. Of the options provided, sinusitis is the most plausible etiology given the clinical presentation. Risk factors in ICU patients for nosocomial sinusitis include endotracheal intubation, nasal colonization with gram-negative organisms, and enteral feeding via a nasogastric tube. Nosocomial sinusitis should be suspected in all intubated patients who have a fever without an obvious source, especially if there is purulent nasal drainage. CT is more sensitive than plan radiography and will show sinus opacification. Culture of sinus fluid is the gold standard for diagnosis. The pathogenic organisms are similar to those causing VAP (*Staphylococcus aureus, Streptococcus, Klebsiella,* and other gram-negative bacilli). Treatment involves systemic antibiotics targeted against the pathogen grown from sinus fluid culture. Initial treatment should broadly target the common pathogens similar to initial antibiotic choices for VAP. Adjunctive therapies include saline irrigation, removal of nasal tubes, and nasal decongestants. Right-upper-quadrant ultrasound would be of little use in this patient as he has had a cholecystectomy and therefore does not have acalculus cholecystitis. He is tolerating tube feeding and has solid, formed stool making *C. difficile* infection extremely less likely. Although deep venous thrombosis may be a cause of persistent fevers, he is already therapeutically anticoagulated with heparin.

**References**

1. Holzapfel L, Chastang C, Demingeon G, et al. A randomized study assessing the systematic search for maxillary sinusitis in nasotracheally mechanically ventilated patients: influence of nosocomial maxillary sinusitis on the occurrence of ventilator-associated pneumonia. *Am J Respir Crit Care Med*. 1999;159:695.
2. Van Zanten AR, Dixon JM, Nipshagen MD, et al. Hospital-acquired sinusitis is a common cause of fever of unknown origin in orotracheally intubated critically ill patients. *Crit Care*. 2005;9:R583.

**5. Correct Answer: A**

**Rationale:**

This patient presents with an infection of the submandibular space (Ludwig angina). This acute condition can progress to critical airway compromise, making intubation extremely difficult. This bacterial infection often occurs after a tooth abscess but can also follow other mouth infections or injuries. It is more common in patients with diabetes and neutropenia. Common presenting signs and symptoms include dysphagia, mouth pain, drooling, and fever. The submandibular tissues are classically described as "woody," not fluctuant, often without any true drainable collection. Typical pathogens include mouth anaerobes (*Fusobacterium*), streptococci, or *Staphylococcus aureus,* and initial antibiotics should broadly target all of these organisms, including MRSA. If untreated, the infection can progress with necrosis of the tongue, aspiration, and death from airway obstruction. If the airway becomes compromised, a surgical airway (tracheotomy or cricothyroidotomy) is typically recommended as first line for airway management. Direct laryngoscopy may be exceedingly difficult and attempting it in a resource-limited environment such as the ICU may lead to further complications. Bronchodilators are unlikely to relieve the airway obstruction. While drainage may be indicated, this patient is acutely decompensating, and the airway should be secured before attempting further procedures.

**References**

1. Reynolds SC, Chow AW. Severe soft tissue infections of the head and neck. *Lung*. 2009;187:271.
2. Joshua J, Scholten E, Schaerer D, Mafee MF, Alexander TH, Crotty Alexander LE. Otolaryngology in critical care. *Ann Am Thorac Soc*. 2018;15:643-654.

# 65

# CARDIOVASCULAR INFECTIONS

Marvin G. Chang

1. A 19-year-old male with no past medical history presented to the emergency room with pelvic fracture after being hit by a car. A central line was placed for administering vasopressors and volume resuscitation. Three days later, the patient became febrile, and blood cultures were obtained revealing *Staphylococcus aureus*. Vancomycin was started, and repeat blood cultures 2 days later are negative. Transthoracic echocardiogram is unremarkable. Which of the following is the next best step?

   A. Transesophageal echocardiogram
   B. Antibiotic lock therapy
   C. Central line removal
   D. Antibiotics for 7 days

2. A 74-year-old male with end-stage renal disease (ESRD) and recent pulmonary embolism on apixaban presents to the intensive care unit from dialysis clinic with a 6-day history of fevers and chills. He received hemodialysis through a tunneled central venous catheter. Blood cultures drawn in the emergency room are all positive for gram-positive cocci that are later identified as coagulase-negative *Staphylcoccus* (CNS). The patient is hemodynamically stable with significant thrombocytopenia to 15 and is methicillin-resistant *Staphylococcus aureus* (MRSA) negative. What is the next best step in this patient's management?

   A. Tunneled dialysis catheter exchange over a guidewire
   B. Obtain transthoracic or transesophageal echocardiogram
   C. Obtain blood cultures every 48 hours until negative
   D. Switch from vancomycin to oxacillin

3. A 67-year-old male with an implantable cardioverter defibrillator (ICD) is admitted with urosepsis. Blood cultures reveal methicillin-sensitive *Staphylococcus aureus*, and transesophageal echocardiogram reveals a 1.9 cm mass on the ICD lead with no evidence of endocarditis. Which of the following is the MOST appropriate management regarding this patient's ICD and leads?

   A. Interventional transvenous lead extraction
   B. Interventional transvenous lead extraction and device explantation
   C. Consider explant only if continued bacteremia
   D. Surgical lead extraction and device explantation

4. A 79-year-old female with ESRD presents to the intensive care unit with 7 days of worsening dyspnea on exertion, lower extremity edema, malaise, and chest pain that radiates toward the left shoulder that is worse with inspiration. Vitals are temperature 38.5°F, blood pressure 105/90 mm Hg, heart rate 95 beats/min, and respiratory rate 21/min. Electrocardiogram (EKG) reveals ST elevations in leads I, II, III, aVF, and aVL. What is the MOST common etiology of this patient's condition?

   A. Viral infection
   B. Myocardial infarction
   C. Bacterial infection
   D. Renal failure

**5.** A 69-year-old female with history of rheumatic mitral stenosis presents to the intensive care unit with 5 days of fevers and night sweats, malaise, and multiple small erythematous lesions on the soles of the feet. The patient develops an escalating pressor requirement, and a bedside echocardiogram reveals severe mitral regurgitation that was not seen a month earlier on a formal echocardiogram. Which of the following is the MOST likely organism to be isolated from blood cultures?

    **A.** CNS
    **B.** *Entercocci*
    **C.** Viridins *Streptococcus*
    **D.** *Staphylococcus aureus*

# Chapter 65 ▪ Answers

**1.** Correct Answer: C.

**Rationale:**

This patient with likely *Staphylococcus aureus* catheter-related blood stream infection (CRBSI) without evidence of endocarditis should have catheters removed and receive antibiotic therapy for 14 days. Salvage therapy using catheter exchange over a guidewire or antibiotic lock therapy should generally be avoided, given increased morbidity, mortality, treatment failure, and recurrence in patients with *Staphylococcus aureus* CRBSI. In spite of a negative transthoracic echocardiogram, a transesophageal echocardiogram is necessary in patients with signs or symptoms of endocarditis, prior history of endocarditis, positive blood cultures after 72 hours despite appropriate antibiotic treatment, a previously placed port or other indwelling vascular device, hemodialysis, a prosthetic valve, cardiac structural and valvular abnormalities, an implantable pacemaker, an intravenous drug abuse, and absence of a reasonable reason for infection.

References

1. Mirrakhimov AE, Jesinger ME, Ayach T, Gray A. When does *S aureus* bacteremia require transesophageal echocardiography? *Cleve Clin J Med*. 2018;85(7):517-520.
2. Chaves F, Garnacho-montero J, Del pozo JL, et al. Diagnosis and treatment of catheter-related bloodstream infection: clinical guidelines of the Spanish Society of Infectious Diseases and Clinical Microbiology and (SEIMC) and the Spanish Society of Spanish Society of Intensive and Critical Care Medicine and Coronary Units (SEMICYUC). *Med Intensiva*. 2018;42(1):5-36.

**2.** Correct Answer: A.

**Rationale:**

This patient likely has CNS CRBSI. Central line removal is often advocated but is controversial in the setting of CNS CRBSI especially in hemodynamically stable and immunocompetent patients without signs of infection and foreign bodies. Salvage therapy using antibiotic lock therapy or a guidewire exchange of his tunneled dialysis catheter can be considered as an alternative treatment for catheter removal especially given this patient's significant coagulopathy and risk for complications related to removing and placing a new central line. For organisms other than *Staphylococcus aureus* and candida, repeat blood cultures are not necessary unless salvage therapy has been used to ensure resolution of bacteremia. Antibiotic course is typically 7 days if the catheter is removed and 14 days if salvage therapy is used. CNS CRBSI should be initially treated with vancomycin until sensitivities return because of the high incidence of resistance to methicillin, cephalosporins, and many other antibiotics. Echocardiogram is not necessary in the setting of CNS CRBSI unless there is persistent bacteremia.

References

1. Raad I, Kassar R, Ghannam D, Chaftari AM, Hachem R, Jiang Y. Management of the catheter in documented catheter-related coagulase-negative staphylococcal bacteremia: remove or retain? *Clin Infect Dis*. 2009;49(8):1187-1194.
2. Chaves F, Garnacho-montero J, Del pozo JL, et al. Diagnosis and treatment of catheter-related bloodstream infection: clinical guidelines of the Spanish Society of Infectious Diseases and Clinical Microbiology and (SEIMC) and the Spanish Society of Spanish Society of Intensive and Critical Care Medicine and Coronary Units (SEMICYUC). *Med Intensiva*. 2018;42(1):5-36.

**3.** Correct Answer: B.

**Rationale:**

Patients with cardiac implantable electronic devices should have complete system (ie, leads and device) explanted if blood cultures are positive, and there are valvular and/or lead vegetations seen on echocardiography. Interventional transvenous lead extractions can be performed for vegetations <2 cm on leads, whereas surgical extraction should be considered if vegetations are >2 cm because of risk for pulmonary embolism. Reimplantation can be considered when blood cultures are negative for at least 72 hours but often times is not necessary, given that many patients no longer meet current criteria for device implantation.

### Reference

1. Döring M, Richter S, Hindricks G. The diagnosis and treatment of pacemaker-associated infection. *Dtsch Arztebl Int.* 2018;115(26):445-452.

**4.** Correct Answer: A.

**Rationale:**

This patient is describing signs and symptoms of acute pericarditis, which most commonly occurs because of a viral infection with patients often recalling a nonspecific prodrome of fever, malaise, and pleuritic chest pain that radiates toward the left shoulder and is worse with inspiration and relieved by leaning forward. The other choices describe other less frequent causes of acute pericarditis. ST elevations are diffusely seen in all or many EKG leads in acute pericarditis and can be differentiated from a ST elevation myocardial infarction by not having ST depressions in reciprocal leads (ie, ST elections in both high lateral leads I and aVL and reciprocal inferior leads II, III, and aVF).

### Reference

1. Goyle KK, Walling AD. Diagnosing pericarditis. *Am Fam Physician.* 2002;66(9):1695-1702.

**5.** Correct Answer: D.

**Rationale:**

This patient satisfies the Duke criteria for the diagnosis of endocarditis with the major criteria satisfied by endocardial involvement assessed with echocardiogram and the three minor criteria satisfied by the patient's fevers, Janeway lesions, and predisposing heart condition of rheumatic heart disease. The most common organisms for endocarditis from most to least common include *Staphylococcus aureus* (31%), viridans *Streptococcus* (17%), CNS (11%), *Enterococci* (11%), *Streptococcus bovis* (7%), other *Streptococci* (5%), fungi (2%), gram-negative HACEK bacilli (2%), and gram-negative non-HACEK bacilli (2%). Endocardial involvement as a major criteria can be satisfied by new valvular regurgitant lesions, vegetations, abscesses, or dehiscence of prosthetic valves.

### Reference

1. Pierce D, Calkins BC, Thornton K. Infectious endocarditis: diagnosis and treatment. *Am Fam Physician.* 2012;85(10):981-986.

# 66

# GASTROINTESTINAL AND INTRA-ABDOMINAL INFECTIONS

Erika Lore Brinson and Kristina Sullivan

1. A 38-year-old man who recently returned from visiting his family in the Philippines presents to the emergency department with 1 week of fatigue, low-grade fever, abdominal pain, and jaundice. Laboratory results include: serum alanine transaminase (ALT) 2,850 U/L, total bilirubin 7.6 mg/dL, and international normalized ratio (INR) of 3.6. Serology comes back as HBsAg negative, anti-HBs positive, anti-HBc IgG positive, and anti-HBc IgM negative. The serology results are most consistent with which of the following?

   A. Acute hepatitis B infection
   B. Chronic hepatitis B infection
   C. Immunity to hepatitis B from prior infection
   D. Immunity to hepatitis B from vaccination
   E. None of the above

2. A 68-year-old woman has been in the ICU for 5 days receiving ceftazidime for *Pseudomonas aeruginosa* meningitis following surgical removal of a meningioma. This morning on rounds her nurse mentions that the patient had three loose stools overnight. Laboratory results show that the patient's white blood cell count jumped from 7,600 to 16,500 cells/μL. Serum creatinine has also increased from 1.2 to 1.9 mg/dL. Nucleic acid amplification test and stool toxin test are both positive for *Clostridium difficile*. What is the recommended management?

   A. Metronidazole 500 mg PO three times daily for 10 days.
   B. Vancomycin 125 mg PO four times daily or fidaxomicin 200 mg PO twice daily for 10 days
   C. Repeat testing for *C. difficile* toxin at 14 days
   D. Both A and C
   E. Both B and C

3. A 45-year-old man with a history of alcoholic cirrhosis and poor medication compliance is dropped off in the emergency department by a friend. He is afebrile, blood pressure 108/56 mm Hg, heart rate 89 beats/min, and oxygen saturation 96% on room air. On examination he is sleepy but rouses to voice. He cannot remember how he got to the hospital and gets irritated with repeated questions. He has asterixis and hyperactive reflexes. His abdomen is moderately distended but not tense or painful. In addition to admitting the patient and starting medical management of his decompensated cirrhosis, what is the best approach to working up and treating a possible infection?

   A. No antibiotics needed at this time, and await results of blood and urine cultures
   B. Send blood and urine cultures, start empiric broad-spectrum antibiotic coverage, and narrow or discontinue based on culture data
   C. Send blood and urine cultures, start empiric broad spectrum antibiotic coverage, and perform diagnostic paracentesis as soon as convenient
   D. Perform diagnostic paracentesis and send blood and urine cultures, and decide whether to start empiric antibiotics based on ascitic fluid cell count or culture results
   E. Perform diagnostic paracentesis and send blood and urine cultures, and decide whether to start empiric antibiotics based on ascitic fluid gram stain or culture results

4. A previously healthy 63-year-old woman presents to the emergency department with 24 hours of severe abdominal pain, nausea, and vomiting. Vital signs include temperature 38.8°C, heart rate 108 beats/min, blood pressure 86/42 mm Hg, and oxygen saturation 93% on room air. On examination, she is in moderate distress with diffuse epigastric pain and diminished bowel sounds. Laboratory results include white blood cell count 18,500 cells/μL, creatinine 2.1 mg/dL, lipase 320 U/L (normal range 7-60 U/L), total bilirubin 2.8 mg/dL, aspartate aminotransferase (AST) 96 U/L, alanine aminotransferase (ALT) 89 U/L, alkaline phosphatase 256 U/L. What is the recommended management?

   A. Start aggressive intravenous fluid repletion, and obtain an abdominal ultrasound, early enteral feeding
   B. Avoid aggressive fluid repletion, and obtain an abdominal ultrasound, early parenteral feeding
   C. Start aggressive intravenous fluid repletion, and obtain an abdominal ultrasound, early parenteral feeding
   D. Avoid aggressive fluid repletion, early enteral feeding
   E. Start aggressive intravenous fluid repletion, and broad spectrum empiric antibiotics, early enteral feeding

5. A previously healthy 24-year-old man presents to the emergency department with severe right lower quadrant pain, anorexia, and nausea. Vital signs include heart rate 126 beats/min, blood pressure 86/43 mm Hg, SpO$_2$ 99% on room air, and temperature 38.7°C. Physical examination is significant for exquisite right lower quadrant tenderness with rebound and guarding. Laboratory test results reveal a white blood cell count of 19,000 cells/μL with a left shift. CT with contrast shows appendiceal wall thickening, periappendiceal fat stranding, and a focal defect in the enhancing wall of the appendix. In addition to IV fluids, what are the next best steps in management?

   A. Start antibiotics with narrower-spectrum, gram-negative, and anaerobic coverage such as ceftriaxone plus metronidazole, urgent surgery
   B. Start antibiotics with broad coverage such as cefepime plus metronidazole, urgent surgery
   C. Start antibiotics with narrower-spectrum gram-negative and anaerobic coverage such as ceftriaxone plus metronidazole, surgery within 24 hours
   D. Start antibiotics with broad coverage such as cefepime plus metronidazole, surgery within 24 hours
   E. Start antibiotics with broad coverage such as cefepime plus metronidazole, no surgery unless the patient does not improve with antibiotics and fluids

6. A 46-year-old woman with newly diagnosed and untreated HIV infection was admitted to the ICU last night with possible pneumocystis pneumonia. Her CD4 count is 42 cells/μL. She is currently intubated and sedated. Since arrival she has had five episodes of bloody loose stools. PCR for *C. difficile* is negative and stool studies for bacteria and parasites are pending. Colonoscopy performed at bedside reveals areas of friable, erythematous mucosa with submucosal hemorrhage and large, deep ulcerations. Biopsies are sent for definitive diagnosis. What empiric antimicrobial should you start while awaiting results?

   A. Ciprofloxacin
   B. Oral vancomycin
   C. Ganciclovir
   D. Nitazoxanide
   E. No need for empiric therapy, await definitive biopsy results

7. A 56-year-old man with a recent diagnosis of acute myeloid leukemia was admitted 10 days ago for induction chemotherapy with cytarabine and anthracycline. Over the past 24 hours he has developed worsening abdominal pain and distension along with a fever of 38.8°C and watery diarrhea. CT shows bowel wall thickening of >10 mm in both the small and large intestine. Which of the following statements is true regarding this patient's likely diagnosis?

   A. Enteral feeding helps to decrease complications
   B. Pneumatosis intestinalis may be seen on CT scan
   C. Early surgical intervention improves outcomes
   D. Antibiotics are not needed at this time
   E. None of these statements are true

8. A previously healthy 36-year-old woman is brought in by ambulance following a seizure. Her husband reports that she has no history of seizures but had been complaining of diarrhea and vomiting for almost a week. She went out of town to a family reunion 10 days ago and had talked to several other family members who also became ill, some even needed to go to the hospital. On examination the patient is confused with diffuse abdominal tenderness. Vitals are within normal limits. Although in the ED she experiences an episode of grossly bloody diarrhea. Significant laboratory results include white blood cell count 12,300 cells/μL, hemoglobin 7.7 g/dL, platelet count 85,000 cells/μL, Cr 5.63. Peripheral blood smear shows a large number of schistocytes. Which of the following statements is true regarding this patient's disease process?

A. Early antibiotics have been shown to improve outcomes
B. Therapeutic plasma exchange is a mainstay of treatment
C. All patients should receive steroids
D. Criteria for renal replacement therapy is the same as that for other causes of acute kidney injury (AKI)
E. None of the above is true

9. A 63-year-old woman with a history of hypertension and dyslipidemia presents to the emergency department with severe right upper quadrant pain. On examination, she is grimacing and agitated with notable jaundice. She is oriented to self only. She has right upper abdominal tenderness, but no peritoneal signs. Vital signs include temperature 38.5°C, heart rate 112 beats/min, blood pressure 92/48 mm Hg, SpO$_2$ 96% on room air. Pertinent laboratory test results include white blood cell count 13,500 cells/µL with a left shift, total bilirubin 4.4 mg/dL, alkaline phosphatase 220 IU/L, AST 846 IU/L, ALT 932 IU/L. Blood cultures are pending. An ultrasound performed at bedside shows biliary dilation. Appropriate initial management includes which of the following:

A. Admission to the general surgical ward
B. Rehydration with enteral fluids
C. A first generation cephalosporin
D. Urgent endoscopic retrograde cholangiopancreatography (ERCP)
E. Urgent surgery

10. A previously healthy 42-year-old man was admitted to the ICU last night with progressive weakness and was intubated early this morning when he became unable to protect his airway. Per his wife, he was in his usual state of health until 2 days ago when he began to complain of weakness, numbness, and pain in his legs. She called an ambulance yesterday when he started having similar symptoms in his arms. On examination he has symmetric weakness in both upper and lower extremities and absence of deep tendon reflexes. CSF studies show a protein level of 110 mg/dL (normal range 15-45 mg/dL) and a white blood cell count of <5 cells/µL. Further history reveals that the whole family had suffered a diarrheal illness a couple of weeks ago. What is the most commonly identified infectious precursor to this patient's syndrome?

A. *Giardia lamblia*
B. *Campylobacter jejuni*
C. *Salmonella enterica*
D. Cytomegalovirus (CMV)
E. *Yersinia pestis*

# Chapter 66 ▪ Answers

1. Correct Answer: C

**Rationale:**
The presence of the combination of anti-HBs and anti-HBc IgG with all other hepatitis B markers being negative suggests immunity from a prior infection. Hepatitis B surface antigen (HBsAg) is a marker of current infection. Hepatitis B surface antibody (anti-HBs) is a marker of immunity through vaccination or previous exposure. Hepatitis B core antibody IgG (anti-HBc IgG) is a marker of previous exposure. Hepatitis B core antibody IgM (anti-HBc IgM) is generally a marker of acute HBV infection, although it can also be positive during spontaneous exacerbation of chronic HBV.

| STATUS | HBsAG | ANTI-HBs | ANTI-HBc IgG | ANTI-HBc IgM |
|---|---|---|---|---|
| Acute HBV Infection | + | – | + | + |
| Chronic HBV Infection | + | – | + | – |
| Resolved HBV infection (immune) | – | + or – | + | – |
| Successful Vaccination | – | + | – | – |
| Susceptible | – | – | – | – |

References
1. Davison SA, Strasser SI. Ordering and interpreting hepatitis B serology. *BMJ*. 2014;348:g2522.
2. Dienstag JL. Acute viral hepatitis. In: Kasper D, Fauci A, Hauser S, Longo D, Jameson J, Loscalzo J, eds. *Harrison's Principles of Internal Medicine*. 19 ed. New York, NY: McGraw-Hill; 2014.

**2.** Correct Answer: B

**Rationale:**

All antibiotics, including vancomycin and metronidazole, carry a risk for *C. difficile* infection (CDI); however, clindamycin, ampicillin, cephalosporins, and fluoroquinolones are associated with the majority of infections. Patients with three or more new, unexplained loose stools in 24 hours should be tested for CDI. All patients with suspected CDI should be placed on contact precautions pending test results and, if positive, these precautions should be continued for at least 48 hours after diarrhea has resolved. Nucleic acid amplification testing, either alone or as part of an algorithm including initial enzyme immunoassay screening for glutamate dehydrogenase antigen and toxins A and B, is now the preferred diagnostic test. Vancomycin or fidaxomicin PO are the recommended antibiotics for the initial episode of both severe and nonsevere disease; however, metronidazole can be used for nonsevere disease if access to oral vancomycin or fidaxomicin is limited. This patient has severe disease based on a leukocytosis of $\geq$15,000 cells/µL and serum creatinine >1.5 mg/dL. Repeat testing following resolution of diarrhea is not indicated because >50% of patients will continue to harbor both the organism and toxin.

References
1. Gerding DN, Johnson S. Clostridium difficile infection, including Pseudomembranous colitis. In: Kasper D, Fauci A, Hauser S, Longo D, Jameson J, Loscalzo J, eds. *Harrison's Principles of Internal Medicine*. 19 ed. New York, NY: McGraw-Hill; 2014.
2. McDonald LC, Gerding DN, Johnson S, et al. Clinical practice guidelines for Clostridium difficile infection in adults and children: 2017 update by the Infectious Diseases Society of America (IDSA) and Society for Healthcare Epidemiology of America (SHEA). *Clin Infect Dis*. 2018;66(7):e1-e48.

**3.** Correct Answer: D

**Rationale:**

All inpatients with ascites should have a diagnostic paracentesis performed at least once during every admission, and it should be repeated if the patient develops new evidence of infection during their stay. The symptoms of spontaneous bacterial peritonitis (SBP) can be subtle, and sending ascitic fluid for culture is a cost-effective way to detect an unexpected infection. The prevalence of SBP in hospitalized patients with cirrhosis and ascites is ~10%. Initial laboratory testing should include ascitic fluid cell count and differential, ascitic fluid total protein, serum-ascites albumin gradient (SAAG), and both aerobic and anaerobic cultures. Cultures should be obtained before the initiation of antibiotics. Other tests may also be indicated based on the clinical scenario. In the presence of cirrhosis a SAAG of $\geq$1.1 g/dL nearly always indicates that the ascites is from portal hypertension. Patients with an ascitic protein concentration of <15 g/L have an increased risk of SBP. An ascitic fluid polymorphonuclear (PMN) leukocyte count greater than 250 cells/mm³ suggests the presence of infection, even if cultures are negative, and empiric antibiotics should be started. Patients with an ascitic fluid PMN count less than 250 cells/mm³, but with signs and symptoms of infection, should also receive empiric antibiotic coverage. Gram stain cannot rule out infection because the concentration of bacteria in the ascitic fluid is often very low (ascitic fluid cultures are positive only ~40% of the time in patients with other clinical evidence of SBP). The most common organisms cultured are *Escherichia coli*, *Klebsiella pneumoniae*, and *Streptococcal pneumoniae*. The preferred treatment for community-acquired SBP is cefotaxime or a similar third-generation cephalosporin. For patients with nosocomial SBP or recent beta-lactam antibiotic exposure, empiric antibiotics should be based on local antibiograms.

References
1. American Association for the Study of Liver Diseases. *Management of Adult Patients with Ascites Due to Cirrhosis: Update 2012*. www.aasld.org/sites/default/files/guideline_documents/141020_Guidelines_Ascites_4UFb_2015.pdf. Accessed September 2, 2018.
2. European Association for the Study of the Liver. EASL clinical practice guidelines on the management of ascites, spontaneous bacterial peritonitis, and hepatorenal syndrome in cirrhosis. *J Hepatol*. 2010;53(3):397-417.

**4.** Correct Answer: A

**Rationale:**

The diagnosis of acute pancreatitis (AP) can be made when patients meet two of the following three criteria: abdominal pain consistent with pancreatitis (constant, generally severe epigastric or left upper quadrant pain that may radiate to the back, chest, or flank), serum amylase or lipase greater than three times the upper limit of normal, and/or characteristic findings on imaging. Serum lipase level is the laboratory test of choice. The American Society for Clinical Pathology even chose testing lipase instead of amylase in cases of suspected AP as one of its recommendations for the Choosing Wisely initiative. ICU admission criteria should be the same as with other patients, but ICU or step-down admission should also be considered for patients who are at high risk of deterioration, such as those at risk of severe AP. Patient characteristics that increase the risk of developing severe AP include age >55 years, BMI >30 kg/m², altered mental status, and presence of comorbid disease. No specific laboratory or imaging results have been able to reliably predict severity in AP, so close monitoring for hypovolemic shock and evidence of organ dysfunction are important. Other risk factors for severe AP include the presence of systemic inflammatory response syndrome, evidence of hypovolemia (elevated BUN or creatinine, hemoconcentration), pleural effusions or pulmonary infiltrates, and presence of multiple or extensive extrapancreatic fluid collections. Death within the first week is usually due to progressive organ dysfunction. Routine use of prophylactic antibiotics is not recommended, even in the presence of severe disease, unless there is evidence of extrapancreatic infection. All patients should receive an abdominal ultrasound to evaluate for cholelithiasis, which is the most common cause of AP (40%-70% of cases). Patients with mild AP can begin eating a low-fat diet as soon as tolerated. Patients with severe AP should be started on enteral nutrition to prevent infectious complications. Parenteral nutrition should only be used if the enteral route is not available, not tolerated, or not meeting caloric requirements.

### References

1. Choosing Wisely. *American Society for Clinical Pathology: Twenty Things Physicians and Patients Should Question.* September 16, 2016. www.choosingwisely.org/societies/american-society-for-clinical-pathology/. Accessed September 3, 2018.
2. Conwell DL, Banks P, Greenberger NJ. Acute and chronic pancreatitis. In: Kasper D, Fauci A, Hauser S, Longo D, Jameson J, Loscalzo J, eds. *Harrison's Principles of Internal Medicine.* 19 ed. New York, NY: McGraw-Hill; 2014.
3. Nathens AB, Curtis JR, Beale RJ, et al. Management of the critically ill patient with severe acute pancreatitis. *Crit Care Med.* 2004;32(12):2524-2536.
4. Tenner S, Baillie J, DeWitt J, et al. American College of Gastroenterology guideline: management of acute pancreatitis. *Am J Gastroenterol.* 2013;108(9):1400-1415.
5. Working Group IAP/APA Acute Pancreatitis Guidelines. IAP/APA evidence-based guidelines for the management of acute pancreatitis. *Pancreatology.* 2013;13(4 suppl 2):e1-e15.

### 5. Correct Answer: A

**Rationale:**

This patient's clinical picture is consistent with perforated appendicitis. Even in the absence of imaging findings, the positive peritoneal signs, hypotension, significantly elevated temperature, and high white blood cell count point to a serious intra-abdominal infection that requires exploration. In the setting of imaging consistent with acute appendicitis, five sensitive and specific CT findings for perforated appendicitis include abscess, phlegmon, extraluminal air, extraluminal appendicolith, and focal defect in the enhancing appendiceal wall. A focal defect in the appendiceal wall is the most sensitive finding. However, up to half of patients with perforated appendicitis will have imaging consistent with simple appendicitis, so imaging by itself cannot rule out perforation.

An intravenous fluid bolus is indicated to treat the patient's hypotension. Because this patient is otherwise healthy and presenting from home, he is not considered to be at an increased risk for resistant or hospital-associated organisms. Coverage of narrower gram-negative and obligate anaerobic organisms is adequate despite the severity of the infection. Recommended single agents include ertapenem and moxifloxacin. Combination regimens could include cefotaxime or ceftriaxone plus metronidazole or ciprofloxacin plus metronidazole. No more than 4 days of antibiotic therapy is recommended for patients with perforated appendicitis who undergo surgery and have adequate source control. Although antibiotics alone have been shown to be successful in simple inflamed appendicitis, 25% to 30% of patients will require readmission or surgery within 1 year. Appendectomy is still recommended for most patients presenting with appendicitis. Patients such as this one with sepsis or peritonitis due to acute appendicitis require urgent surgery. Timing of appendectomy in mild to moderate cases of appendicitis has been more controversial, but delays of 12 to 24 hours have not been associated with increased rates of complications such as perforation.

### References

1. Bhangu A, Søreide K, Di Saverio S, et al. Acute appendicitis: modern understanding of pathogenesis, diagnosis, and management. *Lancet.* 2015;386(10000):1278-1287.
2. Horrow MM, White DS, Horrow JC. Differentiation of perforated from nonperforated appendicitis at CT. *Radiology.* 2003;227(1):46-51
3. Leeuwenburgh MM, Wiezer MJ, Wiarda BM, et al. Accuracy of MRI compared with ultrasound imaging and selective use of CT to discriminate simple from perforated appendicitis. *Br J Surg.* 2014;101(1):e147-e155.
4. Mazuski JE, Tessier JM, May AK, et al. The Surgical Infection Society revised guidelines on the management of intra-abdominal infection. *Surg Infect (Larchmt).* 2017;18(1):1-76.
5. United Kingdom National Research Collaborative, Bhangu A. Safety of short, in-hospital delays in surgery for acute appendicitis: a multicenter cohort study, systematic review, and meta-analysis. *An Surg.* 2014;259(5):894-903.

### 6. Correct Answer: C

**Rationale:**

Although increasingly rare with improvements in antiretroviral therapy, cytomegalovirus colitis is still a concern in HIV-positive patients with CD4 counts <100 cells/µL (usually <50 cells/µL). As the colitis progresses through the full thickness of the bowel, there is a risk for perforation, a life-threatening surgical emergency. Other complications include hemorrhage, infection, and toxic megacolon. Thinning of the bowel wall can lead to bacteremia. Patients with suspected CMV colitis with severe symptoms such as this one should be started on empiric antiviral therapy while awaiting definitive pathologic diagnosis. Endoscopic and biopsy findings confirm the diagnosis. Endoscopy findings are variable and can include diffuse or localized areas of friable, erythematous mucosa with submucosal hemorrhage and mucosal ulcerations. Biopsy shows characteristic intranuclear ("owl's eye") and cytoplasmic inclusion bodies. Recommended treatment is either ganciclovir or foscarnet for 3 to 6 weeks. Relapse is common and maintenance therapy is often required for those with poorly controlled HIV. Prophylaxis with valganciclovir is indicated until the CD4 count is >100 cells/μL for 6 months, and there is no evidence of active CMV disease. PCR for toxigenic genes is highly specific and sensitive for diagnosis of *C. difficile* colitis. So, a negative PCR rules out CDI.

### References

1. Fauci AS, Lane H. Human immunodeficiency virus disease: AIDS and related disorders. In: Kasper D, Fauci A, Hauser S, Longo D, Jameson J, Loscalzo J, eds. *Harrison's Principles of Internal Medicine*. 19 ed. New York, NY: McGraw-Hill; 2014.
2. Lew EA, Poles MA, Dieterich DT. Diarrheal diseases associated with HIV infection. *Gastroenterol Clin North Am*. 1997;26(2):259-290.

---

**7. Correct Answer: B**

**Rationale:**

Neutropenic enterocolitis (NE), also known as necrotizing enterocolitis or ileocecal syndrome, involves inflammation and necrosis of the gut in a neutropenic patient caused by an invasive infection. Patients with an absolute neutrophil count (ANC) <1,500 cells/μL are at risk, although generally the ANC is much lower. Any segment of the gastrointestinal (GI) tract may be involved. Patients being treated for acute leukemia appear to be at highest risk, but it has been documented in most neutropenic and immunocompromised populations. The lack of neutrophils allows overgrowth of gut organisms, particularly gram-negative bacilli. One proposed mechanism of NE is GI distension and impaired perfusion leading to decreased mucosal integrity, allowing entry of these organisms into the bowel wall. Bowel wall integrity can also be compromised by chemotherapy. This can lead to ischemic necrosis, perforation, and/or peritonitis. Signs include lower abdominal tenderness and distension, watery diarrhea, and occasionally GI bleeding. Bacteremia is common and many patients will present with sepsis. Gram-negative bacteria are the usual culprit, but other bacteria and fungi are not uncommon. Most experts suggest that the combination of abdominal pain and fever in a neutropenic patient warrants treatment for presumptive NE with imaging used to help confirm the diagnosis. CT often shows bowel wall thickening and edema, which is also common in *C. diff* colitis; pneumatosis intestinalis is more specific for either NE or ischemia. Other CT findings can include nonspecific ileus, phlegmon, pericecal inflammation, mesenteric stranding, free air, and extraluminal fluid collections. Histologic examination is the gold standard for diagnosis, but due to the risk of perforation and bleeding from colonoscopy in neutropenic, thrombocytopenic patients, tissue samples are rarely obtained. Colonoscopy can show thickened, edematous, hemorrhagic bowel with diffuse ischemic colitis present in the majority of cases. Treatment includes broad-spectrum antibiotics, bowel rest, nasogastric suction, parenteral nutrition, and IV fluids. Myeloid growth factors may also improve outcomes. Surgery is reserved for those with evidence of perforation, peritonitis, gangrenous bowel, or refractory GI hemorrhage. In fact, all febrile neutropenic patients should be started on empiric broad-spectrum antibiotics.

### References

1. Ebert EC, Hagspiel KD. Gastrointestinal manifestations of leukemia. *J Gastroenterol Hepatol*. 2012;27(3):458-463.
2. Gorschlüter M, Mey U, Strehl J, et al. Neutropenic enterocolitis in adults: systematic analysis of evidence quality. *Eur J Haematol*. 2005;75(1):1-13.
3. Gucalp R, Dutcher JP. Oncologic emergencies. In: Kasper D, Fauci A, Hauser S, Longo D, Jameson J, Loscalzo J, eds. *Harrison's Principles of Internal Medicine*. 19 ed. New York, NY: McGraw-Hill; 2014.
4. Ullery BW, Pieracci FM, Rodney JR, et al. *Surg Infect (Larchmt)*. 2009;10(3):307-314.

---

**8. Correct Answer: D**

**Rationale:**

Enterohemorrhagic *Escherichia coli* (EHEC or Shiga toxin producing *E. coli*) is a cause of bloody, infectious diarrhea commonly associated with ingestion of contaminated food such as fresh produce, undercooked beef, or various prepackaged products. Although most infections resolve without complications, occasionally patients go on to develop the triad of nonimmune hemolytic anemia, thrombocytopenia, and AKI known as hemolytic-uremic syndrome (HUS). Although HUS is more commonly associated with children, some newer outbreaks have preferentially affected adults. The most common serotype is *E. coli* O157:H7; however, outbreaks associated with non-O157 serotypes have also been reported. The incubation period is 2 to 12 days. Stool culture is the gold standard for diagnosis, but a presumptive diagnosis can be made based on the presence of bloody diarrhea and the triad of HUS. Central nervous system involvement is common and can include seizures, stroke, coma, hemiparesis, or cortical blindness. Management of the gastroenteritis is generally supportive care including IV fluids. Antimotility agents should not be given and may be associated with increased risk of developing HUS. Antibiotics have not been found to be helpful. For patients who develop HUS, admission with close monitoring is recommended with the use of IV fluids, antihypertensives, renal replacement therapy, and red blood cell transfusions as clinically indicated. Anticoagulation, fresh frozen plasma, steroids, or Shiga toxin binders have not been shown to offer benefit. Unlike with thrombotic thrombocytopenic purpura or nondiarrheal (atypical) HUS, plasmapheresis has also not been shown to improve outcomes. Overall prognosis is good, even for patients that require dialysis. EHEC-associated HUS has a mortality rate of <5%.

### References

1. Nathanson S, Kwon T, Elmaleh M, et al. Acute neurological involvement in diarrhea-associated hemolytic uremic syndrome. *Clin J Am Soc Nephrol.* 2010;5(7):1218-1228.
2. Page AV, Liles WC. Enterohemorrhagic *Escherichia coli* infections and the Hemolytic-Uremic Syndrome. *Med Clin North Am.* 2013;97(4):681-695.
3. Wong CS, Jelacic S, Habeeb RL, et al. The risk of the hemolytic-uremic syndrome after antibiotic treatment of Escherichia coli O157:H7 infectionsThe risk of the hemolytic-uremic syndrome after antibiotic treatment of Escherichia coli O157:H7 infectionsThe risk of the hemolytic-uremic syndrome after antibiotic treatment of Escherichia coli O157:H7 infections. *N Engl J Med.* 2000;342(26):1930-1936.

---

**9.** Correct Answer: D

### Rationale:

Severe acute cholangitis is a life-threatening condition caused by biliary obstruction complicated by infection of the biliary tree. Many patients present with Charcot's triad of right upper quadrant abdominal pain, fever, and jaundice. In cases of severe (suppurative) cholangitis, patients may also have hypotension and altered mental status, which make up Reynold's pentad. Any type of biliary obstruction can lead to acute cholangitis, but biliary calculi are the most common cause. Other causes include benign or malignant biliary stricture and biliary stent obstruction. Enteric bacteria are the most common culprit, and 20% to 80% of patients will have bacteremia. Gram-negative rods such as *E. coli* and *Klebsiella* are often cultured, but gram-positive cocci and anaerobes are not unusual.

The diagnosis of acute cholangitis can be difficult; many patients have a more subtle presentation than this case. Updated Tokyo guidelines for definitive diagnosis include the presence of three criteria: (1) systemic inflammation (fever, leukocytosis, leukopenia, or elevated C-reactive protein, (2) cholestasis (jaundice or liver function tests >1.5 times upper limit of normal), and (3) imaging findings (biliary dilation or evidence of the cause of biliary obstruction on imaging). There are many imaging choices, but ERCP is the most sensitive and has the added benefit of treating the cholangitis through decompression of the biliary tree. However, given the risk associated with sedation/anesthesia for this procedure, noninvasive imaging is usually performed first. Management is focused on treating the infection and relieving obstruction. First steps include rehydration with IV fluids, correction of electrolyte abnormalities and coagulopathy, and broad spectrum antibiotics. Frequently recommended first-line antibiotic regimens include piperacillin/tazobactam or a third- or fourth-generation cephalosporin. Patients with severe acute cholangitis such as this one should be monitored in the ICU because they are at risk for rapid clinical deterioration and mortality is high. Patients managed only conservatively have a mortality approaching 100%, so the next step is biliary decompression, with ERCP preferred over surgery. ERCP has a success rate of 98% and a much lower complication rate compared to surgical decompression. Surgical drainage is now rarely performed because of a very high risk of complications (~66%) and a mortality rate >30%.

### References

1. Kiriyama S, Takado T, Strasberg SM, et al. New diagnostic criteria and severity assessment of acute cholangitis in revised Tokyo Guidelines. *J Hepatobiliary Pancreat Sci.* 2012;19(5):548-556.
2. Kochar R, Banerjee S. Infections of the biliary tract. *Gastrointest Endosc Clin N Am.* 2013;23(2):199-218
3. Lai EC, Mok FP, Tan ES, et al. Endoscopic biliary drainage for severe acute cholangitis. *N Engl J Med.* 1992;326(24):1582-1586.

---

**10.** Correct Answer: B

### Rationale:

Guillain-Barré syndrome (GBS) is the most common cause of acute flaccid paralysis. Patients generally present with progressive, symmetric ascending weakness of the limbs, often accompanied by paresthesia and pain. On examination, patients will have hypo- or areflexia. GBS may progress to involve the facial nerves and respiratory muscles. CSF studies often reveal albuminocytologic dissociation with an elevated protein level, but normal cell counts. *C. jejuni* is the most commonly identified infectious disease preceding the development of GBS, occurring in around 30% of cases. CMV is the second most common and Epstein-Barr virus, varicella-zoster virus, and *Mycoplasma pneumoniae* have also been implicated. *C. jejuni* appears to cause GBS via an autoimmune mechanism involving carbohydrate mimicry between human ganglioside GM1 and *C. jejuni* lipooligosaccharide. Another late onset complication of *C. jejuni* is reactive arthritis, also via an immune mechanism.

### References

1. Bremell T, Bjelle A, Svedhem A. Rheumatic symptoms following an outbreak of campylobacter enteritis: a five year follow up. *Ann Rheum Dis.* 1991;50(12):934-938.
2. Yuki N, Hartung HP. Guillain-Barré syndrome. *N Engl J Med.* 2012;366(24):2294-2304.
3. Yuki N, Susuki K, Koga M, et al. Carbohydrate mimicry between human ganglioside GM1 and Campylobacter jejuni lipooligosaccharide causes Guillain-Barré syndrome. *Proc Natl Acad Sci USA.* 2004;101(31):11404-11409.

# GENITOURINARY INFECTION

Lisa M. Bebell

1. A 67-year-old man has been intubated and sedated in the intensive care unit (ICU) for 6 days. He has a central venous catheter and an indwelling urinary catheter in place. He develops a fever to 38.4°C, and blood, urine, and sputum samples are sent for analysis. His urinalysis is notable for <10 white blood cells, negative for leukocyte esterase and nitrites. Urine culture grows >100,000 *Candida glabrata* after 2 days, susceptible to micafungin, caspofungin, and fluconazole. What is the **MOST** appropriate way to manage the yeast growing in urine culture?

   **A.** Give micafungin
   **B.** Give fluconazole
   **C.** No change in management
   **D.** Remove the existing urinary catheter and replace with a new catheter

2. A 28-year-old pregnant woman is admitted to the ICU, requiring norepinephrine to treat hypotension due to pyelonephritis from highly susceptible, pan sensitive *Escherichia coli*. Ultrasound imaging of the kidneys and bladder on admission was normal. She is treated with ceftriaxone for 2 days, with improvement in her pain, fever, and hypotension. However, on day 3 she develops a fever to 38.4 while still receiving intravenous antibiotic therapy. She has no new symptoms, and no costovertebral angle tenderness to palpation. What is the **MOST** likely cause of her recrudescent fever?

   **A.** Emerging antibiotic resistance to ceftriaxone
   **B.** Drug fever
   **C.** Perinephric abscess
   **D.** Renal abscess

3. A 78-year-old woman with diabetes and hypertension presents to the emergency department with confusion and hypotension. A urinalysis is notable for a white blood cell count of >100,000 and is positive for leukocyte esterase. Urine culture subsequently grows >100,000 *Pseudomonas aeruginosa*, resistant to ciprofloxacin. You begin appropriate antibiotic therapy with a beta-lactam antibiotic. For how long should she be treated?

   **A.** 3 to 5 days
   **B.** 5 to 10 days
   **C.** 10 to 14 days
   **D.** Until her confusion resolves

4. What diagnostic test is **MOST** appropriate to evaluate for perinephric abscess?

   **A.** Abdominal ultrasound
   **B.** Computed tomography (CT) of the abdomen and pelvis
   **C.** Magnetic resonance imaging (MRI) of the abdomen and pelvis
   **D.** All of the above are appropriate depending on the clinical situation

**5.** Which indication below is **NOT** an appropriate indication for indwelling bladder catheterization in the ICU?

   **A.** Management of urinary incontinence
   **B.** Management of immobilized patients
   **C.** Management of patients with neurogenic bladder
   **D.** Hourly urine output measurement in critically ill patients

# Chapter 67 ▪ Answers

**1.** Correct Answer: D

**Rationale:**

Asymptomatic candiduria rarely requires treatment. Patients who should be treated for asymptomatic candiduria include neutropenic patients, very low birthweight infants, and patients with urinary tract (urologic) manipulation. Where possible, when candiduria is detected, it is strongly recommended that indwelling catheters be removed. If catheter removal is not possible, catheter exchange is recommended. Catheter exchange alone can lead to elimination of candiduria in 20% or more of patients with asymptomatic candiduria with no additional therapy.

References

1. Pappas PG, Kauffman CA, Andes DR, et al. Clinical practice guideline for the management of candidiasis: 2016 update by the Infectious Diseases Society of America. *Clin Infect Dis*. 2016;62(4):e1. Epub 2015 Dec 16.
2. Sobel JD, Kauffman CA, McKinsey D, et al. Candiduria: a randomized, double-blind study of treatment with fluconazole and placebo. The National Institute of Allergy and Infectious Diseases (NIAID) Mycoses Study Group. *Clin Infect Dis*. 2000;30(1):19.

**2.** Correct Answer: B

**Rationale:**

Perinephric and renal abscesses are uncommon conditions. Both tend to be insidious in nature with a subacute onset of vague or nonspecific symptoms. Most patients do not report symptoms typical of a urinary tract infection. The majority of patients with renal (Answer D) or perinephric (Answer C) abscesses have fever, chills, flank pain, and costovertebral angle tenderness. Abscesses generally develop over many days to weeks, and it is unlikely that this patient admitted with a normal renal ultrasound (which is common even in pyelonephritis) would develop an abscess within 48 hours, especially while clinically improving. Similarly, antibiotic resistance to ceftriaxone (Answer A) would require time to emerge and is unlikely to occur while on appropriate antibiotics for a short time period with improving clinical parameters. Thus, among the answers given, drug fever to ceftriaxone (Answer B) or another medication is the most likely cause of her fever.

References

1. Lee BE, Seol HY, Kim TK, et al. Recent clinical overview of renal and perirenal abscesses in 56 consecutive cases. *Korean J Intern Med*. 2008;23(3):140.
2. Coelho RF, Schneider-Monteiro ED, Mesquita JL, Mazzucchi E, Marmo Lucon A, Srougi M. Renal and perinephric abscesses: analysis of 65 consecutive cases. *World J Surg*. 2007;31(2):431.

**3.** Correct Answer: C

**Rationale:**

This patient has an acute complicated urinary tract infection. Patients presenting with complicated urinary tract infections should have urine culture performed to confirm the microbiologic cause of the infection and antimicrobial susceptibility of the pathogen(s) causing the infection. Total antibiotic duration depends on the antibiotic class used to treat the infection. Fluoroquinolones are given for 5 to 7 days, trimethoprim/sulfamethoxazole for 7 to 10 days, and beta lactams for 10 to 14 days. Longer durations may be appropriate for patients with an ongoing nidus of infection (eg nonobstructing stone).

References

1. van Nieuwkoop C, van der Starre WE, Stalenhoef JE, et al. Treatment duration of febrile urinary tract infection: a pragmatic randomized, double-blind, placebo-controlled non-inferiority trial in men and women. *BMC Med*. 2017;15(1):70. Epub 2017 Apr 3.
2. Hooton TM. Clinical practice. Uncomplicated urinary tract infection. *N Engl J Med*. 2012;366(11):1028-1037.

**4.** Correct Answer: D

**Rationale:**

The diagnosis of perinephric or renal abscess should be confirmed by imaging. The most commonly used imaging modality is CT scan (Answer B), which has the added advantage of diagnosing extension of infection to adjacent structures, which is more difficult to see on ultrasound imaging (Answer A). MRI (Answer C) is highly sensitive for detecting changes in the urinary tract, but is generally less accessible than CT or ultrasound imaging, and is the least often used. Choice of imaging modality to confirm the diagnosis of renal or perinephric abscess should be tailored to the individual patient and their clinical situation.

References
1. Demertzis J, Menias CO. State of the art: imaging of renal infections. *Emerg Radiol*. 2007;14(1):13. Epub 2007 Feb 21.
2. Rubilotta E, Balzarro M, Lacola V, Sarti A, Porcaro AB, Artibani W. Current clinical management of renal and perinephric abscesses: a literature review. *Urologia*. 2014;81(3):144-147.

**5.** Correct Answer: A

**Rationale:**

Unwarranted urinary catheter placement is very common, occurring in approximately 20% to 50% of hospitalized patients. Urinary catheters should not be placed for the management of urinary incontinence alone (Answer A). Answers B, C, and D represent appropriate indications for catheter placement. Other appropriate indications include management of urinary retention, hematuria associated with clots, open wounds of the sacrum or perineum with associated urinary incontinence, surgery of the genitourinary tract and associated structures, end-of-life care, and occasionally for management of patients with persistent urinary incontinence after conservative, behavioral, pharmacologic, and surgical measures have failed. Regardless of the indication for catheter placement, catheters should be removed as soon as the condition leading to the indication for catheterization has resolved.

References
1. Meddings J, Saint S, Fowler KE, et al. The Ann Arbor criteria for appropriate urinary catheter use in hospitalized medical patients: results obtained by using the RAND/UCLA appropriateness method. *Ann Intern Med*. 2015;162(9 suppl):S1-S34.
2. Gould CV, Umscheid CA, Agarwal RK, Kuntz G, Pegues DA; Healthcare Infection Control Practices Advisory Committee. Guideline for prevention of catheter-associated urinary tract infections 2009. *Infect Control Hosp Epidemiol*. 2010;31(4):319.

# 68

# SOFT-TISSUE, BONE, JOINT INFECTIONS

Ilan Mizrahi

1. A 32-year-old previously healthy man presents with fevers and hypotension. He was bitten by a dog 4 days ago with deep puncture wounds that required operative closure. He has a history of anaphylaxis to penicillin and cephalosporins and has been receiving trimethoprim-sulfamethoxazole since surgery. Tetanus toxoid was administered and his other immunizations are up to date. On examination, his wound shows evidence of cellulitis. Which of the following changes to his antibiotic regimen is most appropriate?

   A. Change trimethoprim-sulfamethoxazole to levofloxacin
   B. Add vancomycin
   C. Add clindamycin
   D. No change necessary

2. A 20-year-old female college student presents with fever and a painful left knee for the last 3 days. She denies any recent trauma and was treated last week for a urinary tract infection. Her vital signs are T 38.8°C, HR 112 beats/min, RR 24 breaths/min, BP 78/42 mm Hg, and $O_2$ saturation 98% on RA. Physical examination reveals a swollen and erythematous knee with decreased range of motion. Joint aspiration demonstrates white blood cell (WBC) 20,000, with 80% neutrophils and calcium pyrophosphate crystals, and no organism are seen on gram stain. In addition to fluid administration, which of the following interventions is most appropriate?

   A. No further treatment warranted
   B. Administer vancomycin and ceftriaxone
   C. Administer intra-articular glucocorticoids
   D. Administer indomethacin

3. A 55-year-old male with non–insulin-dependent diabetes mellitus presents with lower leg swelling and severe pain. He fell while gardening yesterday and has a laceration on his heel. On examination has a fever of 39.4°C and is mildly confused. He has erythema, edema, and crepitus up to the midcalf. Notable laboratory values are a WBC count of 22,000 cells/mm² and lactate 3.9. What is the most appropriate next step in treatment?

   A. Perform surgical debridement
   B. Administer hyperbaric oxygen therapy
   C. Administer intravenous immunoglobulin
   D. Administer AB103, a mimetic of the CD28 T-lymphocyte receptor

4. A 28-year-old woman is admitted to the ICU with septic shock due to a soft-tissue infection. Three days prior to admission, she fell while riding her bicycle and sustained lacerations to her legs which she self-treated. Within the ICU, she undergoes fluid resuscitation, receives vasopressor support and broad-spectrum antibiotics, and is taken for surgical debridement. Tissue and blood cultures grow *Streptococcus pyogenes* and antibiotics are narrowed to penicillin and clindamycin. Two days later, she remains febrile, and vasopressor dependent, has a generalized rash, develops acute kidney injury requiring renal replacement therapy as well as elevated transaminases and jaundice. Sensitivity testing shows no antimicrobial resistance and no further organisms. Which of the following interventions is MOST likely to be beneficial for treatment of this patient?

    **A.** Intravenous immunoglobulin (IVIG) administered for 3 days

    **B.** Hyperbaric oxygen therapy

    **C.** Anti–tumor necrosis factor (TNF) antibody

    **D.** Changing antibiotics to meropenem

**5.** A 61-year-old man presented with fever, malaise, and a blistering red rash 5 days after undergoing a laparoscopic cholecystectomy. Per report, the rash started at his port insertion sites but has progressed and now involves his face, trunk, and extremities. His medical history includes end-stage renal disease on intermittent hemodialysis, hypertension, and diabetes mellitus. Vital signs are T 38.7°C, HR 76 beats/min, BP 150/80 mm Hg, RR 26 breaths/min, and oxygen saturation of 97% on room air. Examination reveals red, blistering, tender skin, warm-to-touch and peels with gentle stroking. The rash is accentuated in the flexor creases. Perioral crusting is present but mucous membranes are spared. What is the MOST likely etiology of this condition?

    **A.** Systemic infection with circulating endotoxins

    **B.** Drug-induced keratinocyte necrosis

    **C.** Staphylococcal infection proliferating exotoxins

    **D.** Bacterial infection invading the fascia

# Chapter 68 ▪ Answers

**1.** Correct Answer: C

**Rationale:**

Prophylactic antibiotics are not typically required after animal bites. However, they reduce the rate of infection of high-risk bites:

- Deep puncture wounds
- Wounds with underlying venous or lymphatic compromise
- Injury to the hands, genitals, face, or wounds near joints
- Wounds needing operative closure
- Wounds in patients who have impaired healing (ie, immunocompromised, diabetes mellitus)

    Amoxicillin-clavulanate for 3 to 5 days is the preferred prophylactic agent. Alternatives in patients with cephalosporin allergies should have activity against both *Pasteurella multocida* (ie, trimethoprim-sulfamethoxazole, doxycycline, levofloxacin) and anaerobes (clindamycin, metronidazole). Thus, this patient has untreated anaerobic infection and would benefit from the addition of clindamycin. Changing to levofloxacin or adding vancomycin would not give the appropriate coverage. Tetanus toxoid should also be administered to all patients who have completed primary immunization but who's booster has been 5 years of greater.

*Reference*

1. Stevens DL, Bisno AL, Chambers HF, et al. Practice guidelines for the diagnosis and management of skin and soft tissue infections: 2014 update by the Infectious Diseases Society of America. *Clin Infect Dis*. 2014;5(9):147.

**2.** Correct Answer: B

**Rationale:**

In patients who present with an acutely painful and swollen joint, prompt identification and treatment of septic arthritis can substantially reduce morbidity and mortality. An associated skin, urinary tract, or respiratory infection should provide insight to the likely pathogen. Definitive diagnosis is established by identification of bacteria in the synovial fluid. Gram stain is positive in many cases, but the absence of bacteria on initial gram stain should be considered conclusive evidence of the absence of infection. Empiric IV antibiotic therapy should be administered while awaiting culture results. Antibiotic therapy should cover (1) methicillin-resistant *Staphylococcus aureus* (which can be treated with vancomycin) and (2) gram-negative organisms such as *Klebsiella pneumoniae* and *Neisseria gonorrhoeae* (which are typically treated with ceftriaxone or third-generation cephalosporin). In addition to antibiotic therapy, patients with septic arthritis should have orthopedic evaluation for irrigation and debridement. Septic arthritis can cause the release of calcium pyrophosphate crystals from cartilage, so the finding of such crystals does not rule out infection. Intra-articular steroids or indomethacin would relieve acute joint inflammation but would not treat the underlying infection nor be immediately appropriate treatment.

## References

1. Sharff KA, Richards EP, Townes JM. Clinical management of septic arthritis. *Curr Rheumatol Rep.* 2013;15:332.
2. Carpenter CR, Schuur JD, Everett WW, Pines JM. Evidence-based diagnostics: adult septic arthritis. *Acad Emerg Med.* 2011;18:781-796.
3. Margaretten ME, Kohlwes J, Moore D, Bent S. Does this adult patient have septic arthritis? *JAMA.* 2007;297:1478-1488.

**3.** Correct Answer: B

**Rationale:**

Necrotizing fasciitis (NF) is a bacterial infection characterized by friability of the superficial fascia, dishwater-gray exudate, and a notable absence of pus. It can occur after major traumatic injuries, as well as after minor breaches of the skin or mucosa or nonpenetrating soft-tissue injuries (eg, muscle strain or contusion). It is more common in immunocompromised patients. Necrotizing infections can result in widespread tissue destruction, which may extend from the epidermis to the deep musculature.

Clinical manifestations of NF include soft-tissue edema, erythema, severe pain and tenderness, fever, and skin bullae or necrosis. Factors that can differentiate NF from cellulitis include pain out of proportion to clinical signs, hypotension, and shock. Patients who are immunosuppressed may present without these typical findings.

NF can be subdivided into three types based on the pathogenic organisms involved:
- Type 1: Polymicrobial, with a heavy burden of anaerobes. Common in immunocompromised patients, with diabetes or peripheral vascular disease.
- Type 2: Monomicrobial, typically group A *Streptococcus* or *S. aureus*. Common in healthy individuals with skin injury as the portal to infection.
- Type 3: Gas gangrene caused by *Clostridium perfringens*.

For patients with aggressive soft-tissue infection, prompt surgical exploration is essential to determine the extent of infection, to assess the need for debridement, and to obtain specimens for gram staining and culture. No single clinical laboratory test or group of tests can adequately replace surgical inspection for diagnosis of these infections. In addition to prompt surgical intervention, appropriate antibiotic treatment and supportive care are essential to reduce morbidity and mortality.

The benefits of hyperbaric oxygen therapy for treatment of NF remain controversial. Surgical debridement should not be delayed in order to pursue hyperbaric oxygen treatment.

The rationale for using IVIG in patients with NF is based on its ability to neutralize extracellular toxins that mediate pathogenesis. Clinical studies supporting its efficacy have had serious limitations, and a consensus supporting its use has not been reached.

Efforts to inhibit bacterial superantigens involved in the pathogenesis of necrotizing infections are ongoing but have not shown clinical success to date.

## References

1. Stevens DL, Bryant AE. Necrotizing soft-tissue infections. *N Engl J Med.* 2017;377(23):2253-2265.
2. Phan HH, Cocanour CS. Necrotizing soft tissue infections in the intensive care unit. *Crit Care Med.* 2010;38:S460.
3. Vincent JL, Abraham E, Moore FA, et al, eds. *Textbook of Critical Care.* 7th ed. Philadelphia, PA: Elsevier; 2017.

**4.** Correct Answer: A

**Rationale:**

Group A Streptococcus (*S. pyogenes*) can produce exotoxins and superantigens that lead to streptococcal toxic shock syndrome characterized by rapidly progressive soft-tissue destruction, shock, and multiple organ failure. Although there is mixed evidence, several studies show benefit of IVIG in cases of streptococcal toxic shock syndrome. IVIG may raise antibody levels by passive immunity in the setting of overwhelming infection. It may contribute neutralizing antibodies against streptococcal exotoxins—however these may differ by specific manufacturer preparations. Hyperbaric oxygen has been studied to varying effect in necrotizing infection, but there is no indication that it would have any direct benefit in this patient. Clinical trials have not demonstrated a benefit of anti-TNF antibody administration in patients with septic shock. There is no role for changing antibiotic regimen in this patient with pansusceptible *S. pyogenes*, and no polymicrobial infection.

## References

1. Darenberg J, Ihendyane N, Sjölin J, et al; StreptIg Study Group. Intravenous immunoglobulin G therapy in streptococcal toxic shock syndrome: a European randomized, double-blind, placebo-controlled trial. *Clin Infect Dis.* 2003;37:333.
2. Poston JT, McSparron JI, Hayes MM, et al. ATS core curriculum 2015: part IV. Adult critical care medicine ATS guidelines. *Ann Am Thorac Soc.* 2015;12:1864.

**5.** Correct Answer: C

**Rationale:**

The patient's presentation is consistent with staphylococcal scalded skin syndrome (SSSS). SSSS is a localized *S. aureus* infection that produces exfoliative exotoxins (exfoliatin). These cause the breakdown of desmosomes and detachment of the epidermal layer. Skin biopsy shows separation within the superficial layer of the epidermis—in contrast to toxic epidermal necrolysis (TEN) which has skin separation at the dermoepidermal junction. SSSS is a disease usually seen in infancy but may appear in older, immunosuppressed patients with renal failure (as the toxins are cleared renally). The skin typically appears burnt, with fluid-filled bullae that easily rupture, with exfoliation of the epidermis under gentle pressure (positive Nikolsky sign). The rash often begins centrally, is sandpaper-like, progressing into a wrinkled appearance, and accentuated in flexor creases. Accompanying signs and symptoms include fever, tenderness and warmth to palpation, facial edema, conjunctivitis, and perioral crusting, but mucous membranes are spared. Dehydration may be present and significant.

Antibiotic treatment depends on whether the isolated pathogen is methicillin-resistant. Supportive treatment includes IV hydration to replace fluid losses, and aggressive skin care with petroleum jelly or similar agent to maintain moisture. A systemic infection with circulating endotoxins is characteristic of bacteremia and sepsis. Drug-induced keratinocyte necrosis is typical of toxic epidermal necrolysis and is noninfectious. Fascial bacterial infection alone would not cause the characteristic skin blistering described here.

References

1. Vincent JL, Abraham E, Moore FA, et al, eds. *Textbook of Critical Care*. 7th ed. Philadelphia, PA: Elsevier; 2017.
2. Murray RJ. Recognition and management of *Staphylococcus aureus* toxin-mediated disease. *Intern Med J*. 2005;35 (suppl 2):S106-S119.

# 69

# ANTIMICROBIAL THERAPY AND RESISTANCE

Lisa M. Bebell

1. A 37-year-old man from Thailand presents to the emergency room with hypoxemia and a 6-week history of coughing, including occasional small-volume hemoptysis. Chest X-ray demonstrates a right lower lobe cavitary lesion. He is placed in a negative-pressure isolation room in the intensive care unit (ICU) and started on rifampicin, isoniazid, ethambutol, pyrazinamide, and clindamycin. Nine days after starting antibiotics, his transaminases are elevated, with alanine aminotransferase 1237 IU/mL and aspartate aminotransferase 964 IU/mL. Which of the following medication(s) is **MOST** likely to have caused his acute hepatic injury?

   **A.** Ethambutol
   **B.** Rifampicin, isoniazid, or pyrazinamide
   **C.** Clindamycin
   **D.** Isoniazid

2. A 46-year-old man living with HIV presents to the emergency room with confusion and quickly becomes obtunded. Lumbar puncture is notable for elevated opening pressure and cerebrospinal fluid with 14 leukocytes/mL. India ink stain is positive. Which of the following therapies is the **BEST** choice for management of his disease?

   **A.** High-dose fluconazole
   **B.** High-dose ketoconazole
   **C.** Liposomal amphotercin B and flucytosine
   **D.** Micafungin or caspofungin 150 mg daily

3. A 19-year-old football player sustains a blunt abdominal injury during practice at a local college. He quickly becomes pale and hypotensive and is rushed to the emergency room, where splenic rupture is confirmed. He undergoes emergent splenectomy, survives, and is now admitted to the ICU for further care. Which vaccines should you give **Immediately**?

   **A.** Meningococcus, *Haemophilus influenzae* type B (HiB), and the 23-valent pneumococcus vaccine, followed by 13-valent pneumococcus vaccine 8 weeks later
   **B.** Meningococcus, seasonal influenza, varicella zoster virus, and shingles
   **C.** HiB, 23-valent pneumococcus vaccine, and 13-valent pneumococcus vaccine
   **D.** No vaccinations now—wait until at least 2 weeks after splenectomy to administer vaccines

4. A bioterrorist attacks your city, sprinkling a white powder over a half-mile-long crowd attending a parade. What antibiotic prophylaxis is **Most** appropriate?

   **A.** Rifampin 1 g orally to all people within a 1-mile radius of the attack
   **B.** Azithromycin 500 mg orally to all people exposed to the powder
   **C.** Ciprofloxacin, levofloxacin, or doxycycline orally to all people older exposed to the powder
   **D.** Ciprofloxacin 500 mg orally to all people over 5 years of age within a 1-mile radius of the attack, rifampin 500 mg to all people under 5 years of age within a 1-mile radius of the attack

5. You admit a 34-year-old woman living with HIV to the ICU after a motor vehicle accident. She sustained blunt abdominal trauma with small bowel injury, requiring removal and re-anastomosis of a section of jejunum. Her CD4 T-cell count 3 weeks before the accident was 273 cells/mL. The surgical team recommends strict avoidance of oral intake and initiating total parenteral nutrition while her bowel heals. The patient is currently taking a three-drug regimen to treat her HIV infection, including dolutegravir, tenofovir, and emtricitabine. What should be done about HIV treatment while the patient remains nil per os?

   A. Stop all HIV medications simultaneously
   B. Continue dolutegravir, tenofovir, and emtricitabine intravenously
   C. Stop tenofovir immediately, but continue tenofovir and emtricitabine intravenously
   D. Stop all HIV medications and start intravenous azithromycin and trimethoprim/sulfamethoxazole prophylaxis against opportunistic infections

6. An 81-year-old woman is transferred to you from another hospital with a history of methicillin-resistant *Staphylococcus aureus* bacteremia that led to prosthetic hardware infection of a recent total hip arthroplasty. Her bacteremia cleared, and rifampin was initiated on the day of transfer, while also continuing vancomycin. She remains intubated and sedated on a ventilator for respiratory failure due to comorbid chronic obstructive pulmonary disease. You consider starting corticosteroids for her exacerbation of her chronic obstructive pulmonary disease. Before starting any new medications for this patient, what should you do?

   A. Check for drug interactions, as rifampin is a potent cytochrome P450 inducer
   B. Use a lower corticosteroid dose than you would usually give
   C. Stop rifampin, give corticosteroids instead
   D. Measure rifampin levels to determine whether cytochrome P450 has already been induced

7. You are caring for an 18-year-old woman undergoing CAR T-cell therapy for relapsed acute lymphoblastic leukemia. She was admitted to the ICU with hypotension and altered mental status. Blood cultures are positive for *S. aureus* in all four bottles collected on the day of admission. Which of the following has been associated with a mortality benefit in *S. aureus* bacteremia?

   A. Removing the implanted vascular access device (port-a-cath) on the day bacteremia is diagnosed
   B. Treating *S. aureus* bacteremia with at least 6 weeks of intravenous antibiotics
   C. Adding rifampin to intravenous antibiotic therapy
   D. Infectious diseases consultation

8. A 56-year-old man is admitted to the ICU for sepsis and meningismus. Eleven days before admission, he had started a corticosteroid burst for severe atopic dermatitis. He is found to have *Streptococcus bovis* meningitis, and polymicrobial bacteremia with *Escherichia coli*, *Enterococcus faecalis*, and *S. bovis*. Of note, he immigrated to the United States from South America 2 years ago. In addition to abdominal imaging with computed tomography and serologic testing, which of the following should you consider treating the patient with?

   A. Ivermectin
   B. Medenbazole
   C. Praziquantel
   D. Tinidazole

9. You are treating a patient for *Klebsiella pneumoniae* bacteremia. Your microbiology laboratory provides you with the following antimicrobial susceptibility data:

| ANTIBIOTIC NAME | MINIMUM INHIBITORY CONCENTRATION (MIC) VALUE IN µg/mL | INTERPRETATION |
|---|---|---|
| Cefepime | ≤2 | Susceptible |
| Ceftriaxone | ≤1 | Susceptible |
| Ciprofloxacin | ≥4 | Resistant |
| Gentamicin | ≤4 | Susceptible |
| Meropenem | ≤0.25 | Susceptible |
| Piperacillin-tazobactam | ≤16 | Susceptible |

Which of the following medications is the **BEST** choice for treatment?

A. Piperacillin-tazobactam
B. Cefepime
C. Imipenem
D. Ceftriaxone

10. You are treating a patient with acute renal failure for *Enterobacter aerogenes* bacteremia. Your microbiology laboratory provides you with the following antimicrobial susceptibility data:

| ANTIBIOTIC NAME | MINIMUM INHIBITORY CONCENTRATION (MIC) VALUE IN μg/mL | INTERPRETATION |
| --- | --- | --- |
| Gentamicin | 8 | Intermediate |
| Ciprofloxacin | ≥4 | Resistant |
| Ceftriaxone | ≤1 | Susceptible |
| Piperacillin-tazobactam | 64 | Intermediate |
| Cefepime | ≤2 | Susceptible |
| Meropenem | ≤0.5 μg/mL | Susceptible |

Of the following medications, which is the **BEST** choice for treatment?

A. High-dose piperacillin-tazobactam
B. Meropenem, imipenem, or ertapenem
C. Cefepime
D. Amikacin

# Chapter 69 ▪ Answers

1. Correct Answer: B

**Rationale:**
Three of the four first-line drugs used to treat tuberculosis (rifampicin, isoniazid, pyrazinamide) can be hepatotoxic. In patients being treated for tuberculosis, the most important step is to determine all potential causes of hepatitis, and stop all nonessential medications that could be causing drug-induced hepatitis. If tuberculosis medications are the suspected culprit(s), it is recommended that all antituberculosis treatment be stopped. If the patient is critically ill from tuberculosis, a nonhepatotoxic regimen can be substituted, including ethambutol, streptomycin, and a fluoroquinolone.

### References
1. Tweed CD, Wills GH, Crook AM, et al. Liver toxicity associated with tuberculosis chemotherapy in the REMoxTB study. *BMC Med.* 2018;16:46.
2. Nahid P, Dorman SE, Alipanah N, et al. Official American Thoracic Society/Centers for Disease Control and Prevention/Infectious Diseases Society of America clinical practice guidelines: treatment of drug-susceptible tuberculosis. *Clin Infect Dis.* 2016;63:e147-e195.
3. WHO. *Treatment of Tuberculosis: Guidelines.* 4th ed. Geneva, Switzerland: World Health Organization; 2010.

2. Correct Answer: C

**Rationale:**
Cryptococcal meningitis is a common central nervous system infection in immunocompromised patients. It is usually diagnosed using India ink stain or detection of cryptococcal antigen in cerebrospinal fluid. When available, the most effective therapy for cryptococcal meningitis is combination liposomal amphotericin B plus flucytosine (Answer C). After an induction period of treatment with combination amphotericin B and flucytosine therapy, fluconazole is often given for six to eighteen more months (Answer A). Although ketoconazole (Answer B) penetrates brain tissue, it is not currently used as first-line therapy for cryptococcal meningitis. Micafungin and caspofungin (Answer D) do not penetrate the central nervous system and thus have no role in treating cryptococcal meningitis or other central nervous system infections.

References

1. Perfect JR, Dismukes WE, Dromer F, et al. Clinical practice guidelines for the management of cryptococcal disease: 2010 update by the infectious diseases Society of America. *Clin Infect Dis.* 2010;50:291-322.
2. WHO Guidelines Approved by the Guidelines Review Committee. *Guidelines for The Diagnosis, Prevention and Management of Cryptococcal Disease in HIV-Infected Adults, Adolescents and Children: Supplement to the 2016 Consolidated Guidelines on the Use of Antiretroviral Drugs for Treating and Preventing HIV Infection.* Geneva: World Health Organization; 2018.

**3.** Correct Answer: D

**Rationale:**

Asplenic and hyposplenic individuals are particularly susceptible to infections caused by encapsulated bacteria, including *Neisseria meningitides*, *Streptococcus pneumoniae*, and *H. influenzae*. It is recommended that all individuals anticipated to become asplenic or hyposplenic be vaccinated against *N. meningitides*, *S. pneumoniae*, *H. influenzae* and seasonal influenza at least 2 weeks before elective splenectomy, or at least 2 weeks after emergent splenectomy. Individuals without evidence of immunity to measles, mumps, rubella, and varicella should also be vaccinated against these viral pathogens, in addition to receiving a booster dose of tetanus, diphtheria, and pertussis vaccine. The order and timing of pneumococcal vaccination is important, and it is generally recommended that the 23-valent pneumococcus vaccine be administered first, with the 13-valent vaccine to be given 8 weeks later. However, individuals who already received the 23-valent vaccine should be given the 13-valent vaccine at least 12 months after receiving the 23-valent vaccine.

References

1. Bonanni P, Grazzini M, Niccolai G, et al. Recommended vaccinations for asplenic and hyposplenic adult patients. *Hum Vaccin Immunother.* 2017;13:359-368.
2. Yorkgitis BK. Primary care of the blunt splenic injured adult. *Am J Med.* 2017;130:365.e1-365.e5.

**4.** Correct Answer: C

**Rationale:**

There are three FDA-approved drugs for *Bacillus anthracis* (anthrax) postexposure prophylaxis for adults 18 years of age and older: ciprofloxacin, levofloxacin, and doxycycline. Current guidelines recommend 60 days of treatment with one of these medications for adults. Although fluoroquinolones are generally not used for infection treatment or prophylaxis in children, and doxycycline is avoided in children younger than 8 years of age, it is generally agreed-upon that the benefits of prophylaxis with these medications in children outweigh potential toxicities in the setting of anthrax exposure. Prophylaxis should be given as soon as possible after exposure, as efficacy diminishes with time since exposure. Three doses of anthrax vaccine adsorbed are also recommended concurrently with antibiotic prophylaxis. Rifampin is often given for prophylaxis to people exposed to *N. meningitides* but is not used for anthrax exposure.

References

1. Hendricks KA, Wright ME, Shadomy SV, et al. Centers for disease control and prevention expert panel meetings on prevention and treatment of anthrax in adults. *Emerg Infect Dis.* 2014;20(2).
2. Sweeney DA, Hicks CW, Cui X, Li Y, Eichacker PQ. Anthrax infection. *Am J Respir Crit Care Med.* 2011;184:1333-1341.
3. Antibiotics for anthrax postexposure prophylaxis. In: Committee on Prepositioned Medical Countermeasures for the Public; Institute of Medicine; Stroud C, Viswanathan K, Powell T, et al, eds. *Prepositioning Antibiotics for Anthrax.* Washington, DC: National Academies Press (US); September 30, 2011:2. Available from https://www.ncbi.nlm.nih.gov/books/NBK190044/

**5.** Correct Answer: A

**Rationale:**

Antiretroviral therapy is life-prolonging in people living with HIV. Research has shown poorer long-term outcomes among people undergoing planned or unplanned treatment interruptions. Nevertheless, there are occasional situations in which a treatment interruption is unavoidable, such as when a patient experiences a severe or life-threatening toxicity or unexpected inability to take oral medications. In this scenario, it is recommended that all antiretroviral medications be stopped simultaneously and restarted together when the patient is again able to take oral medications. Unfortunately, there are currently no FDA-approved intravenous preparations of antiretroviral medications. Certain antiretroviral drugs have long half-lives, including the nonnucleoside reverse transcriptase inhibitors (NNRTIs) efavirenz, etravirine, and rilpivarine. When a patient is taking three-drug antiretroviral regimen containing one of these medications, stopping all antiretroviral medications at once could lead to effective monotherapy with the drug with the longest half-life (often an NNRTI), promoting HIV drug resistance. Because this patient's recent CD4 T-cell count is above 200 cells/mL, antibiotic prophylaxis against opportunistic infections is not indicated. Owing to the complexities of managing patients taking antiretroviral medications with differing half-lives, medication interactions, and increased susceptibility to infections, infectious diseases consultation is recommended whenever discontinuation of antiretroviral medications is considered in a person living with HIV.

### References

1. AIDSinfo. *Guidelines for the use of antiretroviral agents in adults and adolescents living with HIV*. In: *Management of the Treatment-Experienced Patient*. Washington, DC, USA: National Institutes of Health; 2015. https://aidsinfo.nih.gov/contentfiles/lvguidelines/AdultandAdolescentGL.pdf.
2. Aidsmap. *Risks When Stopping NNRTIs*. London, England: NAM; 2018. http://www.aidsmap.com/Risks-when-stopping-NNRTIs/page/1729926/
3. Taylor S, Boffito M, Khoo S, Smit E, Back D. Stopping antiretroviral therapy. *Aids*. 2007;21:1673-1682.

**6.** Correct Answer: A

**Rationale:**

Rifamycins are often used in the management of infections associated with implanted prosthetic materials, and for tuberculosis. Because rifamycins are potent inducers of the cytochrome P450 system (CYP 3A4), it is important to be check for drug-drug interactions and changes in drug metabolism for patients taking these medications. Corticosteroids are metabolized by the cytochrome P450 system, and steroid doses might need to be increased to counteract this increase in metabolism. It is best to work closely with a pharmacist when caring for a patient receiving medications that dramatically alter drug metabolism. Rifampin levels are not useful in indicating the extent to which the cytochrome P450 system has been induced.

### References

1. Baciewicz AM, Chrisman CR, Finch CK, Self TH. Update on rifampin, rifabutin, and rifapentine drug interactions. *Curr Med Res*. 2013;29:1-12.
2. Rothstein DM. Rifamycins, alone and in combination. *Cold Spring Harb Perspect*. 2016;6.

**7.** Correct Answer: D

**Rationale:**

Patients with indwelling central venous catheters (CVCs) are at increased risk of invasive bloodstream infections. *S. aureus* is one of the most common bloodstream infections and is associated with considerable morbidity and mortality. Because of the complexities in management of *S. aureus* bacteremia, infectious diseases consultation is recommended and was shown to provide a mortality benefit in a 2016 systematic review and meta-analysis. Although removal of CVCs early in the course of treatment for *S. aureus* bacteremia is generally recommended, removal on the day of diagnosis is not necessary in most cases and has not been associated with a mortality benefit. Intravenous antibiotic therapy is the mainstay of treatment for *S. aureus* bacteremia, but the duration of therapy is generally 2 to 6 weeks unless there is associated endocarditis or infection of prosthetic material. Adding rifampin is not recommended early in the course of therapy when bacterial burden is high, as there is a low barrier to developing resistance to rifampin.

### References

1. Vogel M, Schmitz RP, Hagel S, et al. Infectious disease consultation for staphylococcus aureus bacteremia – a systematic review and meta-analysis. *J Infect*. 2016;72:19-28.
2. Turner RB, Valcarlos E, Won R, Chang E, Schwartz J. Impact of infectious diseases consultation on clinical outcomes of patients with staphylococcus aureus bacteremia in a community health system. *Antimicrob Agents Chemother*. 2016;60:5682-5687.
3. Jung N, Rieg S. Essentials in the management of S. aureus bloodstream infection. *Infection*. 2018;46:441-442.

**8.** Correct Answer: A

**Rationale:**

This patient likely has *Strongyloides stercoralis* hyperinfection syndrome leading to polymicrobial bacteremia and meningitis. When gastrointestinal organisms are cultured from the cerebrospinal fluid, clinicians should suspect an intestinal source of bacteremia. Common sources include gastrointestinal malignancy, perforation, or intra-abdominal disaster. At least 10% to 40% of people living in tropical and subtropical regions are exposed to the soil helminth *S. stercoralis*, and most infections are asymptomatic, though affected persons may have peripheral eosinophilia. After infection, *S. stercoralis* is normally contained within the gastrointestinal tract by the host immune system, but parasite larvae can escape from the gastrointestinal tract in the setting of high-dose steroid administration or other systemic immune suppression, carrying gastrointestinal bacteria along with the escaped parasite. The larvae can then penetrate multiple sites including the central nervous system, leading to bacterial meningitis with gastrointestinal flora, which is sometimes polymicrobial. The treatment of choice for *S. stercoralis* hyperinfection syndrome is ivermectin. The other antiparasitic medications are not well-established treatments for strongylodiasis.

### References

1. Requena-Mendez A, Buonfrate D, Gomez-Junyent J, Zammarchi L, Bisoffi Z, Munoz J. Evidence-based guidelines for screening and management of strongyloidiasis in non-endemic countries. *Am J Trop Med Hyg*. 2017;97:645-652.
2. Buonfrate D, Requena-Mendez A, Angheben A, et al. Severe strongyloidiasis: a systematic review of case reports. *BMC Infect Dis*. 2013;13:78.

**9.** Correct Answer: D

**Rationale:**

For most bacteremias caused by gram-negative organisms, the antibiotic with the narrowest spectrum and fewest toxicities is generally the best choice for treatment. Both ciprofloxacin and ceftriaxone would be reasonable choices for this patient; however, the minimum inhibitory concentration to ciprofloxacin for this isolate is too high to be considered susceptible. As ciprofloxacin and levofloxacin are the only oral antibiotics commonly used in the United States to treat gram-negative bacteremias, aminoglycosides are associated with greater toxicity, and the other antibiotic choices have a broad spectrum; ceftriaxone is therefore the best of the remaining options.

Reference

1. Dellit TH, Owens RC, McGowan JE Jr, et al. Infectious Diseases Society of America and the Society for Healthcare Epidemiology of America guidelines for developing an institutional program to enhance antimicrobial stewardship. *Clin Infect Dis.* 2007;44:159-177.

**10.** Correct Answer: B

**Rationale:**

*E. aerogenes* is also one of the so-called SPICE or SPACE organisms that exhibit inducible beta-lactamases or stable depression of the chromosomal beta-lactamase. These organisms include bacteria of the genera *Serratia, Pseudomonas*, indole-positive *Proteus, Acinetobacter, Citrobacter*, and *Enterobacter*. These bacteria can develop resistance to third- and fourth-generation cephalosporins (such as Ceftriaxone and Cefepime) during, or shortly after, a course of treatment. The risk of developing resistance is highest in the setting of bacteremia and is estimated at 5% to 20%. The carbapenem antimicrobial class (meropenem, imipenem, or ertapenem) has a low failure rate in this setting, and medications from this class can be safely used in patients with renal failure.

References

1. Macdougall C. Beyond susceptible and resistant, part I: treatment of infections due to gram-negative organisms with inducible beta-lactamases. *J Pediatr Pharmacol.* 2011;16:23-30.
2. Pitout JD, Sanders CC, Sanders WE Jr. Antimicrobial resistance with focus on beta-lactam resistance in gram-negative bacilli. *Am J Med.* 1997;103:51-59.

# 70

# IMMUNE SUPPRESSION: CONGENITAL, ACQUIRED, DRUGS

Rachel C. Frank and Dusan Hanidziar

1. A 52-year-old woman diagnosed with granulomatosis with polyangiitis (Wegener's) 3 months ago and treated with cyclophosphamide and prednisone (40 mg daily) presents to ED due to shortness of breath and dry cough. Last time she noted blood-tinged sputum was more than 2 months ago. Her vitals on arrival are notable for temperature of 39.2°C, heart rate 110 beats/min, blood pressure 104/54, respiratory rate 25 breaths/min, and oxygen saturation 86% on room air. Chest x-ray reveals bilateral infiltrates and cystic-appearing round opacities follow.

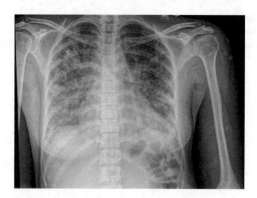

She is placed on high flow nasal cannula at 55 L/min and $FiO_2$ of 0.8, but her respiratory distress continues to worsen, and she requires endotracheal intubation. Her labs are notable for

Arterial blood gas: pH 7.48/$pCO_2$ 23/$pO_2$ 58 (before intubation)
Lactate dehydrogenase (LDH): 664 (normal: 110-210 U/L)

Which of the following treatment regimens would MOST likely improve her condition?

A. Ceftriaxone and azithromycin
B. Trimethoprim/sulfamethoxazole
C. Oseltamivir
D. Isoniazid

2. A 34-year-old male with recently diagnosed Hodgkin lymphoma is admitted to the hospital for induction chemotherapy with doxorubicin, bleomycin, vinblastine, and dacarbazine. On day 7 of the induction, he develops fever as high as 38.4°C and rigors. His blood pressure is 80/52 mm Hg, heart rate is 110 beats/min, respiratory rate is 22 breaths/min, and his oxygen saturation is 92% on 4 L $O_2$ via nasal canula. He is given 2 L of lactated Ringer's after which his blood pressure improves to 98/64. Internal jugular central line site is examined, and no erythema or purulence at the site of insertion is noted. Labs are notable for pancytopenia with a white blood cell count of 0.2 K/μL with 0% neutrophils, hemoglobin of 7.1 g/dL, platelets of 24 K/μL, and lactate of 2.8 mmol/L.

Which of the following interventions is MOST likely to decrease this patient's mortality?

    **A.** Vancomycin and cefepime
    **B.** Neutropenic precautions
    **C.** Granulocyte colony-stimulating factor (filgrastim)
    **D.** Removal of central line

**3.** A 53-year-old man with celiac disease is admitted to hospital from primary physician's office for a workup of weakness and anemia. His hemoglobin is 6.0 g/dL and is suspected to be a result of a slow GI bleed. His vitals are notable for heart rate of 100 beats/min, blood pressure of 92/50 mm Hg, and oxygen saturation of 96% on room air. Two units of cross-matched packed red blood cells are ordered. Ten minutes into the blood transfusion, patient becomes febrile (38.6°C), but other vitals remain unchanged. Transfusion is continued. Fifteen minutes later the patient develops worsening hypotension to 75/40 mm Hg, urticarial rash, and wheezing.

Which of the following is the MOST likely etiology of the patient's decompensation?

    **A.** Bacterial contamination of blood product
    **B.** Hemolytic transfusion reaction related to ABO incompatibility
    **C.** IgA deficiency with exposure to Immunoglobulin A (IgA) in the blood product
    **D.** Worsening GI bleed

**4.** A 52-year-old male with history of end-stage renal disease on hemodialysis is recovering in PACU following deceased donor renal transplant. He is receiving infusion of rabbit antithymocyte globulin (ATG) which was started intraoperatively. On a regular nursing check, he is found to have fever of 38.5°C. His heart rate is 90 beats/min, blood pressure is 110/60 mm Hg (baseline 150/80 mm Hg), CVP is 8, and oxygen saturation is 98% on room air. He is anuric. He has no specific complaints, and his surgical site appears normal.

Which of the following is the next BEST step in management of his condition?

    **A.** Decrease ATG infusion rate, obtain cultures, CBC
    **B.** Start infusion of phenylephrine
    **C.** Administer 2 L of lactated Ringer's
    **D.** Administer 1 U of PRBCs

**5.** A 62-year-old man with refractory non-Hodgkin lymphoma is admitted to hospital for infusion of chimeric antigen receptor T cells (CAR T). On day 3 following the infusion of CAR T cells, he becomes febrile to 38.9°C, hypotensive, and somnolent. Neurological examination is nonfocal. His blood pressure remains 75/40 mm Hg despite quick administration of 2 L lactated Ringer's, and he is transferred to the ICU for further management. The infusion of norepinephrine is initiated. He now requires 6 L/min O$_2$ via nasal cannula to maintain oxygen saturation >90%.

Which of the following is the next BEST step in management?

    **A.** Administration of tocilizumab while ruling out infection
    **B.** Immediate administration of empiric vancomycin and cefepime
    **C.** Fluid and vasopressor management to support hemodynamics while cytokine release syndrome resolves
    **D.** IV hydrocortisone

**6.** A 53-year-old man with history of chronic hepatitis C and acquired immune deficiency syndrome (history of cryptococcal meningitis, last CD4 count 250 cells/μL on antiretroviral therapy with undetectable viral load) presents for open liver resection after he was diagnosed with liver cancer. Following an uncomplicated operation, he is recovering on surgical floor. On postoperative day 3, he develops fever (temperature, 38.9°C). Other vitals are notable for blood pressure of 85/52 mm Hg, heart rate of 110 beats/min, respiratory rate of 26 breaths/min, and oxygen saturation of 92% on 4 L nasal cannula. Abdominal examination is benign. Chest x-ray reveals likely infiltrate and/or atelectasis in the right lower lobe. Lactate level is 3 mmol/L.

Which of the following is the MOST appropriate initial antibiotic regimen for this patient?

    **A.** Vancomycin, cefepime, azithromycin
    **B.** Levofloxacin
    **C.** Trimethoprim and sulfamethoxazole (TMP-SMX)
    **D.** Meropenem

7. A 45-year-old female is admitted to the surgical ICU following liver transplantation. On postoperative day (POD) 3, she develops a tonic-clonic seizure which is terminated by intravenous midazolam. However, she requires intubation for persistently poor mental status. CT scan of the head is obtained immediately and is negative for bleeding or mass lesion. Lumbar puncture is deferred due to coagulopathy (INR 1.9, Plt 50). A brain MRI performed 6 hours later shows left temporal increased signal intensity in T2 and FLAIR weighted images.

Which of the following treatment is most effective to decrease patient mortality?

A. Intravenous acyclovir
B. Gancyclovir
C. Levetiracetam
D. Corticosteroids

8. A 52-year-old female with severe COPD is admitted to the ICU for hypercarbic respiratory failure. She requires mechanical ventilation and is treated with methylprednisolone and azithromycin. She is extubated on ICU day 4. After extubation, she complains of left-sided flank pain, but her examination and labs are normal. On day 6, a vesicular rash with erythematous base develops diffusely across her abdomen, and additional lesions are noted on her face and arms.

Which of the following is the next best step to diagnose her condition?

A. Full ophthalmologic examination
B. Unroofing vesicle and sending varicella-zoster virus and herpes virus direct fluorescence antibody stain (DFA) and reflex culture
C. Punch biopsy for dermatopathology
D. Skin testing for latex allergy

# Chapter 70 ▪ Answers

1. Correct Answer: B

**Rationale:**
Patient has clinical symptoms and laboratory and radiographic signs consistent with pneumocystis jirovecii pneumonia (PJP), an opportunistic infection typically affecting immunocompromised hosts. These may include patients with acquired immune deficiency syndrome (AIDS), those with malignancies, stem cell and solid organ transplant recipients, and patients receiving high-dose corticosteroids and other immunosuppressants. PJP classically presents with fever, dry cough, and hypoxemic respiratory failure with exertional oxygen desaturations.

Positive PJP PCR or silver stain from induced sputum or bronchoalveolar lavage (BAL) samples are confirmatory. LDH elevation is common, particularly in HIV-positive patients in whom the sensitivity is reported to be 100%; however, sensitivity is lower (~60%) in HIV-negative individuals. Radiographic findings include bilateral patchy infiltrates with cystic-appearing opacities on chest x-rays (as seen in the above chest x-ray). On high-resolution CT scans, the most common findings are ground glass opacities with cysts that are seen in approximately one third of patients.

First-line treatment is intravenous trimethoprim/sulfamethoxazole (Bactrim) which should be continued for at least 7 to 10 days or until clinical improvement is seen, when transition to oral antibiotics is considered. Total duration of therapy is typically 3 weeks. PJP prophylaxis should be initiated in patients with CD4 count less than 200 cells/mm³ and those receiving high-dose steroids (>20 mg/d) for more than one month, particularly if the patient is receiving additional cytotoxic agents, as in this clinical vignette.

References
1. Kanne JP, Yandow DR, Meyer CA. Pneumocystis jiroveci pneumonia: high-resolution CT findings in patients with and without HIV infection. *Am J Roentgenol.* 2012;198(6):555-561.
2. Limper AH, Knox KS, Sarosi GA. An Official American Thoracic Society Statement: treatment of fungal infections in adult pulmonary and critical care patients. *Am J Resp Crit Care Med.* 2011;183(1):96-128.
3. Smith DE, Forbes A, Davies S, Barton SE, Gazzard BG. Diagnosis of *Pneumocystis carinii* pneumonia in HIV antibody positive patients by simple outpatient assessments. *Thorax.* 1992;47(12):1005-1009.
4. Vogel MN, Weissgerber P, Goeppert B, et al. Accuracy of serum LDH elevation for the diagnosis of *Pneumocystis jiroveci* pneumonia. *Swiss Med Wkly.* 2011;141:w13184.
5. Wieruszewski PM, Barreto JN, Frazee E, et al. Early corticosteroids for pneumocystis pneumonia in adults without HIV are not associated with better outcome. *Chest.* 2018;154(3):636-644.

**2.** Correct Answer: A

**Rationale:**

This patient has neutropenic fever which is a serious complication of chemotherapy. It is defined by an isolated temperature >38.3°C (101°F) or a temperature of >38.0°C (100.4°F) lasting for >1 hour in a patient with neutropenia. If not treated promptly, sepsis and septic shock can develop. Severe neutropenia is defined as an absolute neutrophil count (ANC) of less than 500 cells/mm³. Neutrophils prevent bacterial and fungal infections; therefore, neutropenic patients are especially prone to these types of infections.

Adequate antibiotic therapy is the key intervention to decrease mortality of this patient. The initial empiric antibiotic therapy for febrile neutropenia is a beta-lactam with pseudomonas coverage (such as ceftazidime, cefepime, piperacillin-tazobactam) or a carbapenem (meropenem, imipenem). While vancomycin is not typically a part of the empiric antibiotic regimen, it should be added in patients with evidence of hemodynamic instability (such as in this patient), pneumonia, skin or soft tissue infection, or catheter-related infection. Vancomycin or alternative gram-positive coverage may be discontinued at 48 hours if there is no confirmation of gram-positive pathogens. Antibiotic therapy should be further tailored to resistance patterns of bacteria previously isolated from a patient and colonization with resistant organisms such as methicillin-resistant *Staphylococcus aureus* (MRSA), vancomycin-resistant enterococcus (VRE), extended-spectrum β-lactamase (ESBL) gram-negative organisms, or carbapenemase-producing organisms.

Patients should be evaluated for the presence of indwelling lines both as a source of infection and for removal depending on the isolated pathogen. In this clinical scenario, immediate removal of central line is not indicated. In patients that are considered to be high risk for infectious complications (hospitalized at the time of fever, age >65 years, expected protracted neutropenia lasting >10 days, or ANC <100/μL, sepsis, pneumonia, or invasive fungal infections), administration of granulocyte colony-stimulating factor should be considered. Neutropenic precautions alone would not be sufficient to decrease this patient's mortality.

References

1. Freifeld AG, Bow EJ, Sepkowitz KA, et al. Clinical practice guideline for the use of antimicrobial agents in neutropenic patients with cancer: 2010 update by the Infectious Diseases Society of America. *Clin Infect Dis*. 2011;52(4):56-93.
2. Thandra K, Salah Z, Chawla S. Oncologic emergencies—the old, the new, and the deadly. *J Intens Care Med*. 2018; [Epub November 9, 2018].

**3.** Correct Answer: C

**Rationale:**

This patient developed anaphylactic reaction to blood product. Anaphylactic reactions to blood products occur in about 1 out of 1.3 million transfusions. These reactions occur most commonly either during or within 4 hours of a transfusion. Anaphylactic reactions should be treated by immediately stopping the blood transfusion, administration of intramuscular epinephrine, intravenous H1 blocker antihistamines (eg, diphenhydramine), H2 blocker antihistamines (eg, ranitidine), intravenous methylprednisolone, and beta-agonists (eg, albuterol) as needed. Adequate respiratory support including supplemental oxygen and/or mechanical ventilatory support should be provided based on the clinical status of the patient.

Isolated IgA deficiency is the most common immunoglobulin deficiency with the prevalence estimated to be between 1 in 200 and 1 in 500. Anti-IgA–mediated anaphylactic reactions occur when patients with IgA deficiency have developed anti-IgA antibodies that can react with IgA in red blood cell products. Sensitization to IgA may occur during prior blood transfusions, pregnancy, or intravenous immunoglobulin infusions. However, some patients do not have a history that suggests prior sensitization. In these cases, it is postulated the anti-IgA antibodies may either occur spontaneously or as a consequence of sensitization either in utero or via breast milk. IgA deficiency is common in patients with celiac disease, such as the patient in this vignette.

Hemolytic blood transfusion reactions occur when there is ABO incompatibility. This is exceptionally rare in the setting of rigorous cross-matching protocols. Symptoms of a hemolytic transfusion reaction include temperature increase >1 or <1°C with associated fevers, chills, hypotension, nausea or vomiting, and evidence of hemolysis. Acute airway compromise and wheezing are not classic signs of hemolytic transfusion reactions.

A diagnosis of septic transfusion is made when bacteria are isolated from both the blood product and the patient. A presumptive diagnosis can be made when bacteria are isolated solely from the blood product in a patient with a clinical syndrome of sepsis. Urticarial rash and respiratory distress would not be consistent with bacterial contamination. Guidelines recommend starting empiric antibiotics (β-lactam or aminoglycoside) with pseudomonas coverage. While a sudden GI bleed could present with worsening hypotension, an urticarial rash and respiratory distress would be atypical.

References

1. Latiff AH, Kerr MA. The clinical significance of immunoglobulin A deficiency. *Ann Clin Biochem*. 2007;44(2):131-139.
2. Delaney M, Wendel S, Bercovitz RS, et al. Transfusion reactions: prevention, diagnosis, and treatment. *Lancet*. 2016;388(10061):2825-2836.
3. Webb C, Norris A, Hands K. An acute transfusion reaction. *Clin Med*. 2018;18(1):95-97.

**4.** Correct Answer: A

**Rationale:**

Antithymocyte globulin (ATG) consists of polyclonal antibodies directed against lymphocytes, therefore depleting them. It is used for induction of immunosuppression and for treatment of acute rejection. ATG use spares early use of nephrotoxic calcineurin inhibitors and also allows for decreased steroid exposure. Common side effects of ATG include fever, hypotension, rash, leukopenia, and thrombocytopenia. Serum sickness and acute respiratory distress syndrome (ARDS) have also been described in the literature.

The patient developed new-onset fever and hypotension in the PACU which could be caused by ATG. The ATG infusion rate should be decreased to see if there is improvement in hypotension, and additional workup should be pursued. Workup of new hypotension in the postoperative period includes repeat laboratory testing (blood counts), culture data (blood culture, urine culture, chest x-ray, sputum culture if available). Should hypotension and fever not improve with decreased rate of ATG infusion, empiric antimicrobials would be reasonable. Administration of volume (crystalloids, blood products) in an anuric patient with a CVP of 8 cm may be harmful by causing volume overload and potentially respiratory failure. Vasopressors may cause arterial constriction and result in ischemic injury of the delicate new renal graft.

## References

1. Bamoulid J, Staeck O, Crépin T, et al. Anti-thymocyte globulins in kidney transplantation: focus on current indications and long-term immunological side effects. *Nephrol Dialysis Transplant.* 2017;32(10):1601-1608.
2. Goligher EC, Cserti-Gazdewich C, Balter M, Gupta V, Brandwein JE. Acute lung injury during antithymocyte globulin therapy for aplastic anemia. *Can Respir J.* 2009;16(2):e3-e5.
3. Hertig A, Zuckermann A. Rabbit antithymocyte globulin induction and risk of post-transplant lymphoproliferative disease in adult and pediatric solid organ transplantation: an update. *Transpl Immunol.* 2015;32(3):179-187.
4. Klipa D, Mahmud N, Ahsan N. Antibody immunosuppressive therapy in solid organ transplant: part II. *MAbs.* 2010;2(6):607-612.
5. Malvezzi P, Jouve T, Rostaing L. Induction by anti-thymocyte globulins in kidney transplantation: a review of the literature and current usage. *J Nephropathol.* 2015;4(4):110-115.

**5.** Correct Answer: B

**Rationale:**

This patient most likely has cytokine release syndrome or sepsis, which are difficult to distinguish clinically.

Cytokine release syndrome (CRS) is a known complication of CAR T cell therapy. This syndrome is a result of the release of proinflammatory cytokines (interleukins 6 and 10 and interferon gamma) during the interaction between genetically engineered CAR T cells and target tumor cells. CRS is reported to occur in up to 50% to 100% of patients receiving CAR T therapy. CRS has many clinical manifestations ranging from minor (fever, fatigue, rash) to severe (hypotension, respiratory failure, coagulopathy, multisystem organ failure, death). Interleukin 6 (IL-6) is thought to be the main inflammatory cytokine in the pathophysiology of CRS. Elevated IL-6 levels are associated with increased vascular leakage, activation of complement, and coagulation cascade as well as myocardial dysfunction. Administration of tocilizumab (IL-6 receptor monoclonal antibody) should be considered in patients with high-grade CRS (requiring vasopressors, $FiO_2 > 40\%$).

Distinguishing CRS from other syndromes with similar presentations, such as septic shock, is challenging. Therefore, broad-spectrum antibiotics should be the first-line therapy administered to each CAR T patients with new-onset hemodynamic or respiratory instability. Delaying antibiotic treatment while awaiting the clinical benefit of tocilizumab or confirming infection results in high mortality rates. Corticosteroids are the mainstay of treatment for high-grade CAR T neurotoxicity. In this patient, somnolence is likely related to hypotension, fever, and CRS, and if improved with fluid, vasopressors, and antibiotics, treatment with corticosteroids is not indicated.

## References

1. Le RQ, Li L, Yuan W, et al. FDA approval summary: tocilizumab for treatment of chimeric antigen receptor T cell-induced severe or life-threatening cytokine release syndrome. *Oncologist.* 2018;23(8):943-947.
2. Neelapu SS, Tummala S, Kebriaei P, et al. Chimeric antigen receptor T-cell therapy—assessment and management of toxicities. *Nat Rev Clin Oncol.* 2018;15(1):47-62.
3. Porter D, Frey N, Wood PA, Weng Y, Grupp SA. Grading of cytokine release syndrome associated with the CAR T cell therapy tisagenlecleucel. *J Hematol Oncol.* 2018;11(35):e1-e12.

**6.** Correct Answer: A

**Rationale:**

This patient most likely developed hospital-acquired pneumonia complicated by sepsis. Initial antimicrobial therapy should be broad while awaiting additional workup with consideration about localizing symptoms (pulmonary). The patient has been admitted to hospital for greater than 48 hours prior to infectious symptom onset, and treatment should cover MRSA and *Pseudomonas.* Therefore, the Correct Answer is A. Initial therapy with vancomycin (MRSA coverage), cefepime (gram-negative including pseudomonas), and azithromycin (atypical coverage) is appropriate.

Although patient previously had an AIDS-defining illness (cryptococcal meningitis), a CD4 count above 200 cells/μL makes him less susceptible to opportunistic infections such as PJP. Based on description, his CXR is not suggestive of PJP pneumonia. Therefore, empiric TMP-SMX is not indicated at this point. Treatment with TMP-SMX alone would leave gaps in gram-negative coverage including pseudomonas and therefore would not be the correct empiric regimen. Meropenem and levofloxacin are not correct treatments for potential MRSA infection.

There are some unique considerations in critically ill patients with HIV/AIDS. Prior antibiotic prophylaxis (ie, azithromycin for mycobacterium avium complex) and the potential for resistance should be considered when choosing an empiric regimen. *Mycobacterium tuberculosis* infection (TB) occurs in patients with HIV/AIDS. If there is clinical concern for TB, empiric fluoroquinolones (ie, levofloxacin) should be avoided. Fluoroquinolones may result in short-term improvement through partial treatment of TB followed by later clinical decompensation and bacterial resistance. Patients with HIV/AIDS and/or intravenous drug use are at greater risk of fungemia. Fungal coverage should be initiated in individuals who fail to improve with initial antimicrobial therapy. Additional caution for drug interactions is needed in patients taking antiretroviral therapy. Azoles and macrolides interact with some forms of antiretroviral therapy and consultation with a pharmacist should occur prior to initiation of these medications.

## References

1. Gade ND, Qazi MS. Fluoroquinolone therapy in Staphylococcus aureus infections: where do we stand? *J Lab Physicians*. 2013;5(2):109-112.
2. Japiassú AM, Amâncio RT, Mesquita EC, et al. Sepsis is a major determinant of outcome in critically ill HIV/AIDS patients. *Crit Care*. 2010;14(4):e1-e8.
3. Panel on Opportunistic Infections in HIV-Infected Adults and Adolescents. *Guidelines for the prevention and treatment of opportunistic infections in HIV-infected adults and adolescents: recommendations from the Centers for Disease Control and Prevention, the National Institutes of Health, and the HIV Medicine Association of the Infectious Diseases Society of America*. Available at http://aidsinfo.nih.gov/contentfiles/lvguidelines/adult_oi.pdf. Accessed 11/3/2018.
4. Silva JM, dos Santos Sde S. Sepsis in AIDS patients: clinical, etiological and inflammatory characteristics. *J Int AIDS Soc*. 2013;16(1):e1-e8.

---

**7.** Correct Answer: A

**Rationale:**

This patient most likely developed herpes simplex virus (HSV) encephalitis—the most common cause of viral encephalitis with significant morbidity and mortality. MRI brain is the most specific imaging modality for encephalitis. Findings consistent with HSV encephalitis on neuroimaging include temporal or inferior frontal lobe edema and increased signal intensity on T2 and fluid-attenuated inversion recovery (FLAIR) images. Suspected HSV is treated with empiric acyclovir while diagnostic CSF studies are pending. In this case, imaging and clinical presentation is highly suggestive and warrants treatment. Patients who are seropositive for HSV prior to transplant are often on HSV prophylaxis with oral acyclovir. In this case, high-dose intravenous acyclovir should be initiated.

Ganciclovir is used to treat viral encephalitis from varicella-zoster virus, human herpes virus 6, and cytomegalovirus (in conjunction with foscarnet) but is not the treatment for HSV. Treatment with levetiracetam may be initiated but would not be alone sufficient to improve patient outcome. Steroids are used to treat some types of encephalitis including Epstein-Barr virus and varicella-zoster virus, but they are not recommended for HSV encephalitis.

## References

1. A Report from the British Society for Antimicrobial Chemotherapy Working Party on Antiviral Therapy; Management of herpes virus infections following transplantation. *J Antimicrob Chemotherapy*. 2000;45(6):729-748.
2. Guenette A, Husain S. Infectious complications following solid organ transplantation. *Crit Care Clin*. 2019;35(1):151-168.
3. Tunkel AR, Glaser CA, Bloch KC, et al. The management of encephalitis: clinical practice guidelines by the Infectious Diseases Society of America. *Clin Infect Dis*. 2008;47(3):303-327.
4. Venkatesan A, Tunkel AR, Bloch KC, et al. Case definitions, diagnostic algorithms, and priorities in encephalitis: consensus statement of the international encephalitis consortium. *Clin Infect Dis*. 2013;57(8):1114-1128.
5. Wilck MB, Zuckerman RA; AST Infectious Diseases Community of Practice. Herpes simplex virus in solid organ transplantation. *Am J Transplant*. 2013;13(4):121-127.

---

**8.** Correct Answer: B

**Rationale:**

Herpes zoster is caused by reactivation of latent varicella-zoster virus in cranial nerves or dorsal root ganglia. Reactivation of the virus is caused by decreased T-cell immunity and may result from increased age, primary infection during the time of an immature immune system, transplantation, immunosuppressive agents (such as steroids), or HIV infection.

A diagnosis of herpes zoster is made by unroofing a vesicle and sending the fluid for direct fluorescent antibody testing and reflex viral culture. Distinguishing reactivation of varicella-zoster virus from the vesicular rash of disseminated herpes virus may pose challenges clinically. Therefore, testing for both is appropriate.

Latex allergies are common with manifestations ranging from contact dermatitis to anaphylaxis. While skin testing is used to diagnose a variety of allergens, a proportion of patients with latex allergy will develop anaphylaxis. Therefore, the best test for suspected latex allergy would be serologic evaluation with IgE-specific latex antibody. The prodromal pain makes a latex allergy less likely. Punch biopsy may be useful in a variety of dermatologic diseases but is not necessary to diagnose herpes zoster. A full dilated eye examination is necessary to rule out herpes zoster ophthalmicus but would not confirm the diagnosis of herpes zoster in the absence of ocular involvement.

## References

1. Cohen JI. Herpes zoster. *N Engl J Med.* 2013;369(3):255-263.
2. Kelly KJ. Skin and serologic testing in the diagnosis of latex allergy. *J Allergy Clin Immunol.* 1993;91(6):1140-1145.
3. Naldi L, Venturuzzo A, Invernizzi P. Dermatological complications after solid organ transplantation. *Clin Rev Allergy Immunol.* 2018;54(1):185-212.
4. Pavlopoulou ID, Poulopoulou S, Melexopoulou C, Papazaharia I, Zavos G, Boletis IN. Incidence and risk factors of herpes zoster among adult renal transplant recipients receiving universal antiviral prophylaxis. *BMC Infect Dis.* 2015;15(1):e1-e8
5. Pergam NA, Limaye AP; AST Infectious Diseases Community of Practice. Varicella zoster virus in solid organ transplantation. *Am J Transplant.* 2013;13(4):138-146.

# 71

# INFECTIONS IN THE IMMUNOCOMPROMISED HOST

Francisco Jesús Marco Canosa, Fatima I Adhi, Ceena N. Jacob, and Teny M. John

1. A 38-year-old female with no significant past medical history was brought to the emergency department with confusion and lethargy. Her family noted that the patient had been complaining of worsening headaches for the last several days. On admission, she was afebrile and hemodynamically stable. Initial laboratory workup showed leukopenia (white blood cell [WBC] count of 3 000 cells/mL) with absolute lymphopenia. Human immunodeficiency virus (HIV) testing was positive with a ribonucleic acid (RNA) viral load of 68 000 copies/mL and CD4 count of 25 cells/μL. Magnetic resonance imaging (MRI) of the brain revealed multiple ring-enhancing lesions of different sizes with surrounding edema and mass effect. What is the NEXT BEST step to diagnose her disease process?

   A. India ink staining
   B. *Toxoplasma gondii* IgG antibody
   C. Stereotactic brain biopsy
   D. Cytomegalovirus CSF polymerase chain reaction (PCR)
   E. Quantiferon tuberculosis testing

2. A 29-year-old male is admitted from the emergency department with fevers. He complained of night sweats and painful cervical lymphadenitis for the last 7 days. He was diagnosed with HIV/AIDS 1 month ago when he was admitted with an episode of community-acquired pneumonia. His CD4 count was 80 cells/μL and HIV RNA viral load was 1 million copies/mL at the time of diagnosis. He was started on anti-retroviral therapy (ART) with tenofovir-emtricitabine and raltegravir. On examination, his blood pressure is 90/45 mm Hg and pulse rate is 106 beats per minute. Blood cultures are in process. He is appropriately fluid resuscitated and started on vancomycin and piperacillin-tazobactam to cover potentially hospital-acquired pathogens. Immune reconstitution inflammatory syndrome (IRIS) secondary to disseminated mycobacterium avium complex (MAC) infection is suspected. What is the NEXT BEST step regarding his ART during this admission?

   A. Hold ART and resume in 1 week
   B. Hold ART and resume in 2 weeks
   C. Continue ART
   D. Optimize ART by increasing the dose of current medications
   E. Optimize ART by changing the ART regimen to include two new medications

**Infections in the neutropenic patient**

3. A 65-year-old male is admitted to the hospital with malaise and fatigue for the past week. His WBC count on admission was 27 000 cells/mL. The patient was ultimately diagnosed with high-grade acute promyelocytic leukemia. A tunneled central venous catheter was placed and the patient was started on all-trans-retinoic acid, daunorubicin, and cytarabine. Four days after initiation of chemotherapy, he developed a fever of 39.1°C (102.3°F) and altered mental status. His blood pressure was 90/54 mm Hg, heart rate 108 beats per minute, respiratory rate 24 breaths per minute, and oxygen saturation 94% on 5 L of supplemental oxygen. Laboratory evaluation was significant for neutropenia (absolute neutrophil count 300 cells/μL). His chest x-ray showed a focal consolidation in the right middle lobe. He was admitted to the intensive care unit and blood cultures were obtained. What is the BEST empiric intravenous antibiotic regimen for this patient?

**A.** Ciprofloxacin and ampicillin-sulbactam
**B.** Meropenem alone
**C.** Piperacillin-tazobactam alone
**D.** Piperacillin-tazobactam and vancomycin
**E.** Meropenem and vancomycin and micafungin

4. A 60-year-old female was admitted to the ICU with acute hypoxic respiratory failure. She endorsed malaise, fevers, and neck swelling for 2 weeks prior to presentation. She received a bilateral lung transplant [cytomegalovirus (CMV) donor negative/recipient negative, Epstein-Barr virus (EBV) donor negative/recipient positive] 4 months ago for idiopathic pulmonary fibrosis and is currently on immunosuppression with azathioprine 200 mg daily and tacrolimus 2 g twice daily. Her antimicrobial prophylaxis includes trimethoprim-sulfamethoxazole one double-strength tablet thrice weekly and itraconazole 200 mg daily. On admission, she was alert and oriented, afebrile, and hemodynamically stable. Cervical lymphadenopathy was present. Her WBC count was 5600 cells/μL, hemoglobin 9.6 g/dL, alkaline phosphatase 125 U/L, aspartate aminotransferase (AST) 100 U/L, and alanine aminotransferase (ALT) 130 U/L. Her chest x-ray showed bilateral diffuse infiltrates. Blood cultures showed no growth on culture at 24 hours of collection. Serum EBV quantitative deoxyribonucleic acid (DNA) PCR was 100 000 copies/mL (undetectable on prior measurement 1 month ago). Posttransplant lymphoproliferative disease is suspected. What is the NEXT BEST step in the management of this patient?

**A.** Start treatment with rituximab
**B.** Reduce the current dose of immunosuppressants
**C.** Start treatment with rituximab and chemotherapy
**D.** Start treatment with acyclovir
**E.** Start treatment with valganciclovir

5. A 62-year-old male who underwent bilateral lung transplantation (CMV donor positive/recipient negative, EBV donor positive/recipient negative) for end-stage lung disease due to chronic obstructive pulmonary disease is admitted to the ICU with left lower quadrant abdominal pain, diarrhea, and hypotension. His symptoms started 5 days ago and have been progressively worsening. Diarrhea is mainly watery and frequency ranges from four to five times per day. On examination, the patient was afebrile with blood pressure 84/60 mm Hg, heart rate of 100 beats per minute, and dry oral mucosa. His abdomen was diffusely tender to palpation. An x-ray of the abdomen demonstrated colonic ileus with no evidence of gas under the diaphragm. Stool *Clostridium difficile* PCR, stool ova and parasites testing, and stool cultures are negative. CMV is undetectable by PCR in the plasma. What is the next BEST step in managing this patient?

**A.** CT scan of the abdomen with contrast
**B.** Colonoscopy and biopsies
**C.** Check serum EBV quantitative viral load
**D.** 24-hour stool fat test
**E.** Empiric treatment with micafungin and valganciclovir

6. A 50-year-old female underwent allogeneic stem cell transplantation for acute myeloid leukemia 10 days ago. She is brought to the ICU with fevers and hypotension. She is neutropenic. She noticed a red rash on her trunk and extremities yesterday. On examination, she appears ill and is febrile (38°C). Her blood pressure is 84/60 mm Hg, heart rate 120 beats per minute, and respiratory rate 36 breaths per minute. Her central venous catheter site is clean and nontender. Physical examination demonstrates grade 3 mucositis of her buccal mucosa, a diffuse erythematous, blanchable rash, and bilateral crackles on auscultation of her posterior lung fields. Her chest x-ray demonstrated bilateral diffuse infiltrates. A bedside echocardiogram showed normal valves with preserved left ventricular function. Her blood cultures grow gram positive cocci in pairs and chains in both sets of aerobic and anaerobic bottles collected on transfer. What is the MOST LIKELY diagnosis?

**A.** Catheter-related infection due to coagulase-negative staphylococci
**B.** Staphylococcal toxic shock syndrome
**C.** Engraftment syndrome
**D.** Infective endocarditis due to *Enterococcus faecalis*
**E.** Septic shock due to *viridans* group *Streptococci*

7. A 39-year-old male who underwent a haploidentical allogeneic hematopoietic stem cell transplantation (HSCT) for acute myeloid leukemia 2 years ago is admitted to the ICU with acute hypoxic respiratory failure requiring supplemental oxygen through a high-flow nasal cannula. His HSCT was complicated by graft-versus-host disease (GVHD) of the skin and gastrointestinal tract 6 weeks ago for which he was treated with pulse dose steroids. He was recovering from an upper respiratory tract infection caused by rhinovirus (nasopharyngeal swab PCR positive) 3 weeks ago when he started to experience shortness of breath that progressively worsened. His WBC count was 4.5 cells/μL with 80% neutrophils on admission. His creatinine was elevated at 2.1 mg/dL (baseline: 1 mg/dL). A CT scan of the chest without contrast revealed multifocal nodular opacities with right-sided predominance. Blood cultures, urine histoplasma antigen, serum cryptococcal antigen, and serum *Aspergillus* galactomannan were negative. His serum β-1,3-D-glucan assay was positive. The patient's sputum culture grew normal respiratory flora. He was started on intravenous vancomycin and piperacillin-tazobactam, but his respiratory status continued to decline eventually requiring intubation 2 days into his admission. Bronchoscopy was performed with bronchoalveolar lavage (BAL). Initial stains on the BAL fluid showed nonpigmented, septate hyphae branching at right angles. What is the NEXT step in the antimicrobial management of this patient?

   A. Add IV micafungin
   B. Add PO voriconazole
   C. Add IV voriconazole
   D. Start IV amphotericin B
   E. Continue current management and wait for final pathogen identification

8. A 26-year-old female with a history of sickle cell disease complicated by multiple sickle cell crises in the past year is admitted to the ICU with acute hypoxic respiratory failure and shock. On arrival to the ICU, she is febrile to 39.1°C with a blood pressure of 82/36 mm Hg and heart rate 110 beats per minute. She is intubated and mechanically ventilated. Initial laboratory evaluation demonstrates a neutrophilic- predominant leukocytosis to 14 000 cells/μL. Her chest x-ray on admission shows a left lower lung infiltrate with an associated pleural effusion. Blood cultures are in process. What would be the NEXT BEST STEP to confirm this patient's diagnosis?

   A. CT scan of the chest with and without IV contrast
   B. Sputum cultures
   C. *Streptococcus pneumoniae* urine antigen
   D. *Legionella* urine antigen
   E. Bronchoscopy with BAL

9. A 45-year-old female who underwent bilateral lung transplantation 6 days ago is brought to the ICU intubated following a seizure episode. Her transplantation was uneventful and she was transferred to a regular nursing floor on postoperative day 4. She was intubated at bedside for airway protection and brought to the ICU. On examination, the patient is sedated and her pupils were mildly dilated but equally reactive to light. Her blood pressure was 110/90 mm Hg and heart rate 120 beats per minute. Mild purulence is noted from the lower part of sternotomy site with no obvious instability or bony crepitations. The output from her chest drains was nonpurulent. An arterial blood gas shows an elevated lactate of 2.5 mmol/L, partial pressure of oxygen of 92 mm Hg, and partial pressure of carbon dioxide of 38 mm Hg. Her laboratory results demonstrate a WBC count of 16 500 cells/μL, hemoglobin of 9.1 g/dL, platelet count of 350 000/μL. Blood cultures are collected. Wound cultures sent from the regular nursing floor prior to transfer show numerous neutrophils but a negative gram stain. A CT scan of the brain did not show any acute abnormalities. Debridement of sternal wound is done and the patient is started on empiric vancomycin and piperacillin-tazobactam. What is the NEXT BEST step in the management of this patient?

   A. Wait for final culture results, no additional antibiotics
   B. Lumbar puncture, empirical IV acyclovir to treat Herpes simplex encephalitis
   C. Check serum ammonia level; start IV doxycycline to cover *Mycoplasma hominis*
   D. Start IV micafungin for empiric fungal coverage
   E. Order an MRI of the brain to rule out posterior reversible leukoencephalopathy

**10.** A 65-year-old former Vietnam War veteran male was admitted to the intensive care unit with shock. He had underwent orthotopic liver transplantation 3 months ago for cirrhosis due to alcohol abuse and hepatitis C infection. His posttransplant course had been complicated by graft-versus-host disease treated with pulse dose methylprednisolone for 3 days followed by prednisone 60 mg daily, which he was currently on. He presented to the emergency room with complaints of headache and wheezing for the last 2 days and was also found to be somnolescent. On the first day of admission, he was noted to have intermittent bouts of cough with two episodes of small volume hemoptysis. Chest x-ray showed bilateral patchy nodular opacities for which he was started on vancomycin and piperacillin/tazobactam. However, on the second day of admission, his condition acutely worsened with tachycardia, hypoxemia, and hypotension requiring vasopressor support. Lactate was elevated raising suspicion of sepsis, and workup for an infectious source was initiated. Urinalysis was unremarkable, stool *Clostridioides difficile* PCR was negative, and CMV PCR was undetectable in blood. CT scan of the head was unremarkable. Two sets of blood cultures were sent. Gram stain of cerebrospinal fluid (CSF) showed gram-negative rods identified later the same day as *Escherichia coli* by PCR, and consequently piperacillin/tazobactam was changed to cefepime. Chest imaging the next day showed marked worsening of opacities on the left upper lobe and right lower lobe, and he was intubated for worsening hypoxia. The tracheal aspirate was sent for culture; however, you received a call from the microbiology lab the same day informing you of an unexpected finding on the gram stain of tracheal aspirate. A representative image follows.

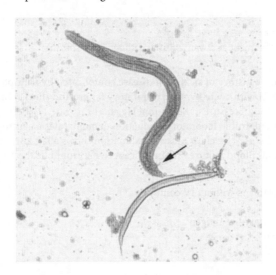

Which of the following describes the best treatment plan for this patient?

**A.** Continue cefepime
**B.** Continue cefepime and add ivermectin
**C.** Discontinue cefepime and start ivermectin
**D.** Discontinue cefepime, reduce the dose of prednisone and start ivermectin
**E.** Continue cefepime, reduce the dose of prednisone and start ivermectin

# Chapter 71 ▪ Answers

**1.** Correct Answer: B

**Rationale:**
This patient with newly diagnosed HIV/AIDS, and a CD4 count <100 cells/μL has central nervous system manifestation of toxoplasmosis. Clues to the diagnosis are compatible clinical features and multiple ring-enhancing lesions with mass effect on MRI.

Toxoplasmosis, caused by the protozoan parasite *Toxoplasma gondii*, is the most common CNS opportunistic infection associated with HIV and is an AIDS-defining illness per the Centers for Disease Control and Prevention (CDC). Incidence of toxoplasmosis varies from 24% to 47% in *T. gondii* seropositive patients with a CD4 count <100 cells/μL. In immunosuppressed patients, disease is caused by the reactivation of latent infection and the CNS is the most common site of reactivation.

Toxoplasma encephalitis presents with fever, headache, mental status changes, focal neurologic deficits, or seizures. Mental status changes can result from global encephalitis and/or increased intracranial pressure.

In the appropriate clinical setting, a presumptive diagnosis can be made if the patient has a positive serology consistent with prior infection—a positive *T. gondii* immunoglobulin G (IgG)—and brain imaging (MRI) with multiple ring-enhancing lesions, often with surrounding edema. A presumptive diagnosis is sufficient to start anti-toxoplasma treatment. Identification of the organism on a tissue biopsy sample can confirm a suspected diagnosis but is not required especially given the morbidity and mortality associated with an invasive brain biopsy. Sulfadiazine-pyrimethamine is the drug of choice. Clinical improvement is expected within 10 to 14 days of treatment initiation; if no improvement is observed by this time period, alternative diagnoses should be considered.

The differential diagnosis for ring-enhancing lesions in the brain in a patient with known HIV includes primary CNS lymphoma, mycobacterial infections, cryptococcosis, and bacterial or fungal abscesses.

### References

1. Renold C, Sugar A, Chave JP, et al. Toxoplasma encephalitis in patients with the acquired immunodeficiency syndrome. *Medicine (Baltimore)*. 1992;71(4):224-239.
2. Luft BJ, Remington JS. Toxoplasmic encephalitis in AIDS. *Clin Infect Dis*. 1992;15(2):211-222.
3. Grant IH, Gold JW, Rosenblum M, Niedzwiecki D, Armstrong D. Toxoplasma gondii serology in HIV-infected patients: the development of central nervous system toxoplasmosis in AIDS. *AIDS*. 1990;4(6):519-521.
4. Zangerle R, Allerberger F, Pohl P, Fritsch P, Dierich MP. High risk of developing toxoplasmic encephalitis in AIDS patients seropositive to Toxoplasma gondii. *Med Microbiol Immunol (Berl)*. 1991;180(2):59-66.

---

**2.** Correct Answer: C

**Rationale:**

This patient's clinical presentation is suggestive of IRIS, an inflammatory disorder manifesting with the emergence or worsening of a preexisting, underlying infection. IRIS usually develops within weeks to months after the initiation of ART during immune recovery. Symptoms and signs relate to the exposed infection.

The diagnosis of IRIS requires the presence of AIDS with a pretreatment CD4 count less than 100 cells/μL, a positive virologic and immunological response to ART, and a temporal association between ART initiation and the onset of clinical features of illness. Common opportunistic infections associated with IRIS are mycobacterial and cryptococcal infections although any infection can present with IRIS.

In this case, the clinical presentation is consistent with MAC infection. Symptoms of MAC are generally nonspecific but often include fevers and diffusely painful lymphadenitis. Laboratory abnormalities include anemia, elevated alkaline phosphatase, and elevated lactate dehydrogenase. The diagnosis is typically confirmed by the isolation of MAC on cultures, although the microorganism burden may be low in IRIS. MAC usually grows on culture within 7 to 10 days.

Management of ART is crucial in IRIS associated with AIDS. Mild manifestations of IRIS usually resolve spontaneously in few days to weeks. Patients with severe symptoms may need adjunctive corticosteroids. Patients on ART who develop IRIS should continue ART alongside appropriate treatment of the exposed opportunistic infection. If the patient presents with MAC at the time of AIDS diagnosis, however, ART should be held until antimicrobial therapy for MAC has been initiated for 2 weeks.

### References

1. Murdoch DM, Venter WD, Feldman C, Van Rie A. Incidence and risk factors for the immune reconstitution inflammatory syndrome in HIV patients in South Africa: a prospective study. *AIDS*. 2008;22(5):601.
2. Manabe YC, Campbell JD, Sydnor E, Moore RD. Immune reconstitution inflammatory syndrome: risk factors and treatment implications. *J Acquir Immune Defic Syndr*. 2007;46(4):456.
3. Breton G, Duval X, Estellat C, et al. Determinants of immune reconstitution inflammatory syndrome in HIV type 1-infected patients with tuberculosis after initiation of antiretroviral therapy. *Clin Infect Dis*. 2004;39(11):1709.
4. Hill AR, Premkumar S, Brustein S, et al. Disseminated tuberculosis in the acquired immunodeficiency syndrome era. *Am Rev Respir Dis*. 1991;144(5):1164.
5. Zolopa A, Andersen J, Powderly W, et al. Early antiretroviral therapy reduces AIDS progression/death in individuals with acute opportunistic infections: a multicenter randomized strategy trial. *PLoS One*. 2009;4(5):e5575. Epub 2009 May 18.

---

**3.** Correct Answer: D

**Rationale:**

Neutropenia can be seen in varying degrees. Mild neutropenia is defined as an absolute neutrophil count (ANC) <1 500 cells/μL, while moderate neutropenia requires an ANC <1 000 cells/μL and severe neutropenia requires an ANC <500 cells/μL or an ANC that is expected to decrease to <500 cells/μL over the next 48 hours. Profound neutropenia is defined by an ANC <100 cells/μL. Fever in neutropenic patients is defined as a single oral temperature of 38.3°C (101°F) or a temperature of 38.0°C (100.4°F) sustained over 1 hour. Patients with prolonged (>7 days) and profound neutropenia are at high risk for complications such as hypotension and in-hospital mortality.

Infections in neutropenic patients are presumed to arise from patient's existent bacterial flora. Although common sites of infection include the skin, lungs, and intestinal tract, the majority of febrile neutropenia episodes do not have an identifiable source of infection.

Empiric antibiotics should be initiated within 120 minutes of patient presentation. Blood cultures should be drawn preferably before antibiotics are initiated. Empiric antimicrobial therapy should include an antipseudomonal beta-lactam agent (cefepime, piperacillin-tazobactam, or a carbapenem). Aminoglycosides and fluoroquinolones may be added as an additional anti-pseudomonal agent. Vancomycin should be added if pneumonia, skin and soft tissue infection, or central venous catheter infection is clinically suspected. Hemodynamic instability is another indication for the addition of vancomycin to a neutropenic patient's initial regimen. Empiric antifungal therapy is only considered in those patients who are persistently febrile and neutropenic on empiric antibacterial therapy for at least 4 days. Candida species–related infections are commonly seen after the first week and mold infections such as aspergillosis are seen after 2 weeks of persistent neutropenia.

In our patient, pneumonia and central venous catheter infection are diagnostic considerations meriting vancomycin in addition to piperacillin-tazobactam for empiric antimicrobial therapy.

### References

1. Taplitz RA, Kennedy EB, Bow EJ, et al. Outpatient management of fever and neutropenia in adults treated for malignancy: American Society of Clinical Oncology and Infectious Diseases Society of America clinical practice guideline update. *J Clin Oncol*. 2018;36:1443-1453.
2. Freifeld AG, Bow EJ, Sepkowitz KA, et al. Clinical practice guideline for the use of antimicrobial agents in neutropenic patients with cancer: 2010 update by the Infectious Diseases Society of America. *Clin Infect Dis*. 2011;52(4):e56-e93.

---

**4.** Correct Answer: B

**Rationale:**

The EBV status and viral load in this solid organ transplant patient point toward a diagnosis of PTLD. Reduction of immunosuppression is a critical step in the management of this condition.

PTLD is the most common malignancy complicating solid organ transplantation. Nine out of ten patients with PTLD have evidence of EBV infection by serologic studies or EBV viral load. PTLD occurs as a consequence of the proliferation of infected B cells in the setting of posttransplant immunosuppression. EBV serostatus and the degree of T-cell immunosuppression are the principal risk factors for the development of disease.

In general, the clinical presentation of PTLD is variable. Initially, the disease may present with a mononucleosis-like syndrome, associated with nonspecific constitutional symptoms such as fever, weight loss, and fatigue as well as peripheral lymphadenophathy. It can also present with tissue infiltrative disease or localized lymphomas. Diagnosis is confirmed by histological examination.

The treatment of PTLD must balance the goals of eradicating disease and maintaining a functional graft. Management strategies are based on the category of disease. Early lesions are managed with careful reduction of immunosuppression alone. Other therapies like rituximab are recommended in addition to the reduction of immunosuppression in patients with polymorphic PTLD (CD20+ PTLD). Rituximab alone or in combination with chemotherapy is used in patients with monomorphic PTLD, and chemotherapy with or without radiation is used in patients with classic Hodgkin lymphoma–like PTLD, which is the least common form.

### References

1. Finberg RW, Fingeroth JD, Finberg RW, Fingeroth JD, Finberg RW, Fingeroth JD. Infections in transplant recipients. In: Jameson J, Fauci AS, Kasper DL, et al. eds. *Harrison's Principles of Internal Medicine*. 20th ed. New York, NY: McGraw-Hill. http://accessmedicine.mhmedical.com/content. aspx?bookid=2129&sectionid=192020844. Accessed November 08, 2018.
2. Straathof KCM, Savoldo B, Heslop HE, Rooney CM. Immunotherapy for post-transplant lymphoproliferative disease. *Br J Haematol*. 2002;118(3):728-740.
3. Heslop HE. How I treat EBV lymphoproliferation. *Blood*. 2009;114(19):4002-4008.

---

**5.** Correct Answer: B

**Rationale:**

This patient with a discordant CMV serology status (donor positive, recipient negative) presenting with diarrhea is most likely to have CMV tissue-invasive disease and colitis despite a negative plasma CMV PCR. Tissue biopsies from multiple sites in the colon showing characteristic histopathology are needed to confirm the diagnosis.

CMV is a member of *Herpesviridae* genus that causes life-threatening infection in both solid organ transplant and hematopoietic stem cell transplant recipients. The virus can cause primary infection that occurs in seronegative patients or secondary infection, usually attributed to reactivation of latent infection. Primary infections are usually more severe than secondary infections.

Plasma CMV PCR can be negative in 15% of tissue-invasive CMV colitis. In patients with compartmentalized CMV disease like colitis, viremia may be very low or transient. Thus, biopsy is needed to confirm the diagnosis. CMV replicates within the nuclei of infected cells which is represented by the large eosinophilic intranuclear inclusion bodies on hematoxylin and eosin staining of tissue samples. There may be associated tissue necrosis and endothelial damage.

However, repeat colonoscopy with biopsy is not required to document clearance after appropriate antimicrobial treatment is completed. A computed tomography (CT) scan of the abdomen is not diagnostic in CMV colitis. Empiric therapy is not indicated in suspected colitis without viremia as ganciclovir treatment is associated with significant marrow toxicity.

### References

1. Razonable RR, Humar AA. Cytomegalovirus in solid organ transplantation. *Am J Transplant.* 2013;13(suppl 4):93-106.
2. Razonable RR, Hayden RT. Clinical utility of viral load in management of cytomegalovirus infection after solid organ transplantation. *Clin Microbiol Rev.* 2013;26(4):703-727.

---

**6.** Correct Answer: E

**Rationale:**

The diffuse erythematous skin rash, fever, and hypotension in a neutropenic patient with mucositis are consistent with septic shock due to *viridans* group *streptocococci* (VGSS).

*Viridans streptococci* are normal inhabitants of oral cavity. They are classified into six major groups. *Streptococcus mitis* is the group of organisms most commonly associated with septic shock. VGSS is a relatively new entity first described in 1990s. The incidence of shock and/or acute respiratory distress syndrome varies from 7% to 39%. Risk factors for bacteremia include profound neutropenia (<100 cells/μL), oral mucositis, and prophylactic fluoroquinolone use. Patients receiving ceftazidime as empiric therapy for febrile neutropenia are also at increased risk. Reduced susceptibility to penicillins and newer beta-lactam agents raise concerns in the management of severe infections due to VGSS. Empiric therapy with vancomycin is suggested until final susceptibilities of the organism are available. Mortality ranges from 6% to 30%.

The identification of gram positive cocci in pairs and chains makes staphylococcal infection unlikely. The clinical scenario is not suggestive of infective endocarditis (IE). Causes for hypotension in IE are septic shock, more common with *Staphylococcus aureus* IE and cardiac failure due to severe valvular regurgitation. Enterococcal IE is rarely implicated in septic shock syndromes, more commonly observed with staphylococcal infection.

### References

1. Freifeld AG, Razonable RR. Editorial commentary: viridans group streptococci in febrile neutropenic cancer patients. What should we fear? *Clin Infect Dis.* 2014;59(2):231-233.
2. Bochud PY, Calandra T, Francioli P. Bacteremia due to viridans streptococci in neutropenic patients: a review. *Am J Med.* 1994;97(3):256-264.
3. Shelburne SA, Lasky RE, Sahasrabhojane P, Tarrand JT, Rolston KVI. Development and validation of a clinical model to predict the presence of β-lactam resistance in viridans group streptococci causing bacteremia in neutropenic cancer patients. *Clin Infect Dis.* 2014;59(2):223-230.
4. Olmos C, Vilacosta I, Fernández C, et al. Contemporary epidemiology and prognosis of septic shock in infective endocarditis. *Eur Heart J.* 2013;34(26):1999-2006.

---

**7.** Correct Answer: C

**Rationale:**

The presence of a positive serum β-1,3-ᴅ-glucan assay and BAL fluid nonpigmented, septate hyphae branching at right angles in a stem cell transplant recipient with recently increased immunosuppression for treatment of GVHD suggests invasive pulmonary aspergillosis. Filamentous fungi are divided into septate and aseptate forms as shown in the following figure. Organisms which characteristically present with septate hyphae include *Aspergillus* and *Fusarium*, but *Fusarium* grows easily in blood cultures, making it less likely in this case.

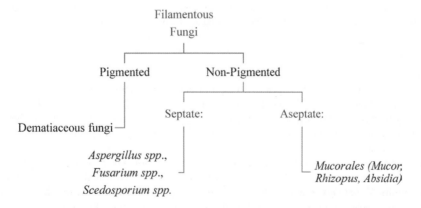

Voriconazole is the first-line treatment for invasive pulmonary aspergillosis. Careful monitoring of serum creatinine is needed in patients receiving intravenous voriconazole due to the potential accumulation of cyclodextrin which is the carrier for the intravenous formulation. The lipid-based formulation of amphotericin B and isavuconazole serve as alternative for patients who cannot tolerate voriconazole due to side effects or drug-drug interactions.

### References

1. Verweij PE, Brandt ME, Murray PR, Baron EJ, Jorgensen JH, Landry ML. Aspergillus, fusarium, and other opportunistic monil-iaceous fungi. *Man Clin Microbiol*. 2007;2:1802-1038.
2. Patterson TF, Thompson GR III, Denning DW, et al. Practice guidelines for the diagnosis and management of aspergillosis: 2016 update by the Infectious Diseases Society of America. *Clin Infect Dis*. 2016;63(4):e1-e60.

## 8. Correct Answer: C

**Rationale:**

In a patient with history of sickle cell disease and multiple sickle cell crises in the past, there is increased suspicion for repeated infarction to the spleen and resultant functional asplenia. Asplenic patients are at increased risk for a fulmi-nant sepsis syndrome usually due to encapsulated organisms such as *Streptococcus pneumoniae*, *Haemophilus influenza*, and *Neisseria meningitides* due to their reduced antibody formation to polysaccharide antigens. (See table that follows.)

| MICROBIOLOGY OF INFECTIONS IN ASPLENIC OR HYPOSPLENIC STATES | INFECTIOUS SYNDROME |
| --- | --- |
| Encapsulated organisms (eg, *S. pneumoniae*, *H. influenzae*, or *N. meningitidis*) | Bacteremia, pneumonia, meningitis |
| *Capnocytophaga* species | Cellulitis, bacteremia |
| *Bordetella holmesii* | Pertussis, bacteremia |
| *Babesia* species | Babesiosis—parasitemia, hemolytic anemia |
| *Plasmodium falciparum* | Malaria |

The risk of sepsis is dependent on the age of the patient and cause of asplenia. In patients with hemoglobinop-athies, the risk of sepsis is greater in children than in adults, but in patients with splenectomy, the risk of sepsis in-creases after the age of 50. Patients with sickle cell anemia or thalassemia major are three to four times more likely to experience sepsis compared with patients with splenectomy secondary to trauma.

Other causes for asplenia/hyposplenism include postsurgical splenectomy, splenic artery thrombosis, graft-ver-sus-host disease, inflammatory bowel disease, SLE, and HIV/AIDS.

Acutely ill patients should undergo appropriate diagnostic evaluation and receive empiric broad-spectrum anti-biotic therapy. The single most valuable diagnostic test in evaluating a patient with suspected postsplenectomy sepsis is blood culture, as the bacterial burden in the blood may be high. In this particular patient, given her increased risk for *S. pneumonia*–related sepsis, obtaining an urine antigen may be helpful to confirm diagnosis.

Recommended empiric antibiotic therapy includes vancomycin and either a third-generation cephalosporin such as ceftriaxone or an extended-spectrum fluoroquinolone such as levofloxacin or ciprofloxacin. Blood cultures and antibiotic susceptibility results will guide subsequent antibiotic selection. Administration of antibiotics should not be delayed pending diagnostic studies, including lumbar puncture if indicated.

### Reference

1. Kyaw MH, Holmes EM, Toolis F, et al. Evaluation of severe infection and survival after splenectomy. *Am J Med*. 2006;119:276. e1-276.e7.
2. Bisharat N, Omari H, Lavi I, et al. Risk of infection and death among post-splenectomy patients. *J Infect*. 2001;43:182-186.
3. Di Sabatino A, Carsetti R, Corazza GR. Post-splenectomy and hyposplenic states. *Lancet*. 2011;378:86-97.

## 9. Correct Answer: C

**Rationale:**

This patient with seizures in the postoperative lung transplant period most likely has hyperammonemia syndrome due to *Mycoplasma hominis* sternal wound infection. Hyperammonemia is a rare but fatal cause of altered mental status in lung transplant recipients, with an incidence of 4.1%. Among infectious causes for this syndrome, *Myco-plasma hominis* and *Ureaplasma* are the two most important culprit organisms and involve the release of ammonia as a by-product of urea metabolism.

*M. hominis* is a fastidious bacteria. Gram stains cannot detect the organism due to the absence of a peptidoglycan cell wall. It is a common colonizer of the urogenital tract in females and usually causes genitourinary infections. In 10% of adults, *M. hominis* colonizes the upper respiratory tract and can cause life-threatening infections after thoracic organ transplantation and other cardiothoracic surgeries, including mediastinitis, pleuro-pericarditis, and sternal osteomyelitis.

*M. hominis* is diagnosed by culture and PCR testing. The organism is usually susceptible to clindamycin or doxy-cycline. The organism is usually resistant to fluoroquinolones, macrolides, and aminoglycosides.

### References

1. Wylam ME, Kennedy CC, Hernandez NM, et al. Fatal hyperammonaemia caused by mycoplasma hominis. *Lancet.* 2013;382(9908):1956.
2. Lichtenstein GR, Yang YX, Nunes FA, et al. Fatal hyperammonemia after orthotopic lung transplantation. *Ann Intern Med.* 2000;132(4):283-287.

**10.** Correct Answer: E

**Rationale:**

This patient's presentation of sepsis with gram-negative meningitis likely from gram-negative bacteremia, rapidly evolving pulmonary infiltrates, and larvae seen in sputum taken together is typical of *Strongyloides* hyperinfection.

*Strongyloides* infection is usually asymptomatic, and when present, the symptoms are typically mild and limited to cutaneous larva migrans rash at the site of penetration of the skin by filariform larvae, intermittent cough or dyspnea during larval migration through the airways, and diarrhea with or without abdominal discomfort. Hyperinfection is a rare syndrome of strongyloidiasis characterized by uncontrolled overproliferation of larvae leading to an exaggeration of the usual symptoms and sometimes causing a dramatic systemic inflammatory response to dissemination and migration of larvae throughout the body. Typical manifestations include fever, wheezing or asthma-like symptoms, hemoptysis, ileus, gastrointestinal bleeding, pneumonitis with or without pneumonia and alveolar hemorrhage, transient bacteremia secondary to translocation along by the larvae penetrating the intestinal mucosa with or without secondary organ seeding, and meningitis. Together these symptoms lead to multiorgan failure with a high rate of mortality.

Hyperinfection has classically been described with corticosteroid use; however, it has been reported with various other immunosuppressive medications and conditions including human immunodeficiency virus (HIV), solid organ, and hematopoietic stem cell transplantation. The underlying mechanism is deemed to be an impairment in cell-mediated immunity. Human T-cell leukemia/lymphoma virus-1 infection, by itself, predisposes to strongyloidiasis and also to hyperinfection without any other immune suppression. Solid-organ transplant recipients who have not been exposed to *Strongyloides* can potentially acquire it from an infected donor's organ; high-risk regions routinely screen for *Strongyloides* in the donor with positive serological screening prompting preemptive treatment of the organ recipients. Eosinophilia, the hallmark of invasive parasitic infections including strongyloidiasis may be absent in hyperinfection syndrome especially if steroids are being used. Of note, even short courses of steroids up to a week and at doses as low as 20 mg per day have been reported to have precipitated hyperinfection within a few days to weeks.

Treatment of strongyloidiasis hyperinfection is a three-pronged approach aimed at (1) targeting the underlying worms while (2) decreasing immunosuppression to allow the body to respond to the infection adequately and at the same time (3) covering for secondary complications like bacteremia with or without seeding. Ivermectin remains the antiparasitic of choice. The oral route is preferred, but if oral absorption is a concern, subcutaneous or intravenous formulations of ivermectin can be used off-label. Albendazole can be added for severe cases although the benefit of this is unclear. Although the presence of larvae or eggs in the stool is not the best diagnostic modality in the setting of chronic infection, in hyperinfection the parasitic is high enough that stool parasites should be ideally monitored for clearance and antiparasitic therapy should be continued for at least 2 weeks after that to cover for autoinfection. All attempts should be made to hold or decrease any immunosuppressive therapies that the patient is on. Antimicrobials targeting gram-negative and gram-positive gut commensals should be used to treat bacteremia. Prophylactic antimicrobials are appropriate even in the absence of microbiological evidence of bacterial infection in the acute setting given the high likelihood of the same.

This patient likely acquired *Strongyloides* during his service in Vietnam and his latent infection became clinically active in the setting of high-dose steroids for graft-versus-host disease of his recently transplanted liver, although it is possible that the infection had become active around the time of his transplant, and the manifestations became more severe with steroid use.

### References:

1. Image taken from www.cdc.gov/dpdx/strongyloidiasis/index.html.
2. Kuriakose K, Carpenter K, Wanjalla C, Pettit A. Case of Strongyloides hyperinfection syndrome. *BMJ Case Rep.* 2017;2017. pii:bcr2016218320.
3. Myint A, Chapman C, Almira-Suarez I, Mehta N. Strongyloides hyperinfection syndrome in an immunocompetent host resulting in bandemia and death. *BMJ Case Rep.* 2017;2017. pii:bcr2016217911.
4. Abanyie FA, Gray EB, Delli Carpini KW, et al. Donor-derived Strongyloides stercoralis infection in solid organ transplant recipients in the United States, 2009-2013. *Am J Transplant.* 2015;15(5):1369-1375.
5. Kassalik M, Monkemuller K. *Strongyloides stercoralis* hyperinfection syndrome and disseminated disease. *Gastroenterol Hepatol (N Y).* 2011;7(11):766.
6. Greaves D, Coggle S, Pollard C, Aliyu SH, Moore EM. Strongyloides stercoralis infection. *BMJ.* 2013;347:f4610.
7. Tuner SA, Maclean JD, Fleckenstein L, et al. Parenteral administration of ivermectin in a patient with disseminated strongyloidiasis. *Am J Trop Med Hyg.* 2005;73:911-914.

# 72

# IMMUNOLOGICAL EFFECTS OF INFECTIONS

Rachel C. Frank and Dusan Hanidziar

1. A 44-year-old female with no known medical history is admitted to the intensive care unit (ICU) with septic shock, presumably from influenza. She is treated with mechanical ventilation, vasopressors, and broad-spectrum antimicrobials including oseltamivir, vancomycin, cefepime, flagyl, and azithromycin. Despite 5 days of treatment, she fails to improve. She has persistent fever to 38.9°C and requires norepinephrine and vasopressin to treat hypotension. Arterial blood gas (ABG) is 7.32/34/98 on FiO$_2$ of 0.5. She is noted to have hepatosplenomegaly, but no rash, asymmetric lower extremity edema, or lymphadenopathy. Laboratory data reveal hemoglobin 7.1 g/dL, platelets 40/µL, and creatinine 0.5 mg/dL.
   Chest x-ray reveals resolving bilateral patchy opacities and mild pulmonary edema. Point of care cardiac ultrasound shows hyperdynamic biventricular function. Culture data are negative to date.

   Which of the following tests would BEST confirm her diagnosis:

   **A.** Ferritin, triglycerides, fibrinogen, soluble IL-2 receptor levels
   **B.** Antineutrophil cytoplasmic antibody (ANCA)
   **C.** Peripheral smear and flow cytometry
   **D.** Platelet factor 4 Ab, serotonin release assay

2. A 68-year-old diabetic man, who had open sigmoidectomy 10 days ago for diverticulitis, is brought to emergency department (ED) after his son found him altered at home. Initial vitals are notable for fever to 40°C, heart rate (HR) of 120 beats per minute, blood pressure 78/42 mm Hg, respiratory rate of 34, O$_2$ and saturation 92% on room air. His blood glucose is normal. Blood cultures, chest x-ray, urinalysis, and urine culture are obtained. He is given vancomycin, cefepime, metronidazole, and 2 L of lactated Ringer's and is subsequently intubated for airway protection. CT scans of the head, chest, abdomen, and pelvis, obtained before the ICU admission, are unremarkable.

   On ICU arrival, detailed physical examination reveals diffuse erythematous blanching rash and hyperemic mucus membranes of the mouth and conjunctiva. His abdominal incision is slightly erythematous but without frank purulence.

   Subsequent management should include which of the following?

   **A.** Intravenous (IV) piperacillin-tazobactam monotherapy
   **B.** Continuation of IV vancomycin, cefepime, metronidazole, and addition of IV clindamycin
   **C.** Discontinuation of vancomycin because of skin reaction
   **D.** IV diphenhydramine and hydrocortisone

3. A 68-year-old man with bronchiectasis and severe pneumonia is mechanically ventilated in the ICU. He is treated with empiric meropenem and vancomycin based on the culture data obtained during prior admission, and his blood pressure is supported with norepinephrine. On ICU day 3, his sputum culture reveals ceftriaxone-susceptible *Streptococcus pneumoniae*. Thirty minutes after the dose of ceftriaxone, he is noted to have worsening hypotension and requires increasing doses of norepinephrine. As ICU physician prepares to perform cardiac ultrasound, he notices urticaria on his chest.

   Which of the following laboratory tests would clarify the diagnosis?

   A. Angiotensin-converting enzyme (ACE) level
   B. Tryptase level
   C. Histamine level
   D. Complete blood count (CBC)

4. A 23-year-old female with refractory acute lymphoblastic leukemia now 28 days postallogeneic hematopoietic stem cell transplant (HSCT) is transferred to the ICU for respiratory distress. On arrival, vital signs are temperature 38.2°C, HR 110 beats per minute, blood pressure 88/52 mm Hg, and respiratory rate 38 breaths per minute. She is saturating 88% on 10 L $O_2$ via nonrebreather. Pulmonary examination is notable for diffuse rales. She does not have a rash, and her sclerae are mildly icteric. She is subsequently intubated and started on norepinephrine infusion for hypotension with improvement in hemodynamics. Broad-spectrum antibiotics are administered for concern of pneumonia. Chest x-ray shows diffuse bilateral patchy opacities.

   The next BEST diagnostic step is:

   A. CT chest and bronchoalveolar lavage
   B. Serum galactomannan, 1-3-beta-D-glucan
   C. No additional workup needed, continue antibiotics
   D. Herpes simplex virus (HSV) and cytomegalovirus (CMV) serum PCR

5. A 65-year-old male who is postoperative day (POD) 3 from right hemicolectomy for cancer is admitted to the ICU for hypoxemia. His HR is 120/min, oxygen saturation is 88% on 15 L oxygen, and he requires intubation. Chest x-ray shows right middle and lower lobe opacities consistent with pneumonia. Mean arterial pressure (MAP) is 65 mm Hg on 5 μg/min of norepinephrine. He is started on broad-spectrum antibiotics including vancomycin, cefepime, and metronidazole. Laboratory results are notable for Hgb of 7.5 g/dL, platelets of 45/μL, and schistocytes in the blood smear. International normalized ratio (INR) is 1.7, activated partial thromboplastin time (aPTT) 45 seconds, D-dimer of 10 000 μg/L, and fibrinogen is undetectable. Physical examination reveals digital necrosis of several fingers and toes.

   What is the most likely cause of his coagulopathy?

   A. Sepsis-induced thrombocytopenia
   B. Thrombotic thrombocytopenic purpura
   C. Disseminated intravascular coagulation (DIC)
   D. Heparin-induced thrombocytopenia (HIT)

# Chapter 72 ▪ Answers

1. Correct Answer: A

   **Rationale:**
   Hemophagocytic lymphohistiocytosis (HLH) is an inflammatory condition characterized by excessive immune activation of macrophages and T cells. This results in elevated levels of inflammatory cytokines including interferon gamma and tumor necrosis factor alpha. Etiologies include genetic mutations, infection, inflammatory disease, and malignancy. Genetic mutations are more common in children. Increasingly, there is evidence that HLH induced by infection is underdiagnosed in the ICU.
      HLH may be diagnosed with five of the following eight criteria:
   • Fever
   • Splenomegaly
   • Cytopenia of >2 lines
   • Hemophagocytosis (bone marrow, spleen, liver, or lymph node)
   • Hypertriglyceridemia (fasting ≥3 mmol/L) or hypofibrinogenemia (<1/5 g/L)
   • Low or absent NK cell activity
   • Ferritin >500 μg/L
   • Soluble CD 25 (soluble interleukin-2 receptor) >2400 U/mL
      Alternatively, diagnosis may be made with a positive genetic testing.
      HLH remains a difficult diagnosis to make in the critically ill, as many of the symptoms are nonspecific and exist in a variety of inflammatory and infectious conditions including sepsis. HLH should be a part of the differential in patients with persistent fever, hepatosplenomegaly, elevated ferritin, cytopenia (without alternative explanation), and failure to improve with appropriate antimicrobials.

In this case, the patient has failed to improve on broad-spectrum antimicrobials. She has pancytopenia, hepato-splenomegaly, and persistent fever, making HLH a possible diagnosis. The next best test to confirm a diagnosis of HLH is to measure ferritin, triglycerides, fibrinogen, and soluble IL-2 receptor levels. Bone marrow biopsy may also be considered but is more invasive.

Platelet factor 4 is a diagnostic test for HIT type II, caused by antibody-mediated destruction of platelets. The confirmatory test is a serotonin release assay. Peripheral smear and flow cytometry are not required to diagnose HLH. ANCA is a laboratory test used for the assessment of vasculitis.

## References

1. Beutel G, Wiesner O, Eder M, et al. Virus-associated hemophagocytic syndrome as a major contributor to death in patients with 2009 influenza A (H1N1) infection. *Crit Care*. 2011;15(2):R80.
2. Bentzer P, Fjell P, Walley KR, et al. Plasma cytokine levels predict response to corticosteroids in septic shock. *Intensive Care Med*. 2016;42(12):1970-1979.
3. Lachmann G, Spies C, Schenk T, et al. Hemophagocytic lymphohistiocytosis: potentially underdiagnosed in intensive care units. *Shock*.2018;50(2):149-155.
4. Rosado FG, Kim AS. Hemophagocytic lymphohistiocytosis: an update on diagnosis and pathogenesis. *Am J Clin Pathol*. 2013;139(6):713-727.
5. Shakoory B, Carcillo JA, Chatham WW, et al. Interleukin-1 receptor blockade is associated with reduced mortality in sepsis patients with features of macrophage activation syndrome: reanalysis of a prior phase III trial. *Crit Care Med*. 2016;44(2):275-281.

## 2. Correct Answer: B

**Rationale:**
Toxic shock syndrome (TSS) is a life-threatening condition because of *Staphylococcus aureus* or group A *Streptococcus* toxin. Patients with surgical and postpartum wounds and, classically, menstruating women are at increased risk. Diagnostic criteria for TSS include fever greater than 38°C, multisystem organ dysfunction including vomiting or diarrhea (often watery), muscular symptoms (myalgias/creatine phosphokinase levels >2× upper limit of normal), mucus membrane involvement, renal dysfunction or pyuria in the absence of urinary tract infection, hepatic dysfunction (elevated bilirubin and aminotransferases), thrombocytopenia, and altered mental status without focal neurologic findings.

The pathophysiology of TSS involves super antigens that cause overwhelming T-cell activation leading to a state of cytokine storm with high levels of IL-1, IL-2, and TNF-alpha and beta, as well as interferon gamma. Super antigens involved in the pathophysiology of TSS include TSST-1 and staphylococcal enterotoxins (A-D).

The best empiric antibiotic management while awaiting culture data is IV clindamycin (to halt toxin synthesis) and vancomycin (methicillin-resistant *Staphylococcus aureus* coverage). Piperacillin-tazobactam is not an optimal antibiotic regimen as it does not have appropriate methicillin-resistant *Staphylococcus aureus* coverage and will not decrease toxin production.

There is currently clinical equipoise regarding the use of intravenous immunoglobulin (IVIg), although observational comparative studies have demonstrated that IVIg is associated with significantly lower mortality at 28 days. The mechanism is thought to include neutralization of the super antigens. This treatment is not ubiquitously used at all institutions.

## References

1. CDC Notifiable Disease Surveillance System. *Toxic Shock Syndrome (Other Than Streptococcal) (TSS) 2011 Case Definition*. Available at https://wwwn.cdc.gov/nndss/conditions/toxic-shock-syndrome-other-than-streptococcal/case-definition/2011/.
2. Schliever PM. Use of intravenous immunoglobulin in the treatment of staphylococcal and streptococcal toxic shock syndromes and related illnesses. *J Allergy Clin Immunol*. 2001;108(4):S107-S110.
3. Sivagnanam S, Deleu D. Red man syndrome. *Crit Care*. 2003;7(2):119-120.
4. Stevens DL, Bisno AL, Chambers HF, et al. Practice guidelines for the diagnosis and management of skin and soft tissue infections: 2014, update by the infectious diseases society of America. *Clin Infect Dis*. 2014;59(2):e10-e52.

## 3. Correct Answer: B

**Rationale:**
Anaphylactic shock is a life-threatening condition that may be difficult to recognize in sedated, intubated patients. Clinical manifestations include increased peak airway pressures, urticarial rash, hypotension, or cardiac arrhythmias. The patient in the vignette has bronchiectasis and history of previous admissions for pneumonia, for which he likely received cephalosporin antibiotics in the past.

Anaphylaxis may either be IgE mediated or non-IgE mediated. In IgE-mediated anaphylaxis, mast cell degranulation, and histamine and protease release (ie tryptase) lead to the clinical manifestations. Non-IgE–mediated anaphylaxis occurs via neutrophil, eosinophil, and complement activation. Common triggers of anaphylaxis include antibiotics, nonsteroidal anti-inflammatory medications, certain anesthetic agents, food and insect venom.

Biomarkers, if positive, are useful in diagnosing anaphylaxis. Tryptase has a plasma half-life of approximately 2 hours. For comparison, a baseline tryptase level should be measured 24 hours after resolution of anaphylaxis to ensure accurate interpretation. Owing to the kinetics of tryptase release, it is the most clinically useful serum marker of anaphylaxis. While histamine is released by mast cells during anaphylactic reactions, peak serum levels occur within 5 to 10 minutes and return to baseline within 1 hour, making it a suboptimal clinical biomarker. ACE level is not a marker of anaphylaxis. Nonspecific changes during anaphylaxis may be seen on CBCs including leukocytosis, neutrophil predominance, and possibly increased eosinophilia. However, this pattern may be seen in a variety of conditions and would not confirm the diagnosis. Further, in a patient with suspected infection, leukocytosis and neutrophil predominance would be expected.

References

1. Kim S-Y, Kim MH, Cho YJ. Different clinical features of anaphylaxis according to cause and risk factors for severe reactions. *Allergol Int.* 2018;67(1):96-102.
2. Reber LL, Hernandez JD, Galli SJ, et al. The pathophysiology of anaphylaxis. *J Allergy Clin Immunol.* 2017;140(2):335-348.

**4.** Correct Answer: A

**Rationale:**

Pulmonary complications following HSCT are common. The differential for pulmonary complications is very broad and includes infection, diffuse alveolar hemorrhage, edema, engraftment syndrome, idiopathic pneumonia syndrome, and graft versus host disease.

Engraftment is defined as recovery of cell counts with absolute neutrophil count > 500/mm³. Engraftment occurs within 2 to 4 weeks of transplantation. Engraftment syndrome is characterized by fever, rash, and evidence of capillary leak including pulmonary edema and weight gain. Other manifestations include dyspnea and noninfectious pulmonary infiltrates on imaging. Hepatic, renal dysfunction, or transient encephalopathy may be present. All symptoms occur within 4 days of reaching an absolute neutrophil count of 500/mm³. Therefore, neutropenia is temporally proximal to symptoms, and empiric antibiotics should be initiated while awaiting culture data. If there is no improvement on appropriate antibiotics after 48 to 72 hours, a diagnosis of engraftment syndrome should be considered. Respiratory failure is the largest contributor to mortality related to engraftment syndrome. Treatment includes steroids (such as methylprednisolone) administered until symptoms resolve (typically 2-3 days), followed by oral prednisone.

Patients are immunocompromised following HSCT and therefore the differential for pulmonary infections includes bacterial, fungal, and viral pathogens. Infections most commonly occur before engraftment during periods of neutropenia but may occur at any time. Viral infections in the early posttransplant period include CMV pneumonia, RSV, influenza A, B, HSV, or varicella-zoster virus (VZV). Fungal infections include aspergillus, pneumocystis and less commonly zygomycetes, rhizopus, and mucor. Treatment is initially broad-spectrum antimicrobials, which can be narrowed based on culture data.

The patient in the above vignette is 28 days post transplant. The differential is extremely broad. Therefore, workup should include bronchoalveolar lavage (BAL) to rule out diffuse alveolar hemorrhage, infectious etiologies, and CT of the chest to evaluate the presence of infection, pulmonary edema, and infiltrates. Steroids are the treatment for several of the conditions on the differential including engraftment syndrome, graft versus host disease (GVHD), and diffuse alveolar hemorrhage. However, empiric steroids without exoneration of infection would not be a correct treatment at this time. HSV and CMV PCR may diagnose viremia, however, would not exclude alternative diagnoses such as diffuse alveolar hemorrhage and GVHD and therefore are not the next best correct test. 1-3-beta-D-glucan is a fungal marker and galactomannan is elevated with invasive aspergillosis. If positive, the test suggests fungal infection. However, it would not rule out nonfungal causes of the patient's respiratory failure.

References

1. Ayha VN. Noninfectious acute lung injury syndromes early after hematopoietic stem cell transplantation. *Clin Chest Med.* 2017;38(4):595-606.
2. Chang L, Frame D, Braun T, et al. Engraftment syndrome after allogeneic hematopoietic cell transplantation predicts poor outcomes. *Biol Blood Marrow Transplant.* 2014;20(9):1407-1417.
3. Panoskaltsis-Morta A, Griese M, Madtes DK, et al. An Official American Thoracic Society research statement: noninfectious lung injury after hematopoietic stem cell transplantation: idiopathic pneumonia syndrome. *Am J Respir Crit Care Med.* 2011;183(9):1262-1279.
4. Spitzer TR. Engraftment syndrome following hematopoietic stem cell transplantation. *Bone Marrow Transplant.* 2001;27(9):893-898.

**5.** Correct Answer: C

**Rationale:**

This patient has septic shock because of hospital-acquired pneumonia and evidence of coagulopathy consistent with DIC. DIC is characterized by hypercoagulability and hyperfibrinolysis resulting in phenotypes ranging from massive bleeding to excessive microvascular thrombosis resulting in multisystem organ failure. Laboratory abnormalities in DIC include prolongation of aPTT, PT/INR, hypofibrinogenemia, decreased platelets, and elevated fibrinogen split products including D-dimer. The treatment of DIC involves treating the underlying cause. Transfusion thresholds typically include platelets ≤50/ µL in bleeding patients and ≤10 to 20/ µL in those whom are not. Fresh frozen plasma may be transfused to correct prolonged aPTT or prothrombin time (PT) and to replenish clotting factors being consumed. In patients who develop hypofibrinogenemia, administration of cryoprecipitate corrects this abnormality. In patients with clotting predominant DIC, heparin or low molecular weight heparin are utilized to prevent further thrombosis.

Sepsis itself may cause thrombocytopenia, which would however not explain global coagulopathy seen in this patient. Although thrombocytopenia and schistocytes are also present in TTP, this syndrome is characterized by normal coagulation times. HIT is not associated with abnormal coagulation times.

## References

1. Koami H, Sakamoto Y, Sakurai R, et al. The thromboelastometric discrepancy between septic and trauma induced disseminated intravascular coagulation diagnosed by the scoring system from the Japanese association for acute medicine. *Medicine*. 2016;95(31):e4514.
2. Okamoto K, Tamura T, Sawatsubashi Y. Sepsis and disseminated intravascular coagulation. *J Intensive Care*. 2016;4(23):e1-e8.
3. Papageorgiou C, Jourdi G, Adjambri E, et al. Disseminated intravascular coagulation: an update on pathogenesis, diagnosis, and therapeutic strategies. *Clin Appl Thromb Hemost*. 2018;24(9S): S8-S28.
4. Simmons J, Pittet JF. The coagulopathy of acute sepsis. *Curr Opin Anaesthesiol*. 2015;28(2):227-236.
5. Wada H, Matsumoto T, Yamashita Y. Diagnosis and treatment of disseminated intravascular coagulation (DIC) according to four DIC guidelines *J Intensive Care*. 2014;2(15):e1-e8.

# 73

# BIOTERRORISM

Jean Kwo

1. A 28-year-old male presents with fever, severe headache, shortness of breath, and altered mental status. While in the emergency room, he develops a seizure and is subsequently intubated and placed on mechanical ventilation. Recent medical history is significant for nonspecific complaints of fever, cough, and malaise. His chest radiograph shows mediastinal widening and pleural effusions. A lumbar puncture reveals grossly bloody CSF with low glucose and elevated white blood cell count. Blood and CSF cultures are growing *Bacillus anthracis*. Which of the following antibiotic combinations should be started?

   A. Ciprofloxacin, Meropenem, and Vancomycin
   B. Doxycycline, Meropenem, and Vancomycin
   C. Ceftriaxone, Ciprofloxacin, and Clindamycin
   D. Trimethoprim-sulfamethoxazole, Meropenem, and Vancomycin

2. A 53-year-old female presents with mydriasis, ptosis, diplopia, dysphagia, dysarthria, and a progressive, symmetric descending flaccid paralysis. She is conscious and has no cardiovascular perturbations. Colleagues at other area hospitals are reporting several similar cases. You recommend to:

   A. Start plasmapheresis or intravenous immunoglobulin and admit her to an intensive care unit (ICU) for close respiratory and cardiovascular monitoring
   B. Administer atropine, pralidoxime, anticonvulsants if seizures occur and admit her to an ICU for close monitoring for respiratory failure and risk of aspiration
   C. Administer antitoxin, supportive care, and admit her to an ICU for close monitoring for respiratory failure and risk of aspiration
   D. Administer edrophonium 2 mg

3. The emergency department calls to inform you that there are multiple patients with symptoms of fever, altered mental status, respiratory failure, and shock that will be transferred to the ICU. Features that the patients may be victims of a biologic attack include all of the following EXCEPT:

   A. Reports of similar cases at other hospitals and clinics
   B. Large numbers of rapidly fatal cases
   C. A rise in a number of patients with similar symptoms over a few hours to days and then a drop off in patients with the symptoms
   D. Patients arriving from a disperse area

4. A 54-year-old postal worker presents with symptoms of chest tightness, cough, dyspnea, and fever. Chest radiograph shows pulmonary edema. He is intubated secondary to severe hypoxia and transferred to the ICU. Per report, he was handling a broken vial containing a white powder, and the post office is currently being decontaminated. Management of this patient includes:

**A.** Respiratory isolation in negative pressure room
**B.** Gut decontamination with activated charcoal
**C.** Supportive treatment with mechanical ventilation
**D.** Administration of an antitoxin

# Chapter 73 ▪ Answers

**1.** Correct Answer: A

**Rationale:**

*B. anthracis* is an encapsulated, gram positive, spore-forming bacterium that can causes pulmonary, meningeal, cutaneous, and gastrointestinal disease. Aerosolized anthrax spores may be used as a biological weapon. The spores are inhaled, phagocytized by alveolar macrophages and carried to mediastinal lymph nodes where they germinate and cause disease through the production of toxins leading to systemic disease and shock.

Early symptoms are nonspecific with fever, cough, myalgia, malaise, and mimic viral illnesses. However, after a short period of apparent recovery, fever, respiratory failure, acidosis, and shock develop. The earliest clue to diagnosis may be radiographic findings of a widened mediastinum and pleural effusions that rapidly progress to a large size. Anthrax meningitis results from hematogenous seeding and occurs in up to 50% of patients with inhalational anthrax. The mortality rate is as high as 67% to 88% even with antimicrobial or antiserum treatment. Diagnostic testing should include blood for culture and polymerase chain reaction assay (PCR), plasma for antitoxin detection, pleural fluid/CSF for culture, and PCR.

The CDC recommends two or more antimicrobial drugs for treatment of *B. anthracis*. In patients with confirmed and probable meningitis, survival was increased in patients who received three or more antimicrobials. The recommended first line drug for treatment of culture-confirmed anthrax meningitis is a fluoroquinolone. Other antibiotics with good CSF penetration and activity against *B. anthracis* include penicillin or ampicillin, meropenem, rifampin, and vancomycin. Although doxycycline has good activity against *B. anthracis*, it has poor CNS penetration and thus, is not recommended for treatment of anthrax meningitis. Because of β-lactam resistance, cephalosporins are contraindicated for the treatment of anthrax.

Patients with anthrax meningitis may need steroids to control cerebral edema and antiepileptic agents to seizures. Early treatment with antibodies directed against anthrax toxins is also recommended.

References

1. Sejvar JJ, Tenover FC, Stephens DS. Management of anthrax meningitis. *Lancet Infect Dis.* 2005;5:287-295.
2. Meyer MA. Neurologic complications of anthrax: a review of the literature. *Arch Neurol.* 2003;60:483-488.
3. Bower WA, Hendricks K, Pillai S, et al. Clinical framework and medical countermeasure use during an anthrax mass-casualty incident: recommendations and reports. *MMWR Morb Mortal Wkly Rep.* 2015 64(RR-04):1-28.

**2.** Correct Answer: C

**Rationale:**

*Clostridium botulinum* produces neurotoxins (types A–G) that block acetylcholine release and affect both nicotinic and muscarinic receptors. Symptoms of botulism include an acute, afebrile, symmetric, descending flaccid paralysis, and prominent bulbar palsies (diplopia, dysarthria, dysphonia, and dysphagia). Blockade of muscarinic receptors result in postural hypotension, nausea, and vomiting from ileus. Respiratory muscle involvement can result in respiratory failure. Mental status is not affected; patients usually have a clear sensorium.

The diagnosis of botulism must be done on a clinical basis as laboratory testing is specialized and requires several days to complete. Differential diagnosis includes Guillain-Barre Syndrome, myasthenia gravis, tick paralysis, organophosphate toxicity, and tick paralysis. Distinguishing features of botulism include prominent cranial nerve palsies initially, symmetric, descending progression, and absence of sensory nerve dysfunction.

Features suggestive of bioterrorism as cause of an outbreak of botulism include a large number of cases, outbreak with an unusual botulinum toxin type, outbreak in a location without a common dietary exposure, and multiple outbreaks at the same time without common source.

Treatment of botulism is largely supportive. Antitoxin should be administered in a timely basis (most effective if given within 24 hours). The antitoxin will limit the severity of disease and subsequent nerve damage but will not reverse existent paralysis.

References

1. Arnon SS, Schechter R, Inglesby TV, et al. Botulinum toxin as a biological weapon: medical and public health management. *JAMA.* 2001;285:1059-1070.
2. Karma M, Currie B, Kvetan V. Bioterrorism: preparing for the impossible or the improbable. *Crit Care Med.* 2005;33:S75-S95.

**3.** Correct Answer: D

**Rationale:**

Bioterrorism refers to the use of biologic agents as weapons to further personal or political agendas. Unlike other methods of terrorism, the effects are not always immediately apparent and can be difficult to distinguish from an outbreak of a naturally occurring infectious disease. Features of a possible bioterrorism-related attack include:

Rapid rise of cases (within hours or days) in a normally healthy population

Number of cases rises and falls during a short period of time (few hours to days) versus more protracted course (weeks to months) seen in natural outbreaks

An unusual increase in number of patients with complaints of fever, respiratory, or gastrointestinal complaints

An endemic disease that occurs in large number of patients at an uncharacteristic time or in an unusual pattern

Lower attack rates among people who were indoors compared to those outdoors

Large number of patients arriving from single locale

Large number of rapidly fatal cases

Patients with uncommon disease with bioterrorism potential (eg anthrax, tularemia, plague)

Increased numbers of sick or dead animals

References

1. Karma M, Currie B, Kvetan V. Bioterrorism: preparing for the impossible or the improbable. *Crit Care Med.* 2005;33:S75-S95.
2. *Bioterrorism Readiness Plan: A Template for Healthcare Facilities.* https://emergency.cdc.gov/bioterrorism/pdf/13apr99APIC-CD-CBioterrorism.pdf. Accessed October 15, 2018.

**4.** Correct Answer: C

**Rationale:**

Ricin is a toxin derived from the castor bean plant. When purified, it is a white powder that is soluble in water. It can be disseminated as an aerosol, by adding to food or water, and by injection. It inhibits protein synthesis leading to cell death. Other mechanisms of toxicity include affecting apoptosis pathways, direct cell membrane damage, and release of cytokines.

Clinical effects depend on the route of exposure. Initial symptoms of ingestion of ricin can mimic gastroenteritis with abdominal pain, nausea, vomiting, and diarrhea. Hematemesis and melena may occur. Severe dehydration, kidney and liver failure, and death may occur. Symptoms of inhalation of ricin include fever, cough, chest tightness, and respiratory distress. Diffuse pulmonary edema can occur leading to respiratory failure. Smaller ricin particles result in higher mortality because they can be deposited deeper into the respiratory tract. Symptoms after injection of ricin may be delayed as much as 10 to 12 hours are initially nonspecific (fever, headache, nausea, abdominal pain, hypotension) and may progress to multiorgan failure.

There is no antidote for ricin and treatment is supportive. Ricin is not contagious, so respiratory isolation is not necessary. To prevent systemic absorption, a single dose of activated charcoal may be given to patients with ricin ingestion. It is not recommended for patients who have inhaled ricin.

Reference

1. Audi J, Belson M, Patel M, et al. Ricin poisoning: a comprehensive review. *JAMA.* 2005;294:2342-2351.

# 74

# HOSPITAL INFECTION CONTROL, HOSPITAL ACQUIRED INFECTIONS

Lisa M. Bebell

1. Which set of precaution measures are **MOST** appropriate for a patient being treated for *Clostridioides* (formerly *Clostridium*) *difficile* colitis?

   A. Mandatory gowns, gloves, and surgical masks for healthcare workers
   B. Mandatory gowns and gloves for healthcare workers, followed by alcohol-based hand cleansing after removing gown and gloves
   C. Mandatory gowns and gloves for healthcare workers, followed by soap-and-water hand cleansing after removing gown and gloves
   D. Mandatory gowns and gloves for healthcare workers, followed by soap-and-water hand cleansing after removing gown and gloves until the patient has fewer than five loose bowel movements daily

2. You are placing a central venous catheter in a 44-year-old patient with unknown identity found down in the street. The patient is intubated and sedated. After multiple attempts to cannulate the vein, you accidentally stick your finger with the finder needle. You remove your glove and see that your finger is bleeding. What should you do next?

   A. Wash your finger with soap and water for 2 minutes, then call your hospital's infection control, infectious diseases consult, or emergency medicine needlestick response team for further assistance
   B. Wash your finger with soap and water for 2 minutes, then order testing for HIV, hepatitis B, and hepatitis C to be sent from the patient's blood
   C. Clean your finger thoroughly with a chlorhexidine swab and then wash with soap and water for 2 minutes
   D. Bandage your finger with an antibiotic ointment and then call your hospital's infection control, infectious diseases consult, or emergency medicine needlestick response team for further assistance

3. A 32-year-old pregnant woman is admitted to your intensive care unit with severe respiratory distress and hypoxemia requiring supplementary oxygen delivered by high-flow nasal cannula. Computed tomography (CT) of the chest demonstrates bilateral perihilar ground-glass and nodular infiltrates. On physical examination, you notice a diffuse erythematous and vesicular rash, with crops of vesicles in different stages of development. The patient tells you the rash is extremely pruritic. Which of the following infection control measures is **MOST** appropriate?

   A. Pregnant and nonimmune healthcare workers should not be assigned to care for this patient; mandatory gowns, gloves, and surgical masks should be worn by healthcare workers
   B. Pregnant and nonimmune healthcare workers should not be assigned to care for this patient; mandatory gowns, gloves, airborne precautions, and N-95 respirator masks should be worn by healthcare workers
   C. Mandatory gowns, gloves, and surgical masks should be worn by healthcare workers
   D. Mandatory gowns, gloves, airborne precautions, and N-95 respirator masks should be worn by healthcare workers

4. Which of the following scenarios represents **INAPPROPRIATE** use of an indwelling urethral catheter?

   A. Monitoring urine output in a man with urinary incontinence
   B. Monitoring urine output in a man with urinary incontinence and urinary retention
   C. Obtaining urine for testing in a patient who can void spontaneously
   D. All of the above are inappropriate uses of an indwelling urethral catheter

**5.** After 4 days of being intubated and sedated on a ventilator, a 62-year-old man develops fever, an increased oxygen requirement, and new infiltrates on chest X-ray. Are these findings sufficient to diagnose the patient with a probable ventilator-associated pneumonia?

A. Yes

B. No, an increase in peripheral blood white blood cell count or increase in respiratory secretions is also needed.

C. No, a lower respiratory tract culture growing a potential pathogen is also needed.

D. No, CT of the chest demonstrating new infiltrates is also needed.

**6.** You admit a 28-year-old woman to the intensive care unit for hypoxemia requiring noninvasive positive-pressure ventilation. She received an allogeneic bone marrow transplant 13 days ago for relapsed acute leukemia and remains neutropenic. What are the **MOST** appropriate infection control measures?

A. Admit to a NEGATIVE-pressure isolation room; all healthcare workers should wear gloves and cleanse hands with alcohol-based hand rub before and after entering patient's room

B. Admit to a NEGATIVE-pressure isolation room; all healthcare workers should wear gloves, N95 respirator masks, and cleanse hands with alcohol-based hand rub before and after entering patient's room

C. Admit to a POSITIVE-pressure isolation room; all healthcare workers should wear gown, gloves, and cleanse hands with alcohol-based hand rub before and after entering patient's room

D. Admit to a POSITIVE-pressure isolation room; all healthcare workers should cleanse hands with alcohol-based hand rub before and after entering patient's room

**7.** You are caring for a patient who underwent right internal jugular central venous catheter placement 36 hours ago. She developed fever 12 hours ago, and blood cultures were sent. No other signs or symptoms of infection are present, and chest X-ray and urinalysis are normal. Five hours after they were drawn, blood cultures are now growing *Staphylococcus aureus* in two of four bottles. What is the **MOST** likely diagnosis?

A. Catheter-related (central line-associated) bloodstream infection (CRBSI/CLABSI)

A. *S. aureus* bacteremia, source unknown

C. Blood culture contamination

D. Methicillin-resistant *S. aureus* bacteremia

**8.** Which of the following is the **MOST** common route(s) of contamination for nonemergently placed central venous catheters?

A. Contamination during catheter placement, for example, by breaches of sterile technique

B. Contaminated infusate leading to catheter contamination

C. Hematogenous seeding from another focus of infection

D. Migration of skin organisms at the catheter insertion site along the catheter with colonization of the catheter tip, and direct contamination of the catheter or catheter hub by contact with hands or contaminated fluids/devices

**9.** A 27-year-old woman with cystic fibrosis is admitted to the intensive care unit with a cystic fibrosis exacerbation due to *Pseudomonas aeruginosa*. Peripheral venous access cannot be obtained, and you plan to place a central venous catheter. What infection control precautions are **MOST** appropriate for the person performing the procedure?

A. Cap, surgical mask, sterile gown, sterile gloves, sterile half-body patient drape, and disposable shoe covers

B. Cap, N95 respirator mask, sterile gown, sterile gloves, sterile full-body patient drape, and disposable shoe covers

C. Cap, surgical mask, sterile gown, sterile gloves, and sterile half-body patient drape

D. Cap, surgical mask, sterile gown, sterile gloves, and sterile full-body patient drape

**10.** A 82-year-old man presents to the emergency department with fever and shortness of breath and is admitted to the intensive care unit for presumed pneumonia requiring high-flow nasal cannula treatment of hypoxemia. On examination, he is awake, alert, conversant in short sentences, and appropriate. His other medical problems include benign prostatic hypertrophy, for which he underwent a remote transurethral resection of the prostate (TURP). Since the procedure, he has been intermittently incontinent of urine, but has not had urinary retention or obstruction. What is the **MOST** appropriate way to manage his urinary incontinence and measure urine output?

A. Placement of an indwelling urethral (Foley) catheter

B. Placement of an external urinary drainage penile sheath ("Texas" or "condom") catheter

C. Keep a portable urinal at bedside and weigh sheets, blankets, and pads soiled with urine to estimate urine output

D. A and B are equally appropriate

# Chapter 74 ▪ Answers

**1.** Correct Answer: C

**Rationale:**

Alcohol-based hand rub does not kill *C.* (formerly *Clostridium*) *difficile* spores, which are more effectively removed by mechanical scrubbing with soap and water. It is recommended that contact precautions and soap-and-water hand washing be continued for at least 48 hours after diarrhea resolves.

References

1. McDonald LC, Gerding DN, Johnson S, et al. Clinical practice guidelines for Clostridium difficile infection in adults and children: 2017 update by the Infectious Diseases Society of America (IDSA) and Society for Healthcare Epidemiology of America (SHEA). *Clin Infect Dis.* 2018;66:987-994.
2. Edmonds SL, Zapka C, Kasper D, et al. Effectiveness of hand hygiene for removal of *Clostridium difficile* spores from hands. *Infect Control Hosp Epidemiol.* 2013;34:302-305.

**2.** Correct Answer: A

**Rationale:**

Soap and water should be used to wash the injured body part after a needlestick injury. The efficacy of chlorhexidine cleansing is not known. The patient on whom the procedure was being performed should be tested for HIV and hepatitis, but only after consent has been obtained from the patient. Because this patient is intubated and sedated, consent for testing cannot currently be obtained, and it is important to discuss postexposure prophylaxis against transmissible infections with your hospital's needlestick team as soon as possible after a needlestick or mucosal exposure occurs.

References

1. Rizk C, Monroe H, Orengo I, Rosen T. Needlestick and sharps injuries in dermatologic surgery: a review of preventative techniques and post-exposure protocols. *J Clin Aesthet Dermatol.* 2016;9:41-49.
2. Riddell A, Kennedy I, Tong CY. Management of sharps injuries in the healthcare setting. *BMJ.* 2015;351:h3733.

**3.** Correct Answer: B

**Rationale:**

Disseminated and severe varicella infection, including varicella pneumonia, is more likely to occur in pregnant and immune-compromised hosts. Primary infection is followed by viral replication in regional lymph nodes for 4 to 6 days, followed by secondary viremia and invasion of the skin tissue leading to rash approximately 2 to 3 weeks later. Varicella is highly transmissible, with secondary attack rates approaching 90% among household contacts in the prevaccine era. Varicella is spread both by contact with virus-filled vesicles and through aerosolized droplets or airborne viral particles, mandating strict infection control precautions. Because varicella is a fetal teratogen, it is recommended that pregnant women not be assigned to care for patients with active varicella infection.

References

1. Weber DJ, Rutala WA, Hamilton H. Prevention and control of varicella-zoster infections in healthcare facilities. *Infect Control Hosp Epidemiol.* 1996;17:694-705.
2. Preventing Varicella in Health Care Settings. Centers for Disease Control and Prevention. 2016. Available at https://www.cdc.gov/chickenpox/hcp/healthcare-setting.html.

**4.** Correct Answer: D

**Rationale:**

Up to half of all indwelling urethral catheters in hospitalized patients are placed for inappropriate indications. Patients who can void spontaneously or collect urine for testing do no need an invasive urethral catheter placed. Men with urinary incontinence without obstruction can have an external penile sheath ("Texas" or "condom" style) catheter placed. Intermittent urethral catheterization can be used for patients with urinary retention or obstruction and must be performed at regular intervals to prevent bladder overdistention.

References

1. Lo E, Nicolle LE, Coffin SE, et al. Strategies to prevent catheter-associated urinary tract infections in acute care hospitals: 2014 update. *Infect Control Hosp Epidemiol.* 2014;35:464-479.
2. Hooton TM, Bradley SF, Cardenas DD, et al. Diagnosis, prevention, and treatment of catheter-associated urinary tract infection in adults: 2009 International Clinical Practice Guidelines from the Infectious Diseases Society of America. *Clin Infect Dis.* 2010;50:625-663.

**5.** Correct Answer: C

**Rationale:**

Ventilator-associated pneumonia is one of several ventilator-associated events (VAE). VAEs can be difficult to diagnose, as patients are often unable to report their symptoms. Diagnostic criteria for probable ventilator-associated pneumonia include new or progressive pulmonary infiltrates on chest X-ray or CT scan, plus one or more clinical signs of infection, including increased oxygen requirement, increased respiratory secretions, increased peripheral blood white blood cell count, and fever. Diagnosis of probable ventilator-associated pneumonia is confirmed when a potential pathogen is identified in a lower respiratory tract sample.

References

1. Kalanuria AA, Ziai W, Mirski M. Ventilator-associated pneumonia in the ICU. *Criti Care.* 2014;18:208.
2. Spalding MC, Cripps MW, Minshall CT. Ventilator-associated pneumonia: new definitions. *Crit Care Clin.* 2017;33:277-292.

**6.** Correct Answer: D

**Rationale:**

Recent hematopoietic stem cell transplant (HSCT) recipients, especially allogeneic bone marrow transplant recipients, are at high risk of bacterial, viral, fungal, and parasitic infection. Current guidelines recommend that HSCT patients be admitted to rooms with HEPA filters, and the rooms be maintained with positive pressure relative to the corridor. Gown, gloves, and mask are not required for healthcare workers or visitors for routine entry into the room. Standard precautions are recommended for healthcare workers and visitors. HSCT patients should wear N95 respirator masks when leaving the positive pressure environment.

References

1. Siegel JD, Rhinehart E, Jackson M, Chiarello L. 2007 Guideline for isolation precautions: preventing transmission of infectious agents in health care settings. *Am J Infect Control.* 2007;35:S65-S164.
2. Centers for Disease Control and PreventionInfectious Disease Society of AmericaAmerican Society of Blood and Marrow Transplantation. Guidelines for preventing opportunistic infections among hematopoietic stem cell transplant recipients. *MMWR Recomm Rep.* 2000;49:1-125, CE1-7.

**7.** Correct Answer: A

**Rationale:**

Catheter-related (also called central line-associated) bloodstream infections (CRBSI or CLABSI) can be challenging to diagnose. Diagnosing CRBSI requires the presence of a bloodstream infection and demonstrating no alternative sources of bacteremia. Diagnosis of CRBSI is supported when the same organism is isolated from at least two blood cultures. Blood cultures should be obtained before initiating antibiotic therapy, and at least one blood culture should be obtained by peripheral venipuncture. Resolution of fever, leukocytosis, hypotension, and other infectious signs and symptoms within 24 hours of removing a central venous catheter also supports this diagnosis. *S. aureus* should not be considered a blood culture contaminant. This scenario presents insufficient information to determine whether the cultured *S. aureus* is methicillin-resistant, as the bacterial species was just identified, and susceptibility information will follow later. Lastly, this scenario meets criteria for CRBSI, and as such, the source of bacteremia is not unknown.

References

1. Mermel LA, Allon M, Bouza E, et al. Clinical practice guidelines for the diagnosis and management of intravascular catheter-related infection: 2009 update by the Infectious Diseases Society of America. *Clin Infect Dis.* 2009;49:1-45.
2. Miller JM, Binnicker MJ, Campbell S, et al. A guide to utilization of the microbiology laboratory for diagnosis of infectious diseases: 2018 update by the Infectious Diseases Society of America and the American Society for Microbiology. *Clin Infect Dis.* 2018;67:813-816.

**8.** Correct Answer: D

**Rationale:**

Although all of the answers listed are potential ways in which central venous catheters can become contaminated, the two most common are migration of skin organisms along the catheter from the skin surface to the catheter tip, and direct contamination of the catheter hub itself (Answer D). Hematogenous seeding (Answer C) occurs but is rare, and contaminated infusates (intravenous medications, Answer B) are also uncommon. Lastly, owing to improvements in sterile technique, contamination of the catheter during nonemergent placement is rare (Answer A).

References

1. O'Grady NP, Alexander M, Burns LA, et al. Guidelines for the prevention of intravascular catheter-related infections. *Am J Infect Control.* 2011;39:S1-S34.
2. Anaissie E, Samonis G, Kontoyiannis D, et al. Role of catheter colonization and infrequent hematogenous seeding in catheter-related infections. *Eur J Clin Microbiol Infect Dis.* 1995;14:134-137.

**9.** Correct Answer: D

**Rationale:**

Maximal sterile barrier precautions should be used when placing central venous catheters to reduce the risk of catheter-related bloodstream infection and other complications. A half-body patient drape is not considered a maximal sterile barrier. N95 respirator masks and disposable shoe covers are not necessary or recommended for central venous catheter placement.

References

1. O'Grady NP, Alexander M, Burns LA, et al. Guidelines for the prevention of intravascular catheter-related infections. *Am J Infect Control*. 2011;39:S1-S34.
2. Raad II, Hohn DC, Gilbreath BJ, et al. Prevention of central venous catheter-related infections by using maximal sterile barrier precautions during insertion. *Infect Control Hosp Epidemiol*. 1994;15:231-238.

**10.** Correct Answer: B

**Rationale:**

Indwelling urethral catheters are overused, and 20% to 50% of catheters placed in hospitalized patients are unwarranted. Because indwelling urethral catheters confer a higher risk of urinary tract infection than other methods of collecting urine, noninvasive or intermittently invasive measures are preferred, where appropriate. External penile sheath catheters are associated with a lower risk of infection when the patient does not have urinary retention, the sheath is placed correctly (not too tight), and the patient does not excessively manipulate the catheter. Patients with normal mental status and no evidence of urinary retention are therefore good candidates for an external penile sheath catheter. Patients with urinary retention are better candidates for intermittent urethral catheterization. Although a portable urinal at bedside combined with weighing sheets, blankets, and pads soiled with urine is logistically possible, this is not the most appropriate way to manage the patient's urinary incontinence, as sitting or lying in urine-soaked linens could lead to skin breakdown.

References

1. Lo E, Nicolle LE, Coffin SE, et al. Strategies to prevent catheter-associated urinary tract infections in acute care hospitals: 2014 update. *Infect Control Hosp Epidemiol*. 2014;35:464-479.
2. Hooton TM, Bradley SF, Cardenas DD, et al. Diagnosis, prevention, and treatment of catheter-associated urinary tract infection in adults: 2009 International Clinical Practice Guidelines from the Infectious Diseases Society of America. *Clin Infect Dis*. 2010;50:625-663.

# 75

# IMMUNOLOGICAL DISEASES

Jamie Sparling

1. A 72-year-old woman with hypertension, hypothyroidism, and a history of giant cell arteritis (GCA) presents with acute onset of chest pain. Computed tomography (CT) angiography in the emergency department reveals a type B aortic dissection, and she is brought to the surgical intensive care unit (ICU) for close hemodynamic monitoring and medical management of the dissection. Which of the following factors most increased her risk for thoracic aortic dissection?

   A. Hypertension
   B. Gender
   C. Age
   D. GCA
   E. Hypothyroidism

2. A 65-year-old male presents with new onset thyrotoxicosis, and he is found to be in atrial fibrillation with rapid ventricular response and is hypotensive. He is currently being treated with propylthiouracil and steroids and awaiting total thyroidectomy for definitive therapy, while his cardiovascular status is optimized. During his hospitalization, he develops massive hemoptysis. He is intubated for airway protection and brought to the ICU where serial bronchoalveolar lavage (BAL) reveals progressively more hemorrhagic specimens with each aliquot. Laboratory analysis reveals a positive antineutrophil cytoplasmic antibody (ANCA) in a cytoplasmic pattern and a positive antiproteinase 3 (anti-PR3) antibody. Which of the following medications is most associated with drug-induced ANCA vasculitis?

   A. Furosemide
   B. Amiodarone
   C. Propylthiouracil
   D. Propranolol
   E. Heparin

3. A 56-year-old woman with a history of hypertension, hyperlipidemia, mixed connective tissue disease (MCTD), and hypothyroidism presents with respiratory failure secondary to influenza A and *Staphylococcus aureus* pneumonia. She is admitted to the ICU for invasive mechanical ventilation. Titers of which of the following antibodies do you most expect to be positive?

   A. Anti-La
   B. Anti-double stranded DNA (anti-dsDNA)
   C. Anti-PR3
   D. Anti-U1-ribonucleoprotein (anti-U1-RNP)
   E. Antimyeloperoxidase (anti-MPO)

4. A 47-year-old woman with MCTD presents from home with fever and dyspnea. In the emergency room, she is found to have hypoxemia with a room air saturation of 87% and a right upper lobe opacity on chest x-ray. Her oxygenation improves with supplemental oxygen and then she is transported to the CT scanner. There she acutely decompensated with worsened hypoxemia and hypotension prompting endotracheal intubation, presumably after a gastric aspiration event. Which is the most common site of gastrointestinal involvement of MCTD?

A. Esophagus
B. Stomach
C. Duodenum
D. Cecum
E. Sigmoid colon

5. A 68-year-old woman, who immigrated to the United States from Peru 7 years ago, with a history of rheumatoid arthritis (RA), maintained on adalimumab, presents to the emergency department with fever, arthralgias, dyspnea, and a productive cough. Physical examination is notable for distended abdomen with splenomegaly and ascites. Chest x-ray shows bilateral micronodular opacities, seen on subsequent chest CT scan with mediastinal lymphadenopathy and lymph node calcifications. Despite empiric antibiotic and antifungal coverage, her clinical condition worsened and was transferred to the ICU where intubation and mechanical ventilation instituted. Diagnostic bronchoscopy and paracentesis are performed. Rapid tuberculosis (TB) testing shows positivity in both the sputum and ascitic fluid samples, and both develop positive mycobacterial cultures at day 14. Which of the following statements is true of her disseminated TB?

A. Completion of 9 months of chemoprophylaxis eliminates the risk of reactivation of TB among purified protein derivative (PPD)–positive patients started on adalimumab.
B. Immunosuppression may result in a false-negative PPD test, but QuantiFERON-TB Gold assay is unaffected.
C. Adalimumab's mechanism of action is by competitively binding to the IL-6 receptor.
D. The risk of TB is 4X higher in patients on anti-tumor necrosis factor α (anti-TNFα) therapies.

6. A 56-year-old woman with systemic lupus erythematosus (SLE), who is maintained on prednisone 20 mg daily, presents for open right hemicolectomy for colon cancer. She is admitted to the surgical ICU postoperatively for refractory hypotension. Which of the following is true regarding perioperative stress dose steroid supplementation?

A. Before an elective surgical case, preoperative adrenocorticotropic hormone (ACTH) stimulation testing is warranted in this patient to determine need for stress dose steroid administration.
B. The dose and duration of perioperative steroid administration are the same regardless of the type of surgery.
C. Stress dose steroids should be administered similarly regardless of the duration of this patient's prednisone use.
D. Dexamethasone may alternatively be used for stress dose steroid administration, as it has higher relative glucocorticoid activity compared with hydrocortisone.
E. Stress dose steroids should be administered only in the event of intraoperative hypotension refractory to intravenous fluids and vasopressors.

7. Which of the diffuse connective tissue disorders (DCTDs) has the highest rate of pulmonary involvement?

A. Systemic lupus erythematosus (SLE)
B. Systemic sclerosis (SS)
C. Polymyositis (PM)
D. Dermatomyositis (DM)
E. Rheumatoid arthritis (RA)

8. A 54-year-old woman with SLE, maintained on chronic prednisone, and complicated by stage III chronic kidney disease presents with acute anuric kidney injury. Which of the following statements is most correct regarding this patient's renal failure?

A. Following treatment, renal biopsy is unlikely to show pathologic changes despite clinical improvement.
B. In the longer term, cyclophosphamide, mycophenolate mofetil, or calcineurin inhibitors may be used alone or in combination to improve disease remission.
C. Azathioprine reduces rate of progression to end-stage renal disease.
D. High-dose corticosteroids are contraindicated.
E. When renal replacement therapy is initiated in the acute setting, patients will invariably require long-term hemodialysis.

9. Which of the following is most consistent with a diagnosis of Takayasu arteritis (TAK)?

A. Immediate revascularization should be pursued during active flares to prevent ischemic complications.
B. Blood pressure discrepancy ≥10 mm Hg between the contralateral upper extremities is a diagnostic criterion.
C. Corticosteroids alone achieve remission in >90% cases.
D. Angiography demonstrates stenosis of the aorta, its branches, and/or large arteries of the upper or lower extremities.
E. Pulmonary arteries are spared.

**10.** A 64-year-old gentleman with hypertension, hyperlipidemia, and mild asthma presents to the emergency department from home with massive hemoptysis. He is intubated for airway protection, and chest CT scan shows diffuse bilateral alveolar ground-glass opacities with inter- and intralobular thickening. He is admitted to the ICU where bronchoscopy and BAL is performed and consistent with diffuse alveolar hemorrhage (DAH). During his ICU course, he develops worsening acute renal failure with hematuria. Anti–glomerular basement membrane (anti-GBM) antibody is positive. Which of the following statements is most likely correct regarding his disease?

**A.** The cause of this patient's pulmonary-renal syndrome is a type of vasculitis.
**B.** Patients must have both pulmonary and renal manifestations in order to be diagnosed with anti-GBM disease.
**C.** A positive ANCA precludes diagnosis of anti-GBM disease.
**D.** Anti-GBM antibodies are directed at smooth muscle cells of medium-sized arteries.
**E.** Urinalysis will likely show dysmorphic red cells, red cell casts, and proteinuria.

# Chapter 75 ▪ Answers

**1.** Correct Answer: D

**Rationale:**
GCA is an inflammatory vasculopathy affecting predominantly elderly patients, with a mean age of 70 to 80 years. 65% to 75% diagnoses are made in females. GCA affects medium and large arteries, specifically, those that have well-defined layers and in which vaso vasorum are present. It preferentially affects the external carotid arteries and its branches and thus typically presents with headache. The American College of Rheumatology (ACR) requires three of the following criteria for diagnosis of GCA:

- Age at disease onset ≥50 years
- New headache, either new onset or new type of localized pain in the head
- Abnormal temporal artery, with tenderness to palpation or decreased pulsation
- Elevated ESR >50 mm/h during first hour of testing (Westergren method)
- Biopsy evidence of vasculitis with predominance of mononuclear-cell infiltration or granulomatous inflammation, usually with multinucleated giant cells

Aortitis was previously thought to occur in 3% to 18% of patients with GCA, but these diagnoses were only made when aortic aneurysm formation or dissection became clinically apparent. Now, the true rate of aortic involvement is thought to be much higher, and thus regular screening of the aorta is recommended for patients with GCA to exclude aortitis and presence of an asymptomatic aneurysm. The screening modalities recommended are either the combination of chest radiograph, echocardiogram, and abdominal Doppler ultrasound or a CT scan of the chest and abdomen with intravenous contrast.

Although increasing age and hypertension are both risk factors for aortic dissection, the diagnosis of GCA is a much stronger risk factor for thoracic aneurysm formation and aortic dissection. In one population-based cohort study, patients with giant GCA were 17 times more likely to develop thoracic aortic aneurysm and 2.4 times more likely to develop isolated abdominal aortic aneurysm. Male gender, not female, increases risk for aortic dissection.

References
1. Weyand CM, Goronzy JJ. Giant-cell arteritis and polymyalgia rheumatica. *N Engl J Med*. 2014;371:50-57.
2. Bossert M, Prati C, Balblanc JC, Lohse A, Wendling D. Aortic involvement in giant cell arteritis: current data. *Joint Bone Spine*. 2011;78(3):246-251.
3. Martínez-Valle F, Solans-Laqué R, Bosch-Gil J, Vilardell-Tarrés M. Aortic involvement in giant cell arteritis. *Autoimmun Rev*. 2010;9(7):521-524.
4. Kermani TA, Warrington KJ, Crowson CS, et al. Predictors of dissection in aortic aneurysms from giant cell arteritis. *J Clin Rheumatol*. 2016;22(4):184-187.

**2.** Correct Answer: C

**Rationale:**
This patient exhibits DAH, which occurs because of the accumulation of red blood cells into the alveolar space. It is diagnosed with BAL by observation of progressively more hemorrhagic aliquots. DAH generally presents with dyspnea, hemoptysis, chest infiltrates, and a fall in hemoglobin, though surprisingly, hemoptysis is absent in up to one-third of cases.

New diagnosis of DAH should prompt a diagnostic workup including serologies for the common forms of small-vessel vasculitis. Small-vessel vasculitis is defined as vasculitis that affects vessels smaller than arteries, such as arterioles, venules, and capillaries. ANCAs bind to antigens in neutrophil and monocyte lysosomes and occur in two staining patterns: cytoplasmic (c-ANCA) and perinuclear (p-ANCA). A positive ANCA is seen in granulomatosis with polyangiitis (GPA, formerly known as Wegener granulomatosis), eosinophilic granulomatosis with polyangiitis (EGPA, formerly known as Churg-Strauss syndrome), microscopic polyangiitis (MPA), and renal-limited ANCA vasculitis. Most patients with GPA have a c-ANCA pattern and antibodies to anti-PR3, whereas most patients with EGPA or MPA have a p-ANCA pattern and antibodies to anti-MPO.

Antithyroid drugs, including methimazole and propylthiouracil, are well-known to be associated with the development of ANCA-associated small-vessel vasculitis. Other drugs known to cause small-vessel vasculitis, with or without ANCA positivity, include hydralazine and levamisole (an agent found in adulterated cocaine).

Treatment for DAH secondary to drug-induced ANCA vasculitis includes withdrawal of the offending agent, high-dose corticosteroids, cyclophosphamide, and rituximab. Plasmapheresis is recommended in severe cases.

### References

1. Jennette JC, Falk RJ. Small-vessel vasculitis. *N Engl J Med.* 1997;337:1512-1523.
2. Nasser M, Cottin V. Alveolar hemorrhage in vasculitis (primary and secondary). *Semin Respir Crit Care Med.* 2018;39(4): 482-493.
3. Balavoine AS, Glinoer D, Dubucquoi S, Wémeau JL. Antineutrophil cytoplasmic antibody-positive small-vessel vasculitis associated with antithyroid drug therapy: how significant is the clinical problem? *Thyroid.* 2015;25(12):1273-1281.
4. Arai N, Nemoto K, Oh-Ishi S, et al. Methimazole-induced ANCA-associated vasculitis with diffuse alveolar haemorrhage. *Respirol Case Rep.* 2018;6(5):e00315.

**3.** Correct Answer: D

**Rationale:**

There are five diffuse connective tissue disorders (DCTDs):
- Systemic lupus erythematosus (SLE)
- Systemic sclerosis (SS)
- Polymyositis (PM)
- Dermatomyositis (DM)
- Rheumatoid arthritis (RA)

However, up to 25% of patients experience symptoms that may evolve from one disorder into another over time or have characteristics of several disorders at presentation, and thus are said to have an "overlap syndrome." MCTD, also known as Sharp syndrome, is one such "overall syndrome" and shares clinical similarities with SLE, SS, and PM. Several sets of diagnostic criteria exist for MCTD, but the requirement for a positive Anti-U1-RNP antibody is universal among them. The Kasukawa criteria are one such, well-accepted, diagnostic criteria:
- Presence of Raynaud phenomenon and/or finger edema
- Positive anti-U1-RNP antibody
- Presence of symptoms of two among three of the following connective tissue diseases:
  - SLE (polyarthritis, pericarditis/pleuritis, lymphadenopathy, facial erythema, or leukopenia/thrombocytopenia)
  - SS (sclerodactyly, pulmonary fibrosis, or esophageal dysmotility)
  - PM (proximal muscle weakness, high creatine phosphokinase, or myopathic electromyography pattern)

Aside from musculoskeletal manifestations (above), other clinical features of MCTD include pulmonary hypertension (affecting 10%-50% patients), interstitial lung disease (ILD) (affecting 47%-78% patients), oroesophageal involvement (affecting 64% patients), cardiovascular involvement (13%-65% patients), and renal involvement (5%-36% patients).

Among the other answer choices, anti-La is seen in primary Sjogren syndrome, anti-dsDNA is seen in SLE, and anti-PR3 and anti-MPO are seen in ANCA vasculitis.

### References

1. Orsi D, Correa-Lopez W, Cavagnaro J. Rheumatologic and inflammatory conditions in the ICU. In: Oropello JM, Pastores SM, Kvetan V, eds. *Critical Care.* New York, NY: McGraw-Hill. http://accessanesthesiology.mhmedical.com/content.aspx?book-id=1944&sectionid=143518884. Accessed March 14, 2019.
2. Kasukawa R. Mixed connective tissue disease. *Intern Med.* 1999;38:386-393.
3. Gunashekar S, Prakash M, Minz RW, et al. Comparison of articular manifestations of mixed connective tissue disease and systemic lupus erythematosus on clinical examination and musculoskeletal ultrasound. *Lupus.* 2018;27:2086-2092.

**4.** Correct Answer: A

**Rationale:**

MCTD, also known as Sharp syndrome, is considered an "overall syndrome" and shares clinical similarities with SLE, SS, and PM. MCTD is characterized by positive anti-U1-RNP antibody. Aside from the musculoskeletal system, the cardiovascular system, gastrointestinal tract, lungs, hematologic system, renal system, and central nervous system may all be involved.

Among gastrointestinal manifestations, approximately 85% involve the esophagus. Of all patients with MCTD, 45% to 85% may experience esophageal dysmotility, which may be subclinical at the time of diagnosis. As in SS, esophageal studies including manometry or barium swallow may show reduced peristalsis of the lower third of the esophagus and deceased pressure of the lower esophageal sphincter. Whether esophageal dysmotility and subsequent aspiration of gastric contents in MCTD is related to the manifestation of ILD is an area of debate. In MCTD patients with normal esophageal motility, only 20% experience dyspnea, versus over 70% of those with moderately reduced esophageal peristalsis or aperistalsis.

Although esophageal involvement is the most common, MCTD may also affect nearly every component of the GI system, including delayed gastric emptying, slow intestinal transit, malabsorption, and colonic pseudodiverticula and colonic perforations.

### References

1. Orsi D, Correa-Lopez W, Cavagnaro J. Rheumatologic and inflammatory conditions in the ICU. In: Oropello JM, Pastores SM, Kvetan V, eds. *Critical Care*. New York, NY: McGraw-Hill. http://accessanesthesiology.mhmedical.com/content.aspx?bookid=1944&sectionid=143518884. Accessed March 14, 2019.
2. Nica AE, Alexa LM, Ionescu AO, et al. Esophageal disorders in mixed connective tissue diseases. *J Med Life*. 2016;9(2):141-143.
3. Marie I, Dominique S, Levesque H, et al. Esophageal involvement and pulmonary manifestations in systemic sclerosis. *Arthritis Rheum*. 2001;45(4):346-354.
4. Caleiro MT, Lage LV, Navarro-Rodriguez T, et al. Radionuclide imaging for the assessment of esophageal motility disorders in mixed connective tissue disease patients: relation to pulmonary impairment. *Dis Esophagus*. 2006;19(5):394-400.

---

**5.** Correct Answer: D

**Rationale:**

RA affects 5 in 1000 individuals worldwide, with 2 to 3× as many women as men affected and peak incidence in the sixth decade of life. Treatment of RA has evolved over the last 2 decades with the advent of biologic therapies targeted at stopping or substantially slowing the joint destruction seen in RA. Modern therapy for RA includes disease-modifying antirheumatic drugs (DMARDs), which refer to medications that reduce the signs and symptoms of RA, improve physical function, and inhibit progression of joint destruction. Methotrexate, together with steroid therapy, is the first-line DMARD. Biological agents are second-line therapy.

Biologic agents for RA include the TNFα-inhibitors (etanercept, infliximab, adalimumab, golimumab, certolizumab), IL-6 receptor antibodies (tocilizumab, sarilumab), the anti-CD20 antibody rituximab, and the anti-CD80/86 antibody abatacept. The TNFα antibodies place patients at increased risk for infection, reactivation of TB, drug-induced lupus, exacerbation of demyelinating diseases, nonmelanoma skin cancer, psoriaform skin changes, and injection or infusion site reactions. The risk for reactivation of TB is present for all biologic DMARDs except rituximab and perhaps abatacept. Thus, patients must be screened for latent TB before initiation of therapy and treated if positive. Despite this, false negatives are possible for both PPD and QuantiFERON-Gold tests; in addition, patients may develop new TB infection during therapy. The DMARDs targeted at the janus kinase (JAK) pathway, tofacitinib and baricitinib, increase risk for herpes zoster reactivation, not the anti-TNFα medications.

In patients maintained on anti-TNFα therapy, there is a fourfold increased risk of active TB infection, and in those who develop TB, extrapulmonary and disseminated TB are increased even when compared with other immunocompromised populations such as human immunodeficiency virus (HIV)–infected patients.

### References

1. Aletaha D, Smolen JS. Diagnosis and management of rheumatoid arthritis a review. *JAMA*. 2018;320(13):1360-1372.
2. Cantini F, Nannini C, Niccoli L, Petrone L, Ippolito G, Goletti D. Risk of tuberculosis reactivation in patients with rheumatoid arthritis, ankylosing spondylitis, and psoriatic arthritis receiving non-anti-TNF-targeted biologics. *Mediators Inflamm*. 2017;2017:8909834.
3. Dantes E, Tofolean DE, Fildan AP, et al. Lethal disseminated tuberculosis in patients under biological treatment – two clinical cases and a short review. *J Int Med Res*. 2018;46(7):2961-2969.
4. Liote H, Liote F. Review: role for interferon-gamma release assays in latent tuberculosis screening before TNF-α antagonist therapy. *Joint Bone Spine*. 2011;78(4):352-357.

---

**6.** Correct Answer: D

**Rationale:**

Patients with rheumatologic disease requiring long-term steroid supplementation for maintenance often exhibit secondary adrenal insufficiency, which may manifest as adrenal crisis during periods of perioperative stress. In the past, these patients may have indiscriminately received stress dose steroids, without preoperative risk stratification to determine which patients would benefit from such supplementation. Emerging literature suggests that it may even be safe to continue many patients' baseline steroid dosage without supplementation for more minor procedures. Both the risk of secondary adrenal insufficiency and the level of surgical stress must be considered when determining which patients to administer stress dose steroids:

- Patients with diagnosed secondary adrenal insufficiency, confirmed by prior laboratory evaluation, should receive stress dose steroids.

- Patients receiving doses equivalent to prednisone 20 mg/d or higher, for at least 3 weeks, or those exhibiting clinical evidence of Cushing syndrome should receive stress dose steroids (unless recent ACTH stimulation test has demonstrated integrity of hypothalamic axis [HPA]).
- Patients receiving less than 5 mg/d of prednisone or its equivalent, or any dose for less than 3 weeks, do not require stress dose steroid supplementation.
- Patients not clearly falling into one of these categories may benefit from preoperative evaluation of their HPA if time allows; if testing is not able to be completed, discretion is left to the treating physician. A low threshold to initiate rescue dosing is advised for any suspicion of adrenal crisis.

This type of surgery must also be considered, as the endogenous steroid secretion rate varies considerably between superficial (8-10 mg/d cortisol), minor (50 mg/d), moderate (75-150 mg/d), and major (75-150 mg/d) surgeries. Open abdominal surgery such as a colectomy qualifies as a moderate surgery, and thus this patient should receive stress dose steroid administration beginning preoperatively and continuing for at least the first postoperative day.

Hydrocortisone is the steroid of choice for stress and rescue steroid administration, given its relationship to endogenous cortisol. However, it is the glucocorticoid effect that is deficient in secondary adrenal insufficiency, and as doses rise, patients may experience adverse mineralocorticoid effects from high-dose hydrocortisone including edema, fluid retention, and hypokalemia. In these cases, it is reasonable to substitute a steroid with a higher relative glucocorticoid: mineralocorticoid activity, such as methylprednisolone or dexamethasone.

### References

1. Liu MM, Reidy AB, Saatee S, Collard CD. Perioperative steroid management: approaches based on current evidence. *Anesthesiology*. 2017;127(1):166-172.
2. Yong SL, Coulthard P, Wrzosek A. Supplemental perioperative steroids for surgical patients with adrenal insufficiency. *Cochrane Database Syst Rev*. 2012;12:CD005367.

---

**7.** Correct Answer: B

**Rationale:**

Of the five DCTDs; SLE, SS, PM, DM, and RA, SS has the highest rate of pulmonary involvement, affecting up to 80% of patients. ILD and pulmonary arterial hypertension (PAH) are the most common features; together, these are the most common causes of death in SS, together accounting for up to 60%. ILD tends to affect patients with diffuse cutaneous sclerosis subtype, whereas PAH tends to affect patients with limited cutaneous sclerosis, though there is considerable overlap.

Aspiration due to incompetent lower esophageal sphincter and esophageal dysmotility may further complicate SS patients' pulmonary function. Because of the importance of early treatment, monitoring with pulmonary function testing and high-resolution chest CT scan is recommended at regular intervals.

### References

1. Orsi D, Correa-Lopez W, Cavagnaro J. Rheumatologic and inflammatory conditions in the ICU. In: Oropello JM, Pastores SM, Kvetan V, eds. *Critical Care*. New York, NY: McGraw-Hill. http://accessanesthesiology.mhmedical.com/content.aspx?bookid=1944&sectionid=143518884. Accessed March 14, 2019.
2. Giacomelli R, Liakouli V, Berardicurti O, et al. Interstitial lung disease in systemic sclerosis: current and future treatment. *Rheumatol Int*. 2017;37(6):853-863.

---

**8.** Correct Answer: B

**Rationale:**

Lupus nephritis affects approximately 50% of patients with SLE and is a risk factor for both morbidity and mortality associated with SLE. Approximately 10% of patients with SLE go on to develop end-stage renal disease. As such, patients should be evaluated at the time of diagnosis and at least annually thereafter with a urinalysis and metabolic panel. When there is clinical evidence of renal impairment, a kidney biopsy is recommended. The most common type of renal involvement in SLE is immune complex–mediated glomerulonephritis. However, other types of injury including thrombotic microangiography and lupus podocytopathy may also occur.

The types of lupus nephritis are defined by the International Society of Nephrology/Renal Pathology Society (ISN/RPS) nomenclature. Depending on the class of injury, patients may benefit from potent immunosuppression with steroids and/or immunosuppressive agents. Traditionally, cyclophosphamide has been used, but increasingly mycophenolate mofetil and calcineurin inhibitors are being used with comparable or improved disease remission. Azathioprine, on the other hand, may increase disease relapse.

During an acute flare of lupus nephritis, it may be appropriate to re-biopsy to determine whether histology has changed in an effort to tailor therapy. Similarly, in patients who clinically respond to induction therapy, repeat biopsy will guide the required duration of maintenance therapy before a taper is started.

References

1. Almaani S, Meara A, Rovin BH. Update on lupus nephritis. *CJASN.*2017;12(5):825-835.

2. Tunnicliffe DJ, Palmer SC, Henderson L, et al. Immunosuppressive treatment for proliferative lupus nephritis. *Cochrane Database Syst Rev.* 2018;6:CD002922.

3. Ponticelli C, Imbasciati E, Brancaccio D, Tarantino A, Rivolta E. Acute renal failure in systemic lupus erythematosus. *Br Med J.* 1974;3(5933):716-719.

**9.** Correct Answer: D

**Rationale:**

TAK is a large-vessel vasculitis affecting both adults and children; it is the most frequent cause of large vessel vasculitis in children. TAK causes intramural granulomatous inflammation of the aorta and its major branches, which are demonstrated as narrowing or stenosis on angiography of these vessels in the absence of atherosclerosis or fibromuscular dysplasia. The most common clinical presentations include malaise, weight loss, fever, headache, arthralgia, and claudication of the extremities; however, more acute presentations may include syncope, stroke, and aortic dissection. Clinical examination may reveal a discrepancy in systolic blood pressure between the limbs (present in 67% of patients in one series) and/or a bruit over the large arteries (present in 56% in one series). Pulmonary arteries are affected in 70% of cases, which may lead to pulmonary hypertension and/or pulmonary infarction.

Corticosteroids are the mainstay of remission induction, but approximately half of the patients require additional immunosuppression with either conventional or biologic DMARDs.

Morbidity and mortality from TAK are often because of ischemic complications of the large vessel involvement. Either surgical or endovascular revascularization is indicated to relieve critical, symptomatic stenoses, but these interventions are best undertaken during inactive disease. Acute therapy consists primarily of prompt immunosuppression to induce remission.

References

1. Orsi D, Correa-Lopez W, Cavagnaro J. Rheumatologic and inflammatory conditions in the ICU. In: Oropello JM, Pastores SM, Kvetan V, eds. *Critical Care.* New York, NY: McGraw-Hill. http://accessanesthesiology.mhmedical.com/content.aspx?bookid=1944&sectionid=143518884. Accessed March 14, 2019.

2. Aeschlimann FA, Eng SWM, Sheikh S, et al. Childhood Takayasu arteritis: disease course and response to therapy. *Arthritis Res Ther.* 2017;19(1):255.

3. Misra DP, Wakhlu A, Agarwal V, Danda D. Recent advances in the management of Takayasu arteritis. *Int J Rheum Dis.* 2019;22(suppl 1):60-68.

**10.** Correct Answer: E

**Rationale:**

This patient's pulmonary-renal syndrome is caused by anti-GBM disease, formerly known as Goodpasture disease, in which there is the presence of antibodies directed against the α3 chain of type IV collagen, found in the renal GBMs and the alveolar capillaries. Patients may present with glomerulonephritis, pulmonary hemorrhage, or both, but the most common manifestation is rapidly progressive renal failure.

Urinalysis in anti-GBM disease will show dysmorphic red cells, red cell casts, and proteinuria. Renal biopsy is necessary for confirmation of the disease and will show crescenteric glomerulonephritis and linear deposition of IgG along the GBM. When hemoptysis is present, chest x-ray may show bilateral alveolar infiltrates, greater in the perihilar areas and lower lobes. Chest CT is more sensitive and will detect ground-glass opacities, mainly in the middle lung fields.

Anti-GBM disease is caused by immune complex deposition, not a vasculitis. However, in up to 20% to 30% of patients with anti-GBM disease, patients may also have a positive ANCA.

Treatment of anti-GBM disease consists of high-dose steroids, cyclophosphamide, and plasmapheresis. Poor prognostic factors include >50% crescents on renal biopsy, serum creatinine >7 mg/dL, and requirement of renal replacement therapy within 72 hours of presentation.

References

1. Orsi D, Correa-Lopez W, Cavagnaro J. Rheumatologic and inflammatory conditions in the ICU. In: Oropello JM, Pastores SM, Kvetan V, eds. *Critical Care.* New York, NY: McGraw-Hill. http://accessanesthesiology.mhmedical.com/content.aspx?bookid=1944&sectionid=143518884. Accessed March 14, 2019.

2. Cortese G, Nicali R, Placido R, Gariazzo G, Anrò P. Radiological aspects of diffuse alveolar haemorrhage. *Radiol Med.* 2008;113(1):16-28.

# HEMATOLOGIC AND
# ONCOLOGIC DISORDERS

# 76

# RBC DISORDERS

Jean Kwo

1. Which of the following statements regarding anemia in hospitalized patients is MOST correct?

   A. A low serum iron, normal or low serum ferritin, and normal or high total iron-binding capacity are associated with iron-deficiency anemia.
   B. Blood draws for diagnostic studies is an infrequent cause of anemia in hospitalized patients.
   C. Microcytic anemia is commonly associated with acute blood loss.
   D. The reticulocyte percentage can be artificially decreased in severe anemia.

2. A 57-year-old man has been in the ICU for 10 days with acute respiratory distress syndrome (ARDS) and sepsis due to pneumonia. His hemoglobin level is 7.5 g/dL. Which of the following statements is MOST correct regarding management of his anemia associated with critical illness?

   A. Use of recombinant human erythropoietin (EPO, epoetin alfa) will reduce his need for red-cell transfusion.
   B. Iron supplementation will reduce his need for red-cell transfusion.
   C. He should be transfused with red blood cells as patients with sepsis have better outcomes with a target hemoglobin >9.
   D. Strategies to minimize blood loss associated with phlebotomy such as use of pediatric tubes, point-of-care testing, or use of blood conservation devices can decrease blood loss and transfusion requirements.

3. Which of the following statements regarding red blood cell transfusion in critically ill patients is MOST correct?

   A. Transfusion of leukoreduced red blood cells (RBCs) is associated with decreased risk of ARDS in trauma patients.
   B. Transfusion of RBCs that have been stored for a longer period of time is associated with increased infection, organ dysfunction, and mortality.
   C. A liberal transfusion goal may be associated with an increased risk of nosocomial infections.
   D. Patients with coronary artery disease should have a transfusion threshold of hemoglobin 10 g/dL.

4. A 63-year-old man is admitted to the ICU after exploratory laparotomy, superior mesenteric artery (SMA) thrombectomy, and small bowel resection. He received 2 L of crystalloid resuscitation in the operation room, and his estimated blood loss was 150 mL. He did not receive transfusion in the operating room. His white blood count is 20,000 cells/microL with 90% neutrophils, hemoglobin 19.1 g/dL, hematocrit 57%, and platelet count 265,000 platelets/microL. Which of the following statements regarding his laboratory data is MOST correct?

   A. His complete blood count (CBC) likely reflects a volume depleted state and no further workup is necessary.
   B. He cannot have polycythemia vera (PV) if the JAK2V617F mutation is not detected.
   C. If he has PV, he should be treated with aspirin alone.
   D. His serum EPO level should be low if he has PV.

**5.** Which of the following statements regarding hemoglobinopathies is MOST correct?

**A.** Deoxygenation of sickle hemoglobin (HbS) results in polymerization that produces sickling of the red cell which is reversible.

**B.** The alpha-thalassemias are usually caused by the deletion of one or more beta-globin genes.

**C.** Fetal hemoglobin (HbF) increases the polymerization of HbS and promotes sickling of RBCs.

**D.** Pulmonary embolism is the most common cause of death in β-thalassemia major (TM).

# Chapter 76 ▪ Answers

**1.** Correct Answer: A

**Rationale:**

Reasons for anemia in hospitalized patients are myriad and can include exacerbation of an underlying disease, blood loss from procedures, hemodilution from fluid administration, and impaired erythropoiesis. Phlebotomy for diagnostic purposes is also major cause of anemia. One study showed that 74% of patients developed anemia during their hospitalization.

Evaluation of the RBC indices can help determine the cause of anemia. The mean corpuscular volume (MCV) is the average volume of the patient's RBC and can be low, normal, or elevated. Microcytic RBCs are formed because of decreased production of hemoglobin, which can be due to abnormal globin (thalassemias) or heme (sideroblastic anemias) production or lack of iron (iron-deficiency, anemia of inflammation). Iron studies can help elucidate the cause of microcytic anemias. Iron-deficiency anemia is characterized by low serum iron, a high transferrin, and low ferritin levels. Anemia of inflammation is associated with low iron levels due to reduced iron absorption from the gastrointestinal tract as well as decreased release of iron from body stores. The serum transferrin is usually normal to low and serum ferritin is usually normal to high. Serum iron and ferritin levels are usually normal to high in sideroblastic anemias and thalassemias.

An elevated MCV (macrocytic) is usually due to red cell membrane defects or DNA synthesis defects. Defects in DNA synthesis is associated with folate or vitamin B12 (cobalamine) deficiency, abnormal RBC maturation (eg myelodysplastic syndrome), or certain chemotherapeutic medications. Liver disease or hypothyroidism can cause red cell membrane defects.

However, the RBCs are normal sized (normocytic) in many cases. In these cases, it may be helpful to determine the mechanism underlying the anemia. Mechanisms leading to anemia include decreased RBC production, increased RBC destruction, and blood loss. These mechanisms are not mutually exclusive and can be operating at the same time in a patient.

The reticulocyte count can help distinguish between decreased RBC production and increased RBC destruction. However, because the reticulocyte count is often reported as a percentage of all RBCs, it can be falsely elevated in anemia. Furthermore, younger reticulocytes with a longer lifespan are released into the circulation in the setting of anemia. The reticulocyte production index is a calculated index that corrects for both hematocrit and reticulocyte lifespan.

### References

1. Cascio MJ, DeLoughery TG. Anemia. *Med Clin North Am.* 2017;101:263-284
2. DeLoughery TG. Microcytic anemia. *N Engl J Med.* 2014;371:1324-1331.
3. Koch CG, Li L, Sun Z, et al. Hospital-acquired anemia: prevalence, outcomes, and healthcare implications. *J Hosp Med.* 2013;8:506-512.
4. Thavendiranathan P, Bagai A, Ebidia A, et al. Do blood tests cause anemia in hospitalized patients? The effect of diagnostic phlebotomy on hemoglobin and hematocrit levels. *J Gen Intern Med.* 2005;20:520-524.

**2.** Correct Answer: D

**Rationale:**

Anemia is common in ICU patients. Ninety-seven percent of critically ill patients are anemic by day 8. Anemia results from RBC loss from injury, phlebotomy, procedures, etc., and decreased RBC production. Hepcidin plays a central role in iron homeostasis. Its synthesis is upregulated by inflammatory cytokines, resulting in decreased iron absorption and decreased release of iron from body stores creating an iron-deficiency–like state. Decreased renal function and proinflammatory cytokines decrease EPO production.

In a prospective, multicenter, randomized, double-blind, placebo-controlled trial involving 1460 patients, the use of recombinant human EPO (epoetin alfa) to treat anemia in critically ill patients was not associated with decreased red transfusions using a target hemoglobin concentration between 7 and 9 g/dL. In this study, patients who received

EPO had a higher rate of thrombotic events if they did not receive prophylactic or therapeutic doses of heparin. Overall mortality was the same between the group that received EPO and the group that received placebo.

The use of iron supplementation is controversial in critically ill patients because it can promote bacterial growth and infection. Hepcidin's upregulation by inflammatory cytokines may be protective. One multicenter, randomized, placebo-controlled trial of intravenous iron supplementation in critically ill trauma patients showed no difference between groups in hemoglobin concentration, packed red blood cell transfusion requirement, risk of infection, length of stay, or mortality at 14 days. A meta-analysis of five randomized controlled trials involving 665 patients showed iron supplementation did not reduce RBC transfusion. However, the strength of this conclusion is limited by moderate heterogeneity between the studies.

In a study comparing a transfusion threshold of 9 versus 7 g/dL in patients with septic shock, there was no difference in 90-day mortality, rates of ischemic events, or use of life support between the two groups. Patients assigned to the lower transfusion group received fewer transfusions. The Surviving Sepsis guidelines recommend not transfusing RBCs in adults with sepsis until the hemoglobin falls below 7.0 g/dL.

Phlebotomy can result in a daily loss of 40 to 70 mL of blood in a critically ill patient exceeding the basal RBC formation rate of 15 to 20 mL/d under normal conditions. Strategies to minimize blood loss such as use of small volume phlebotomy tubes, point-of-care testing, reinfusion of discard sample from indwelling lines, and reducing the number of laboratory studies obtained can decrease this source of blood loss.

## References

1. Corwin HL, Gettinger A, Fabian TC, et al. Efficacy and safety of epoetin alfa in critically ill patients. *N Engl J Med*. 2007;357:965-976.
2. Hayden SJ, Albert TJ, Watkins TR, Swenson ER. Anemia in critical illness: insights into etiology, consequences, and management. *Am J Respir Crit Care Med*. 2012;185:1049-1057.
3. Holst LB, Haase N, Wetterslev J, et al. Lower versus higher hemoglobin threshold for transfusion in septic shock. *N Engl J Med* 2014;371:1381-1391.
4. Shah A, Roy NB, McKechnie S, et al. Iron supplementation to treat anemia in adult critical care patients: a systematic review and meta-analysis. *Crit Care*. 2016;20:306-316.

---

**3.** Correct Answer: C

**Rationale:**

The primary goal of red blood cell transfusion is to improve oxygen delivery. However, potential adverse effects include transfusion reactions, infection, transfusion-related acute lung injury (TRALI), transfusion-related circulatory overload (TRCO), and transfusion-related immunomodulation (TRIM).

Transfusions are associated with immunosuppression (TRIM) and may result in an increased risk of nosocomial infections in hospitalized patients. One small, retrospective study found a dose-related response between the number of transfusions, and the risk for infection showed a dose-response relation such that the risk of infection increased by a factor of 1.5 for each unit transfused. A meta-analysis of 17 randomized trials comparing restrictive versus liberal RBC transfusion strategies involving 7456 patients found an increased risk of serious infections among patients treated with a liberal transfusion strategy with a number needed to treat (NNT) of 48 with a restrictive strategy in order to prevent serious infections.

Leukoreduction not only removes donor leukocytes from packed RBCs but also filters inflammatory mediators (eg, tumor necrosis factor [TNF-α], interleukin-1 [IL-1]) and viruses transmitted via leukocytes (eg, Epstein-Barr virus [EBV], cytomegalovirus [CMV]), and reduces human leukocyte antigen (HLA) alloimmunization. Multiple studies have been performed looking at the effect of transfusion leukoreduced RBCs on infection, organ dysfunction scores, mortality, and risk of ARDS. Many of these studies are limited by size and study design but show no advantage to using leukoreduced RBCs.

The maximum storage period for RBC units is 42 days as mandated by the US Food and Drug Administration. However, the storage of blood for longer periods results in changes in the RBC membrane, which can impede microvascular flow and trigger inflammation, decreased 2,3-DPG concentrations, which can make red cells ineffective as oxygen carriers, and increased concentrations of proinflammatory cytokines. Two recent studies have looked at the effect of age of transfused blood in critically ill patients. The Age of Blood Evaluation (ABLE) trial was a multicenter trial that randomized 2430 critically ill patients (mean APACHE score 21.8 ± 7.6) to receive either fresh red cells (stored a mean of 6.1 ± 4.9 days) or standard-issue red cells (stored a mean of 22 ± 8.4 days). There was no difference in 90-day mortality (primary outcome) or duration of respiratory, hemodynamic, or renal support, hospital length of stay, and transfusion reactions (secondary outcomes) between the two groups. The Standard Issue Transfusion versus Fresher Red-Cell Use in Intensive Care (TRANSFUSE) trial randomized 4994 critically ill patients (mean APACHE III score 72.9 ± 29.4, median APACHE III risk of death of 21.5%) to receive either blood that was stored for a mean of 11.8 days or blood that was stored for a mean of 22.4 days. There was no difference between the two groups in the primary outcome of 90-day mortality and secondary outcomes of organ dysfunction, need of mechanical ventilation and renal replacement therapy, blood stream infection, transfusion reactions, and ICU and hospital length of stay.

The Transfusion Requirements in Critical Care (TRICC) trial found no difference in 30-day mortality in 838 euvolemic patients with normal baseline hemoglobin and no active ischemia or bleeding randomized to either a restrictive or liberal transfusion strategy (threshold hemoglobin, 7 vs 10 g/dL). However, there was a higher mortality that was not statistically significant in patients with coronary artery disease receiving a restrictive transfusion strategy. Although not done in critically ill patients, two studies suggest that a transfusion threshold of a hemoglobin of 8 is safe in patients with cardiovascular disease. The Transfusion Requirements after Cardiac Surgery (TRACS) showed that a restrictive transfusion strategy (maintain hematocrit ≥24%) was noninferior to a liberal transfusion strategy (maintain hematocrit ≥30%) in terms of a composite end-point consisting of 30-day all-cause mortality and severe morbidity (cardiogenic shock, ARDS, or acute renal injury requiring dialysis or hemofiltration). A second study randomized 2016 patients with either a history of or risk factors for cardiovascular disease undergoing hip fracture surgery, either a liberal transfusion strategy (if hemoglobin <10 g/dL) or a restrictive transfusion strategy (symptoms of anemia with a hemoglobin <8 g/dL). There was no difference between the groups in the primary outcome of death or functional disability on 60-day follow-up. Furthermore, there was no difference between the groups in the rates of in-hospital acute myocardial infarction, unstable angina, or death.

### References

1. Cooper DJ, McQuilten ZK, Nichol A, et al. Age of red cells for transfusion and outcomes in critically ill adults. *N Engl J Med.* 2017;377:1858-1867.
2. Hajjar LA, Vincent JL, Galas FR, et al. Transfusion requirements after cardiac surgery: the TRACS randomized controlled trial. *JAMA.* 2010;304:1559-1567.
3. Hebert PC, Wells G, Blajchman MA, et al. A multicenter, randomized, controlled clinical trial of transfusion requirements in critical care. *N Engl J Med.* 1999;340:409-417.
4. Lacroix J, Hebert PC, Fergusson DA, et al. Age of transfused blood in critically ill adults. *N Engl J Med.* 2015;372:1410-1418.
5. Rohde JM, Dimcheff DE, Blumberg N, et al. Health care–associated infection after red blood cell transfusion: a systematic review and meta-analysis. *JAMA.* 2014;311:1317-1326.
6. Watkins TR, Rubenfeld GD, Martin TR, et al. Effects of leukoreduced blood on acute lung injury after trauma: a randomized controlled trial. *Crit Care Med.* 2008;36:1493-1499.

**4.** Correct Answer: D

**Rationale:**

Although the differential diagnosis of an elevated RBC mass is large including volume contraction, chronic hypoxia, and exogenous EPO, PV should be suspected in a patient with unusual thrombosis, thrombocytosis and/or leukocytosis, or splenomegaly. PV is a chronic myeloproliferative neoplasm characterized by an increased RBC mass. It is associated with an increased risk of thrombosis (both arterial and venous), leukemic transformation, and myelofibrosis. Workup for PV should include EPO level and peripheral blood mutation screening for JAK2 V617F. The World Health Organization diagnostic criteria for PV are listed in Table 76 1. Either all three major criteria or the first two major criteria plus the minor criterion is needed for the diagnosis of PV.

The presence of the JAK2 V617F mutation is 97% sensitive and 100% specific for PV. The addition of a low EPO level confirms the diagnosis. Additional mutational analysis for the JAK2 exon 12 mutation should be pursued if the EPO level is low and the JAK2 V617F mutation is not present as 3% of patients with PV are JAK2 V617F-negative.

All patients with PV require phlebotomy to a hematocrit target of <45%. Other treatment depends on risk stratification based on age, history of prior thrombosis, and cardiovascular risk factors. Patients younger than 60 years of age without history of thrombosis can be treated with observation alone or aspirin depending on cardiovascular risk factors. Patients older than 60 years of age or with a history of thrombosis should be treated with aspirin and a cytoreductive agent. Hydroxyurea, interferon alfa, and busulfan are all acceptable initial therapies for PV.

**TABLE 76.1 2016 World Health Organization Diagnostic Criteria for Polycythemia Vera**

| | | |
|---|---|---|
| Major criteria | 1. | Hemoglobin >16.5 g/dL in men, >16 g/dL in women OR Hematocrit >49% in men, >48% in women OR Red cell mass >25% above normal predicted value |
| | 2. | Hypercellular bone marrow with trilineage myeloproliferation and pleomorphic mature megakaryocytes |
| | 3. | Presence of JAK2 V617F or JAK2 exon 12 mutation |
| Minor criteria | 1. | Subnormal serum erythropoietin level |

### References

1. Khan FA, Khan RA, Iqbai M, et al. Polycythemia vera: essential management protocols. *Anaesth Pain Intensive Care.* 2012;16:91-97.
2. Tefferi A, Barbul T. Polycythemia vera and essential thrombocythemia: 2017 update on diagnosis, risk-stratification, and management. *Am J Hematol.* 2017;92:95-108.
3. Tefferi A, Vannucchi A, Barbui T. Polycythemia vera treatment algorithm 2018. *Blood Cancer J.* 2018;8:3.

**5.** Correct Answer: A

**Rationale:**

Hemoglobin is the major protein responsible for oxygen transport and is usually composed of two alpha-globin chains and two beta-globin chains. The synthesis of alpha and beta chains must also be closely matched as free globin units are toxic to red cells. Hemoglobinopathies arise from either (1) a quantitative defect (either reduction or total absence) in the production of one of the globin chains or (2) a structural defect in one of the globin chains. Quantitative disorders of globin chain synthesis result in the thalassemia syndromes. Most mutations that result in structural defects in the one of the globin chains are clinically silent and are discovered as an incidental finding. Those that are clinically relevant can cause the sickle cell disorders, anemia due to hemolysis, changes in oxygen affinity resulting in polycythemia or cyanosis, or methemoglobinemia.

The thalassemia syndromes are inherited disorders that result in either decreased or absence of either the alpha- or beta-globin chains. Under normal circumstances, the synthesis of alpha- and beta-globin chains is highly regulated to prevent excess of one or the other chain. If synthesis of one globin chain is decreased or absent, there is accumulation of the unaffected globin chain that precipitates and leads to hemolysis and decreased red cell survival. The clinical manifestations of the thalassemia syndromes range from asymptomatic carrier status to profound abnormalities including severe anemia, extramedullary hematopoiesis, and skeletal and growth deficits.

The alpha-thalassemias are usually caused by the deletion of one or more alpha-globin genes. Deletion of one or two alpha-globin genes is not associated with severe hematologic abnormalities; a mild hypochromic, microcytic anemia is seen with deletion of two alpha-globin genes. Deletion of three alpha-globin genes (eg, hemoglobin H [HbH] disease) results in a microcytic, hypochromic anemia with hemoglobin levels between 8 and 10 g/dL. The anemia can be exacerbated by acute infections, oxidative stress, and pregnancy and is treated with transfusions as needed. Deletion of all four alpha-globin chains results in hydrops fetalis and is usually fatal during late pregnancy or shortly after birth.

There are two beta-globin genes and beta-thalassemias are usually caused by point mutations in one or both genes. The mutations can result in decreased production or absence of beta-globin. Severity of disease depends on how much beta-globin is made with the most severe disease in homozygotes that make no beta-globin (TM). These patients have severe anemia (Hb range 1-7 g/dL), hemolysis, and ineffective erythropoiesis, resulting in skeletal abnormalities due to expanded marrow cavities and extramedullary hematopoiesis. Iron overload occurs because of increased intestinal iron uptake secondary to ineffective erythropoiesis and from transfusions. Excess iron stores can cause toxicity in the liver, heart, and endocrine organs, with resulting organ dysfunction. Heart failure is the most common cause of death in TM and primarily results from cardiac iron accumulation.

HbS results from an amino acid substitution on the beta-globin chain. Patients with sickle cell disease are homozygous for HbS. Deoxygenation of HbS results in polymerization that distorts the shape of the red cell, which is reversible with reoxygenation of HbS. Sickled RBCs increase blood viscosity and obstruct capillary flow causing vaso-occlusion and pain. Furthermore, repeated cycles of sickling damage the RBC membrane, resulting in premature destruction of RBCs and a chronic hemolytic anemia. The polymerization of deoxygenated HbS is inhibited by HbF. Treatment of sickle cell disease includes pain medications to treat pain associated with vaso-occlusive crises, transfusions, hydroxyurea to increase HbF concentrations, and hematopoietic stem cell transplantation.

References

1. Bunn HF. Pathogenesis and treatment of sickle cell disease. *N Engl J Med*. 1997;337:762-769.
2. Forget BG, Bunn HF. Classification of the disorders of hemoglobin. *Cold Spring Harb Perspect Med*. 2013;3:a011684.
3. Pennell DJ, Udelson JE, Arai AE, et al. Cardiovascular function and treatment in β-thalassemia major: a consensus statement from the American Heart Association. *Circulation*. 2013;128:281-308.
4. Rachmilewitz EA, Giardina PJ. How I treat thalassemia. *Blood* 2011;118:3479-3488.
5. Yawn BP, Buchanan GR, Afenyi-Annan AN, et al. Management of sickle cell disease: summary of the 2014 evidence-based report by expert panel members. *JAMA*. 2014;312:1033-1048.

# 77

# WHITE BLOOD CELL DISORDERS

Jean Kwo

1. A 57-year-old male with history of alcohol abuse is admitted to the intensive care unit after a fall from a ladder. He has sustained a left ankle fracture and several rib fractures. His white blood cell count is 1600/µL. Initial workup for possible causes of leukopenia includes all of the following EXCEPT:

   A. Obtain complete blood count (CBC) with differential
   B. Review patient's medications
   C. Obtain screening studies for rheumatologic disorders
   D. Review results of CBCs/differential counts from prior hospitalizations and the ambulatory setting

2. A 52-year-old female presents with fever of 38.3°C (101°F) and malaise. Her white blood cell count is 710/µL with 70% neutrophils. She was recently diagnosed with an urinary tract infection and is currently taking trimethoprim-sulfamethoxazole. Which of the following statements is TRUE?

   A. Her neutropenia is unlikely to be due to idiosyncratic drug–induced acute neutropenia because her absolute neutrophil count (ANC) is <500/µL.
   B. Use of granulocyte colony-stimulating factor (G-CSF) is contraindicated.
   C. Her prognosis is poor as mortality associated with idiosyncratic drug–induced acute neutropenia is over 50%.
   D. Vancomycin is not recommended for initial therapy of neutropenic patients with fever.

3. A 62-year-old male is admitted with fatigue and new-onset shortness of breath. His white blood count is 85,000/µL and bone marrow biopsy shows 35% myeloblasts. He is started on induction chemotherapy for acute myeloid leukemia. During treatment, his creatinine rises and he develops hyperuricemia. Which of the following statements is FALSE regarding his management?

   A. He should receive hydration with intravenous fluids with a target urine output of at least 2 mL/kg/h.
   B. He should have continuous cardiac monitoring and measurement of electrolytes, creatinine, and uric acid every 4 to 6 hours.
   C. Rasburicase is contraindicated if he has a glucose-6-phosphate dehydrogenase deficiency.
   D. His uric acid level will decrease rapidly after starting allopurinol.

4. A 22-year-old female with a history of bilateral lung transplantation for cystic fibrosis 9 months ago now presents with fever, weight loss, and lymphadenopathy. Lymph node biopsy shows diffuse large B-cell lymphoma. Treatment includes all of the following EXCEPT:

   A. Reduction of immunosuppression
   B. Ganciclovir
   C. Chemotherapy with cyclophosphamide, doxorubicin, vincristine, and prednisone (CHOP)
   D. Rituximab

5. All the following are possible long-term complications of treatment of non-Hodgkin lymphoma (NHL) EXCEPT:

   A. Breast cancer
   B. Stroke
   C. Congestive heart failure
   D. Adrenal insufficiency

6. A 62-year-old male with a history of acute myeloid leukemia and allogeneic hematopoietic stem cell transplantation (HSCT) 2 months ago presents with cough, dyspnea on exertion, and fevers for 1 week. On examination, his temperature was 100.9°F, heart rate 100 beats/min, respiratory rate 20 breaths/min, and blood pressure 120/80 mm Hg. He appeared chronically ill with bibasilar crackles on auscultation. His white blood cell count was 3400 cells/μL and his chest radiograph showed bilateral lower lobe infiltrates. Differential diagnosis includes all of the following EXCEPT:

   A. Periengraftment respiratory distress syndrome
   B. Bacterial pneumonia
   C. Radiation pneumonitis
   D. Idiopathic pneumonia syndrome

7. A 67-year-old male who presented with severe back pain and bilateral lower extremity weakness is admitted to the intensive care unit after emergent surgical spinal decompression and fixation. Bone marrow biopsy shows >10% clonal plasma cells. Other criteria for the diagnosis of multiple myeloma include all the following EXCEPT:

   A. MRI showing two or more focal bone or bone marrow lesions at ≥5 mm in size
   B. Hypercalcemia
   C. Recurrent infections
   D. Creatinine clearance <40 mL/min

8. A 73-year-old male with a history of multiple myeloma presents with symptoms of nausea, abdominal pain, and lethargy. His serum calcium is 15 mg/dL. Which of the following statements about the management of hypercalcemia is FALSE?

   A. Risedronate is not recommended for the treatment of severe hypercalcemia.
   B. Calcitonin decreases bone resorption but takes 48 hours to see a decrease in serum calcium levels.
   C. Denosumab limits bone resorption by inhibiting receptor activator of nuclear factor kappa-B (RANKL).
   D. Dialysis may be needed if he has renal failure due to hypercalcemia or multiple myeloma or both.

# Chapter 77 ▪ Answers

**1.** Correct Answer: C

**Rationale:**
Leukopenia is a reduction in the circulating white blood cells below the normal range. It is often used interchangeably with neutropenia as the neutrophils are the most abundant white blood cells. The pathophysiology of neutropenia involves decreased production, increased destruction, or sequestration of neutrophils in the spleen or vascular endothelium. Medications, infection/inflammation, and genetics are more common causes of neutropenia.

   Initial workup for neutropenia includes obtaining a CBC including a differential to calculate the ANC. A history and physical examination should be performed looking for possible causes. This patient's history of trauma may point to inflammation as a possible cause of neutropenia. Other possible causes based on his history include nutritional deficiencies or liver disease because of alcohol abuse. Reviewing results of CBCs/differential counts from prior hospitalizations and the ambulatory setting will help determine whether the neutropenia developed during hospitalization or is chronic. The patient's medication list should be reviewed for medications that may cause neutropenia and should be stopped if the ANC <1000 cells/μL or continues to drop. Though rheumatological disorders can cause rarely cause leukopenia, it is unlikely in this patient presenting with trauma.

References
1. Berliner N. Approach to the adult with unexplained neutropenia. In: Newburger P, ed. *UpToDate*. Waltham, MA: UpToDate, Inc. http://www.uptodate.com. Accessed on September 25, 2018.
2. Dale D. How I diagnose and treat neutropenia. *Curr Opin Hematol*. 2016;23:1-4.

**2.** Correct Answer: D

**Rationale:**

The incidence of idiosyncratic drug reactions is estimated to be between 1/10,000 and 1/100,000. Diagnostic criteria include an ANC of <500/μL and onset of agranulocytosis during treatment with the offending drug and resolution of neutropenia within 1 to 3 weeks after stopping the drug though recovery may take longer. Reexposure to the drug results in recurrence of neutropenia.

Patients with drug-induced agranulocytosis are at risk for infection. The mortality rate is 5%. Older age (>65 years), an ANC <100/μL, development of severe infection, and preexisting comorbidities (renal disease, cardiac disease, pulmonary disease, systemic inflammatory diseases) are associated with worse prognosis.

In patients with neutropenia, fever is defined as a single oral temperature of ≥38.3°C (101°F) or a temperature of ≥38.0°C (100.4°F) sustained over a 1-hour period. Broad-spectrum antibiotics should be initiated after obtaining blood, urine, sputum, and any other relevant cultures. The Infectious Diseases Society of America (IDSA) recommends starting an antipseudomonal beta-lactam agent such as cefipime, meropenem, or piperacillin-tazobactam. Vancomycin is not recommended unless there is a catheter-related infection, skin or soft-tissue infection, pneumonia, or hemodynamic instability.

While the use of G-CSF has not been studied in large, randomized trials, its use is associated with shorter times to recovery of neutrophil count, lower rate of infectious and fatal complications, and shorter duration of antibiotic therapy and hospitalization. Because growth factors have minimal toxicity, the benefits outweigh the risks in drug-induced agranulocytosis patients with infection.

### References

1. Coates TD. Drug-induced neutropenia and agranulocytosis. In: Newburger P, ed. *UpToDate*. Waltham, MA: UpToDate, Inc. http://www.uptodate.com. Accessed on September 6, 2018.
2. Andres E, Maloisel F. Idiosyncratic drug-induced agranulocytosis or acute neutropenia. *Curr Opin Hematol*. 2008;15:15-21.
3. Freifeld AG, Bow EJ, Sepkowitz KA, et al. Clinical practice guideline for the use of antimicrobial agents in neutropenic patients with cancer: 2010 update by the Infectious Diseases Society of America. *Clin Infect Dis*. 2011;52(4):e56.
4. Dale D. How I diagnose and treat neutropenia. *Curr Opin Hematol*. 2016;23:1-4.

**3.** Correct Answer: D

**Rationale:**

Tumor lysis syndrome arises from massive tumor cell death. Cell lysis results in release of potassium, phosphorus, and nucleic acids causing metabolic derangements including hyperuricemia, hyperkalemia, hypocalcemia, and hyperphosphatemia. Diagnostic criteria for tumor lysis syndrome include having two or more of these abnormalities occurring within 3 days before or up to 7 days after initiation of cancer therapy. Tumor lysis syndrome is an oncologic emergency, and treatment must begin immediately as complications including renal failure, seizures, cardiac arrhythmias, and death may ensue. Continuous cardiac monitoring should be started along with frequent measurement of electrolytes, creatinine, and uric acid.

Treatment includes intravenous hydration with a target urine output of at least 2 mL/kg/h. Diuretics may be given if enough fluid has been administered and target urine output has not been reached. Hyperkalemia may be treated with oral sodium polystyrene sulfonate though hemodialysis may be needed with severe hyperkalemia, especially in the setting of acute kidney injury. Hyperphosphatemia may be treated with phosphate binders.

Allopurinol and rasburicase both reduce the level of uric acid. Allopurinol blocks the xanthine oxidase enzyme and prevents the formation of uric acid. However, the uric acid level may take several days to decrease because any existing uric acid must still be excreted. Rasburicase breaks down uric acid to allantoin which is easily excreted renally and can reduce uric acid levels within hours. It is contraindicated in patients with glucose-6-phosphate dehydrogenase deficiency because of a high risk of hemolysis and methemoglobinemia.

### References

1. Howard SC, Jones DP, Pui CH. The tumor lysis syndrome. *N Engl J Med*. 2011;364:1844-1854.
2. Mirrakhimov AE, Voore P, Khan M, Ali AM. Tumor lysis syndrome: a clinical review. *World J Crit Care Med*. 2015;4:130-138.

**4.** Correct Answer: B

**Rationale:**

Posttransplantation lymphoproliferative disorders (PTLDs) are lymphomas that occur after solid-organ or allogenic HSCTs due to immunosuppression and infection or reactivation of Epstein-Barr virus (EBV), though up to 50% of cases of PTLD may be EBV-negative.

Reduction of immunosuppression is the first-line treatment of PTLD. Calcineurin inhibition should be reduced by at least 50% and antimetabolic agents stopped. Since response to immunosuppression reduction occurs early, restaging of lymphoma can be performed at 2 to 4 weeks. For patients who do not have a response to reduced immunosuppression, rituximab may be added. Chemotherapy, radiotherapy, surgical excision, and adoptive immunotherapy may also be indicated depending on the response to reduced immunosuppression and rituximab, and the subtype of PTLD.

Since PTLD is associated with EBV-seropositive donor organs transplanted into EBV-seronegative recipients, prophylactic ganciclovir and EBV monitoring may reduce to risk of PTLD.

References

1. Dierickx D, Habermann TM. Post-transplantation lymphoproliferative disorders in adults. *N Engl J Med*. 2018;378:549-562.
2. Dierickx D, Tousseyn T, Gheysens O. How I treat posttranplanst lymphoproliferative disorders. *Blood*. 2015;126:2274-2283.

---

**5.** Correct Answer: D

**Rationale:**

Improvements in therapy for NHL have resulted in increasing numbers of long-term survivors of this disease. Because NHL is a heterogeneous group of diseases, there are multiple treatment options including radiation therapy, chemotherapy, immunotherapy, and any combination of these. The treatment a patient receives depends on the histologic subtype of NHL and disease stage. Complications resulting from treatment include second malignancies, cardiovascular disease, endocrine dysfunction, and neurologic complications.

Second malignancies occurring after treatment of NHL include breast cancer, lung cancer, cancers of the gastrointestinal tract, as well as leukemia and skin cancers. Cardiovascular complications including cardiomyopathy, heart failure, valvular heart disease, and coronary artery disease may arise from either chemotherapy or radiation therapy or both. The risk of stroke is increased after neck irradiation. Pulmonary fibrosis may occur after lung irradiation or as a result of certain chemotherapeutic agents. Hypothyroidism and infertility due to gonadal dysfunction may also occur after treatment for NHL.

The adrenal gland involvement in disseminated lymphoma or as primary adrenal NHL may result in adrenal insufficiency.

References

1. Boyne DJ, Mickle AT, Brenner DR, et al. Long-term risk of cardiovascular mortality in lymphoma survivors: a systematic review and meta-analysis. *Cancer Med*. 2018;7:4801-4813.
2. Ng AK, LaCasce A, Travis LB. Long-term complications of lymphoma and its treatment. *J Clin Oncol*. 2011;29:1885-1892.

---

**6.** Correct Answer: A

**Rationale:**

Allogeneic HSCT is used to treat a variety of hematologic malignancies and nonmalignant disorders. Pulmonary complications occur in up to one-third of patients after HSCT and may be either infectious or noninfectious. The types of complications also vary based on the time after HCST.

Pulmonary complications associated with the preengraftment phase (<30 days after HSCT) can occur because of neutropenia, mucositis, cardiotoxic effects of medications, and copious fluid administration. These include bacteria, viral, and fungal pneumonia. Patients are also at increased risk for aspiration as mucositis from the conditioning regimen can lead to swallowing difficulties. Pulmonary edema may occur due to cardiac dysfunction (from chemotherapy or chest irradiation) or be of noncardiac origin (sepsis, aspiration, viral infection, hyperacute graft-versus-host disease). Periengraftment respiratory distress syndrome typically develops 7 to 11 days after HSCT and is characterized by fever, rash, noncardiogenic pulmonary edema, and hypoxemia. It is more frequently seen in autologous HSCT and is believed to be due to diffuse capillary leakage associated with the release of cytokines and influx of neutrophils into the lungs with engraftment. Treatment is supportive though consideration should be given to using high-dose corticosteroids in symptomatic patients.

In the immediate postengraftment phase (30-100 days after HSCT), cellular immunity is impaired. Patients continue to be at risk for bacterial, fungal, and viral infections. The median onset time of *Aspergillus* infection is 100 days post HSCT. Infection with *Pneumocystis jirovecii* should be suspected in patients with a lapse in their prophylaxis. Diffuse alveolar hemorrhage (DAH) and idiopathic pneumonia syndrome (IPS) are two causes of respiratory failure after HSCT that should be considered once infection is ruled out. Chemotherapeutic agents (eg, busulfan, cyclophosphamide, sirolimus) and radiation used for preparative conditioning can cause lung toxicity and injury. Acute radiation pneumonitis can develop 4 to 12 weeks after chest or whole-body radiation. Late or fibrotic radiation pneumonitis can develop 6 to 12 months after radiation.

Late pulmonary complications are those that occur >100 days post HSCT. Humoral and cellular immunity are impaired. Patients are at risk for infection with encapsulated bacteria (*Haemophilus influenzae*, *Streptococcus pneumoniae*) as well as *Nocardia*, *Legionella*, and *Actinomyces*. The risk of cytomegalovirus (CMV) pneumonitis is highest in CMV-seropositive recipients with seronegative donors. Late noninfectious pulmonary complications include bronchiolitis obliterans, cryptogenic organizing pneumonia, and posttransplant lymphoproliferative disorder.

References

1. Chi AK, Soubani AI, White AC, et al. An update on pulmonary complications of hematopoietic stem cell transplantation. *Chest*. 2013;144:1913-1922.
2. Elias AD, Mark EJ. A 60-year-old man with pulmonary infiltrates after a bone marrow transplantation. *N Engl J Med*. 1997;337:480-489.
3. Kaner RJ, Zappetti D. Pulmonary complications after allogeneic hematopoietic cell transplantation. In: King TE, ed. *UpToDate*. Waltham, MA: UpToDate, Inc. http://www.uptodate.com. Accessed on December 6, 2018.

**7.** Correct Answer: C

**Rationale:**

Multiple myeloma is a neoplasm of plasma cells resulting in a monoclonal immunoglobulin. It is distinguished from premalignant forms, monoclonal gammopathy of undetermined significance (MGUS), and smoldering multiple myeloma (SMM), by the presence of certain clinical features. Clinical symptoms of multiple myeloma result from the infiltration of plasma cells into bone or other organs or kidney damage from excess light chains.

To make the diagnosis of multiple myeloma (see Table 77.1 for diagnostic criteria for multiple myeloma), a bone marrow biopsy or aspirate must show >10% clonal plasma cells or biopsy-proven plasmacytoma plus presence of organ or tissue damage related to the plasma cell proliferative disorder. The myeloma-defining clinical features are hypercalcemia, renal failure, anemia, and bone lesions (CRAB).

**TABLE 77.1 Diagnostic Criteria for Multiple Myeloma**

**Clonal bone marrow plasma cells ≥ 10% of biopsy-proven bone or soft tissue plasmacytoma AND one or more myeloma-defining events:**

- End-organ damage due to plasma cell proliferative disorder:
  - Hypercalcemia: Serum calcium >1 mg/dL higher than upper limit of normal or >11 mg/dL
  - Renal insufficiency: Creatinine clearance <40 mL/min or serum creatinine >2 mg/dL
  - Anemia: Hemoglobin <10 or >2 g/dL below normal
  - Bone lesions: One or more osteolytic lesions ≥5 mm in size. MRI, CT, or PET/CT is preferred over skeletal survey for detection of bone lesions.
- Biomarker associated with progression to malignancy and end-organ damage
  - ≥60% clonal plasma cells in bone marrow
  - Involved:uninvolved free light chain ratio >100
  - MRI with more than one bone or bone marrow focal lesion

In 2014, the International Myeloma Working Group updated the diagnostic criteria for multiple myeloma with three biomarkers to identify those patients who are at imminent risk of progression of their malignancy to intervene prior to the development of end-organ damage. The biomarkers are:

1. Bone marrow plasma cells of 60% or greater.
2. Involved:uninvolved light chain ratio of >100 and involved free light chain ≥100 mg/dL.
   - Excess production of one free light chain type (κ or λ) due to clonal plasma cell disorder results in increased light chain ratio.
3. MRI with two or more focal bone or bone marrow lesions that are 5 mm in size or greater.

References

1. Rajkumar SV. Updated diagnostic criteria and staging system for multiple myeloma. *Am Soc Clin Oncol Educ Book*. 2016;35:e418-e423.
2. Rajkumar SV, Dimopoulos MA, Palumbo A, et al. International myeloma working group updated criteria for the diagnosis of multiple myeloma. *Lancet Oncol*. 2014;15:e538-e548.

**8.** Correct Answer: B

**Rationale:**

Hypercalcemia is one of the myeloma-defining events and is caused by the osteolytic tumor lesions. Symptoms of hypercalcemia include nausea, vomiting, weakness, abdominal pain, constipation, confusion. Severe hypercalcemia (defined at serum calcium >14 mg/dL) can result in cardiac arrhythmias and coma.

Treatment of hypercalcemia includes hydration with isotonic saline with possible use of loop diuretics to both augment excretion of calcium as well as inhibit calcium reabsorption in the thick ascending limb. Calcitonin decreases bone resorption and works within 4 to 6 hours to lower calcium levels. However, because of tachyphylaxis, its efficacy is limited to about 48 hours. Bisphosphonates also decrease bone resorption by inhibiting osteoclasts but its onset of action is 24 to 72 hours. Zoledronic acid or pamidronate are can be given intravenously and are recommended for hypercalcemia due to malignancy. Oral third-generation bisphosphonates such as risedronate and alendronate are not recommended for the treatment of severe or acute hypercalcemia. Denosumab is a monoclonal antibody that inhibits RANKL and decreases osteoclast activity. It is recommended for the treatment of hypercalcemia in patients who do not respond to bisphosphonates. Unlike bisphosphonates, it is not cleared by the kidney and can be used in patients with kidney disease. Its onset of action is 4 to 10 days. Hemodialysis may be needed in patients with severe hypercalcemia and neurologic symptoms (eg, coma) or in patients with renal failure or heart failure who cannot tolerate aggressive volume expansion.

References

1. Cicci JD, Buie L, Bates J, et al. Denosumab for the management of hypercalcemia of malignancy in patients with multiple myeloma and renal dysfunction. *Clin Lymphoma Myeloma Leuk*. 2014;14:e207-e211.
2. Goldner W. Cancer-related hypercalcemia. *J Oncol Pract*. 2015;12:426-432.
3. Shane E, Berenson JR. Treatment of hypercalcemia. In: Rosen CJ, ed. *UpToDate*. Waltham, MA: UpToDate, Inc. http://www.uptodate.com. Accessed on December 28, 2018.

# 78

# PLATELET DISORDERS

Sean M. Baskin and Kunal Karamchandani

1. A 72-year-old male is admitted to the intensive care unit after undergoing aortic valve replacement for severe aortic stenosis. He was successfully weaned from bypass, required no blood products, and received appropriate protamine reversal. In the intensive care unit, he has been having persistent drainage from the thoracotomy tubes. A complete blood count (CBC) shows a hematocrit of 40% and platelet count of 150,000/mm³. Coagulation studies including a thromboelastogram (TEG) are sent.

   TEG results:

   Prothombin Time: 11 seconds (11-13.5 seconds)
   Partial Thromboplastin Time: 38 seconds (30-40 seconds)
   R-time: 8 minutes (5-10 minutes)
   K-time: 4 minutes (3-6 minutes)
   Alpha angle: 52° (45-55°)
   Maximum Amplitude (MA): 37 mm (50-70 mm)
   Based on the results of the TEG, which of the following would be the best treatment option

   A. Platelet
   B. Protamine
   C. Fibrinogen
   D. Fresh Frozen Plasma

2. A 63-year-old female with known lower-extremity deep vein thrombosis (DVT) is admitted to the intensive care unit after presenting with shortness of breath and chest pain. Imaging is negative for a pulmonary embolism, and blood tests including a CBC and serum electrolytes are normal. She is started on supplemental oxygen and a heparin infusion titrated to aPTT of 60 to 90 seconds. On admission day 7, her platelet count is found to have decreased from 150,000/mm³ to 62,000mm/³ over a 24-hour period. To assist in making the diagnosis, you calculate the patient's 4-T score. Which of the following is NOT a part of the 4-T score?

   A. Timing of Platelet decrease
   B. Presence of Thrombosis
   C. Severity of thrombocytopenia
   D. Tachycardia

3. After calculating a 4-T score of 6, you proceed to obtain confirmatory testing to support your diagnosis. A Heparin PF-4 antibody test is positive, and heparin-induced serotonin release assay (SRA) is under process. Given the presumptive diagnosis, which of the following treatment strategies would be most appropriate?

   A. Discontinue Heparin and start low-molecular weight Heparin
   B. Discontinue Heparin and start Argatroban
   C. Discontinue Heparin and transfuse platelets
   D. Start warfarin

4. A 32-year-old male presents to the hospital complaining of progressive fatigue, productive cough, and intermittent epistaxis. His initial evaluation is significant for left lower lobe consolidation on chest X-ray and a temperature of 38.7°C. During attempts to obtain peripheral venous access, he bruises easily and missed attempts bleed for over 2 minutes. A CBC and coagulation studies are obtained and are as follows:

WBC: 1.2 K/μL
Hgb: 6.5 mg/dL
Hct: 19.5%
Platelet count: 74000/μL
PT: 22 seconds (normal 10-14)
aPTT: 56 seconds (normal 25-40)
Fibrinogen: 65 mg/dL (normal 140-400 mg/dL)

He is subsequently admitted to the ICU where broad spectrum antibiotics are initiated, and a bone marrow aspirate (BMA) is obtained, which shows finding consistent with acute myeloid leukemia. Which of the following is the best **initial** treatment option for this patient?

A. Platelet transfusion
B. All-trans-retinoic acid (ATRA)
C. Packed RBC transfusion
D. Administer IV Vitamin K and Fresh Frozen Plasma

5. A 29-year-old male is admitted to the intensive care unit after undergoing an uncomplicated laparoscopic splenectomy for idiopathic thrombocytopenic purpura. On post-op day 2, he is recovering well, is afebrile, is hemodynamically stable, and has no complaints. Routine laboratory test results are sent, which are significant for a platelet count of 654,000/μL. What is the most likely cause of thrombocytosis in this patient?

A. Sepsis
B. Reactive thrombocytosis
C. Cancer
D. Lab error

# Chapter 78 ▪ Answers

1. Correct Answer: A

**Rationale:**
Thomboelastogram, or TEG, is a whole blood, point-of-care test that analyses viscoelastic proprieties of evolving clot in the patient's whole blood and can provide information about fibrin formation, platelet activation, and clot retraction, therefore assisting in identifying the cause of coagulopathy. Unlike the more traditional laboratory tests such as PT and PTT, which give a general state of the extrinsic and intrinsic pathways, TEG provides distinct values as well as a graphical representation of various stages in clot formation (Figure 1).

R-time is the duration of time from the application of the blood sample until the clot reaches a graphical amplitude of 2 mm, in other words, the time elapsed between clot formation and a predetermined and consistent size. The initiation of clot formation is dependent on circulating, function clotting factors from both the intrinsic and extrinsic pathways. A normal R-time is 5 to 10 minutes, whereas a value less than 5 minutes implies hypercoagulability, and conversely, a value greater than 10 minutes indicates either a quantitative or qualitative deficiency in clotting factors. Treatment for prolonged R-time typically is Fresh Frozen Plasma, or factor concentrate in the setting of known factor deficiency (ie Hemophilia).

K-time represents the time elapsed between the conclusion of R-time and a graphical amplitude of 20 mm. Because the K-time is the duration between an initial amplitude (2 mm) and final amplitude (20 mm), this provides a quantitate assessment of the speed of clot formation. Thrombin catalyzes the conversion of fibrinogen to fibrin, which adheres the platelet plug, strengthening it, and finalizing the clot formation. A prolonged K-time indicates inadequate circulating fibrin and is treated with either fibrinogen concentrate, or cryoprecipitate.

Alpha angle is a measurement of the speed of clot strengthening via fibrin cross-linking. It is formed by a tangential line originating from the start of K-time and intersecting the upward slope of the graph. A decreased alpha angle is similar to a prolongation of K-time and is treated in a similar manner.

MA is the greatest width between the two arms of the curve and represents overall clot strength. As the available platelets continue to form clot, which is subsequently stabilized by fibrin cross-links, the strength of the clot increases and the arms of the curve move farther apart. Eventually, the clot begins to degrade and the arms start sloping downwards. This transition point marks the MA. MA is a surrogate for platelet function, where a decreased MA suggests either inadequate supply (ie postcardiac bypass thrombocytopenia) or suboptimal function (ie liver disease). A decreased MA is treated with platelets.

This patient has a decreased MA suggesting poor clot strength likely from platelet deficiency. So, the best treatment option based on the TEG would be to administer platelets.

Sample TEG demonstrating normal coagulation morphology with normal values:

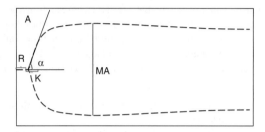

| R-Time | 5-10 minutes |
| K-Time | 3-6 minutes |
| Alpha Angle | 45-55 degrees |
| Maximum Amplitude | 50-70mm |

### References

1. Scarpelini S, Rhind SG, Nascimento B, et al. Normal Range values for thromboelastography in healthy adult volunteers. *Braz J Med Biol Res.* 2009;42(12):1210-1217.
2. Verma A, Hemlata. Thromboelastography as a novel viscoelastic method for hemostatis monitoring: its methodology, applications and constraints. *Glob J Transfus Med.* 2017;2:8-18.

**2.** Correct Answer: D

**3.** Correct Answer: B

**Rationale:**

Under normal conditions, Heparin binds to Antithrombin III (AT-3), which inactivates thrombin and Factor Xa causing a relative state of hypocoagulability. Intermittent bolus dosing is beneficial for patients at risk for thromboembolic events such as patients undergoing prolonged surgery. For patients with known DVT/PE, or other vascular thrombi, a continuous infusion may be utilized to prevent additional clot formation as well as enhance existing clot degradation. However, exposure to heparin may cause an autoimmune reaction where IgG-mediated antibodies bind to Heparin-PF4 complexes resulting in platelet activation and the formation of microthrombi and eventual thrombosis. The microthrombi consume existing platelets and results in thrombocytopenia. This entity is referred to as Heparin-induced thrombocytopenia/thrombosis (HIT).

One of the ways to predict the likelihood of HIT is to calculate the 4-T score. The 4-T score consists of four criteria graded on a 0 to 2 scale as shown in the table below. Scores of 0 to 3, 4 to 5, and 6 to 8 correspond to low, moderate, and high risk for HIT respectively. The negative predictive value of a low 4-Ts score has been found to be as high as 99%; meanwhile the positive predictive value of a high score is only 64%. For patients with thrombocytopenia and a moderate or high 4-Ts score, further testing is necessary to establish the diagnosis of HIT.

**Estimating the likelihood of HIT: the "4-Ts" score**

| CATEGORY | 2 POINTS | 1 POINT | 0 POINT |
| --- | --- | --- | --- |
| Thrombocytopenia | >50% fall, or nadir of 20-100 × 10⁹/L | 30%-50% fall, or nadir of 10-19 × 10⁹/L | 30% fall, or nadir of <10 × 10⁹/L |
| Timing of platelet count fall | Days 5-10 or ≤1 d if prior heparin exposure within the last 30 d | Onset after day 10 or unclear (but fits with HIT) or ≤1 d if heparin exposure within past 30-100 d | ≤1 d (no recent heparin) |
| Thrombosis or other sequelae | Proven thrombosis, skin necrosis, or, after heparin bolus, acute systemic reaction | Progressive, recurrent, or silent thrombosis; erythematous skin lesions | None |
| Other causes of thrombocytopenia | None evident | Possible | Definite |

Adapted from Ahmed I, Majeed A, Powell R. Heparin induced thrombocytopenia: diagnosis and management update. *Postgrad Med J.* 2007;83(983):575-582.

All patients with a presumptive diagnosis of HIT should have laboratory testing for HIT antibodies. This testing is challenging because HIT immunoassays (eg, enzyme-linked immunosorbent assay for antiplatelet factor 4 [PF4] antibodies) are readily available but not very sensitive or specific. Functional assays such as a SRA and Heparin-induced Platelet aggregation (HIPA), which measure the ability of patient serum to activate test platelets in the presence of heparin, are definitive but may take several days to return. The SRA is more sensitive than HIPA (95% vs 35%-85%), but is a more technically challenging test to perform.

Given the morbidity associated with HIT, prompt treatment is required to prevent further thrombus formation and worsening thrombocytopenia. Regardless of the likelihood of diagnosis, the first step in treatment is to immediately discontinue any heparin infusion, or heparin-coated products. Because HIT causes a functional hypercoagulable state, platelet transfusions should be withheld unless clinically indicated for significant bleeding or operative risk. Although awaiting the normalization of the platelet count, patients should be initiated on nonheparin anticoagulants, such as direct thrombin inhibitors (eg Argatroban, bivalirudin), fondaparinux, or factor Xa inhibitors (apixaban, rivaroxaban, etc.). Patients should be watched closely for bleeding as well as complications of thrombosis.

### References

1. Cuker A, Gimotty PA, Crowther MA, et al. Predictive value of the 4Ts scoring system for heparin induced thrombocytopenia: a systematic review and meta-analysis. *Blood*. 2012;120(20):4160-4167.
2. Jang IK, Hursting MJ. When heparins promote thrombosis: review of heparin-induced thrombocytopenia. *Circulation*. 2005;111:2671-2683.
3. Ahmed I, Majeed A, Powell R. Heparin induced thrombocytopenia: diagnosis and management update. *Postgrad Med J*. 2007;83(983):575-582.

## 4. Correct Answer: B

**Rationale:**

This patient most likely has Acute promyelocytic leukemia (APL), a variant of Acute Myelogeneous Leukemia (AML) given his presentation with bleeding diathesis and the elevated PT and aPTT with BMA findings of AML. APL can cause acute Disseminated Intravascular Coagulopathy (DIC), which may be life-threatening. DIC is a consumptive coagulopathy; activation of the clotting cascade results in the development of thrombi, which in turn activate the fibrinolytic pathway resulting in accumulation of fibrin degradation products (FDP). FDP inhibits further fibrin clot formation and bleeding ensues.

It is critical to start treatment with ATRA without delay as soon as the diagnosis is suspected, and before definitive confirmation of the diagnosis has been made. If the diagnosis is not confirmed, ATRA can be discontinued and treatment changed to that used for other types of AML. Transfusion of blood products, specifically platelets may be ineffective owing to the high rate of platelet consumption caused by DIC. Administration of red blood cells may be indicated for patients experiencing large volume blood loss, although this is rarely seen in the absence of trauma. Fresh Frozen Plasma may be given to replenish clotting factors and Vitamin K can cause an increase in Vitamin-K–dependent clotting factors that can further assist in reversing the coagulopathy. However, the initial therapy that can be lifesaving in these patients is administration of ATRA.

### References

1. Tallman MS, Altman JK. How I treat acute promyelocytic leukemia. *Blood*. 2009;114(25):5126-5135.
2. Park JH, Qiao B, Panageas KS, et al. Early death rate in acute promyelocytic leukemia remains high despite all-trans retinoic acid. *Blood*. 2011;118(5):1248-1254. doi:10.1182/blood-2011 to 04 to 346437. Epub 2011 Jun 8.
3. Carlson KB. Acute leukemia. In: Hall JB, Schmidt GA, Kress JP, eds. *Principles of Critical Care*. 4th ed. New York, NY: McGraw-Hill; 2014:chap 29.

## 5. Correct Answer: B

**Rationale:**

Thrombocytosis is defined as platelet levels more than 450,000/µL and can be seen in sepsis, hematologic malignancy, or postsplenectomy. This patient most likely has a postsplenectomy-reactive thrombocytosis. As the spleen is a major site for platelet regulation and removal, thrombocytosis is seen in the acute postsplenectomy period and normalizes over time, typically reaching normal levels within 1 month.

Complications arising from the thrombocytosis have been reported and are most commonly thrombotic events in the mesenteric and hepatic vasculature, although rare cerebral and cardiac occlusions have been reported. Treatment of thrombocytosis is dependent on the presentation and patient's risk factors. Antiplatelet agents such as hydroxyurea and anagrelide have been used with positive results, although side effects such as leukemic transformation and anemia have been reported respectively. In a situation where thrombocytosis is posing a threat to life, plasmapheresis can be utilized for rapid reduction.

### References

1. Supe A, Parikh M, Prabhu R, Kantharia C, Farah J. Post-splenectomy response in adult patients with immune thrombocytopenic purpura. *Asian J Transfus Sci*. 2009;3(1):6-9. doi:10.4103/0973-6247.45255.
2. Khan PN, Nair RJ, Olivares J, Tingle LE, Li Z. Post-splenectomy reactive thrombocytosis. *Proc (Bayl Univ Med Cent)*. 2009;22(1):9-12.

# 79

# COAGULOPATHIES

Phillip Ramirez and Somnath Bose

1. A 67-year-old woman with a recent history of deep vein thrombosis treated with apixaban 5 mg BID was admitted to the ICU for postoperative respiratory insufficiency following elective ventral hernia repair. She was extubated successfully on postoperative day 2. Her anticoagulation was bridged appropriately and home apixaban restarted on day 3 in anticipation of discharge. She suddenly became altered, hemodynamically unstable, and her bed was filled with melena. Vital signs were noted as follows: BP 60/45 mm Hg, HR 125 beats/min, and $SpO_2$ 92% on 10 L oxygen via non-rebreather. What is the most effective form of anticoagulation reversal for this patient?

   A. Fresh Frozen Plasma
   B. Adnexanet Alpha
   C. Prothrombin complex concentrate (PCC)
   D. Idarucizumab

2. A 52-year-old male with alcoholic cirrhosis, Na-MELD score of 19, and esophageal varices was admitted to the ICU for altered mental status and suspected sepsis. He had been admitted to the hospital for 3 weeks before this ICU admission. The patient was placed on prophylactic subcutaneous heparin on admission per standard protocol. The next day, he had significant left arm edema with grimacing on palpation. Ultrasound later that day showed acute brachial vein thrombosis. Laboratory test results that morning showed his platelet count dropped to 60,000 from 150,000/mm³ on the day of his admission. Renal function is within normal limits. Which of the following medications is the best choice for the prevention of clot propagation?

| CATEGORY | 2 POINTS | 1 POINT | 0 POINTS |
|---|---|---|---|
| Thrombocytopenia | >50% fall or nadir ≥20 K | 30%-50% fall or nadir 10-19 K | <30% fall or nadir <10 K |
| Timing of platelet decrease | Days 5-10 or ≤1 d if heparin exposure in past 30 d | >10 d or timing unclear, or <1 d with heparin exposure in past 30-100 d | <4 d with no recent heparin exposure |
| Thrombosis or other sequelae | Proven thrombosis, skin necrosis, or acute systemic reaction after heparin bolus | Progressive, recurrent, or silent thrombosis; erythematous skin lesions | None |
| Other causes of thrombocytopenia | None | Possible | Definite |

   A. Bivalirudin
   B. Apixaban
   C. Dabigatran
   D. Argatroban

3. A 28-year-old female with a past medical history significant for Crohn disease status post multiple bowel resections who was admitted to the hospital 10 days ago was transferred to the ICU with a diagnosis of sepsis. Her blood cultures were positive for Vancomycin-resistant enterococcus, and nasal swab was also positive for MRSA. A chest X-ray from a week ago showed a right middle lobe infiltrate for which she was started on antibiotics. She had been on the appropriate antibiotics for 7 days. Trending her laboratory test results, you notice her platelet count has decreased from 180,000 on admission to 9,800 today. Which of the following antibiotics is most commonly implicated in drug-induced thrombocytopenia?

A. Linezolid
B. Daptomycin
C. Piperacillin tazobactam
D. Vancomycin

4. A 75-year-old male with a past medical history significant for severe aortic stenosis is admitted to the surgical intensive care unit for acute posthemorrhagic anemia secondary to a lower GI bleed. Lower endoscopy reveals angiodysplasias of the ascending colon that were subsequently cauterized. The next day the patient has additional bloody bowel movements. Laboratory test results show a platelet count of 120,000, hemoglobin of 7.2, and PTT of 42. What is the most definitive treatment for this patient?

A. FFP
B. Desmopressin
C. Repeat Endoscopy with cauterization
D. Aortic Valve Replacement

5. A 24-year-old male was admitted to the surgical ICU following open reduction and internal fixation of a tibial fracture after symptoms consistent with a transient ischemic attack in phase II of recovery. All workup thus far has remained inconclusive of a cause to include MRI/MRA, echocardiogram, telemetry, and EEG. The next day he has downtrending hemoglobin and platelets, an increase in serum creatinine, and a temperature of 38.8 without leukocytosis or leukopenia. His surgical site is without any obvious sign of infection. Physical examination is remarkable for petechiae seen all over his body. Blood smear reveals schistocytes. ADAMTS13 levels were noted to be <10%. What is the most appropriate treatment for this condition?

A. Discontinue all antibiotics
B. Stop all heparin products and start argatroban
C. Plasma exchange
D. IVIG and high-dose corticosteroids

# Chapter 79 ▪ Answers

1. Correct Answer: B

**Rationale:**
When life-threatening hemorrhage or bleed in a critical area occurs in the setting of anticoagulation, rapid reversal is crucial. The efficacy of FFP for the reversal of Xa inhibitors is modest at best. FFP has an INR of ~1.4, must be blood group specific, needs to be thawed before administration, and a volume of 10 to 15 mL/kg is needed. The delay in administration, potential for volume overload, transfusion related acute lung injury, and more effective options make this a less than ideal treatment.

PCC may be useful in anticoagulation reversal but not the best option. PCC comes in two types, 4 factor and 3 factor. The 4 factor PCC contains all of the vitamin K–dependent coagulation factors—II, VII, IX, and X. The 3 factor PCC does not contain factor VII and would not be good for vitamin K antagonists. Current consensus guidelines suggest 50 μg/kg of 4 factor PCC should be given to those on a factor Xa inhibitor with life-threatening bleeding or bleeding in a critical area.

Adnexanet Alfa is a decoy factor Xa with no active site. It has shown promise in phase III clinical trials. The AN-NEXA-4 (Adnexanet Alfa for Acute Major Bleeding Associated with Factor Xa Inhibitors) clinical trial is currently underway and shows effective reversal. If available, this is the best option. Recent FDA fast-track approval will likely bring this to the frontline for reversal of factor Xa inhibitors.

Because of its short half-life and the NOACs differing pharmacology, dosage varies by drug. Adnexanet alfa bolus is no longer effective 2 hours after it is administered and requires an infusion. Patients on apixaban 5 mg

BID require a 400 mg bolus followed by a continuous infusion of 4 mg/min for 2 hours. Those on rivaroxaban 20 mg daily require an 800 mg bolus followed by a continuous infusion of 8 mg/min for 2 hours.

Idarucizumab is a monoclonal antibody specific to dabigatran. Axiomatically, it is not an appropriate reversal agent for apixaban.

## References

1. Barnes GD. Consensus for management of bleeding on oral anticoagulants. *J Am Coll Cardiol.* 2017;(2):4-6. Available at https://www.acc.org/latest-in-cardiology/ten-points-to-remember/2017/11/29/17/23/2017-acc-expert-consensus-of-bleeding-on-oacs.
2. Raval AN, Cigarroa JE, Chung MK, et al. Management of patients on non–vitamin k antagonist oral anticoagulants in the acute care and periprocedural setting: a scientific statement from the American Heart Association. *Circulation.* 2017;135(10). Available at https://www.ahajournals.org/doi/10.1161/CIR.0000000000000477.
3. Kaatz S, Bhansali H, Gibbs J, Lavender R, Mahan CE, Paje DG. Reversing factor Xa inhibitors – clinical utility of andexanet alfa. *J Blood Med.* 2017;8:141-149. Available at http://www.ncbi.nlm.nih.gov/pubmed/28979172.

---

**2.** Correct Answer: A

**Rationale:**

The patient is most likely suffering from Heparin-induced Thrombocytopenia (HIT). HIT is due to an autoimmune reaction triggered by heparin against antiplatelet factor 4. Treatment consists of cessation of all heparin products, including LMWH, and beginning anticoagulation with a different agent.

The screening test of choice is the 4T score. It has a 99% sensitivity at a cut-off of 3 points. The 4T score is shown in Table 79.1:

**TABLE 79.1  4T Score**

| CATEGORY | 2 POINTS | 1 POINT | 0 POINTS |
| --- | --- | --- | --- |
| **Thrombocytopenia** | >50% fall or nadir ≥20 K | 30-50% fall or nadir 10-19 K | <30% fall or nadir <10 K |
| **Timing of platelet decrease** | Days 5-10 or ≤1 day if heparin exposure in past 30 d | >10 d or timing unclear, or <1 d with heparin exposure in past 30-100 d | <4 d with no recent heparin exposure |
| **Thrombosis or other sequelae** | Proven thrombosis, skin necrosis or acute systemic reaction after heparin bolus | Progressive, recurrent or silent thrombosis; erythematous skin lesions | None |
| **Other causes of thrombocytopenia** | None | Possible | Definite |

Our patient's 4 T score is 6: new thrombosis, ≤1 day after initiating heparin with exposure within the past 30 days (previous admission), with a possible cause being sepsis and liver failure, with a platelet count fall >50% that is greater than 20,000.

Confirmatory tests include anti-PF4 ELISA with or without platelet activation serotonin assay. In the presence of thrombosis, it is advised that a patient be treated as though they have HIT with a 4T score of 3 or greater until confirmatory testing is complete.

Xa inhibitor, apixaban, is appropriate for treatment of HIT in the outpatient setting, but is not recommended in patients with severe liver dysfunction. Dabigatran is a direct thrombin inhibitor that is also useful in HIT. However, patients with liver dysfunction have been found to have an exaggerated response to dabigatran, increasing their risk of bleeding. Hence, dabigatran is not recommended in cirrhotic patients or patients with elevated transaminases.

Argatroban is also a direct thrombin inhibitor. The half-life is about 1 hour. However, argatroban is hepatically metabolized. There has been successful use with dose reductions, but there is no specific reversal agent for this medication. It may be an appropriate choice, but not the best choice. Bivalirudin is a direct thrombin inhibitor that has a half-life of 25 minutes. It is easily titratable and is cleared renally. Given the patient's critical illness, preserved renal function and likely need for further interventions bivalirudin would be the best choice.

## References

1. Lo GK, Juhl D, Warkentin TE, Sigouin CS, Eichler P, Greinacher A. Evaluation of pretest clinical score (4 T's) for the diagnosis of heparin-induced thrombocytopenia in two clinical settings. *J Thromb Haemost.* 2006;4(4):759-765. Available at https://onlinelibrary.wiley.com/doi/full/10.1111/j.1538-7836.2006.01787.x.
2. Graff J, Harder S. Anticoagulant therapy with the oral direct factor Xa inhibitors rivaroxaban, apixaban and edoxaban and the thrombin inhibitor dabigatran etexilate in patients with hepatic impairment. *Clin Pharmacokinet.* 2013;52(4):243-254. Available at http://link.springer.com/10.1007/s40262-013-0034-0.
3. Levine RL, Hursting MJ, McCollum D. Argatroban therapy in heparin-induced thrombocytopenia with hepatic dysfunction. *Chest.* 2006;129(5):1167-1175. Available at http://www.ncbi.nlm.nih.gov/pubmed/16685006.

**3.** Correct Answer: A

**Rationale:**

Thrombocytopenia occurs in 15% to 58% of ICU patients, of which 19% to 25% is attributable to drug-induced thrombocytopenia (DIT). Three general mechanisms of thrombocytopenia are consumption, decreased production, and sequestration. Medications cause thrombocytopenia via bone marrow suppression and immunologically driven consumption; the latter is termed Drug Induced Immune Thrombocytopenia (DITP). DITP is believed to be the most common cause of DIT. HIT is the most common form of DITP, but, antibiotics are also commonly implicated.

There is no reported cut-off for percent drop from baseline or absolute platelet count. However, a platelet count <20,000 is highly suggestive of DIT. Onset within 5 to 7 days after initiation of a new medication when no other cause of declining platelets is identifiable is also suggestive. If a patient had previous exposure to a medication, the onset could be within 1 day. After cessation of the offending medication, any bleeding diathesis acquired from DIT should resolve in about 1 day, and platelets should return to baseline within approximately 1 week. This rapid resolution is attributable to its pathogenesis.

Though debated, it is hypothesized that antibiotics lead to hapten formation or drug-induced conformational change of proteins (Immunoglobulin/receptor) that expose different epitopes capable of triggering abnormal antibody-antigen formations. There are reports of continued thrombocytopenia when stopping a presumed offending drug. However, consistent with its pathogenesis, it is not common to have persistent thrombocytopenia with DIT even after the offending drug is removed.

Linezolid is reported to cause thrombocytopenia in 2.5% to 47% of patients and is the most cited antibiotic. Clinically, linezolid is associated with thrombocytopenia after 10 to 14 days of use. Vancomycin-induced thrombocytopenia appears to be under recognized. Though it may be as prevalent a cause as linezolid, it is not cited as much as Linezolid. Current studies suggest a minor difference or no difference in incidence of thrombocytopenia when compared to linezolid. With vancomycin, risk increases as total exposure (dose x time) increases. Incidence of thrombocytopenia with piperacillin is reported at 1% to 4%. Daptomycin has not been associated with thrombocytopenia.

### References

1. Priziola JL, Smythe MA, Dager WE. Drug-induced thrombocytopenia in critically ill patients. *Crit Care Med*. 2010;38(6 suppl):S145-S154. Available at https://insights.ovid.com/crossref?an=00003246-201006001-00008.
2. Visentin GP, Liu CY. Drug-induced thrombocytopenia. *Hematol Oncol Clin North Am*. 2007;21(4):685-696, vi. Available at http://www.ncbi.nlm.nih.gov/pubmed/17666285.
3. Aster RH, Bougie DW. Drug-induced immune thrombocytopenia. *N Engl J Med*. 2007;357(6):580-587. Available at http://www.nejm.org/doi/abs/10.1056/NEJMra066469.
4. Aster RH, Curtis BR, McFarland JG, Bougie DW. Drug-induced immune thrombocytopenia: pathogenesis, diagnosis, and management. *J Thromb Haemost*. 2009;7(6):911-918. Available at http://www.ncbi.nlm.nih.gov/pubmed/19344362.
5. Rondina MT, Walker A, Pendleton RC. Drug-induced thrombocytopenia for the hospitalist physician with a focus on heparin-induced thrombocytopenia. *Hosp Pract (1995)*. 2010;38(2):19-28. Available at http://www.ncbi.nlm.nih.gov/pubmed/20469610.
6. Loo AS, Gerzenshtein L, Ison M. Antimicrobial drug-induced thrombocytopenia: a review of the literature. *Semin Thromb Hemost*. 2012;38(8):818-829. Available at https://www.ncbi.nlm.nih.gov/pubmed/23081819.
7. Rao N, Ziran BH, Wagener MM, Santa ER, Yu VL. Similar hematologic effects of long-term linezolid and vancomycin therapy in a prospective observational study of patients with orthopedic infections. *Clin Infect Dis*. 2004;38(8):1058-1064. Available at https://academic.oup.com/cid/article-lookup/doi/10.1086/382356.
8. Nasraway SA, Shorr AF, Kuter DJ, O'Grady N, Le VH, Cammarata SK. Linezolid does not increase the risk of thrombocytopenia in patients with nosocomial pneumonia: comparative analysis of linezolid and vancomycin use. *Clin Infect Dis*. 2003;37(12):1609-1616. Available at https://academic.oup.com/cid/article-lookup/doi/10.1086/379327.

**4.** Correct Answer: D

**Rationale:**

The patient's presentation is most likely Heyde syndrome. First noticed in 1958, the triad includes moderate to severe aortic stenosis or calcified aortic valves, bleeding from arteriovenous malformations in the colon, and acquired von Willebrand disease (vWD). The different vWD Types are shown in Table 79.2.

**TABLE 79.2 von Willebrand Disease Types**

| VON WILLEBRAND DISEASE TYPES | |
| --- | --- |
| Type 1 | Partial Quantitative Deficiency |
| Type 3 | Complete Quantitative Deficiency |
| Type 2 | Qualitative Deficiency |
| Type 2A | Decreased platelet-dependent function because of small multimers |

## VON WILLEBRAND DISEASE TYPES

| | |
|---|---|
| Type 2B | Increased affinity for GPIb |
| Type 2M | Decreased function not of 2A |
| Type 2N | Decreased affinity for FVIII |

Acquired vWD or vWD 2A occurs in numerous disease processes. The various etiologies include hematologic cancers, solid tumors (Wilm's), and extremely turbulent areas of blood flow with a sufficient proportion of total blood flow to cause significant disruption of total circulating von Willebrand Factor (vWF) (eg aortic stenosis).

The pathogenesis of vWD IIA in aortic stenosis is uncoiling of the vWF multimer. When uncoiled by shear stress the site at which ADAMTS13 (vWF cleaving protease) cleaves the vWF multimer is exposed, resulting in shorter vWF strands with decreased function in primary hemostasis and enhanced clearance. The clinical impact is persistent bleeding from mucosal tissues, in this case, from colonic angiodysplasia.

Laboratory test result values will be mostly normal with either a normal or slightly prolonged PTT due to the physical association of vWF and factor VIII. However, the PTT cannot be used to rule-out vWF deficiency. Temporizing measures include administration of FFP or desmopressin. Although data are limited in the case of recurrent bleeding from Heyde syndrome, aortic valve replacement could offer definitive management.

### References

1. Pate GE, Mulligan A. An epidemiological study of Heyde's syndrome: an association between aortic stenosis and gastrointestinal bleeding. *J Heart Valve Dis.* 2004;13(5):713-716. Available at http://www.ncbi.nlm.nih.gov/pubmed/15473467.
2. Godino C, Lauretta L, Pavon AG, et al. Heyde's syndrome incidence and outcome in patients undergoing transcatheter aortic valve implantation. *J Am Coll Cardiol.* 2013;61(6):687-689. Available at https://www.sciencedirect.com/science/article/pii/S0735109712057130?via%3Dihub.
3. Loscalzo J. From clinical observation to mechanism – heyde's syndrome. *N Engl J Med.* 2012;367(20):1954-1956. Available at http://www.nejm.org/doi/abs/10.1056/NEJMcibr1205363.

## 5. Correct Answer: C

**Rationale:**

Antibiotic-related side effects have not been reported to cause the myriad of symptoms presented in this case. IVIG and high-dose corticosteroids are not used for the management of TTP but can be used for various other immunologic reactions including idiopathic thrombocytopenic purpura (ITP). ITP is autoimmune destruction of platelets without activation of platelets, would cause bleeding, would result in petechiae/purpura but would not cause symptoms of organ ischemia as in this patient, schistocytes, or decreased vWF. Argatroban would be appropriate if the patient had HIT. The patient's 4T score is not consistent with HIT. His symptoms are most consistent with a thrombotic microangiopathic anemia.

Thrombotic Microangiopathic Anemias (TMAs) present with a classic triad or pentad of symptoms. The triad consists of fever, anemia, and thrombocytopenia, whereas the pentad includes renal and neurologic dysfunction. The three common etiologies of TMA are Hemolytic Uremic Syndrome (HUS), atypical Hemolytic Uremic Syndrome (aHUS), and Thrombocytopenic Thrombotic Purpura (TTP). There are but a few findings that can reliably differentiate among them (Table 79.3).

**TABLE 79.3 Rapid Review of High Yield Differences in Hemolytic Uremic Syndrome (HUS), Thrombocytopenic Thrombotic Purpura (TTP), and atypical Hemolytic Uremic Syndrome (aHUS)**

| | ETIOLOGY | H&P | TREATMENT | DIAGNOSIS |
|---|---|---|---|---|
| HUS | • Shiga-toxin | • Hemorrhagic enterocolitis<br>• Renal dysfunction universal | • Supportive<br>• Antibiotics<br>• +/– Eculizumab | • Renal Biopsy<br>• STEC/Shiga-Toxin |
| aHUS | • Numerous associations | • History not associated with diarrhea | • Supportive<br>• Treat underlying cause<br>• +/– Eculizumab | • TMA not consistent with TTP without HUS prodome |
| TTP | • Genetic<br>• Acquired autoantibodies to ADAMTS13 | • Neuro symptoms more likely<br>• Renal symptoms possible | • Plasma Exchange<br>• Recurrent or refractory: splenectomy +/– eculizumab | • ADAMTS13 <10%<br>• vWF length analysis |

TTP is a result of abnormal, absent, or autoimmune disruption of ADAMTS13 (vWF-cleaving protease). Antibodies to ADAMTS13 are responsible for >90% of the diagnosed cases of TTP. Known causes of autoimmune TTP include ticlopidine and HIV. TTP is also associated with malignancies and various infectious processes. Most cases of acquired ADAMTS13 deficiency are idiopathic.

The pathophysiology of TTP is a result of dysfunction of ADAMTS13, resulting in dysfunctional vWF. vWF is excreted from Weibel-Palade as a long-coiled chain. ADAMTS13 cleaves this chain into smaller molecules. As a result of ADAMTS13 deficiency, longer vWF more readily provokes platelet aggregation. Ultimately, the inability of ADAMTS13 to properly process vWF results in abnormal clot formation in microvasculature and subsequent organ ischemia.

Consistent with its pathophysiology, confirmation relies upon ADAMTS13 levels <10% and analysis of vWF showing a greater proportion of long vWF multimers compared to controls. However, these tests are unusual and may have an unacceptably long processing time. Relying on history, symptoms and rule-out of other disease processes is crucial for timely treatment. Furthermore, improvement in symptoms will be seen with plasma exchange in TTP, will not affect HUS outcomes, and may help with aHUS. There may also be a role for eculizumab in the treatment of TTP.

Untreated, TTP is mostly fatal in 10 to 14 days. Plasma exchange is the treatment of choice. The exchange provides ADAMTS13 and reduces circulating autoantibodies. Giving plasma can be a temporizing measure. Various immunosuppressive regimens have been reported, though data do not support their use at this time. Splenectomy is a last resort for those who are unresponsive to plasma exchange or are reliant on plasma exchange due to repeated occurrence; data on outcomes are sparse.

## References

1. Kaur H, Sasapu A, Fox MH, Motwani P. Successful eculizumab therapy in thrombotic thrombocytopenic purpura (TTP) refractory to plasma exchange, steroids and rituximab. *Blood.* 2014;124(21):2794. Available at http://www.bloodjournal.org/content/124/21/2794?sso-checked=true.
2. George JN. How I treat patients with thrombotic thrombocytopenic purpura: 2010. *Blood.* 2010;116(20):4060-4069. Available at http://www.ncbi.nlm.nih.gov/pubmed/10942361.
3. Tsai H-M. Thrombotic thrombocytopenic purpura: a thrombotic disorder caused by ADAMTS13 deficiency. *Hematol Oncol Clin North Am.* 2007;21(4):609-632. Available at https://www.sciencedirect.com/science/article/pii/S0889858807000706?via%-3Dihub.
4. Dubois L, Gray DK. Case series: splenectomy: does it still play a role in the management of thrombotic thrombocytopenic purpura? *Can J Surg.* 2010;53(5):349-355. Available at http://www.ncbi.nlm.nih.gov/pubmed/20858382.
5. Schwartz J, Eldor A, Szold A. Laparoscopic splenectomy in patients with refractory or relapsing thrombotic thrombocytopenic purpura. *Arch Surg.* 2001;136(11):1236. Available at http://archsurg.jamanetwork.com/article.aspx?doi=10.1001/archsurg.136.11.1236.

# 80

# HYPERCOAGULABLE STATES

Hassan Farhan

1. A 39-year-old woman with nephrotic syndrome presents to the emergency department with 1 week history of headaches and nausea. She develops an acute deterioration in her mental status and is intubated and mechanically ventilated. Imaging reveals cerebral venous sinus thrombosis of the sagittal and transverse sinuses. Heparin anticoagulation is prescribed; however activated partial thromboplastin time (aPTT) is 46 seconds after multiple boluses and infusion per hospital protocol. Which of the following is the MOST appropriate next step in managing this patient's condition?

    A. Use a new batch of heparin and notify the manufacturer of inefficacy of this batch
    B. Switch to bivalirudin
    C. Transfuse packed red blood cells
    D. Cease further boluses, but rather double the infusion rate

2. Which of the following is LEAST likely to be a manifestation of factor V Leiden?

    A. Superficial vein thrombosis
    B. Deep vein thrombosis (DVT)
    C. Cerebral vein thrombosis
    D. Arterial thrombosis

3. A 58-year-old obese man with pancreatic cancer recently started neoadjuvant chemotherapy before a planned surgical resection. He presents to the emergency department with shortness of breath and chest pain. His hemoglobin is 11.5 g/dL, platelets are $550 \times 10^9$/L, and white blood cell count is $10.5 \times 10^9$/L.

    He is hemodynamically stable. He had noticed swelling of his left lower extremity a week prior. He denies family history of "clots." Computed tomography (CT) angiogram revealed pulmonary embolism, and therapeutic anticoagulation is initiated. Which of the following is a component of the Khorana score that has been validated as a risk factor for the development of venous thromboembolism (VTE) in a patient receiving chemotherapy?

    A. Age >55
    B. Body mass index (BMI) >30
    C. Prechemotherapy platelet count $>350 \times 10^9$/L
    D. Thyroid cancer

4. The combined oral contraceptive pill is associated with an increased risk of developing VTE. Which of the following factors has been demonstrated to reduce the risk of VTE?

    A. <50 μg of ethinyl estradiol
    B. First-generation progestins
    C. Oral contraceptive use of <1 year
    D. Age >39 years

**5.** Which of the following laboratory findings is MOST likely to be found in a patient diagnosed with antiphospholipid syndrome?

**A.** Platelets $65 \times 10^9$/L
**B.** Hgb 15 g/dL
**C.** Leukocytes $23 \times 10^9$/L
**D.** aPTT 35 seconds

# Chapter 80 ▪ Answers

**1.** Correct Answer: B

**Rationale:**

This patient's resistance to heparin is likely because of an acquired antithrombin deficiency. Heparin resistance has been defined as a requirement of greater than 35 000 IU/d to achieve therapeutic anticoagulation. Nephrotic syndrome is one of the causes of acquired antithrombin deficiency. Antithrombin is a natural anticoagulant that inhibits thrombin, factor Xa, and other serine proteases. Heparin works by binding to antithrombin, causing a conformational change that results in a 1000-fold increase in the anticoagulant activity of antithrombin III (ATIII).

Hereditary antithrombin deficiency is very rare (1 in 5000 to 1 in 10 000). It is inherited in an autosomal dominant with variable penetrance. Patient's with hereditary ATIII deficiency often have family members with a history of VTE. Acquired causes include acute thrombosis, liver disease, extracorporeal membrane oxygenation (ECMO), hemodialysis, and asparaginase therapy (treatment of acute lymphocytic leukemia). A functional antithrombin assay can help with the diagnosis of antithrombin deficiency.

Management options include transfusion with fresh frozen plasma (FFP, contains ATIII, which will allow heparin to exert its anticoagulant effect), infusion of ATIII concentrates, or using an alternative anticoagulant such as a direct thrombin inhibitor (bivalirudin).

References

1. Cosgriff TM, Bishop DT, Hershgold EJ, et al. Familial antithrombin III deficiency: its natural history, genetics, diagnosis and treatment. *Medicine (Baltimore)*. 1983;62:209.
2. Di Minno MN, Ambrosino P, Ageno W, et al. Natural anticoagulants deficiency and the risk of venous thromboembolism: a meta-analysis of observational studies. *Thromb Res*. 2015;135:923.

**2.** Correct Answer: D

**Rationale:**

Factor V Leiden is a mutated form of coagulation factor V that results in resistance to the anticoagulant effects of protein C. As a result, individuals with this factor V mutation are at increased risk for VTE. Heterozygosity for factor V Leiden is the most common inherited thrombophilia in Caucasian individuals with VTE. Factor V Leiden should be considered in a patient presenting with VTE at a young age, VTE in an unusual location (eg portal vein, cerebral vein), or recurrent VTE. Diagnosis can be made by DNA analysis or a functional coagulation test for activated protein C resistance. There is data associating factor V Leiden mutation with superficial vein thrombosis, pulmonary embolism, cerebral vein thrombosis (especially in women taking the oral contraceptive pill), and portal or hepatic vein thrombosis. Current data associating factor V Leiden mutation with arterial thromboembolism is weak, and the effect is small, if present.

References

1. Dahlback B. Anticoagulant factor V and thrombosis risk (editorial). *Blood*. 2004;103:3995.
2. Cushman M, Rosendaal FR, Psaty BM, et al. Factor V Leiden is not a risk factor for arterial vascular disease in the elderly: results from the cardiovascular health study. *Thromb Haemost*. 1998;79:912.

**3.** Correct Answer: C

**Rationale:**

Cancer induces a hypercoagulable state that puts patients at risk for thrombotic complications. Up to 10% of patients with cancer may develop VTE. Certain tumor types are associated with higher risk: for example, 30% to 50% of patients with pancreatic cancer have evidence of thrombosis.

The Khorana risk score for VTE in cancer patients is a validated scoring tool intended to be used in patients undergoing chemotherapy to stratify patients in terms of their future risk of VTE. The tool can be used to identify patients who are high risk and select those patients for ultrasound screening to diagnose DVT early. Data regarding use of the score for selecting patients for thromboprophylaxis are pending.

Components of the score are cancer type (stomach, and pancreas get two points, lung, lymphoma, gynecologic, bladder, and testicular cancers get one point), prechemotherapy platelet count of $\geq 350 \times 10^9$/L, hemoglobin level <10 g/dL, and prechemotherapy leukocyte count >11 $\times 10^9$/L and BMI $\geq 35$ kg/m$^2$. A score of $\geq 3$ infers a 6.7% to 7.1% risk of VTE in 2.5 months.

### References
1. Chew HK, Wun T, Harvey D, et al. Incidence of venous thromboembolism and its effect on survival among patients with common cancers. *Arch Intern Med*. 2006;166:458.
2. Lyman GH, Khorana AA, Kuderer NM, et al. Venous thromboembolism prophylaxis and treatment in patients with cancer: American Society of Clinical Oncology clinical practice guideline update. *J Clin Oncol*. 2013;31(17):2189-2204. doi:10.1200/JCO.2013.49.1118. Epub 2013 May 13.
3. Khorana AA, Kuderer NM, Culakova E, et al. Development and validation of a predictive model for chemotherapy-associated thrombosis. *Blood*. 2008;111:4902-4907.
4. Dutia M, White RH, Wun T. Risk assessment models for cancer-associated venous thromboembolism. *Cancer*. 2012;118:3468-3476.

---

### 4. Correct Answer: A

**Rationale:**

VTE is the most common vascular complication of combined oral contraception (COC) use. Although the risk is higher than in nonusers, the absolute risk is low and much less than the risk of VTE in pregnancy and early postpartum.

Studies have demonstrated that the risk of VTE is reduced by use of lower doses of ethinyl estradiol (<50 µg) and second-generation progestins (levonorgestrel). The risk of VTE is actually highest in the first year of COC use. The risk of VTE rises sharply after the age of 39 years in women taking COC. Women who smoke also have a greater risk.

### References
1. Lidegaard Ø, Løkkegaard E, Svendsen AL, Agger C. Hormonal contraception and risk of venous thromboembolism: national follow-up study. *BMJ*. 2009;339:b2890.
2. van Hylckama Vlieg A, Helmerhorst FM, Vandenbroucke JP, et al. The venous thrombotic risk of oral contraceptives, effects of oestrogen dose and progestogen type: results of the MEGA case-control study. *BMJ*. 2009;339:b2921.
3. de Bastos M, Stegeman BH, Rosendaal FR, et al. Combined oral contraceptives: venous thrombosis. *Cochrane Database Syst Rev*. 2014;(3):CD010813.
4. Nightingale AL, Lawrenson RA, Simpson EL, et al. The effects of age, body mass index, smoking and general health on the risk of venous thromboembolism in users of combined oral contraceptives. *Eur J Contracept Reprod Health Care*. 2000;5:265.

---

### 5. Correct Answer: A

**Rationale:**

Antiphospholipid syndrome is a systemic autoimmune disorder leading to a hypercoagulable state characterized by venous or arterial thrombosis in the presence of evidence of persistent antiphospholipid antibodies (anticardiolipin, anti-beta-2-glycoprotein, lupus anticoagulant). Antiphospholipid syndrome can occur as a primary condition or in the presence of another systemic autoimmune disease.

Diagnosis is made by a combination of clinical factors and laboratory tests:

1. The occurrence of one or more otherwise unexplained arterial or venous thrombotic events, especially in young patients.
2. Adverse pregnancy outcomes including fetal death after 10 weeks gestation, premature birth due to severe preeclampsia or placental insufficiency, or multiple embryonic losses (<10 weeks gestation).
3. Persistent detection of one or more of the antiphospholipid antibodies on two occasions at least 12 weeks apart.

Other laboratory findings include thrombocytopenia, prolonged aPTT in patients not receiving anticoagulation, and a history of false-positive serologic test for syphilis (antigen used in venereal disease research laboratory [VDRL] and rapid plasma reagin [RPR] tests contains cardiolipin). Leukocyte count and hemoglobin are not specifically associated with antiphospholipid syndrome.

### References
1. Ruiz-Irastorza G, Crowther M, Branch W, Khamashta MA. Antiphospholipid syndrome. *Lancet*. 2010;376:1498.
2. Giannakopoulos B, Passam F, Ioannou Y, Krilis SA. How we diagnose the antiphospholipid syndrome. *Blood*. 2009;113:985.

# 81

# TRANSFUSION MEDICINE

Nandini C. Palaniappa and Kevin C. Thornton

1. A patient with a history of prior transfusions is receiving a unit of packed red blood cells following a lengthy surgery and has a temperature increase from 37.0° to 38.3°. The patient is otherwise not in distress and has stable vital signs. The nurse stops the transfusion and asks you what he should do next. What is the BEST next course of action *and* which blood management modality could have prevented this reaction?

   A. Stop transfusion, evaluate patient, rule out infectious etiology and acute hemolytic reaction, and administer antipyretics; leukoreduction
   B. Stop transfusion; evaluate patient, rule out infectious etiology and acute hemolytic reaction, and administer antipyretics; washed RBCs
   C. Continue transfusion without further intervention or evaluation; leukoreduction
   D. Continue transfusion after ruling out an infectious source and acute hemolytic reaction and administration of antipyretics; washed RBCs

2. A patient presents with a subdural hematoma with midline shift and was noted to be on warfarin. The patient's INR is 3.5, and he is scheduled for an emergent decompressive craniotomy. Which of the following is the best treatment for his coagulopathy?

   A. Fresh Frozen Plasma
   B. Cryoprecipitate
   C. Platelets
   D. Prothrombin complex concentrate (PCC)

3. A 32-year-old woman with a history of a ruptured ectopic pregnancy who underwent a laparoscopic salpingectomy 4 days ago presents to the hospital after 1 day of feeling short of breath. In the ED, her examination is significant for labored breathing and her vital signs show a heart rate of 105 bpm, blood pressure of 98/65 mm Hg, $SpO_2$ of 88%, with respiratory rate of 22/min. Her chest X-ray is clear. Her laboratory test results are notable for a NT proBNP of 600 pg/mL and troponin I of 0.5 ng/mL. CT angiogram of her chest demonstrates large, central pulmonary embolus (PE), and RV/LV ratio of 1. You are called for admission to the ICU given the patient's newly diagnosed PE. Which of the following interventions is contraindicated in this patient?

   A. IVC filter
   B. Heparin anticoagulation only
   C. Directed catheter therapy
   D. Systemic tPA

4. A 38-year-old woman with no prior medical history presents to the ED with altered mental status and a temperature of 38.3°C. Physical examination reveals petechiae on both arms but is otherwise unremarkable. Her vital signs are normal and labs are significant for platelets of 30,000/μL, normal INR, normal aPTT, normal fibrinogen, a mildly elevated Creatinine, normal liver enzymes, and the appearance of schistocytes on peripheral blood smear. What is the most likely diagnosis?

**A.** Heparin induced thrombocytopenia (HIT)

**B.** Idiopathic thrombocytopenic purpura (ITP)

**C.** Disseminated intravascular coagulation (DIC)

**D.** Thrombotic thrombocytopenic purpura (TTP)

5.  A 65-year-old man with end-stage renal disease on hemodialysis is transferred to the ICU with new onset hematemesis. After adequate IV access is established, he is transfused four units of packed red blood cells, four units of fresh frozen plasma, and one apheresis unit of platelets. His vital signs improve though he still is having episodes of hematemesis. As you await the GI consult for possible endoscopy, what is the next best step in management?

**A.** PCC

**B.** Desmopressin

**C.** Fresh frozen plasma

**D.** Additional packed red blood cells

# Chapter 81 ▪ Answers

**1.** Correct Answer: A

**Rationale:**
Febrile nonhemolytic transfusion reactions are common and generally benign, but require ruling out other possible reactions such as an acute hemolytic reaction. They are the most common type of transfusion reaction, with an incidence of 0.5% to 2%. Their main feature is an increase in temperature of at least one degree. The fever may be accompanied by chills and rigors.

Several mechanisms have been proposed for this type of reaction including stimulation of donor leukocytes by recipient antibodies that were induced after prior transfusions; and cytokine accumulation in stored blood products. When a transfusion reaction is suspected, evaluation should include checking the blood for clerical error, examining for signs of hemolysis, and obtaining a direct antiglobulin test. It is important to rule out an acute hemolytic reaction and transfusion of a contaminated unit. Treatment of this type of reaction includes administration of antipyretics.

Leukoreduction of donor blood can reduce the incidence of febrile nonhemolytic reactions and transmission of cytomegalovirus. It may be preferred in certain patient populations such as potential transplant patients and chronically transfused patients. Washing donor blood can reduce the incidence of allergic reactions and is preferred for those with known IgA deficiency and at high risk for anaphylactic reactions. Irradiation of RBCs destroys donor T-lymphocytes and is used to prevent graft versus host disease in transplant patients and severely immunocompromised patients.

References
1. Eder A, ed. *Chapter 29 – Febrile Nonhemolytic Transfusion Reactions, Handbook of Transfusion Medicine.* 2001:253-257.
2. Yazer MH, Podlosky L, Clarke G, Nahirniak SM. The effect of prestorage WBC reduction on the rates of febrile nonhemolytic transfusion reactions to platelet concentrates and RBC. *Transfusion.* 2004;44(1):10-15.
3. King KE, Shirey RS, Thoman SK, Bensen-Kennedy D, Tanz WS, Ness PM. Universal leukoreduction decreases the incidence of febrile nonhemolytic transfusion reactions to RBCs. *Transfusion.* 2004;44(1):25-29.

**2.** Correct Answer: D

**Rationale:**
PCC can normalize the INR in 30 minutes. Dosing of PCC is based on the patient's INR and ranges between 25 to 50 units per kilogram. Additionally, PCC is advantageous in that its administration constitutes a much smaller volume load compared to FFP. PCC is the recommended reversal agent for warfarin-induced INR elevation in the setting of intracranial hemorrhage.

FFP can take much longer to correct an elevated INR, and some studies found a median time of 30 hours for normalization of INR in patients with intraparenchymal bleeds. Moreover, the required volume of FFP can cause pulmonary edema, transfusion-related acute lung injury, and transfusion-associated circulatory overload.

Indications for cryoprecipitate include: hypofibrinogenemia, tPA-related life-threatening bleeding, von Willebrand's disease, uremic bleeding, massive transfusion, and hemophilia A. Platelets may be transfused if the patient is thrombocytopenic.

### Reference

1. Frontera JA, Lewin JJIII, Rabinstein AA, et al. Guideline for reversal of antithrombotics in intracranial hemorrhage: a statement for healthcare professionals from the Neurocritical Care Society and Society of Critical Care Medicine. *Neurocrit Care.* 2016;24(1):6-46.

**3.** Correct Answer: D

**Rationale:**

There are several risk stratification tools for patients presenting with an acute PE. Given patient's relative hemodynamic stability (with a systolic blood pressure >90 mm Hg), her PE can be classified as submassive. Her elevated BNP, troponin, and RV/LV ratio greater than 0.9 are signs of RV dysfunction. She can thus be further classified as having an intermediate-high risk PE.

Data surrounding treatment of submassive PEs are controversial. The decision of whether to administer systemic tPA in these patients should entail a discussion between care team members and the patient regarding the risks and benefits. Generally, however, recent surgery (defined as having surgery less than 3 weeks prior) is a contraindication to systemic tPA.

**Key point:** Contraindications to systemic tPA include:

- hemorrhagic stroke or stroke of unknown origin at any point in time
- Ischemic stroke within past 6 months
- CNS damage or neoplasm
- major surgery/trauma within past 3 weeks
- GI bleeding within past 1 month
- active bleeding
- bleeding diathesis

### References

1. ESC Committee for Practice Guidelines. 2014 ESC guidelines on the diagnosis and management of acute pulmonary embolus: the task force for the diagnosis and management of acute pulmonary embolism of the European Society of Cardiology (ESC). *Eur Heart J.* 2014;35(43):3033-3073.
2. Konstantinides SV, Barco S, Lankeit M, Meyer G. Management of pulmonary embolism: an update. *J Am Coll Cardiol.* 2016;67(8):976-990.

**4.** Correct Answer: D

**Rationale:**

TTP is a thrombotic microangiopathy caused by platelet binding to abnormal von Willebrand factor on the microvascular endothelium. The classic pentad presentation includes: fever, altered mental status, acute renal failure, thrombocytopenia, and microangiopathic hemolytic anemia. Diagnosis requires thrombocytopenia and microangiopathic hemolytic anemia (as evidenced by schistocytes on peripheral smear). It can be distinguished from DIC since INR, aPTT, and fibrinogen levels are normal. Treatment is early plasma exchange until platelet count is over 50,000 for at least 48 hours and avoidance of platelet transfusions because it can lead to further thrombosis. Left untreated, TTP is almost always fatal.

HIT occurs when heparin binds to platelet factor 4 and triggers the formation of IgG antibodies that bind to platelets and causes the promotion of thrombosis. It generally occurs 5 to 10 days after the first heparin exposure but can appear in 1 day if heparin exposure occurred within the prior 30 days. Venous thrombosis is more common than arterial thrombosis. Diagnosis requires high clinical score on the 4T score and a positive antibody test. Treatment includes discontinuing all heparin and heparin-containing products and anticoagulation with a direct thrombin inhibitor such as argatroban.

ITP is caused by autoantibody-mediated platelet clearance and usually results in a severe thrombocytopenia. Physical examination can reveal petechiae and the peripheral smear may show large platelets. Treatment of ITP includes glucocorticoids, IVIG, and rituximab in those who are unresponsive to initial corticosteroid therapy.

DIC is caused by release of tissue factor that activates clotting factors that lead to widespread microvascular thrombosis and consumption of platelets and clotting factors. Clinically, DIC can lead to multiorgan failure along with bleeding. Laboratory test results will show an elevation of INR and aPTT, low fibrinogen, and elevated D-dimer, whereas a peripheral smear will show schistocytes. Treatment is primarily supportive and addressing the underlying cause inciting DIC.

### Reference

1. Scully M, Hunt BJ, Benjamin S, Liesner R, Rose P, Peyvandi F; British Committee for Standards in Haematology. Guidelines on the diagnosis and management of thrombotic thrombocytopenic purpura and other thrombotic microangiopathies. *Br J Haematol.* 2012;158(3):323-335. http://doi.org/10.1111/j.1365-2141.2012.09167.x.

**5.** Correct Answer: B

**Rationale:**

Patients with renal dysfunction often have impaired platelet function and abnormal platelet-endothelial interaction that can lead to increased bleeding. Uremic bleeding can present as ecchymoses, purpura, epistaxis, and GI bleeding and intracranial bleeding. Treatment options include administration of desmopressin, which is thought to reduce bleeding by increasing the release of factor VIII:von Willebrand factor multimers. Bleeding time is reduced in an hour and its effects typically last 4 to 8 hours. Dosing of desmopressin is 0.3 μg/kg IV or subcutaneously.

PCC and Fresh frozen plasma would be indicated in the setting of an elevated INR, while tranexamic acid would be indicated in the setting of hyperfibrinolysis.

References

1. Galbusera M, Remuzzi G, Boccardo P. Treatment of bleeding in dialysis patients. *Semin Dial*. 2009;22(3):279-286.
2. Hedges SJ, Dehoney SB, Hooper JS, Amanzadeh J, Busti AJ. Evidence-based treatment recommendations for uremic bleeding. *Nat Clin Pract Nephrol*. 2007;3(3):138-153.

# 82

# SOLID TUMORS

Milad Sharifpour and Ofer Sadan

1. A 67-year-old man with past medical history of hypertension, diabetes mellitus, smoking, and recent diagnosis of small cell lung cancer is admitted to the ICU presents with complaints of nausea, vomiting, weakness, and altered mental status. On examination he is somnolent but opens his eyes to voice. He is not oriented to person or place. He appears well hydrated and his vital signs are within normal limits. His basic metabolic panel is notable for serum sodium level of 119 mmol/L, creatinine of 0.65 mg/dL, and serum osmolality of 260 mOsm/kg. The patient has a seizure as you are examining him. After ensuring adequate oxygenation and ventilation the most appropriate next treatment is ?

   A. Fluid Restriction
   B. Intravenous furosemide
   C. Intravenous 3% NS
   D. Tolvaptan

2. A 63-year-old woman with a recent diagnosis of lung cancer is admitted to the ICU with hypotension, acute onset of chest pain, cough, and shortness of breath. Her vital signs are T 37.6, HR 123, RR 40, BP 87/65 mm Hg, and oxygen saturation of 88% on 6 L NC. Chest X-ray is notable for a right lower lobe consolidation, as well as widened mediastinum. Chest computed tomography with contrast reveals a large pericardial effusion and transthoracic echocardiography shows a large pericardial effusion with diastolic collapse of the right ventricle. Which of the following is next most appropriate therapeutic intervention at this time?

   A. Noninvasive positive pressure ventilation
   B. Emergent endotracheal intubation
   C. Echocardiography guided pericardiocentesis
   D. Emergent radiation therapy

Questions 3 & 4 are a part of a two-question scenario:

3. A 57-year-old woman with history of breast cancer treated with L. mastectomy and chemotherapy and radiation presents with a 1-week history of headaches, gait instability, progressive confusion, and a new onset seizure. On physical examination she is somnolent and only opens her eyes in response to voice. She is only oriented to person (knows her own name) but is not oriented to place or date. She does not follow commands but does withdraw from painful stimuli. Emergent noncontrast head CT is performed, which reveals multiple masses with surrounding edema and no evidence of blood. Based on the data provided what is the patient's Glasgow Coma Score?

   A. 11
   B. 8
   C. 12
   D. 9

4. What is the most appropriate intervention for this patient at this time?

   **A.** Endotracheal intubation
   **B.** IV dexamethasone therapy
   **C.** Radiation therapy
   **D.** Extra ventricular drain placement

5. A 47-year-old man with recent diagnosis of pheochromocytoma is admitted to the ICU for management of hypertensive crisis. A radial arterial catheter is placed, and the patient is started on sodium nitroprusside with goal systolic blood pressure of 140 to 160 mm Hg. During rounds on the second day following ICU day, the bedside nurse notifies you that the patient's blood pressure has been progressively increasing despite up titration of the nitroprusside infusion. On examination, the patient is complaining of headache and appears anxious and confused. His skin is flushed and he is tachycardic and hypertensive. The sodium nitroprusside is discontinued, oxygen administered, and a nicardipine infusion is started. What is the most appropriate to administer for treatment of this patient?

   **A.** Silver nitrate
   **B.** Sodium thiosulfate
   **C.** Methylene blue therapy
   **D.** Fenoldopam

# Chapter 82 ▪ Answers

**1.** Correct Answer: C

**Rationale:**
The patient presents with hyponatremia (serum Na <135 mEq/L) most likely secondary to syndrome of inappropriate antidiuretic hormone (SIADH) resulting from his lung cancer. Patients with hyponatremia and severe neurological symptoms (seizures, coma, inability communicate) should be treated with hypertonic saline. Left untreated, severe hyponatremia can lead to potentially lethal cerebral edema.

The SIADH is characterized by euvolemic hyponatremia, low serum osmolality (<280 mOsm/kg), and increased urine osmolality. Hyponatremia is secondary to antidiuretic hormone–induced retention of ingested water. Common causes of SIADH include malignancies (highest among patients with small-cell lung cancer), infections (pneumonia, meningitis, AIDS), medications, hormone deficiencies (hypothyroidism, adrenal insufficiency), neurological injuries (subarachnoid hemorrhage), and surgery.

Treatment of hyponatremia depends on the severity of the symptoms and the rapidity with which they develop. In asymptomatic patients, treatment of the underlying cause can correct hyponatremia. Fluid restriction is the mainstay of therapy in patients with SIADH without any neurological symptoms. Patients with neurological symptoms, and those with resistant hyponatremia, should be treated with intravenous hypertonic saline.

### References
1. Sterns RH, Hix JK, Silver SM. Management of hyponatremia in the ICU. *Chest*. 2013;144:672-679.
2. Gross P. Clinical management of SIADH. *Ther Adv Endocrinol Metab*. 2012;3:61-73.

**2.** Correct Answer: C

**Rationale:**
The patient presents with respiratory distress and hypotension secondary to pericardial effusion with tamponade physiology. Emergent echocardiography–guided pericardiocentesis will evacuate the pericardial effusion and relieve symptoms.

Pericardial effusions are common in patients with metastatic cancer. However, most cancer patients with pericardial effusions are asymptomatic. Symptoms develop in patients with large pericardial effusions or those with rapid fluid accumulation. Typical symptoms include cough, dyspnea, and chest pain. Physical examination findings are notable for hypotension, tachypnea, tachycardia, respiratory distress, jugular venous distension, and pulsus paradoxus. Chest X-ray may show widened mediastinum and EKG may show sinus tachycardia, low voltage, nonspecific ST/T changes, and electrical alternans. Echocardiography is the gold standard for diagnosing pericardial effusion. Tamponade physiology is characterized by diastolic collapse of the right ventricle, dilatation of inferior vena cava, and loss of respiratory variability in IVC diameter as well as pronounced ventricular interdependence with respiration.

Positive pressure ventilation reduces venous return (cardiac preload) and can lead to hemodynamic collapse (choices A and B are incorrect). Although radiation therapy may reduce the risk of recurrence, it has no role in acute management of pericardial effusion with tamponade physiology.

### References

1. Maisch B, Ristic A, Pankuweit S. Evaluation and management of pericardial effusion in patients with neoplastic disease. *Prog Cardiovasc Dis.* 2010;53:157-163.
2. Thorvardur R, Hogan WJ, Madsen BE, et al. Emergencies in hematology and oncology. *Mayo Clin Proc.* 2017;92:609-641.

---

**3.** Correct Answer: A

**Rationale:**
The Glasgow Coma Scale provides a practical method for assessment of impairment of conscious level in response to defined stimuli. The scale measures the mental status of patients according to three categories of responsiveness: eye opening, motor, and verbal responses (Table 82.1).

**TABLE 82.1 Glasgow Coma Scale Score**

| EYE OPENING | | VERBAL RESPONSE | | MOTOR RESPONSE | |
|---|---|---|---|---|---|
| Spontaneous | 4 | Oriented, converses normally | 5 | Follows command | 6 |
| To voice | 3 | Confused/disoriented | 4 | Localizes to pain | 5 |
| To pain | 2 | Inappropriate words | 3 | Withdraws from pain | 4 |
| None | 1 | Incomprehensible sounds | 2 | Decorticate (abnormal flexion) | 3 |
| | | None | 1 | Decerebrate (abnormal extension) | 2 |
| | | | | No movements | 1 |

The patient in this scenario opens her eyes to voice (3 points), withdraws from painful stimulus (4 points), and is confused and disoriented (4 points) and therefore has a Glasgow Coma Score of 11.

---

**4.** Correct Answer: B

**Rationale:**
Brain metastases occur in up to 20% of the patients with cancer and indicate poor prognosis. Lung cancer, breast cancer, renal cell carcinoma, and melanoma are the most common types of cancer that metastasize to brain. Contrast-enhanced magnetic resonance imagining is the study of choice for diagnosing brain metastases.

IV glucocorticoids are indicated in symptomatic patients with brain metastases and surrounding edema and can be symptomatically effective within hours of administration.

The patient in the question is able to protect her airway, and therefore at this point there is no indication for endotracheal intubation (choice A is incorrect). Although radiation therapy may play a role in long-term management of brain metastases, there is no role for radiation therapy in acute management (choice C is incorrect). Although the patient does have evidence of increased intracranial pressure (headache, nausea/vomiting), conservative measures such as glucocorticoids should be attempted first. In comatose patients or those with severely increased intracranial pressure (TBI, obstructive hydrocephalus, intracranial hemorrhage), hyperventilation, hyperosmolar therapy with osmotic diuretics, and extra ventricular drainage of cerebrospinal fluid may be utilized to reduce intracranial pressure.

### References

1. Kaal EC, Vecht CJ. The management of brain edema in brain tumors. *Curr Opin Oncol.* 2004;16:593-600.
2. Halfdanarson TRHogan WJMadsen BE. Emergencies in hematology and oncology. *Mayo Clin Proc.* 2017;92:609-641.
3. Lin X, DeAngelis LM. Treatment of brain metastases. *J Clin Oncol.* 2015;33:3475-3484.

---

**5.** Correct Answer: D

**Rationale:**
Sodium nitroprusside interacts with oxyhemoglobin and releases cyanide, methemoglobin, and nitric oxide. Prolonged infusions of sodium nitroprusside or doses exceeding 2 µg/kg/min increase the risk of cyanide toxicity as cyanide avidly binds ferric iron of cytochrome oxidase, inhibiting oxidative phosphorylation and leading to anaerobic metabolism and lactic acidosis. The patient in this scenario has developed tachyphylaxis to sodium nitroprusside, which is a sign of cyanide toxicity. Sodium nitroprusside should be promptly discontinued and therapy with sodium thiosulfate initiated.

Addition of a fenoldopam infusion to the nicardipine infusion may help to control the patient's blood pressure but will not fix the underlying cyanide toxicity (choice D is wrong). Methylene blue is the therapeutic agent of choice for management of methemoglobinemia, which can develop in association with nitroprusside or nitroglycerine infusion. However, the patient in this scenario suffers from cyanide toxicity not methemoglobinemia (choice C is incorrect).

Silver nitrate is an inorganic chemical with antiseptic activity. It also is used as a cauterizing or sclerosing agent. It is not a treatment for cyanide poisoning (choice A is incorrect)

## References

1. Lockwood A. Sodium nitroprusside associated cyanide toxicity in adult patients – fact or fiction? A critical review of the evidence and clinical relevance. *Open Access J Clin Trials*. 2010;2010:133-148.
2. Friederich JA, Butterworth JFIV. Sodium nitroprusside: twenty years and counting. *Anesth Analg*. 1995;81:152-162.
3. Hottinger DG, Beebe DS, Kozhimannil T, Prielipp RC, Belani KG. Sodium nitroprusside in 2014: a clinical concepts review. *J Anaesthesiol Clin Pharmacol*. 2014;30:462-471.

# 83

# ONCOLOGICAL SYNDROMES

Milad Sharifpour and Ofer Sadan

1. A 19-year-old man with acute lymphoblastic leukemia is found to be lethargic and complains of nausea and muscle cramps after receiving cytotoxic therapy. A basic metabolic panel is notable for a potassium level of 6.9 mEq/L, plasma phosphate of 5.5 mg/dL, and uric acid level is 17 mg/dL. An ECG is notable for peaked T waves and frequent premature ventricular complexes. Which one of the following treatment options is MOST appropriate at this time?

   A. Rasburicase
   B. Allopurinol
   C. Hemodialysis
   D. IV fluid therapy

2. A 65-year-old man with a diagnosis of small-cell lung cancer presents to the emergency with complaints of hoarseness, shortness of breath, and swelling of his face and right arm. His vital signs are T 36.4°C, RR 42 breaths/min, HR of 122 beats/min, BP 100/67 mm Hg, and SpO$_2$ 87% on 4L nasal cannula. On examination, he is stridorous and unable to speak in full sentences. ECG is notable for sinus tachycardia and a chest x-ray reveals widened mediastinum. What is the most appropriate next step in management?

   A. Endotracheal intubation
   B. Catheter-based venography
   C. CT venography
   D. Radiation therapy

3. A 54-year-old woman with breast cancer is brought to the emergency room with progressive confusion, anorexia, constipation, weight loss, and weakness. Vital signs are temperature 36.7°C, BP 94/57 mm Hg, HR 87 beats/min, and SaO$_2$ 96% on RA. On examination, she is drowsy but easily arousable and oriented to person. Her neurologic examination is otherwise unremarkable. Lab studies are notable for a creatinine level of 1.78 mg/dL (baseline 0.8 mg/dL) and serum calcium of 13.7 mg/dL. What is the most appropriate initial treatment?

   A. 0.9% normal saline infusion with furosemide
   B. 0.9% normal saline infusion
   C. Bisphosphonate therapy
   D. Calcitonin

4. A 57-year-old woman with a history of breast cancer treated with mastectomy and radiation therapy is admitted with a 4-week history of progressive low back pain. She reports decreased sensation over her buttocks, perineal region, and posterior superior thighs and occasional difficulty with voiding. Her physical examination is noticeable for decreased anal sphincter tone. What is the most appropriate next step in management?

   A. Emergent decompressive surgery
   B. CT scan of the spine with and without contrast
   C. MRI of full spine
   D. Intravenous dexamethasone

**5.** A 63-year-old man is admitted to the ICU with epistaxis, blurred vision, and altered mental status. His medical history includes hypertension, diabetes mellitus, and Waldenstrom macroglobulinemia. Vital signs are T 37.3°C, HR 102 beats/min, RR 44 breaths/min, BP 112/57 mm Hg, and SaO$_2$ 80% on 100% nonrebreathing mask. His physical examination is notable for bloody nostrils, and he is somnolent but responsive to verbal stimuli. Laboratory studies are notable for a Hgb of 9.8 mg/dL, platelet count of 87,000, and a large monoclonal spike on serum protein electrophoresis. Which one of the following interventions is not indicated at this time?

**A.** Red blood cell (RBC) transfusion
**B.** Plasma exchange
**C.** Endotracheal intubation
**D.** IV fluid therapy

# Chapter 83 ▪ Answers

**1.** Correct Answer: C

**Rationale:**
The patient has symptomatic hyperkalemia, evidence by peaked T waves and a plasma potassium level of 6.9 mEq/L, which is an indication for emergent dialysis.

Tumor lysis syndrome (TLS) is an oncologic emergency caused by release of large amounts of potassium, phosphate, and uric acid into the plasma in response to tumor cell lysis resulting from cytotoxic therapy, radiation therapy, immunotherapy, or glucocorticoid therapy. Patients with high-grade lymphomas (Burkitt lymphoma) or acute lymphoblastic leukemia, those with large tumor burdens, or highly proliferative tumors are at higher risk for TLS. TLS can also occur spontaneously in highly proliferative tumors due to high cell turnover.

Hyperuricemia leads to precipitation of uric acid crystals in the renal tubules and can cause acute kidney injury (AKI). Hyperphosphatemia and deposition of calcium phosphate crystals in the renal tubules can also lead to AKI. Hyperkalemia can lead to arrhythmias, including ventricular fibrillation and cardiac arrest.

The signs and symptoms of TLS occur from metabolic abnormalities (hyperkalemia, hyperphosphatemia, hyperuricemia) and associated development of AKI and include lethargy, nausea, vomiting, diarrhea, anorexia, muscle cramps, tetany, hematuria, arrhythmias, and cardiac arrest.

Aggressive intravenous fluid therapy to increase renal perfusion and prevent precipitation of uric acid and calcium phosphate crystals in the renal tubules is the mainstay of TLS prophylaxis. Recommended urine output is 2 mL/kg/h. Rasburicase is the first-line hypouricemic agent for patients at high risk for TLS, especially those with renal or cardiac dysfunction, while allopurinol, a xanthine oxidase inhibitor which blocks the metabolism of hypoxanthine and xanthine to uric acid, is the first-line prophylactic agent in patients at intermediate risk for TLS.

References
1. Thandra K, Salah Z, Chawla S. Oncological emergencies – The old, the new, the deadly. *J Intensive Care Med.* 2018; [Epub ahead of print].
2. Coiffier B, Altman A, Pui CH, Younes A, Cairo MS. Guidelines for the management of pediatric and adult tumor lysis syndrome: an evidence-based review. *J Clin Oncol.* 2008;26:2767-2778.

**2.** Correct Answer: A

**Rationale:**
The patient has superior vena cava syndrome (SVCS) from malignancy with life-threatening symptoms (eg, stridor, respiratory distress) and require immediate stabilization (endotracheal intubation to secure the airway, circulatory support), followed by definitive intervention (endovenous recanalization, mechanical thrombectomy, SVC filter placement).

Radiation therapy is no longer recommended as the first-line treatment.

SVCS occurs in response to mechanical obstruction of the SVC due to external compression, tumor invasion into the vessel, or internal obstruction. Malignancy is the most common cause of SVCS, with lung cancer and non-Hodgkin lymphoma as the most common types of associated malignancy. Dyspnea is the most common presenting symptom. Other symptoms may include facial, neck, and arm swelling, hoarseness, stridor, chest pain, and dysphagia. Physical examination findings in patients with SVCS include facial, neck, and arm edema, engorged neck veins, stridor, and in severe cases, obtundation due to increased intracranial pressure and brain swelling.

Chest radiography and ECG provide nonspecific information in patients with SVCS. Chest radiograph may show widened mediastinum and ECG commonly shows sinus tachycardia. CT venography provides information about the location and extent of the obstruction, and catheter-mediated thrombolysis can be performed concurrently with the imaging.

References
1. Zimmerman S, Davis M. Rapid fire: superior vena cava syndrome. *Emerg Med Clin North Am.* 2018;36:577-584.
2. Breault S, Doenz F, Jouannic AM, Qanadli SD. Percutaneous endovascular management of chronic superior vena cava syndrome of benign causes: long term follow-up. *Eur Radiol.* 2017;1:97-104.
3. McCurdy MT, Shanholtz CB. Oncologic emergencies. *Crit Care Med.* 2012;40:2212-2222.

**3.** Correct Answer: B

**Rationale:**

Hypercalcemia accounts for 0.6% of hospital admissions. It can present with a variety of nonspecific symptoms that affect multiple organ systems. Symptoms include neurological disturbances (ranging from anxiety and confusion, to lethargy and coma), gastrointestinal disturbances (anorexia, nausea, constipation, and pancreatitis), renal dysfunction (polyuria, dehydration, AKI), and musculoskeletal abnormalities (weakness, cramping). ECG may show a shortened QT interval, and in severe cases of hypercalcemia, arrhythmias and ventricular tachycardia may be present. Severity of symptoms correlates with the severity of hypercalcemia.

Up to 90% of the cases of hypercalcemia are due to hyperparathyroidism and malignancy (lung cancer, multiple myeloma, and renal cell). Other causes, however, include medications (thiazide diuretics, antacids such as calcium carbonate, vitamin A and D supplements, and lithium), immobilization, granulomatous diseases (sarcoidosis), and thyrotoxicosis.

When an elevated plasma calcium level is identified, it should be confirmed to ensure true hypercalcemia (serum calcium level is affected by albumin concentration, and hypoalbuminemia falsely elevates the serum calcium level). In addition ionized calcium levels should be interpreted in the context of the patient's pH. Parathyroid hormone level and serum phosphorus level should also be measured.

Treatment of hypercalcemia depends on the severity of the patient's symptoms. While asymptomatic patients can be treated on an outpatient basis, symptomatic patients and those with significantly elevated calcium levels should be hospitalized for IV fluid therapy. If a malignancy is detected as the underlying cause of hypercalcemia, the patient should undergo definitive treatment for malignancy, if possible.

IV fluid therapy with 0.9% NS is the cornerstone of treatment of patients with hypercalcemia. Dehydration is secondary to decreased intake (anorexia, nausea) and increased urine output (polyuria). Calcitonin is quick acting and can be given for initial stabilization in addition to IV fluids. Bisphosphonates take 48 hours to work and are utilized for long-term management of hypercalcemia. Furosemide is no longer recommended due to the risk of dehydration and lack of evidence of benefit.

References
1. Carrick AI, Costner HB. Rapid fire: hypercalcemia. *Emerg Med Clin North Am.* 2018;36:549-555.
2. Naganathan S, Badireddy M. *Hypercalcemia. StatPearls* [Internet]. Treasure Island, FL: StatPearls Publishing; 2018.
3. Goldner W. Cancer related hypercalcemia. *J Oncol Practice.* 2016;12:426-432.
4. Maier JD, Levine SN. Hypercalcemia in the intensive care unit: a review of pathophysiology, diagnosis, and modern therapy. *J Intensive Care Med.* 2015;30:235-252.

**4.** Correct Answer: C

**Rationale:**

Malignant spinal cord compression (MSCC) is a devastating complication of cancer. Cancers of prostate, breast, and lung account for most cases of vertebral metastases; however cancer of any origin can metastasize to the spine.

Back pain occurs in 95% of patients for up to 2 months before signs related to MSCC appear. Pain can be localized or radicular in nature and the severity of pain often increases over time. A higher index of suspicion is required in patients with a known history of cancer and those presenting with unremitting pain or pain localized to middle or upper spine. Motor deficits (eg, weakness, unsteady gait, difficulty walking or standing, etc.) that has progressed over days or few weeks is the second most common symptom in patients with MSCC. Sensory symptoms (eg, parasthesias, numbness, decreased sensation) are less common than motor deficits. Autonomic dysfunction (bowel or bladder incontinence) is a late complication of MSCC. Cauda equina syndrome, characterized by low back pain, unilateral or bilateral radicular pain, saddle anesthesia, erectile dysfunction, loss of bladder or bowel continence, and lower extremity weakness, may be the first presentation of MSCC in patients with metastasis to lumbar spine.

An MRI of full spine within 24 hours of presentation is the imaging study of choice in patients presenting with pain and autonomic dysfunction (bowel/bladder incontinence). CT scan is used for surgery or radiation therapy planning.

Definitive therapy for MSCC includes decompressive surgery and radiation therapy. In absence of contraindications, all patients with MSCC should receive corticosteroids as adjunctive therapy.

References
1. Al-Qurainy R, Collis E. Metastatic spinal cord compression: diagnosis and management. *BMJ.* 2016;353:i2539.
2. Quaile A. Cauda equina syndrome – the questions. *Int Orthop.* 2018; [Epub ahead of print].
3. McCurdy MT, Shanholtz CB. Oncologic emergencies. *Crit Care Med.* 2012;40:2212-2222.

**5.** Correct Answer: A

**Rationale:**

Hyperviscosity syndrome (HVS) is an oncological emergency characterized by the triad of neurological symptoms, visual disturbances, and mucosal bleeding and is an oncological emergency. HVS is caused by a pathological increase in serum proteins, RBCs, white blood cells (WBCs), and/or platelets, or by deformed RBCs. Waldenstrom macroglobulinemia is the most common cause of HVS. Other causes include multiple myeloma, rheumatoid disease, polycythemia, sickle cell disease, leukemia, and spherocytosis.

Diagnosis is established by clinical evidence of elevated serum viscosity. Additional laboratory tests to confirm the diagnosis include complete blood count (CBC), peripheral blood smear, and coagulation profile. Measurement of serum immunoglobulins is not necessary for establishing diagnosis of HVS.

Timely treatment can prevent catastrophic ischemic sequalae such as myocardial infarction, stroke, thromboembolic events, and multiorgan system dysfunction. Supportive care in addition to plasma exchange or plasmapheresis is the mainstay of managing HVS. In cases where emergent plasmapheresis cannot be arranged, phlebotomy can be performed (removing 1-2 units of the patient's blood) as a temporizing measure. Dehydration increases plasma viscosity and should be treated with IV fluids. Chemotherapy for the underlying malignancy is the definitive therapy. RBC transfusion can increase blood viscosity and worsen the thrombotic/ischemic effects.

References

1. Stone MJ, Bogen SA. Evidence based focused review of management of hyperviscosity syndrome. *Blood.* 2012;119:2205-2208.
2. Lewis MA, Hendrickson AW, Moynihan TJ. Oncologic emergencies: pathophysiology, presentation, diagnosis, and treatment. *CA Cancer J Clin.* 2011;61:287-314.
3. Perez Rogers A, Estes M. *Hyperviscosity Syndrome. StatPearls* [Internet]. Treasure Island, FL: StatPearls Publishing; 2018.
4. Gertz MA. Acute hyperviscosity: syndromes and management. *Blood.* 2018;132:1379-1385.

# 84

# HEMOPOIETIC CELL TRANSPLANTATION

Jeffrey Gotts

1. A 34-year-old woman presents to the ED with several days of worsening abdominal pain, anorexia, nausea, and copious diarrhea. Three months ago, she had underwent matched unrelated-donor allogeneic stem cell transplant for acute lymphocytic leukemia (ALL). Examination reveals an afebrile woman with a maculopapular rash over her neck, shoulders, and palms, HR 140, BP 70/40, RR 14 100% RA. She is given 30 mL/kg IVF and SBP remains in the 80s, prompting ICU admission. Laboratory test results are notable for WBC 6,000/μL, plt 150,000/μL, Cr 1.6 mg/dL, and BUN 3 mg/dL. Which of the following statements about the most likely diagnosis is true?

   A. Liver biopsy should be a high priority
   B. The extent of skin and gut involvement predicts a higher mortality
   C. Initial treatment in this case would be topical steroids
   D. The pathology is primarily neutrophil-driven
   E. Aggressive treatment will reduce the probability of relapsed ALL

2. A 23-year-old man with pre-B ALL who had an allogeneic stem cell transplant 1 week ago is transferred to the ICU for close monitoring with neutropenic fever and mild septic shock. He improves on antibiotics, has count recovery, and discussions begin about transferring back to the floor 5 days after ICU transfer. However, the oncologists are concerned about rising direct bilirubin (up to 8 mg/dL) associated with epigastric/RUQ pain and weight gain. RUQ ultrasound reveals hepatomegaly and ascites but does not show evidence of biliary obstruction. Which of the following is the most likely diagnosis?

   A. Ascending cholangitis
   B. Acalculous cholecystitis
   C. Acute hepatitis B
   D. Cholestasis of sepsis
   E. Hepatic sinusoidal obstruction syndrome

3. A 35-year-old woman who had an allogeneic BMT 10 years ago for pre-B ALL complicated by GVHD of the skin (controlled with topical steroids) presents to the ED with several months of worsening dyspnea. PFTs done a month ago revealed FEV1 of 24% predicted, FVC of 70% predicted, and FEV1/FVC of 0.35. She is afebrile, normotensive, and not hypoxemic but becomes severely dyspneic with mild activity. Chest X-ray is clear. High-resolution chest CT reveals mosaic perfusion and evidence of extensive air-trapping on expiratory views.

   Which of the following statements is correct?

   A. Lung biopsy is indicated
   B. Azithromycin given posttransplant is effective for prevention of this condition
   C. Lung transplantation has been reported to be an option in this type of patient
   D. Bone marrow biopsy is likely to reveal recurrent leukemia
   E. Reduced immunosuppression is indicated

4. A 58-year-old man with a new diagnosis of AML receives induction chemotherapy with cytarabine and doxorubicin on the Oncology ward. About 10 days later he develops neutropenic fever in association with worsening hypoxemic respiratory failure. A chest CT is performed (see figure that follows) and Infectious Disease and Pulmonary are consulted, with bronchoscopy performed the following day notable for friable-appearing airways but with minimal mucous. Gram stain of BAL is unrevealing. Postbronchoscopy the patient has worsening hypoxemic respiratory failure and is transferred to the ICU and intubated. Despite the administration of vancomycin, cefepime, and voriconazole, fevers persist and hypoxemia continues to worsen, requiring high levels of ventilator support. Serial plain films of the chest show progressive whiteout on the right side. Three days postintubation the patient develops massive hemoptysis and cannot be ventilated, resulting in cardiac arrest and subsequent transition to comfort measures after discussion with family.

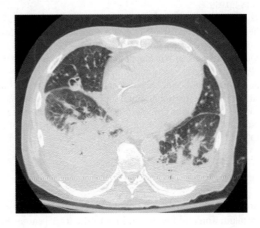

The BAL cultures are most likely to show:

A. *Staphylococcus aureus*
B. *Streptococcus pneumoniae*
C. *Pseudomonas aeruginosa*
D. *Aspergillus fumigatus*
E. Influenza A

5. A 63-year-old man develops acute respiratory failure after autologous stem cell transplant for lymphoma. His initial posttransplant course was notable for mucositis. Approximately 2.5 weeks posttransplant, following count recovery, he develops a dry cough and worsening arterial hypoxemia. Chest CT reveals diffuse ground glass opacities, and he is transferred to the ICU, given diuretics, and placed on high flow nasal cannula oxygen and broad-spectrum antibiotics. On ICU day 2 he is intubated for worsening work of breathing and fatigue. Bronchoscopy is unremarkable, and microbiologic studies of BAL including respiratory viral PCR are unrevealing. His ventilatory settings escalate despite low-tidal volume ventilation, and after another week of mechanical ventilation, his course is complicated by multiorgan failure. Care is transitioned to comfort measures only. Which of the following is the most likely diagnosis?

A. Invasive pulmonary aspergillosis (IPA)
B. *P. aeruginosa* bronchopneumonia
C. Idiopathic pneumonia syndrome
D. Acute graft-versus-host disease
E. Cardiogenic pulmonary edema

# Chapter 84 ▪ Answers

1. Correct Answer: B

**Rationale:**
The most likely diagnosis here is acute graft-versus-host disease (GVHD), a multisystem inflammatory attack on the host's tissues by the grafted immune system. Risk factors include the degree of HLA mismatch and the prophylactic regimen employed posttransplant. The pathogenesis involves T lymphocytes primarily, though neutrophils and activated macrophages contribute to a lesser extent. The most common sites of acute GVHD are the GI tract, skin,

and liver, and presentation typically occurs within the first few months of transplant. A grading system exists based on the extent of skin involvement, severity of diarrhea, and bilirubin elevations, with higher grades associated with reduced survival. Diagnosis may be made on clinical grounds along with the classic rash of GVHD (maculopapular, involving palms/soles), though biopsy of skin or the distal GI tract (typically not liver) may be performed in cases where infection is higher in the differential diagnosis. Although topical steroids may be effective in GVHD limited to the skin, for any signs of systemic involvement systemic glucocorticoids are indicated as first line treatment. Notably, intense immunosuppression over a prolonged period exposes the host to many risks, including a reduction in the graft-versus-malignancy effect that helps allogeneic stem cell recipients maintain long-term remissions.

### References

1. Kuba A, Raida L. Graft versus host disease: from basic pathogenic principles to DNA damage response and cellular senescence. *Mediators Inflamm.* 2018;2018:9451950.
2. Cahn J-Y, Klein JP, Lee SJ, et al. Prospective evaluation of 2 acute graft-versus-host (GVHD) grading systems: a joint Société Française de Greffe de Moëlle et Thérapie Cellulaire (SFGM-TC), Dana Farber Cancer Institute (DFCI), and International Bone Marrow Transplant Registry (IBMTR) prospective study. *Blood.* 2005;106:1495-1500.
3. Firoz BF, Lee SJ, Nghiem P, Qureshi AA. Role of skin biopsy to confirm suspected acute graft-vs-host disease: results of decision analysis. *Arch Dermatol.* 2006;142:175-182.
4. Ross WA, Ghosh S, Dekovich AA, et al. Endoscopic biopsy diagnosis of acute gastrointestinal graft-versus-host disease: rectosigmoid biopsies are more sensitive than upper gastrointestinal biopsies. *Am J Gastroenterol.* 2008;103:982-989.
5. Rashidi A, DiPersio JF, Sandmaier BM, Colditz GA, Weisdorf DJ. Steroids versus steroids plus additional agent in frontline treatment of acute graft-versus-host disease: a systematic review and meta-analysis of randomized trials. *Biol Blood Marrow Transplant.* 2016;22:1133-1137.

---

**2.** Correct Answer: E

**Rationale:**

Hepatic sinusoidal obstruction syndrome (SOS, also known as veno-occlusive disease) is an unusual complication of hematopoietic stem cell transplantation and involves injury to the liver venous endothelium likely from the conditioning chemotherapeutic regimen. Fibrin and factor 8 have been found in the vein walls and sinusoids, suggesting the existence of a pro-coagulant state. Risk factors include preexisting liver disease and certain chemotherapeutic agents. Most patients develop the syndrome within 3 weeks of transplant, and the clinical diagnosis is made by a combination of elevated direct bilirubin, hepatomegaly, and sudden weight gain. Important differentials to consider include Budd-Chiari, acute GVHD, viral hepatitis, and cholestatic drug reactions. Some evidence supports the use of prophylaxis with ursodiol or heparin. Management for severe disease includes the use of defibrotide, which increases plasmin activity and decreases vWF expression, though we await completion of the first phase 3 randomized controlled trial for this indication.

### References

1. Scrobohaci ML, Drouet L, Monem-Mansi A, et al. Liver veno-occlusive disease after bone marrow transplantation changes in coagulation parameters and endothelial markers. *Thromb Res.* 1991;63:509-519.
2. Carreras E, Bertz H, Arcese W, et al. Incidence and outcome of hepatic veno-occlusive disease after blood or marrow transplantation: a prospective cohort study of the European Group for Blood and Marrow Transplantation. European Group for Blood and Marrow Transplantation Chronic Leukemia Working Party. *Blood.* 1998;92:3599-3604.
3. Essell JH, Schroeder MT, Harman GS, et al. Ursodiol prophylaxis against hepatic complications of allogeneic bone marrow transplantation. A randomized, double-blind, placebo-controlled trial. *Ann Intern Med.* 1998;128:975-981.
4. Attal M, Huguet F, Rubie H, et al. Prevention of hepatic veno-occlusive disease after bone marrow transplantation by continuous infusion of low-dose heparin: a prospective, randomized trial. *Blood.* 1992;79:2834-2840.
5. Richardson PG, Riches ML, Kernan NA, et al. Phase 3 trial of defibrotide for the treatment of severe veno-occlusive disease and multi-organ failure. *Blood.* 2016;127:1656-1665.

---

**3.** Correct Answer: C

**Rationale:**

This patient suffers from postallogeneic stem cell transplant bronchiolitis obliterans syndrome (BOS) resulting from the destruction of small airways by scarring inflammation, a form of chronic GVHD in the lung. A similar disease occurs in lung transplant patients (mismatch between lung and immune system). Patients may present with symptoms of moderate to severe airflow obstruction, though many patients postallogeneic SCT have mild obstructive lung disease without symptoms. BOS is diagnosed based on new airflow obstruction (FEV1/FVC <0.7 with FEV1 <75% predicted) in the absence of acute infection, with the most specific feature on high-resolution CT of extensive air trapping. Lung biopsy is typically not pursued if imaging does not suggest an alternative diagnosis, especially if the patient has other evidence of GVHD. Although no high-quality RCT evidence exists, most clinicians prescribe inhaled glucocorticoids and beta-agonists. Unfortunately, BOS is often irreversible and lung transplantation is sometimes pursued. Extrapolating from the experience in lung transplant, some physicians used to administer azithromycin post-BMT for prophylaxis. However, a recent RCT showed harm, although there may still be a role for azithromycin in the *treatment* of newly diagnosed BOS.

## References

1. Gunn MLD, Godwin JD, Kanne JP, Flowers ME, Chien JW. High-resolution ct findings of bronchiolitis obliterans syndrome after hematopoietic stem cell transplantation. *J Thorac Imaging.* 2008;23:244-250.
2. Chien JW, Duncan S, Williams KM, Pavletic SZ. Bronchiolitis obliterans syndrome after allogeneic hematopoietic stem cell transplantation – an increasingly recognized manifestation of chronic graft-versus-host disease. *Biol Blood Marrow Transplant.* 2010;16:S106-S114.
3. Holm AM, Riise GC, Hansson L, et al. Lung transplantation for bronchiolitis obliterans syndrome after allo-SCT. *Bone Marrow Transplant.* 2013;48:703-707.
4. Bergeron A, Chevret S, Granata A, et al. Effect of azithromycin on airflow decline–free survival after allogeneic hematopoietic stem cell transplant: the ALLOZITHRO randomized clinical trial. *JAMA.* 2017;318:557-566.
5. Yadav H, Peters SG, Keogh KA, et al. Azithromycin for the Treatment of obliterative bronchiolitis after hematopoietic stem cell transplantation: a systematic review and meta-analysis. *Biol Blood Marrow Transplant.* 2016;22:2264-2269.

**4.** Correct Answer: D

**Rationale:**

The chest CT reveals a cavitary nodule, which in neutropenic patients (severely immunocompromised as in this patient who recently received cytotoxic chemotherapy) is highly concerning for a fungal infection. Although lung cavitation may be seen with bacterial infection (especially *Staph*, *Klebsiella*, *Nocardia*, and occasionally *Pseudomonas*), with such a high burden of disease Gram stain is likely to be positive and the patient would likely be producing more airway secretions than described (though notably with systemic neutropenia secretions are less purulent than in an immunocompetent host.) *A. fumigatus* is a ubiquitous mold that causes a spectrum of disease ranging from allergic airway disease to IPA as in this case. KOH stains of respiratory secretions may reveal fungal elements; however, identification of the species requires sporulation and typically takes several days. Galactomannan is a component of *Aspergillus* (and other mold) cell walls and may be tested in blood and BAL. While awaiting the definitive diagnosis of species and susceptibility, some experts recommend broadening from voriconazole to liposomal amphotericin; though with the introduction of the newer antifungal azoles posaconazole and isavuconazole, this decision should involve expert consultation. Regardless of the mold drug sensitivities, drug penetration into areas of lung destruction by angioinvasive molds is poor and mortality is very high. Notably, lung resection in cases of invasive mold disease in bone marrow transplant patients has been described.

## Reference

1. Bernard A, Caillot D, Couaillier JF, et al. Surgical management of invasive pulmonary aspergillosis in neutropenic patients. *Ann Thorac Surg.* 1997;64:1441-1447.

**5.** Correct Answer: C

**Rationale:**

Idiopathic pneumonia syndrome is a dreaded complication of hematopoietic stem cell transplantation, defined as diffuse alveolar injury in the absence of evidence of respiratory tract infection. Although the pathogenesis remains unclear, it is thought most likely to be an inflammatory reaction to the pre-transplant conditioning regimen, which may involve high-dose chemotherapy and radiotherapy. Differential considerations include viral pneumonia and diffuse alveolar hemorrhage. Many clinicians administer high-dose steroids; etanercept (TNF-alpha inhibitor) has also been studied, though no high quality evidence exists to support either treatment and the prognosis remains very poor. This patient had an autologous stem cell transplant and so cannot have developed GVHD. Infectious causes are possible despite the negative workup (eg, a viral pathogen not tested for with multiplex PCR), but fungal and bacterial infections are unlikely given the imaging and unrevealing BAL.

## References

1. Clark JG, Hansen JA, Hertz MI, et al. NHLBI workshop summary. Idiopathic pneumonia syndrome after bone marrow transplantation. *Am Rev Respir Dis.* 1993;147:1601-1606.
2. Panoskaltsis-Mortari A, Griese M, Madtes DK, et al. An official American Thoracic Society research statement: noninfectious lung injury after hematopoietic stem cell transplantation: idiopathic pneumonia syndrome. *Am J Respir Crit Care Med.* 2011;183:1262-1279.
3. Yanik GA, Horowitz MM, Weisdorf DJ, et al. Randomized, double-blind, placebo-controlled trial of soluble tumor necrosis factor receptor: enbrel (etanercept) for the treatment of idiopathic pneumonia syndrome after allogeneic stem cell transplantation: blood and marrow transplant clinical trials network protocol. *Biol Blood Marrow Transplant.* 2014;20:858-864.

# 85

# COMPLICATIONS OF IMMUNOSUPPRESSIVE DRUGS AND CHEMOTHERAPY

Jeffrey Gotts

1. Which of the following statements about glucocorticoid toxicity is incorrect?

   A. Effects on the eye include cataracts and glaucoma
   B. Gastritis and ulcers resulting from glucocorticoids are much more common in patients also taking NSAIDs
   C. Immune suppression is dose-dependent
   D. Steroid-induced psychosis should prompt a gradual taper
   E. A patient taking 8 mg of prednisone a day may be at risk for HPA axis suppression

2. Which of the following statements about methotrexate toxicity is correct?

   A. Folate supplementation prevents pulmonary toxicity
   B. Approximately 15% of patients may experience an erythematous morbilliform drug rash
   C. Hepatotoxicity is not a significant concern
   D. The drug is primarily metabolized by the liver
   E. Leucovorin is typically administered 72 to 96 hours after high-dose methotrexate

3. A 52-year-old woman with a history of depression, diabetes, and hypertension, and who has had kidney transplantation 1.5 years ago, presents to the ED with confusion. Laboratory test results (with recent baseline) are notable for Cr 2.4 mg/dL (0.8 mg/dL), platelet count 35 k/mm³ (240 k/mm³), and hemoglobin 7 g/dL (11 g/dL). LDH is elevated at 1,600, and peripheral smear reveals reticulocytosis and evidence of schistocytes. UA shows mild protein but >50 WBC/hpf.

   Which of the following medications is the most likely culprit?

   A. Amlodipine
   B. Lexapro
   C. Metoprolol
   D. Insulin
   E. Sirolimus

4. Which of the following side effects is not commonly associated with tacrolimus?

   A. Nephrotoxicity
   B. Glucose intolerance
   C. Neurotoxicity
   D. Adrenal insufficiency
   E. Increased likelihood of squamous cell cancer

**5.** A 63-year-old man with multiple myeloma is admitted to the ICU with neutropenic fever following melphalan treatment in advance of autologous stem cell treatment. Which of the following toxicities are not commonly associated with alkylating agents?

    **A.** Enterocolitis
    **B.** Pancytopenia
    **C.** Elevated transaminases
    **D.** Mucositis
    **E.** Cardiac toxicity

# Chapter 85 ▪ Answers

**1.** Correct Answer: D

**Rationale:**

Glucocorticoids have widespread effects on a diverse array of tissue types. Ophthalmologic effects include cataracts and increased intraocular pressure. GI effects include gastritis and ulcer formation and occur synergistically with NSAIDs. Glucocorticoids exert broad immunosuppressive effects on both innate and adaptive immunity in a dose-dependent manner. Psychiatric effects range from confusion to psychosis. Serious psychiatric effects occur in approximately 6% of patients, with the most important risk factor being the steroid dose, though notably the dose is not predictive of the time of onset, type, or duration of symptoms. Treatment of steroid psychosis involves expedited dose reduction when possible and the use of antipsychotic medications as needed. Hypothalamic-pituitary axis suppression is unlikely when patients have received less than 5 mg of prednisone daily for any length of time, likely when patients have received more than 20 mg of prednisone daily for 3 or more weeks, and otherwise is uncertain.

References

1. Skalka HW, Prchal JT. Effect of corticosteroids on cataract formation. *Arch Ophthalmol.* 1980;98:1773-1777.
2. Tripathi RC, Parapuram SK, Tripathi BJ, Zhong Y, Chalam KV. Corticosteroids and glaucoma risk. *Drugs Aging.* 1999;15:439-450.
3. Piper JM, Ray WA, Daugherty JR, Griffin MR. Corticosteroid use and peptic ulcer disease: role of nonsteroidal anti-inflammatory drugs. *Ann Intern Med.* 1991;114:735-740.
4. Franchimont D. Overview of the actions of glucocorticoids on the immune response: a good model to characterize new pathways of immunosuppression for new treatment strategies. *Ann N Y Acad Sci.* 2004;1024:124-137.
5. Dubovsky AN, Arvikar S, Stern TA, Axelrod L. The neuropsychiatric complications of glucocorticoid use: steroid psychosis revisited. *Psychosomatics.* 2012;53:103-115.
6. Ross DA, Cetas JS. Steroid psychosis: a review for neurosurgeons. *J Neurooncol.* 2012;109:439-447.
7. Broersen LHA, Pereira AM, Jørgensen JOL, Dekkers OM. Adrenal insufficiency in corticosteroids use: systematic review and meta-analysis. *J Clin Endocrinol Metab.* 2015;100:2171-2180.

**2.** Correct Answer: B

**Rationale:**

Rapidly dividing cells require high amounts of folates for DNA synthesis. Methotrexate competitively inhibits an enzyme that reduces folate derivatives into molecules suitable for thymidine synthesis, thus preferentially affecting cells in s-phase. Up to 90% of methotrexate is excreted unchanged in the urine. Leucovorin is a reduced folate that bypasses the enzyme inhibited by methotrexate and can rescue cells that have not suffered severe DNA damage from high-dose methotrexate. To be effective, leucovorin must be initiated approximately 24 to 36 hours after methotrexate. In one study, up to 16% of patients receiving high-dose methotrexate develop an erythematous rash. Hepatotoxicity ranging from asymptomatic elevations in transaminases to cirrhosis can occur with high- or low-dose methotrexate, and alcohol and other hepatotoxic medications should be avoided. Similarly, pulmonary toxicity that typically takes the form of hypersensitivity pneumonitis may occur with low-dose chronic use of methotrexate or after high doses of the drug, in which case leucovorin does not appear to reduce the risk.

References

1. Howard SC, McCormick J, Pui C-H, Buddington RK, Harvey RD. Preventing and managing toxicities of high-dose methotrexate. *Oncologist.* 2016;21:1471-1482.
2. Hansen HH, Selawry OS, Holland JF, McCall CB. The variability of individual tolerance to methotrexate in cancer patients. *Br J Cancer.* 1971;25:298-305.
3. Bath RK, Brar NK, Forouhar FA, Wu GY. A review of methotrexate-associated hepatotoxicity. *J Dig Dis.* 2014;15:517-524.
4. Lateef O, Shakoor N, Balk RA. Methotrexate pulmonary toxicity. *Expert Opin Drug Saf.* 2005;4:723-730.

**3.** Correct Answer: E

**Rationale:**

This patient is presenting with evidence of a thrombotic microangiopathy, most likely hemolytic uremic syndrome (HUS). HUS following organ transplantation is commonly due to calcineurin inhibitors (cyclosporine, tacrolimus) and/or mTOR inhibitors (sirolimus, everolimus).

Reference

1. Langer RM, Van Buren CT, Katz SM, Kahan BD. De novo hemolytic uremic syndrome after kidney transplantation in patients treated with cyclosporine a sirolimus combination. *Transplant Proc.* 2001;33:3236-3237.

**4.** Correct Answer: D

**Rationale:**

The calcineurin inhibitors cyclosporine and tacrolimus impair the transcription of interleukin-2 and other T cell cytokines. Both drugs exhibit multiple organ toxicities but not adrenal insufficiency. In addition to A-C and E above, these drugs are associated with hypertension, hyperkalemia, hyperlipidemia, infections, nausea/vomiting, and an increased risk of posttransplant lymphoproliferative disorder.

Reference

1. Magnasco A, Rossi A, Catarsi P, et al. Cyclosporin and organ specific toxicity: clinical aspects, pharmacogenetics and perspectives. *Curr Clin Pharmacol.* 2008;3:166-173.

**5.** Correct Answer: E

**Rationale:**

Alkylating agents include a broad array of chemically diverse drugs that cause cross-linking of DNA in all cells, but have their greatest effect in rapidly dividing cells. Common side effects include pancytopenia, infertility, mucosal injury, alopecia, and increased risk of malignancy. Less common toxicities include hepatic veno-occlusive disease (hepatomegaly, RUQ pain, jaundice, and ascites), pulmonary fibrosis, and hemorrhagic cystitis. Cardiac toxicity occurs but is rare in comparison to the anthracyclines. The dose-limiting toxicity of the alkylating agents is to the bone marrow, with the nadir of neutropenia between 8 and 16 days postadministration followed by recovery at approximately 21 days.

References

1. Colvin M. *Alkylating agents. Holland-Frei Cancer Medicine.* 6th ed. 2003.
2. Chatterjee K, Zhang J, Honbo N, Karliner JS. Doxorubicin Cardiomyopathy. *Cardiology.* 2010;115:155-162.

# GASTROINTESTINAL, NUTRITION AND GENITOURINARY DISORDERS

# 86

# ESOPHAGUS

Irfan Qureshi and Yuk Ming Liu

1. A 65-year-old man with a history of reflux disease experiences chest discomfort after undergoing an upper endoscopy for surveillance. The patient is hemodynamically stable and a gastrografin esophagram confirms a small contained perforation in the mid esophagus with minimal contamination in the mediastinum. The most appropriate initial therapy consists of:

   A. Thoracotomy with primary repair and appropriate drainage
   B. Esophagectomy with immediate reconstruction
   C. Esophageal stent placement
   D. Diversion cervical esophagostomy

2. A 70-year-old woman undergoes upper endoscopy, which reveals a distal esophageal mass. Biopsy of the mass confirms adenocarcinoma with invasion into the mucularis propria. Whole body PET scan shows the distal esophageal mass with no lymphadenopathy and no distal metastases. Which statement regarding treatment with chemoradiation therapy is most correct for this patient?

   A. Preoperative chemoradiation increases postoperative mortality.
   B. Preoperative chemoradiation before surgical resection improves survival compared to surgery alone.
   C. Preoperative radiation in addition to chemotherapy improves survival.
   D. Preoperative chemoradiation commonly results in esophageal perforation.

3. A 60-year-old male with a history of coronary artery disease and Barrett disease completes a surveillance upper endoscopy. A 1-cm flat plaque is identified with pathology confirming low-grade dysplasia (LGD). Endoscopic ultrasound shows no lymphadenopathy and the tumor is confined to the mucosa. What is an appropriate next step in treatment?

   A. Photodynamic therapy
   B. Neoadjuvant chemotherapy
   C. Transhiatal esophagectomy
   D. Repeat endoscopic surveillance with biopsy in 1 year

4. A 40-year-old man with a history of gastroesophageal reflux disease (GERD) undergoes esophageal sampling for Barrett esophagus (BE). An increase in the presence of which biomarker would indicate the presence of this condition?

   A. Trefoil factor 1 (TFF1)
   B. Fructose-bisphosphatase 1 (FBP1)
   C. Forkhead box A3 (FOXA3)
   D. Trefoil factor 3 (TFF3)
   E. Flavin-containing monooxygenase 5 (FMO5)

**5.** A 60-year-old man with a history of heart failure with reduced ejection fraction (HFrEF), chronic obstructive pulmonary disease (COPD) requiring home oxygen, and GERD presents with dysphagia of solid and liquid foods, which has worsened over the last year. An esophagogastroduodenoscopy (EGD) is performed is performed, which reveals normal esophageal mucosa with negative biopsy results. High-resolution manometry reveals an integrated relaxation pressure of 20 mm Hg and a distal contractile integral (DCI <100 mm Hg/s/cm) of 100%. Esophagram demonstrates a dilated esophagus with poor emptying of barium. Which of the following therapies would be the most appropriate for this patient?

**A.** Nissen fundoplication
**B.** Botulinum toxin injection
**C.** Esophageal pneumatic dilation (PD)
**D.** Peroral endoscopic myotomy (POEM)

# Chapter 86 ▪ Answers

---

**1.** Correct Answer: C

**Rationale:**
Iatrogenic esophageal perforation can be a catastrophic complication of upper endoscopy. The incidence of perforation due to rigid endoscopy approaches 0.1% to 0.4% while that of flexible endoscopy varies from 0.01% to 0.06%. Perforation rates increase when additional interventions are performed such as balloon dilation. The timing of perforation is critical in managing the morbidity and mortality of this complication. Initial operative mortality rates approach 12% to 50%; however, a delay in management of 12 to 24 hours can significantly increase morbidity and mortality. The postoperative suture breakdown rate can reach 50% if repair is delayed beyond 24 hours.

Treatment of esophageal perforation requires multimodal therapy with intravenous antibiotics, nothing per mouth (NPO), isolating the area of the leak, and providing adequate nutrition either enterally via gastrostomy or intravenous therapy. Blind nasogastric tube insertion is discouraged as it may further damage the injured esophagus.

Hemodynamically stable patients with a contained perforation can be treated endoscopically with the placement of an esophageal stent to contain the leak and prevent further contamination. Depending on the location of the esophageal perforation, success rates with stent placement approach 80% to 90% in some series, allowing healing of the injured esophagus. Furthermore, stenting carries the lowest morbidity and mortality of all options available for treatment of esophageal perforation, challenging the old dogmatic teaching of primary repair as the "gold standard."

References
1. Fischer A, Thomusch O, Benz S, von Dobschuetz E, Baier P, Hopt UT. Nonoperative treatment of 15 benign esophageal perforations with self-expandable covered metal stents. *Ann Thorac Surg.* 2006;81:467-472.
2. Dasari BV, Neely D, Kennedy A, et al. The role of esophageal stents in the management of esophageal anastomotic leaks and benign esophageal perforations. *Ann Surg.* 2014;259:852-860.

---

**2.** Correct Answer: C

**Rationale:**
Esophageal adenocarcinoma (EA) is a highly lethal disease with a 5-year survival rate of approximately 10%. The ideal timing, treatment sequence, and dose of therapy remain an active area of investigation and controversy. Multiple studies have shown improved outcomes with the addition of neoadjuvant chemoradiation before surgical resection. This form of treatment has now become the standard approach in Europe and the United States for patients with locally advanced disease such as this patient with stage II disease (T2, N0, M0).

No current studies have definitively shown that the addition of radiation to chemotherapy improves overall survival over chemotherapy alone. Chemotherapy and radiation are each active against different forms of the cancer cell population with chemotherapy most effective against micrometastatic disease and radiation targeting the locoregional tumor mass. Esophageal perforation is a rare event after neoadjuvant chemoradiation occurring in less than 0.5% of patients evaluated.

References
1. Van Hagen P, Hulshof MC, van Lanschot JJ, et al. Preoperative chemoradiotherapy for esophageal or junction cancer. *N Engl J Med.* 2012;366:2074-2084.
2. Shapiro J, van Lanschot JJB, Hulshhof MCCM, et al. Neoadjuvant chemoradiotherapy plus surgery versus surgery alone for esophageal or junctional cancer (CROSS): long-term results of a randomized controlled trial. *Lancet Oncol.* 2015;16:1090-1098.
3. Swisher SG, Hofstetter W, Komaki R, et al. Improved long-term outcome with chemoradiotherapy strategies in esophageal cancer. *Ann Thorac Surg.* 2010;90:892-898; discussion 898-9.

**3.** Correct Answer: D

**Rationale:**

BE is a premalignant condition with an increased risk of developing EA. Dysplasia continues to be the best clinically available marker of malignancy risk in patients with BE. In fact, the risk of progression for patients with nondysplasia is 0.2% to 0.5% per year but increases to 0.7% for patients afflicted with LGD and 7% in high-grade dysplasia. Definitive diagnosis of dysplasia can be challenging with slight variations in the interpretation of "indefinite for dysplasia" and LGD and thus requiring verification from a second pathologist with expertise in BE for confirmation of dysplasia. Patients with LGD should receive aggressive antisecretory therapy for reflux disease with a proton pump inhibitor to decrease changes associated with inflammation.

Current guidelines for management of LGD recommend annual surveillance with a protocol of four-quadrant biopsies at 1 cm intervals until two examinations in a row are negative for dysplasia, after which time surveillance intervals for nondysplastic BE can be followed. Six-month interval surveillance is advised for those with a diagnosis of "indefinite for dysplasia" who require further confirmation.

All other therapies are reserved for a locally advanced symptomatic disease rather than a tumor confined to the mucosa (Tis, N0, M0).

### References

1. Kerkhof M, Van Dekken H, Steyerberg EW, et al. Grading of dysplasia in Barrett's oesophagus: substantial interobserver variation between general and gastrointestinal pathologists. *Histopathology*. 2007;50:920-927.
2. Shaheen NJ, Falk GW, Iyer PG, et al. ACG clinical guideline: diagnosis and management of Barrett's esophagus. *Am J Gastroenterol*. 2015;111:30-50.

**4.** Correct Answer: D

**Rationale:**

BE is defined as intestinal metaplasia from squamous to columnar epithelium and is a risk factor for the development of EA. However, the majority of EA occurs de novo, and the prevalence of BE is reported to be between 1% and 8% calling into question the cost-effectiveness of routine endoscopy screening programs. Consequently, nonendoscopic methods for screening are also being employed. One method uses a device called a capsule sponge combined with an immunohistochemical biomarker (TFF3). The patient ingests the capsule that is attached to a string and contains a compressed mesh. The mesh is exposed when the gelatin capsule dissolves in the stomach. The mesh is then withdrawn through the esophagus where it collects samples of the cells lining the esophageal lumen. The biomarker is then used to differentiate Barrett epithelial cells from gastric columnar and esophageal squamous cells. An increase in the biomarker trefoil factor indicates an increase in columnar epithelium with intestinal metaplasia compared to normal esophagus. The expression of the biomarkers TFF1, FBP1, FMO5, and FOXA3 is increased in BE, but the levels are similar to those observed in the gastric mucosa.

### References

1. Pera M. Trends in incidence and prevalence of specialized intestinal metaplasia, Barrett's esophagus, and adenocarcinoma of the gastroesophageal junction. *World J Surg*. 2003;27:999-1006.
2. Lao-Sirieix P, Boussioutas A, Kadri SR, et al. Non-endoscopic screening biomarkers for Barrett's esophagus: from microarray analysis to the clinic. *Gut*. 2009;58:1451-1459.

**5.** Correct Answer: C

**Rationale:**

Achalasia is a primary esophageal disorder with a pathologic consequence of degeneration of ganglion cells in the myenteric plexus of the esophageal body and the lower esophageal sphincter (LES) of unknown etiology. The degeneration leads to insufficient relaxation of the LES. Esophagraphy typically reveals esophageal aperistalsis with proximal dilation and minimal LES opening resulting in a "bird's beak" appearance. At present, achalasia is incurable and management consists of palliation of symptoms. In patients who are felt to be good surgical candidates, laparoscopic myotomy with partial fundoplication is an effective strategy for long-term resolution of symptoms. However, in patients who are high-risk surgical candidates, initial treatment with graded PD is recommended. A prospective randomized multicenter European trial comparing graded PD to surgical myotomy in 200 patients revealed no difference in success rate after 2 years of follow-up (92% for PD vs 87% for surgical myotomy).

Complete 360-degree fundoplication would exacerbate the symptoms of dysphagia and is not an appropriate intervention for achalasia. Botulinum toxin is an attractive and user-friendly approach which interrupts the release of acetylcholine from presynaptic vesicles causing an interruption of a neurogenic component but has no effect on the myogenic component of the LES. Although the initial 1-month response rate is close to 75%, the therapeutic effect wears off and approximately 50% of patients relapse and require repeat treatment at 6- to 24-month intervals. POEM is a novel method of endoluminal myotomy performed by traversing the esophageal mucosa. Although the technique is promising, it requires advanced endoscopic skills. In addition, POEM has been shown in 50% of patients to promote further acid reflux.

## References

1. Vaezi MF, Richter JE. Diagnosis and management of achalasia. American College of Gastroenterology Practice Parameter Committee. *Am J Gastroenterol*. 1999;94:3406-3412.
2. Boeckxstaens GE, Annese V, des Varannes SB, et al.Pneumatic dilation versus laparoscopic Heller's myotomy for idiopathic achalasia. *N Engl J Med*. 2011;364:1807-1816.
3. Annese V, Bassotti G, Coccia G, et al. A multicentre randomised study of intrasphincteric botulinum toxin in patients with esophageal achalasia. GISMAD Achalasia Study Group. *Gut*. 2000;46:597-600.

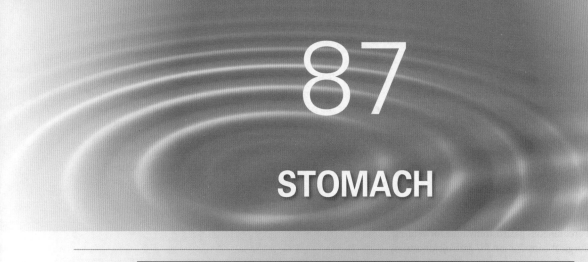

# STOMACH

Margaret R. Connolly and Peter Fagenholz

1. A 65-year-old woman with a history of smoking and osteoarthritis is recovering well after a cosmetic plastic surgery procedure. On postoperative day 2 she has resumed her home medications including daily aspirin and is being prepared for discharge; however, she becomes newly hypotensive. She is transferred to the ICU with 1 L of normal saline infusing and a blood pressure of 92/60 mm Hg with heart rate 118 beats/min. She is pale, diaphoretic, and agitated. Her incision is clean and dry. Her laboratory test results on arrival to the ICU are notable for Hgb 6.5 mg/dL from 12 mg/dL, last checked two days prior. She then has an episode of hematemesis and her blood pressure drops to 70/40 mm Hg. Transfusion of packed red blood cells is initiated. Which of the following is the **MOST** appropriate next step in management of this patient?

   A. STAT CT angiogram of the abdomen
   B. Interventional radiology consultation for possible angioembolization
   C. Urgent surgical exploration
   D. Upper GI endoscopy
   E. PRBC transfusion to Hgb ≥10 with no further intervention

2. A 25-year-old man is the unrestrained driver in a head-on motor vehicle collision. He arrives with a Glasgow Coma Score of 5 and is intubated in the trauma bay. CT head demonstrates skull fractures with subdural and subarachnoid hemorrhage requiring craniotomy. Postoperatively he is admitted to the ICU intubated and sedated. On postoperative day 6 his nurse notices that his orogastric tube aspirate has become red-brown with coffee-ground appearance. What is the **BEST** way to avoid this complication?

   A. Avoid prophylactic heparin
   B. Avoid gastric tube placement
   C. Administer an H2 blocker or proton pump inhibitor
   D. Administer *Helicobacter pylori* treatment
   E. Avoid enteral nutrition

3. A 65-year-old man with a history of hypertension, GERD, and chronic low back pain presents with vague chest pain. He takes oxycodone, gabapentin, and ibuprofen daily. He is admitted for observation and cardiac workup. EKG shows nonspecific T-wave changes and laboratory test results are unremarkable. On hospital day 2 he has sudden acute onset abdominal pain with temperature 100.5°F, heart rate 122/min, blood pressure 85/60 mm Hg, respiratory rate 30/min, SpO$_2$ 95% on room air. His abdomen is distended with tap tenderness and guarding on mild palpation in all four quadrants. Upright chest X-ray demonstrates free air under the diaphragm. Which of the following is the **MOST** appropriate next step in management?

   A. Repeat EKG and troponins
   B. Obtain CT abdomen with IV and PO contrast
   C. Place NGT and perform serial abdominal examinations
   D. Consult gastroenterology for endoscopic evaluation
   E. Consult surgery for exploratory laparotomy

**4.** A 55-year-old man with hypertension, anxiety, and type 1 diabetes mellitus recently adjusted his medication regimen and began taking clonidine. He presents now with abdominal pain and nausea. This has been associated with occasional episodes of emesis of gastric contents over the past few weeks. His weight is unchanged. His vital signs are within normal limits. On physical examination, his abdomen is distended with moderate tenderness in the epigastrium, but no rebound or guarding. His electrolytes are unremarkable and his finger stick glucose is 350 mg/dL. Upper endoscopy and CT scan show large amount of gastric contents with no evidence of mechanical obstruction. In addition to reviewing his medication list, what is the BEST next step in caring for this patient?

**A.** Nasogastric decompression
**B.** Dietary modification and optimization of glycemic control
**C.** PPI treatment
**D.** Percutaneous gastrostomy tube for venting
**E.** Surgical consultation for gastrojejunostomy

# Chapter 87 ▪ Answer

**1.** Correct Answer: D

**Rationale:**

This patient with hematemesis became hemodynamically unstable because of an upper GI bleed. Smoking, aspirin, and NSAID use (common in patients with osteoarthritis) are among the most important risk factors for peptic ulcer disease (PUD), and in this case the patient likely has an acute bleed from an ulcer. Up to 50% of peptic ulcers are asymptomatic until bleeding occurs, which may present as hematemesis or melena.

Upper GI endoscopy is the gold standard for diagnosis of PUD and the first-line therapy for bleeding ulcers. This should be performed urgently in the hemodynamically unstable patient as it allows for both diagnosis and treatment (clipping, cautery, or injection of a bleeding vessel). CT angiogram of the abdomen may identify a source of bleeding; however, it is less sensitive than endoscopy for identifying a source of bleeding and does not allow therapeutic intervention. Surgical exploration is associated with a higher risk of complications than endoscopic management and so should not be pursued initially. Angiographic embolization is an alternative to repeat endoscopy or surgical intervention but does not replace the initial endoscopic management of upper GI bleed and may have a higher risk of rebleeding than surgery.

Intravenous fluid resuscitation and transfusion of blood products are essential in the early management of this patient with hypotension and evidence of bleeding. Although resuscitation goals for acute upper GI bleeding vary, restrictive strategies recommend transfusion for hemoglobin <7.0 mg/dL. Transfusion to higher hemoglobin goals (>10 mg/dL) is associated with higher rates of mortality and rebleeding and therefore not recommended (E).

### References

1. Li LF, Chan RL, Lu L, et al. Cigarette smoking and gastrointestinal diseases: the causal relationship and underlying molecular mechanisms (review). *Int J Mol Med.* 2014;34:372-380.
2. Lanas A, Chan FKI. Peptic ulcer disease. *Lancet.* 2017;390:613-624.
3. Villanueva C, Colomo A, Bosch A, et al. Transfusion strategies for acute upper gastrointestinal bleeding. *N Engl J Med.* 2013;368:11-21.
4. Lau JY, Barkun A, Fan DM, Kuipers EJ, Yang YS, Chan FK. Challenges in the management of acute peptic ulcer bleeding. *Lancet.* 2013;381:2033-2043.

**2.** Correct Answer: C

**Rationale:**

This patient is critically ill with traumatic brain injury and has been intubated for over 48 hours. Greater than 40% of mechanically ventilated patients may develop evidence of GI bleeding. Traumatic brain or spinal cord injury has also been associated with stress ulcer development. Stress ulcers are generally attributed to an imbalance in mucosal protection and gastric acid production. There is not clear evidence for superiority of histamine H2-receptor antagonists versus proton pump inhibitors for stress ulcer prophylaxis and either may be used. The use of prophylactic heparin is not associated with an increased risk of upper GI bleeding. Critically ill intubated patients frequently require gastric decompression and/or enteral feeding access, and orogastric tube is a reasonable choice. Early enteral feeding is protective against stress ulcer development, and in addition provides nutritional support necessary in critically ill patients, and should not be withheld. Although *H. pylori* may contribute to stress ulcer development, there is nothing to suggest that this patient has a peptic ulcer related to *H. pylori* infection, and he should not be treated prophylactically.

References

1. Cook DJ, Fuller HD, Guyatt GH, et al. Risk factors for gastrointestinal bleeding in critically ill patients. *N Engl J Med.* 1994;330:377-381.
2. Chu Y, Jiang Y, Meng M, et al. Incidence and risk factors of gastrointestinal bleeding in mechanically ventilated patients. *World J Emerg Med.* 2010;1(1):32-36.
3. Toews I, George AT, Peter JV, et al. Interventions for preventing upper gastrointestinal bleeding in people admitted to intensive care units. *Cochrane Database Syst Rev.* 2018;6:CD008687.
4. Maury E, Tankovic J, Ebel A, Offenstadt G. An observational study of upper gastrointestinal bleeding in intensive care units: is Helicobacter pylori the culprit? *Crit Care Med.* 2005;33(7):1513-1518.

**3.** Correct Answer: E

**Rationale:**

This patient's chronic NSAID use puts him at risk of developing PUD. Patients with PUD may be asymptomatic or have a history of dyspepsia. Nearly half of patients with PUD also experience acid regurgitation symptoms. This patient's presenting complaint was chest pain, but his cardiac workup is unremarkable. Acid reflux and epigastric pain are frequently confused with chest pain, as was likely in this case. When the patient subsequently developed acute abdominal pain with hypotension, peritoneal signs, and evidence of free air, a perforated ulcer should be high on the differential. Repeating the cardiac workup would delay care and potentially have distracting findings related to cardiac demand. With free air on upright chest X-ray, taking a hemodynamically unstable patient to the CT scanner is an unnecessary delay. Similarly, monitoring him with serial abdominal examinations would be unsafe. Although upper endoscopy is the most accurate diagnostic test for PUD with up to 90% sensitivity in detecting a lesion, in this unstable patient, it would not allow for definitive management of his perforated ulcer. This patient needs a surgical consultation for identification and repair of his perforated peptic ulcer.

References

1. Barkun A, Leontiadis G. Systematic review of the symptom burden, quality of life impairment and costs associated with peptic ulcer disease. *Am J Med.* 2010;123:358-366.
2. Solis CV, Chang Y, DeMoya MA, Velmahos GC, Fagenholz PJ. Free air on plain film: do we need a computed tomography too? *J Emerg Trauma Shock.* 2014;7(1):3-8.

**4.** Correct Answer: B

**Rationale:**

Gastroparesis, or delayed gastric emptying, is the motility disorder in which food remains in the stomach for a prolonged period of time. This typically presents with postprandial fullness, nausea, vomiting, pain, and/or bloating. It may be due to a variety of factors. Medications that prolong gastric emptying include alpha-2-adrenergic agonists (such as clonidine, which this patient is taking), narcotics, calcium channel blockers, tricyclic antidepressants, and incretin-based diabetes medications. Diabetes mellitus is also a risk factor for gastroparesis, with type 1 diabetics at greater risk than type 2. Once mechanical obstruction has been ruled out, the first-line therapy in gastroparesis is dietary modification and optimization of glycemic control. Large meals and foods high in fat or fiber should be avoided. In this patient, there is no mechanical obstruction and there is no current complaint of emesis, making nasogastric decompression unnecessary. Similarly, there is no mention of ulcerative disease on his endoscopy and therefore no indication for proton pump inhibitors. Gastrostomy tube is very rarely indicated in gastroparesis, and certainly not in this patient with recent onset of mild symptoms who has not yet tried lifestyle or medical management. Gastrojejunostomy can be used to bypass a mechanical gastric outlet obstruction but will not improve the motility of the stomach.

References

1. Choung RS, Locke GR, Schleck CD, Zinsmeister AR, Melton LJ, Talley NJ. Risk of gastroparesis in subjects with type 1 and 2 diabetes in the general population. *Am J Gastroenterol.* 2012;107(1):82-88.
2. Camilleri M, Parkman HP, Shafi MA, Abell TL, Gerson L. Clinical guideline: management of gastroparesis. *Am J Gastroenterol.* 2013;108(1):18-38.

# 88

# SMALL INTESTINE

Lydia R. Maurer and Peter Fagenholz

1. A 50-year-old man with a history of hypertension, active smoking, and a laparoscopic Roux-en-Y gastric bypass 5 years prior presents to the emergency department with 4 weeks of upper abdominal pain that acutely worsened on the morning of presentation. He is toxic appearing, temperature 100°F, heart rate 120/min, blood pressure 90/50 mm Hg, respiratory rate 25/min, oxygen saturation 98% on room air. His abdomen is diffusely tender and he is guarding. He has WBC 20,000/mm³, Hgb 12 mg/dL, and lactate 4 mg/dL. Blood cultures are sent and broad-spectrum antibiotics administered. A CT scan shows a moderate amount of free fluid in the upper abdomen. What is the BEST definitive management of this patient?

   A. Admission to the intensive care unit for serial abdominal examinations and intravenous antibiotics
   B. Nasogastric tube placement
   C. Consult to gastroenterology for urgent endoscopy
   D. Urgent operation
   E. Consult to interventional radiology for angioembolization

2. A 66-year-old man presents to the emergency department with melanotic stools, dizziness, and hypotension. He is admitted to the ICU, his hemoglobin and blood pressure normalize after three units of packed red blood cells, and his melena slows down. Upper GI endoscopy and colonoscopy are performed, which do not show any source of bleeding. Shortly thereafter he develops more melena and a drop in hemoglobin. A repeat endoscopy, tagged RBC study, and CT angiogram all fail to identify a bleeding source, but hemoglobin again normalizes with two more units of packed red blood cells. The following day he again develops hematochezia, with a worsening transfusion requirement and associated hypotension. Which of the following is the next best step to managing this bleeding?

   A. Continued transfusion, hold subcutaneous heparin, observe
   B. Repeat tagged RBC study
   C. Mesenteric angiogram
   D. Urgent exploratory laparotomy
   E. Video capsule endoscopy (VCE)

3. A 75-year-old woman presents to the emergency department with perforated diverticulitis and undergoes emergent surgery in which there is diffused fecal contamination. She is admitted to the ICU postoperatively, where she remains on broad-spectrum antibiotics and is hemodynamically stable. She is started on clear liquids on postoperative day 2. On postoperative day 4 her abdomen is distended, and she is vomiting and has no ostomy output. An abdominal X-ray shows diffusely dilated loops of small bowel. What is the best next step in management of this patient?

   A. Nasogastric tube placement
   B. Urgent surgical re-exploration
   C. Mineral oil enema
   D. Initiate pro-motility agents and antiemetics
   E. GI consult for EGD

4. A 34-year-old man with a history of Crohn disease presents with foul-smelling drainage from his abdominal wall. He has experienced malaise and poor oral intake over the preceding 3 weeks and had been having worsening abdominal pain for 5 days. In the last 3 days, he noticed swelling of his abdominal wall superior to his umbilicus, in an area that began to drain foul-smelling, greenish drainage. The area has become erythematous and very tender. The drainage has increased in volume over the past 24 hours to the point that it saturates his clothes, and he has started to develop fevers, chills, and dark urine. On arrival he has the following vitals: temperature 102°F, heart rate 110 beats/min, blood pressure 95/50 mm Hg, respiratory rate 18/min, and oxygen saturation 98% on room air. A CT scan shows oral contrast extravasation from the small bowel that exits at the site of drainage, but no drainable fluid collection in the abdominal wall. Which is the most appropriate management at this time?

**A.** Take the patient to the OR urgently for exploratory laparotomy
**B.** Start broad spectrum antibiotics, monitor fluid and electrolyte status closely, nutritional support
**C.** Perform incision and drainage at the bedside
**D.** Percutaneous jejunostomy tube placement, initiate tube feeding
**E.** Consult gastroenterology for endoscopy

# Chapter 88 ▪ Answers

1. Correct Answer: D

**Rationale:**
The patient in this scenario has a perforated marginal ulcer. A marginal ulcer is a known complication of Roux-en-Y gastric bypass surgery at the anastomosis between the gastric pouch and the jejunum. An ulcer is usually formed on the jejunal side, and the greatest risk factor for marginal ulcer formation is smoking. As with all patients who present with intestinal perforation, a perforated marginal ulcer must be recognized promptly. As in this situation, patients with intestinal perforation may not present with the classic finding of "free air" on CT scan or abdominal X-ray. Instead, they may have free fluid or fat stranding. In patients who present with peritonitis and manifest the hemodynamic effects of sepsis, even with more subtle CT findings, clinical suspicion for perforation must be high and these patients should be taken to the operating room urgently.

In this case, the patient has peritonitis and is septic, and solely admission to the ICU with serial examinations and antibiotics is not appropriate in the absence of operative intervention. Although nasogastric tube placement is reasonable, this is not sufficient to treat the underlying problem of a perforation. Endoscopy is appropriate for outpatient evaluation of a suspected marginal ulcer in a patient with occult anemia or pain, but it is not indicated in the setting of perforation. Finally, while the patient is tachycardic, she has no melena or hematochezia to suggest that she is bleeding. Although marginal ulcers can present with bleeding, particularly in patients on anticoagulation, those patients generally do not also present with peritonitis. Because this patient is not bleeding, a consult to interventional radiology for angioembolization would not be helpful.

References
1. Coblijn UK, Goucham AB, Lagarde SM, et al. Development of ulcer disease after Roux-en-Y gastric bypass, incidence, risk factors, and patient presentation: a systematic review. *Obes Surg.* 2014;24:299-309.
2. Wendling MR, Linn JG, Keplinger KM, et al. Omental patch repair effectively treats perforated marginal ulcer following Roux-en-Y gastric bypass. *Surg Endosc.* 2013;27:384-389.

2. Correct Answer: C

**Rationale:**
The general approach to GI bleeding should start with the ABCs, including confirming that the patient has large bore IV access and is in the appropriate clinical setting for close hemodynamic monitoring. Evaluation should begin with upper GI endoscopy and colonoscopy. When these tests are negative, it is possible that (1) the site of bleeding is located between the ligament of Treitz and the ileocecal valve, and thus not visualized on endoscopy, (2) there is an intermittent source of bleeding that may be in the stomach, duodenum, or colon but was not visualized at the time of the test, (3) the lesion was small and/or hard to see and was therefore missed, or (4) the bleeding has stopped. If bleeding persists, a repeat endoscopy can be considered to catch an intermittent source of bleeding that may have been missed. If these are unrevealing, other diagnostic tests can be considered. GI bleeding is often intermittent, and in many cases does require multiple tests to identify and treat the site of bleeding.

The patient in this scenario has an intermittent, brisk bleed resulting in hemodynamic instability requiring continued transfusion. At this point, continued transfusion and just observing the patient is not appropriate given that the bleeding is ongoing, brisk, and now resulting in hemodynamic instability. A tagged RBC study can assist in locating slow, occult bleeds, but will only grossly localize bleeding when more brisk and will not allow intervention. It is generally not useful in hemodynamically unstable patients. Once blood pools in the small bowel, the study carries a false positive rate at downstream locations. In the patient above with a brisk bleed, a repeat tagged RBC study would be unlikely to yield new, helpful information. VCE has the potential to identify a bleeding source in the small bowel, but has many limitations. There is no way to mark the site of bleeding, the information is reviewed retrospectively, and in many cases the intestinal mucosa cannot be completely visualized. Other techniques available at some centers to evaluate the small bowel include push endoscopy, in which a pediatric endoscope is used to examine 50 to 70 cm past the ligament of treitz, or single or double balloon endoscopy that allows an endoscope to be advanced deep into the small bowel. Surgically, there is very limited ability to localize GI bleeding intraoperatively. Occasionally, intraoperative enteroscopy can also be used to look intraluminally at the small bowel but is difficult to perform and invasive. Surgery should very rarely be performed on patients with GI bleeding that is unlocalized preoperatively, as the capacity to identify the site of bleeding intraoperatively is very limited.

An angiogram has both diagnostic and therapeutic potential. A standard angiogram will demonstrate active extravasation if bleeding is greater than a rate of 0.5 mL/min. Most hemodynamically unstable patients are bleeding at this rate or higher. An angiogram can also be done in a "provocative" fashion with anticoagulants, vasodilators, and antifibrinolytics to encourage bleeding and assist with identifying the site. This does come with the risk of exacerbating hemorrhage, and a surgery team is available to assist in the event of uncontrolled hemorrhage. If the site of bleeding is identified at a focal area, embolization of the area of active extravasation can be performed. For this patient who is hemodynamically unstable and has already undergone multiple other diagnostic procedures, an angiogram gives the best chance of identifying and treating the bleeding source.

### References

1. Barkun AN, Bardou M, Kuipers EJ, et al. International consensus recommendations on the management of patients with non-variceal upper gastrointestinal bleeding. *Ann Intern Med.* 2010;152:101-113.
2. Gralnek IM. Obscure-overt gastrointestinal bleeding. *Gastroenterology.* 2005;128:1424-1430.
3. Tavakkoli A, Ashley S. Acute gastrointestinal hemorrhage. In: Townsend C, Beauchamp RD, Evers M, Mattox K, eds. *Sabiston Textbook of Surgery: The Biological Basis of Modern Surgical Practice.* 20th ed. Philadelphia: Elsevier Saunders; 2017.

---

**3.** Correct Answer: A

**Rationale:**

This patient has a postoperative ileus. Following any operation, there is a risk of postoperative ileus, and diffuse contamination is another risk factor. Additionally, opiates administered postoperatively may contribute to ileus. An ileus usually presents a few days after the operation with increased abdominal distention, nausea, and vomiting, along with minimal to no bowel function. The management of an ileus involves placement of a nasogastric tube for decompression, initiating intravenous fluids for resuscitation, minimizing narcotics, and electrolyte monitoring and repletion as needed. Often these will resolve on their own in several days, but if not resolving, particularly in the setting of a rising WBC or fevers, it may also be important to look for an underlying cause, such as abscess.

At this point, there is no need for urgent reexploration. Enemas, while effective in the management of constipation, are not effective in helping resolve an ileus, as the issue is primarily one of reduced small bowel motility. Promotility agents are not effective in the management of ileus, and any delay in placement of a nasogastric tube (ie with attempted management solely with antiemetics) not only fails to resolve the ileus but may increase the risk of aspiration if the patient continues to vomit. Also, endoscopy is not necessary for diagnosis or treatment of ileus.

### Reference

1. Harris JW, Evers M. Small intestine. In: Townsend C, Beauchamp RD, Evers M, Mattox K, eds. *Sabiston Textbook of Surgery: The Biological Basis of Modern Surgical Practice.* 20th ed. Philadelphia: Elsevier Saunders; 2017.

---

**4.** Correct Answer: B

**Rationale:**

This patient presents with a new enterocutaneous fistula (ECF). Patients with inflammatory bowel disease (IBD) are particularly prone to ECF formation. These often present following a prior operation but can also appear spontaneously, particularly in patients with IBD. When patients first present with an ECF, they are often volume depleted with electrolyte disarray from intestinal losses and can have sepsis. This requires broad-spectrum antibiotics and drainage of any associated intra-abdominal abscesses if present. Depending on how proximal the fistula is, nutritional losses can be considerable. Patients should be started on TPN until the anatomy of the fistula is defined and output can be controlled. The anatomy can usually be defined with a CT scan with enteral and IV contrast, which has the added benefit of defining any undrained intra-abdominal fluid collections. If the anatomy is unclear, a fistulagram can be performed, in which water soluble contrast is injected into the fistula's external opening to identify the location of the fistula and any communication with any additional fistulas or abscess pockets. Wound care and control of the fistula effluent to minimize skin breakdown and manage output can be complex and may require the assistance of an enterostomal therapy or wound nurse.

In addition to identifying the location of the fistula, the cause and any factors that would inhibit closure should be identified. In this case, underlying IBD is the cause, and in these patients, medical treatment of the underlying Crohn disease should be optimized. Factors that can impair fistula closure include the presence of a foreign body (eg mesh used in herniorrhaphy), prior radiation exposure, undrained or untreated intraabdominal infection, malignancy as the cause of the fistula, distal intestinal obstruction, or immunosuppression. Whenever possible these perpetuating factors should be minimized or eradicated. When underlying factors cannot be addressed (for example prior radiation exposure), their recognition can at least allow accurate prognostication about the chances of spontaneous fistula closure and the need for surgery.

In any patient population—with or without IBD—principles of managing a new ECF include sepsis control, nutritional support, fluid and electrolyte repletion, and defining the anatomy and cause of the fistula. It is not recommended to take the patient to the OR urgently. The majority of ECFs will heal on their own, and if needed, surgery should be performed in a delayed manner when the patient has been well resuscitated, nutritional status is optimized, and intra-abdominal inflammation has subsided somewhat, often many months after the initial presentation. In this case incision and drainage is not needed as there is no drainable fluid collection in the abdominal wall on CT scan, but it is important to perform imaging with CT to evaluate undrained intra-abdominal or abdominal wall collections. Percutaneous jejunostomy tube would not be appropriate before fully defining the anatomy of the fistula. In this case, neither upper GI endoscopy nor colonoscopy would be beneficial, as we suspect this fistula to be located in the small bowel and there are more effective methods of localization that better depict the small bowel.

## References

1. Kulaylat MN, Dayton MT. Surgical complications – intestinal fistulas. In: Townsend C, Beauchamp RD, Evers M, Mattox K, eds. *Sabiston Textbook of Surgery: The Biological Basis of Modern Surgical Practice*. 20th ed. Philadelphia: Elsevier Saunders; 2017.
2. Orangio GR. Enterocutaneous fistula: medical and surgical management including patients with Crohn's disease. *Clin Colon Rectal Surg*. 2010;23:169-175.

# 89

# LARGE INTESTINE

Maryam Bita Tabrizi and Martin G Rosenthal

1. An 80-year-old male patient is recovering from a 3-vessel CABG he underwent 2 weeks prior when he develops abdominal pain with distension and obstipation. His heart rate is 115 bpm and his laboratory test results are notable for a WBC of 15 and potassium of 2.6. He is on a scheduled narcotic regimen prescribed by pain medicine for chronic back pain and ciprofloxacin for a UTI. He denies any history of melena and states his last screening colonoscopy was 4 months ago, which was normal. An obstructive series is ordered demonstrating the following findings:

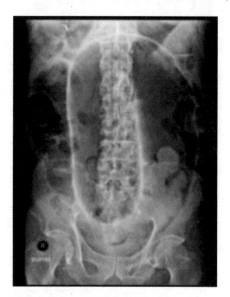

What is the next BEST step in the management of this patient?

A. Administer neostigmine with atropine available as needed
B. Obtain a CT of the abdomen/pelvis with a surgical consult
C. Start PO vancomycin and IV metronidazole
D. Place a nasogastric tube with serial abdominal examinations
E. Start a bowel regimen including enemas

2. A 60-year-old male with no significant past medical history presents with sigmoid diverticulitis diagnosed by CT scan, which demonstrated microperforation and phlegmon. His vitals on presentation are within normal limits, laboratory test results are only significant for a leukocytosis, and abdominal examination demonstrates mild left lower quadrant abdominal tenderness without rebound or guarding. He is admitted to the hospital, kept NPO, and started on IV ciprofloxacin and metronidazole. On hospital day 4 he is transferred to the ICU with atrial fibrillation with rapid ventricular rate but remains normotensive. He is started on metoprolol with successful rate control. Laboratory test results demonstrate an acute kidney injury. His abdomen is distended and tender diffusely to palpation. What is the next BEST step in his management?

A. Change antibiotics to meropenem
B. Noncontrast CT abdomen/pelvis
C. Start anticoagulation
D. Exploratory laparotomy and colectomy
E. Amiodarone bolus and infusion

3. A 38-year-old male presents after a bout of hematemesis at home and subsequently vomits another 400 mL of bright red blood in the emergency room. He is tachycardic and hypotensive. Large bore IVs are obtained and he receives 2 units of packed red blood cells. He is intubated for airway protection and admitted to the ICU. On chart review he is found to have a significant alcohol abuse history and several admissions for alcoholic pancreatitis, but his liver function studies and coagulation parameters are within normal limits. A recent MRI of the abdomen and liver biopsy show no evidence of cirrhosis. The patient is started on an IV proton pump inhibitor and IV octreotide. Bedside ultrasound showed no signs of ascites. He subsequently undergoes an EGD that demonstrates oozing gastric varices that were sclerosed with cyanoacrylate, and EUS shows thrombosis of the splenic vein and calcification of the pancreas. He remains hemodynamically stable and is extubated after the procedure. Six hours later he has another large volume hematemesis and becomes hypotensive. He receives an additional 3 units or packed red blood cells and it stabilizes his blood pressure.

What is the next BEST step?

A. Transjugular Intrahepatic Portosystemic Shunt (TIPS)
B. Nadolol
C. Continue massive transfusion protocol
D. Splenectomy
E. Catheter-directed tPA to splenic vein

4. A 70-year-old male with a history of diabetes, hypertension, and colon cancer status post a left hemicolectomy 10 years prior is brought to the emergency room from an outside hospital with a contained ruptured abdominal aortic aneurysm (AAA). On arrival he was hypotensive with a heart rate 115 bpm and blood pressure 85/55 mm Hg. He is taken emergently for endovascular aneurysm repair, which was uncomplicated. Postoperatively he is transferred to the surgical intensive care unit and remains stable overnight. Twelve hours later you are called to bedside as the patient is complaining of severe abdominal pain and distension. His vitals are as follows: temperature 101.5°F, heart rate 110 bpm, blood pressure 100/70 mm Hg, and urine output <15 mL/h over the last 4 hours. Laboratory test results are significant for a leukocytosis of 15,000 cell/mL, serum lactate of 3.1 mmol/L, and creatinine is 2 mg/dL. The hemoglobin has remained stable from preoperative levels. Which is the MOST likely reason for the patients decline?

A. Endoleak with bleeding
B. Abdominal compartment syndrome
C. Hypovolemia with significant third spacing
D. Colonic ischemia
E. Retroperitoneal hematoma

5. A 55-year-old female is admitted to the surgical intensive care unit with severe abdominal pain, nausea, vomiting, and diarrhea for the last 3 days. Her vitals at arrival are as follows: heart rate 122 bpm, blood pressure 100/50 mm Hg, temperature 102°F. On examination her abdomen is diffusely tender with voluntary guarding. Laboratory test results are notable for a leukocytosis of 18,000 cells/mL and hypokalemia. A thorough medical history is significant for a recent diagnosis of ulcerative colitis treated with sulfasalazine and a recent urinary tract infection of which she completed a 7-day course of ciprofloxacin. A CT of the abdomen and pelvis is performed, which demonstrates a significantly dilated colon up to 6 cm in diameter and diffuse colonic wall thickening with patent vasculature. What additional testing is required before full medical management can be initiated.

A. CT angiography of the mesenteric vessels
B. Colonoscopy with biopsies
C. *Clostridium difficile* stool test
D. Serum CMV test
E. Barium enema

# Chapter 89 ▪ Answers

**1.** Correct Answer: B

**Rationale:**

This patient has imaging findings concerning for a large bowel obstruction that is most likely caused by a sigmoid volvulus as seen by the presence of an inverted U-shaped colon that is distended and extending from the pelvis to the right upper quadrant along with paucity of air in the rectum. Abdominal radiographs can only diagnose sigmoid volvulus in 60% of cases and usually require CT imaging or contrast enema. The most appropriate next step requires CT of the abdomen/pelvis and surgical consultation. CT is useful to rule out other causes of obstruction such as a tumor, impacted stool, or foreign body. The management of sigmoid volvulus requires sigmoidoscopy to evaluate the mucosa, and if no signs of ischemia are present, the next step would be an attempt at endoscopic detorsion with elective sigmoidectomy, as there is a 60% recurrence rate of nonsurgical management. If the mucosa is ischemic the patient would require an emergent sigmoidectomy. The patient's age and history of recent antibiotic exposure places him at risk of *C. difficile* colitis and toxic megacolon, and occasionally *C. difficile* colitis presents with ileus but empiric treatment without a positive stool sample is unlikely to improve the patient's symptoms. Nasogastric tubes function even in large bowel obstructions independent of a competent ileocecal valve but serial abdominal examinations would lead to perforated sigmoid colon in this patient. The obstructive series shows no significant stool burden, and constipation is unlikely to be driving this process. Intestinal pseudo-obstruction (Ogilvie syndrome) is a diagnosis of exclusion and usually involves dilation of the entire colon. It is more common in cardiac surgery patients and supportive care including correction of electrolytes, especially hypokalemia, and avoidance of narcotics are beneficial. Neostigmine can be used for treatment of patients refractory to supportive care. However, neostigmine can cause significant bradycardia (which can be treated with atropine), and thus needs to be administered in a monitored setting. However, a mechanical obstruction must be ruled out before administration of neostigmine, as this can lead to proximal colonic perforation. Further management includes colonic decompression.

## References

1. Halabi WJ, Jafari MD, Kang CY, et al. Colonic volvulus in the United States: trends, outcomes and predictors of mortality. *Ann Surg.* 2014;259:293.
2. Mangiante EC, Croce MA, Fabian TC, et al. Sigmoid volvulus. A four-decade experience. *Am Surg.* 1989;55:41.

**2.** Correct Answer: B

**Rationale:**

The patient has complicated diverticulitis as evidenced by microperforation and phlegmon. Patients who are hemodynamically stable are treated with parenteral antibiotics and NPO status. They are assessed daily for improvement in vital signs, abdominal examination, and diet toleration. Most improve within 2 to 3 days. This patient is showing signs of worsening abdominal pain, new onset atrial fibrillation, and end organ damage all concerning for sepsis. Failure to improve should prompt repeat imaging to evaluate for complications of diverticulitis such as abscess, frank perforation, or obstruction. As the patient has an acute kidney injury, contrast would place the patient at increased risk for worsening renal failure although it would surely increase the sensitivity of the CT scan. However, complications of diverticulitis such as frank perforation, free air and large abscesses, and distended bowel and obstruction will likely be evident on noncontrast CT scans. The patient with no past medical history and no recent hospital exposure is likely not at high risk for resistant organisms, such as extended spectrum beta lactamases. Thus, changing antibiotics to meropenem is less likely to improve the patient's course. The patient has new onset atrial fibrillation, which began a few hours earlier and is responding well to rate control, which is the preferred strategy for initial management over rhythm control. His $CHA_2DS_2$-VASc score is 0 and no valvular disease, lowering his risk for thromboembolism and not likely to require anticoagulation. The patient may require surgery based on the CT scan results; however, intra-abdominal abscesses related to diverticulitis respond well to percutaneous drainage and antibiotics.

## References

1. Paterson DL, Bonomo RA. Extended-spectrum beta-lactamases: a clinical update. *Clin Microbiol Rev.* 2005;18:657.
2. January CT, Wann LS, Alpert JS, et al. 2014 AHA/ACC/HRS guideline for the management of patients with atrial fibrillation: a report of the American College of Cardiology/American Heart Association Task Force on Practice Guidelines and the Heart Rhythm Society. *J Am Coll Cardiol.* 2014;64:e1.

**3.** Correct Answer: D

**Rationale:**

The patient has a history significant for chronic pancreatitis, which carries an 8% risk of splenic vein thrombosis. Splenic vein thrombosis can lead to left-sided (sinistral) portal hypertension. The majority of patients with splenic vein thrombosis have no gastrointestinal bleeding, and splenectomy is no longer considered the ideal treatment in asymptomatic patients. Patients typically have normal liver function tests and no signs of cirrhosis. Management includes EGD for diagnosis and management with banding and sclerotherapy/obliteration. However, in the acutely bleeding patient who has failed endoscopic management, splenectomy is the ideal choice to control gastric variceal bleeding. Nadolol is useful to decrease the portal pressures for chronic management but is not useful in the acutely bleeding patient. TIPS will not decrease the portal pressure within the splenic vein as the obstruction is proximal to the portal vein. The patient has now stabilized after receiving 2 units or pRBCs thus ongoing massive transfusion protocol would not be useful. tPA is currently not indicated for portal vein thrombosis.

References

1. Agarwal AK, Raj Kumar K, Agarwal S, Singh S Significance of splenic vein thrombosis in chronic pancreatitis. *Am J Surg.* 2008;196:149-154.
2. Fernandes A, Almeida N, Ferreira A, et al. Left-sided portal hypertension: a sinister entity. *GE Port J Gastroenterol.* 2015;22(6):234-239.

**4.** Correct Answer: D

**Rationale:**

Colonic ischemia complicates 1% to 3% of elective AAA repairs but up to 10% of ruptured AAA repairs. Physicians must have a high index of suspicion as no laboratory values are pathognomonic for colonic ischemia. Patients commonly develop abdominal pain with fever, elevated lactate, and leukocytosis, while only 30% will have the classic finding of bloody diarrhea. Colonic ischemia can occur in both open and endovascular repairs of AAA. Inferior mesenteric ligation (IMA) in open repairs and coverage of IMA with endovascular repairs likely leads to insufficient blood flow, and prior colon resections likely lead to decreased collaterals between the superior and inferior mesenteric arteries. Atheromatous embolization is also believed to be a culprit in colonic ischemia. Additional risk factors for colonic ischemia include longer operative time, renal insufficiency, and hypotension. Flexible sigmoidoscopy is the diagnostic modality of choice to confirm diagnosis and plan subsequent treatment. Mild forms of colonic ischemia limited to the mucosa may be treated with antibiotics, bowel rest, and serial sigmoidoscopies; however, transmural necrosis requires colectomy and carries a high mortality rate. Retroperitoneal hematoma and endoleak are complications of endovascular surgery and should be kept high on the differential; however, with a stable hemoglobin and signs of colonic ischemia, they are less likely. Ruptured AAAs can result in a large retroperitoneal hematoma before bleeding is controlled and can lead to significant third spacing resulting in abdominal compartment syndrome with signs of hypovolemia or shock; however, this would be unlikely to manifest as fever and leukocytosis.

References

1. Brewster DC, Franklin DP, Cambria RP, et al. Intestinal ischemia complicating abdominal aortic surgery. *Surgery.* 1991;109:447-454.
2. Bjorck M, Troeng T, Bergqvist D. Risk factors for intestinal ischemia after aortoiliac surgery: a combined cohort and case-control study of 2824 operations. *Eur J Vasc Endovasc Surg.* 1997;13:531-539.

**5.** Correct Answer: C

**Rationale:**

This patient has findings concerning for toxic megacolon based on the following criteria: radiologic evidence of colonic distension, plus at least three of the following: fever >38°C, heart rate >120 bpm, neutrophilic leukocytosis >10,500 or anemia; plus at least one of the following: dehydration, altered sensorium, electrolyte disturbances, hypotension. In contrast to ulcerative colitis where inflammation is limited to the mucosa, toxic megacolon is characterized by extension of severe of inflammation to the smooth muscle layer, which is thought to lead to the colonic distension. Although toxic megacolon is most commonly recognized as a complication of inflammatory bowel disease (IBD), it can also occur with infectious and ischemic colitides. Toxic megacolon most commonly occurs during the first several months after diagnosis of IBD and not infrequently is the first manifestation of the disease. IBD is also a risk factor for *C. difficile* colitis and so is her recent antibiotic exposure. Medical treatment for IBD versus *C. difficile* differs in the choice of antibiotics and the use of corticosteroids. Steroids have not been found to increase the risk of colonic perforation; however, they will significantly suppress the immune systems response to infectious colitides such as cytomegalovirus (CMV), amebic, and bacterial (*Shigella, Salmonella, Campylobacter*, and *C. difficile*). This patient has no prior history of immunosuppression, and thus CMV is unlikely and the diagnosis of CMV colitis often requires endoscopic biopsies, which is too risky in toxic megacolon. Barium enemas to rule out distal obstruction are also high risk for perforation and should be avoided if possible.

References

1. Gan SI, Beck PL. A new look at toxic megacolon: an update and review of incidence, etiology, pathogenesis and management. *Am J Gastroenterol.* 2003;98:2363.
2. Dieterich DT, Rahmin M. Cytomegalovirus colitis in AIDS: presentation in 44 patients and a review of the literature. *J Acquir Immune Defic Syndr.* 1991;4(suppl 1):S29.

# 90

# LIVER

Daniel P Walsh and Somnath Bose

1. A 53-year-old male with past medical history significant for alcoholic cirrhosis complicated by esophageal varices presents to the intensive care unit (ICU) with hypoxia. He has noticed dyspnea on exertion that has been worsening over the last several months and complains of platypnea (shortness of breath relieved by lying down). Breath sounds are clear. Chest radiography is normal and contrast chest CT is negative for pulmonary embolus.

   Which of the following is the MOST definitive treatment option for his disease?

   A. Broad spectrum antibiotics
   B. Therapeutic paracentesis
   C. Nebulized bronchodilators
   D. Listing for liver transplantation
   E. Bronchoscopy

2. A patient presents with elevated aminotransferases approximately 15 times the upper limit of normal. Other laboratory values include international normalized ratio of 1.9, creatinine 0.9 mg/dL, and lactate of 1.9 mmol/L. The systemic arterial blood pressure is 90/50 mm Hg and the central venous pressure is 6 mm Hg.

   Which of the following is LEAST likely to be the etiology of the liver dysfunction?

   A. Acute viral hepatitis
   B. Ischemic hepatitis
   C. Acetaminophen toxicity
   D. Portal vein thrombosis
   E. HELLP syndrome

3. A 63-year-old female with history of cirrhosis complicated by ascites requiring previous paracentesis presents with fever, abdominal pain, and hypotension. Diagnostic paracentesis shows gram-negative bacteria on Gram stain and neutrophil count of 400 cells/mm$^3$.

   Which of the following is the BEST next step in management?

   A. Abdominal CT scan
   B. Initiate therapy with cefotaxime
   C. Right upper quadrant ultrasound
   D. Initiate therapy with vancomycin
   E. Large volume paracentesis

4. A 63-year-old male is in the ICU waiting to be listed for liver transplantation. He has become increasingly agitated and combative. His white blood cell count is 8200 cells/µL, sodium is 132 mEq/L, potassium is 3.1 mEq/L, creatinine is 0.9 mg/dL, and blood urea nitrogen is 15 mg/dL. Head CT reveals mild cerebral edema with no bleed or focal abnormality. He is receiving lactulose and having bowel movements three times daily.

   Which of the following is MOST LIKELY to improve his agitation?

   **A.** Intermittent midazolam
   **B.** Bisacodyl suppository
   **C.** Soft restraints
   **D.** Broad spectrum antibiotics
   **E.** Potassium repletion

5. A 62-year-old male with a history of hepatic cirrhosis complicated by ascites and esophageal varices presents with decreased urine output. His creatinine is elevated at 1.4 mg/dL. Investigation of the urine reveals fractional excretion of sodium <1%, no casts or blood cells, no protein, and renal ultrasound was normal. No improvement in urine output or creatinine is achieved after several doses of albumin. His white blood cell count is 7600 cells/μL, diagnostic paracentesis was not suggestive of infection, and his blood pressure is 98/62 mm Hg.

   Which of the following is the MOST effective next treatment?

   **A.** Norepinephrine infusion
   **B.** 2 L of normal saline bolus
   **C.** Broad spectrum antibiotics
   **D.** Corticosteroids
   **E.** Diuretics

6. A 42-year-old female presented with anorexia and fatigue. Workup revealed elevated aminotransferases approximately 10 times the upper limit of normal. Immunoglobulin G levels are elevated, and she is found to have positive titers for antinuclear antibodies. Liver biopsy reveals inflammation at the boundaries of the hepatocytes and portal triad. The patient is started on therapy with prednisone.

   The addition of which medication would be MOST helpful?

   **A.** Hydrocortisone
   **B.** Tenofovir
   **C.** Azathioprine
   **D.** Warfarin
   **E.** Cefotaxime

7. A 62-year-old man with history of ethanol use and hepatic cirrhosis presents with upper gastrointestinal bleeding. Endoscopy reveals multiple varices with signs of recent bleeding. Bands are placed on the varices and the patient is started on an octreotide infusion. His hemoglobin responds well to the single unit of packed red blood cells he was given before endoscopy. Thirty hours later large amount of blood is suctioned out of his nasogastric tube, he becomes hypotensive, and his hemoglobin does not increase despite transfusion of packed red blood cells.

   What is the MOST effective additional treatment option?

   **A.** Fresh frozen plasma transfusion
   **B.** Placing additional bands on varices
   **C.** Permissible hypotension
   **D.** Transjugular intrahepatic portosystemic shunt (TIPS)
   **E.** Increase octreotide infusion

8. A 52-year-old female presents with jaundice and right upper quadrant pain. Obstruction of her hepatic vein was found on ultrasonography. After anticoagulation and interventional angioplasty her aminotransferases and bilirubin remain elevated and she is now developing ascites.

   Which treatment option should be considered next?

   **A.** TIPS
   **B.** Liver transplantation
   **C.** Increase therapeutic range of anticoagulation
   **D.** Placement of an inferior vena cava filter
   **E.** Paracentesis

9. A patient with no history of chronic liver disease is in the ICU with acute fulminant hepatic failure. Their family is asking you if they will survive. You tell them they are very ill and that based on their liver failure alone the chances they will still be alive in three weeks is around:

A. Less than 10%
B. 33%
C. 70%
D. Greater than 90%

10. Which of the following is NOT a risk factor for the development of significant cerebral edema in the setting of liver failure?

A. Hyperacute (0-7 d) presentation
B. Older individuals (>40 y)
C. High-grade hepatic encephalopathy (HE)
D. Serum ammonia >150 µmol/L
E. Concurrent infection

# Chapter 90 ▪ Answers

1. Correct Answer: D

**Rationale:**
The history of dyspnea on exertion over a period of months in a patient with cirrhosis with portal hypertension (as evidenced by history of esophageal varices) makes hepatopulmonary syndrome a possible diagnosis. Platypnea and orthodeoxia affect up to 66% and 88% of patients with hepatopulmonary syndrome, respectively. Hepatopulmonary syndrome is progressive, and the only definitive treatment of hepatopulmonary syndrome is liver transplantation.

   Normal chest radiography and absence of symptoms such as fever, cough, or sputum production make infection less likely as the etiology of hypoxia in this case and thus antibiotics are not indicated. Although this patient may have ascites, increased abdominal pressure from ascites causing dyspnea should improve with upright positioning and worsen with supine positioning. This makes tense ascites a less likely etiology of hypoxia in this case. A normal chest radiograph and CT make a process of bronchial obstruction that could be cleared with bronchoscopy less likely.

References

1. Rodriques-Roisin R, Krowka MJ. Hepatopulmonary syndrome – a liver-induced lung vascular disorder. *N Engl J Med.* 2008;358(22):2378.
2. Younis I, Sarwar S, Butt Z, Tanveer S, Qaadir A, Jadoon NA. Clinical characteristics, predictors, and survival among patients with hepatopulmonary syndrome. *Ann Hepatol.* 2015;14(3):354-360.
3. Gomez FP, Martínez-Pallí G, Barberà JA, et al. Gas exchange mechanism of orthodeoxia in hepatopulmonary syndrome. *Hepatology.* 2004;40(3):660-666.
4. Gupta S, Castel H, Rao RV, et al. Improved survival after liver transplantation in patients with hepatopulmonary syndrome. *Am J Transplant.* 2010;10(2):354.

2. Correct Answer: B

**Rationale:**
Although markedly elevated aminotransferases are often from ischemic or hypoxic hepatitis, other causes for marked elevations include acute viral hepatitis, hepatic toxins or drug reaction, autoimmune hepatitis, focal arterial or venous obstruction, or HELLP syndrome. Ischemic or hypoxic hepatitis is generally associated with global hypoperfusion or hypoxia. The normal creatinine and lactate in this case do not support global hypoperfusion or hypoxia. Hypotension from nonhepatic trauma (and hypovolemia) rarely causes ischemic hepatitis, but cardiogenic shock with elevated cardiac filling pressures (high CVP, leading to hepatic venous congestion) has been shown to promote development of ischemic hepatitis. Thus, despite the borderline low systemic blood pressure, normal central venous pressure makes ischemic hepatitis less likely. When ischemic hepatitis is suspected other etiologies should be investigated by testing for acetaminophen levels, acute viral hepatitis serologies, autoimmune markers, and right upper quadrant ultrasound with doppler.

References

1. Tapper EB, Sengupta N, Bonder A. The incidence and outcomes of ischemic hepatitis: a systemic review with meta-analysis. *Am J Med.* 2015;128(12):1314-1321.
2. Seeto RK, Fenn B, RockeyDC. Ischemic hepatitis: clinical presentation and pathogenesis. *Am J Med.* 2000;109(2):109.
3. Gitlin N, Serio KM. Ischemic hepatitis: widening horizons. *Am J Gastroenterol.* 1992;87(7):831.

**3.** Correct Answer: B

**Rationale:**

This presentation of fever, abdominal pain, and ascitic fluid neutrophils >250 cells/mm$^3$ in a patient with history of cirrhosis and ascites is highly suggestive of spontaneous bacterial peritonitis (SBP). Depending on other aspects of the patient's history and presentation other workup could be warranted for secondary peritonitis, but this presentation is suspicious enough for SBP that treatment should be initiated regardless of additional ongoing workup. Empiric treatment is generally a third-generation cephalosporin, but cefotaxime has especially good penetration into the ascitic fluid so is preferred except when high rates of local resistance is present. A large volume paracentesis could put the patient at increased risk of hypotension in the setting of a current infection.

References

1. Dever JB, Sheikh MY. Review article: spontaneous bacterial peritonitis – bacteriology, diagnosis, treatment, risk factors and prevention. *Aliment Pharmacol Ther*. 2015;41(11):1116-1131.
2. Chavez-Tapia NC, Soares-Weiser K, Brezis M, Leibovici L. Antibiotics for spontaneous bacterial peritonitis in cirrhotic patients. *Cochrane Database Syst Rev*. 2009;21(1).
3. Runyon BA, Akriviadis EA, Sattler FR, Cohen J. Ascitic fluid and serum cefotaxime and desacetyl cefotaxime levels in patients treated for bacterial peritonitis. *Dig Dis Sci*. 1991;36(12):1782.

**4.** Correct Answer: E

**Rationale:**

This patient has HE. Around 30% to 40% of patients with cirrhosis will at some point have HE. HE can be precipitated by a number of factors including infection, constipation, GI bleeding, and electrolyte disorders among others. Identifying and treating precipitating factors is an important component of treatment. Hypokalemia increases the production of ammonia within the kidney through an effect mediated by changes in pH within the renal tubule cells. Midazolam can precipitate and worsen delirium in general and may worsen HE specifically. Soft restraints may be useful in maintaining safety but will not improve the agitation. Broad spectrum antibiotics could be useful if there was a precipitating infection, but this patient has a normal white blood cell count and no other indication of infection. Lactulose is one of the most often used treatments and this patient is already stooling regularly, so the addition of a suppository is unlikely to be helpful.

References

1. Vilstrup H, Amodio P, Bajaj J, et al. Hepatic encephalopathy in chronic liver disease: 2014 Practice Guideline by the American Association for the Study of Liver Diseases and the European Association for the Study of the Liver. *Hepatology*. 2014;60(2):715.
2. Tizianello A, Garibotto G, Robaudo C, et al. Renal ammoniagenesis in humans with chronic potassium depletion. *Kidney Int*. 1991;40(4):772.
3. Gabduzda GJ, Hall PW III. Relation of potassium depletion to renal ammonium metabolism and hepatic coma. *Medicine (Baltimore)*. 1966;45(6):481.
4. Artz SA, Paes IC, Faloon WW. Hypokalemia-induced hepatic coma in cirrhosis. Occurrence despite neomycin therapy. *Gastroenterology*. 1966;51(6):1046.

**5.** Correct Answer: A

**Rationale:**

This patient likely has hepatorenal syndrome (HRS). This is a diagnosis of exclusion that appears clinically very similar to prerenal acute kidney injury but fails to improve with administration of volume, such as albumin. Infection in patients with portal hypertension can increase the risk of HRS, but this patient has no signs of infection so would likely not be helpful in this case. Increasing the mean arterial pressure by 10 mm Hg in patients with HRS has been shown to increase urine output and decrease creatinine even if the patient is not initially hypotensive.

References

1. Testino G, Ferro C. Hepatorenal syndrome: a review. *Hepatogastroenterology*. 2010; 57(102-103):1279-1284.
2. Nanda A, Reddy R, Safraz H, et al. Pharmacological therapies for hepatorenal syndrome: a systematic review and meta-analysis. *J Clin Gastroenterol*. 2018;52(4):323-330.
3. Gupta K, Rani P, Rohatgi A, et al. Noradrenaline for reverting hepatorenal syndrome: a prospective, observational, single-center study. *Clin Exp Gastroenterol*. 2018;11:317-324.

**6.** Correct Answer: C

**Rationale:**

This patient has autoimmune hepatitis with classic features such as elevated IgG and positive ANA (this is most common autoantibody present in autoimmune hepatitis, but there are other multiple possible autoantibodies), and inflammatory changes on biopsy. Initial treatment is either prednisone monotherapy or combined therapy with azathioprine. Often azathioprine is added to prednisone monotherapy as the dose of steroid is tapered. More steroids would not necessarily be helpful. Tenofovir is a treatment for hepatitis B virus. Cefotaxime is used for SBP prophylaxis.

References

1. Lohse AW, Chazouilleres O, Dalekos G, et al. EASL clinical practice guidelines: autoimmune hepatitis. *J Hepatol*. 2015;63(4):971-1004.
2. Cropley A, Weltman M. The use of immunosuppression in autoimmune hepatitis: a current literature review. *Clin Mol Hepatol*. 2017;23(1):22-26.

**7.  Correct Answer: D**

**Rationale:**

Elevated portal pressure is the primary reason for variceal bleeds. Transjugular intrahepatic portosystemic shunt (TIPS) allows for decompression of the elevated portal venous system pressures. This can stop bleeding in up to 90% of cases of variceal hemorrhage and is a commonly recommended second line treatment for variceal hemorrhage.

References

1. Habib A, Sanyal AJ. Acute variceal hemorrhage. *Gastrointest Endosc Clin N Am*. 2007;17(2):223-252.
2. Nelms DW, Pelaez CA. The acute upper gastrointestinal bleed. *Surg Clin North Am*. 2018;98(5):1047-1057.

**8.  Correct Answer: A**

**Rationale:**

Budd–Chiari syndrome is caused by hepatic venous outflow obstruction. The majority of patients have an underlying disorder putting them at risk for thrombosis. The venous outflow obstruction causes ischemia to the hepatocytes and increases liver sinusoidal pressure causing liver congestion and portal hypertension. TIPS may increase survival in patients refractory to anticoagulation or angioplasty/stenting from around 45% to around 70%. Liver transplantation may still be required, but TIPS would generally be attempted prior. Increasing the anticoagulation will likely only increase the risk of bleeding. Placement of an inferior vena cava filter can help prevent clots from transmitting to the pulmonary vasculature but will not affect the hepatic vein. Paracentesis may relieve complications directly related to ascites but will not treat the underlying cause.

Reference

1. Valla DC. Budd-Chiari syndrome/hepatic venous outflow obstruction. *Hepatol Int*. 2018;12(1):168-180.

**9.  Correct Answer: D**

**Rationale:**

Although there are many variables that go into predicting survival/mortality for any individual patient, patients with acute liver failure overall have around a 70% survival rate at 21 days.

References

1. Reuben A, Tillman H, Fontana RJ, et al. Outcomes in adults with acute liver failure between 1998 and 2013: an observational cohort study. *Ann Intern Med*. 2016;164(11):724-732.
2. Ostapowicz G, Fontana RJ, Schiødt FV, et al. Results of a prospective study of acute liver failure at 17 tertiary care centers in the United States. *Ann Intern Med*. 2002;137(12):947-954.

**10.  Correct Answer: B**

**Rationale:**

Elevated intracranial pressures related to cerebral edema in 20% or more of patients with acute liver failure. Risk factors associated with developing significant cerebral edema in the setting of liver failure are hyperacute presentation, younger individuals (<35 years), high-grade HE, serum ammonia >150 μmol/L, presence of systemic inflammatory response syndrome or concurrent infection, high Sequential Organ Failure Assessment score, and requirement for vasopressors or renal replacement therapy. In addition, older individuals are protected against development of intracranial hypertension with cerebral edema due to reduction in cerebral volume with age.

Reference

1. Kok B, Karvella CJ. Management of cerebral edema in acute liver failure. *Semin Respir Crit Care Med*. 2017;38(6):821-829.

# 91

# GALLBLADDER AND BILIARY TRACT

Casey McBride Luckhurst and Peter Fagenholz

1. A 71-year-old male with past medical history of hypertension, hyperlipidemia, congestive heart failure with 20% ejection fraction, and chronic obstructive pulmonary disease on 3 L home oxygen presents to the emergency department from his nursing home with complaints of: 5 days of fever, nausea, and right upper quadrant abdominal pain. His vital signs are as follows: temperature 101°F, heart rate 115/min, blood pressure 90/60 mm Hg, respiratory rate 18/min, oxygen saturation 95% of 3 L oxygen via nasal canula. He undergoes an ultrasound that shows cholelithiasis, gallbladder wall thickening with pericholecystic fluid, and a positive sonographic Murphy sign, consistent with a diagnosis of acute calculous cholecystitis. What is the most appropriate management?

   A. IV antibiotics alone
   B. Endoscopic Retrograde Cholangiopancreatography
   C. Laparoscopic Cholecystectomy
   D. Open Cholecystectomy
   E. Percutaneous Cholecystostomy Tube

2. A 65-year-old male is now 10 days status post coronary artery bypass grafting with a postoperative course complicated by bleeding-requiring reoperation, and ventilator-associated pneumonia. After being afebrile for 2 days he spikes a temperature to 102°F and his laboratory test results demonstrate a new leukocytosis. An abdominal ultrasound is obtained that shows a distended gallbladder with wall thickening and pericholecystic fluid. A computed tomography scan of his abdomen confirms the aforementioned findings and is otherwise unremarkable. From the following choose the correct diagnosis and treatment.

   A. Acalculous cholecystitis—laparoscopic cholecystectomy
   B. Acalculous cholecystitis—percutaneous cholecystostomy tube
   C. Acalculous cholecystitis—endoscopic retrograde cholangiopancreatography
   D. Acute calculous cholecystitis—laparoscopic cholecystectomy
   E. Acute calculous cholecystitis—percutaneous cholecystostomy tube

3. A 45-year-old female with a past medical history of obesity and cholelithiasis presents to the emergency department with 2 days of right upper quadrant abdominal pain, fevers, and emesis. She is febrile to 102°F and her systolic blood pressure in the 80s mm Hg. Her systolic blood pressure improves to the 100s with 2 L lactated ringers. Her laboratory test results are notable for a WBC count of 19,000/mm³ (85% neutrophils), total bilirubin 6 mg/dL, and amylase 130 U/L. An abdominal ultrasound is obtained in the emergency department that shows cholelithiasis, a common bile duct measuring 8 mm and an otherwise normal gallbladder. In addition to continued resuscitation with IV fluids, what is the most appropriate next step in management?

   A. Laparoscopic cholecystectomy
   B. IV antibiotics alone
   C. Percutaneous cholecystostomy tube
   D. Endoscopic Retrograde Cholangiopancreatography
   E. Percutaneous Transhepatic Cholangiography

4. A 50-year-old male with a past medical history of hypertension presents to the emergency department with right upper quadrant abdominal pain, nausea, and fevers. He is noted to have an elevated white blood cell count and total bilirubin of 5 mg/dL. Further evaluation with an abdominal ultrasound shows a dilated common bile duct to 8 mm with a visualized obstructing gallstone within the lumen. All of the following are appropriate antibiotic choices EXCEPT:

   A. Pipercillin-Tazobactam 3.375 g IV every 6 hours
   B. Ertapenem 1 g IV once daily
   C. Cefazolin 1 to 2 g IV every 8 hours and Metronidazole 500 mg IV every 8 hours
   D. Ceftriaxone 2 g IV once daily

# Chapter 91 ▪ Answers

1. Correct Answer: E

**Rationale:**

Acute calculous cholecystitis is inflammation of the gallbladder in the presence of gallstones and obstruction of the cystic duct. Typical management involves initiation of antibiotic therapy and surgical cholecystectomy if the patient is an appropriate candidate. The patient presented above is a high surgical risk candidate given his multiple comorbidities and poor baseline functional status. Therefore, it would not be advisable to proceed with operative intervention at this time including laparoscopic or open cholecystectomy. In the setting of sepsis and presentation >72 hours after onset of symptoms it is unlikely that intravenous antibiotics alone will lead to resolution, although initiation of antibiotic therapy within 6 hours is recommended, or within 1 hour in patients presenting in septic shock. Endoscopic retrograde cholangiopancreatography is a procedure performed for a variety of reasons, including common bile duct obstruction in choledocholithiasis or cholangitis, but it is not typically used to address cystic duct obstruction in the setting of acute cholecystitis. The most appropriate management of this patient would include placement of a percutaneous cholecystostomy tube under ultrasound guidance. This allows for decompression of the gallbladder and can be done under local anesthesia and thus places minimal physiologic strain on this unstable and comorbid patient. The success rate for percutaneous cholecystostomy tube for the treatment of calculous cholecystitis is over 90% with a complication rate (most importantly bleeding and bile leakage) of less than 10%. Typically, these tubes remain in place for a minimum of 4 to 6 weeks, at which time further evaluation is performed with cholangiography, and a decision can be made about the need for elective cholecystectomy.

References

1. Baron TH, Grimm IS, Swanstrom LL. Interventional approaches to gallbladder disease. *N Engl J Med*. 2015;373(4):357-365.
2. Gomi H, Solomkin JS, Schlossberg D, et al. Tokyo Guidelines 2018: antimicrobial therapy for acute cholangitis and cholecystitis. *J Hepatobiliary Pancreat Sci*. 2018;25:3-16.
3. Little MW, Briggs JH, Tapping CR, et al. Percutaneous cholecystostomy: the radiologist's role in treating acute cholecystitis. *Clin Radiol*. 2013;68(7):654-660.
4. Alvino DM, Fong ZV, McCarthy CJ, et al. Long-term outcomes following percutaneous cholecystostomy tube placement for treatment of acute calculous cholecystitis. *J Gastrointest Surg*. 2017;21(5):761-769.

2. Correct Answer: B

**Rationale:**

Acalculous cholecystitis is an inflammatory disease of the gallbladder, which occurs in the absence of gallstones and is multifactorial in etiology. Acalculous cholecystitis accounts for approximately 10% of cases of acute cholecystitis and is typically seen in critically ill patients, such as the one described above. Risk factors for acalculous cholecystitis include, but are not limited to, major trauma, burns, sepsis, prolonged total parenteral nutrition, and congestive heart failure. Diagnosis involves high clinical suspicion of the clinician in the appropriate clinical setting and can be confirmed with standard laboratory evaluation and imaging studies including either ultrasonography or computed tomography. In cases where the diagnosis is still uncertain, cholescintigraphy (HIDA scan) can be used. Delay in treatment can result in bacterial superinfection and potential gallbladder perforation. In addition to initiation of antibiotic therapy, definitive therapy with either cholecystectomy or gallbladder drainage is warranted. Of the above choices, Answer B provides the correct diagnosis (acalculous cholecystitis) and the most appropriate method of gallbladder drainage (percutaneous cholecystostomy tube) in the setting of recent cardiac surgery and critical illness. Endoscopic retrograde cholangiopancreatography does not provide appropriate gallbladder decompression as mechanical obstruction is not the cause in acalculous cholecystitis.

References
1. Afdhal NH. *Acalculous Cholecystitis: Clinical Manifestations, Diagnosis, and Management.* UpToDate. Updated July 18, 2018.
2. Barie PS, Fischer E. Acute acalculous cholecystitis. *J Am Coll Surg.* 1995;180(2):232.

**3. Correct Answer: D**

**Rationale:**

Acute cholangitis, or ascending cholangitis, is the result of stasis and subsequent infection of the biliary tract typically due to mechanical obstruction. The most common etiology of obstruction is biliary calculi, although other causes include benign and malignant strictures and biliary stent obstruction. Charcot triad of fever, abdominal pain, and jaundice is the classic presentation, with the addition of hypotension and altered mental status forming Reynold Pentad, which is indicative of more severe cholangitis with associated septic shock. Diagnosis is made with a high clinical suspicion, laboratory values including a leukocytosis with neutrophil predominance and a cholestatic pattern of liver tests (predominantly conjugated bilirubinemia) and imaging with biliary ductal dilatation or visualization of the underlying cause of obstruction. Imaging modalities include ultrasound, computed tomography, or magnetic resonance cholangiopancreatography. In addition to resuscitation with isotonic crystalloid solution and initiation of antibiotic therapy, it is important to address the need for biliary ductal decompression or resolution of persistent biliary obstruction. In the patient above presenting with acute cholangitis and concerns for persistent biliary obstruction (total bilirubin 6 mg/dL, common bile duct measuring 8 mm) antibiotics alone will not be sufficient. Although a percutaneous cholecystostomy tube will aid in decompression of the biliary tree, it does not address the distal common bile duct obstruction and therefore is not the best first line option. Given that the patient's cholangitis is likely due to choledocholithiasis (gallstones obstructing the common bile duct), she may eventually benefit from a cholecystectomy to prevent recurrent episodes of choledocholithiasis, but cholecystectomy at this time will not address her ongoing bile duct obstruction. Although percutaneous transhepatic cholangiography performed by Interventional Radiology decompresses the biliary tree and may be able to address more distal obstructions, it is a technically difficult procedure that typically requires intrahepatic ductal dilatation and is not currently first line therapy when a gastroenterologist is available to perform endoscopic retrograde cholangiopancreatography and the patient's anatomy is amenable to it.

References
1. Kavanagh PV, vanSonnenberg E, et al. Interventional radiology of the biliary tract. *Endoscopy.* 1997;29(6):570
2. Kimura Y, Takada T, Kawarada Y, et al. Definitions, pathophysiology, and epidemiology of acute cholangitis and cholecystitis: Tokyo Guidelines. *J Hepatobiliary Pancreat Surg.* 2007;14(1):15-26.

**4. Correct Answer: D**

**Rationale:**

Empiric antibiotic choices should include those with coverage of enteric pathogens, which can later be narrowed based on culture data. Most common pathogens include gram negative aerobic enteric organisms (*Escherichia coli*, *Enterobacter* species, *Klebsiella* species), gram positive organisms (*Streptococcus* and *Enterococcus* species) and anaerobes. Though unlikely in this patient, history of healthcare-associated infections or infection with drug-resistant organisms may require additional empiric coverage. All choices except ceftriaxone are effective against the spectrum of common pathogens relevant in ascending cholangitis. Though ceftriaxone is effective against various gram positive and negative organisms, it is not effective against anaerobes.

Reference
1. Solomkin JS, Mazuski JE, Bradley JS, et al. Diagnosis and management of complicated intra-abdominal infection in adults and children: guidelines by the Surgical Infection Society and the Infectious Diseases Society of America. *Clin Infect Dis.* 2010;50(2):133-164.

# 92

# PANCREAS

Casey McBride Luckhurst and Peter Fagenholz

1. A 30-year-old female with no past medical history presents to the emergency department complaining of severe abdominal pain after a night of binge drinking. She is noted to have a low-grade temperature of 100.4°F with the following vital signs: heart rate 115/min, blood pressure 95/60 mm Hg, respiratory rate 18/min, oxygen saturation 99% on room air. On examination, she has focal moderate to severe tenderness in her mid-epigastrium without peritoneal signs. Her laboratory test results are notable for a WBC 15 000/mm³, lipase 5000 U/L, and creatinine 1.3 mg/dL from a baseline of 0.6 mg/dL. An abdominal ultrasound shows no evidence of cholelithiasis. She is diagnosed with acute alcoholic pancreatitis and admitted to the hospital. All of the following are important initial steps in the management of moderate-severe acute pancreatitis EXCEPT:

   A. Admission to a monitored hospital bed
   B. Initial resuscitation with lactated ringers at a rate of 5 to 10 mL/kg/h with close monitoring for markers of end organ perfusion
   C. Initiation of broad spectrum antibiotics
   D. Pain control with multimodal pain therapy
   E. Early initiation of oral feeding as tolerated

2. All of the following statements are true regarding nutrition in patients with moderate to severe acute pancreatitis EXCEPT:

   A. Oral feeding can be initiated early in the setting of improving abdominal pain and decreasing inflammatory markers
   B. If oral feeding cannot be tolerated, it is recommended to start enteral nutrition by day 5 to 7
   C. Enteral nutrition is preferred over total parenteral nutrition if it can be tolerated
   D. Enteral nutrition likely helps to maintain the intestinal mucosal barrier, thereby reducing bacterial translocation and infectious complications of acute pancreatitis
   E. Nasojejunal feeding is preferred over nasogastric feeding because of deceased pancreatic stimulation

3. A 45-year-old male was admitted to the intensive care unit (ICU) 2 days ago with a diagnosis of acute pancreatitis secondary to alcohol abuse. After initial resuscitation with large volume isotonic crystalloid solution for persistent hypotension, he developed worsening pulmonary edema with an increased oxygen requirement ultimately requiring intubation. In addition to Acute Respiratory Distress Syndrome, another potential complication seen in severe pancreatitis requiring large volume resuscitation is abdominal compartment syndrome. All of the following are signs/symptoms of abdominal compartment syndrome EXCEPT:

   A. Intra-abdominal pressure = 10 mm Hg
   B. Tense, distended abdomen
   C. Progressive oliguria
   D. Hypotension that is temporarily relieved with volume administration
   E. Increased peak inspiratory and mean airway pressures

4. A 35-year-old male is hospitalized following a first episode of acute severe gallstone pancreatitis. Initially, he presented to the emergency department with tachycardia, hypotension, and signs of end organ dysfunction. After aggressive resuscitation and supportive management in the ICU he showed signs of improvement. On hospital day 18 he develops new fevers and an associated leukocytosis. A computed tomography (CT) abdomen/pelvis is obtained that showed new air in areas of previously noted pancreatic necrosis. Which of the following statements is true regarding this patient's condition?

   A. Use of prophylactic antibiotics has been shown to decrease the rate of infection in necrotizing pancreatitis
   B. Primary management is urgent surgical debridement to attain source control
   C. Mortality associated with infected pancreatic necrosis ranges from 70% to 80%
   D. Current management involves initiation of antibiotic therapy and a step-up approach utilizing minimally invasive and endoscopic techniques
   E. Diagnostic Fine Needle Aspiration is required for a diagnosis of infected pancreatic necrosis

5. A 30-year-old obese female with a past medical history of cholelithiasis presents to the emergency room with progressive abdominal pain, nausea, and emesis for 2 days. While in the emergency department, she was noted to be afebrile with the following vital signs: heart rate 85/min, blood pressure 120/70 mm Hg, respiratory rate 18/min, oxygen saturation 99% in room air. Her laboratory evaluation was notable for WBC 14 000/ mm³, lipase 2000 U/L, total bilirubin 1 mg/dL. An abdominal ultrasound shows cholelithiasis without secondary signs of cholecystitis and a common bile duct measuring 5 mm. She is admitted for supportive management and the following day her total bilirubin is 0.6 mg/dL, lipase is 500 U/L, and her pain and nausea are significantly improved. What is the best next step in management?

   A. Endoscopic Retrograde Cholangiopancreatography (ERCP)
   B. Laparoscopic cholecystectomy during this admission
   C. IV antibiotics alone
   D. No further intervention necessary
   E. Magnetic Resonance Cholangiopancreatography (MRCP)

6. A 55-year-old male with pancreatic adenocarcinoma is now 3 weeks status post an uncomplicated pancreaticoduodenectomy (Whipple procedure). He was discharged home 7 days following his procedure and has been feeling well until yesterday morning when he developed gradually worsening abdominal discomfort and recent onset of nausea. Although in the emergency department he is noted to be afebrile, tachycardic with heart rate 105/min, and a blood pressure of 110/70 mm Hg. His laboratory evaluation is notable for a white blood cell count of 8000/mm³ and a hemoglobin (Hgb) of 6.0 g/dL. His Hgb at discharge was 9 g/dL. While in the emergency department, he vomits a small amount of bloody emesis. He is admitted to the ICU, has large bore peripheral intravenous access established, is transfused 2 U PRBC, and his Hgb increases to 8.0 g/dL. A CT scan is ordered for further evaluation. That night, before the CT scan is done, he starts vomiting large amounts of bright red blood and becomes hypotensive. What is the most likely cause for his presentation?

   A. Gastroduodenal artery pseudoaneurysm
   B. Bleeding esophageal varices
   C. Aortoenteric fistula
   D. Bleeding gastric ulcer
   E. Mallory-Weiss Syndrome

7. Choose the correct statement regarding acute pancreatitis from the list below:

   A. The diagnosis of gallstone pancreatitis is made by a combination of laboratory test results, imaging, and ERCP
   B. Alcohol is responsible for 70% of cases of acute pancreatitis in the United States
   C. Routine evaluation for all patients presenting with a first episode of pancreatitis includes a social history with specific inquiry about ethanol consumption, serum triglyceride levels, serum calcium, liver biochemical tests, and an abdominal ultrasound
   D. A diagnosis of post-ERCP pancreatitis is made by checking serum amylase and lipase levels the day following the procedure
   E. Hypertriglyceridemia-induced pancreatitis is treated with initiation of statin therapy

8. A 50-year-old male with a past medical history of hypertension and recent hospitalization for acute pancreatitis presents to the emergency department with complaints of increasing abdominal discomfort, anorexia, and intermittent emesis. He reports that he had been feeling well since his discharge from the hospital 3 weeks ago but has noticed the gradual onset of symptoms that have now increased in severity. All of the following are true regarding the diagnosis and management of a suspected pancreatic pseudocyst EXCEPT:

A. Pancreatic pseudocysts are fluid-filled cavities that lack a true epithelial layer and most commonly arise in the setting of pancreatitis or trauma

B. CT and MRI cross-sectional imaging are the best modalities for diagnosis and routine evaluation of pseudocysts

C. Nutritional assessment and initiation of nasoenteric feeding may be beneficial in symptomatic patients

D. Modalities for intervention include endoscopic drainage, percutaneous catheter drainage, and surgical drainage

E. Most pancreatic pseudocysts eventually require invasive intervention to achieve resolution

# Chapter 92 ▪ Answers

**1.** Correct Answer: C

**Rationale:**

Acute pancreatitis is an inflammatory disease of the pancreas with a variety of etiologies but is most commonly caused by gallstones or alcohol use. The resultant systemic inflammatory response and potential resultant organ failure are currently used in the severity assessment of individual cases. Initial management of a patient presenting with moderate to severe acute pancreatitis involves admission to a monitored bed including consideration for admission to an ICU if appropriate, as well as initiation of isotonic crystalloid resuscitation with Lactated Ringer solution. CT at the time of initial presentation rarely alters management and thus is not required when the diagnosis is clear based on clinical and biochemical grounds. Early initiation of oral feeding is strongly recommended given multiple studies demonstrating the safety of early enteral feeding in addition to reduced rates of infectious complications, multisystem organ failure, and mortality. Current guidelines recommend against the use of prophylactic antibiotics. This is based on review of the literature including 10 randomized control trials that showed no difference in infectious outcomes or mortality.

References

1. Crockett SD, Wani S, Gardner TB, Falck-Ytter Y, Barkun AN; American Gastroenterological Association Institute Clinical Guidelines Committee. American gastroenterological association institute guideline on initial management of acute pancreatitis. *Gastroenterology.* 2018;154(4):1096-1101.

2. Petrov MS, Pylypchuck RD, Uchugina AF. A systematic review of the timing of artificial nutrition in acute pancreatitis. *Br J Nutr.* 2009;101(6):787-793.

**2.** Correct Answer: E

**Rationale:**

Historically, patients presenting with moderate to severe episodes of acute pancreatitis were made nil per os in an attempt to provide bowel rest and avoid further pancreatic stimulation. Multiple studies looking at all severities of acute pancreatic have demonstrated that not only is initiation of early enteral feeding safe, but it also has favorable effects on infectious outcomes and mortality. It is believed that early enteral nutrition maintains the integrity of the gut mucosal barrier, thereby limiting bacterial overgrowth and intestinal atrophy, which may play a role in bacterial gut translocation. If oral feeding can be tolerated, it is recommended to resume an oral diet within 24 hours and allowing up to 3 to 5 days before initiating enteral feeding with nasogastric or nasojejunal feeding tube placement. In general, enteral nutrition is preferred over total parenteral nutrition for the aforementioned reasons, and thus the role of total parenteral nutrition is limited to those patients who are unable to tolerate any form of enteral nutrition despite maximal support. Despite the theoretical reasons to avoid gastric feeding, including avoidance of pancreatic stimulation, multiple studies have shown that there are no differences in nasogastric and nasojejunal feeding.

References

1. Crockett SD, Wani S, Gardner TB, Falck-Ytter Y, Barkun AN; American Gastroenterological Association Institute Clinical Guidelines Committee. American gastroenterological association institute guideline on initial management of acute pancreatitis. *Gastroenterology.* 2018;154(4):1096-1101.

2. Working Group IAP/APA Acute Pancreatitis Guidelines. IAP/APA evidence-based guidelines for the management of acute pancreatitis. *Pancreatology.* 2013;13 e1-e15.

**3.** Correct Answer: A

**Rationale:**

Abdominal compartment syndrome (ACS) is defined as end organ dysfunction related to sustained intra-abdominal hypertension (IAH). The average intra-abdominal pressure in critically ill patients is 5 to 7 mm Hg, not including patients with obesity or pregnancy, which may predispose them to slightly higher baseline pressures. IAH is defined as sustained pressures >12 mm Hg and is further subdivided into Grades I-IV based on escalating pressure intervals. ACS is defined as sustained IAH with new IAH-induced organ dysfunction, which includes increased peak inspiratory and mean airway pressures leading to alveolar barotrauma, renal impairment both from renal vein compression and renal artery vasoconstriction, decreased cardiac output secondary to cardiac compression and decreased venous return, and decreased mesenteric perfusion causing intestinal mucosal ischemia. There is no set intra-abdominal pressure that defines ACS, but sustained intra-abdominal pressures >20 mm Hg is typically required to cause the physiologic disturbances described above. Because of these relatively high pressures, these patients present with a tense and distended abdomen (Answer B). Although intra-abdominal compartment pressures can be measured through a number of indirect methods (intragastric, intracolonic, inferior vena cava), the standard method is intra-vesicular via a foley catheter.

References

1. Kirkpatrick AW, Roberts DJ, De Waele J, et al. Intra-abdominal hypertension and the abdominal compartment syndrome: updated consensus definitions and clinical practice guidelines from the World Society of the Abdominal Compartment Syndrome. *Intensive Care Med.* 2013;39(7):1190-1206.
2. Papavramidis TS, Marinis AD, Pliakos I, et al. Abdominal compartment syndrome – intra-abdominal hypertension: defining, diagnosing, and managing. *J Emerg Trauma Shock.* 2011;4(2):279-291.

**4.** Correct Answer: D

**Rationale:**

Acute pancreatitis is an acute inflammatory reaction caused by a variety of etiologies. A subset of patients with acute pancreatitis develops necrosis of a portion of the pancreatic parenchyma and surrounding tissues, which is termed necrotizing pancreatitis. In the acute setting, these necrotic collections are comprised of fluid and necrotic tissue, which over time organize into walled off pancreatic necrosis. Initially presumed sterile, 15% to 30% of collections eventually become infected, which is manifested by clinical deterioration, usually several weeks after an episode of acute pancreatitis. This patient likely has infected pancreatic necrosis. CT imaging demonstrates the presence of gas or air within the collections. Gas within necrosis is due either due to the presence of gas-forming microorganisms or fistulization into the gastrointestinal tract. This is diagnostic of infection and Fine Needle Aspiration is not required for the diagnosis of infected pancreatic necrosis. The first step in management is initiation of intravenous antibiotic therapy. In patients who fail to respond to IV antibiotic therapy alone, a step-up approach is used, which involves percutaneous or endoscopic drainage followed by minimally invasive or endoscopic necrosectomy. With the widespread utilization of minimally invasive approaches rather than traditional open necrosectomy, mortality associated with infected necrotizing pancreatitis has significantly decreased from 40%-60% to 10%-20%. Prophylactic use of antibiotics has not been shown to prevent superinfection of initially sterile pancreatic necrosis and thus is not recommended.

References

1. Banks PA, Freeman ML; Practice Parameters Committee of the American College of Gastroenterology. Practice guidelines in acute pancreatitis. *Am J Gastroenterol.* 2006;101(10):2379-2400.
2. Beger HG, Rau BM. Severe acute pancreatitis: clinical course and management. *World J Gastroenterol.* 2007;13(38):5043-5051.
3. van Santvoort HC, Besselink MG, Bakkar OJ, et al. A step-up approach or open necrosectomy for necrotizing pancreatitis. *N Engl J Med.* 2010;362:1491-1502.

**5.** Correct Answer: B

**Rationale:**

This patient's presentation is consistent with mild gallstone pancreatitis. After initial resuscitation, her laboratory test results improved (normalizing total bilirubin and lipase). With no evidence of ongoing biliary obstruction and no signs/symptoms of cholangitis, there is no indication to proceed with further imaging (MRCP) or ERCP. Current recommendations are for laparoscopic cholecystectomy during the same admission for patients who present with gallstone pancreatitis. This is based on the clear reduction in risk for recurrent gallstone-related events and that surgical outcomes do not differ in same admission versus delayed cholecystectomy. There is no evidence to support the use of prophylactic antibiotics in patients with gallstone pancreatitis, regardless of severity. The patient presented in this question has no evidence of ongoing or active infection to warrant antibiotic therapy.

References

1. Crockett SD, Wani S, Gardner TB, Falck-Ytter Y, Barkun AN, American Gastroenterological Association Institute Clinical Guidelines Committee. American gastroenterological association institute guideline on initial management of acute pancreatitis. *Gastroenterology.* 2018;154(4):1096-1101.
2. Fogel EL, Sherman S. ERCP for gallstone pancreatitis. *N Engl J Med.* 2014;370:150-157.

**6.** Correct Answer: A

**Rationale:**

The patient above is presenting 3 weeks after a Whipple procedure with a bleeding visceral artery pseudoaneurysm, likely from the gastroduodenal artery stump. Although the other four answer choices are in the differential diagnosis for a patient presenting with an acute upper gastrointestinal bleed, given the patient's history, classic presentation, and recent Whipple procedure, a ruptured visceral artery pseudoaneurysm is the most likely etiology. A delay in diagnosis in this situation is life-threatening. Management is time sensitive and requires placement of adequate venous access, transfusion as indicated, and emergent angioembolization. Visceral artery pseudoaneurysms typically present with a "sentinel bleed" in which a small amount of upper GI bleeding occurs before rupture of the pseudoaneurysm and massive hemorrhage ensues. If this entity is not recognized and time is wasted performing an upper GI endoscopy as would be performed for most patients with upper gastrointestinal bleeding, the window of time for intervention may be lost and the patient may exsanguinate. When a pseudoaneurysm is suspected, even in a stable patient, diagnosis and treatment must proceed urgently. A CT angiogram can diagnose a pseudoaneurysm before frank rupture.

### Reference

1. Fuji Y, Shimada H, Endo I, et al. Management of massive arterial hemorrhage after pancreatobiliary surgery: does embolotherapy contribute to successful outcome? *J Gastrointest Surg.* 2007;11(4):432-438.

---

**7.** Correct Answer: C

### Rationale:

A diagnosis of gallstone pancreatitis is made with the appropriate clinical history, evidence of cholelithiasis on imaging, and elevated serum lipase in the setting of acute onset abdominal pain. ERCP is not indicated in the routine diagnosis and evaluation of gallstone pancreatitis unless there is evidence of ongoing biliary obstruction or concomitant cholangitis. Although alcohol is one of the two leading causes of acute pancreatitis in the United States, it accounts for approximately 30% of cases. A diagnosis of post-ERCP pancreatitis is made in patients with signs and symptoms of acute pancreatitis in addition to elevations in serum amylase and lipase. In patients with acute pancreatitis secondary to hypertriglyceridemia, initial treatment is with apheresis and intravenous insulin therapy. Long-term therapy with lifestyle modification and initiation of pharmacologic therapy, typically gemfibrozil, is recommended for prevention of future episodes. It is important to note that hypertriglyceridemia is often a consequence of acute pancreatitis and is much less commonly the inciting cause. Routine evaluation for all patients presenting with a first episode of pancreatitis includes serum triglyceride levels, serum calcium, liver biochemical tests, and an abdominal ultrasound. In cases of acute pancreatitis of unclear etiology or recurrent episodes, initial evaluation with endoscopic ultrasound is recommended given the ability to detect small pancreatic cancers, periampullary masses, strictures, and microlithisias with fewer associated risks when compared to ERCP.

### References

1. Forsmark CE, Baillie J, AGA Institute Clinical Practice and Economics Committee; AGA Institute Governing Board. AGA institute technical review on acute pancreatitis. *Gastroenterology.* 2007;132(5):2022.
2. Scherer J, Singh VP, Pitchumoni CS, Yadav D. Issues in hypertriglyceridemic pancreatitis: an update. *J Clin Gastroenterol.* 2014;48(3):195.
3. Vege SS. *Etiology of Acute Pancreatitis.* UpToDate. Updated April 12, 2018

---

**8.** Correct Answer: E

### Rationale:

Acute peripancreatic fluid collections that form in the setting of acute pancreatitis or pancreatic trauma usually resolve, but can eventually form a well-defined wall, maturing into a pancreatic pseudocyst. Pancreatic pseudocysts lack a true epithelial layer and typically contain fluid without the presence of solid material or pancreatic necrosis. This process takes approximately 4 to 6 weeks after the initial episode of pancreatitis and is best identified on cross-sectional imaging using CT and MRI. Initial management of pancreatic pseudocysts includes monitoring and supportive care in the absence of symptoms. The majority of patients experience decrease in pseudocyst size and does not require further intervention. Nutritional assessment is recommended in all patients, with supplemental enteral feeding if necessary. Indications for invasive intervention on pancreatic pseudocysts include symptomatic patients not responsive to medical therapy, rapidly enlarging pseudocysts, and infected pseudocysts not responsive to antibiotics alone. Drainage into the gastrointestinal tract is the first choice of treatment for pseudocyst, as any ongoing leakage of pancreatic fluid is controlled without the need for external drains. Internal drainage is usually performed endoscopically but can be performed surgically. Occasionally pseudocysts can be drained percutaneously, but this runs the risk of resulting in a pancreatic fistula requiring prolonged drain placement.

### References

1. ASGE Standards of Practice Committee; Muthusamy VR, Chandrasekhara V, Acosta RD, et al. The role of endoscopy in the diagnosis and treatment of inflammatory pancreatic fluid collections. *Gastrointest Endosc.* 2016;83:481-488.
2. Banks PA, Bollen TL, Dervenis C, et al; Acute Pancreatitis Classification Working Group. Classification of acute pancreatitis–2012: revision of the Atlanta classification and definitions by international consensus. *Gut.* 2013;62(1):102.
3. Cui ML, Kim KH, Kim HG, et al. Incidence, risk factors and clinical course of pancreatic fluid collections in acute pancreatitis. *Dig Dis Sci.* 2014;59:1055-1062.

# 93

# GENITOURINARY

Maryam Bita Tabrizi and Martin G Rosenthal

1. A 38-year-old male suffered two gunshot wounds to the abdomen and was admitted to the ICU after an exploratory laparotomy with small bowel resection, sigmoid colon resection, and one intra-abdominal drain placement. Postoperatively, the patient is extubated in the ICU without complications. On postoperative day # 1, he acutely develops decreasing urine output, rising creatinine, and drain output with moderate serous output. The ICU team suspects Acute Kidney Injury. They obtain a fractional excretion of urine sodium, which is between 1% to 2%, and a bedside renal ultrasound demonstrates a normal collecting duct system. What is the BEST next step?

   A. Continue to monitor and discuss fluid balance
   B. Intra-abdominal drain studies
   C. CT abdomen and pelvis
   D. Patient is stable, send to the floor, and have the surgical team obtain a nephrology consult

2. A 65-year-old patient 12 hours status post renal biopsy presents to the ICU with gross hematuria, acute blood loss anemia, and tachycardia. After two units of packed RBCs and DDAVP, with a normal INR and platelet counts, the patient continues to have significant gross hematuria with continued tachycardia and downtrending hemoglobin with a systolic blood pressure of 90 mm Hg. What is the next BEST step?

   A. Surgical and Interventional radiology consultation
   B. CT angiography of the abdomen
   C. Continue to monitor and transfuse as needed
   D. Start Levophed

3. A 25-year-old male was involved in a motor vehicle crash in which he was clearly intoxicated. On presentation to the emergency department he is tachycardic and hypotensive and has suffered bilateral superior and inferior pubic rami fractures, with resulting acute blood loss anemia. He is transfused two units of packed RBCs. On presentation to the ICU, his blood pressure remains 100/70 mm Hg. On complete evaluation of the patient, you notice a small amount of blood at the penile meatus and no foley had been placed in the ED. What is the NEXT appropriate management of this patient?

   A. No need for foley placement as he is alert with stable vital signs. Once he voids, send for urinalysis
   B. Place a foley and obtain a urinalysis
   C. CT Cystogram
   D. Retrograde Urethrogram

4. All the medications below can lead to acute urinary retention EXCEPT:

   A. Dopamine
   B. Diltiazem infusion
   C. Phenylephrine
   D. Hydralazine

# Chapter 93 ▪ Answers

**1.** Correct Answer: B

**Rationale:**

Early diagnosis of urinary tract obstruction or ureteral injury is important and should be corrected as soon as possible, as delay in diagnosis could lead to kidney injury. All patients with AKI should have a workup for urinary tract obstruction. Ultrasound is the preferred imaging test for this diagnosis. It is important to recognize this patient's injury and the moderate to high drain serous output with an acute decrease in urine output. This patient had a gunshot wound to the abdomen involving the sigmoid colon, which also should hint the reader to a missed ureteral injury during the abdominal exploration as they are in close proximity. A negative ultrasound has 98% negative predictive value. It is great at ruling out a chronic and acute obstruction. However, it has a false positive rate of 26%. The positive predictive is only 70%. Although this patient's bedside ultrasound was negative for dilated collecting duct system, you cannot rule out a ureteral injury and must have a high index of suspicion. A urinoma may not be obvious in this case because there is a drain in place draining the serous fluid. If the urinoma does not build up to compress the collecting system, then it is unlikely to see a dilated collecting duct in this acute setting. The next most best step is to send the drain output for creatinine levels and notify the surgical team.

References

1. Ellenbogen PH, Scheible FW, Talner LB, et al. Sensitivity of gray scale ultrasound in detecting urinary tract obstruction. *AJR Am J Roentgenol.* 1978;130(4):731.
2. Kamholtz RG, Cronan JJ, Dorfman GS. Obstruction and the minimally dilated renal collecting system: US evaluation. *Radiology.* 1989;170(1 Pt 1):51.

**2.** Correct Answer: A

**Rationale:**

It is important to recognize that bleeding is a primary complication of renal biopsy. Renal biopsy tends to have the highest bleeding risk compared to other biopsy sites with a rate of 1.2%. Bleeding after renal biopsy will most likely occur at three locations. One site of bleeding is into the collecting system, which can lead to microscopic or gross hematuria as seen in the patient above. The other two sites would be beneath the renal capsule presenting with pain post procedure or in the peri-nephric space in the retroperitoneum. The patient above has been given DDAVP and has a normal coagulation panel and a normal platelet count but continues to have gross hematuria with signs of shock. This patient should not be transported to the CT scanner as the patient is currently showing signs of shock. Although the CT angiography of the abdomen would be an ideal study to evaluate for active extravasation, this patient has gross hematuria with continued bleeding. Monitoring the patient and continuing transfusion is reasonable after the surgical service has evaluated the patient. In bleeding patients, it is reasonable to allow "permissive hypotension." It is better to gently resuscitate than start vasopressors in a bleeding patient. The sudden rise in the mean arterial pressure and systolic blood pressures could lead to increased bleeding or reactivation of bleeding. The best decision for this patient is to get a surgical consultation and have interventional radiology on standby for angiogram, which can be both diagnostic and therapeutic in this patient while the patient is being monitored closely and transfused with appropriate transfusion ratios.

References

1. Appel GB, Madaio MP. Renal biopsy: how effective, what technique, and how safe. *Kidney Int.* 1990;38(3):529.
2. Atwell TD, Spanbauer JC, McMenomy BP, et al. The timing and presentation of major hemorrhage after 18,947 image-guided percutaneous biopsies. *AJR Am J Roentgenol.* 2015;205(1):190-195.
3. Whittier WL, Korbet SM. Timing of complications in percutaneous renal biopsy. *J Am Soc Nephrol.* 2004;15(1):142.
4. Redfield RR, McCune KR, Rao A, et al. Nature, timing, and severity of complications from ultrasound-guided percutaneous renal transplant biopsy. *Transpl Int.* 2016;29(2):167.
5. Shidham GB, Siddiqi N, Beres JA, et al. Clinical risk factors associated with bleeding after native kidney biopsy. *Nephrology (Carlton).* 2005;10(3):305.
6. Corapi KM, Chen JL, Balk EM, Gordon CE. Bleeding complications of native kidney biopsy: a systematic review and meta-analysis. *Am J Kidney Dis.* 2012;60(1):62-73. Epub April 24, 2012.

**3.** Correct Answer: D

**Rationale:**

Bladder injury occurs in approximately 3.4% of patients with pelvic trauma, whereas urethral injury occurs in only 1% of these patients. Males are 10 times more likely to have a urethral injury in such situations. If the physical examination reveals any signs of genital bruising, blood at meatus, high riding prostate, and gross hematuria, urethral injury should be suspected and ruled out. Advance Trauma Life Support recommends ruling out a urethral injury before inserting a Foley to avoid further injury, although the data on this are sparse. A systematic review of a thousand pediatric patients revealed the total incidence of genitourinary injury to be approximately 11% to 12%. Of these patients, 26.4% had urethral injury. As the severity of the pelvic injury worsened, the percentages appropriately increased. It is important to recognize this and have a high suspicion of injury during the examination of such patients. The first two choices involve placing a Foley catheter before any investigative work. CT Cystogram is ideal to rule out bladder injury. Retrograde Urethrogram is the test of choice to rule out urethral injury.

### References
1. Shlamovitz GZ, McCullough L. Blind urethral catheterization in trauma patients suffering from lower urinary tract injuries. *J Trauma.* 2007;62(2):330.
2. Gänsslen A, Hildebrand F, Heidari N, et al. Pelvic ring injuries in children. Part I: epidemiology and primary evaluation. A review of the literature. *Acta Chir Orthop Traumatol Cech.* 2012;79(6):493.

**4.** Correct Answer: B

**Rationale:**

**Pharmacologic agents associated with urinary retention**

| | |
|---|---|
| Sympathomimetics (alpha-adrenergic agents) | Ephedrine sulfate (Marax, Tedral) |
| | Phenylephrine HCl (Neo-Synephrine) |
| | Phenylpropanolamine HCL (Conlac) |
| | Pseudoephedrine HCl (Sudafed, Actifed) |
| Sympathomimetics (beta-adrenergic agents) | Isoproterenol |
| | Metaproterenol |
| | Terbutaline |
| Antidepressants | Imipramine (Tofranil) |
| | Nortriptyline (Aventyl) |
| | Amitriptyline (Elavil) |
| | Doxepin (Adapin) |
| | Amoxapine (Asendin) |
| | Maprotiline (Ludiomil) |
| Antiarrhythmics | Quinidine |
| | Procainamide |
| | Disopyramide |
| Anticholinergics (selected) | Atropine |
| | Scopolamine hydrobromide |
| | Clidinium bromide (Quarzan) |
| | Glycopyrrolate (Robinul) |
| | Mepenzolate bromide (Cantil) |
| | Oxybutynin (Ditropan) |
| | Flavoxate HCl (Urispas) |
| | Hyoscyamine sulfate (Anaspaz) |
| | Belladonna |
| | Homatropine methylbromide |
| | Propantheline bromide (Probanthine) |
| | Dicyclomine HCl (Bentyl) |

| | |
|---|---|
| Antiparkinsonian agents | Trihexyphenidyl HCl (Arlane) |
| | Benztropine Mesylate (Cogentin) |
| | Amantadine HCl (Symmetrel) |
| | Levodopa (Sinemet) |
| | Bromocriptine Mesylate (Parlodel) |
| Hormonal agents | Progesterone |
| | Estrogen |
| | Testosterone |
| Antipsychotics | Haloperidol (Haldol) |
| | Thiothixene (Navane) |
| | Thioridazine (Mellaril) |
| | Chlorpromazine (Thorazine) |
| | Fluphenazine (Prolixin) |
| | Prochlorperazine (Compazine) |
| Antihistamines (selected) | Diphenhydramine HCl (Benadryl) |
| | Chlorpheniramine (Chlor-Trimeton) |
| | Brompheniramine (Dimetane) |
| | Cyproheptadine (Periactin) |
| | Hydroxyzine (Atarax, Vistaril) |
| Antihypertensives | Hydralazine (Apresoline) |
| | Nifedipine (Procardia) |
| Muscle relaxants | Diazepam (Valium) |
| | Baclofen (Lioresal) |
| | Cyclobenzaprine (Flexeril) |
| Miscellaneous | Indomethacin (Indocin) |
| | Carbamazepine (Tegretol) |
| | Amphetamines |
| | Dopamine |
| | Vincristine |
| | Morphine sulfate and other opioids |
| | Anesthetic agents |

## Reference

1. Curtis LA, Dolan TS, Cespedes RD. Acute urinary retention and urinary incontinence. *Emerg Med Clin North Am.* 2001;19:591.

# 94

# DIAGNOSTIC AND MANAGEMENT MODALITIES

Maryam Bita Tabrizi and Martin G Rosenthal

1. A 55-year-old male is brought to the intensive care unit (ICU) after an exploratory laparotomy because of a motor vehicle collision where he suffered a liver laceration. He is intubated with an open abdomen and a negative pressure abdominal wound dressing. He remains hypotensive on norepinephrine infusion of 1 μg/kg/min and was transfused 16 units of packed RBCs, 8 units of fresh frozen plasma, 8 packs of platelets, 2 bags of cryoprecipitate. Repeat laboratory tests show a stable hemoglobin postoperatively. However, his urine output starts to decline, and his pressor requirements start to rise. On examination, the abdomen is distended and tight. In the case of intra-abdominal hypertension (IAH), what is the minimum ideal abdominal perfusion pressure (APP) correlating to improved survival?

   **A.** 90 mm Hg
   **B.** 80 mm Hg
   **C.** 70 mm Hg
   **D.** 60 mm Hg

2. A 48-year-old male who is 1 month status postorthotopic liver transplant for NASH Cirrhosis is transferred to the ICU with abdominal distention, pain, and septic shock. He has a known history of duodenal ulcer. A computed tomography (CT) of the abdomen and pelvis does not show any obvious free air or perforation. Sepsis guidelines are followed, and the decision is to proceed with a diagnostic paracentesis. The fluid drained does not contain any bile staining. Which one of the answers below supports a spontaneous bacterial peritonitis rather than a secondary bacterial peritonitis?

   **A.** Ascites protein concentration of less than 1 g/dL
   **B.** Glucose concentration of 25 mg/dL
   **C.** LDH level of 200 units/L
   **D.** Elevated Amylase in the fluid

3. An 85-year-old male who was recently treated for an upper respiratory tract infection presented 2 days ago with abdominal pain. On abdominal examination, he has tenderness to palpation with mild distention but no signs of peritonitis. On admission, the WBC was 25 cell/mL and now it is 18 cell/mL. Urinalysis does show bacteria and the initial diagnosis is a UTI. Cultures have been sent. Chest X-ray does not show any evidence of pneumonia. He starts to develop hypotension on the floor with oliguria requiring 2 L of crystalloid. A request is made to transfer the patient to the ICU. The nurse notes that in the past 24 hours, he has had four episodes of diarrhea. Stool was sent for GDH (glutamate dehydrogenase) and Toxin A and B. GDH was negative, but the Toxin A/B was positive. She asked the intern on the floor to start IV Flagyl for a presumed *Clostridium difficile* infection, but the intern has not started it yet. Aside from the sepsis guidelines and ICU care, what is the NEXT step to address a possible *C. difficile* infection?

   **A.** Hydration, bowel rest, continuing current empiric antibiotics, and monitoring her symptoms
   **B.** Start IV Flagyl because the patient is positive for Toxins and obtain a KUB
   **C.** Send stool for nucleic acid amplification testing then start IV Flagyl and obtain a KUB
   **D.** Start IV Flagyl and PO Vancomycin and obtain a KUB

4. Which one of the following immunosuppressants is in the macrolide family?

    A. Mycophenolate
    B. Tacrolimus
    C. Sirolimus
    D. Cyclosporine

5. A 35-year-old otherwise healthy female status post Roux-en-Y gastric bypass surgery presents to the ICU with abdominal pain mainly in the epigastric region with temperature of 101.5°F, blood pressure of 84/60 mm Hg with altered mental status after 4 L of crystalloid in the ED. A CT scan that does not demonstrate any bowel obstruction or internal hernia however a mildly dilated common bile duct with gallstones is visualized without signs of cholecystitis. On examination, she is jaundiced with epigastric tenderness to palpation. She has a slight elevation in her AST and ALT and direct bilirubin of 5 mg/dL. Aside from appropriate intensive care resuscitation, what is the next BEST step in the management of this patient?

    A. IV antibiotics and emergent surgical and gastroenterology consultation
    B. IV antibiotics, MRCP, and consult to interventional radiology
    C. Stat bedside right upper quadrant ultrasound
    D. Stat head CT for altered mental status and ammonia laboratory test results

6. A 55-year-old male who is POD # 3 status post a Whipple procedure suddenly begins to have worsening tachycardia, tachypnea, and destruction with abdominal distention. Surgically placed intra-abdominal drains are in place. Chest X-ray shows bilateral patchy infiltrates, $PaO_2/FiO_2$ ratio is 150, and he has sinus tachycardia with heart rate 130 bpm and stable blood pressures. How would you diagnose and confirm a pancreatic leak in a post Whipple patient?

    A. CT abdomen and pelvis with PO and IV contrast
    B. Reexploration in the operating room
    C. Send drain fluid for Amylase level, diagnostic if the abdominal drain fluid Amylase level is 2× the upper limit of normal serum Amylase
    D. Send drain fluid and serum for Amylase level, diagnostic if the abdominal drain fluid Amylase level is 3× the upper limit of normal serum Amylase

7. A 64-year-old male with no significant past medical history has recently immigrated to the United States from Peru and now presents with severe abdominal pain and sinus tachycardia, with otherwise stable vital signs. CT of the abdomen and pelvis shows a 14-cm liver cyst in the right lobe with multiple daughter cysts, intermittent minute calcifications, and small pockets of gas. Liver enzyme tests show a slight elevation of AST and ALT but no elevation of alkaline phosphatase or total and direct bilirubin. No evidence of biliary obstruction is noted. Owing to concerns for impending rupture, the patient is sent to the ICU for close monitoring. What is the BEST next step?

    A. Start Albendazole and monitor the patient closely
    B. Start Flagyl and monitor the patient closely
    C. Start Albendazole and consideration for puncture, aspiration, injection, reaspiration, (PAIR) versus surgical treatment
    D. Start metronidazole and consideration for PAIR versus surgical treatment

8. Which is the BEST test to detect the gastrointestinal bleeding rate of 0.3 to 0.5 mL/min in a hemodynamically labile patient in the ICU?

    A. CT angiography of the abdomen and pelvis
    B. Radionuclide Imaging
    C. Capsule endoscopy
    D. Formal interventional radiology Angiogram

# Chapter 94 ▪ Answers

**1.** Correct Answer: D

**Rationale:**

Patients with an open abdomen and a negative pressure wound dressing can still develop IAH and abdominal compartment syndrome (ACS). Intra-abdominal pressure (IAP) of 5 to 7 mm Hg is considered a normal steady state pressure within the abdominal space. Morbidly obese patients may have a higher baseline IAP. APP is calculated as the mean arterial pressure minus the IAP. Studies have showed that an APP of at least 60 mm Hg is correlated with improved survival from IAH and ACS. This resuscitation end point was found to be more important than arterial pH, base deficit, lactate, and hourly urine output in regression model analysis. IAH is defined as IAP greater than or equal to 12 mm Hg. There are four grades of IAH. ACS is defined as IAP greater than or equal to 20 mm Hg with signs of end organ dysfunction. The standard method of measuring IAP is measurement of bladder pressures. Care must be taken to make these measurements with consistent head and body positioning, ideally with a paralyzed patient at end expiration.

### References

1. Schein M, Ivatury R. Intra-abdominal hypertension and the abdominal compartment syndrome. *Br J Surg*. 1998;85(8):1027.
2. Caldwell CB, Ricotta JJ. Changes in visceral blood flow with elevated intraabdominal pressure. *J Surg Res*. 1987;43(1):14.
3. Iberti TJ, Lieber CE, Benjamin E. Determination of intra-abdominal pressure using a transurethral bladder catheter: clinical validation of the technique. *Anesthesiology*. 1989;70(1):47.

**2.** Correct Answer: A

**Rationale:**

When there is a clinical concern for the diagnosis of primary versus secondary bacterial peritonitis, cell counts and cultures often do not help to differentiate. In these diagnostic dilemmas examination of fluid chemistries may help with the diagnosis. Although when the serum-ascites albumin gradient (SAAG) is greater than 1.1 g/dL is highly suggestive of portal hypertension with 97% accuracy, it does not help differentiate between primary versus secondary bacterial peritonitis alone. Measure of the ascites fluid total protein concentration can often provide additional diagnostic clues. Patients with the most "dilute" ascites have the lowest level of opsonins, which puts them at the highest risk of spontaneous bacterial peritonitis. Ascites fluid protein concentration less than 1 g/dL correlates inversely with higher risk of developing spontaneous bacterial peritonitis. Additionally, neutrophils consume large amounts of glucose and thus ascites glucose concentration generally remains above 50 mg/dL in spontaneous bacterial peritonitis. But this number often falls below this level in secondary bacterial peritonitis, which can help with the diagnosis. In bowel perforations, the levels may fall to as low as zero. Ascites fluid lactate dehydrogenase (LDH) in the ascites fluid is released when the PMNs have been lysed. The LDH numbers rise in spontaneous bacterial peritonitis, but their numbers increase even further in secondary bacterial peritonitis. The upper limit varies but LDH levels in sterile ascites generally range between 40 ± 20 units/L. Amylase levels are elevated in the ascites fluid with pancreatitis and bowel perforation supporting a secondary bacterial peritonitis.

### References

1. Runyon BA. Low-protein-concentration ascitic fluid is predisposed to spontaneous bacterial peritonitis. *Gastroenterology*. 1986;91(6):1343.
2. Runyon BA. Patients with deficient ascitic fluid opsonic activity are predisposed to spontaneous bacterial peritonitis. *Hepatology*. 1988;8(3):632.
3. Soriano G, Castellote J, Alvarez C, et al. Secondary bacterial peritonitis in cirrhosis: a retrospective study of clinical and analytical characteristics, diagnosis and management. *J Hepatol*. 2010;52(1):39.
4. Akriviadis EA, Runyon BA. Utility of an algorithm in differentiating spontaneous from secondary bacterial peritonitis. *Gastroenterology*. 1990;98(1):127.
5. Runyon BA. Amylase levels in ascitic fluid. *J Clin Gastroenterol*. 1987;9(2):172.

**3.** Correct Answer: C

**Rationale:**

The laboratory approaches to diagnosis of *C. difficile* is followed when there is a suspicion for *C. difficile* infection. Generally, this infection is suspected when there is acute onset, and clinically significant diarrhea (≥ three loose stools over 24 hours) and risk factures such as recent antibiotic use, hospitalization, and advanced age. This patient has all the criteria for a suspected *C. difficile* infection. The stool was appropriately sent for ELISA Immunoassay for GDH antigen and Toxins A and B. If both are positive, then testing is consistent with *C. difficile* infection. If both are negative, then testing is not consistent with *C. difficile* infection. However, if one test is positive and the other is negative, then that is considered an intermediate test result. Then the stool must be sent for Nucleic acid amplification test (NAAT). The laboratory will then perform a NAAT for tcdB and tcdC genes. If this test is positive, then the patient is considered to have *C. difficile* infection. If this test is negative, then the patient is considered to not have the infection. It is important to note that the NAAT testing should ideally be sent before *C. difficile* infection treatment. However, if there is a high suspicion for the infection and the patient is showing signs sepsis, then early treatment is essential. With the abdominal pain and signs of early septic shock, it is important to get a KUB to rule out signs of toxic megacolon on imaging. A patient with signs of peritonitis will need an urgent surgical evaluation.

### References

1. Kelly CP, Pothoulakis C, LaMont JT. Clostridium difficile colitis. *N Engl J Med*. 1994;330(4):257.
2. McDonald LC, Gerding DN, Johnson S, et al. Clinical practice guidelines for clostridium difficile infection in adults and children: 2017 update by the Infectious Diseases Society of America (IDSA) and Society for Healthcare Epidemiology of America (SHEA). *Clin Infect Dis*. 2018;66(7):e1.
3. Kufelnicka AM, Kirn TJ. Effective utilization of evolving methods for the laboratory diagnosis of clostridium difficile infection. *Clin Infect Dis*. 2011;52(12):1451-1457.
4. Luo RF, Banaei N. Is repeat PCR needed for diagnosis of Clostridium difficile infection? *J Clin Microbiol*. 2010;48(10):3738.
5. Bélanger SD, Boissinot M, Clairoux N, et al. Rapid detection of clostridium difficile in feces by real-time PCR. *J Clin Microbiol*. 2003;41(2):730.
6. Sunkesula VC, Kundrapu S, Muganda C, et al. Does empirical clostridium difficile infection (CDI) therapy result in false-negative CDI diagnostic test results? *Clin Infect Dis*. 2013;57(4):494.

---

**4.** Correct Answer: C

**Rationale:**

Sirolimus is a macrolide antibiotic with potent immunosuppressant and antifungal properties. Tacrolimus and cyclosporine are calcineurin inhibitors. Mycophenolate is a nucleotide blocking agent.

### Reference

1. Suthanthiran M, Morris R, Strom T. Immunosuppressants: cellular and molecular mechanisms of action. *Am J Kidney Dis*. 1996;28(2):159-172.

---

**5.** Correct Answer: A

**Rationale:**

Acute cholangitis should be suspected in patients with fever, abdominal pain, and jaundice (Charcot triad) and abnormal liver enzyme tests with signs of obstructive jaundice. This patient already has a CT scan that shows a mildly dilated common bile duct. CT imaging has a high sensitivity for bile duct dilation but low sensitivity for bile duct stones. A follow-up ultrasound is not necessary for this patient. Abdominal ultrasound has a high specificity for bile duct dilation and bile duct stones but variable sensitivity for bile duct dilation and bile duct stones. In a patient with Charcot triad and elevated liver enzymes with a normal CT scan and/or ultrasound, and MRCP is ordered with a higher diagnostic accuracy in identifying causes of biliary obstruction. However, this patient has evidence of Reynold Pentad defined by Charcot triad along with signs of end organ dysfunction such as altered mental status and hypotension consistent with signs of severe cholangitis. Patients with mild and moderate cholangitis generally respond well to early antibiotic therapy and biliary decompression within 24 to 48 hours. Patients with mild to moderate cholangitis who fail to respond to conservative management within 24 hours or those patients with severe (suppurative) cholangitis require biliary decompression urgently (within 24 hours). Endoscopic sphincterotomy with stone extraction and/or stent insertion is the treatment of choice. Endoscopic decompression is successful in 90% to 95% of patients after sphincterotomy. Endoscopic drainage has a significantly improved mortality and morbidity compared to surgical decompression. Percutaneous transhepatic biliary drainage can be performed when ERCP is unavailable or unsuccessful. Surgical decompression is used in patients whom ERCP and drainage have failed. Laparoscopic or open common bile duct exploration with decompression with or without placement of T-tube is the surgical choice. In this patient who is showing signs of hemodynamic instability and end organ dysfunction, both the surgical team and gastrointestinal team should get involved urgently. CT head is not the next best step as this patient's clinical examination, imaging, and laboratory test results support cholangitis as the reason for the altered mental status with no lateralizing symptoms.

### References

1. Lai EC, Mok FP, Tan ES, et al. Endoscopic biliary drainage for severe acute cholangitis. *N Engl J Med*. 1992;326(24):1582.
2. Chijiiwa K, Kozaki N, Naito T. Treatment of choice for choledocholithiasis in patients with acute obstructive suppurative cholangitis and liver cirrhosis. *Am J Surg*. 1995;170(4):356.
3. Leese T, Neoptolemos JP, Baker AR, et al. Management of acute cholangitis and the impact of endoscopic sphincterotomy. *Br J Surg*. 1986;73(12):988.
4. Lai EC, Tam PC, Paterson IA, et al. Emergency surgery for severe acute cholangitis. The high-risk patients. *Ann Surg*. 1990;211(1):55.

**6.** Correct Answer: D

**Rationale:**
Acute postoperative pancreatic leak can lead to signs of SIRS, abdominal pain, and respiratory insufficiency. A CT abdomen and pelvis may show postoperative free fluid, but it does not give the physician a definitive diagnosis as the free fluid can be nonspecific. The diagnostic test of choice for the diagnosis of postoperative pancreatic leak or fistula is diagnosed when the amylase content of the intra-abdominal fluid from the surgical drain on or after post-operative day 3 is greater than three times the upper limit of normal serum amylase content based on the International Study Group of Pancreatic Fistulas. These pancreatic leaks/fistulas postoperatively occur at an incidence of 20% but become clinically significant in 5% to 10 % of the patients. Patients with higher body mass index and preoperative comorbidities such as jaundice, soft pancreas, and smaller pancreatic duct are at higher risk of postoperative pancreatic leak.

**References**
1. Butturini G, Daskalaki D, Molinari E, et al. Pancreatic fistula: definition and current problems. *J Hepatobiliary Pancreat Surg.* 2008;15(3):247.
2. Bassi C, Dervenis C, Butturini G, et al. Postoperative pancreatic fistula: an international study group (ISGPF) definition. *Surgery.* 2005;138(1):8.

**7.** Correct Answer: C

**Rationale:**
Cystic Hydatidosis is a significant public health problem in South America, the Middle East and eastern Mediterranean regions, some sub-Saharan African countries, western China, and the former Soviet Union territories. In the United States, transmission has been seen in California, Arizona, New Mexico, Utah, and Alaska. CT has higher overall sensitivity (95%-100%) compared to ultrasound in this diagnosis. It is superior to ultrasonography for evaluation of complications such as infection and intrabiliary rupture and fistula. Intrahepatic biliary rupture and fistula can lead to severe cholangitis and septic shock. Among the serological testing for the diagnosis of Cystic Hydatidosis, ELISA is accepted as the most sensitive and specific test. Liver and lungs are the most common sites for this disease process and the prevalence of liver and pulmonary hydatic cysts increase with age. Surgery or puncture, aspiration, injection, and re-aspiration otherwise known as PAIR are the treatments of choice. The choice between surgery or PAIR will depend on specific criteria and the complexity of the cyst and disease process. Albendazole is generally started one week before the operation and/or procedure and continued at least 4 weeks postoperatively. Metronidazole is the agent of choice for Amebic liver abscesses not Echinococcal cysts.

**References**
1. Dhar P, Chaudhary A, Desai R, et al. Current trends in the diagnosis and management of cystic hydatid disease of the liver. *J Commun Dis.* 1996;28(4):221.
2. Safioleas M, Misiakos E, Manti C, et al. Diagnostic evaluation and surgical management of hydatid disease of the liver. *World J Surg.* 1994;18(6):859.
3. Xynos E, Pechlivanides G, Tzortzinis A, et al. Hydatid disease of the liver. Diagnosis and surgical treatment. *HPB Surg.* 1991;4(1):59.
4. Kervancioglu R, Bayram M, Elbeyli L. CT findings in pulmonary hydatid disease. *Acta Radiol.* 1999;40(5):510.
5. al Karawi MA, el-Shiekh Mohamed AR, Yasawy MI. Advances in diagnosis and management of hydatid disease. *Hepatogastroenterology.* 1990;37(3):327.
6. Nasseri Moghaddam S, Abrishami A, Malekzadeh R. Percutaneous needle aspiration, injection, and reaspiration with or without benzimidazole coverage for uncomplicated hepatic hydatid cysts. *Cochrane Database Syst Rev.* 2006;(2):CD003623.
7. Neumayr A, Troia G, de Bernardis C, et al. Justified concern or exaggerated fear: the risk of anaphylaxis in percutaneous treatment of cystic echinococcosis-a systematic literature review. *PLoS Negl Trop Dis.* 2011;5(6):e1154.

**8.** Correct Answer: A

**Rationale:**
Colonoscopy and upper endoscopy have certain advantages and disadvantages compared to any other test for lower gastrointestinal bleeding. Colonoscopy can localize the bleeding site specifically no matter the etiology or the rate of bleeding and it can be therapeutic at the same time. In this question, capsule endoscopy is a type of endoscopy however, not the ideal test for a hemodynamically labile patient in the ICU and generally used in the outpatient setting. Radionuclide imaging can detect bleeding at the lowest rate of 0.1 to 0.5 mL/min. It is considered the most sensitive radiographic test for gastrointestinal bleeding. This test is also not the ideal test for a patient with concerns of labile hemodynamics in the ICU as it can take from 90 minutes to 24 hours and perhaps multiple visits to the nuclear medicine department and away from close hemodynamic monitoring. CT angiography is an appealing diagnostic modality as it is fast and minimally invasive. It can detect bleeding at rates of 0.3 to 0.5 mL/min but offers no therapeutic benefit. A formal angiography requires active blood loss of 0.5 to 1.0 mL/min. This test is reserved for patients for whom endoscopy cannot be done or with severe bleeding causing hemodynamic instability. The question above is specifically focused on which test would be ideal for a patient with hemodynamic concerns detecting a slow rate of bleeding of 0.3 to 0.5 mL/min. CT angiography is the ideal test for this patient.

### References

1. Nicholson ML, Neoptolemos JP, Sharp JF, et al. Localization of lower gastrointestinal bleeding using in vivo technetium-99m-labelled red blood cell scintigraphy. *Br J Surg.* 1989;76(4):358.
2. Olds GD, Cooper GS, Chak A, et al. The yield of bleeding scans in acute lower gastrointestinal hemorrhage. *J Clin Gastroenterol.* 2005;39(4):273.
3. Hunter JM, Pezim ME. Limited value of technetium 99m-labeled red cell scintigraphy in localization of lower gastrointestinal bleeding. *Am J Surg.* 1990;159(5):504.
4. Scheffel H, Pfammatter T, Wildi S, et al. Acute gastrointestinal bleeding: detection of source and etiology with multi-detector-row CT. *Eur Radiol.* 2007;17(6):1555.
5. Yoon W, Jeong YY, Shin SS, et al. Acute massive gastrointestinal bleeding: detection and localization with arterial phase multi-detector row helical CT. *Radiology.* 2006;239(1):160.
6. Martí M, Artigas JM, Garzón G, et al. Acute lower intestinal bleeding: feasibility and diagnostic performance of CT angiography. *Radiology.* 2012;262(1):109-116.
7. Jacovides CL, Nadolski G, Allen SR, et al. Arteriography for lower gastrointestinal hemorrhage: role of preceding abdominal computed tomographic angiogram in diagnosis and localization. *JAMA Surg.* 2015;150(7):650-656.
8. García-Blázquez V, Vicente-Bártulos A, Olavarria-Delgado A, et al. Accuracy of CT angiography in the diagnosis of acute gastrointestinal bleeding: systematic review and meta-analysis. *Eur Radiol.* 2013;23(5):1181.

# 95

# NUTRITION IN CRITICAL ILLNESS

Galen Royce-Nagel

1. A 22-year-old female who has sustained a 50% total body surface area burn in a house fire is intubated in the ICU. She is scheduled for serial debridements in the OR. The best management for perioperative nutrition includes:

   A. Begin TPN to ensure adequate nutrition despite intermittent NPO periods
   B. Place a postpyloric feeding tube to allow continuation of tube feeds intraoperatively
   C. Stop tube feeds 8 hours before the OR start time
   D. Stop tube feeds at midnight before the OR

2. A 39-year-old 80-kg trauma patient is intubated and sedated in the ICU. You are planning to start enteral nutrition. What is his daily calorie goal that you need to meet with tube feeding?

   A. 2100 kcal/d
   B. 1800 kcal/d
   C. 2600 kcal/d
   D. 1500 kcal/d

3. Which of the following patients should have enteral nutrition advanced to goal within the first 24 to 48 hours of hospitalization instead of waiting up to 1 week before instituting enteral nutrition?

   A. 24-year-old with history of type I diabetes mellitus now post multitrauma motorcycle crash
   B. 39-year-old G1P1 with ROSC after arrest due to postpartum hemorrhage
   C. 76-year-old with a history of COPD and hypertension with urosepsis and renal failure
   D. 85-year-old with a history of a lung nodule now post right lower lobe lobectomy

4. A patient's calculated nitrogen balance is 4 g/d. What change to the patient's nutrition would you make?

   A. Increase protein intake
   B. Decrease protein intake
   C. No change needs to be made to the protein content
   D. Begin 25% albumin every 8 hours

5. A frail appearing 82-year-old male is admitted to the ICU with respiratory insufficiency due to pneumonia. A nasogastric tube is placed as there are concerns for dysphagia and tube feeds are started. Approximately 24 hours after admission the patient develops signs and symptoms of left heart failure. The most likely cause of this patient's sudden cardiac dysfunction is:

   A. Low systemic phosphorous
   B. Cor pulmonale
   C. Pulmonary embolism
   D. Vitamin B3 deficiency

6. A 63-year-old female with a BMI of 55 is admitted to the ICU with a necrotizing soft tissue infection. She is intubated and enteral tube feeds are started. If indirect calorimetry is not available, how should her calorie requirements be estimated?

   A. Indirect calorimetry
   B. 22 to 25 kcal/kg/d of ideal body weight
   C. 11 to 14 kcal/kg/d of actual body weight
   D. 25 to 30 kcal/kg/d of ideal body weight

7. Indirect calorimetry determines energy expenditure by measuring:

   A. The $O_2$ consumption and $CO_2$ production over 24 hours
   B. The $O_2$ consumption via measurements from a pulmonary artery catheter
   C. The $O_2$ consumption and $CO_2$ production at rest
   D. The heat released by the body and steam released via the skin and respiration

8. A 56-year-old male is admitted with severe acute pancreatitis due to alcohol ingestion. Appropriate management of his nutrition includes:

   A. Complete bowel rest until resolution of symptoms
   B. Parenteral nutrition until recovery
   C. Enteral nutrition via jejunal route only
   D. Enteral nutrition via gastric or jejunal routes

# Chapter 95 ■ Answers

1. Correct Answer: B

   **Rationale:**
   A metaanalysis in 2003 did not find a decreased risk for aspiration with prolonged NPO. Protein-calorie malnutrition has been linked to worse outcomes with respect to ventilator-free days, ICU and hospital LOS, wound healing, and mortality. Continuing tube feeds despite trips to the OR is the best choice for nutrition management in this scenario. There is no indication to initiate TPN at this time.

   ### References
   1. Peev MP, Yeh DD, Quraishi SA, et al. Causes and consequences of interrupted enteral nutrition: a prospective observational study in critically ill surgical patients. *JPEN J Parenter Enteral Nutr.* 2015;39(1):21-27.
   2. Abunnaja S, Cuviello A, Sanchez JA. Enteral and parenteral nutrition in the perioperative period: state of the art. *Nutrients.* 2013;5(2):608-623.

2. Correct Answer: A

   **Rationale:**
   The American Society of Enteral and Parenteral Nutrition recommends the usage of a simple formula to predict calorie needs when indirect calorimetry is not available. Using 25 to 30 kcal/kg/d with the patient's dry or usual body weight allows easy calculation of an appropriate calorie range.

   ### Reference
   1. McClave SA, Taylor BE, Martindale RG, et al. Guidelines for the provision and assessment of nutrition support therapy in the adult critically ill patient. *JPEN J Parenter Enteral Nutr.* 2016;40:159-211.

3. Correct Answer: C

   **Rationale:**
   The American Society of Enteral and Parenteral Nutrition recommends that patients with a NUTRIC score ≥5 should be rapidly advanced to goal enteral nutrition within the first 24 to 48 hours. NUTRIC scores are based on age, comorbidities, APACHE score, SOFA score, and days from hospital to ICU admission (IL-6 level can also be included if available).

   ### References
   1. McClave SA, Taylor BE, Martindale RG, et al. Guidelines for the provision and assessment of nutrition support therapy in the adult critically ill patient. *JPEN J Parenter Enteral Nutr.* 2016;40:159-211.
   2. Heyland DK, Stephens KE, Day AG, McClave SA. The success of enteral nutrition and ICU-acquired infections: a multicenter observational study. *Clin Nutr.* 2011;30(2):148-155.

**4.** Correct Answer: C

**Rationale:**

Calculating the nitrogen balance requires a 24-hour urine collection and can be derived using the following formula: (total protein intake [g/d]/6.25) − (urinary urea nitrogen − 4). A standard goal for nitrogen balance is (+) 4 to 6 g/d.

Reference

1. Dickerson RN. Using nitrogen balance in clinical practice. *Hosp Pharm*. 2005;40(12):1081-1085.

**5.** Correct Answer: A

**Rationale:**

Elderly patients are particularly at risk for refeeding syndrome owing to unrecognized under nutrition. The electrolyte abnormalities that accompany refeeding syndrome include hypophosphatemia, hypomagnesemia, hypokalemia, and thiamine deficiency. All of the above are depleted during periods of malnutrition, but plasma levels drop precipitously when the body switches from catabolism during starvation to anabolism during refeeding. Cor pulmonale and pulmonary embolism are unlikely as this patient has evidence of left ventricle dysfunction. Niacin (vitamin B3) deficiency is associated with rash, vomiting/diarrhea, and dementia.

References

1. Aubry E, Friedli N, Schuetz P, et al. Refeeding syndrome in the frail elderly population: prevention, diagnosis and management. *Clin Exp Gastroenterol*. 2018;11:255-264.
2. Mehanna H, Moledina J, Travis J. Refeeding syndrome: what is it, and how to prevent and treat it. *BMJ*. 2008;336(7659):1495-1498.

**6.** Correct Answer: A

**Rationale:**

Indirect calorimetry is the gold standard for predicting calorie needs. In obese ICU patients this is particularly true as predictive formulas do not come within 10% of actual resting energy expenditure as measured by IC. In the absence of IC, ASPEN guidelines recommend using a weight-based formula of 22 to 25 kcal/kg/d of ideal body weight for patients with a BMI >50, providing 65% to 75% of caloric requirements, to allow for steady weight loss and some of the associated benefits of weight loss including decreased insulin resistance. For patients with a BMI of 30 to 50 the recommended predictive formula is 11 to 14 kcal/kg/d.

Reference

1. McClave SA, Taylor BE, Martindale RG, et al. Guidelines for the provision and assessment of nutrition support therapy in the adult critically ill patient. *JPEN J Parenter Enteral Nutr*. 2016;40:159-211.

**7.** Correct Answer: C

**Rationale:**

Indirect calorimetry takes minutes to perform and measures diluted concentrations of $O_2$ and $CO_2$ of a patient breathing at rest. A pulmonary artery catheter and arterial line can be used to estimate $O_2$ consumption, but this has been shown to underestimate the absolute number when compared to the gold standard of respiratory indirect calorimetry. Measuring the heat and steam released by the body is how direct calorimetry is performed and presents a significant cost challenge.

References

1. Pinheiro Volp AC, Esteves de Oliveira FC, Duarte Moreira Alves R, et al. Energy expenditure: components and evaluation. *Nutr Hosp*. 2011;26(3):430-440.
2. McClave SA, Taylor BE, Martindale RG, et al. Guidelines for the provision and assessment of nutrition support therapy in the adult critically ill patient. *JPEN J Parenter Enteral Nutr*. 2016;40:159-211.

**8.** Correct Answer: D

**Rationale:**

Multiple studies have indicated the benefits of continued enteral nutrition during severe acute pancreatitis. When compared to parenteral nutrition, enteral nutrition reduces infectious morbidity, multi-system organ failure, and mortality.

References

1. Seres DS, Valcarcel M, Guillaume A. Advantages of enteral nutrition over parenteral nutrition. *Therapy Adv Gastroenterol*. 2013;6(2):157-167.
2. McClave SA, Taylor BE, Martindale RG, et al. Guidelines for the provision and assessment of nutrition support therapy in the adult critically ill patient. *JPEN J Parenter Enteral Nutr*. 2016;40:159-211.

# SURGERY, TRAUMA, AND TRANSPLANTATION

# 96

# CARDIOTHORACIC AND VASCULAR SURGERY

Mina Khorashadi, Daniel Austin, Wendy Smith, Revati Nafday, Steven Hur, and Lundy Campbell

1.  A 70-year-old male is admitted to the ICU following esophagectomy for esophageal carcinoma via laparotomy and right thoracotomy. He has a history of former tobacco use (40 pack-years), hypertension, type 2 diabetes, non–obstructive coronary artery disease, and stage 3 chronic kidney disease.

    A thoracic epidural was placed preoperatively and started during the surgery. Postoperatively, the epidural infusion consists of ropivacaine 0.1% with fentanyl 2 µg/mL at 6 mL/h. Initially, the patient complained of right-sided shoulder pain that was relieved with addition of scheduled acetaminophen. On postoperative day 1, the patient is comfortable at rest, but complains of a small area of distal abdominal incisional pain that is uncontrolled when he moves or coughs. He has minimal chest wall pain. Which of the following is the most appropriate initial change to his pain regimen?

    A.  Add scheduled intravenous morphine and ketorolac
    B.  Change the epidural opioid from fentanyl to hydromorphone
    C.  Replace the epidural with a right-sided paravertebral catheter
    D.  Double the concentration of ropivacaine in the epidural solution and halve the rate of infusion

2.  A 48-year-old female with no significant past medical history presents to the emergency department (ED) with 7 days of dyspnea, fatigue, and 2 days of coughing up frank blood. Chest CT shows a large right pulmonary arteriovenous malformation (PAVM) extending the width of the right middle lobe, which is thought to be the source of bleeding. The patient is admitted to the ICU for monitoring and while in the ICU she has an episode of large volume hemoptysis (more than 300 mL) associated with desaturation to 83%, which improves to 98% with deep suctioning and oxygen delivery via non-rebreather face mask.

    The patient is intubated using a 39F left-sided double lumen tube (DLT) and the endobronchial cuff is inflated to isolate her right lung and prevent blood from entering the left lung. Immediately after intubation her vital signs are: HR 110, BP 125/68, $SaO_2$ 99% on 100% $FiO_2$.

    After confirming appropriate tube position with bronchoscopy, left-sided one lung ventilation is initiated. Approximately 10 minutes after start of one lung ventilation, her vital signs are as follows: HR 101 bpm, BP 100/62, $SaO_2$ 92% on 100% $FiO_2$.

    Which of the following factors correlates with increased risk of hypoxemia during one lung ventilation?

    A.  Right-sided one lung ventilation
    B.  Normal baseline spirometry
    C.  Normal $PaO_2$ during two lung ventilation
    D.  Lateral position

3. A 76-year-old female who is a former smoker with a 30 pack-year history is admitted to the ICU with new productive cough, fevers, dyspnea, and hypoxia. She is started on high flow nasal cannula, steroids, and antibiotics with workup initiated for COPD exacerbation versus pneumonia. Her admission chest X-ray reveals a new focal lesion in the left upper lobe (LUL); follow-up CT shows a solitary tumor involving a portion of the LUL with PET scan finding no evidence of metastases. The patient's recent pulmonary function testing demonstrates a forced expiratory volume in one second (FEV1) and diffusion capacity (DLCO) of 100%. She is being evaluated by your thoracic surgery team for possible left upper lobectomy. Using the lung segment model, what is her predicted postoperative (PPO) FEV1 and DLCO and what additional testing is necessary to further stratify her operative risk?

   A. Her predicted postoperative (ppo)-FEV1 and ppo-DLCO are approximately 75%; no further testing is necessary as she is considered low risk for anatomic lung resection

   B. Her ppo-FEV1 and ppo-DLCO are approximately 50%; no further testing is necessary as she is considered low risk for anatomic lung resection

   C. Her ppo-FEV1 and ppo-DLCO are approximately 75%; low technology exercise testing is necessary (either stair climb or shuttle walk)

   D. Her ppo-FEV1 and ppo-DLCO are approximately 50%; low technology exercise testing is necessary (either stair climb or shuttle walk)

4. A 67-year-old female with a 50 pack-year of smoking history, COPD, hypertension, and type II diabetes is admitted to the ICU following a right middle lobectomy for resection of non–small-cell adenocarcinoma. The patient has required positive pressure ventilation since her operation because of persistent hypoxemia and inadequate ventilation on pressure support. On postoperative day 5, she develops a new persistent air leak through her right-sided chest tube. Bronchoscopy confirms the presence of a bronchopleural fistula (BPF) on the right side. The ventilator repeatedly alarms for low minute ventilation (less than 0.8 L/min) despite increasing tidal volumes and RR. The latest ABG shows the following: pH 7.15, $PCO_2$ 82, $PO_2$ 63, $HCO_3$ 27 on ventilator settings of VC, TV 520, RR 24, PEEP 6, $FiO_2$ 100%. Blood pressure and heart rate have remained stable.

   Which of the following ventilation strategies is most appropriate until surgical repair of BPF can take place?

   A. Pressure control ventilation
   B. Single lung ventilation
   C. High Frequency Oscillator ventilation
   D. Synchronized Intermittent Mandatory Ventilation

5. A 54-year-old female with HTN, IDDM, obesity, and postintubation tracheal stenosis underwent a 4.3 cm tracheal resection with a pedicle flap. She is extubated after the surgery and maintained with head elevation, neck flexion, voice rest, and NPO. Routine bronchoscopy reveals a small anterior separation at the anastomosis site. Which of the following is **not** a risk factor for tracheal anastomosis complications?

   A. Age less than 18
   B. Diabetes
   C. Obesity BMI >35 kg/m²
   D. Length of tracheal resection
   E. Reoperation

6. A 72-year-old female is admitted to the ICU following a right upper lobectomy for squamous cell carcinoma that was found incidentally on workup of a thoracic vertebral compression fracture. Her past medical history is significant for 35 pack-year smoking history. She underwent preoperative PFTs that showed no evidence of significant pulmonary disease with a normal FEV1 and DLCO. Otherwise, she has an old compression fracture at T10, osteoarthritis, and mild peripheral vascular disease. She arrived to the ICU extubated, pain-free with epidural analgesia, and on 10 L oxygen delivered via facemask with an oxygen saturation of 88%. An arterial blood gas is drawn, which reveals a pH of 7.34, $pCO_2$ of 48, and a $pO_2$ of 64. Given her age, smoking history, and right upper lobectomy, you are concerned about postoperative respiratory failure. Which of the following is the best method during operative one lung ventilation to decrease the incidence of post-op acute lung injury?

   A. Ensure tidal volume of 8 to 10 mL/kg ideal body weight (IBW) to prevent atelectasis in the ventilated lung and to ensure adequate oxygenation

   B. Maintain 100% $FiO_2$ throughout one lung ventilation to avoid hypoxia and hypoxic vasoconstriction

   C. Avoid the use of PEEP in the ventilated lung to allow the use of higher tidal volume ventilation while reducing the risk of barotrauma

   D. Ensure tidal volume of 4 to 6 mL/kg IBW combined with 5 to 10 cm $H_2O$ PEEP to reduce overdistention of the ventilated single lung and maintain adequate oxygenation

7. A 29-year-old male with a history of two spontaneous pneumothoraces in the past year, and mild exercise-induced asthma, is admitted to the ICU for monitoring after a video assisted thoracoscopic surgery for resection of a 6 × 10 cm bleb in the right lower lobe. The procedure was uncomplicated and the patient was extubated without difficulty in the operating room before transport to the ICU.

   Per the anesthesiologist's note, to facilitate surgical exposure on the operative lung, the patient was intubated with a left-sided DLT after induction of anesthesia. Single lung ventilation (of the nonoperative lung) was then initiated following conformation of proper position of the DLT using a flexible fiberoptic bronchoscope.

   Which of the following is an advantage of a DLT over a bronchial blocker (BB)?

   A. DLT is preferred in patients who require postoperative mechanical ventilation
   B. Selective lobar isolation can only be achieved using a DLT
   C. Bronchial suctioning of the nonventilated lung is only possible when using a DLT
   D. DLT is the preferred method to isolate the lung in a tracheostomized patient who has had a laryngectomy.

8. A 46-year-old previously healthy male who was recently diagnosed with lymphoma is transferred to your ICU from an outside hospital in septic shock due to presumed pneumonia. On arrival he is developing worsening hypoxemic, hypercarbic respiratory failure, and will need to be intubated. A CXR is significant for bilateral, patchy opacities, and a widened superior mediastinum. Which of the following tests would be most helpful in determining the patient's risk for airway compromise during induction of general anesthesia (GA) and intubation?

   A. Normal, recent pulmonary function tests
   B. Ability to lie supine without orthopnea or cough
   C. Lung and airway auscultation
   D. Echocardiogram

9. A 46-year-old female with a history of atrial fibrillation presents with a left atrial appendage clot, despite being on oral anticoagulation therapy. She was admitted to the ICU from the electrophysiology laboratory following left atrial appendage isolation with the LARIAT procedure. She received 5000 units of heparin before trans-septal puncture. Following successful left atrial appendage exclusion, she received protamine and all procedural catheters were removed. Over the course of her first hour in the ICU she has become progressively more hypotensive and tachycardic, and she remains in atrial fibrillation. On physical examination she is tachypneic with jugular venous distension and muffled heart sounds. What is the next best step in confirming her diagnosis?

   A. Assessing for the presence of pulsus paradoxus
   B. Cardiac MRI
   C. Echocardiogram
   D. Cardiac catheterization

10. A 68-year-old male with a thoracic aortic aneurysm underwent thoracic endovascular aortic stent graft repair (TEVAR). A lumbar spinal drain was placed at the start of the case for spinal cord protection and cerebral spinal fluid (CSF) pressure was maintained at less than 15 mm Hg by intermittent CSF drainage as needed throughout the case. The procedure went well and lasted approximately 6 hours. At the end of the case, the patient was extubated and was admitted to the ICU for post-op management.

   The spinal drain was kept in place, and the CSF pressure was maintained in the 10 to 12 mm Hg range for the first 24 hours with intermittent CSF drainage as needed. On postoperative day #2, the patient remained neurologically intact and the drain was clamped. The following day, he was noted to have bilateral lower extremity weakness. The ICU team was called urgently to evaluate him. He was hemodynamically stable with a heart rate of 65, blood pressure of 110/55 with a MAP of 73, respiratory rate of 12 on room air with an oxygen saturation of 98%. Laboratory test results revealed a white blood cell count of 10, hemoglobin of 8, and platelets of 220. Physical examination was remarkable only for symmetric bilateral lower extremity weakness of 2/5.

   Which of the following interventions would be the least helpful to restore neurologic function in the patient?

   A. Reopen the spinal drain and drain off CSF to a pressure of approximately 10 mm Hg. Do not exceed 10 to 15 mL of CSF drainage per hour
   B. Increase MAP to 90 mm Hg or greater using vasopressors as needed
   C. Transfuse patient to a hemoglobin of 10 or greater
   D. Reopen the spinal drain and immediately drain 30 mL CSF per hour as needed to restore neurologic function and achieve a CSF pressure of less than 10 mm Hg

**11.** A 66-year-old female with a history of peripheral vascular disease, hypertension, prior stroke, and insulin-dependent diabetes is found to have expansion of her abdominal aortic aneurysm (AAA) on interval surveillance imaging and is scheduled for elective AAA open repair. As part of her preoperative workup, she has a positive nuclear stress test, leading to a cardiac catheterization showing 80% stenosis of the distal left anterior descending (LAD) artery. She undergoes elective AAA repair and is admitted to the ICU afterward. During her recovery, a family member is upset to learn that her coronary artery disease was not fixed before such a large surgery. How do you answer?

    **A.** This was a major oversight—coronary artery revascularization should be performed before most elective major vascular surgery, as this has been shown to decrease long-term mortality

    **B.** Coronary artery revascularization should not be performed before major elective surgery as it has been shown to increase long-term mortality

    **C.** Coronary artery revascularization should not be performed before major elective vascular surgery as it has not been shown to provide any long-term mortality benefit

    **D.** There have not been any large clinical trials assessing coronary revascularization before elective major vascular surgery to help answer this family member's question

**12.** A 63-year-old female who initially presented to the ED with chest pain radiating to her back was found to have a Stanford type B (descending only) aortic dissection and was admitted to the ICU for acute medical management. Her urine output is adequate (1 mL/kg/min), is neurologically intact, and has normal metabolic laboratories. To decrease the shear stress on her aortic dissection she was started on IV metoprolol and IV labetolol with good initial results. Her heart rate is 60 bpm, her blood pressure is 110/70, and she is pain-free.

On her third ICU day she develops increasing pain and becomes progressively more hypertensive with BP 150/90, on metoprolol and labetolol. Considering her worsening condition, what course of therapy has been shown to most improve her overall survival?

    **A.** Increase her antihypertensive medications with the addition of iv sodium nitroprusside

    **B.** Proceed with endovascular aortic stent graft repair

    **C.** Increase her pain medications to better control pain and associated hypertension

    **D.** Proceed with emergent open repair of her type B dissection

**13.** You are called to the ED to evaluate a 54-year-old female who presented with sudden onset chest pain, which began while exercising at the gym, described as "tearing," with radiation to her upper back. She is a former smoker with a history of hypertension, hyperlipidemia, and diabetes. On presentation her heart rate is 112 and blood pressure is 182/93; she is taking shallow breaths at 18 and her oxygenation saturation is 98% on 2 L NC. Physical examination is significant for a middle-aged woman, mildly diaphoretic, with a diastolic, decrescendo murmur, best heard at the left upper sternal border, and equal breath sounds with crackles at the bases. Chest CT shows an aortic dissection originating in the ascending aorta. What is the next best step in her management?

    **A.** Transesophageal echo

    **B.** Start a nitroprusside infusion

    **C.** Consult cardiology

    **D.** Start an esmolol infusion

**14.** A 72-year-old male was brought into the ED with crushing substernal chest pain while mowing his lawn with EKG changes showing T-wave inversions and elevated serum troponins. His symptoms resolve with sublingual nitroglycerin, and he is hemodynamically stable throughout his workup. He undergoes cardiac catheterization shortly thereafter and is found to have multivessel coronary artery disease and is scheduled for coronary-artery bypass graft (CABG) surgery with the use of cardiopulmonary bypass (CPB) (on-pump) the next day. He is admitted to the ICU on a heparin infusion for closer monitoring. Which of the following statements is correct with regard to off-pump versus on-pump CABG?

    **A.** Off-pump CABG decreases all-cause mortality compared with on-pump CABG

    **B.** Off-pump CABG increases all-cause mortality compared with on-pump CABG

    **C.** Across many clinical trials, no significant mortality differences have been shown between on-pump and off-pump CABG

    **D.** There have not been adequate randomized clinical trials comparing off-pump versus on-pump CABG

15. A 59-year-old male who underwent an aortic valve replacement for congenital bicuspid aortic stenosis is admitted to the ICU post-op. The case went well, with a short bypass and cross-clamp time, minimal blood loss, and no blood products given. At the end of the case, an intraoperative TEE showed good biventricular function and a small amount of air in the apex of the left ventricle. For medications during the case, the patient received 1500 µg fentanyl; 100 mg of Propofol for induction; 100 mg of rocuronium, heparin, and protamine for bypass; and tranexamic acid for antifibrinolysis, and he was placed on dexmedetomidine post-op for sedation in the ICU.

He was extubated without difficulty 5 hours after his arrival from the operating room. Shortly after extubation, he had a witnessed generalized myoclonic seizure. The seizure was terminated within a few minutes after one dose of intravenous lorazepam. A stat head CT was obtained, which was read as normal with no acute changes. He was seen by neurology and had no further seizure activity throughout his hospital stay.

Other than air from the surgical procedure, which of the following medications that the patient received are most likely associated with postoperative risk of seizure?

A. Propofol
B. Dexmedetomidine
C. Rocuronium
D. Tranexamic acid
E. Fentanyl

# Chapter 96 ▪ Answers

1. Correct Answer: B

**Rationale:**
Pain following thoracic surgery can be a serious issue for patients, not only because of its intensity and duration but also because of its adverse effects on pulmonary function and recovery.

Opioids are considered a mainstay of significant postoperative pain management. However, a narrow therapeutic range and potential for sedation and respiratory depression are general limitations of this class of drugs. Morphine (A) in particular should be used with caution in elderly patients and patients with renal disease due to its active metabolites and long-lasting effects. Although addition of an intravenous opioid might improve this patient's pain control, his major complaint has to do with pain with activity, and scheduling morphine is not the most appropriate first step.

NSAIDs are reversible COX inhibitors that can be very effective for treating the inflammatory component of postoperative pain. In general, meta-analyses of randomized controlled trials report improved pain scores and reduced analgesic use when intravenous morphine combined with ketorolac is compared with intravenous morphine alone. With respect to thoracotomy pain, the addition of NSAIDs as part of a multimodal pain regimen can be especially effective to treat shoulder pain that is refractory to epidural anesthesia, as well as to reduce overall opioid requirements. However, NSAIDs have also been associated with decreased platelet function, gastric erosions, increased bronchial reactivity, and decreased renal function. NSAIDs should be used with caution in patients who are elderly or have known risk factors for postoperative renal failure, including hypertension, diabetes, and preexisting renal disease. This patient's shoulder pain has already been relieved by acetaminophen, which is a weak COX inhibitor. Although NSAIDs may also improve his incisional pain, scheduled ketorolac (A) would not be the best option given his age and comorbidities.

Currently, in the absence of contraindications, a thoracic epidural may be considered the "standard" of analgesia for open thoracotomy. Coverage of dermatomes far from the site of insertion can be achieved by increasing volume of local anesthetic or replacing epidural fentanyl with a hydrophilic opioid such as hydromorphone (B) or morphine, as highly lipid-soluble agents are associated with narrower dermatomal spread, and given his pain is concentrated to a small area, the fentanyl may be spreading too much.

Paravertebral catheters (C) have been shown to have similar efficacy to epidurals following thoracic surgery and are a reasonable alternative. However, this patient's epidural appears to be functioning, given that he has no chest wall pain and only a small distal area of pain. Before proceeding with another invasive procedure, it is more appropriate to attempt to augment the existing epidural by changing the solution or increasing the rate.

Increasing the concentration of ropivacaine in the epidural while halving the rate (D) would potentially increase the density of the blockade, but not the spread.

References

1. American Society of Anesthesiologists Task Force on Acute Pain Management. Practice guidelines for acute pain management in the perioperative setting: an updated report by the American Society of Anesthesiologists Task Force on Acute Pain Management. *Anesthesiology.* 2004;100:1573-1581.

2. Gottschalk A, Cohen SP, Yang S, Ochroch EA. Preventing and treating pain after thoracic surgery. *Anesthesiology.* 2006;104:594-600.

3. Kavanagh BP, Katz J, Sandler AN. Pain control after thoracic surgery: a review of current techniques. *Anesthesiology.* 1994;81:737-759.

4. Miller RD. *Miller's Anesthesia.* 8th ed. Philadelphia, PA: Elsevier Churchill Livingstone; 2015.

## 2. Correct Answer: B

**Rationale:**

During one lung ventilation while both lungs are perfused only one lung is ventilated. This invariably leads to transpulmonary shunting and impairment in oxygenation. Hypoxemia typically occurs within the first 10 to 30 minutes of initiation of OLV and stabilizes or slightly increases as hypoxic pulmonary vasoconstriction (HPV) increases over the next 2 hours.

A number of factors may be helpful in predicting oxygenation during OLV:

Side of ventilation—The right lung is larger and 10% better perfused than the left lung. Thus, it is not surprising that right-sided OLV is better tolerated than left-sided OLV. The overall mean $PaO_2$ is 100 mm Hg higher during stable right-sided OLV than during left-sided OLV (A).

Baseline Spirometry—Studies consistently show that patients with better spirometric lung function are more likely to desaturate during OLV. This is due to a dramatic increase in shunt fraction on initiation of one lung ventilation. Oxygenation often improves as HPV diverts blood flow to the ventilated lung with decreasing shunt fraction over time.

Typically, patients with an obstructive spirometric pattern tolerate OLV very well. In a chronically diseased lung, perfusion to areas with poor function is decreased because of chronic HPV. Thus, there is a less dramatic change in shunt fraction when OLV is initiated (B).

Baseline $PaO_2$—Abnormally low arterial oxygen tension ($PaO_2$) as found by blood gas analysis during two lung ventilation is a reliable indicator of abnormal lung function and a predictor of hypoxemia during OLV. $PaO_2$ levels during two lung ventilation are strongly and positively correlated with $PaO_2$ during OLV (C)

Position—Patient's position during OLV is a factor in oxygenation. Positioning ventilated lung in the dependent position decreases VQ mismatch as perfusion to the ventilated lung increases because of gravity, whereas blood flow to the nonventilated lung is decreased (D).

References

1. Karzai W, Schwarzkopf K. Hypoxemia during one-lung ventilation: prediction, prevention, and treatment. *Anesthesiology.* 2009;110(6):1402-1411.

2. Guenoun T, Journois D, Silleran-Chassany J, et al. Prediction of arterial oxygenation during one-lung ventilation: analysis of preoperative and intraoperative variables. *J Cardiothorac Vasc Anesth.* 2004;16:199-203.

## 3. Correct Answer: A

**Rationale:**

It is vital to understand the role of preoperative testing and risk stratification in lung resection surgery candidates, as poor candidate selection can lead to profound morbidity and mortality. There are evidence-based guidelines to help clinicians risk stratify individual patients and pursue further testing for higher risk candidates based on PPO function. According to the American College of Chest Physicians (ACCP): "In patients with lung cancer being considered for surgery, it is recommended that both $FEV_1$ and DLCO be measured in all patients and that both PPO $FEV_1$ and PPO DLCO are calculated" (Brunelli et al 2013, pg. e173S).

The anatomic lung segment model divides the lungs into 19 total segments; the left upper and left lower lobe each respectively contain 5 and 4 segments while the right upper, middle, and lower lobes respectively contain 3, 2, and 5 segments. To calculate the PPO FEV1 or DLCO, first determine the percent reduction in lung volume; in your patient, a left upper lobectomy would eliminate 5 of the 19 segments, or roughly 25% (5/19 = 0.26). Therefore, the new FEV1 (or DLCO) would be:

$$\text{ppo-FEV1\%} = \text{Patient's Baseline FEV1} - \left[ \left( 1 - \text{resected lung segment fraction} \right) \times 100 \right]$$

$$= 100 - \left[ \left( 1 - 0.26 \right) \times 100 \right] = 74\%$$

According to ACCP Guidelines, "In patients with lung cancer being considered for surgery, if both PPO FEV1 and PPO DLCO are >60% predicted, no further tests are recommended" (Brunelli et al 2013, pg e175S). For those whose ppo-FEV1 and/or ppo-DLCO is less than 60%, additional testing is required and depends on the severity of disease (see Brunelli et al 2013, pg e179S).

### Reference

1. Brunelli A, Kim AW, Berger KI, et al. Physiologic evaluation of the patient with lung cancer being considered for resectional surgery. *Chest.* 2013;143(5 suppl):e166S-e190S.

---

**4.** Correct Answer: B

**Rationale:**

BPF occurs when air from a lobar or segmental bronchus leaks into the pleural space. This is most commonly encountered after lung resection surgery with a frequency ranging from 4.5% to 20% after pneumonectomy and 0.5% to 1% after lobectomy.

In most cases BPF is present in the early postoperative period (<2 weeks) following lung resection. BPF should be suspected in the postoperative lung resection patient who presents with sudden onset of dyspnea, chest pain, subcutaneous emphysema, and hemodynamic instability (ie symptoms of tension pneumothorax). Symptoms may be less abrupt, however, in patients whose chest tube is still in place. In such patients, presence of persistent or new air leak may be the only presenting sign. Bronchoscopy is often used to confirm the diagnosis.

BPFs are associated with significant morbidity and a mortality that ranges from 16% to 72%. BPFs do not typically resolve spontaneously and almost always require surgical or bronchoscopic intervention. Supportive measures should be taken to maintain hemodynamic and ventilatory stability. The first intervention is insertion of a chest tube (if not already in place) on the ipsilateral side, to drain air and fluid from the pleural space. Positive pressure and PEEP should be minimized as higher airway pressures worsen air leak and may result in impairment in ventilation and gas exchange. If adequate ventilation is not achieved using minimal positive pressure and low PEEP, isolated ventilation of the contralateral lung is indicated to maintain adequate gas exchange until definitive correction of BPF can take place.

### References

1. Farkas EA, Detterbeck FC. Airway complications after pulmonary resection. *Thorac Surg Clin.* 2006;16:243.
2. Wright CD, Wain JC, Mathisen DJ, Grillo HC. Postpneumonectomy bronchopleural fistula after sutured bronchial closure: incidence, risk factors, and management. *J Thorac Cardiovasc Surg.* 1996;112:1367.
3. Li SJ, Zhou XD, Huang J, et al. A systematic review and meta-analysis-does chronic obstructive pulmonary disease predispose to bronchopleural fistula formation in patients undergoing lung cancer surgery? *J Thorac Dis.* 2016;8:1625.

---

**5.** Correct Answer: C

**Rationale:**

The most frequent indication for tracheal resection is postintubation tracheal stenosis. Other indications include tumor, idiopathic laryngotracheal stenosis, and tracheoesophageal fistula. Operative complications can be divided into anastomotic (granulation tissue, restenosis, and separation) and nonanastomotic (infection, laryngeal dysfunction, edema, post-op hoarseness, and fistula). Based on the largest case series published on postoperative outcomes from Massachusetts General Hospital from 1975 to 2003, anastomotic complications occurred in 9% of patients, with separation occurring in 4% of patients. Risk factors for anastomotic complications were identified as reoperation, diabetes, tracheal resection ≥4 cm, laryngotracheal resection, and age <18. Interestingly, neither obesity (BMI >35) or steroid use was a risk factor. The most important postoperative goal is to minimize anastomotic tension. That is accomplished by early extubation (if possible), neck flexion, minimizing coughing and vomiting, voice rest, careful swallow evaluation, and routine bronchoscopy to detect issues before occurrence of symptoms. Careful attention should be paid toward stridor, voice changes, secretions, subcutaneous air, and neck swelling. Should timely extubation be difficult, a small tracheostomy at least 2 cm distal to the anastomosis should be considered.

### References

1. Auchincloss HG, Wright CD. Complications after tracheal resection and reconstruction: prevention and treatment. *J Thorac Dis.* 2016;8(suppl 2):S160-S167.
2. Auchincloss HG, Mathisen DJ. Tracheal stenosis—resection and reconstruction. *Ann Cardiothorac Surg.* 2018;7(2):306-308.

---

**6.** Correct Answer: D

**Rationale:**

This topic remains somewhat controversial, as there is no clear evidence that ventilation with low tidal volumes in all patients undergoing one lung ventilation is universally beneficial. However, based on patients with acute lung injury, and on animal models where low tidal volume ventilation has been shown to improve survival, it has become accepted practice to reduce tidal volumes to 4 to 6 mL/Kg of IBW and apply moderate PEEP in the 5 to 10 cm $H_2O$ range to maintain adequate oxygenation in this patient population.

It is thought that lower tidal volumes during one lung ventilation may be protective against postoperative respiratory complications due to inflammation of the ventilated lung leading to postoperative injury such as pulmonary edema. This reduction in inflammation was demonstrated in a study of patients undergoing esophagectomy with single lung ventilation. In that study, ventilation with 5 mL/Kg of IBW and application of 5 cm $H_2O$ PEEP resulted in reduced levels of the inflammatory markers IL-1B, IL-6, and IL-8, compared to patients who were ventilated at 9 mL/Kg IBW without PEEP during one lung ventilation. Any maneuver that will increase tidal volume is likely to be harmful during single lung ventilation. Excessively high inspired oxygen levels are associated with oxygen free radical injury and should be avoided if at all possible.

A recent meta-analysis demonstrated higher postoperative $PaO_2/FiO_2$ ratios in patients who were ventilated with low tidal volumes, versus conventional (8-10 mL/kg ventilation) during one lung ventilation. This same meta-analysis also demonstrated a decreased incidence of postsurgical pulmonary infiltrates and acute lung injury in patients ventilated with a low tidal volume strategy.

### References

1. Michelet P, D'Journo X-B, Roch A, et al. Protective ventilation influences systemic inflammation after esophagectomy. A randomized controlled study. *Anesthesiology*. 2006;105:911-919.
2. El Tahan MR, Pasin L, Marczin N, et al. Impact of low tidal volumes during one-lung ventilation. A meta-analysis of randomized controlled trials. *J Cardiothorac Vasc Anesth*. 2017;31:1767-1773.
3. Yang M, Ahn HJ, Kim K, et al. Does a lung protective ventilation strategy reduce the risk of pulmonary complications after lung cancer surgery? A randomized controlled trial. *Chest*. 2011;139:530-537.
4. Blank RS, Colquhoun DA, Durieux ME, et al. Management of one-lung ventilation. Impact of tidal volume on complications after thoracic surgery. *Anesthesiology*. 2016;124:1286-1295.
5. Slinger PD. Do low tidal volumes decrease lung injury during one-lung ventilation? *J Cardiothorac Vasc Anesth*. 2017;31:1774-1775.

---

**7.  Correct Answer: C**

**Rationale:**

There are a number of indications for lung isolation. In practice, the most common indications are for surgical exposure during thoracic, mediastinal, vascular, or esophageal procedures. Lung isolation is also used to prevent contamination to the contralateral lung from bleeding, pus, or saline lavage as in the case of hemoptysis, abscess, and whole lung lavage. In addition, lung isolation can be used for differential pattern of ventilation in cases of unilateral reperfusion injury (unilateral lung transplant or pulmonary thromboendarterectomy), trauma, and BPFs.

Lung isolation can be achieved by three different techniques: DLTs, BBs, or mainstem intubation using a single lumen endotracheal tube. The most common method is with a DLT, which is a bifurcated tube with both an endotracheal and an endobroncheal lumen and is used to isolate the right or the left lung. DLTs may be inserted by direct laryngoscopy or by guiding the endobronchial lumen to the mainstem bronchus using a flexible fiberoptic bronchoscope. Auscultation alone is not reliable to confirm proper positioning and bronchoscopic verification should be used, in addition to auscultation, to confirm placement every time a DLT is placed or when the patient is repositioned. DLT cannot be used for selective lobar isolation because both tracheal and endobronchial cuffs are positioned proximal to the lobar bronchi. Thus, ventilation through either lumen will result in inflation of all the lobes in that lung (B). DLTs are not ideal for placement in a tracheal stoma owing to their size. In a tracheostomized patient who cannot be intubated orally (eg post laryngectomy), BBs may be used to achieve one lung ventilation (D).

Lung isolation with a BB is achieved by occluding a mainstem bronchus and allowing lung collapse distal to the occlusion. These devices are most commonly placed within a single lumen tube, and a fiberoptic bronchoscope is required to position the blocker in the appropriate bronchus. They can also be placed in a lobar bronchus to selectively isolate a lobe (B). Suctioning of the nonventilated lung (or lobe) is not possible when using a BB because the bronchus is completely occluded by the device (C).

Another advantage of the BB is when postoperative mechanical ventilation is being considered after prolonged thoracic or esophageal surgery. These patients often have significant airway edema at the end of the procedure. If a BB is used, there is no need to change the endotracheal tube and there is no compromise of the airway if mechanical ventilation is needed in the postoperative period (A). Prolonged use of DLT without an indication for OLV is not recommended.

### References

1. Clayton-Smith A, Bennett K, Alston RP, et al, A comparison of the efficacy and adverse effects of double-lumen endobronchial tubes and bronchial blockers in thoracic surgery: a systematic review and meta-analysis of randomized controlled trials. *J Cardiothorac Vasc Anesth*. 2015;29:955-966.
2. Miller RD. *Miller's Anesthesia*. 8th ed. Philadelphia, PA: Elsevier Churchill Livingstone; 2015.

---

**8.  Correct Answer: B**

**Rationale:**

Given this patient's recent diagnosis of lymphoma and widened superior mediastinum on CXR, there is concern for an anterior mediastinal mass, which may lead to airway compromise during induction of GA. During spontaneous ventilation, extrinsic intrathoracic airway compression is mitigated by bronchial smooth muscle tone and airway distension as a result of the normal transpleural pressure gradient during inspiration. These protective mechanisms are blunted or eliminated during GA, and tracheobronchial diameters are further reduced as a result of decreased lung volumes and through possible compression from the anterior mediastinal mass. In light of this, a methodical induction and intubation plan must be formulated for these patients. Ideally, in a patient such as this, available chest CT images should be reviewed before proceeding with intubation. This is done to better characterize the size and location of the mass and any airway displacement or narrowing to determine the difficulty of passing an endotracheal tube distal to the obstruction. As this patient is heading toward emergent intubation because of his concomitant respiratory failure, the decision to intubate will have to proceed without this information.

In the presence of an anterior mediastinal mass, a patient's ability to lie flat without orthopnea or coughing has been found to be the best predictor of airway compromise during induction of anesthesia. These symptoms can be classified as mild, moderate, or severe. Patients with severe symptoms will be unwilling to lie flat, even for short periods of time, and carry the highest risk of airway compromise.

Though abnormalities in air flow patterns on pulmonary function tests do accompany severe tracheal obstruction in patients with mediastinal masses, the classical blunting of the expiratory limb does not appear to be pathognomonic for variable intrathoracic airway obstruction in the setting of anterior mediastinal mass and has not been shown to predict airway complications during induction and intubation. However, the presence of a mixed restrictive/obstructive pattern may predict postoperative pulmonary complications including atelectasis and pneumonia as it implies the compression of lung parenchyma.

If chest imaging, physical examination and or vital sign changes indicate pericardial effusion or compression of cardiac chambers or major vessels, an echocardiogram is indicated to further evaluate for the risk of hemodynamic compromise on induction of GA but will not predict the risk of airway compromise.

Lung auscultation should always be performed before intubation however; it will not provide a reliable prediction of airway compromise in this patient.

### References

1. Blank RS, De Souza DG. *Can J Anesth*. 2011;58:853-867.
2. Hnatiuk OW, Corcoran PC, Sierra A. Spirometry in surgery for anterior mediastinal masses. *Chest*. 2001;120:1152-1156.
3. Kaplan JA, Augoustides JGT, Manecke GR, et al. *Kaplan's Cardiac Anesthesia: For Cardiac and Noncardiac Surgery*. Philadelphia, PA: Elsevier; 2017:Chap 49.
4. Vander Els NJ, Sorhage F, Bach AM, et al. Abnormal flow volume loops in patients with intrathoracic Hodgkin's disease. *Chest*. 2000;117:1256-1261.

---

**9.** Correct Answer: C

**Rationale:**
This patient has risk factors for and signs of cardiac tamponade. Noninvasive procedures involving trans-septal puncture carry the risk of bleeding into the pericardium should the proceduralist mistakenly exit and reenter the heart when traveling from the right to left atrium rather than directing their catheter through the fossa ovalis. The gold standard for identifying pericardial effusions causing tamponade is echocardiography, which allows assessment of the size and location of the effusion and also the pathognomonic signs of late diastolic right atrial collapse and early diastolic right ventricular collapse. Although pulsus paradoxus is often present in cardiac tamponade it may be absent in many instances leading to a false negative test. These conditions include: the presence of a large ASD, severe aortic regurgitation, loculated effusions, left-ventricular hypertrophy, hypovolemic shock, severe LV dysfunction, low-pressure tamponade, right ventricular hypertrophy, positive pressure ventilation, and arrhythmias such as atrial fibrillation. A cardiac MRI will also provide information regarding the size and location of effusion but could lead to an inappropriate delay in diagnosis or management in an unstable patient. Although this patient may ultimately go to the cardiac catheterization laboratory where hemodynamic parameters can be confirmed and the effusion can be drained via pericardiocentesis, an echo should first be performed to confirm the diagnosis.

### References

1. Parrillo JE, Dellinger RP. *Critical Care Medicine: Principles of Diagnosis and Management in the Adult*. Philadelphia, PA: Elsevier; 2014:Chap 24.
2. Adler Y, Charron P, Imazio M, et al. 2015 ESC guidelines for the diagnosis and management of pericardial diseases. *Eur Heart J*. 2015;36:2921-2964.

---

**10.** Correct Answer: D

**Rationale:**
Spinal cord injury following TEVAR has been reported to occur in up to 12% of cases. This is comparable to open surgical repair; however, with endovascular procedures, there is a greater percentage of patients who present with delayed onset paraplegia. In a few randomized clinical trials and multiple retrospective studies, CSF drainage has been shown to reduce the risk of postoperative spinal cord injury.

In TEVAR procedures, spinal cord injury is believed to occur via occlusion of spinal cord perfusing intercostal arteries by the covered stent graft. Essentially the treatment goal to prevent postoperative paraplegia is to increase oxygen delivery to the partially ischemic spinal cord. Oxygen delivery is maximized by increasing the hemoglobin level in the blood as well as by improving blood flow to the cord through optimization of the spinal cord perfusion pressure (SPP). This pressure is the difference between MAP and spinal fluid pressure (SFP) and is demonstrated by the following formula.

$$SPP = MAP - SFP$$

Therefore, by both raising MAP and reducing SFP, SPP is optimized. Current consensus guidelines recommend a MAP of at least 80 mm Hg, and a CSF pressure between 10 to 12 mm Hg for at least 48 hours in the perioperative period to improve cord perfusion pressure. Over drainage of the CSF with pressures below 10 mm Hg, or removing more than 10 to 15 mL per hour may cause intracranial hypotension resulting in intracranial hemorrhage. In addition to optimizing SPP, consensus guidelines also recommend keeping hemoglobin levels at 10 or greater to increase the oxygen carrying capacity of the blood that is reaching the spinal cord, thereby improving oxygen delivery.

Excessive drainage of CSF (such as draining 30 mL/h to drive CSF pressure to less than 10 mm Hg) risks intracranial hemorrhage.

## References

1. Coselli JS, LeMaire SA, Köksoy C, et al. Cerebrospinal fluid drainage reduces paraplegia after thoracoabdominal aortic aneurysm repair: results of a randomized clinical trial. *J Vasc Surg.* 2002;35:631-639.
2. Kakinohana M. What should we do against delayed onset paraplegia following TEVAR? *J Anesth.* 2014;28:1-3.
3. Fedorow CA, Moon MC, Mutch AC, et al. Lumbar cerebrospinal fluid drainage for thoracoabdominal aortic surgery: rationale and practical considerations for management. *Anesth Analg.* 2011;111:46-58.
4. Scott DA, Denton MJ. Spinal cord protection in aortic endovascular surgery. *Br J Anaesth.* 2016;117(S2):ii26-ii31.
5. Riambau V, Capoccia L, Mestres G, Matute P. Spinal cord protection and related complications in endovascular management of B dissection: LSA revascularization and CSF drainage. *Ann Cardiothorac Surg.* 2014;3(3):336-338.
6. Weigang E, Hartert M, Siegenthaler MP, et al. Perioperative management to improve neurologic outcome in thoracic or thoracoabdominal aortic stent-grafting. *Ann Thorac Surg.* 2006;82:1679-1687.
7. Hamdy A, Ramadan ME, El Sayed HF, et al. Spinal cord injury after thoracic endovascular aortic aneurysm repair. *Can J Anaesth.* 2017;64(12):1218-1235.

---

**11.** Correct Answer: C

**Rationale:**

The Coronary Artery Revascularization Prophylaxis Trial, published in the New England Journal of Medicine in 2004, completed a multicenter randomized clinical trial to assess whether preemptive coronary revascularization (either percutaneous coronary intervention or coronary artery bypass graft [CABG] surgery) conferred any mortality benefit before elective major vascular surgery (either AAA repair or arterial occlusive disease of the lower extremities). Five hundred patients with stable cardiac symptoms and known coronary artery disease were randomized to either receive coronary revascularization, followed by elective vascular surgery, or proceed directly to the planned vascular surgery. The study measured mortality up to 2.7 years after randomization and found no significant difference in mortality between the two groups. Both groups also had equivalent rates of postoperative myocardial infarction (within 30 days of surgery). Based on these findings, it is generally recommended to proceed directly with vascular surgery in patients with stable coronary artery disease.

## Reference

1. McFalls EO, Ward HB, Moritz TE, et al. Coronary-artery revascularization before elective major vascular surgery. *N Engl J Med.* 2004;351(27):2795-2804.

---

**12.** Correct Answer: B

**Rationale:**

Type B aortic dissections that demonstrate a good response to medical therapy alone with alleviation of pain and heart rate below 60 and systolic blood pressure between 100 to 120 are classified as uncomplicated. Typically, patients with uncomplicated dissections are medically managed with beta blockers and antihypertensive agents to decrease the shear forces on the aortic wall and prevent further dissection. Optimal medical management is associated with a 90% to 99% long-term survival in this patient group.

Refractory pain or worsening hypertension in patients with uncomplicated type B aortic dissection denotes failure of medical management. Worsening pain may indicate progression of the dissection flap, and worsening hypertension may be due to renal malperfusion from an extending dissection. In this case, the type B dissection should then be classified as a complicated dissection. Continued medical management alone in this patient group is associated with significantly increased mortality (approximately 30%-40% in-hospital mortality compared with 1%-2% in-hospital mortality in patients with uncomplicated dissections).

Patients with complicated dissections should be treated with surgical intervention to halt further dissection of the aorta. Traditionally this was performed via an open surgical approach, but the in-hospital mortality associated with open repair has remained consistently high, around 20% to 30% since the first operation of this type was performed.

Conversely, endovascular repair of type B aortic dissection is associated with a much lower in-hospital mortality of approximately 3% to 10%. Therefore, to give this patient the best chance of survival, an endovascular repair of her complicated type B aortic dissection should be performed.

### References

1. Suzuki T, Mehta RH, Ince H, et al. Clinical profiles and outcomes of acute type B aortic dissection in the current era: lessons from the international registry of aortic dissection (IRAD). *Circulation.* 2003;108:II-312-II-317.
2. Umana JP, Lai DT, Mitchell RS, et al. Is medical therapy still the optimal treatment strategy for patients with acute type B aortic dissections? *J Thorac Cardiovasc Surg.* 2002;124:896-910.
3. Trimarchi S, Eagle KA, Nienaber CA, et al. Importance of refractory pain and hypertension in acute type B aortic dissection. Insights from the international registry of acute aortic dissection (IRAD). *Circulation.* 2010;122:1283-1289.
4. Hughes GC. Management of acute type B aortic dissection; ADSORB trial. *J Thorac Cardiovasc Surg.* 2015;149:S158-S162.
5. Tsai TT, Nienaber CA, Eagle KA. Acute aortic syndromes. *Circulation.* 2005;112:3802-3813.
6. Nienaber CA, Rousseau H, Eggebrecht H, et al. Randomized comparison of strategies for type B aortic dissection. The INvestigation of STEnt grafts in Aortic Dissection (INSTEAD) trial. *Circulation.* 2009;120:2519-2528.
7. Estrera AL, Miller CC, Safi HJ, et al. Outcomes of medical management of acute type B aortic dissection. *Circulation.* 2006;114(suppl I):I-384-I-389.
8. Scott AJ, Bicknell CD. Contemporary management of acute type B dissection. *Eur J Vasc Endovasc Surg.* 2016;51:452-459.

---

**13.** Correct Answer: D

**Rationale:**

This patient has clear evidence of type A aortic dissection with high risk features, which will require immediate surgical intervention. While awaiting definitive treatment, your priority must be to reduce the risk of dissection propagation by decreasing shearing forces. This is best achieved by controlling heart rate (goal 60-75 bpm), decreasing contractile force and lowering blood pressure. Although Nitroprusside will lower this patient's blood pressure, it may lead to reflex tachycardia and should only be started once heart rate control has been achieved with an easily titratable agent such as Esmolol. If the patient had been unstable and inappropriate for transport to the CT scanner, a transesophageal echo would have been an acceptable alternative imaging modality, but given that you already have evidence of a type A dissection in a patient with high-risk features, no further imaging is necessary. Given this patient's presentation, part of your initial assessment should have been to differentiate between acute coronary syndrome and aortic dissection. Had the question indicated that the EKG was consistent with a STEMI, a consult to cardiology for emergency revascularization therapy would have been appropriate. However, given the need for immediate surgical invention in this case, a consult to CT Surgery is needed.

### References

1. Hiratzka LF, Bakris GL, Beckman JA, et al. Guidelines for the diagnosis and management of patients with thoracic aortic dissection. *Circulation.* 2010;121:e266-e369.
2. Parrillo JE, Dellinger RP. *Critical Care Medicine: Principles of Diagnosis and Management in the Adult.* Philadelphia, PA: Elsevier; 2014:Chap 33.

---

**14.** Correct Answer: B

**Rationale:**

CABG surgery can be performed both without and with CPB for multivessel coronary artery disease. Although CPB with cardioplegia is thought to provide optimal surgical conditions for coronary anastomoses, off-pump CABG avoids the many negative consequences of subjecting the human body to CPB. There have been numerous well-designed multicenter randomized control trials comparing the two methods. The four largest clinical trials to date comparing the two methods include CORONARY, DOORS, GOPCABE, and ROOBY included more than 10 000 patients in total looking at outcomes up to 5 years from surgery. In 2012, a Cochrane Review showed that off-pump CABG is associated with increased all-cause mortality versus on-pump CABG. Although on-pump CABG shows improved mortality benefit, there are cases necessitating off-pump CABG, and it is ultimately an individual decision based on surgeon preference and a discussion with each patient.

### References

1. Møller CH, Penninga L, Wetterslev J, et al. Off-pump versus on-pump coronary artery bypass grafting for ischaemic heart disease. *Cochrane Database Syst Rev.* 2012;(3):CD007224.
2. Shroyer AL, Grover FL, Hattler B, et al. On-pump versus off-pump coronary-artery bypass surgery. *N Engl J Med.* 2009;361:1827-1837.
3. Diegeler A, Börgermann J, Kappert U, et al. Off-pump versus on-pump coronary-artery bypass grafting in elderly patients. *N Engl J Med.* 2013;368:1189-1198.
4. Houlind K, Kjeldsen BJ, Madsen SN, et al. On-pump versus off-pump coronary artery bypass surgery in elderly patients: results from the Danish on-pump versus off-pump randomization study. *Circulation.* 2012;125:2431-2439.
5. Lamy A, Devereaux PJ, Prabhakaran D, et al. Five-year outcomes after off-pump or on-pump coronary-artery bypass grafting. *N Engl J Med.* 2016;375:2359-2368.

**15.** Correct Answer: D

**Rationale:**

Tranexamic acid (TXA) is an antifibrinolytic drug that binds to plasminogen and blocks the interaction of plasmin with fibrin, thereby stabilizing the fibrin clot. TXA is a lysine analog and crosses the blood-brain barrier and is thought to affect the central nervous system (CNS) by competitively binding to GABA-A receptors in a dose-dependent fashion. GABA-A receptors, which function in inhibition of CNS transmission, are thereby blocked, resulting in decreased inhibitory activity and increased neuronal excitation in the brain.

In a meta-analysis of seizure risk associated with TXA use in open chamber cardiac procedures, the cumulative incidence rate of seizures was 2.7%, which was much higher than the average 1% risk when TXA was not used. Because TXA inhibits GABA-A in a dose-dependent fashion, the incidence of seizures was shown to increase from 1.4% in the low-dose (25-50 mg/kg) range, to 2.4% incidence in a middle dose of approximately 60 mg/kg, up to an incidence of 5.3% in the high-dose (80-110 mg/kg) range.

Note that propofol can cause myoclonus but is very unlikely to produce actual seizure activity. Fentanyl has been associated with seizures, but this is more typically seen with intrathecal use, and dexmedetomidine is also highly unlikely to affect the seizure threshold. Neuromuscular blocking agents such as rocuronium have no effect on seizure activity.

References

1. Manji RA, Grocott HP, Leake J, et al. Seizures following cardiac surgery: the impact of tranexamic acid and other risk factors. *Can J Anesth*. 2012;59:6-13.
2. Lin Z, Xiaoyi Z. Tranexamic acid-associated seizures: a meta analysis. *Seizure*. 2016;36:70-73.
3. Montes FR, Pardo DF, Carreño M, et al. Risk factors associated with postoperative seizures in patients undergoing cardiac surgery who received tranexamic acid: a case controlled study. *Ann Card Anesth*. 2012;15:6-12.
4. Martin K, Knorr J, Breuer T, et al. Seizures after open heart surgery: comparison of epison-aminocaproic acid and tranexamic acid. *J Cardiothorac Vasc Anesth*. 2011;25:20-25.

# ABDOMINAL AND GASTROINTESTINAL SURGERY

April E. Mendoza

1. A 33-year-old male from South Asian presents with acute abdominal pain and several weeks of constipation. He had undergone cholecystectomy 2 months ago for similar symptoms with some resolution of the pain. He now presents with nausea, vomiting, and pain localized to the epigastrium. His laboratory test results are significant for hemoglobin of 8 µg/dL and white blood cell count of 9 µg/dL. He reports taking Ayurvedic home remedies. What additional tests should be considered to diagnose the cause of his acute abdomen?

   A. Serum heavy metal screen
   B. Lipid profile
   C. Serum troponin
   D. CMV antibody

2. A 28-year-old male who is an avid outdoorsman presents approximately 2 weeks after a hike in New Hampshire to the emergency department with severe abdominal pain. He is hypotensive with a distended abdomen. He denies recent trauma or falls. The focused assessment with sonography for trauma (FAST) is positive on the left for free fluid around the spleen. An exploratory laparotomy reveals a ruptured spleen. What is the MOST likely explanation for his presentation?

   A. Trauma
   B. Malaria
   C. Tuberculosis
   D. Babesiosis

3. A 34-year-old morbidly obese male with a past medical history of intravenous drug abuse, HCV, lymphedema, and obstructive sleep apnea has now been in the intensive care unit (ICU) for 2 weeks for acute respiratory failure secondary to sepsis from a soft tissue infection. He develops a new fever with associated hypotension requiring vasopressor support. On physical exam he is intubated and sedated, with coarse breath sounds that are unchanged; however, an increase in peak airway pressures are noted, and his abdominal exam is notable only for severe obesity. What imaging study would you request NEXT?

   A. Three-view abdominal radiographs
   B. Right upper quadrant ultrasound
   C. KUB
   D. Chest, abdomen, and pelvis computed tomography (CT)

4. A 63-year-old obese female undergoes a robotic low anterior resection for rectal cancer, which goes well. On postoperative day 7, it is noted that she has become somnolent and febrile. You are called bedside to evaluate her for an ICU admission. On examination, she is lethargic and tachypneic with clear breath sounds. Her abdomen is mildly distended with moderate pain on palpation. Her vitals reveal her temperature is 39°C, oxygen saturation is 90%, respiratory rate is 45 breaths per minute, heart rate is 130 bpm with a blood pressure of 100 mm Hg systolic. In addition to the standard septic workup including chest radiograph and culture data, you NEXT proceed to:

A. Transfer to ICU and start IV cefepime and vancomycin to cover for hospital-acquired pneumonia

B. Transfer to ICU, start zosyn and vancomycin, and request urgent CT

C. Transfer to ICU, start Rocephin and vancomycin at meningeal dosing, and request stat lumbar puncture

D. Call the surgeon and prepare the OR for emergent exploratory laparotomy

5. Two weeks after a Whipple procedure, a 66-year-old male presents to the emergency department with severe abdominal pain. On evaluation, he is in moderate distress and is obviously uncomfortable. His vitals are notable for tachycardia of 120 bpm and hypotension with systolic blood pressure of 95 mm Hg. He is afebrile. A FAST reveals free fluid in all quadrants. Blood transfusion of blood products are initiated and his blood pressure responds to resuscitation. The NEXT best management option is:

A. Emergent exploratory laparotomy

B. Stat head, chest, abdomen, and pelvis CT

C. Emergent consultation of interventional radiology

D. Admission to the ICU with emergent consultation for pan-endoscopy

6. A 47-year-old female undergoes bilateral mastectomy with immediate reconstruction with free TRAM flap. She is admitted to the ICU for flap monitoring. When you evaluate her, she is complaining of shortness of breath and is intermittently unresponsive. How do you proceed?

A. Immediately start CPR and request STAT echo

B. Immediately start CPR and decompress bilateral chests by needle thoracostomy

C. Call surgery bedside for resuscitative thoracotomy

D. Immediately start CPR, and call cardiac to consider ECPR (extracorporeal cardiopulmonary resuscitation)

7. A 77-year-old female presents with acute worsening of abdominal pain. She describes nausea and vomiting along with some diarrhea after a recent trip to Florida, but states that these symptoms were improving when she suddenly developed severe acute abdominal pain. She denies similar abdominal complaints in the past and reports no prior abdominal surgeries. Past medical history is significant for atrial fibrillation of which she takes rivaroxaban, although she does report she may missed a few doses earlier in the week. What would be the test of choice to confirm the diagnosis?

A. Echocardiogram

B. Abdominal ultrasonography

C. CT angiography

D. CT with contrast

8. Which of the following is NOT considered a risk factor for nonocclusive mesenteric ischemia (NOMI)?

A. Infrarenal aortic bifemoral bypass surgery (ABF)

B. Hemodialysis

C. Acute myocardial infarction

D. Burn injury

9. A 79-year-old female with a past medical history of COPD is admitted to the ICU for community-acquired pneumonia. She develops fever, and blood-tinged diarrhea. She remains KUB reveals air-fluid levels within the small bowel. A CT demonstrates fat-stranding involving the colon and colonic wall thickening. The BEST method to confirm the diagnosis and begin treatment is:

A. Obtain stool cultures and start IV antibiotics.

B. Request an emergent surgical consultation for exploratory laparotomy

C. Barium enema and IV antibiotics

D. Nasogastric decompression, IV antibiotics, and request urgent colonoscopy

10. Which scenario is MOST consistent with abdominal compartment syndrome (ACS)?

A. A 34-year-old obese male (120 kg), mechanically ventilated with abdominal distension and bladder pressures of 22 cm $H_2O$. Fraction of inspired oxygen is 35%; positive end-expiratory pressure is 12 mm Hg. Peak inspiratory pressures are 28 cm $H_2O$.

B. A 55-year-old female (75 kg) is admitted preoperatively for surgical resection of a pelvic mass. She is breathing spontaneously on 4 L. Bladder pressure is 22 cm $H_2O$.

C. An 18-year-old (70 kg) gunshot-wound victim with multiple of injuries involving the chest, abdomen, and extremities. He received 22 units of packed red blood cells, 18 units of fresh frozen plasma, and 2 packs of platelets intraoperatively. He has an open abdomen with a vacuum-assisted dressing in place. He is mechanically ventilated with fraction of inspired oxygen at 60% and positive end-expiratory pressure of 18 mm Hg. Peak inspiratory pressures are 40 cm $H_2O$. Urine output has been minimal. Bladder pressure is 22 cm $H_2O$.

D. A 38-year-old (85 kg) burn victim with 20% total body surface area of partial-thickness wounds involving the flank and left lower extremity. He has received 8 L of resuscitation over the first 24 hours. The bladder pressure is 22 mm Hg. He is breathing comfortably on 2 L nasal cannula. Urine output is 60 mL/h.

11. To obtain the MOST accurate intravesicular bladder pressure readings, the following must be true:

A. The head of bed must be 45°, with the transducer at the axillary line and 50 mL of saline instillation

B. The patient must be supine, paralyzed, with transducer at the iliac crest, with maximum of 25 mL of saline instillation.

C. The temperature of fluid instillation does not affect intra-abdominal pressure (IAP) readings

D. No more than a single reading should be obtained every 8 hours

12. A 66-year-old male presents to the emergency department with hypotension and severe abdominal and back pain. He was found to have a ruptured abdominal aortic aneurysm, and the massive transfusion protocol was initiated. He is now s/p EVAR in the ICU. The nurse notifies you that his urine output continues to decline. Which laboratory and/or examination finding is the MOST suggestive of ACS?

A. Abdominal distension with bladder pressure of 25 cm $H_2O$, increasing oxygen requirements

B. Abdominal distension with bladder pressure of 15 cm $H_2O$, unchanged oxygen requirements, unchanged peak inspiratory pressures, urine sodium of 80 Meq/L

C. Mixed venous oxygen saturation 70%

D. Cardiac ultrasound demonstrating obliteration of the left ventricle cavity. Repeat CBC demonstrated a hemoglobin of 4 g/dL from prior

# Chapter 97 ▪ Answers

**1.** Correct Answer: A

**Rationale:**
Ayurvedic medications are known to contain heavy metals and in particular lead, and many of these remedies have been associated with lead poisoning. The acute abdomen has a multitude of causes. Many require surgical intervention, but some are related to medical conditions including endocrine, hematologic, and toxins including lead poisoning. It is important to elicit travel, medication, and work history. It is also important to consider environmental endemic conditions affecting the local community that the patient may be unaware such as the presence of lead paint or contaminated water supply.

Reference
1. Breyre A, Green-McKenzie J. Case of acute lead toxicity associated with ayurvedic supplements. *BMJ Case Rep.* 2016:bcr2016215041.

**2.** Correct Answer: D

**Rationale:**
Spontaneous rupture of the spleen is rare and is usually caused by a discrete pathology such as malaria, Ebstein-Barr virus or other disorders associated with splenomegaly. Babesiosis is relatively common in the northeastern United States and is also known as "Nantucket fever." Its incidence continues to rise in this part of the country. Splenic rupture has been reported more often in men with babesiosis, and this population tends to be healthy without previous trauma. Spleen conservation can be attempted in this population if they remain hemodynamically stable. Diagnosis is by blood smear or PCR. Treatment includes either atovaquone plus azithromycin or clindamycin plus quinine. Antibiotic management should be guided by an infectious disease specialist.

References
1. Li S, Goyal B, Cooper JD, Abdelbaki A, Gupta N, Kumar Y. Splenic rupture from babesiosis, an emerging concern? A systematic review of current literature. *Ticks Tick Borne Dis.* 2018;9(6):1377-1382. doi:10.1016/j.ttbdis.2018.06.004.
2. Sanchez E, Vannier E, Wormser GP, Hu LT. Diagnosis, treatment, and prevention of lyme disease, human granulocytic anaplasmosis, and babesiosis: a review. *JAMA.* 2016;315(16):1767-1777. doi:10.1001/jama.2016.2884.

**3.** Correct Answer: A

**Rationale:**

In this scenario, there is an acute decompensation in a critically ill patient. He is now hemodynamically compromised making CT imaging challenging, but not impossible. In most cases, it is usually easy and faster to obtain plain radiographs. They are extremely helpful in detecting free air. The three-view abdominal radiographs include an upright chest film, upright abdominal film, and supine abdominal film. The chest film is helpful in this patient as it will detect evidence of pneumonia, effusion, or ARDS, but can be detect as little of 1 mL of free air below the diaphragm. Abdominal radiographs can identify abnormal calcifications such as appendicoliths or gallstones, but they are less sensitive in establishing these diagnoses. They are more helpful in diagnosing gastric outlet obstruction, bowel obstruction, or large bowel volvulus. Owing to the ease and efficiency, plain radiographs would be the preferred next imaging obtained as it diagnosed this patient's free air and expedited the time to operative intervention.

Reference

1. Squires R, Carter SN, Postier RG. Acute abdomen. In: Townsend CM, Beauchamp RD, Evers BM, Mattox KL, eds. *Sabiston Textbook of Surgery*. 20th ed. Elsevier 2017:Chap 45.

**4.** Correct Answer: B

**Rationale:**

This patient is 7 days after surgery, which makes the differential for sepsis quite wide. Important thing to consider is presence of lines or catheters. Other things to evaluate are the presence of drains. Risk factors for anastomotic leaks remain debated, but obesity, preoperative radiation, and lower rectal anastomoses are generally accepted risk factors. Pelvic drains can be placed intraoperatively, and this is a point of contention in the literature as far as their utility. There is some evidence of intraoperatively placed drains, which may in fact be a risk factor for anastomotic leaks. If they are present, the color and character can be helpful especially in the above clinical situation when purulent, feculent, or grossly blood output is noted. In the above scenario, anastomotic leak should be high on the differential and imaging should be obtained urgently.

References

1. Kulaylat MN, Dayton MT. Surgical complications. In: Townsend CM, Beauchamp RD, Evers BM, Mattox KL, eds. *Sabiston Textbook of Surgery*. 20th ed. Elsevier; 2017:Chap 12.
2. Zhang HY, Zhao CL, Xie J, et al. To drain or not to drain in colorectal anastomosis: a meta-analysis. *Int J Colorectal Dis*. 2016;31:951-960.

**5.** Correct Answer: C

**Rationale:**

Major hemorrhage after pancreaticoduodenectomy is uncommon, but is associated with a high mortality. Gastroduodenal stump pseudoaneurysms are the most common site of bleeding. They are classified based on timing of presentation. Early hemorrhage can occur 24 hours after surgery, and immediate return to the operating room is the typical management of choice. This is usually the result of a technical failure. Delayed hemorrhage can occur days to weeks after initial surgery and is thought to be due to erosion of vessels by biliary or pancreatic leaks. Typically this type of bleeding is best managed by interventional radiology.

Reference

1. Hur S, Yoon CJ, Kang S-G, et al. Transcatheter arterial embolization of gastroduodenal artery stump pseudoaneurysms after pancreaticoduodenectomy: safety and efficacy of two embolization techniques. *J Vasc Interv Radiol*. 2011;22(3):294-301.

**6.** Correct Answer: B

**Rationale:**

The incidence of pneumothorax after breast reconstruction is extremely rare (0.55%). However, it should be considered in any patient who presents with respiratory complaints in the perioperative period. Other nonthoracic procedures that carry a risk for inadvertent pneumothorax include open nephrectomy, and robotic or laparoscopic surgery regardless of the indication.

References

1. Shneider LF, Albornoz CR, Huang J, Cordeiro PG. Incidence of pneumothorax during tissue expander-implant reconstruction and algorithm for intraoperative management. *Ann Plast Surg*. 2014;73(3):279-281.
2. Huynh RK, Ross AS. Delayed pneumothorax after laparoscopic sigmoid colectomy in a patient without underlying lung disease. *SAGE Open Med Case Rep*. 2014;2:2050313X14554940. Published online October 16, 2014. doi:10.1177/2050313X14554940.

**7. Correct Answer: C**

**Rationale:**

Acute mesenteric ischemia (AMI) is characterized into arterial or venous occlusion. There is also a form of AMI that is associated with vasocontriction or low-flow states termed NOMI. Arterial occlusion by emboli used to be the most common cause of AMI, but with the widespread use of anticoagulants the cause of AMI is more evenly split between embolic and thrombotic sources. Although echocardiogram as well CT of the chest may prove essential in identifying the source of embolic phenomenon, the initial chest of choice to confirm the diagnosis is a CT angiography of the abdomen and pelvis as this test is relatively quick and readily available. The diagnostic gold standard remains conventional angiography, but this study is more often utilized after the diagnosis of AMI has been established and catheter-based interventions appear warranted.

**Reference**

1. Cloud A, Dussel JN, Webster-Lake C, Indes J. Mesenteric ischemia. In: Yeo CJ, ed. *Shackelford's Surgery of the Alimentary Tract.* 8th ed. Elsevier; 2019:Chap 87.

**8. Correct Answer: A**

**Rationale:**

All the above are considered risks for NOMI except for infrarenal ABF. ABF bypass is associated with ischemic colitis as the inferior mesenteric artery is typically sacrificed. NOMI results in local malperfusion due to splanchnic vasospasm. This can be the result of vasoconstrictive medications, shock, cardiac arrest with ROSC, or ACS as can been seen after aggressive resuscitation (ie burn injury resuscitation). Cardiopulmonary bypass, extracorporeal membrane oxygenation, and hemodialysis are associated with NOMI and should be considered in patients with a concerning clinical picture. Many patients with NOMI are critically ill, which makes examination findings difficult to follow. The classic "pain out of proportion" is nearly impossible to appreciate thereby making a high clinical suspicion important for early identification and management. Symptoms can be nonspecific, which can include but not limited to abdominal distension, new or worsening feeding intolerance, or unexplained metabolic acidosis. Mesenteric ischemia is an emergency, and there should be no delays in obtaining a diagnosis.

**References**

1. Lo RC, Schermerhorn ML. Mesenteric arterial disease: epidemiology, pathophysiology, and clinical evaluation. In: Sidawy AN, Perler BA, eds. *Rutherford's Vascular Surgery and Endovascular Therapy.* 9th ed. Elsevier; 2019:Chap 131.
2. Khorsandi M, Dougherty S, Bouamra O, et al. Extra-corporeal membrane oxygenation for refractory cardiogenic shock after adult cardiac surgery: a systematic review and meta-analysis. *J Cardiothorac Surg.* 2017;12(1):55.

**9. Correct Answer: D**

**Rationale:**

Risk factors for ischemic colitis are older age (>65 years), constipation, vasculitis, sickle cell disease, and COPD. Infrarenal aortic aneurysms and aortic surgery are also common causes of left-sided ischemic colitis. Often, this can be managed expectantly, but colonoscopy can confirm the diagnosis. However, it can be difficult to determine partial-thickness from full-thickness ischemia by endoscopy alone. Hypotension and worsening metabolic acidosis require emergent surgical consultation, but the majority of ischemic colitis can be managed medically. Medical management includes adequate resuscitation, nasogastric decompression, avoidance of hypotension, serial abdominal examinations, and IV antibiotics. Barium and contrast enemas should be avoided as there is a risk for perforation. Symptoms that do not improve within 24 to 48 hours should prompt a reevaluation either with endoscopy, CT, or both.

**References**

1. Mahmoud NN, Bleier JIS, Aarons CB, Paulson C, Shanmugan S, Fry RD. Colon and rectum. In: Townsend CM, Beauchamp RD, Evers BM, Mattox KLA, eds. *Sabiston Textbook of Surgery.* 20th ed. Elsevier; 2017Chap 51.
2. Yadav S, Dave M, Edakkanambeth VJ, et al. A population-based study of incidence, risk factors, clinical spectrum, and outcomes of ischemic colitis. *Clin Gastroenterol Hepatol.* 2015;13(4):731-738.

**10. Correct Answer: C**

**Rationale:**

ACS is defined by intra-abdominal hypertension in conjunction with organ dysfunction. An elevated IAP by indirect measurement with bladder pressure is insufficient to prompt management especially surgical decompression. Usually, a constellation of symptoms occur, which include respiratory insufficiency and notably reduced pulmonary compliance, hypotension from reduced venous return, and decreased urine output. In addition, increased intracranial pressure is observed with ACS, and this can be observed in patients with ICP monitors in place. In general, an intra-abominal pressure of >25 mm Hg warrants surgical compression, but the overall clinical picture should correspond with ACS to maximize benefits of an open abdomen and reduce morbidity. It is important to note that even with an open abdomen, ACS can occur, and it is important to remain vigilant when the constellation of symptoms exist.

## Reference

1.  Ferreira JD. *Chapter: abdominal compartment syndrome*. In: Ferri FF, ed. *Ferri's Clinical Advisor*. Elsevier; 2019.

---

**11.** Correct Answer: B

**Rationale:**

To obtain accurate IAP measurements, the needed steps must be performed correctly. The patient must be pharmacologically paralyzed, therefore preventing abdominal contractions. The patient must be completely supine, with the IAP transducer leveled at the mid-axillary line. This usually correlates at the level of the iliac crests. It is important to obtain multiple readings at the time of measurement and wait at least 30 to 60 seconds after instillation of room temperature of saline as cold fluids cause detrusor contractions. A maximum of 25 mL of sterile saline should be used as larger amounts will falsely elevate IAP.

## References

1.  McBeth PB, Zygun DA, Widder S, et al. Effect of patient positioning on intra-abdominal pressure monitoring. *Am J Surg*. 2007;193:644-647.
2.  De Waele J, Pletinckx P, Blot S, Hoste E. Saline volume in transvesical intra-abdominal pressure measurement: enough is enough. *Intensive Care Med*. 2006;32:455-459.
3.  Chiumello D, Tallarini F, Chierichetti M, et al. The effect of different volumes and temperatures of saline on the bladder pressure measurement in critically ill patients. *Crit Care*. 2007;11:R82.

---

**12.** Correct Answer: A

**Rationale:**

ACS encompasses an increased IAP in conjunction with the presence of end-organ dysfunction notably decreased renal function, decreased pulmonary function, and reduced preload. Typically, urine sodium in ACS is reduced in addition to decreased mixed venous saturation, which correspond to the reduced cardiac output. Cardiac ultrasound should correspond with hypovolemia in the setting of ACS, but a significant drop of hemoglobin complicates the picture as the patient has ongoing bleeding. Therefore, the best answer is A.

## References

1.  Malbrain ML, De Iaet IE. Intra-abdominal hypertension: evolving concepts. *Clin Chest Med*. 2009;30(1):45-70.
2.  Ke L, Tong Z, Ni H, et al. The effect of intra-abdominal hypertension incorporating severe acute pancreatitis in a porcine model. *PLoS One*. 2012;7(3):e33125. doi:10.1371/journal.pone.0033125.

# 98

# SKIN, SOFT TISSUE, AND EXTREMITIES

Casey McBride Luckhurst and April E. Mendoza

1. A 25-year-old male with no significant past medical history presents to the emergency department complaining of pain and "redness" of his left lower extremity. He denies any history of trauma or injury to the area. His vital signs are notable for Temp: 102.2F, HR 110, BP 95/65, RR 25, Sat 100% on room air. On examinaton, he is clearly agitated and in pain. His left lower extremity is erythematous and tender to palpation without any noticeable skin breakdown, crepitus, or evidence of external trauma. All of the following statements about the evaluation and diagnosis of a necrotizing soft tissue infection (NSTI) are true EXCEPT:

   A. Clinical manifestations of a NSTI can include erythema, edema, pain out of proportion to examination, overlying skin changes, and systemic signs of infection including fever and hypotension
   B. Symptoms are typically acute in onset and rapidly progressive over a short period of time
   C. The LRINEC score, developed specifically to aid in differentiation of NSTI from other soft tissue infections, has high sensitivity and specificity and thus a negative score rules out NSTI
   D. If clinical suspicion for a NSTI is high, surgical intervention should not be delayed for further diagnostic evaluation
   E. Computed Tomography (CT) is the best radiographic imaging modality in the evaluation of a NSTI

2. A 55-year-old male with a history of methicillin-resistant *Staphylococcus aureus* (MRSA) colonization presents to the emergency department with complaints of purulent drainage from his surgical incision. He is now 7 days postop from his sigmoid colectomy. On examination, his temperature is 102°F and hemodynamically within normal limits. His incision has skin staples in place and moderate surrounding erythema extending >5 cm from the wound edge and associated induration. Purulent drainage is easily expressed from the most inferior aspect of the incision. Which of the following is the most appropriate management of this patient?

   A. Open the incision, obtain a fluid culture, and start on an empiric course of IV Vancomycin and Piperacillin-Tazobactam
   B. Open the incision, obtain a fluid culture and start on an empiric course of IV Vancomycin alone
   C. Discharge home on a 7-day course of oral Cephalexin
   D. Open the incision, obtain a fluid culture, and start on an empiric course of IV Piperacillin-Tazobactam alone
   E. Open the incision, obtain a fluid culture, and hold off on starting antimicrobial therapy until culture data returns

3. A 30-year-old male presents with significant erythema overlying his right arm and a fever to 101.0°F. He explains that he sustained an abrasion over the affected area while at work, and when the redness started 2 days ago he was prescribed a course of antibiotics by the Urgent Care Clinic, which he has been taking without improvement of his symptoms. An ultrasound shows edema and a phlegmon without an obvious abscess collection. He is admitted to the hospital and started on IV cefoxitin. Over the next 48 hours it is noted that even though there is some regression of the erythema, a firm, fluctuant area can be palpated in the subcutaneous tissue measuring >2 cm. What is the most appropriate next step in management?

A. Broaden antibiotics to IV Piperacillin-Tazobactam
B. Broaden antibiotics to IV Vancomycin
C. Repeat ultrasound
D. CT scan of the arm
E. No change in current management

4. A patient is admitted to the surgical critical care unit after being found down for an unknown period of time following presumed assault. The patient was intubated at the scene. In addition to a multitude of other injures, the patient is noted to have an acute kidney injury (AKI) with an elevated creatine kinase (CK) to 10,000. On examination, all extremity compartments are soft. With regards to the management of AKI from traumatic rhabdomyolysis, which of the following statements is true?

A. In the absence of other indications for renal replacement therapy, prophylactic hemodialysis is recommended in the setting of elevated CK above 5,000 U/L
B. Commonly seen laboratory abnormalities include elevated CK, hypocalcemia, hypokalemia, and hypophosphatemia
C. Resuscitation with sodium bicarbonate solution, titrated to urine pH, can prevent acute renal failure
D. If the patient is oligo-anuric, the addition of mannitol is recommended
E. Early, aggressive resuscitation with normal saline solution fundamental to treatment

5. A 60-year-old male with a past medical history notable for obesity, hypertension, hyperlipidemia, and type 2 diabetes presents to the emergency department with complaints of significant scrotal and perineal pain with associated drainage. He explains that the symptoms started about 24 hours before presentation and have been rapidly progressive since. His vital signs are as follows: Temp 102.5°F, HR 102 bpm, BP 90/65 mm Hg, RR 18, Sat 100% on room air. On examination, he is diaphoretic and noticeably uncomfortable. His scrotum and perineum are diffusely erythematous and tender to palpation, with a pinpoint area draining dishwasher color fluid that is malodorous. All of the following are appropriate next steps in the management of a patient presenting with Fournier's gangrene EXCEPT:

A. Aggressive fluid resuscitation to markers of end organ perfusion as dictated by early goal-directed therapy
B. After acquiring appropriate culture data, initiation of broad spectrum antimicrobial therapy with empiric coverage for NSTI causing organisms
C. Obtaining radiographic imaging to delineate the extent of infection and to aid in operative planning D. Early surgical consultation for urgent evaluation and operative debridement
E. Postoperative admission to a surgical intensive care unit for ongoing monitoring and hemodynamic support

6. In addition to aggressive fluid resuscitation and urgent surgical intervention, the initiation of appropriate antimicrobial therapy is crucial in the setting of a NSTI. Which of the following represents an appropriate antibiotic regimen for the given clinical situation?

A. A 25-year-old male presenting with clinical findings concerning for NSTI of his left arm: Vancomycin, Piperacillin-Tazobactam
B. A 25-year-old male with penicillin allergy, presenting with clinical findings concerning for NSTI of his left arm: Vancomycin, Meropenem, Clindamycin
C. A 25-year-old male presenting with documented group A streptococcus NSTI: Piperacillin-Tazobactam
D. A 30-year-old fisherman presenting with findings concerning for an NSTI of his left leg: Vancomycin, Ceftriaxone, Clindamycin
E. A 30-year-old fisherman presenting with findings concerning for an NSTI of his left leg: Vancomycin, Doxycycline

7. A 34-year-old female with a history of IV substance abuse presents to the hospital via EMS after being found down for some unknown amount of time. While in the ED, she was treated with naloxone for presumed IV heroin overdose. On further examination, she was noted to have stigmata of recent IV drug use, and her right forearm is significantly swollen with tense compartments. When asked to move her fingers she is able to do so, but reports decreased sensation over the dorsal aspect of her hand as well as significant pain in her forearm with passive range of motion of her wrist. All of the following statements regarding the diagnosis and management of acute compartment syndrome (ACS) are true EXCEPT:

A. Mechanisms of development of ACS include fracture, thermal burns, prolonged compression, crush injuries, and revascularization following procedures
B. Muscle breakdown leads to elevations in serum CK
C. Although not necessary for diagnosis of ACS, compartmental pressures can be used to aid in the diagnosis, specifically when used to calculated extremity perfusion pressures
D. Management involves early surgical consultation for compartmental decompression with fasciotomies
E. Clinical diagnosis is classically made with the "five Ps": Pain, Pallor, Paresthesias, Poikilothermia, Pulselessness

8. A 20-year-old male presents with a closed fracture of his left tibia and fibula sustained while playing basketball. He undergoes splinting by Orthopedic Surgery and 3 hours later he begins to complain of pain in his distal lower extremity. His pain is worsened with passive range of motion, and he notes decreased sensation over the dorsal aspect of his foot. His pulse examination is symmetric over bilateral lower extremities but his capillary refill time is delayed. What is the most appropriate next step in the management of this patient?

A. Increase dose of IV morphine to provide pain relief
B. Remove splint and if symptoms are not improved, proceed to the operating room for emergent fasciotomies
C. Invasive measurement of compartment pressures
D. Computed tomography angiography (CTA) of the affected extremity
E. Elevate lower extremity and serial examinations

# Chapter 98 ▪ Answers

---

**1.** Correct Answer: C

**Rationale:**
NSTIs are severe infections that can be found in any layer of soft tissue and are associated with a high mortality rate. These infections can be classified based on imaging findings, specifically the presence of gas in the tissues, as well as microbiology (polymicrobial vs monomicrobial). Clinically, NSTIs classically present with erythema, edema, pain out of proportion to examination, overlying skin changes, and systemic signs of infection including fever and hypotension (Answer A). Symptoms are typically acute in onset and rapidly progressive over a short period of time, making the time from presentation to diagnosis crucial in the overall outcome of the patient (Answer B). When clinical suspicion is high, surgical consultation should be obtained immediately with a low threshold to proceed to the operating room for surgical evaluation and extensive debridement as indicated (Answer D). More commonly, the differentiation between NSTI and severe cellulitis is not clear. The Laboratory Risk Indicator for Necrotizing Fasciitis (LRINEC) score was developed to aid in differentiation between a severe cellulitis and NSTI with initial studies showing high negative predictive value. Of note, subsequent evaluation has called into question the sensitivity of the scoring system, which includes white cell count, hemoglobin, sodium, glucose, creatinine, and C-reactive protein. Although helpful in the evaluation, a negative score does not replace clinical evaluation and alone cannot rule out the presence of an NSTI (Answer C). Other diagnostic tools CT imaging with intravenous contrast, which has been deemed the best radiographic imaging modality in the evaluation of a NSTI. Findings include gas in the soft tissues, fluid collections, heterogeneous tissue enhancement, and inflammatory changes beneath the fascia (Answer E).

References
1. Stevens DL, Bisno AL, Chambers HF, et al. Practice guidelines for the diagnosis and management of skin and soft tissue infections: 2014 update by the Infectious Diseases Society of America. *Clin Infect Dis.* 2014;59(2):147.
2. Wong CH, Khin LW, Heng KS, Tan KC, Low CO. The LRINEC (Laboratory Risk Indicator for Necrotizing Fasciitis) score: a tool for distinguishing necrotizing fasciitis from other soft tissue infections. *Crit Care Med.* 2004;32(7):1535.
3. Zacharias N, Velmahos GC, Salama A, et al. Diagnosis of necrotizing soft tissue infections by computed tomography. *Arch Surg.* 2010;145:452.

---

**2.** Correct Answer: A

**Rationale:**
Surgical site infection following an abdominal operation can be further classified as superficial or deep infections. Common features include peri-incisional tenderness, erythema, and induration, with purulent drainage present at the site of the incision. More significant infections can present with systemic signs including fever, tachycardia, and hypotension in addition to the localized findings. Once diagnosed, the treatment of a surgical site infection involves opening the incision to allow for adequate irrigation and drainage, obtaining a fluid culture of the purulent fluid and initiation of antibiotic therapy if there is evidence of extension of the infection into the surrounding tissues or systemic signs of infection (Answer E). Choice of antimicrobial therapy depends on the type of operation (in this case an abdominal operation involving the colon, which would be considered a clean contaminated case) and risk factors for MRSA (prior colonization or infection, recent hospitalization, recent antibiotics). In this case, it would be appropriate to cover for gram negative organisms as well as anaerobes. Given his recent hospitalization and known MRSA colonization status, the most appropriate choice listed above would be Vancomycin and Piperacillin-Tazobactam. Of the other choices listed above, Vancomycin alone and Cephalexin alone do not provide appropriate gram negative and anaerobic coverage (Answer B, Answer C). Although Piperacillin-Tazobactam does provide appropriate coverage for gram negative and anaerobic organisms, the addition of MRSA coverage is

recommended given that he is MRSA colonized and his recent hospitalization (Answer D). Answer A is best answer given that it recommends opening the incision, culturing the purulent fluid obtained, and initiating appropriate antimicrobial therapy.

### References
1. Stevens DL, Bisno AL, Chambers HF, et al. Practice guidelines for the diagnosis and management of skin and soft tissue infections: 2014 update by the infectious diseases society of America. *Clin Infect Dis.* 2014;59(2):147.
2. Mizell JS. *Complications of Abdominal Surgical Incisions.* UpToDate; May 15, 2018.

---

### 3. Correct Answer: C

**Rationale:**

An initial presentation of presumed uncomplicated cellulitis can be treated with a trial of oral antibiotic therapy, with or without coverage for MRSA as indicated. Failure of improvement in symptoms and systemic signs of infection (including fever greater than 100.5°F) are indications for parenteral antibiotic therapy. In the patient above, an ultrasound was obtained that showed no underlying abscess collection initially, but his new examination findings are concerning for interval development of an abscess. The most appropriate next step listed above would be to repeat an ultrasound to assess for the formation of an abscess or drainable fluid collection (Answer C, Answer E). There is no indication to further broaden the antibiotic regimen given that the cellulitis is improving and the treatment for an abscess is drainage (Answer A, Answer B). Although a CT scan will provide a more detailed image, it is not necessary in this scenario and subjects the patient to unnecessary radiation (Answer D).

### References
1. Stevens DL, Bisno AL, Chambers HF, et al. Practice guidelines for the diagnosis and management of skin and soft tissue infections: 2014 update by the Infectious Diseases Society of America. *Clin Infect Dis.* 2014;59(2):147.
2. Raff AB, Kroshinsky D. Cellulitis: a review. *JAMA.* 2016;316(3):325-337.

---

### 4. Correct Answer: E

**Rationale:**

AKI following rhabdomyolysis is one of the more serious complications and is seen in an estimated 20% to 33% of patients. Accumulation of myoglobin from muscle injury combined with hypovolemia can lead to a mixed acute tubular necrosis picture and resultant AKI. Causes of rhabdomyolysis are not limited to, but include traumatic injury or compression, exertional (metabolic myopathies, hyperthermia) and infections, toxins, or pharmacologic agents. Commonly seen laboratory abnormalities include elevated CK, hypocalcemia, hyperphosphatemia, and hyperkalemia, which can be potentially life threatening (Answer B). The only effective treatment of rhabdomyolysis-induced AKI is aggressive fluid resuscitation with treatment of the associated metabolic and electrolyte abnormalities as they arise (Answer E). Adjuncts such as the addition of mannitol and sodium bicarbonate solution have not been shown to be effective and are currently not recommended as mainstays of treatment (Answer C, D). Additionally, the use of mannitol in the oligo-anuric patient is contraindicated, and in that setting, consideration for the need for renal replacement therapy should be undertaken. The indications for dialysis are no different than the usual indications, including severe acidosis, uremia, volume overload, and refractory hyperkalemia. There has been no convincing evidence to show the benefit of prophylactic initiation of hemodialysis in the setting of rhabdomyolysis (Answer A).

### References
1. Torres PA, Helmstetter JA, Kaye AM, Kaye AD. Rhabdomyolysis: pathogenesis, diagnosis and treatment. *Ochsner J.* 2015;15(1): 58-69.
2. Brown CV, Rhee P, Chan L, et al. Preventing renal failure in patients with rhabdomyolysis: do bicarbonate and mannitol make a difference? *J Trauma.* 2004;56(6):1191-1196.

---

### 5. Correct Answer: C

**Rationale:**

NSTIs are rapidly progressive, life-threatening bacterial infections that can present following trauma, a surgical procedure, or even minor breaches of the skin. NSTIs can be further classified as Type 1 (polymicrobial) or Type II (monomicrobial) with Type 1 infections being more common. Diagnosis is made with a high index of suspicion and can be aided with use of the LRINEC Score. Initial management involves initiation of fluid resuscitation, starting broad spectrum antibiotic coverage with empiric coverage for NSTI-causing organisms after obtaining culture data, and early surgical consultation for emergent operative debridement (Answer A, Answer B, Answer D). Postoperatively, these patients require close hemodynamic monitoring and support, typically requiring an ICU setting (Answer E). Given the rapidly progressive nature of NSTIs, operative debridement should not be delayed. Once a diagnosis is made, there is no indication to obtain further imaging and delay operative intervention (Answer C).

### Reference
1. Stevens DL, Bryant AE. Necrotizing soft-tissue infections. *N Engl J Med.* 2017;377(23):2253.

**6.** Correct Answer: B

**Rationale:**

When a patient presents with signs and symptoms of an aggressive infection and associated systemic toxicity, concern for an aggressive NSTI must be high. In addition to intravenous fluid resuscitation and urgent surgical consultation, initiation of broad spectrum antibiotic therapy is prudent. Initial coverage with broad spectrum antibiotic therapy is recommended given that infections may be polymicrobial (Type 1 NSTI) or monomicrobial (Type 2 NSTI) in nature. Initial coverage includes vancomycin or linezolid plus piperacillin-tazobactam or a carbapenem. Addition of Clindamycin provides antitoxin coverage should the pathogen include a toxin-producing strain of streptococcus or staphylococcus. Of the choices above, Answer B provides appropriate broad coverage, which can later be de-escalated based on culture data. Although the vignette in Answer E raises concern for *Vibrio vulnificus*, which would be appropriately covered with Doxycycline, it would be remiss to not empirically treat for a polymicrobial infection until further culture data are obtained.

**Reference**

1. Stevens DL, Bisno AL, Chambers HF, et al. Practice guidelines for the diagnosis and management of skin and soft tissue infections: 2014 update by the Infectious Diseases Society of America. *Clin Infect Dis*. 2014;59(2):147.

**7.** Correct Answer: E

**Rationale:**

Acute compartment syndrome (ACS) of an extremity occurs when elevated pressures within a fascial compartment result in compromised circulation and muscle death. The causes of ACS of the extremity are varied, but include trauma, specifically following long bone fractures, ischemia-reperfusion injuries, thermal burns, and crush injuries, among others (Answer A). The resultant muscle necrosis and breakdown can be measured by increases in serum CK (Answer B). The diagnosis is clinical, and an early high index of suspicion is critical. Early signs and symptoms include pain out of proportion that is worsened with passive range of motion and swollen, tense compartments. Decreased sensation and muscle weakness are later findings, suggestive of nerve and muscle ischemia. The "classic findings" associated with ACS, the "five Ps" are overall inaccurate, and waiting for these symptoms before intervention will result in irreversible damage and morbidity (Answer E). Instead, diagnosis is made by performing serial physical exam and may be aided by the measurement of compartmental pressures, specifically when used to calculate extremity perfusion pressures rather than used as an absolute number (Answer C). Management involves early surgical consultation for compartmental decompression and fasciotomies (Answer D).

**References**

1. Via AG, Oliva F, Spoliti M, Maffulli N. Acute compartment syndrome. *Muscles Ligaments Tendons J*. 2015;5(1):18-22.
2. Velmahos GC, Toutouzas KG. Vascular trauma and compartment syndromes. *Surg Clin North Am*. 2002;82(1):125-141.

**8.** Correct Answer: B

**Rationale:**

The patient above is presenting with acute compartment syndrome (ACS) of his lower extremity following a closed, traumatic fracture. Although rare, it is important to remember that these patients are at risk of developing ACS and delays in diagnosis can result in irreversible damage, morbidity, and potential limb loss. The patient above has developed increased pain hours after splinting of his lower extremity, which is not relieved by pain medication and is worsened with passive range of motion. These signs, in conjunction with his decreased sensation and prolonged capillary refill time, are all clinical signs concerning for the development of ACS. It would be inappropriate to treat his symptoms with increased doses of narcotic pain medication, which may mask his symptoms and does not address the underlying problem (Answer A). Similarly, elevating the extremity will not address the underlying problem, and although serial examinations are important for monitoring, the patient above requires more aggressive intervention to avoid irreversible damage (Answer E). Invasive measurement of compartment pressures may aid in the diagnosis when it is not clinically apparent and should not delay surgical intervention in cases where clinical suspicion is sufficiently high (Answer C). There is no role in this clinical situation for obtaining a CTA and doing so would only delay the necessary intervention (Answer D).

**References**

1. Shadgan B, Pereira G, Menon M, et al. Risk factors for acute compartment syndrome of the leg associated with tibial diaphyseal fractures in adults. *J Orthop Traumatol*. 2015;16(3):185-192.
2. Frink M, Hildebrand F, Krettek C, Brand J, Hankemeier S. Compartment syndrome of the lower leg and foot. *Clin Orthop Relat Res*. 2010;468(4):940-950.

# 99

# POLYTRAUMA

Casey McBride Luckhurst, and April E. Mendoza

1. A 40-year-old male is admitted to the Surgical Intensive Care Unit (SICU) following a high-speed motor vehicle collision with an extensive trauma burden. He has no significant past medical history, and on arrival to the SICU he is noted to be hemodynamically stable. However, his respirations are shallow and he is currently requiring 4 L nasal cannula to maintain an oxygen saturation above 92%. On review of his imaging, you note multiple right-sided rib fractures including ribs 2 to 8 with fractures of ribs 3 to 6 in two places. Which of the following statements is true regarding the diagnosis and management flail chest?

   A. Flail chest is primarily a radiographic diagnosis
   B. A flail segment has minimal impact on overall pulmonary mechanics and thoracic volume
   C. Rib fixation and plating is indicated in all diagnosed cases of flail chest
   D. The diagnosis of flail chest is made with radiographic evidence of fractures of three or more ribs in two or more places and clinically apparent paradoxical chest movement
   E. Flail chest is most commonly seen in blunt trauma and has equal prevalence in the adult and pediatric populations

2. A 50-year-old male with a past medical history of hypertension and long-standing tobacco use is being admitted to the SICU after being involved in a motorcycle accident resulting in multiple bilateral rib fractures with underlying pulmonary contusions. On arrival to the ICU the patient is noted to be in obvious discomfort, taking in shallow breaths and requiring 4 L nasal cannula for oxygen supplementation. All of the following statements about the management of a polytrauma with pulmonary contusions are true EXCEPT:

   A. Colloid is preferred over crystalloid in the resuscitation of trauma patients with pulmonary contusions
   B. Pulmonary contusions may not be present on initial plain radiograph but can develop in days following the initial trauma
   C. Initial management involves judicious use of IVF fluid resuscitation and multimodal pain management
   D. Pulmonary contusions secondary to blunt trauma result in decreased lung compliance and ventilation-perfusion inequalities
   E. Pulmonary contusions may be present in certain patient populations without associated overlying rib fractures

**Hemothorax:**

3. All of the following are appropriate methods to evaluate for the presence of an acute traumatic hemothorax in the setting of blunt thoracic trauma EXCEPT:

   A. Chest tube placement
   B. Plain film chest X-ray
   C. Computed Tomography (CT)
   D. Ultrasound
   E. Magnetic Resonance Imaging (MRI)

4. A 25-year-old male is brought to the emergency department after being involved in a multiple vehicle motor collision. On primary survey his ABCs are intact and his initial vital signs are as follows: Temp 99°F, HR 100 bpm, BP 130/70 mm Hg, RR 19, Sat 95% on room air. On completion of his trauma workup he is noted to have an extensive trauma burden, including a traumatic right sided hemo-pneumothorax with associated overlying rib fractures for which a tube thoracostomy is performed. Which of the following statements regarding acute traumatic hemothoraces and pneumothoraces is true?

   A. All traumatic hemothoraces should be evaluated further via chest tube thoracostomy and Video-Assisted Thorascopic Surgery (VATS)
   B. Diagnosis of an occult pneumothorax is an indication for chest tube placement
   C. Persistent air-leak and/or recurrent pneumothorax should prompt evaluation for intrathoracic tracheobronchial injury
   D. Given the risk of progression, patients requiring positive pressure ventilation in the presence of a pneumothorax require chest tube placement
   E. Chest tube output >250 mL on initial placement is an indication to proceed to the operating room for thoracotomy

5. A 55-year-old female is the unrestrained passenger in a rollover motor vehicle accident. Among other injuries, she sustains multiple facial fractures, fractures involving C2-4 and multiple rib fractures bilaterally. According to the Denver Criteria, which of the following is NOT an indication for Computed Tomography Angiography (CT Angiography or CTA) as part of the comprehensive trauma evaluation?

   A. High-impact mechanism resulting in significant polytrauma
   B. Neurological examination not congruent with findings on noncontrast CT of the head
   C. LeFort Fracture type 2 or 3
   D. Base of skull fractures involving the carotid canal
   E. Cervical spine fractures involving C1-3 vertebrae

6. In a patient presenting with blunt trauma and obvious head involvement, a CT angiography of the head is obtained based on the Denver Modification Screening Criteria for blunt cerebrovascular injury (BCVI). The patient is subsequently diagnosed with a Grade 3 injury. Which of the following below correctly describes a Grade 3 BCVI according to the widely accepted Biffl scale?

   A. Transection
   B. Complete Occlusion
   C. Dissection or intramural hematomas with ≥25% luminal narrowing
   D. Pseudoaneurysm or hemodynamically insignificant arteriovenous fistula
   E. Intimal irregularity or dissection with <25% luminal narrowing

7. A 30-year-old male with no significant medical history is brought to the emergency department via EMS after sustaining a fall from an estimated 20 feet onto the pavement below. On arrival to the ED, he is alert and oriented with stable vital signs. The portable chest X-ray obtained in the trauma bay is concerning for a widened mediastinum. He is taken to the CT scanner for further evaluation of his injuries. All of the following statements regarding blunt thoracic aortic injury (BTAI) are true EXCEPT:

   A. The mechanism of injury typically involves a rapid deceleration event
   B. If clinically suspected, definitive evaluation with Transthoracic Echocardiography (TTE) or Transesophageal Echocardiography (TEE) is recommended
   C. The majority of blunt thoracic aortic injuries occur at the aortic isthmus, or just distal to the left subclavian
   D. A normal plain film in the trauma bay does not exclude the presence of a BTAI
   E. Initial management in the hemodynamically stable patient involves obtaining large bore IV access and maintaining SBP (~100 mm Hg) and HR (<100 bpm) control to prevent extension

8. Blunt aortic injuries in hemodynamically stable patients can be classified based on radiographic appearance. Which of the following terms is not used in the classification of blunt thoracic aortic injuries?

   A. Intimal tear
   B. Intramural hematoma
   C. Pseudoaneurysm
   D. True aneurysm
   E. Rupture

9. A 31-year-old male presents to the emergency department following a mountain biking accident. He has an obvious deformity to his right thigh, which appears to be an expanding hematoma. Aside from some otherwise superficial abrasions, he has no other significant trauma burden. He is taken to the operating room that day for Orthopedic surgery and undergoes an uneventful procedure. The following day, on postoperative day 1, the physician is called to his room where the patient is noted to have altered mental status and dyspnea with associated hypoxemia. On closer inspection, he is noted to have a fine petechial rash covering his neck and anterior trunk. All of the following statements about the underlying diagnosis are true EXCEPT:

   A. Most commonly associated with long bone fractures and pelvic fractures
   B. Typically presents 24 to 72 hours after the initial injury
   C. The classic triad includes neurologic changes, respiratory distress, and a nondependent petechial rash
   D. Diagnosis is made with aid of radiographic imaging, specifically CT of the chest
   E. Treatment is largely supportive, including fluid resuscitation, oxygenation, and mechanical ventilation if indicated

10. A young appearing male with an unknown past medical history is transported to the emergency department by EMS after being involved in a motor vehicle accident in which he was the unrestrained driver. The patient required a prolonged extrication from his vehicle, which was severely damaged, and EMS noted that the steering wheel was grossly deformed. The patient was intubated at the scene and vital signs on admission included the following: Temp: 98.0°F, HR 120 bpm, BP 110/60 mm Hg. In addition to a complete evaluation given the extent of his trauma, what additional testing would be the most helpful initially in ruling out a blunt cardiac injury (BCI)?

   A. Electrocardiogram (ECG), cardiac biomarkers, transthoracic echocardiogram, and continuous cardiac monitoring
   B. Continuous cardiac monitoring and cardiac biomarkers
   C. Continuous cardiac monitoring, cardiac biomarkers, and cardiology consultation
   D. ECG, cardiac biomarkers, and continuous cardiac monitoring
   E. Transthoracic echocardiogram alone

11. A 50-year-old male presents as a trauma following a motor vehicle accident. He has a Glasgow Coma Scale (GCS) score of 15 and is complaining of abdominal pain. His vital signs are as follows: Temp 99.0°F, HR 99 bpm, BP 110/70 mm Hg, Sat 100% on room air. On examination, he has significant tenderness to palpation over his mid-abdomen, and an ecchymosis is present in a bandlike distribution. A FAST examination is negative. He is taken for a CT scan that reveals no evidence of solid organ injury, no free air, and moderate free fluid on the pelvis and a mesenteric hematoma. He continues to have significant pain on abdominal examination. What is the most appropriate next step in management?

   A. Surgical consultation and exploratory laparotomy
   B. Admission to the floor for serial abdominal examinations
   C. Repeat FAST examination
   D. Administer IV morphine for pain control
   E. Place a nasogastric tube for decompression

12. A 55-year-old female presents to a Level 1 Trauma center following a motor vehicle collision with CT findings of an AAST (American Association for the Surgery of Trauma) Grade III liver laceration with a small "blush" identified by radiology. The patient has a GCS score of 15, is hemodynamically stable, and has only mild abdominal discomfort on examination. What is the most appropriate next step in the management of this patient?

   A. Admit to the floor for serial abdominal examinations
   B. Place two large bore IVs and administer 3 L crystalloid for trauma resuscitation
   C. Trend liver function tests (LFTs)
   D. Admit to a surgical critical care unit with interventional radiology consultation
   E. Exploratory laparotomy

13. A 27-year-old male presents to the Emergency Department after sustaining a fall from a third-story balcony. On primary survey, the patient is noted to have an intact airway and bilateral, symmetric breath sounds. His pulses are palpable, but weak, and his initial vital signs are as follows: HR 50, BP 80/40, Sat 100% on room air. EMS reports that he was given 3 L crystalloid in the field for persistent hypotension without significant improvement in his vital signs. On examination, he has no obvious source of bleeding, and he is noted to have decreased sensation at the level of the mid chest extending to bilateral lower extremities with 0/5 strength bilaterally. All of the following are appropriate in the initial evaluation and management of a patient with suspected neurogenic shock EXCEPT?

A. Evaluation for concomitant causes of shock including hypovolemic, cardiogenic, and other subtypes of distributive shock
B. Immobilization of the neck using a cervical collar and log roll precautions
C. Initiation of resuscitation with appropriate crystalloid/blood transfusion followed by use of vasoactive medications
D. Obtain CT imaging of the head and neck to look for cervical spine fractures
E. Admission to a SICU for monitoring of potential life-threatening complications including respiratory failure and cardiovascular instability

14. A 45-year-old female is hypotensive following a motorcycle accident. She is taken to the trauma bay where she is noted to be hypotensive. An abdominal FAST examination is negative for intraperitoneal fluid. On examination, she has no abdominal tenderness and her pelvis is grossly deformed. A chest radiograph is obtained that demonstrates no obvious hemothorax, and a pelvis film shows a severe open book deformity. In addition to resuscitation, what is the most appropriate next step in management of this patient?

A. Proceed to the operating room for exploratory laparotomy
B. Obtain CT scan with IV contrast of the abdomen and pelvis
C. Application of a pelvic binder and Interventional Radiology consultation for angiography
D. Admit to the surgical ICU for hemodynamic monitoring
E. Placement of a sheath introducer (ie Cordis) in the femoral vein for large volume resuscitation

15. A 4-year-old male is brought to the emergency department by his parents after swallowing a coin. On presentation, the child has a cough but otherwise appears comfortable, interacting with his parents and with oxygenation saturation readings 100% on room air. A plain radiograph is obtained that shows a radiopaque foreign body in the proximal right mainstem bronchus. What is the most appropriate next step in management of this patient?

A. CT scan
B. Perform the Heimlich maneuver
C. Upper GI swallow study
D. Provide education for prevention of future aspiration events
E. Flexible and/or rigid bronchoscopy

# Chapter 99 ▪ Answers

1. Correct Answer: D

**Rationale:**
Radiographically, a flail segment is defined as fractures of three or more ribs in two or more places. This can be seen on plain film imaging or more commonly on cross-sectional CT. Clinically, a diagnosis of flail chest is made when a patient has the radiographic findings consistent with the diagnosis, as well as a clinically apparent chest wall segment with paradoxical movement (Answer A). During normal inspiration, the chest wall expands while the diaphragm contracts, causing a strong negative pressure force within the pleural cavity. When a flail segment is present, this negative pressure causes a paradoxical movement of the segment inward, rather than outward with the remainder of the chest wall. This has many implications on underling pulmonary physiology, including hypoventilation, worsening atelectasis, and increased work of breathing, all of which contribute to respiratory failure (Answer B). The majority of patients presenting with rib fractures and flail chest are treated nonoperatively with pain control, aggressive pulmonary toilet, and ventilator support as indicated. No prospective randomized-controlled trials exist comparing surgical rib fixation to standard pain control with multimodal analgesia, including epidural catheter placement. Currently there is no hard set of indications for surgical rib fixation, and the clear majority of patients are management nonoperatively with multimodal analgesia and aggressive pulmonary toilet (Answer C). Flail chest is more commonly seen with blunt trauma compared to penetrating trauma. Owing to the pliability of the pediatric chest wall, rib fractures in the setting of blunt thoracic trauma are much more uncommon compared to the adult population (Answer E).

References
1. Dehghan N, de Mestral C, McKee MD, Schemitsch EH, Nathens A. Flail chest injuries: a review of outcomes and treatment practices from the National Trauma Data Bank. *J Trauma Acute Care Surg.* 2014;76(2):462-468.
2. Simon B, Ebert J, Bokhari F, et al. Management of pulmonary contusion and flail chest: an Eastern Association for the Surgery of Trauma practice management guideline. *J Trauma Acute Care Surg.* 2012;73(5 suppl 4):S351-S361.

**2.** Correct Answer: A

**Rationale:**

Pulmonary contusions result from blunt thoracic trauma, which may or may not be associated with overlying rib fractures, particularly in children (Answer E). Pulmonary contusions can develop over the first 24 to 48 hours, even if they are not seen on the initial trauma radiograph (Answer B). The pathophysiology involves direct impact injury to the lung parenchyma, resulting in leakage of blood and plasma into the alveoli. This results in decreased compliance and impaired diffusion. (Answer D). Initial management involves adequate resuscitation with either an isotonic crystalloid solution or colloid solution to maintain adequate tissue perfusion, initiation of multimodal pain management, and aggressive pulmonary toilet (Answer C). Although no studies have ever shown the benefit of colloid over crystalloid in the initial trauma resuscitation phase, there is evidence to support the negative effects of over-resuscitation, with any fluids, including worsening of oxygenation and development of Acute Respiratory Distress Syndrome. (Answer A).

**References**

1. Simon B, Ebert J, Bokhari F, et al. Management of pulmonary contusion and flail chest: an Eastern Association for the Surgery of Trauma practice management guideline. *J Trauma Acute Care Surg*. 2012;73(5 suppl 4):S351-S361.
2. Wanek S, Mayberry JC. Blunt thoracic trauma: flail chest, pulmonary contusion, and blast injury. *Crit Care Clin*. 2004;20(1):71.

**3.** Correct Answer: E

**Rationale:**

In the setting of acute blunt thoracic trauma, one must rule out the presence of an acute hemothorax. Typically, a plain film portable chest X-ray is obtained in the trauma bay to evaluate for the presence of a hemothorax or pneumothorax that would require urgent placement of a chest tube (Answer B). More recently, ultrasound has become a widely accepted method of initial evaluation of the thoracic cavity, specifically to determine the presence of a significant pleural effusion/hemothorax or pneumothorax (Answer D). Both of these modalities provide a quick, real time assessment of the patient in the trauma bay. In stable patients, a CT of the chest can be obtained, in addition to other indicated trauma imaging, which can help further identify the presence of a hemothorax and other concomitant thoracic injuries (Answer C). In the unstable trauma patient who arrives to the trauma bay, early evaluation with tube thoracostomy may be indicated if there is concern for possible hemothorax (Answer A). Although MRI of the chest can identify the presence of a hemothorax, the test itself requires significantly more time to perform and does not provide additional necessary information in the setting of acute thoracic trauma (Answer E).

**References**

1. ATLS Subcommittee; American College of Surgeons' Committee on Trauma; International ATLS working group. Advanced trauma life support (ATLS®): the ninth edition. *J Trauma Acute Care Surg*. 2013;74(5):1363-1366.
2. Broderick SR. Hemothorax: etiology, diagnosis, and management. *Thorac Surg Clin*. 2013;23(1):89-96.

**4.** Correct Answer: C

**Rationale:**

Following blunt trauma in the hemodynamically stable patient, the diagnosis of an acute hemothorax or pneumothorax can be made using portable plain chest X-ray, ultrasound, or CT of the chest. An occult pneumothorax is defined as an asymptomatic pneumothorax that is not seen on chest radiograph but is present on CT imaging. Stable patients with an occult pneumothorax may be observed without need for immediate intervention, regardless of whether or not they require positive pressure ventilation (Answer B and Answer D). Although the presence of a traumatic hemothorax should prompt consideration for tube thoracostomy placement, it is necessary to note the clinical stability of the patient and the size of the hemothorax. All traumatic hemothoraces do not necessarily require drainage with a chest tube, and not all patients requiring a tube thoracostomy require further evaluation with VATS (Answer A). In general, indications to consider operative intervention rely on patient physiology rather than any absolute numbers. In addition to patient physiology, situations prompting consideration to proceed to the operating room include persistent retained hemothorax, persistent air-leak on post-injury day 3, and >1500 mL via the chest tube in a 24-hour period (Answer E). Tracheobronchial injuries resulting from blunt thoracic trauma are rare, occurring in less than 1% of patients presenting with blunt thoracic trauma. Classically, these patients present with significant air leak on tube thoracostomy placement, as well as pneumothorax or pneumomediastinum that reaccumulates despite chest tube placement (Answer C).

**References**

1. Mowery NT, Gunter OL, Collier BR, et al. Practice management guidelines for management of hemothorax and occult pneumothorax. *J Trauma*. 2011;70(2):510.
2. Legome E. *Initial Evaluation and Management of Blunt Thoracic Trauma In Adults*. UpToDate; March 29, 2018.
3. Moonsamy P, Sachdeva UM, Morse CR. Management of laryngotracheal trauma. *Ann Cardiothorac Surg*. 2018;7(2):210-216.

**5.** Correct Answer: A

**Rationale:**

The Denver Criteria for screening for BCVI in the setting of trauma is a set of criteria (see below) that was created to guide clinicians on the need for obtaining further imaging, specifically CT angiography, when there is concern for a BCVI. Mechanisms of injury that lead to BCVI most commonly involve cervical hyperextension, flexion, and rotation, as well as direct injury to the boney structures involving the vascular foramen. Approximately 1% of hospitalized blunt trauma patients in the United States have a BCVI, but unfortunately the majority are diagnosed when they become symptomatic. Therefore, a push was made to screen asymptomatic patients who sustained a significant blunt trauma. Several studies by Biffl et al. and Cothren et al. aided in creating screening criteria for evaluation of the trauma patient at risk for BCVI. Table 99.1 shows the Denver Modification of Screening Criteria for BCVI (Answers B-E). While many of these injuries are sustained during a high impact trauma, the mechanism of the blunt trauma itself is not an indication for further imaging to rule out BCVI (Answer A).

**TABLE 99.1 Denver Modification of Screening Criteria for BCVI**

| SIGNS/SYMPTOMS OF BCVI: | RISK FACTORS FOR BCVI: |
|---|---|
| Arterial hemorrhage | High-energy impact with: |
| Cervical bruit | Lefort II or III fracture |
| Expanding cervical hematoma | Cervical spine fracture patterns: subluxation, fractures extending into the transverse foramen, fractures of C1-C3 |
| Focal neurological deficit | Basilar skull fracture with carotid canal involvement |
| Neurologic examination incongruous with CAT scan findings | Diffuse axonal injury with GCS = 6 |
| Ischemic stroke on secondary CAT scan | Near hanging with anoxic brain injury |

References

1. Bromberg WJ, Collier BC, Diebel LN, et al. Blunt cerebrovascular injury practice management guidelines: the Eastern Association for the Surgery of Trauma. *J Trauma*. 2018;68:471-477.
2. Biffl WL, Moore EE, Offner PJ, et al. Optimizing screening for blunt cerebrovascular injuries. *Am J Surg*. 1999;178:517-522.
3. Cothren CC, Moore EE, Biffl WL, et al. Anticoagulation is the gold standard therapy for blunt carotid injuries to reduce stroke rate. *Arch Surg*. 2004;139:540-545.

**6.** Correct Answer: D

**Rationale:**

The Biffl scale, first described in 1999, has been used to describe the spectrum of vascular injuries seen on angiography following blunt trauma to the head and neck. This scale provides prognostic information based on the injury grade in addition to helping guide monitoring and therapeutic strategies. The table below provides descriptive information on the grading scale, as well as the corresponding risk of stroke associated with the involved vessel.

| GRADE | DESCRIPTION | BCI INCIDENCE OF STROKE (%) | BVI INCIDENCE OF STROKE (%) |
|---|---|---|---|
| 1 | Intimal irregularity or dissection with <25% luminal narrowing | 8% | 6% |
| 2 | Dissection or intramural hematomas with ≥25% luminal narrowing, intraluminal clot, or a visible intimal flap | 14% | 38% |
| 3 | Pseudoaneurysm or hemodynamically insignificant arteriovenous fistula | 26% | 27% |
| 4 | Complete occlusion | 50% | 28% |
| 5 | Transection with active extravasation (hemorrhage) or hemodynamically significant arteriovenous fistula | 100% | |

BCI, Blunt carotid artery injury; BVI, Blunt vertebral artery injury.

### References

1. Bromberg WJ, Collier BC, Diebel LN, et al. Blunt cerebrovascular injury practice management guidelines: the Eastern Association for the Surgery of Trauma. *J Trauma*. 2018;68:471-477.
2. Biffl WL, Ray CE Jr, Moore EE, et al. Treatment-related outcomes from blunt cerebrovascular injuries: importance of routine follow-up arteriography. *Ann Surg*. 2002;235(5):699.

### 7. Correct Answer: B

**Rationale:**

An estimated 1.5% to 2% of all patients sustaining blunt thoracic trauma have a blunt aortic injury (BAI). The main risk factor for this type of injury is a mechanism that involves a rapid deceleration event, with the most common cause being involvement in a motor vehicle collision (Answer A). The majority of blunt thoracic aortic injuries occur at the aortic isthmus, or just distal to the left subclavian. Although multiple theories exist to explain this phenomenon, anatomically this area represents the transition from the mobile ascending aorta to the fixed descending aorta, thereby predisposing it to injury in rapid deceleration events (Answer C). Diagnosis begins with a high clinical suspicion, followed by initial evaluation involving plain film of the chest in the trauma bay. A normal plain film in the trauma bay does not exclude the presence of a BTAI (Answer D). The imaging modality of choice is contrast-enhanced CT angiography of the chest. The NEXUS criteria was developed as a guideline to help determine which patients, based on mechanism and presentation, warranted further evaluation with CT of the chest for further evaluation for BAI. Subsequent modifications have been made, with the most recent guidelines, when used in the appropriate clinical context, serving to reduce the need for unnecessary imaging studies. While TEE can be used to evaluate the thoracic aorta, it requires the patient to be intubated, is typically less available in the acute setting in the trauma bay, and is not interchangeable with TTE (Answer B). On diagnosis, initial management of a BAI in a hemodynamically stable patient involves obtained adequate vascular access and maintaining adequate heart rate (<100 bpm) and blood pressure control (<100 mm Hg), typically with a beta blocker if not contraindicated (Answer E). Hemodynamically unstable trauma patients require an emergent trip to the operating room.

### References

1. Lee WA, Matsumura JS, Mitchell RS, et al. Endovascular repair of traumatic thoracic aortic injury: clinical practice guidelines of the Society for Vascular Surgery. *J Vasc Surg*. 2011;53(1):187.
2. Richens D, Field M, Neale M, Oakley C. The mechanism of injury in blunt traumatic rupture of the aorta. *Eur J Cardiothorac Surg*. 2002;21:288-293.
3. Neschis DG, Scalea TM, Flinn WR, Griffith BP. Blunt aortic injury. *N Engl J Med*. 2008;359:1708-1716.
4. Rodriguez RM, Langdorf MI, Nishijima D, et al. Derivation and validation of two decision instruments for selective chest CT in blunt trauma: a multicenter prospective observational study (NEXUS Chest CT). *PLoS Med*. 2015;12(10):e1001883.

### 8. Correct Answer: D

**Rationale:**

The evaluation of BTAI following trauma is best done by obtaining a CT of the chest with intravenous contrast. Findings on imaging can then be used to classify individual BTAIs as Grade 1 to 4 in severity, which is then used in the management algorithm including both serial imaging studies and invasive intervention either by endovascular or open techniques. According to the widely accepted grading scale, Grade 1 is an intimal tear, Grade 2 is an intramural hematoma, Grade 3 is a pseudoaneurysm, and Grade 4 is a free rupture (Answer A, B, C, and E). By definition, a pseudoaneurysm, also known as a false aneurysm, where intraluminal blood dissects into the walls of the vessel, thereby creating an area that is only contained by the arterial adventitia or surrounding tissues. Pseudoaneurysm formation commonly occurs following trauma but can also occur in the setting of other pathological processes including vasculitis and other inflammatory processes. In contrast, a true aneurysm is a local dilation of an artery that involves all three layers (intima, media, and adventitia) of the arterial wall. True aneurysm formation is not seen in the setting of BTAIs.

### Reference

1. Lee WA, Matsumura JS, Mitchell RS, et al. Endovascular repair of traumatic thoracic aortic injury: clinical practice guidelines of the Society for Vascular Surgery. *J Vasc Surg*. 2011;53(1):187.

### 9. Correct Answer: D

**Rationale:**

Fat embolism syndrome (FES) is a rare clinical syndrome that classically presents with the triad of neurological changes, respiratory distress (dyspnea, tachypnea, hypoxemia), and a nondependent petechial rash (Answer C). Interestingly, although part of the classic triad, the petechial rash is only present in an estimated 33% of patients. Although reports exist of FES occurring following nonorthopedic trauma (eg Isolated soft tissue injury), nonorthopedic operations (eg Liposuction, lipo-injection), and nontrauma-related conditions (eg Pancreatitis), the majority of cases present in 24 to 72 hours following long bone and pelvic fracture injuries (Answer A, B). A diagnosis of FES is typically a diagnosis of exclusion that is made in the appropriate clinical setting. Although laboratory evaluation and imaging (CT head and chest) should be obtained to rule out other diagnoses in the differential for altered mental status and respiratory distress, none of these tests can individually confirm the diagnosis of FES (Answer D). Once a diagnosis is made, treatment is largely supportive, including fluid resuscitation, oxygenation, and mechanical ventilation if indicated (Answer E).

References
1. Mellor A, Soni N. Fat embolism. *Anesthesia*. 2001;56(2):145.
2. Stein PD, Yaekoub AY, Matta F, Kleerekoper M. Fat embolism syndrome. *Am J Med Sci*. 2008;336(6):472-427.

**10.** Correct Answer: D

**Rationale:**

The true incidence of BCI in high impact trauma is unknown but is most commonly seen following motor vehicle collisions. BCI sustained during high-impact trauma can present in a variety of ways ranging from new arrhythmias to devastating structural injuries. Interestingly, the majority of BCIs are silent on presentation, with patients asymptomatic at the time of presentation. Given the wide variety of presentations and manifestations of BCI, there is no clear diagnostic criteria. Therefore, the appropriate diagnostic evaluation begins with a high degree of clinical suspicion. Evaluation should begin with a baseline ECG and cardiac biomarkers. The role of cardiac biomarkers alone is still a topic of much debate, but when used in conjunction with ECG, they may play an important role in ruling out BCI (Answer B, C). Alone, a negative ECG has a reported negative predictive value of up to 95%, which is increased to 100% with the addition of negative biomarker testing. Continued cardiac monitoring, specifically in the setting of new ECG findings, is recommended. For patients with new ECG findings or hemodynamic instability on presentation, an echocardiogram is recommended for further structural and functional evaluation (Answer E). Of the answers above, Answer D represents a thorough initial evaluation for BCI in a patient who is hemodynamically stable on presentation. There is no indication at present to obtain an echocardiogram (Answer A)

References
1. Clancy K, Velopulos C, Bilaniuk JW, et al. Screening for blunt cardiac injury: an eastern association for the surgery of trauma practice management guideline. *J Trauma*. 2012;73(5):S301-S306.
2. Moore EE, Malangoni MA, Cogbill TH, et al. Organ injury scaling. IV: thoracic vascular, lung, cardiac, and diaphragm. *J Trauma*. 1994;36(3):299.
3. Salim A, Velmahos GC, Jindal A, et al. Clinically significant blunt cardiac trauma: role of serum troponin levels combined with electrocardiographic findings. *J Trauma*. 2001;50(2):237.

**11.** Correct Answer: A

**Rationale:**

Gastrointestinal injury following blunt abdominal trauma occurs in an estimated 3.1% of patients being evaluated followed blunt abdominal trauma. Most commonly, these injuries are seen the following motor vehicle collisions, where the mechanism involves crushing of the bowel between solid structures (ie the spine and a steering wheel). The definitive diagnosis of hollow viscus injury is made by abdominal exploration, with physical examination and CT imaging being used to help make the decision to go to the operating room. The patient presented above has a concerning abdominal examination, which in combination with the CT findings of free fluid in the absence of solid organ injury, is concerning for a hollow viscus injury. Although the finding of free intraperitoneal air on CT imaging has high specificity for a hollow viscus injury, the lack of pneumoperitoneum on imaging does not rule out a diagnosis of hollow viscus perforation. The next appropriate step would be to obtain urgent surgical consultation and proceed with exploratory laparotomy (Answer A). Admission to the floor for serial examinations and administering IV narcotic pain medication both fail to address the underlying diagnosis and could lead to life-threatening complications (Answer B, D). CT scans are more sensitive for the identification of free intraperitoneal fluid, thus there is no benefit at this point of repeating a FAST ultrasound examination (Answer C). There is no role here in placing a nasogastric tube for gastric decompression (Answer E).

References
1. Fakhry SM, Watts DD, Luchette FA; EAST Multi-Institutional Hollow Viscus Injury Research Group. Current diagnostic approaches lack sensitivity in the diagnosis of perforated blunt small bowel injury: analysis from 275,557 trauma admissions from the EAST multi-institutional HVI trial. *J Trauma*. 2003;54(2):295-306.
2. Atri M, Hanson JM, Grinblat L, Brofman N, Chughtai T, Tomlinson G. Surgically important bowel and/or mesenteric injury in blunt trauma: accuracy of multidetector CT for evaluation. *Radiology*. 2008;249(2):524-533.

**12.** Correct Answer: D

**Rationale:**

The liver is the most commonly injured abdominal organ in the setting of blunt abdominal trauma. Historically, liver injuries required operative intervention but based on multiple studies, current consensus recommendations have shifted to the nonoperative management of liver injuries in the hemodynamically stable patient who do not otherwise have an indication for surgical intervention (Answer D, E). Additionally, these patients, should they require an intervention, may benefit from selective vascular embolization via Interventional Radiology, rather than operative intervention. When nonoperative management is pursued, the patient requires close hemodynamic monitoring in a critical care unit as well as serial abdominal examinations should their examination evolve (Answer A). While it is important to maintain adequate access for large volume resuscitation should need arise, there is no role for the prophylactic administration of large volume crystalloid in the trauma patient (Answer B). There is no clinically relevant role for monitoring LFTs in the setting of known blunt hepatic injury (Answer C). Patients who are hemodynamically unstable or who have diffuse peritonitis on examination differ greatly in their management, as they do require urgent operative intervention.

### Reference

1. Stassen NA, Bhullar I, Cheng JD, et al. Nonoperative management of blunt hepatic injury: an Eastern Association for the Surgery of trauma practice management guideline. *J Trauma Acute Care Surg.* 2012;73(5):S299-S293.

---

**13.** Correct Answer: D

### Rationale:

Neurogenic shock is a form of distributive shock that is seen in patients with severe traumatic brain injury and spinal cord injury (cervical and upper thoracic spine). It differs from spinal shock in the sense that not all spinal cord injuries cause a distributive shock picture, and rarely is it seen in spinal cord injuries below the level of T6. In a trauma patient presenting with signs/symptoms concerning for neurogenic shock, it is important to rule out concomitant causes of shock including hypovolemic shock (hemorrhagic and nonhemorrhagic), cardiogenic shock, obstructive shock, and other forms of distributive shock (Answer A). Initial management involves completing a thorough physical examination, close hemodynamic monitoring, initiation of resuscitation with crystalloid or blood products as indicated, and initiation of vasopressor therapy if hypotension persists despite adequate resuscitation (Answer C). Until imaging is obtained that can rule out an unstable spine injury, it is pertinent to maintain Cervical spine stabilization with use of a C collar and spinal precautions to avoid worsening an injury (Answer B). Initial imaging with CT is indicated to evaluate the spine as well as any other concomitant injuries, with the need for further imaging being dictated by a spine specialist. It is important to note though that imaging of the head and C spine is inadequate given that upper thoracic spine injuries (above T6) can also cause neurogenic shock and its sequelae (Answer D). Following diagnosis, admission to a SICU is recommended for continued monitoring and treatment given the potential life-threatening complications including cardiovascular collapse and respiratory failure (Answer E).

### References

1. Piepmeier JM, Lehmann KB, Lane JG. Cardiovascular instability following acute cervical spinal cord trauma. *Cent Nerv Syst Trauma.* 1985;2(3):153-160.
2. ATLS Subcommittee; American College of Surgeons' Committee on Trauma; International ATLS Working Group. Advanced trauma life support (ATLS®): the ninth edition. *J Trauma Acute Care Surg.* 2013;74(5):1363-1366.

---

**14.** Correct Answer: C

### Rationale:

This patient is presenting after a motorcycle accident with hypotension and an obvious pelvic deformity. In addition to obtaining large bore peripheral access and initiating resuscitation, it is recommended that a temporary pelvic binder is applied to reapproximate the pelvic ring (Answer C). Emergent Orthopedic surgery consultation allows for the evaluation for external pelvic fixation in addition to ongoing hemorrhage control maneuvers. As in any trauma patient presenting with hypotension, it is important to obtain adequate intravenous access for resuscitation. If peripheral access cannot be obtained, central venous access is an option, although in a patient presenting with a pelvic fracture the femoral veins should be avoided (Answer E). Hemorrhage associated with pelvic fractures is most commonly from the sacral venous plexus, although occasionally an arterial source may be involved. Pelvic angiography by Interventional Radiology allows for localization of the source of bleeding, as well as intervention in the form of selective embolization or internal iliac embolization, which decreases overall pelvic inflow. It would be inappropriate to send this patient to the CT scanner or the ICU without first addressing the hypotension and presumed ongoing hemorrhage (Answer B, D).

### References

1. Cullinane DC, Schiller HJ, Zielinski MD, et al. Eastern association for the surgery of trauma practice management guidelines for hemorrhage in pelvic fracture – update and systematic review. *J Trauma.* 2011;71(6):1850-1868
2. Velmahos GC, Chahwan S, Falabella A, Hanks SE, Demetriades D. Angiographic embolization for intraperitoneal and retroperitoneal injuries. *World J Surg.* 2000;24:539-545.

---

**15.** Correct Answer: E

### Rationale:

The child above is presenting after a witnessed aspiration event of a small object with signs of a partial airway obstruction. In children presenting with signs of a complete airway obstruction, including severe respiratory distress, cyanosis, and altered mental status, attempts at object dislodgement can be made including back blows, chest compressions, and the Heimlich maneuver. In cases of partial obstruction in the stable patient, these maneuvers should be avoided for fear that they may convert a partial obstruction to a complete airway obstruction (Answer B). In the stable patient, a CT scan can provide additional information if the diagnosis is unclear, but in the case mentioned above, no additional necessary information is needed before therapeutic intervention (Answer A). The next appropriate step in management of this patient would be to proceed to the operating room for a flexible and/or rigid bronschoscopy for evacuation of the foreign body and visual evaluation of the airways (Answer C). The majority of foreign body ingestions/inhalations occur while under adult supervision, and education may be helpful in reducing the incidence; this is not the most appropriate next step in management of this child (Answer D). An upper GI swallow does not add any value to the management of this patient (Answer C).

### References

1. Sahin A, Meteroglu F, Eren S, Celik Y. Inhalation of foreign bodies in children: experience of 22 years. *J Trauma Acute Care Surg.* 2013;74(2):658-663.
2. Ruiz FE. *Airway foreign bodies in children.* UpToDate; June 25, 2018.

# 100

# HEMORRHAGE AND RESUSCITATION

Rachel Steinhorn and Galen Royce-Nagel

1. A 24-year-old male was involved in a motor vehicle accident. On arrival to the trauma bay, he is noted to have an open tibia-fibula fracture with significant blood loss. His systolic blood pressure (BP) is 65 mm Hg. Appropriate resuscitation includes

   A. Administering a 10 mL/kg intravenous (IV) fluid bolus
   B. Transfusing red blood cells, plasma, and cryoprecipitate in equal numbers
   C. Transfusing red cells, plasma, and platelets in equal numbers
   D. Transfusing red cells, plasma, and platelets in a 4:1:1 ratio

2. A 45-year-old male with open bilateral femur fractures is brought in with a systolic BP of 58 mm Hg. He has delayed capillary refill, and heart rate (HR) is 168. Based on his clinical presentation, he has likely lost

   A. 20% to 30% of blood volume
   B. 10% to 20% of blood volume
   C. 5% to 10% of blood volume
   D. >30% of blood volume

3. A 23-year-old male is brought to the emergency department by emergency medical services (EMS) with a penetrating abdominal wound. Initial vital signs are HR 127 and BP 84/36. One unit of uncrossmatched blood is given as he is sent emergently to the operating room (OR) for exploratory laparotomy. During the procedure, 2 L of blood is evacuated immediately and ongoing bleeding is appreciated. What is the best initial fluid resuscitation strategy?

   A. Transfusion with packed red blood cells (PRBCs), platelets, and fresh frozen plasma (FFP) in a 1:1:1 ratio until hemodynamic stability is achieved
   B. Resuscitate with lactated ringers, check labs frequently, and transfuse PRBCs for Hgb <7, platelets for <100, and FFP for international normalized ratio (INR) >1.7
   C. Resuscitate with albumin 5%, check labs frequently, and transfuse PRBCs for Hgb <7, platelets for <100, and FFP for INR >1.7
   D. Transfuse PRBCs until hemodynamic stability is achieved, transfuse platelets for <100 and FFP for INR >1.7

4. A 44-year-old, 70 kg female with a history of insulin-dependent diabetes, nonobstructive coronary artery disease (CAD), heart failure with preserved ejection fraction, and chronic kidney disease with a baseline Cr 1.6 is admitted to the intensive care unit (ICU) intubated after a laparoscopic appendectomy complicated by rupture of the appendix during resection. Blood loss was minimal, per surgical hand off. First set of ICU vital signs: HR 119, BP 83/36, respiratory rate (RR) 18 on volume control ventilation, and temperature 38.6°C. Preliminary set of labs are remarkable for WBC 17, Hgb 7.8, platelets 54, pH 7.3, lactate 3, and all electrolytes within normal limits. After a 1 L crystalloid bolus and initiation of a norepinephrine drip at 4 μg/min, BP is now 96/54. What is the best strategy for ongoing resuscitation?

A. Transfuse PRBCs for goal Hgb >9 g/dL
B. Transfuse platelets for goal >100 000/mm³
C. No further fluid resuscitation; titrate norepinephrine drip to maintain mean arterial pressure (MAP) >65
D. Repeat 1 L crystalloid bolus

5. An 83-year-old male with a history of chronic kidney disease, hypertension, and insulin-dependent diabetes is admitted to the floor with a small bowel obstruction. After 2 days of conservative therapy, HR is now 118 with MAP <65 despite repeated crystalloid boluses, and he has peritonitic signs on abdominal examination. The plan is to go to the OR for an exploratory laparotomy and small bowel resection. What is the goal platelet count before surgery?

   A. 10 000/mm³
   B. 20 000/mm³
   C. 50 000/mm³
   D. 100 000/mm³

6. A 76-year-old female with a history of hepatitis C cirrhosis and CAD status post three-vessel coronary artery bypass grafting (CABG) 2 years prior is admitted to the ICU with 1 day of melena and hematemesis. She has another episode of hematemesis on arrival to the ICU, with 50 mL bright red blood collected in a basin. Initial vital signs are HR 105, BP 96/45, RR 14, and SpO₂ 99% on room air. Labs return with Hgb 7.8, platelets 76, electrolytes within normal limits, and lactate 1.8. Large bore IV access is established, and the plan is made for an esophagogastroduodenoscopy (EGD). What is the best transfusion threshold in this patient?

   A. Transfuse for Hgb <9 g/dL
   B. Transfuse for Hgb <7 g/dL
   C. Transfuse for platelets <100 000/mm³
   D. Transfuse for MAP <65

7. A 34-year-old female with no significant past medical history is now gravida 2, para 2 (G2P2) after cesarean section of a term neonate for placenta accreta. Large bore IV access was established preoperatively, and a type and screen was sent in anticipation of intraoperative blood loss. The patient's blood type is O, and she is RhD−. Which blood product is most suitable to transfuse?

   A. FFP, type AB, RhD+
   B. Platelets, type AB, RhD+
   C. FFP, type O, RhD−
   D. Platelets, type O, RhD−

8. A 34-year-old male with a history of Hodgkin lymphoma and atrial fibrillation on warfarin presents after a 5-foot fall from a ladder. He was intubated in the field because of obtundation, and a noncontrast head computed tomography (CT) on arrival demonstrates a left subdural hematoma with midline shift. Other trauma burden on primary survey includes left-displaced radial fracture and contusions to the left side of the thorax. The patient is sent to the OR for emergent craniotomy for decompression. Vital signs on arrival to the OR are HR 95, BP 96/47, SpO₂ 95% on 100% FiO₂, and labs show Hgb 6.5 g/dL and platelets 56 000/mm³. How should blood products be prepared for this patient?

   A. Leukoreduction
   B. Washing
   C. Irradiation
   D. No special preparation needed

9. A 19-year-old male who sustained two gunshot wounds to the chest is brought in by ambulance. His initial vitals are BP 75/30 and HR 144. While securing the airway, large bore IV access is established. Which of the following catheters is the best choice for rapid volume resuscitation?

   A. 18G 45 mm catheter
   B. 16G 50 mm catheter
   C. 18G port on a triple lumen central line
   D. 16G port on a triple lumen central line

**10.** A 45-year-old female with no past medical history is brought in via ambulance after a motor vehicle accident. Her initial vitals are BP 62/30 and HR 157. On primary survey, she is noted to have significant ecchymosis across her abdomen. Focused assessment with sonography in trauma (FAST) is positive, and she is taken emergently to the OR for ex-lap. In the OR, they find multiple liver lacerations with diffuse bleeding. Along with volume resuscitation, what would be a useful adjunct to obtain hemostasis?

A. Cryoprecipitate in equal numbers with PRBCs
B. Prothrombin complex concentrate
C. Vitamin K
D. Tranexamic acid

# Chapter 100 ▪ Answers

**1.** Correct Answer: C

**Rationale:**
Studies assessing transfusion ratios found that patients who were transfused in a 1:1:1 ratio were more likely to have adequate hemostasis and have fewer exsanguination deaths at 24 hours, and in some cases lower mortality at 30 days. Given he has "significant" blood loss and is hypotensive, a fluid bolus would be less than adequate. Cryoprecipitate should be administered when a patient has hypofibrinogenemia.

### References
1. Holcomb JB, Tilley BC, Baraniuk S, et al. Transfusion of plasma, platelets, and red blood cells in a 1:1:1 vs a 1:1:2 ratio and mortality in patients with severe trauma: the PROPPR randomized clinical trial. *JAMA*. 2015;313(5):471.
2. Borgman MA, Spinella PC, Perkins JG, et al. The ratio of blood products transfused affects mortality in patients receiving massive transfusions at a combat support hospital. *J Trauma*. 2007;63(4):805.
3. Holcomb JB, Wade CE, Michalek JE, et al. Increased plasma and platelet to red blood cell ratios improves outcome in 466 massively transfused civilian trauma patients. *Ann Surg*. 2008;248(3):447.

**2.** Correct Answer: D

**Rationale:**
Class 3 hemorrhage is distinguished from less severe forms of hemorrhage by the development of hypotension and is associated with >30% of blood volume loss.

**ATLS classification of hemorrhagic shock**

|  | CLASS 1 | CLASS 2 | CLASS 3 | CLASS 4 |
|---|---|---|---|---|
| Blood loss | <15% | 15%-30% | 30%-40% | >40% |
| Pulse (beats/min) | <100 | 100-120 | 120-140 | >140 |
| Blood pressure (mm Hg) | Normal | Normal | Decreased | Much decreased |
| Pulse pressure | Normal or increased | Decreased | Decreased | Decreased |
| Respiratory rate (breaths/min) | 14-20 | 20-30 | 30-40 | >40 |
| Mental status | Slightly anxious | Mildly anxious | Anxious, confused | Confused, lethargic |
| Urine output (mL/hr) | >30 | 20-30 | 5-15 | Minimal |

### Reference
1. ATLS Subcommittee: American College of Surgeons' Committee on Trauma; International ATLS Working Group. Advanced trauma life support (ATLS®): ninth edition. *J Trauma Acute Care Surg*. 2013;74(5):1363-1366.

**3.** Correct Answer: A

**Rationale:**

This patient meets the criteria for hemorrhagic shock, the second most frequent cause of death in trauma patients and a leading cause of early in-hospital trauma mortality. Resuscitation of patients with massive hemorrhage has moved from reactive strategies based on laboratory values to proactive, standardized massive transfusion protocols (MTPs). A lab-based approach to transfusion in hemorrhage can lead to a delay in the recognition and treatment of a rapidly developing anemia and coagulopathy. Additionally, excessive crystalloid or nonblood colloid should be avoided to limit hemodilution and coagulopathy exacerbation.

The Prospective, Observational, Multicenter, Major Trauma Transfusion (PROMMTT) study found that patients transfused with ratios of plasma:PRBCs or platelets:PRBCs of 1:1 or higher were less likely to die in the first 24 hours than those with ratios less than 1:2. This is especially notable, as most hemorrhagic deaths occur in the first 6 hours of admission.

### References

1. Sauaia A, Moore FA, Moore EE, et al. Epidemiology of trauma deaths: a reassessment. *J Trauma*. 1995;38(2):185-193.
2. Tien H, Nascimento B, Callum J, Rizoli S. An approach to transfusion and hemorrhage in trauma: current perspectives on restrictive transfusion strategies. *Can J Surg*. 2007;50(3):202-209.
3. Spinella PC, Holcomb JB. Resuscitation and transfusion principles for traumatic hemorrhagic shock. *Blood Rev*. 2009;23(6):231-240.
4. Patil V, Shetmahajan M. Massive transfusion and massive transfusion protocol. *Indian J Anaesth*. 2014;58(5):590-595.
5. Holcomb JB, del Junco DJ, Fox EE, et al. The prospective, observational, multicenter, major trauma transfusion (PROMMTT) study: comparative effectiveness of a time-varying treatment with competing risks. *JAMA Surg*. 2013;148(2):127-136.

**4.** Correct Answer: D

**Rationale:**

Anemia is a common condition in the ICU, with studies showing that two-thirds of ICU patients have a Hgb <12 on the day of admission, and 97% of patients become anemic after a week in the ICU. The etiology is often multifactorial and is associated with worse outcomes.

The Transfusion Requirements in Critical Care (TRICC) trial examined differences in mortality between euvolemic, critically ill patients randomized to a liberal transfusion strategy with goal Hgb >10 g/dL or a restrictive transfusion strategy with goal Hgb >7 g/dL. A restrictive transfusion strategy was associated with significantly lower in-hospital mortality. The benefit was most prominent among the younger (age <55 years) and less critically ill (APACHE score <20) subset. Other studies have demonstrated no difference in mortality, ischemic events, or life support requirements in patients with septic shock transfused to goal Hgb >7 or >9.

In this patient with septic shock, the Surviving Sepsis guidelines recommend initial resuscitation of 30 mL/kg, or 2.1 L in this 70 kg patient, and she would benefit most from a second 1 L crystalloid bolus. Platelets should not be used for expansion of the circulatory volume in a patient without signs of active bleeding and platelets >50 000/mm³.

### References

1. Hébert PC, Wells G, Blajchman MA, et al; Transfusion Requirements in Critical Care Investigators, Canadian Critical Care Trials Group. A multicenter, randomized, controlled clinical trial of transfusion requirements in critical care. *N Engl J Med*. 1999;340:409-417.
2. Hayden SJ, Albert TJ, Watkins TR, Swenson ER. Anemia in critical illness: insights into etiology, consequences, and management. *Am J Respir Crit Care Med*. 2012;185(10):1049-1057.
3. Rawal G, Kumar R, Yadav S, Singh A. Anemia in intensive care: a review of current concepts. *J Crit Care Med (Targu Mures)*. 2016;2(3):109-114. doi:10.1515/jccm-2016 to 0017.
4. Salpeter SR, Buckley JS, Chatterjee S, et al. Impact of More Restrictive Blood Transfusion Strategies on Clinical Outcomes: A Meta-analysis and Systematic Review. *Am J Med*. 2014;127(2):124-131.e3.
5. Holst LB, Haase N, Wetterslev J, et al. Lower versus higher hemoglobin threshold for transfusion in septic shock. *N Engl J Med*. 2014;371(15):1381-1391.

**5.** Correct Answer: C

**Rationale:**

Thrombocytopenia is common in the critically ill population, and it serves as an independent predictor of mortality. Critical illness–associated thrombocytopenia is multifactorial; it often results from a combination of bone marrow suppression, consumption of coagulation factors, and increased turnover. Few randomized trials of prophylactic platelet transfusion thresholds mean to prevent, rather than treat, bleeding in critically ill patients, and recommendations are based largely on expert opinion and institution-specific guidelines. Most of the current guidelines have been extrapolated from oncology patients with chemotherapy-associated thrombocytopenia. Current consensus guidelines recommend prophylactic platelet transfusion for counts <10 000/mm³ in the absence of bleeding or for counts <20 000/mm³ for patients at high-risk of bleeding. Platelet counts >50 000/mm³ are recommended for active bleeding, surgery, or other invasive procedures. Surgery at critical sites, such as ocular surgery and neurosurgery, often requires counts >100 000/mm³.

References

1. Hui P, Cook DJ, Lim W, Fraser GA, Arnold DM. The frequency and clinical significance of thrombocytopenia complicating critical illness: a systematic review. *Chest.* 2011;139(2):271-278.
2. Estcourt L, Stanworth S, Doree C, et al. Prophylactic platelet transfusion for prevention of bleeding in patients with haematological disorders after chemotherapy and stem cell transplantation. *Cochrane Database Syst Rev.* 2012;5:CD004269.
3. Liumbruno G, Bennardello F, Lattanzio A, Piccoli P, Rossetti G; Italian Society of Transfusion Medicine and Immunohaematology (SIMTI) Work Group. Recommendations for the transfusion of plasma and platelets. *Blood Transfus.* 2009;7(2):132-150.
4. Rhodes A, Evans LE, Alhazzani W, et al. Surviving sepsis campaign: international guidelines for management of sepsis and septic shock: 2016. *Intensive Care Med.* 2017;43:304.
5. Miller Y, Bachowski G, Benjamin R, et al. *Practice Guidelines for Blood Transfusion. A Compilation from Recent Peer-Reviewed Literature.* 2nd ed. American National Red Cross; 2007. Available at http://www.redcross.org/wwwfiles/Documents/Working-WiththeRedCross/practiceguidelinesforbloodtrans.pdf.

**6.** Correct Answer: B

**Rationale:**

TRICC trial found that patients had a lower in-hospital mortality when transfused for a restrictive threshold of Hgb <7 g/dL as opposed to a liberal threshold of Hgb <9 g/dL. The trial excluded actively bleeding patients, however, including those with gastrointestinal bleeding. A randomized controlled trial of patients with active upper GI bleeding demonstrated that a restrictive transfusion threshold (Hgb <7 g/dL) was likewise associated with decreased mortality compared to a liberal transfusion threshold (Hgb <9 g/dL). In addition, the study demonstrated a shorter length of stay, fewer adverse events, and fewer rebleeding events in the restrictive group.

Transfusion guidelines for platelets in the setting of active bleeding are typically for count <50 000/mm$^3$. Counts >75 000/mm$^3$ may be required for massive trauma and central nervous system (CNS) injury with the risk for bleeding, whereas surgery at high-risk sites such as ocular surgery and neurosurgery can require platelets >100 000/mm$^3$. This patient has active bleeding, but her platelets are already >50 000/mm$^3$. Hemodynamic stability, including MAP >65, is a more suitable criterion for transfusion in patients with severe, ongoing hemorrhage, as lab values will lag behind the rapidly evolving clinical picture.

References

1. Hébert PC, Wells G, Blajchman MA, et al; Transfusion Requirements in Critical Care Investigators, Canadian Critical Care Trials Group. A multicenter, randomized, controlled clinical trial of transfusion requirements in critical care. *N Engl J Med.* 1999;340:409-417.
2. Villanueva C, Colomo A, Bosch A, et al. Transfusion strategies for acute upper gastrointestinal bleeding [Erratum, *N Engl J Med.* 2013;368:2341]. *N Engl J Med.* 2013;368:11-21.
3. Liumbruno G, Bennardello F, Lattanzio A, Piccoli P, Rossetti G; Italian Society of Transfusion Medicine and Immunohaematology (SIMTI) Work Group. Recommendations for the transfusion of plasma and platelets. *Blood Transfus.* 2009;7(2):132-150.
4. Spinella PC, Holcomb JB. Resuscitation and transfusion principles for traumatic hemorrhagic shock. *Blood Rev.* 2009;23(6):231-240.

**7.** Correct Answer: A

**Rationale:**

In red blood cell transfusion reactions, recipient plasma antibodies react against antigens on donor cells. Conversely, the concern with transfusing plasma-containing products such as FFP and platelets is for antibodies in donor plasma to react against recipient red blood cell antigens. As a result, the recommendation is for FFP to be ABO compatible with the recipient, with AB being the universal plasma donor and O, the universal plasma recipient. FFP does not need to be RhD compatible, and anti-D prophylaxis is not needed in RhD– recipients of RhD+ FFP.

Platelet concentrates should likewise be as ABO compatible as possible to ensure an appropriate increase in platelet count, as ABO-incompatible platelets have reduced efficacy. Group O platelet concentrates can be used in patients of a different blood type if resuspended in additive/preservative solutions or if the plasma suspension is negative for high anti-A/B titers. In contrast to FFP, RhD– patients, particularly women of childbearing age, should receive only RhD– platelets if possible or should also be treated with anti-D immunoglobulin.

References

1. Liumbruno G, Bennardello F, Lattanzio A, Piccoli P, Rossetti G; Italian Society of Transfusion Medicine and Immunohaematology (SIMTI) Work Group. Recommendations for the transfusion of plasma and platelets. *Blood Transfus.* 2009;7(2):132-50.
2. O'Shaughnessy DF, Atterbury C, Bolton Maggs P, Murphy M, Thomas D, Yates S, Williamson LM; British Committee for Standards in Haematology; Blood Transfusion Task Force. Guidelines for the use of fresh-frozen plasma, cryoprecipitate and cryosupernatant. *Br J Haematol.* 2004;126(1):11-28.
3. Herman JH, King KE. Apheresis platelet transfusions: does ABO matter? *Transfusion.* 2004;44:802-804.

**8.** Correct Answer: C

**Rationale:**

Both adults and children diagnosed with Hodgkin lymphoma should receive irradiated red cells and platelets for life because of the risk for transfusion-associated graft-versus-host disease (TA-GvHD). Donor T lymphocytes in cellular blood products react against host antigens, manifesting as multiorgan system dysfunction. Unlike GvHD associated with hematopoietic cell transplant, TA-GvHD also impacts the bone marrow, and the resultant aplastic anemia is the most frequent cause of death. Other immunosuppressed populations that should receive irradiated cell-containing products include

1. Severe T-lymphocyte immunodeficiency syndromes
2. Recipients of allogeneic stem cell transplants during conditioning chemotherapy, throughout the 6 month posttransplant prophylaxis and as long as immunosuppression is required
3. Recipients of autologous stem cell transplant during conditioning chemotherapy and throughout 3 to 6 months of posttransplant prophylaxis
4. Patients undergoing bone marrow harvest during and 7 days before the procedure
5. Patients treated with purine analogue immunosuppressive agents
6. All intrauterine fetal transfusions

It is not typically necessary to use irradiated products for patients with human immunodeficiency virus (HIV), solid tumors, autoimmune disease, or after solid organ transplantation. Leukoreduction decreases the number of donor T lymphocytes but does not completely eliminate them. Leukoreduced products minimize the incidence of febrile nonhemolytic reactions and human leukocyte antigen (HLA) alloimmunization, in addition to decreasing transmission of Epstein-Barr virus (EBV) and cytomegalovirus (CMV). Patients with IgA deficiency often develop anti-IgA antibodies that can result in an anaphylactic transfusion reaction. Blood cells and platelets for these patients should be washed to decrease the amount of IgA present, and FFP should be from IgA-deficient donors.

References
1. Treleaven J, Gennery A, Marsh J, et al. Guidelines on the use of irradiated blood components prepared by the British Committee for Standards in Haematology blood transfusion task force. *Br J Haematol.* 2011;152:35-51.
2. Sharma RR, Marwaha N. Leukoreduced blood components: advantages and strategies for its implementation in developing countries. *Asian J Transfus Sci.* 2010;4(1):3-8.
3. Vassallo RR. Review: IgA anaphylactic transfusion reactions. Part I. Laboratory diagnosis, incidence, and supply of IgA-deficient products. *Immunohematology.* 2004;20(4):226-233.

**9.** Correct Answer: B

**Rationale:**

Poiseuille's law establishes the relationship between catheter size and length and the importance of each. $Q = (\pi P r^4)/(8 n L)$, where Q = flow, P = pressure, r = radius, n = viscosity, and l = length. It is important to note that increasing the radius dramatically increases flow, whereas increasing length decreases flow in much smaller proportion. Each manufacturer publishes the flow rate for their catheters. Reddick et al, however, studied catheters in real-life situations and found that Poiseuille's law still holds. Options C and D are incorrect since a central line is at least 18 cm long, which reduces flow. Though option A has a marginally shorter length, the larger radius on option B will have a greater impact on flow.

Reference
1. Reddick AD, Ronald J, Morrison WG. Intravenous fluid resuscitation: was Poiseuille right? *Emerg Med J.* 2011;28:201-202.

**10.** Correct Answer: D

**Rationale:**

In this patient with hemodynamically significant bleeding, tranexamic acid would be the best adjunct to achieve hemostasis. In the CRASH-2 trial, they found in patients with hemorrhage or at significant risk for hemorrhage that tranexamic acid when given within the first 8 hours reduced all-cause mortality. Prothrombin complex and vitamin K are inappropriate in a patient without a history of taking anticoagulants. Currently there is no evidence for transfusing cryoprecipitate in equal parts with PRBCs.

Reference
1. CRASH-2 Trial Collaborators. Effects of tranexamic acid on death, vascular occlusive events, and blood transfusion in trauma patients with significant haemorrhage (CRASH-2): a randomised, placebo-controlled trial. *Lancet.* 2010;376:23-32.

# 101

# ENVIRONMENTAL INJURY

Lydia R. Maurer and April E. Mendoza

1. A 65-year-old male is admitted to the hospital after he was found down in his kitchen during a house fire. On admission to the hospital, he was somnolent, had singed nasal hairs, and carbonaceous material in his mouth. He was hypoxic to the 80s and hoarse and was intubated for airway protection. His carboxyhemoglobin in the ED was 10%. He had no cutaneous burns identified. He was admitted to the ICU. On the ventilator, his settings are volume control, tidal volume 6 mL/kg, PEEP 10, RR 18, $FiO_2$ 70% with plateau pressure 25, and $O_2$ sat 99% with last ABG pH 7.4, $pCO_2$ 45, $pO_2$ 80. On bronchoscopy, he had moderate erythema and carbonaceous deposits. What is the **BEST** management of this patient's inhalation injury?

   **A.** Start broad-spectrum antibiotics
   **B.** Continue lung protective ventilation and wean $FiO_2$ as tolerated
   **C.** Extubate patient and transition to BiPAP
   **D.** Increase tidal volume to 10 mL/kg

2. A 19-year-old male is brought in by ambulance to the ED after a near-drowning episode in which he was caught in a rip tide. Rescuers extracted him from the water within 20 minutes. On the scene, he was coughing and mildly confused. On arrival to the ED he is found to be awake and alert, with initial oxygen saturation 85% on room air. Supplemental oxygen is administered via aerosol face mask at 10 L/min, and after 30 minutes, his oxygen saturation rises to 90%. He remains awake and is in no distress. What is the **BEST** next step in management?

   **A.** An oxygen saturation of 90% is sufficient. Trial him off face mask in preparation for discharge from the ED
   **B.** Use the Heimlich maneuver to extract additional fluid from his lungs
   **C.** Intubate the patient and perform bronchoscopy to clear the aspirated fluid
   **D.** Initiate noninvasive positive pressure ventilation such as BiPAP

3. A 34-year-old woman female fell off a dam into a lake while intoxicated. She was extracted approximately 10 minutes after the incident. She is unresponsive at the scene, and rescue breathing was initiated by onlookers. On EMS arrival, she has a pulse and is her respiratory rate is 10. Supplemental oxygen is administered and she is brought to the ED. On arrival, her GCS is 8, and her oxygen saturation is 85% on 15L non-rebreather. She is intubated. Which of the following is **TRUE** regarding freshwater versus saltwater drowning?

   **A.** Patients who suffer near-drowning in salt- versus freshwater should be managed similarly
   **B.** Saltwater ingestion results in a hyperosmolar load, and patients benefit from desmopressin administration
   **C.** Freshwater ingestion results in a hypoosmolar load, and these patients benefit from diuresis with furosemide
   **D.** Patients with saltwater ingestion are more prone to developing pneumonia

4. A 45-year-old male ascends to 16 000 feet on an ice climbing expedition. He initially develops some headaches, and then becomes increasingly confused. Two days into the trip, he becomes unable to walk straight and trips over his feet. His climbing partners become increasingly concerned and administer supplemental oxygen and dexamethasone they have with them. They assist him with descent to a safe location where he is transported by helicopter to the local emergency department, where he is found to be interactive with improved mental status and only mild ataxia. Which of the following is the **MOST** appropriate management for this patient?

   A. Lumbar puncture and administration of empiric antibiotics
   B. Treat with acetazolamide exclusively
   C. Supplemental oxygen administration and continuation of dexamethasone therapy
   D. Discharge patient with outpatient follow-up

5. A 28-year-old painter is working on an aluminum ladder when the ladder he is working on comes in contact with high-voltage power lines (~14 000 V). He has immediate pain to his bilateral hands, forearms, and feet but is able to lower himself to the ground. He presents to the ED, where he has a normal ECG, but continues to complain of arm and foot pain. He has superficial partial-thickness burns to his bilateral hands, but full sensation and range of motion. Volume resuscitation with 150 mL/h of LR (lactated Ringer's) is initiated. Three hours later, the patient is complaining of bilateral forearm swelling, hand numbness, and limited ability to move his fingers. Which of the following is the **BEST** next step in management of this patient?

   A. Elevate bilateral arms above the level of the heart
   B. Wrap bilateral arms to provide compression
   C. Take patient to OR for forearm fasciotomies and carpal tunnel release
   D. Perform CTA to examine upper extremity flow

6. A 42-year-old farmer is working in a field when the tractor he is operating is struck by lightning. He loses consciousness at the scene and is subsequently confused. He is brought in to the ED by his colleagues. On arrival, he is hemodynamically stable but remains confused. Which of the following is **TRUE** about this patient's lightning injury?

   A. This patient suffered a direct current electrical injury, which is associated with greater tissue damage than alternating current injuries
   B. This patient is at high risk of a permanent paralysis
   C. He should be evaluated by ophthalmology given the risk of developing cataracts with high-energy electrical and lightning injuries
   D. This patient suffered a "contact injury," which refers to when lightning strikes the ground and spreads through it to injure the victim

7. An 80-year-old female is found down at a bus stop. The outdoor temperature is 25°. She is unresponsive with shallow breathing and is intubated on the scene. She has palpable carotid pulses and is brought in by ambulance to the ED. Her core temperature is 78°F. Her initial blood pressure obtained is 90/45. Two large bore IVs are placed. Wet clothes are removed and active external rewarming is initiated. On recheck of her temperature 2 hours in, it is only 82. What is the **RECOMMENDED** technique for rewarming of this patient?

   A. Continue gradual, active external rewarming
   B. Initiate active internal rewarming with infusion of heated IV fluids and warmed, humidified oxygen
   C. Initiate intraperitoneal rewarming
   D. Cannulate patient for ECMO and initiate rewarming via V-V ECMO

8. A group of five people present to the emergency department after an unknown substance was released in the subway. They have headaches, blurry vision, rhinorrhea, and are mildly short of breath, and some are vomiting. It is believed that sarin gas was released. Which of the following is the BEST management of patients with the most severe symptoms from sarin gas?

   A. IV fluid resuscitation and close monitoring in the ICU
   B. Atropine administration
   C. Atropine and pralidoxime administration
   D. Hydroxocobalamin administration

**9.** A 45-year-old male is working at a nuclear facility when there is a radioactive leak. He goes to the ED where his clothing is removed and he is washed with soap and water. At the time, he was not manifesting any signs or symptoms of radiation exposure. He follows up with his PCP a month later, where he is found to be pancytopenic with white blood cell count 1.5 (absolute neutrophil count 1000), hemoglobin 6.0, and platelet count 50. He is transferred to the ED. Which of the following is **TRUE** about the management of this patient's radiation injury?

A. Start empiric antibiotics
B. Initiate transfusion with irradiated, leukoreduced blood and administer G-CSF
C. Perform hematopoietic stem cell transplant
D. Continue to trend labs monthly with no additional intervention

**10.** A 78-year-old female with a history of alcohol abuse is found down on a park bench in the middle of a summer day, in which the external temperature is 95° Fahrenheit. She is found to be able to answer yes or no questions and follow commands but is listless and lethargic. She is brought in by ambulance, and on arrival her temperature is 105, HR 130, BP 90/50, and her oxygen saturation is 98% on room air. Her GCS is 13, and she smells of alcohol. What is the **BEST** next step in the management of this patient?

A. Administer dantrolene
B. Initiate peritoneal lavage with cold water
C. Initiate treatment with acetaminophen around the clock
D. Use evaporative and convective cooling techniques including lukewarm mist and ice packs to axilla, groin, and neck

# Chapter 101 ▪ Answers

**1.** Correct Answer: B

**Rationale:**
The bronchoscopy findings and clinical history suggest this patient has a moderate (Grade 2) inhalation injury. Some centers will obtain a CT chest for additional information about the extent of inhalation injury, in which increased interstitial markings and ground glass opacities correlate with a more severe injury. Early intubation has long been one of the tenets of managing inhalation injury, because of the risk of progressive upper airway edema and airway compromise in these patients. For patients on the ventilator, lung protective ventilation is generally recommended, with tidal volume goal less than 7 mL/kg, maintaining plateau pressures less than 30 with the minimum $FiO_2$ necessary to effectively oxygenate. Providers often follow $PO_2/FiO_2$ ratios to follow the progression of inhalation injury with these different methods. When a sufficient $PO_2/FiO_2$ ratio cannot be maintained with the above guidelines, patients may need increased sedation, paralysis, less conventional ventilator settings, or even in severe cases ECMO to effectively oxygenate and ventilate, minimizing barotrauma.

Although inhalation injury does place this patient at higher risk of developing pneumonia, there is no indication that this patient has an active infection currently, so (A), broad-spectrum antibiotics are not indicated. (C) It would be inappropriate to extubate the patient in this situation, given that he is still on an assist-control setting on the ventilator with an $FiO_2$ 70%, and therefore requires considerable weaning on the ventilator before he will be ready for extubation. As described above, tidal volumes between 6 and 8 mL/kg are advised in accordance with lung protective guidelines, and (D) there is no indication to increase the tidal volume to 10 mL/kg.

Reference
1. Walker PF, Buehner MF, Wood LA, et al. Diagnosis and management of inhalation injury: an updated review. *Crit Care.* 2015;19:351.

**2.** Correct Answer: D

**Rationale:**
In a near-drowning situation, symptomatic patients can be hypoxic on arrival to the ED. In this case, supplemental oxygen should be administered in order to maintain the patient's oxygen saturation greater than 94%, or greater than a $PaO_2$ of 60. When initial supplemental oxygen is not sufficient, as long as the patient can maintain their airway and does not have another contraindication to noninvasive positive pressure ventilation, CPAP, BiPAP, or high-flow nasal cannula can be attempted prior to deciding to intubate the patient.

(A) An oxygen saturation of 90% is not sufficient. It is recommended to target an oxygen saturation of >94%, and it would not be appropriate to deescalate supplemental oxygen at this time. Although in the past, performing (B) the

Heimlich maneuver was recommended in the prehospital setting to evacuate water from a patient's lungs, it is no longer recommended, as it delays the assisted ventilation (rescue breaths) that should be initiated as soon as possible. It has no role in the hospital setting. (C) Intubation should be considered in near-drowning patients with depressed neurologic status and concern for ability to maintain an airway, and in patients who are persistently hypoxic with $SpO_2$ <90% or $PaO_2$<60.

### References

1. Schmidt AC, Sempsrott JR, Hawkins SC. Wilderness medical society practice guidelines for the prevention and treatment of drowning. *Wilderness Environ Med*. 2016;2:236-251.
2. Orlowski JP, Szpilman D. Drowning: rescue, resuscitation, and reanimation. *Pediatr Clin North Am*. 2001;3:627-646.

**3.** Correct Answer: A

**Rationale:**

Near-drowning in saltwater versus freshwater was previously thought to cause different effects on the lung parenchyma, but it has now been demonstrated that (A) there is unlikely to be a significant difference between salt- and freshwater ingestion, and therefore the two groups should be managed similarly. It was previously thought that ingesting saltwater resulted in a hyperosmolar load to the lung parenchyma, not only increasing the amount of pulmonary edema but also contributing increased osmolarity to the plasma. It has since been demonstrated that the amount of water usually ingested during a near-drowning incident is not generally enough to confer this type of effect, whether that water is hyperosmolar or hypoosmolar (in the case of freshwater ingestion). Therefore, neither (B) desmopressin administration nor (C) furosemide administration is indicated in the acute setting. Although there are different organisms that tend to reside in salt- versus freshwater, (D) ingestion of one or the other is not particularly associated with increased risk of pneumonia.

### Reference

1. Orlowski JP, Szpilman D. Drowning: rescue, resuscitation, and reanimation. *Pediatr Clin North Am*. 2001;3:627-646.

**4.** Correct Answer: C

**Rationale:**

This patient is presenting with high-altitude cerebral edema (HACE), as defined by altered mental status in the setting of high altitude exposure. HACE is on the spectrum with acute mountain sickness, which can start with headaches and light-headedness, ataxia, and severe confusion are an indication that the patient has progressed to HACE. Initial management involves descending to a lower-altitude location, supplemental oxygen, and if available dexamethasone administration as well. If symptoms are severe and the ability to descend is limited, portable hyperbaric chambers can be helpful if they are available. This patient, while improving, would not be appropriate for (D) discharge with outpatient follow-up. Instead, because this patient is still ataxic and confused, (C) supplemental oxygen should be administered along with continuation of dexamethasone therapy. (B) Acetazolamide is generally used as prophylaxis to help with acclimatization to high altitude, as opposed to treatment for acute mountain sickness or HACE. Finally, there is no indication this patient has a CNS infection, so (A) lumbar puncture and administration of empiric antibiotics would not be indicated.

### Reference

1. Luks AM, McIntosh SE, Grissom CK, et al. Wilderness medical society practice guidelines for the prevention and treatment of acute altitude illness: 2014 update. *Wilderness Environ Med*. 2014;4:S4-S14.

**5.** Correct Answer: C

**Rationale:**

This patient has sustained a high-voltage electrical injury, as defined by voltage greater than 1000 V. These patients are at high risk of extensive tissue damage, often which is not immediately visible. They will often present with relatively small cutaneous burns like this patient, but extension through the tissue can result in tissue breakdown beyond the site of injury. Volume resuscitation is indicated in these patients, and it is imperative to pay close attention to affected extremities given the risk of compartment syndrome. This patient has loss of sensation and motor capacity in the hands, indicating a compartment syndrome of the forearms, and likely the carpal tunnel, and therefore (C) should go to the OR for forearm fasciotomies and carpal tunnel release. In a patient with this degree of neurovascular compromise, the answer is compartment release, and there is never an indication for purely (A) elevation or (B) wrapping the bilateral arms. We have enough clinical suspicion for compartment syndrome that there is no role for further workup including (D) CTA.

### References

1. Mann R, Gibran N, Engrav L, et al. Is immediate decompression of high voltage electrical injuries to the upper extremities always necessary? *J Trauma*. 1996;4:584-587.
2. Brandao C, Vaz M, Brito IM, et al. Electrical burns: a retrospective analysis over a 10-year period. *Ann Burns Fire Disasters*. 2017;4:268-271.

**6.** Correct Answer: C

**Rationale:**

Lightning injuries are high-energy direct current injuries. These high-energy injuries confer considerable morbidity and mortality, ranging from cutaneous burns, neurologic injury, cardiopulmonary insult, blast effect (trauma), and others. Patients who sustain high-energy electrical and lightning injuries are (C) at higher risk of developing cataracts and should be evaluated by ophthalmology on presentation. Choice (A) is incorrect because high-voltage alternating current injuries, such as those in most industrial or household settings, are more likely to cause extensive tissue damage and cutaneous burns than direct current injuries. Lightning strike injuries can have considerable neurologic effects. Choice (B) is incorrect because paralysis that occurs from a lightning strike injury most commonly affects the lower extremities and is transient, lasting a few hours, after which sensory and motor function returns to normal. A "contact injury" (D) refers to when a patient is in contact with a structure or object that has been struck by lightning. A "ground current" refers to when lightning strikes the ground near a victim and transfers current to the patient.

Reference

1. Ritenour AE, Morton MJ, McManus JG, et al. Lightning injury: a review. *Burns*. 2007;5:585-594.

**7.** Correct Answer: B

**Rationale:**

This patient has severe hypothermia, as defined by a core temperature of less than 82° Fahrenheit. These patients are often unconscious. The complications of severe hypothermia can include coma, hypotension, bradycardia and other arrhythmias, and pulmonary edema. For patients who are severely hypothermic, active rewarming should be initiated in a stepwise fashion after all wet clothes have been removed and active external rewarming is initiated. First, warmed IV crystalloid can be delivered along with warmed, humidified oxygen. If additional measures are needed, (C) irrigation with warmed fluids to the peritoneum or thorax can be considered, although this comes with possible complications. If these measures all fail, (D) ECMO can be considered in extreme cases but is not the first step of rewarming.

References

1. Dalton HR. The management of accidental hypothermia. *BMJ*. 2009;338:b2085.
2. Brown DJ, Brugger H, Boyd J, Paal P. Accidental Hypothermia. *N Engl J Med*. 2012;367:1930-1938

**8.** Correct Answer: C

**Rationale:**

The mechanism of action of sarin gas is as an acetylcholinesterase inhibitor, in which acetylcholine accumulates in the neuromuscular junction, resulting in a cholinergic syndrome, with miosis, rhinorrhea, wheezing, vomiting, and diarrhea. Treatment is indicated, and (A) IV fluid resuscitation and close monitoring in the ICU alone would not be appropriate. The severity of the symptoms can vary. For patients with mild effects, including miosis alone or miosis and severe rhinorrhea without other effects, (B) the anticholinergic agent atropine should be administered, but this is not sufficient for patients with moderate effects from sarin gas. For patients with moderate effects, including respiratory distress, nausea, vomiting, weakness, or fasciculations, (C) both atropine and pralidoxime should be administered. (D) Hydroxocobalamin should be administered to patients with cyanide poisoning but is not indicated in sarin gas poisoning.

References

1. Madsen JM. *Chemical Terrorism: Rapid Recognition and Initial Medical Management*. 2018. https://www.uptodate.com/contents/chemical-terrorism-rapid-recognition-and-initial-medical-management.
2. Lee EC. Clinical manifestations of sarin nerve gas exposure. *JAMA*. 2003;5:659-662.

**9.** Correct Answer: B

**Rationale:**

Patients who sustain radiation injury do not always immediately manifest symptoms. After decontamination, patients may not begin to show effects for 1 to 2 weeks. Cytopenias are a common manifestation and should be managed with supportive care, including (B) blood product transfusion with irradiated, leukoreduced products and G-CSF in the case of leukopenia. Transfusion thresholds are similar to those used in oncology patients, with goal hemoglobin of at least 7 to 8 in asymptomatic patients. (A) Empiric antibiotics are not recommended unless the patient is significantly neutropenic (ANC<500). Although these patients are at increased risk of infection, antibiotics should only be started when there is clinical evidence of infection. (C) Stem cell transplant can be indicated as a treatment for profound cytopenias, but initial management is supportive and stem cell transplant is not the first step. Finally (D) trending labs with no intervention would not be appropriate, and supportive care should be initiated.

Reference

1. Waselenko JK, MacVittie TJ, Blakely WF, et al. Medical management of the acute radiation syndrome: recommendations of the Strategic National Stockpile Radiation Working Group. *Ann Intern Med*. 2004;12:1037-1051.

**10.** Correct Answer: D

**Rationale:**

This patient is presenting with severe hyperthermia (or heatstroke). The elderly are at an increased risk for developing heatstroke, as are patients who have ingested alcohol and other drugs. This tends to occur particularly when the external temperature is elevated, and in patients who have increased susceptibility due to being elderly or having other medical conditions that make them increasingly susceptible. Diagnosis is based on elevated core temperature (generally greater than 104°F), in addition to altered mental status, in the setting of extreme heat exposure. Initial management for severely ill patients can even involve intubation, volume resuscitation, and vasopressors if needed. The patient described above does not need to be intubated, but rapid cooling should be initiated. Cooling should involve (D) evaporative and convective cooling techniques, which can include spraying the patient with a mist of lukewarm water, and in the setting of this benzodiazepines can be used to control shivering as needed. In addition, ice packs should be applied to the axilla, groin, and neck to cool the core areas at the location of major blood vessels. (A) Dantrolene has not been shown to be of benefit in the case of nonmalignant hyperthermia. (B) Although peritoneal lavage is an option for cooling, it is preferable to start with less invasive options, and only escalate if absolutely necessary. (C) Treatment with acetaminophen around the clock has not been shown to be beneficial in the management of heatstroke.

References

1. Bouchama A, Cafege A, Devol EB, et al. Ineffectiveness of dantrolene sodium in the treatment of heatstroke. *Crit Care Med.* 1991;19:176.
2. Bouchama A, Knochel JP. Heat stroke. *N Engl J Med.* 2002;346:1978-1988.

# 102

# BURNS

John Andre, Kevin E. Galicia, and Yuk Ming Liu

1. An 18-year-old female suffers a 4% superficial partial-thickness burn to her right arm. At an outpatient burn clinic, she is treated with silver sulfadiazine and sent home. She presents to the emergency department 2 days later with increasing tenderness and erythema at the burn site. On examination, the wound appears dark brown and blood is present underneath the eschar. Viable tissue surrounding the eschar is biopsied, revealing >105 viable microorganisms per gram. What is the most appropriate treatment for this patient?

   A. IV antibiotics only
   B. IV antibiotics and silver sulfadiazine
   C. Surgical excision of infected tissues
   D. Application of sodium hypochlorite 0.025%

2. A 9-year-old male sustains 45% mixed superficial and deep partial-thickness burns after falling into a campfire. During a prolonged ICU stay, he is persistently hyperglycemic, requiring regular insulin administration. Which of the following correctly identifies two physiologic changes that are associated with the use of insulin within the burn population?

   A. Improves muscle protein synthesis and exerts proinflammatory effects
   B. Attenuates lean body mass and exerts anti-inflammatory effects
   C. Reduced infection rates and exerts proinflammatory effects
   D. Increases donor-site healing time and exerts anti-inflammatory effects

3. A 53-year-old female presents after being found unconscious in her house during a fire. Upon physical examination, you note that the patient has singed nasal hairs, carbonaceous sputum, and burns to her chin/forehead and is stridorous. You place her on 100% oxygen via a nonrebreather; however, her $SpO_2$ remains in the low 80s, and she is tachypneic to 35. You are concerned for an inhalation injury. What is the MOST sensitive test for diagnosing an inhalation injury?

   A. Physical examination and high clinical suspicion
   B. Chest radiograph
   C. Ventilation and perfusion scan
   D. Bronchoscopy

4. An 8-year-old male presented to your burn unit after sustaining 25% TBSA (total body surface area) superficial and deep partial-thickness scald burns to his torso and legs after a pot of boiling water fell onto him. After you complete your primary survey of the patient and adequate fluid resuscitation has begun, you evaluate the wound and note that the genitalia has been spared. You decide on silver nitrate soaks for your dressing as it is painless and readily available at your institution. What side effect must you be worried about with this dressing?

   A. Methemoglobinemia
   B. Hyponatremia
   C. Metabolic acidosis
   D. Neutropenia

5. A 47-year-old, 70 kg male presents as a transfer to the burn unit after sustaining a roughly 10% superficial burn, 30% superficial partial- and deep-thickness burn, and a 20% full-thickness burn after being in a warehouse fire. There is no concern for inhalation injury. With the help of EMS and records from the outside hospital, you estimate that the time of injury was at 2 hours prior to arrival at your institution. En route to the outside hospital the patient receives 500 mL of lactated Ringer's solution. At the outside facility and en route to your burn unit the patient receives an additional 1 L of lactated Ringer's solution. What would the additional 24-hour resuscitation requirements entail using the Parkland formula?

   A. 688 mL/h for an additional 6 hours, then 263 mL/h for remaining 16 hours
   B. 875 mL/h for an additional 8 hours, then 438 mL/h for remaining 16 hours
   C. 917 mL/h for an additional 6 hours, then 438 mL/h for remaining 16 hours
   D. 583 mL/h for an additional 8 hours, then 583 mL/h for remaining 16 hours

6. Your previously described 47-year-old burn patient is in the midst of being appropriately resuscitated based on your Parkland formula. The patient's hourly urine output is measured to be about 1 mL/kg. During the last couple of hours of your initial 24-hour postinjury resuscitation, you note that the patient's urine output starts to decrease. In addition, you note that the patient is having difficulty breathing with frequent episodes of desaturation despite being on a nonrebreather. Your physical examination reveals a distended abdomen with increased abdominal girth. The patient is intubated, and you note elevated peak airway pressures at 45 mm Hg. You ask the nurse to perform a bladder pressure, which is noted to be 25 mm Hg. What is your diagnosis, and what is the appropriate treatment?

   A. Intra-abdominal hypertension, continue to monitor for signs of end-organ dysfunction
   B. Intra-abdominal hypertension, decrease fluid resuscitation
   C. Abdominal compartment syndrome, escharotomies
   D. Abdominal compartment syndrome, decompressive laparotomy

7. A 24-year-old male is admitted to the ICU after suffering 54% deep partial- and full-thickness burns to his face, torso, and arms after being involved in a house fire. At 72 hours post burn, his heart rate and cardiac output remain significantly elevated. Which of the following would best treat this patient's tachycardia and prevent subsequent cardiac stress and myocardial dysfunction?

   A. Propranolol
   B. Verapamil
   C. Crystalloid resuscitation
   D. Disopyramide

8. A 66-year-old male sustains a 25% second-degree scald burn when a large pot of boiling water is spilled onto his torso and lower extremities. He is immediately transferred to a burn center. During his course of treatment, he is started on 5 mg oxandrolone PO BID. Which of the following physiologic changes has been associated with the administration of this drug?

   A. Improved muscle protein catabolism
   B. Reduced weight loss
   C. Increased donor-site wound healing
   D. All of the above

# Chapter 102 ▪ Answers

1. Correct Answer: C

   **Rationale:**
   Aggressive surgical debridement and excision of infected tissues has substantially decreased the incidence of invasive burn wound infection and secondary sepsis. Burn wound infections are most often recognized based on the gross appearance of the burn and/or skin graft donor site and the rapid systemic changes (like signs of sepsis or new-onset enteral feeding intolerance). The presence of localized pain, erythema, color change, and premature separation of the burn eschar are all highly indicative of a burn wound infection.

The spectrum of microorganisms causing infections in burn patients varies with time and location. Immediately after thermal injury, primarily gram-positive bacteria from the patient's endogenous flora or the external environment start to colonize the burn wound. The predominant gram-positive organisms found in burn wound infections remain *Staphylococcus aureus*, followed by *Enterococcus* species. Endogenous gram-negative bacteria from the gastrointestinal flora also rapidly colonize the burn wound surface in the first few days after injury. Given their wide range of virulence factors and antimicrobial resistance traits, gram-negative bacteria have emerged as the most common etiologic agents of invasive infection. *Pseudomonas aeruginosa* remains the most frequent gram-negative microorganism isolated from burn wounds, followed by *E. coli*. Fungi (eg, *Candida*, *Aspergillus*, *Fusarium*, *Mucor* species) and multiresistant organisms (eg, methicillin-resistant *Staphylococcus aureus* [MRSA], vancomycin-resistant *Enterococcus* [VRE], *Acinetobacter*) appear late and typically occur after use of broad-spectrum antibiotics and/or a prolonged hospital stay. *Candida* sp. is the most common fungus isolated from burn wounds, and HSV-1 remains the most common viral organism.

## References

1. Church D, Elsayed S, Reid O, Winston B, Lindsay R. Burn wound infections. *Clin Microbiol Rev*. 2006;19(2):403-434.
2. Greenhalgh DG, Saffle JR, Holmes JHIV, et al. American Burn Association consensus conference to define sepsis and infection in burns. *J Burn Care Res*. 2007;28:776.
3. Pruitt BA, McManus AT, Kim SH, Goodwin CW. Burn wound infections: current status. *World J Surg*. 1998;22(2):135-145.

## 2.  Correct Answer: B

**Rationale:**

In severely burned patients, insulin administered during acute hospitalization improves muscle protein synthesis, accelerates donor-site healing time, attenuates lean body mass loss and the acute phase response, and reduces infection and mortality rates. In addition to its anabolic actions, insulin exerts anti-inflammatory effects, potentially neutralizing the proinflammatory actions of glucose.

## References

1. Williams FN, Jeschke MG, Chinkes DL, et al. Modulation of the hypermetabolic response to trauma: temperature, nutrition, and drugs. *J Am Coll Surg*. 2009;208:489-502.
2. Sabiston DC, Townsend CM, eds. *Sabiston Textbook of Surgery: The Biological Basis of Modern Surgical Practice*. Philadelphia, PA: Elsevier Saunders; 2012.
3. Dellinger RP, Levy MM, Carlet JM, et al. Surviving sepsis campaign: International guidelines for management of severe sepsis and septic shock: 2008. *Crit Care Med*. 2008;36:296-327.
4. Jeschke MG, Abdullahi A, Burnett M, et al. Glucose control in severely burned patients using metformin: an interim safety and efficacy analysis of a phase II randomized controlled trial. *Ann Surg*. 2016;264:518.

## 3.  Correct Answer: D

**Rationale:**

There are many reasons for intubating a burn patient, which includes concern for possible inhalation injury. Inhalation injury includes both direct, thermal injury to the airway as well as inflammation-induced injury to the parenchyma. Despite an overall decrease in burn mortality over the past couple of decades, inhalational injury remains one of the most critical injuries in this population with a mortality rate between 25% and 50%. The tenet of inhalation injury management is early diagnosis, which is critical to the survival of burn patients. Although singed nasal hairs, carbonaceous sputum, facial burns, and a history of closed space exposure can be found in patients with inhalation injury, they cannot be used alone to discriminate between patients with and those without inhalation injury. However, seeing these signs in addition to being found unconscious at the scene, stridor, and an overall high clinical suspicion should prompt the diagnosis of potential inhalation injury. The current accepted standard for diagnosis of inhalation injury is bronchoscopy. Endor and Gamelli created a grading system of inhalation injury based on bronchoscopic findings. These authors also demonstrated that survival was worse in those patients with higher grades of injury based on the bronchoscopic criteria in the figure that follows.

| Grade 0 | Absence of carbonaceous deposits, erythema, edema, bronchorrhea, or obstruction |
|---------|------------------------------------------------------------------------------------|
| Grade 1 | Minor or patchy areas of erythema, carbonaceous deposits in proximal or distal bronchi (any or combination) |
| Grade 2 | Moderate degree of erythema, carbonaceous deposits, bronchorrhea with or without compromise of the bronchi (any or combination) |
| Grade 3 | Severe inflammation with friability, copious carbonaceous deposits, bronchorrhea, bronchial obstruction (any or combination) |
| Grade 4 | Evidence of mucosal sloughing, necrosis, endoluminal obliteration (any or combination) |

Grading of inhalation injury.

### References

1. Flint L, ed. Wound healing and burn injuries. *Selected Readings in General Surgery*. 2017;43(8):1-58.
2. Sabiston DC, Townsend CM, eds. *Sabiston Textbook of Surgery: The Biological Basis of Modern Surgical Practice*. Philadelphia, PA: Elsevier Saunders; 2012.
3. Ching JA, Shah JL, Doran CJ, Chen H, Payne WG, Smith DJJr. The evaluation of physical exam findings in patients assessed for suspected burn inhalation injury. *J Burn Care Res*. 2015;36(1):197-202.
4. Endorf FW, Gamelli RL. Inhalation injury, pulmonary perturbations, and fluid resuscitation. *J Burn Care Res*. 2007;28:80-83.

### 4. Correct Answer: B

**Rationale:**

Burn wounds are complicated, and their appropriate management is essential to the survival of the patient. If left untreated, the burn wound quickly becomes colonized by bacteria and fungi, which subsequently invade into the surrounding viable tissue and blood vessels, causing a systemic infection that will lead to death. Therefore, early treatment of these wounds is imperative to the health and survival of burn patients. The type of antimicrobial dressing is based on the characteristics of the wound.

Superficial (first-degree) burns result in minimal loss of the skin barrier; therefore, these wounds are usually treated with topical salves to help with pain and moisture control. Superficial partial-thickness (superficial second-degree) burns result in a higher loss of skin barrier than superficial burns. Despite this, the majority are able to be treated with dressing changes and do not require surgical excision. These wounds are treated with topical antibiotics and at least daily dressing changes. Sometimes, superficial partial-thickness burns can be treated with temporary biologic or synthetic dressings to help with burn wound healing. In cases of deep partial-thickness (deep second-degree) and full-thickness (third-degree) burns, surgical excision and grafting should be performed depending on the size and location of the wound. For these patients, the dressing regimen of choice should be based on helping to prevent infection until the burn can be excised.

Topical dressings can be divided into two broad groups: salves and soaks. Salves include 1% silver sulfadiazine (Silvadene), 11% mafenide acetate (Sulfamylon), polymyxin B, neomycin, bacitracin, mupirocin, and nystatin. Silvadene and bacitracin are the most commonly used given their broad antimicrobial coverage, as well as their easy applicability and high patient tolerance. The side effects of Silvadene include neutropenia and thrombocytopenia. Sulfamylon is also frequently used, as it is penetrates eschar (Silvadene does not), and is especially useful against *Pseudomonas* and *Enterococcus* species. Sulfamylon cream is primarily used in cartilaginous areas (such as the nose, ears), as well as areas where the tendons are exposed. A potential disadvantage of Sulfamylon is that sometimes patients complain of pain with application. Soaks include 0.5% silver nitrate solution, 5% mafenide acetate solution (Sulfamylon), and rarely 0.025% sodium hypochlorite solution (Dakin's). Silver nitrate has complete antimicrobial effectiveness and is painless; however, this solution can cause staining of tissue. A potential complication of this product includes electrolyte leaching (as the solution is hypotonic). Methemoglobinemia is a very rare complication of silver nitrate. Sulfamylon is a carbonic anhydrase inhibitor; therefore, it can lead to metabolic acidosis.

### References

1. Flint L, ed. Wound healing and burn injuries. *Selected Readings in General Surgery*. 2017;43(8):1-58.
2. Sabiston DC, Townsend CM, eds. *Sabiston Textbook of Surgery: The Biological Basis of Modern Surgical Practice*. Philadelphia, PA: Elsevier Saunders; 2012.
3. Sheridan RL, Chang P. Acute burn procedures. *Surg Clin North Am*. 2014;94(4):755-764.
4. Fiser SM. The ABSITE Review; 2017.

### 5. Correct Answer: C

**Rationale:**

While institutions may have various different protocols for resuscitation (crystalloid, albumin) with differing end points (mean arterial pressure, urine output), fluid resuscitation remains the essential pillar of burn care. Children with >10% TBSA and adults with >15% TBSA require intravenous fluid resuscitation. The initial fluid used should be isotonic crystalloid, more specifically lactated Ringer's. The use of albumin during fluid resuscitation has been debated.

The Parkland formula has become one of the most commonly used tools for guiding fluid resuscitation in a burn patient. In adult patients who have greater than 15% to 20% TBSA burns, initial 24-hour total fluid requirement is 4 mL/kg/%TBSA burned. Half of the total volume should be given within the first 8 hours post injury, with the remaining half given over the subsequent 16 hours (completing a 24-hour postinjury fluid resuscitation). It must be noted that superficial burns (previously known as first-degree burns) should not be used in the calculation of necessary fluid resuscitation when using these formulas. For children with greater than 10% TBSA burns, initial 24-hour total fluid requirement is 3 mL/kg/%TBSA burned. In addition, children usually require an additional maintenance rate based on their weight.

The American Burn Association recommends fluid resuscitation to begin at 2 to 4 mL/kg per TBSA burn percentage. A study performed by Chung et al. that was published in the *Journal of Trauma and Acute Care Surgery* in 2009 compared resuscitation of severely burned military casualties based on the modified Brooke formula (2 mL/kg) with the Parkland formula (4 mL/kg). Although the objective of the study was to evaluate the relationship between estimated volumes calculated and actual volumes received, the study found that patients who received resuscitation based on the modified Brooke formula received significantly less 24-hour fluid with similar morbidity and mortality. They suggested that patients who receive resuscitation based on the Parkland formula are at risk of excessive fluid and the implications that come with fluid overload.

With regard to the calculation for this question, the Parkland formula of 4 mL/kg per TBSA burn percentage is used. As mentioned previously, only partial- and full-thickness burns are included in the calculation of fluid resuscitation (30% for superficial partial- and deep-thickness burn, 20% for full-thickness burn, equaling 50% total in this patient's case). The patient's total fluid requirement for the first 24 hours post injury would be (4 mL) (70 kg) (50%) = 14,000 L. The patient must receive half of the resuscitation (7000 L) in the first 8 hours post injury. By the time the patient has presented to you, he is already 2 hours post injury. Therefore, he must receive the remainder of his resuscitation for this time period in 6 hours. In addition, he has already received a total of 1500 mL prior to his presentation to your hospital. For the remaining 6 hours post injury, he requires a rate of roughly 917 mL/h (7000 L − 1500 L = 5500 L); (5500 L/6 h = 917 mL/h). The remaining half of his total 24-hour postinjury resuscitation (7000 L) is given over the following 16 hours (7000 L/16 h = 438 mL/h).

### References

1. Flint L, ed. Wound healing and burn injuries. *Selected Readings in General Surgery.* 2017;43(8):1-58.
2. Haberal M, Sakallioglu Abali AE, Karakayali H. Fluid management in major burn injuries. *Indian J Plast Surg.* 2010;43(suppl):S29-S36.
3. Baxter CR, Marvin JA, Curreri PW. Early management of thermal burns. *Postgrad Med.* 1974;55(1):131-139.
4. Chung KK, Wolf SE, Cancio LC, et al. Resuscitation of severely burned military casualties: fluid begets more fluid. *J Trauma.* 2009;67(2):231-237.
5. Sabiston DC, Townsend CM, eds. *Sabiston Textbook of Surgery: The Biological Basis of Modern Surgical Practice.* Philadelphia, PA: Elsevier Saunders; 2012.

**6.** Correct Answer: D

**Rationale:**

A clinician who is guiding the management of a burn patient must be privy to the complications of aggressive fluid resuscitation. Peripheral edema, pulmonary edema/effusions, and abdominal hypertension with subsequent abdominal compartment syndrome are a few of the problems that may arise despite what would be considered adequate fluid resuscitation.

Burn patients, in addition to any other patient requiring aggressive fluid resuscitation, are susceptible to secondary abdominal compartment syndrome (ACS). Patients who present with ACS will have preceding intra-abdominal hypertension (IAH), which is defined as an intra-abdominal pressure (IAP) greater than 12 mm Hg that is measured at least three times, 4 to 6 hours apart. When the IAP is greater than or equal to 20 mm Hg and there is at least failure of one organ system not previously failing, the diagnosis of ACS is confirmed.

The treatment of abdominal compartment syndrome is a formal laparotomy. The treatment of secondary ACS in a burn patient is not escharotomy, as the issue is from intra-abdominal fluid causing increased intra-abdominal pressure.

### References

1. Flint L, ed. Wound healing and burn injuries. *Selected Readings in General Surgery.* 2017;43(8):1-58.
2. Sabiston DC, Townsend CM, eds. *Sabiston Textbook of Surgery: The Biological Basis of Modern Surgical Practice.* Philadelphia, PA: Elsevier Saunders; 2012.

**7.** Correct Answer: A

**Rationale:**

The patient in this question has a large body-surface-area burn and is exhibiting signs of sustained sympathetic surge. Such patients develop marked tachycardia, 150% higher than predicted, and may remain elevated for up to 2 years after the burn. Likewise, cardiac output has been shown to be 150% higher than predicted for healthy adults and remains high at time of discharge. Increased cardiac stress and myocardial dysfunction may be main contributors to mortality in large burns, implying the therapeutic need to improve cardiac stress and function.

To reduce the risk of cardiac failure, judicious fluid resuscitation should be performed upon a patient's arrival to the hospital. For the cardiac dysfunction or hyperdynamic state that occurs in almost all patients with burns >40% TBSA, nonselective ß-blockade is recommended. Propranolol, a nonselective ß-receptor antagonist, used at a dose titrated to reduce the heart rate by 15% to 20%, has been found to diminish cardiac work in the burn population.

### References

1. Sabiston DC, Townsend CM, eds. *Sabiston Textbook of Surgery: The Biological Basis of Modern Surgical Practice.* Philadelphia, PA: Elsevier Saunders; 2012.
2. Greenhalgh DG, Saffle JR, Holmes JHIV, et al. American Burn Association consensus conference to define sepsis and infection in burns. *J Burn Care Res.* 2007;28:776.
3. Chung KK, Wolf SE. Critical care in the severely burned: organ support and management of complications. In: Herndon DN, ed. *Total Burn Care.* 4th ed. Saunders Elsevier; 2012.

4. Clark A, Imran J, Madni T, Wolf SE. Nutrition and metabolism in burn patients. *Burns Trauma*. 2017;5:11.

5. Moiemen N, Joory K, Moiemen NS. History of burns: the past, present and the future. *Burns Trauma*. 2014;2(4):169.

6. Williams FN, Herndon DN, Kulp GA, Jeschke MG. Propranolol decreases cardiac work in a dose-dependent manner in severely burned children. *Surgery*. 2011;149:231.

7. Jeschke MG, Celeste F. The hepatic response to thermal injury. In: Herndon DN, ed. *Total Burn Care*; 2012.

**8.** Correct Answer: D

**Rationale:**

The hypermetabolic response to burn injury is associated with increased substrate turnover, cachexia, and poor clinical outcomes. Therefore, management of hypermetabolism remains a clinical priority. Treatment with oxandrolone, a testosterone analogue with a low level of virilizing androgenic effect, improves muscle protein catabolism, reduces weight loss, and increases donor-site wound healing. For adults with moderate to severe burns, 10 mg PO BID is recommended. In older patients >65 years of age, the recommended dose is 5 mg PO BID.

Oxandrolone, a synthetic analogue, administered orally, offers only 5% of the masculinizing effects of testosterone and is safe for both genders. Oxandrolone, when administered at a dose of 0.1 mg/kg twice daily, improved net muscle protein synthesis and protein metabolism in severely burned patients.

During the acute phase post burn and up to 1 year of treatment, oxandrolone increased lean body mass, bone mineral content, and muscle strength. In addition, it decreased length of stay by decreasing time between operations for patients randomized to receive oxandrolone plus standard of care. Oxandrolone results in considerable improvements in lean body mass, protein synthesis, and overall growth in burn patients, mitigating the 1% risk of hirsutism and hepatic dysfunction that can be seen with treatment.

It must be noted that although anabolic steroids can increase lean body mass, exercise is essential to developing strength.

### References

1. Porter C, Tompkins RG, Finnerty CC, Sidossis LS, Suman OE, Herndon DN. The metabolic stress response to burn trauma: current understanding and therapies. *Lancet*. 2016;388(10052):1417-1426.

2. Sabiston DC, Townsend CM, eds. *Sabiston Textbook of Surgery: The Biological Basis of Modern Surgical Practice*. Philadelphia, PA: Elsevier Saunders; 2012.

3. Lam NN, Tien NG, Khoa CM. Early enteral feeding for burned patients – an effective method which should be encouraged in developing countries. *Burns*. 2008;34:192.

4. Branski LK, Herndon DN, Barrow RE, et al. Randomized controlled trial to determine the efficacy of long-term growth hormone treatment in severely burned children. *Ann Surg*. 2009;127:145-154.

5. Williams FN, Jeschke MG, Chinkes DL, et al. Modulation of the hypermetabolic response to trauma: temperature, nutrition, and drugs. *J Am Coll Surg*. 2009;208:489-502.

6. Langouche L, Van den Berghe G. Glucose metabolism and insulin therapy. *Crit Care Clin*. 2006;22:119-129.

# 103

# DISASTER MANAGEMENT

Todd A. Jaffe and Jarone Lee

1. A 57-year-old government employee who works to counter bioterrorism without any pertinent medical history is exposed to a small amount of an unknown white powder on his skin. Over 4 days, he develops a flulike illness with symptoms including malaise, fever, and fatigue. On presentation to the emergency department, he has a temperature of 38.5°C (101.3°F), HR of 102/min, BP of 148/86 mm Hg, and O$_2$ of saturation of 98% on room air. Physical examination is notable for the skin lesion figure that follows.

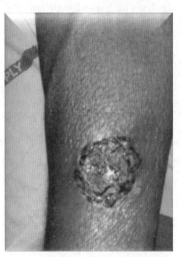

Image courtesy of Balachandrudu B, Amrutha Bindu SS, Kuman CN, Malakondaiah P. An outbreak of cutaneous anthrax in a tribal area of Visakhapatnam district, Andhra Pradesh. *J NTR Univ Health Sci.* 2018;7:49-53.

Laboratory studies are notable for a WBC of 10,800. Gram staining of the substance reveals large, spore-forming, gram-positive bacilli.

The patient is placed in isolation and admitted to the general medical service. Twelve hours after admission, the patient becomes increasingly altered. He endorses nuchal rigidity and photophobia, is unable to formulate complete sentences, and is transferred to the ICU. Lumbar Puncture demonstrates amber colored fluid, an opening pressure of 35 cm H$_2$O, 4800 WBCs/mm$^3$ with 85% PMNs, 30 RBCs/mm, protein of 400 mg/dL, and a glucose of 24 mg/dL. In addition to antitoxin, which of the following antibiotic(s) should be empirically started on this patient in the ICU?

A. Moxifloxacin and clindamycin
B. Ciprofloxacin, meropenem, and linezolid
C. Cefepime and vancomycin
D. Levofloxacin and acyclovir

2. Twelve employees of a clothing factory are transported to the emergency department after a fire at their factory. The factory utilizes wool, silk, and multiple other clothing products. The group was in the building for 2 hours while the fire was ablaze. A 55-year-old male who was found located close to the fire presents with headache, vomiting, and altered mental status. He also reports a "bitter almond" smell. Initial examination is notable for T37.0°C (98.6°F), HR 121/min, BP 160/96 mm Hg, $O_2$ saturation of 92% on room air. The patient appears flushed. His clothing is removed, and his skin is rinsed with soap and water.

As laboratory test results are pending, the patient has multiple episodes of convulsions and is intubated for airway protection. Laboratory test results are shown in the table that follows. Which of the following treatments for cyanide toxicity should be AVOIDED in this patient?

| LAB | PATIENT VALUE |
| --- | --- |
| Hgb | 13.6 g/dL |
| Hct | 44% |
| WBC | 14 000/μl (H) |
| Platelets | 420 000/μl |
| Sodium | 142 mEq/L |
| Chloride | 101 mEq/L |
| Glucose | 121 mg/dL |
| Potassium | 4.2 mEq/L |
| BUN | 16 mg/dL |
| Creatinine | 1.1 mg/dL |
| Cyanide | 32 μmol/L (H) |
| Methemoglobin | 18% (H) |

**A.** Sodium nitrite
**B.** Sodium thiosulfate
**C.** Hydroxocobalamin
**D.** 100% Oxygen

3. Multiple villagers in a war-torn Middle Eastern country are exposed to an unknown toxic agent. They present to a medical facility complaining of abdominal pain, diarrhea, frequent urination, and excessive tearing in their eyes. Physical examination is notable for bradycardia, miosis, and salivary secretions. Which of the following is the most likely agent and what is the appropriate antidote?

**A.** Sarin Nerve Gas; Atropine and pralidoxime
**B.** Atropa belladonna; Physostigmine
**C.** Benzodiazepines; Flumazenil
**D.** Arsenic; Dimercaprol

4. A 56-year-old male who was working at a nuclear power plant presents to the emergency department complaining of significant nausea and vomiting. Initial vitals are temperature of 36.8°C (98.2°F), HR of 108/min, BP of 118/76 mm Hg, $O_2$ saturation of 96% on room air. Physical examination is otherwise unremarkable. He is decontaminated, placed in isolation, and admitted to the ICU for further management. It is estimated that he was exposed to 4 -6 Gy of radiation.

On day 8 of admission, his laboratory studies are notable for WBC of 1500/μl with ANC of 300/μl, Hgb of 5.8 g/dL, Hct of 23%, and Plt of 23000/μL.

In patients with hematopoietic radiation injury, which of the following is NOT a recommended component of treatment?

**A.** Granulocyte colony-stimulating factor for patients exposed to >2 Gy
**B.** Empiric antibiotics for patients with ANC <500
**C.** Hematopoietic cell transplantation for individuals exposed to >10 Gy
**D.** Administration of blood products that have undergone leukoreduction and irradiation

**5.** A 55-year-old male presents to an emergency department in China with a 5-day history of cough, fever, and myalgias. On presentation, his temperature of 39.8°C (103.6°F), HR of 112/min, BP of 98/66 mm Hg, $O_2$ saturation of 88% on room air, which improves to 94% on 2 L of nasal cannula. Chest X-ray demonstrates a left lower lobe pneumonia. He receives 2 L of lactated ringers, is started on empiric broad spectrum antibiotics with cefepime and vancomycin, and is admitted to an isolated bed on the general medicine floor for further management. Two days after admission, he develops a worsening oxygen requirement, is transferred to the ICU, where he is ultimately intubated for hypoxic respiratory failure. His CXR just before intubation is shown below.

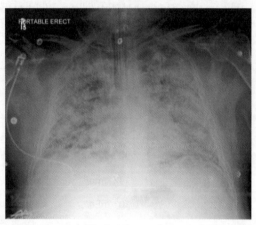

Image adapted from: Fan E, Brodie D, Slutsky AS. Acute respiratory distress syndrome: advances in diagnosis and treatment. *JAMA*. 2018;319:698-710.

A nasopharyngeal aspirate and endotracheal aspirate are ultimately positive for Avian Influenza A H7N9. Which of the following is true regarding the management of H7N9?

**A.** Inhaled zanamivir should be reserved for patients with underlying airway disease
**B.** Treatment with an antiviral agent such as oseltamivir or zanamivir is recommended, even if more than 48 hours have elapsed since illness onset
**C.** Treatment with IV zanamivir is preferred over PO oseltamivir
**D.** Antiviral administration should be held until laboratory testing has confirmed the viral pathogen

**6.** A tropical storm strikes a town with a large nuclear reactor, and there is concern for ongoing leaking of radioactive material, with potential exposure to both the building inhabitants and nearby population. Representatives from the police force, fire rescue, medical personnel, and public health arrive on the scene to coordinate a response. The responders utilize the National Incident Management System (NIMS) and Incident Command System (ICS). When utilizing these guidelines, which of the following roles is responsible for managing the overall response to the potential emergency described above?

**A.** Operations Section Chief
**B.** Incident Commander
**C.** Logistics Section Chief
**D.** Safety Officer

# Chapter 103 ▪ Answers

**1.** Correct Answer: B

**Rationale:**
This patient likely has been exposed to anthrax. *Bacillus anthracis* is a gram-positive, aerobic, capsulated, spore-forming, rod-shaped bacterium. It can be transmitted through cutaneous exposure, inhalation, ingestion, and injection, with each transmission method posing the potential for systemic progression. Patients first develop a prodromal flulike illness. However, there are fatal complications of anthrax, most notably hemorrhagic mediastinitis and meningitis.

Anthrax meningitis is almost invariably fatal. Patients may present with fever, neck rigidity, altered mental status, and with LP findings consistent with bacterial meningitis: elevated opening pressure, elevated WBCs with neutrophil predominance, elevated protein, and low glucose. In addition, the presence of frank blood or RBCs is also common given that anthrax meningitis may have a hemorrhagic component. Anthrax meningitis requires broad spectrum antibiotics with multiple antibiotic modalities and CSF penetration (B). This treatment should include at least one protein synthesis inhibitor to reduce exotoxin production.

Moxifloxacin and clindamycin (A) would be appropriate empiric coverage for cutaneous anthrax without evidence of meningitis. However, linezolid has significantly better CNS penetration compared with clindamycin. Cefepime and vancomycin (C) are broad spectrum antibiotics with strong gram-positive and -negative coverage; however, studies have demonstrated that cephalosporins, including cefepime, have unreliable coverage of *B. anthracis*. Levofloxacin and other fluoroquinolones are often first line treatment for cutaneous anthrax; however, they would not be adequate coverage for anthrax meningitis.

### References

1. Lanska DJ. Anthrax meningoencephalitis. *Neurology*. 2002;59:327-334.
2. Sejvar JJ, Tenover FC, Stephens DS. Management of anthrax meningitis. *Lancet Infect Dis*. 2005;5:287-295.
3. Hendricks KA, Wright ME, Shadomy SV, et al. Centers for disease control and prevention expert panel meetings on prevention and treatment of anthrax in adults. *Emerg Infect Dis*. 2014;20.
4. Bakici MZ, Elaldi N, Bakir M, Dokmetas I, Erandac M, Turan M. Antimicrobial susceptibility of Bacillus anthracis in an endemic area. *Scand J Infect Dis*. 2002;34:564-566.

**2.** Correct Answer: A

**Rationale:**
This patient presents with headache, vomiting, and altered mental status after prolonged smoke exposure, which is concerning for cyanide toxicity. Initial treatment for cyanide toxicity includes removal from the exposure, decontamination, and airway protection. Patients with inhalation cyanide toxicity secondary to smoke exposure often copresent with carbon monoxide poisoning. There are multiple modalities to definitively treat cyanide toxicity, including sodium nitrite, sodium thiosulfate, hydroxocobalamin, and 100% or hyperbaric oxygen.

Sodium nitrite (A) is effective in treating cyanide by inducing methemoglobinemia. This leads to the oxidation of iron in hemoglobin to form the ferric ion. Cyanide can bind with the formed methemoglobin structure, which creates cyanomethemoglobin, which is less toxic than other cyanide products. However, the formation of methemoglobin shifts the oxygen dissociation curve to the left, which can be harmful for patients with concurrent carbon monoxide poisoning. As such, the induction of methemoglobinemia in patients with both cyanide poisoning and carbon monoxide poisoning has the potential to be lethal and should be avoided in these patients.

Sodium thiosulfate (B) works by providing sulfur donors, which can convert cyanide to thiocyanate. Thiocyanate is readily excreted through the kidneys and is a reasonable treatment for this patient. Hydroxocobalamin works by binding to intracellular cyanide with greater affinity than cytochrome oxidase and forms cyanocobalamin. This structure can be excreted in the urine and works rapidly. Studies have found that 100% oxygen and hyperbaric oxygen can improve outcomes in cyanide poisoning. This patient may have concomitant carbon monoxide poisoning, with which 100% oxygen would be a cornerstone of treatment.

### References

1. Bryson PD. *Comprehensive Review in Toxicology for Emergency Clinicians*. 3rd ed. Denver: Taylor and Francis; 1996:352.
2. Dumestre D, Nickerson D. Use of cyanide antidotes in burn patients with suspected inhalation injuries in North America: a cross-sectional survey. *J Burn Care Res*. 2014;35:e112-e117.
3. Dries DJ, Endorf FW. Inhalation injury: epidemiology, pathology, treatment strategies. *Scand J Trauma Resusc Emerg Med*. 2013;21:31.
4. Takano T, Miyazaki Y, Nashimoto I, Kobayashi K. Effect of hyperbaric oxygen on cyanide intoxication: in situ changes in intracellular oxidation reduction. *Undersea Biomed Res*. 1980;7:191-197.

**3.** Correct Answer: A

**Rationale:**
These patients are presenting with cholinergic toxidrome consistent with organophosphate poisoning. Sarin nerve gas is a colorless and odorless nerve agent that blocks the acetylcholinesterase enzyme that leads to the accumulation of acetylcholine at the neuromuscular junction. This can lead to a cholinergic crisis with the symptomatology described above. Symptoms include salivation, lacrimation, urination, diarrhea, GI pain, and emesis. The extreme of organophosphate poisoning is the sequelae of bradycardia, bronchorrhea, and bronchospasm, which can be fatal. The villagers in the question stem would likely need close monitoring of their airway with a low threshold for intubation, as they have evidence of increased secretions on physical examination.

Atropa belladonna (B) is also known as deadly nightshade and contains atropine, hyocyamine, and scopolamine. It can lead to an anticholinergic toxidrome characterized by tachycardia, dry and flushed skin, altered mental status, and mydriasis, with the potential for significant neurologic dysfunction at high doses. Benzodiazepine overdose (C) would be characterized by lethargy, ataxia, and respiratory depression. It is unlikely in this group of people, and the clinical symptoms would differ from those described in this question. Arsenic ingestion (D) is characterized by prominent GI symptoms as well as jaundice, hematuria, and altered mental status. Subacute poisoning would present with anemia and peripheral neuropathy, which are not characterized by the individuals in the given question.

### References

1. Chai PR, Boyer EW, Al-Nahhas H, Erickson TB. Toxic chemical weapons of assassination and warfare: nerve agents VX and sarin. *Toxicol Commun.* 2017;1:21-23.
2. Mundy SW. Arsenic. In: *Goldfrank's Toxicologic Emergencies.* In: Hoffman RS, Lewin NA, Howland MA, et al, eds. 10th ed. New York: Mcgraw-Hill Education; 2015:1169.
3. Kwakye GF, Jimenez J, Jimenez JA, Aschner M. Atropa belladonna neurotoxicity: implications to neurological disorders. *Food Chem Toxicol.* 2018;116:346-353.

**4.** Correct Answer: C

**Rationale:**

Radiation injuries are largely dependent on the exposure burden for patients, and a patient's clinical course can often be predicted based on exposure. Patients exposed to 0 -2 Gy are unlikely to have significant complications from their radiation exposure. Patients with 2 -9 Gy may have significant sequelae from their exposure and require significant monitoring and care. Hematopoietic cell transplantation has been described as potentially beneficial for patients with Gy exposure between 2 and 9. Exposure greater than 10 Gy is almost invariably fatal (see Radiation Injury Doses and Syndromes and Phases of Radiation Injury tables). Considering the fatality rates of greater exposures and the limited resources available for transplantation, it has been documented that it is unwise to transplant patients with greater exposure (C).

Granulocyte colony-stimulation factor (A) has been shown to be beneficial for patients with significant exposure. Recommendations include daily administration of G-CSF until neutropenia resolves. For patients with significant cytopenia, including those with ANCs <500, empiric antibiotics (B) are highly recommended as a cornerstone of therapy. Recommended prophylactic therapy would likely include the use of a penicillin with beta-lactamase inhibition or the use of fluoroquinolones that have been shown to improve mortality in neutropenic patients. Regarding the administration of blood products, patients with hematopoietic radiation injury benefit greatly from supportive care and routine administration of blood products for anemia and thrombocytopenia. It is critical that these blood products undergo leukoreduction and irradiation (D) to limit significant transfusion reactions, most notably graft-versus-host disease.

### Radiation Injury Doses and Syndromes

| DOSE (GY) | SYNDROME | PROGNOSIS |
|---|---|---|
| 8 and above | Neurovascular syndrome onset | (>10 Gy) Multiple organ failure probable death |
| | | (8-10 Gy) Consider stem cell transplant |
| 3-7 Gy | GI syndrome onset | (6-7 Gy) LD50/60 with supportive care |
| | | (3-5 Gy) LD50/60 without treatment |
| 0-2 Gy | Hematopoietic syndrome onset | (0-2 Gy) ~100% survival without treatment |

Adapted from Lopez M, Martin M. Medical management of the acute radiation syndrome. *Rep Pract Oncol Radiother.* 2011;16:138-146.

### Phases of Radiation Injury

| DOSE RANGE, GY | PRODROME | MANIFESTATION OF ILLNESS | PROGNOSIS (WITHOUT THERAPY) |
|---|---|---|---|
| 0.5-1.0 | Mild | Slight decrease in blood cell counts | Almost certain survival |
| 1.0-2.0 | Mild to moderate | Early signs of bone marrow damage | Highly probably survival (>90% of victims) |
| 2.0-3.5 | Moderate | Moderate to severe bone marrow damage | Probable survival |
| 3.5-5.5 | Severe | Severe bone marrow damage; slight GI damage | Death within 3.5-6 wk (50% of victims) |
| 5.5-7.5 | Severe | Pancytopenia and moderate GI damage | Death probable within 2-3 wk |
| 7.5-10.0 | Severe | Marked GI and bone marrow damage, hypotension | Death probable within 1-2.5 wk |
| 10.0-20.0 | Severe | Severe GI damage, pneumonitis, altered mental status, cognitive dysfunction | Death certain within 5-12 d |
| 20.0-30.0 | Severe | Cerebrovascular collapse, fever, shock | Death certain within 2-5 d |

Adapted from Waselenko JK, MacVittie TJ, Blakely WF, et al. Medical management of the acute radiation syndrome: recommendations of the Strategic National Stockpile Radiation Working Group. *Ann Intern Med.* 2004;140:1037-1051.

References

1. Dainiak N. Medical management of acute radiation syndrome and associated infections in a high-casualty incident. *J Radiat Res.* 2018;59:ii54-ii64.
2. Dainiak N, Gent RN, Carr Z, et al. First global consensus for evidence-based management of the hematopoietic syndrome resulting from exposure to ionizing radiation. *Disaster Med Public Health Prep.* 2011;5:202-212.
3. Gafter-Gvili A, Fraser A, Paul M, Leibovici L. Meta-analysis: antibiotic prophylaxis reduces mortality in neutropenic patients. *Ann Intern Med.* 2005;142:979-995.

**5.** Correct Answer: B

**Rationale:**

As confirmed by laboratory testing, this patient has avian bird flu, H7N9. H7N9 is highly virulent form of influenza with the first cases of this new strain of influenza reported in 2013 in China. Patient's clinical presentations may vary but have often included the acute onset and rapid progression of common influenza symptoms. In addition, many patients have presented with leukopenia, lymphopenia, and thrombocytopenia. The severity of the illness often correlates with the baseline health of the infected patient; however, over 75% of patients were reported to be admitted to the ICU while hospitalized, and over 25% of patients have died.

The CDC published interim guidelines in 2013 regarding treatment for patients with H7N9. For those admitted to the hospital, antiviral treatment with neuroaminidase inhibitors (oseltamivir or zanamivir) is recommended. It is recommended that these antiviral agents are included in treatment even after 48 hours of illness onset, especially for patients admitted to the hospital. For other forms of influenza, it is debated whether oseltamivir should be included in treatment after 48 hours.

Inhaled Zanamivir should be avoided in patients with underlying airway disease (A), and instead oseltamivir or IV formulations should be used. There is no difference in outcomes when comparing IV zanamivir and PO oseltamivir (C). Zanamivir would only be preferred if the patient is unable to tolerate PO medications. Additionally, for patients with presumed avian flu, antivirals should be included in treatment even while laboratory testing is pending. The recommended test for H7N9 is the utilization of real-time reverse-transcriptase polymerase chain reaction for avian influenza A H7N9 on an oropharyngeal or nasopharyngeal aspirate. This study will likely include send-out laboratory testing, and treatment should not be delayed while results are pending.

References

1. Emerging pathogens: influenza - H7n9. *Dis Mon.* 2017;63:251-256.
2. Gao HN, Lu HZ, Cao B, et al. Clinical findings in 111 cases of influenza A (H7N9) virus infection. *N Engl J Med.* 2013;368:2277-2285.
3. Centers for Disease Control and Prevention. *Interim Guidance on the Use of Antiviral Agents for Treatment Of Human Infections With Avian Influenza A (H7n9) Virus.* http://www.cdc.gov/flu/avianflu/h7n9-antiviral-treatment.htm.
4. Jefferson T, Jones MA, Doshi P, et al. Neuraminidase inhibitors for preventing and treating influenza in healthy adults and children. *Cochrane Database Syst Rev.* 2014:CD008965.
5. Centers for Disease Control and Prevention. *Interim Guidance For Specimen Collection, Processing, and Testing For Patients Who May Be Infected With Avian Influenza A (H7N9) Virus.* http://www.cdc.gov/flu/avianflu/h7n9/specimen-collection.htm?s_cid=-seasonalflu-govd-003.

**6.** Correct Answer: B

**Rationale:**

The ICS is a component of the NIMS and serves to guide the response to public crises. Since 2004, the federal government has mandated that organizations utilize this system to conduct emergency management activities. ICS is one aspect of the broader NIMS, the latter being a national initiative to standardize emergency medicine activities across the entire United States. ICS functions as the executional component of NIMS related to specific incidents and has the aim of streamlining multiple aspects of disaster response including organizational structure, communication patterns, and resource allocation. The system is designed to be adaptable for localized incidents and large, regional crises.

One major component of the ICS is the role of an incident commander, whose function is to manage the overall response to an incident. This may be one individual or could include representation from multiple affected organizations (eg police commissioner and public health representative). Furthermore, the role may change depending on the magnitude of the incident, with incident commanders playing more of a hands-on role in smaller-scale incidents. The typical organizational structure of the ICS is included in Figure 103.1 below.

Medical professionals are often a key component of ICS in multiple facets. This can vary from acting as incident commander to safety officer or technical specialist as warranted by the nature of specific instances. Within medical facilities, there exists a Hospital ICS, which is geared toward addressing hospital-related incidents such as infection control, power outages, and security concerns.

The operations section chief (A) and logistics section chief (C) may directly report to the incident commander or other officers. They are responsible for directing actions to accomplish objectives and resource management, respectively. The safety officer (D) is responsible for ensuring the safety of personnel involved in the incident as well as those responding to the incident.

**Incident Command System Organizational Structure**

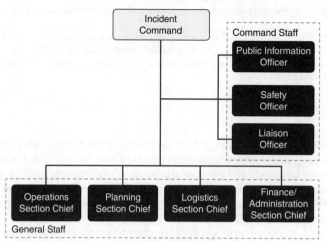

FIGURE 103.1 Incident command system organizational structure.

## References

1. Jensen J, Thompson S. The incident command system: a literature review. *Disasters.* 2016;40:158-182.
2. Adapted from "*National Incident Management System*". FEMA. December 2008:53. https://www.fema.gov/pdf/emergency/nims/NIMS_core.pdf. Accessed September 18, 2018.
3. Furin M, Goldstein S. *EMS, Incident Command System (ICS).* Treasure Island, FL: StatPearls;2018.
4. Rogers FB, McCune W, Jammula S, et al. Emergency operations program is an excellent platform to deal with in-hospital operation disaster. *Am J Disaster Med.* 2017;12:267-273.
5. Federal Emergency Management Agency "FEMA Glossary". FEMA; October 28, 2010. https://training.fema.gov/emiweb/is/ics-resource/assets/icsglossary.pdf. Accessed September 18, 2018.

# 104

# TRANSPLANTATION

Reem Almuqati, Sandeep Khanna, and Roshni Sreedharan

1. 30-year-old multiparous female with left ventricular noncompaction cardiomyopathy presents to the intensive care unit (ICU) from the operating room after undergoing an orthotopic cardiac transplantation. The donor organ was retrieved from a 20-year-old brain dead man. Preoperatively, the recipient was on chronic intravenous dobutamine therapy. Intravenous basiliximab was administered immediately prior to her transplant for induction of immunosuppression. Post termination of cardiac bypass in the operating room, temporary pacing was initiated in view of persistent bradyarrhythmia. The MOST likely cause of her posttransplant bradyarrhythmia is:

   A. Basiliximab induction
   B. Surgical trauma
   C. Donor age and gender
   D. Preoperative dobutamine therapy

2. A 40-year-old male with known nonischemic cardiomyopathy and pulmonary hypertension returns to the ICU intubated and sedated after undergoing an orthotopic heart transplant. Graft ischemia time was 4 hours. On arrival, he is on high-dose intravenous vasopressor support including 0.5 µg/kg/min norepinephrine, 0.5 µg/kg/min epinephrine, and 0.1 units/h of vasopressin. He is receiving inhaled nitric oxide 40 ppm. Monitoring reveals the following: Cardiac index of 1.6 L/min/m², invasive arterial pressure of 80/40 mm Hg, central venous pressure of 18 mm Hg, and heart rate 130 beats/min. The LEAST likely cause of his cardiogenic shock is:

   A. T-lymphocyte–mediated rejection of allograft
   B. Mediastinal bleeding with regional cardiac tamponade
   C. Ischemia-reperfusion injury–related primary graft failure
   D. Acute on chronic pulmonary hypertension

3. 50-year-old male with end-stage lung disease and pulmonary hypertension secondary to emphysema is admitted to ICU after undergoing bilateral lung transplantation on cardiopulmonary bypass. His body mass index (BMI) is 22 kg/m². The lungs were retrieved from a 25-year-old brain dead man. The donor was a nonsmoker. On POD 2, the recipient's PaO$_2$/FiO$_2$ ratio is 150 and bilateral lung opacities consistent with pulmonary edema are noted on chest x-ray suggesting a diagnosis of grade 3 primary graft dysfunction (PGD). The risk factor MOST likely associated with PGD in this scenario is:

   A. Donor's nonsmoker status
   B. Recipient and donor age mismatch
   C. BMI less than 25 kg/m²
   D. Preexisting pulmonary hypertension

4. 40-year-old male underwent liver transplant 20 years ago due to biliary cirrhosis. He is now listed for a redo liver transplant in view of recurrent cirrhosis. He is admitted to the ICU with upper gastrointestinal variceal bleeding requiring massive transfusion. He is intubated and on mechanical ventilation. Bedside echocardiography reveals an ejection fraction of 70% and absence of diastolic dysfunction. Electrocardiogram exhibits sinus tachycardia with a normal QT interval. Chest x-ray appears normal. Patient's invasive arterial pressure is 100/60 mm Hg and central venous pressure is 8 mm Hg. A pulmonary artery catheter is inserted and the following values are obtained: Cardiac output of 10 L/min, mean pulmonary artery pressure of 30 mm Hg, and pulmonary artery occlusion pressure of 10 mm Hg. This is MOST likely due to:

   A. Porto pulmonary hypertension
   B. Hyper dynamic circulation
   C. Transfusion-associated circulatory overload
   D. Cirrhotic cardiomyopathy

5. A 45-year-old male with hepatitis C–related cirrhosis presents to the ICU from the operating room after undergoing orthotopic liver transplantation. At reperfusion, he suffered a brief asystolic arrest due to hyperkalemia. The donor liver was MOST likely preserved in which preservative solution:

   A. Celsior
   B. Histidine-tryptophan-ketoglutarate (HTK)
   C. Institut Georges Lopez-1 (IGL-1)
   D. University of Wisconsin

6. 50-year-old male received a kidney transplant 3 months ago and is on immunosuppression with prednisone, tacrolimus, and mycophenolate. Antiviral prophylaxis includes valganciclovir. He recently attended a wedding in Mexico and was noncompliant with his medication regimen. He now presents with persistent diarrhea, nausea, and abdominal pain. He is admitted to ICU in view of need for ongoing fluid resuscitation. Nuclear acid testing is suggestive of cytomegalovirus (CMV) disease. Treatment of this condition MOST likely includes:

   A. Reduction in doses of all immunosuppressants
   B. Initiation of oral valganciclovir
   C. Initiation of intravenous ganciclovir
   D. Initiation of intravenous cidofovir

7. After initiation of appropriate drug therapy, the patient in the above stem demonstrates clinical improvement but develops leukopenia. He will MOST likely benefit from:

   A. Discontinuation of antiviral treatment
   B. Discontinuation of tacrolimus
   C. Addition of foscarnet
   D. Addition of filgrastim

8. 40-year-old male arrives to ICU from the operating room after undergoing an orthotopic combined liver kidney transplant. Intraoperative course was complicated by severe vasoplegic shock necessitating initiation of high-dose norepinephrine infusion. Which of the following is LEAST likely to increase mean arterial pressure (MAP) in this patient?

   A. Angiotensin I
   B. Hydroxocobalamin
   C. Methylene blue
   D. Vasopressin

9. 30-year-old female is admitted to the ICU in view of progressive shortness of breath and increasing oxygen requirements. She had bilateral lung transplant secondary to cystic fibrosis 3 month ago. The LEAST likely cause for this presentation is:

   A. Opportunistic infection
   B. Acute rejection
   C. Bronchial airway stenosis
   D. Pulmonary vein stenosis

10. 25-year-old male undergoes a combined pancreas kidney transplant. Maintenance immunosuppression includes tacrolimus, mycophenolate, and prednisone. Infection prophylaxis includes valganciclovir and trimethoprim-sulfamethoxazole. Two months later, he presents to the emergency department with seizures necessitating intubation for airway protection. Per his family, recent medication changes include the addition of pantoprazole and diltiazem; they are unaware if he has been compliant. He has also been drinking grapefruit juice for the last 1 week instead of orange juice. He is admitted to the ICU for further workup. Computed tomography reveals hypodensity in the posterior white matter. Elevations in plasma levels of which drug is MOST likely responsible for this condition?

**A.** Tacrolimus
**B.** Pantoprazole
**C.** Valganciclovir
**D.** Trimethoprim-sulfamethoxazole

# Chapter 104 ▪ Answers

1. Correct Answer: B

**Rationale:**
Sinus node dysfunction occurs in up to 50% of patients following cardiac transplantation. Such dysfunction commonly manifests as bradycardia, is usually temporary, and spontaneously resolves in a majority of patients within the first 3 months of transplantation. Temporary atrial pacing often suffices in the early postoperative period as atrioventricular (AV) node conduction is usually preserved. Unlike sinus node dysfunction, AV nodal conduction abnormalities are uncommon and tend to occur late after cardiac transplantation.

Various risk factors for developing sinus node dysfunction and ensuing posttransplant bradycardia have been described. These include surgical trauma to the sinus node, perinodal atrial tissue, or sinoatrial artery; ischemia-reperfusion injury; pretransplant use of amiodarone; older donors; and rejection. While robust evidence for most risk factors is lacking, the most likely cause of sinus node dysfunction is surgical trauma at the time of transplantation. Use of bicaval anastomotic technique instead of the biatrial surgical approach for orthotopic cardiac transplantation has substantially decreased the incidence of posttransplant bradyarrhythmia and nearly eliminated the need for permanent pacing. Donor gender and choice of immunosuppressive induction agent are not risk factors for sinus node dysfunction.

**Key point**: Sinus node dysfunction commonly occurs early after cardiac transplantation and is often related to surgical trauma.

References
1. DiBiase A, Tse TM, Schnittger I, et al. Frequency and mechanism of bradycardia in cardiac transplant recipients and need for pacemakers. *Am J Cardiol.* 1991;67:1385.
2. Heinz G, Hirschl M, Buxbaum P, et al. Sinus node dysfunction after orthotopic cardiac transplantation: postoperative incidence and long-term implications. *Pacing Clin Electrophysiol.* 1992;15:731.
3. Heinz G, Kratochwill C, Koller-Strametz J, et al. Benign prognosis of early sinus node dysfunction after orthotopic cardiac transplantation. *Pacing Clin Electrophysiol.* 1998;21:422.
4. Melton IC, Gilligan DM, Wood MA, Ellengbogen KA. Optimal cardiac pacing after heart transplantation. *Pacing Clin Electrophysiol.* 1999;22:1510-1527.

2. Correct Answer: A

**Rationale:**
Early allograft dysfunction after orthotopic heart transplant can be apparent in the intraoperative period or can develop within 24 hours after transplant surgery. It can manifest as left ventricular (LV) dysfunction, isolated right ventricular (RV) dysfunction, or biventricular dysfunction. It is associated with significantly increased 30-day and 1-year mortality. Multiple factors can contribute to early graft dysfunction and include hyperacute rejection, pulmonary hypertension, prolonged graft ischemic time, cardiac tamponade, and suboptimal donor heart.

PGD is defined as ventricular dysfunction that occurs within 24 hours after surgery and is not associated with a discernible cause. Hyperacute cellular rejection can present with immediate cardiogenic shock post transplantation and is commonly mediated by preformed B-cell antibodies. Acute rejection commonly occurs weeks to months after transplantation and is mediated by T-lymphocyte activation. Most cases of acute rejection are diagnosed by routine surveillance endomyocardial biopsy at a time when the patient is asymptomatic and ventricular function is normal.

Acute rejection commonly occurs weeks to months after transplantation, is mediated by T-lymphocyte activation, and is NOT a cause for cardiogenic shock in the immediate postoperative period. Differentials for immediate posttransplant cardiogenic shock include PGD, exacerbation of pulmonary hypertension, cardiac tamponade, and hyperacute rejection.

### References

1. Kobashigawa J, Zuckermann A, Macdonald P, et al. Report from a consensus conference on primary graft dysfunction after cardiac transplantation. *J Heart Lung Transplant.* 2014;33(4):327-340.
2. McNamara D, Di Salvo T, Mathier M, Keck S, Semigran M, Dec GW. Left ventricular dysfunction after heart transplantation: incidence and role of enhanced immunosuppression. *J Heart Lung Transplant.* 1996;15(5):506-515.
3. Michaels PJ, Espejo ML, Kobashigawa J, et al. Humoral rejection in cardiac transplantation: risk factors, hemodynamic consequences and relationship to transplant coronary artery disease. *J Heart Lung Transplant.* 2003;22(1):58.

### 3. Correct Answer: D

**Rationale:**

PGD after lung transplantation develops in the first 72 hours after transplantation and is characterized by hypoxemia with radiographic appearance of diffuse pulmonary opacities. Multiple risk factors for PGD have been identified. Donor and recipient characteristics, presence of preoperative disease, and intraoperative risk factors may contribute to PGD.

Donor risk factors include smoking, aspiration, lung contusion, undersized donor relative to recipient, heavy alcohol use, fat embolism, and thromboembolism.

Recipient factors include female gender, elevated recipient BMI ($\geq$25 kg/m$^2$), and being African American.

Pretransplant diseases with increased risk of PGD include idiopathic pulmonary fibrosis, sarcoidosis, and pulmonary arterial hypertension (PAH).

Intraoperative risk factors include large volume intraoperative blood product transfusion, prolonged ischemic time, and use of cardiopulmonary bypass (CPB).

PGD post lung transplantation is characterized by hypoxemia and the radiographic appearance of diffuse pulmonary opacities. Multiple risk factors for this condition exist.

### References

1. Snell GI, Yusen RD, Weill D, et al. Report of the ISHLT working group on primary lung graft dysfunction, part I: definition and grading-A 2016 consensus group statement of the International Society for Heart and Lung Transplantation. *J Heart Lung Transplant.* 2017;36(10):1097.
2. Liu Y, Su L, Jiang SJ. Recipient-related clinical risk factors for primary graft dysfunction after lung transplantation: a systematic review and meta-analysis. *PLoS One.* 2014;9(3):e92773.
3. Bermudez CA, Shiose A, Esper SA, et al. Outcomes of intraoperative venoarterial extracorporeal membrane oxygenation versus cardiopulmonary bypass during lung transplantation. *Ann Thorac Surg.* 2014;98(6):1936-1942

### 4. Correct Answer: B

**Rationale:**

Portopulmonary hypertension (PoPH) is PAH arising in the setting of portal hypertension with or without liver cirrhosis.

The definition of PoPH comprises three essential elements:

1. Mean pulmonary arterial pressure (mPAP) greater than 25 mm Hg
2. Pulmonary vascular resistance (PVR) greater than 240 dynes/s/cm$^5$ or 3 Wood Units
3. Pulmonary arterial occlusion pressure (PAOP) less than or equal to 15 mm Hg

The cause of PoPH is unknown. It has been hypothesized that humoral substances such as interleukin-1, endothelin-1, glucagon, secretin, thromboxane B2, and vasoactive intestinal peptide, which would normally be metabolized by the liver, are able to access the pulmonary circulation through portosystemic collaterals, resulting in PoPH. In the stem above, calculated PVR is 2 Wood Units. Although our patient's mPAP is greater than 25 mm Hg with a PAOP less than 15 mm Hg, he would not meet the criteria for PoPH given his current PVR.

Cirrhotic cardiomyopathy is a cardiac condition observed in patients with end-stage liver disease regardless of etiology. It is characterized by normal to increased cardiac output and contractility at rest but impaired systolic response to stress. It is commonly associated with diastolic dysfunction and electrophysiological abnormalities such as QT interval prolongation. Diagnosis of cirrhotic cardiomyopathy requires presence of both systolic and diastolic dysfunction with or without electrophysiological abnormalities. Our patient in the stem would not qualify.

Transfusion-associated circulatory overload commonly presents with respiratory distress and hypertension within 6 hours of receiving transfusion. Evidence of fluid overload is often present in a chest x-ray. Although our patient received massive blood transfusion, he has no evidence of circulatory overload. A hyperdynamic circulation can lead to increased mean pulmonary artery pressures in the presence of a normal PVR.

Elevated mean pulmonary artery pressures can occur for various reasons in cirrhosis with portal hypertension and should be cautiously interpreted.

## References

1. Badesch DB, Champion HC, Sanchez MA, et al. Diagnosis and assessment of pulmonary arterial hypertension. *J Am Coll Cardiol.* 2009;54:S55.
2. Mandell MS, Groves BM. Pulmonary hypertension in chronic liver disease. *Clin Chest Med.* 1996;17(1):17.
3. Rodríguez-Roisin R, Krowka MJ, Hervé P, Fallon MB. Highlights of the ERS Task Force on pulmonary-hepatic vascular disorders (PHD). *J Hepatol.* 2005;42(6):924-927.
4. Zardi EM, Abbate A, Zardi DM, et al. Cirrhotic cardiomyopathy. *Am Coll Cardiol.* 2010;56(7):539.
5. Chayanupatkul M, Liangpunsakul S. Cirrhotic cardiomyopathy: review of pathophysiology and treatment. *Hepatol Int.* 2014;8(3):308-315.

## 5. Correct Answer: D

### Rationale:

The University of Wisconsin solution is the standard criterion static cold preservation for the procurement of liver, kidney, pancreas, and intestine. Other preservation solutions include HTK, IGL-1, and Celsior.

University of Wisconsin solution is a potassium-rich (125 mmol/L), sodium-depleted, osmotically active fluid, with ion composition comparable with the intracellular milieu.

Potential disadvantages of using University of Wisconsin solution include:

a. Its high viscosity that may impede flushing of organs
b. Potential for hyperkalemic cardiac arrest given its high-potassium content
c. Increased incidence of ischemic-type biliary complications

HTK solution is cheaper, has low viscosity, and a low-potassium content (9 mmol/L).

Celsior is another cold storage solution, which has been studied as an alternative to University of Wisconsin solution. Celsior has less viscosity and greater buffering potential for acidosis than University of Wisconsin solution. Celsior solution has high-sodium and low-potassium content (15 mmol/L), with impermeants lactobionate and mannitol which limit cellular edema.

IGL-1 is a new preservation solution, with a composition resembling that of UW with inversed potassium/sodium concentrations and hydroxyethyl starch substituted with polyethylene glycol. It has 30 mmol/L of potassium.

University of Wisconsin solution is a potassium-rich, sodium-depleted, osmotically active fluid and can potentially precipitate hyperkalemic cardiac arrest during reperfusion in patients undergoing liver transplantation.

### References

1. Kalayoglu M, Sollinger HW, Stratta RJ, et al. Extended preservation of the liver for clinical transplantation. *Lancet.* 1988;1:617-619.
2. Voigt MR, Delario GT. Perspectives on abdominal organ preservation solutions: a comparative literature review. *Prog Transplant.* 2013;23:383-391.
3. Schneeberger S, Biebl M, Steurer W, et al. A prospective randomized multicenter trial comparing histidine–tryptophane–ketoglutarate versus University of Wisconsin perfusion solution in clinical pancreas transplantation. *Transpl Int.* 2009;22:217-224.
4. Karam G, Compagnon P, Hourmant M, et al. A single solution for multiple organ procurement and preservation. *Transpl Int.* 2005;18:657-663.

## 6. Correct Answer: C

### Rationale:

CMV can lead to either active CMV infection or CMV disease in transplant patients.

Active CMV infection is defined as detection of CMV replication in the blood regardless of whether signs or symptoms are present. Tissue-invasive CMV disease is defined as the demonstration of CMV in tissue biopsy specimens by histopathology in the presence of clinical symptoms and signs of end-organ disease (enteritis, colitis, hepatitis, nephritis, pneumonitis, meningitis, encephalitis, and retinitis). CMV disease can lead to allograft loss and mortality. Kidney transplant patients commonly receive CMV prophylaxis with oral valganciclovir for 3 to 6 months after transplantation. Oral valganciclovir has great bioavailability unlike oral ganciclovir. Oral ganciclovir is not available in the United States.

Patients with life-threatening CMV disease, high viral loads, or moderate to severe gastrointestinal disease are preferably treated with intravenous ganciclovir. While reduction of immunosuppression is reasonable in patients with CMV disease, it does increase the risk of rejection. Commonly, the antimetabolite mycophenolate is stopped during treatment of CMV disease while tacrolimus is usually continued.

Patients with mild CMV disease are often treated with oral valganciclovir. Patients with ganciclovir-resistant CMV may require intravenous foscarnet or cidofovir. These drugs are intensely nephrotoxic and have a worse side-effect profile as compared to ganciclovir.

Life-threatening CMV disease with high viral loads or moderate to severe gastrointestinal disease should be treated with intravenous ganciclovir.

### References

1. Razonable RR, Humar A. Cytomegalovirus in solid organ transplantation. *Am J Transplant.* 2013;13(S4):93-106.
2. Beam E, Razonable RR. Cytomegalovirus in solid organ transplantation: epidemiology, prevention, and treatment. *Curr Infect Dis Rep.* 2012;14:633-641.

**7.** Correct Answer: D

**Rationale:**

Ganciclovir and valganciclovir may lead to bone marrow suppression and leukopenia. Caution is advised if the absolute neutrophil count is under 500 cells/μL or when the platelet count is under 25,000/μL. CMV disease in itself can suppress bone marrow production, but antiviral therapy with ganciclovir typically results in improvement of hematologic parameters. Worsening or unchanged leukopenia during ongoing anti-CMV treatment with ganciclovir necessitates use of hematopoietic growth factors such as granulocyte colony-stimulating factor (G-CSF) or filgrastim to stabilize neutrophil counts. Growth factors also reduce the risk of bacterial infections which may be secondary to improved neutrophil chemotaxis and phagocytosis. Hematopoietic growth factors such as G-CSF or granulocyte-macrophage colony-stimulating factor, GM-CSF, are widely used to counter the effects of myelosuppressive drugs.

References

1. Markham A, Faulds D. Ganciclovir. An update of its therapeutic use in cytomegalovirus infection. *Drugs*. 1994;48(3):455.
2. Kotton CN, Kumar D, Caliendo AM, et al. Updated international consensus guidelines on the management of cytomegalovirus in solid-organ transplantation. *Transplantation*. 2013;96:333.

**8.** Correct Answer: A

**Rationale:**

Vasoplegic syndrome during liver transplantation is potentially lethal. It is characterized by hypotension, normal or elevated cardiac index, decreased systemic vascular resistance, and an attenuated response to vasoactive medications. The incidence of vasoplegic syndrome in end-stage liver disease is unknown, but its etiology is most likely multifactorial.

Vasodilation of the splanchnic circulation in liver failure reduces systemic vascular resistance and contributes to a hyperdynamic cardiovascular profile. Patients with liver failure also have a deficiency of endogenous vasopressin when compared to healthy subjects. Vasopressin is a potent vasoconstrictor that binds to receptors on vascular smooth muscle and can be added to increase MAP. Abnormal nitric oxide (NO) metabolism also has been shown to play a prominent role in vasoplegic syndrome. Methylene blue has gained widespread use for the treatment of vasoplegic syndrome in both cardiac surgery and liver transplant patients because of its actions as an NO synthase inhibitor and guanylate cyclase inhibitor. Hydroxocobalamin (Vitamin $B_{12a}$) is used for the treatment of acute cyanide toxicity and often leads to hypertension. The exact mechanism is not well defined, but it is believed it may act as a scavenger of NO. Utility of hydroxocobalamin for vasoplegia has been demonstrated in patients undergoing cardiac surgery and liver transplantation. Angiotensin I has minimal hemodynamic effects. Angiotensin-converting enzyme converts angiotensin I to angiotensin II. The latter is a potent vasoconstrictor. Hydroxocobalamin may be a suitable alternative treatment of vasoplegic syndrome when methylene blue is ineffective or contraindicated.

References

1. Roderique JD, VanDyck K, Holman B, et al. The use of high-dose hydroxocobalamin for vasoplegicsyndrome. *Ann Thorac Surg*. 2014;97:1785-1786.
2. Burnes ML, Boetthcer BT, Woehlck HJ, et al. Hydroxocobalamin as a rescue treatment for refractory vasoplegic syndrome after prolonged cardiopulmonary bypass. *J Cardiothorac Vasc Anesth*. 2017;31:1012-1014.
3. Boettcher BT, Woehlck HJ, Reck SE, et al. Treatment of vasoplegic syndrome with intravenous hydroxocobalamin during liver transplantation. *J Cardiothorac Vasc Anesth*. 2017;31:1381-1384.

**9.** Correct Answer: D

**Rationale:**

The differential diagnosis of a decline in allograft function after initial recovery includes infection, humoral rejection, airway complications (including stenosis at the bronchial anastomosis, bronchomalacia, and granulation tissue), chronic rejection (bronchiolitis obliterans syndrome), thromboembolism, and recurrent primary disease.

Anastomotic pulmonary arterial stenosis (PAS) is a rare complication with a reported incidence of less than 2%. A mild degree of stenosis at the arterial anastomosis without hemodynamic significance is a normal finding after transplantation secondary to donor-receptor size discordance or secondary to the suture technique.

Pulmonary venous stenosis (PVS) is a rare complication that occurs usually in early postoperative period (first 48 hours) after lung transplantation. If left untreated PVS may lead to venous thrombosis and transplant failure. Thrombus formation at the pulmonary venous/left atrial anastomotic suture line carries the risk of systemic embolization and cerebrovascular accident. The incidence of venous thrombosis is about 15%. The inferior pulmonary veins and particularly the left lower pulmonary vein are most commonly involved secondary to their anatomical position and predisposition to suture stenosis.

Complications of pulmonary arterial and venous anastomoses are less frequently seen than airway anastomotic complications. Pulmonary venous vascular complications including stenosis and thrombosis typically occur in early postoperative period.

References

1. Machuzak M, Santacruz JF, Gildea T, Murthy SC. Airway complications after lung transplantation. *Thorac Surg Clin*. 2015;25:55.
2. Anaya-Ayala JE, Loebe M, Davies MG. Endovascular management of early lung transplant-related anastomotic pulmonary artery stenosis. *J Vasc Interv Radiol*. 2015;26(6):878-882.

**10.** Correct Answer: A

**Rationale:**

The clinical syndrome of reversible posterior leukoencephalopathy syndrome (RPLS) is characterized by headaches, altered consciousness, visual disturbances, and seizures. Although the pathogenesis of RPLS has not been completely elucidated, acute hypertension is often the precipitating event. Acute hypertension leads to disordered cerebral autoregulation and endothelial dysfunction resulting in vasogenic edema. Drugs that have commonly been implicated include cyclosporine, tacrolimus, sirolimus, cisplatin, and bevacizumab.

Tacrolimus is a potent calcineurin inhibitor currently used for prophylaxis and treatment of allograft rejection. Tacrolimus metabolism occurs via the cytochrome P450-3A4 (CYP3A4) and coadministration of drugs that inhibit this enzyme lead to increased plasma levels of tacrolimus. Such drugs include protease inhibitors, diltiazem, and most proton pump inhibitors with the exception of pantoprazole. Transplant recipients are instructed to avoid grapefruit juice as it is a potent inhibitor of CYP3A4 enzyme. Tacrolimus often causes renal artery vasoconstriction leading to hypertension. Diltiazem is commonly employed to treat hypertension in this setting as it reverses the renal vasoconstriction and allows for a lower dose of tacrolimus for immunosuppression. Trimethoprim-sulfamethoxazole does not have significant interactions with tacrolimus, diltiazem, pantoprazole, and grapefruit juice.

Tacrolimus has multiple drug interactions. Increased plasma levels have been associated with RPLS.

References

1. Singh N, Bonham A, Fukui M. Immunosuppressive associated leukoencephalopathy in organ transplant recipients. *Transplantation*. 2000;69(4):467-472.
2. Li XQ, Andersson TB, Ahlstrom M, et al. Comparison of inhibitory effects of the proton pump-inhibiting drugs Omeprazole, Esomeprazole, Lansoprazole, Pantoprazole, and Rabeprazole on human cytochrome P450 activities. *Drug Metab Dispos*. 2004;32:821-827.
3. Kothari J, Nash M, Zaltzman J, et al. Diltiazem use in tacrolimus-treated renal transplant recipients. *J Clin Pharm Ther*. 2004;29(5):425-430.
4. Peynaud D, Charpiat B, Vial T, et al. Tacrolimus severe overdosage after intake of masked grapefruit in orange marmalade. *Eur J Clin Pharmacol*. 2007;63:721-722.
5. Liu C, Shang YF, Zhang XF, et al. Co-administration of grapefruit juice increases bioavailability of tacrolimus in liver transplant patients: a prospective study. *Eur J Clin Pharmacol*. 2009;65(9):881-885.

# PHARMACOLOGY AND TOXICOLOGY

# 105

# BASIC PHARMACOLOGIC PRINCIPLES

Sarah Welch and Avneep Aggarwal

1.  A 52-year-old woman is admitted to the ICU, who is s/p orthotopic liver transplant 2 weeks ago, for septic shock requiring vasopressor support. Pertinent past medical history includes an unprovoked pulmonary embolism 3 months ago for which she takes apixaban 5 mg twice daily at home. Review of systems reveals normal renal function, active bowel sounds with two recent bowel movements, and a Glasgow Coma Score of 15. In the presence of distributive shock requiring vasopressor support, with regard to absorption, which scheduled medications would you be most concerned about?

    A. Subcutaneous enoxaparin
    B. Sublingual tacrolimus
    C. Intravenous hydrocortisone
    D. Oral mycophenolate

2.  A 49-year-old man is admitted to the ICU for hemodynamic instability and ventilator weaning following surgery for a bowel perforation. His past medical history includes Crohn disease for which he takes adalimumab 40 mg once weekly. He was hospitalized 2 weeks ago for medical management of a bowel obstruction. He is started empirically on piperacillin/tazobactam and vancomycin, and 5 μg/min of norepinephrine to maintain a mean arterial pressure of at least 65 mm Hg. Over next 24 hours, the patient decompensates and is now requiring 37 μg/min of norepinephrine and 0.03 units/min of vasopressin to maintain a mean arterial pressure of 65 mm Hg, despite fluid resuscitation with 3 L of lactated ringers. He is currently anuric, is not responsive to fluids, and appears volume overloaded. Given his risk factors for multidrug-resistant organisms, his antibiotic regimen is broadened to meropenem, amikacin, daptomycin, and micafungin. When determining dose of amikacin for this patient, what considerations should be made?

    A. Decrease the dose because of diminished renal clearance
    B. Increase the dosing frequency because of the increased volume of distribution
    C. Increase the dose because of the increased volume of distribution
    D. Decrease the dose because of decreased protein binding

3.  Which pathophysiological change seen in critically ill patients most frequently makes medication dosage adjustment necessary?

    A. Decreased plasma protein binding
    B. Decreased renal clearance
    C. Diminished GI or subcutaneous perfusion
    D. Inhibition of hepatic enzymes

4.  Fentanyl, a drug with a high extraction ratio, will be most influenced by which critical illness–related metabolic abnormality?

    A. Decreased hepatic blood flow
    B. Decreased intrinsic clearance
    C. Decreased protein binding
    D. Decreased functional hepatocytes

5. Phenytoin, a drug with a low extraction ratio, will be most influenced by which critical illness–related metabolic abnormality?

   A. Decreased hepatic blood flow
   B. Decreased intrinsic clearance
   C. Decreased protein binding
   D. Decreased acetylation

6. A 76-year-old woman is admitted to the ICU for atrial fibrillation with rapid ventricular rate after an exploratory laparotomy. You elect to use Drug A for rate control. The oral formulation of Drug A undergoes significant first-pass metabolism. With this knowledge, what dosage adjustment should be made to the intravenous form of Drug A?

   A. Increase the dose
   B. Decrease the dose
   C. Make no dosage adjustment
   D. Increase the dosing interval

7. A patient is admitted to the cardiac ICU after suffering a cardiac arrest. She is nonresponsive and therapeutic hypothermia is initiated. In addition to cooling, she receives a midazolam infusion for sedation, intermittent hydromorphone boluses for pain, and an atracurium infusion for shivering. What is your concern with this patient's current medication regimen?

   A. Therapeutic hypothermia may affect CYP450 activity decreasing the metabolism of midazolam and therefore prolong its sedative affect
   B. Therapeutic hypothermia may affect CYP450 activity decreasing the metabolism of atracurium and therefore prolong its neuromuscular blocking affects
   C. Therapeutic hypothermia may affect Hofmann elimination decreasing the metabolism of hydromorphone and therefore prolong its sedative affect
   D. Therapeutic hypothermia may affect Hofmann elimination decreasing the metabolism of midazolam and therefore prolong its sedative affect

8. A 43-year-old woman is admitted to the ICU with community-acquired pneumonia. She is mechanically intubated and requires vasopressor support. Pertinent past medical history includes seizure disorder for which she takes phenytoin 100 mg by mouth three times daily. On day 3 in the ICU, patient remains intubated, is off vasopressors, and enteral tube feeding is started. Pertinent lab values on day 3 are as follows: ALT 154 U/L, AST 95 U/L, albumin 1.5 g/dL, SCr 2.3 mg/dL. On day 5 in the ICU patient suffers a seizure. What is the most likely cause of her seizure?

   A. Kidney dysfunction
   B. Enteral tube feeds
   C. Elevated liver enzymes
   D. Hypoalbuminemia

9. On ICU day 3, the patient grows a multidrug-resistant *Klebsiella pneumoniae* from her bronchoscopy culture. She is initiated on a recently approved drug to treat carbapenem-resistant enterobacteracieae. She is given a reduced dose based on a calculated creatinine clearance of less than 20 mL/min. On ICU day 4, she is started on continuous veno-venous hemodialysis (CVVHD). You cannot find any dosing recommendations for CVVHD; however, you're able to find that this new drug is 60% renally eliminated as unchanged drug, volume of distribution is 3 L/kg, its ~25% bound to protein, and has a small molecular weight. What change should you make to the dosing regimen?

   A. Increase the dose because of low protein binding and small molecular weight
   B. Increase the dose because of large volume of distribution
   C. Maintain current dose because of low protein binding and small molecular weight
   D. Maintain current dose because of large volume of distribution

10. A 23-year-old man is admitted to the ICU for management of salicylate toxicity. His arterial blood gas on arrival shows the following: pH 7.54, $PaCO_2$ 22 mm Hg, $PaO_2$ 93 mm Hg, $HCO_3^-$ 18 mEq/L, oxygen saturation 90%. Sodium bicarbonate 100 mEq IV push is administered followed by a continuous infusion of sodium bicarbonate 150 mEq/L at 250 mL/h. Hypokalemia is corrected as appropriate. What physiochemical property of aspirin counters or supports sodium bicarbonate therapy?

A. Sodium bicarbonate therapy is contraindicated because of a pH of 7.54
B. In cases of salicylate toxicity, metabolic acidosis follows respiratory alkalosis. Sodium bicarbonate therapy can prevent severe acidemia
C. Salicylic acid is a weak acid. Sodium bicarbonate will alkalinize the urine, enhancing renal tubular excretion
D. Salicylic acid is a weak acid; therefore sodium bicarbonate therapy is contraindicated as urine alkalization will enhance renal tubular reabsorption

# Chapter 105 ▪ Answers

1. Correct Answer: A

**Rationale:**
Critically ill patients receiving vasopressors may have reduced subcutaneous absorption of drugs. Presence of shock and/or use of vasopressors decrease peripheral tissue perfusion, resulting in impaired subcutaneous absorption. Studies evaluating low-molecular-weight heparins demonstrate lower antifactor Xa levels in critically ill patients receiving vasopressors when compared with critically ill patients not on vasopressors or those who are not critically ill. Sublingual absorption is not impaired in states of critical illness, and intravenous therapy always results in 100% bioavailability. Although blood is shunted to vital organs in states of hypotension and shock, the impact of splanchnic perfusion on drug absorption has not been well studied.

References
1. Joachleberger S, Mayr V, Luckner G, et al. Anitfactor Xa activity in critically ill patients receiving antithrombotic prophylaxis with standard dosages of certoparin: a prospective, clinical study. *Crit Care.* 2005;9(5):R541-R548.
2. Dorffler-Melly J, de Jonge E, Pont AC, et al. Bioavailability of subcutaneous low-molecular weight heparin to patients on vasopressors. *Lancet.* 2002;359(9309):849-850.

2. Correct Answer: C

**Rationale:**
Hydrophilic molecules, such as amikacin, generally remain in the plasma water volume. Capillary leak due to septic shock and exogenous volume administration will contribute to an increase in the volume of distribution. Studies evaluating aminoglycosides in states of critical illness report increases in the volume of distribution anywhere from 25% to 50%. Additionally, aminoglycosides are concentration-dependent agents that are most effective at concentrations 10 times the minimal inhibitory concentration of the offending pathogen. Therefore, the pharmacokinetic properties of the drug should lead the clinician to administering an increased dose. Although clearance of aminoglycosides will be decreased with impaired renal function, the initial dose should not be decreased because of the increased volume of distribution. Increasing the dosing frequency will increase the time above the minimal inhibitory concentration, but not result in target peak concentrations for some time. Amikacin is not protein bound, so will not be affected by decreased protein.

References
1. Taccone FS, Laterre PF, Spapen H, et al. Revisiting the loading dose of amikacin for patients with severe sepsis and septic shock. *Crit Care.* 2010;14:R53.
2. Rhonda R, CapitanoB, BiesR, et al. Suboptimal aminoglycoside dosing in critically ill patients. *Ther Drug Monit.* 2008;30:674-681.

3. Correct Answer: B

**Rationale:**
Medications that undergo renal elimination generally have dosing recommendations based on GFR (glomerular filtration rate) estimated using the Cockroft-Gault formula. For renally eliminated medications, modifying dose regimens is essential in patients with acute or chronic kidney injury to prevent adverse drug events. Conversely, conditions such as sepsis, trauma, surgery, burns, and use of vasopressors can lead to an increase in renal blood flow, resulting in increased renal drug clearance. No empiric changes for augmented renal clearance are recommended by drug manufacturers. Although a decrease in plasma proteins can increase the free concentration of highly protein bound drugs, there are no empiric dosing changes that are recommended based on the degree of protein decrease. Similarly, although both enteral

and subcutaneous absorption of medications is diminished in states of critical illness, no dosing adjustments exist for any medication empirically. Finally, there is no biomarker readily available in the clinical setting that can be used to determine the degree of liver impairment for the purposes of drug dosing. Although the Child-Pugh classification uses patient-specific data to assess severity of hepatic disease, its purpose was to predict mortality. Although some drug manufacturers include dosing adjustment recommendations based on Child-Pugh score, such recommendations are neither available for many drugs nor are they validated in critically ill patients.

### References

1. Cantu TG, Ellerbeck EF, Yun SW, et al. Drug prescribing for patients with changing renal function. *Am J Hosp Pharm.* 1992;49(12):2944-4948.
2. Brown R, Babcock R, Talbert J, et al. Renal function in critically ill postoperative patients: sequential assessment of creatinine osmolar and free water clearance. *Crit Care Med.* 1980;8(2):68-72.
3. Marin C, Eon B, Saux P, et al. Renal effects of norepinephrine used to treat septic shock patients. *Crit Care Med.* 1990;18(3):282-285.
4. Pugh RN, Murray-Lyon IM, Dawson JL, et al. Transection of the esophagus for bleeding esophageal varices. *Br J Surg.* 1973;60(8):646-649.

### 4. Correct Answer: A

**Rationale:**

The hepatic extraction ratio is the fraction of drug that is removed from the blood after one pass through the liver. Hepatic clearance of drugs with high extraction ratio (>0.7) primarily depends on liver blood flow and is less affected by changes in liver function (ie, intrinsic clearance or function hepatocytes). Conversely, hepatic clearance of drugs with low extraction ratio (<0.3) is more sensitive to changes in liver function. Protein binding can be an important determinant of a drug's hepatic extraction ratio; however, changes to plasma protein binding are only relevant for drugs with high extraction ratios.

### References

1. Benet LZ, Hoener BA. Changes in plasma protein binding have little clinical relevance. *Clin Pharmacol Ther.* 2002;71(3):115-121.
2. Smith B, Yogaratnam D, Levasseur-Franklin KE, et al. Introduction to drug pharmacokinetics in the critically ill patient. *Chest.* 2012;141(5):1327-1336.

### 5. Correct Answer: B

**Rationale:**

The hepatic extraction ratio is the fraction of drug that is removed from the blood after one pass through the liver. Hepatic clearance of drugs with low extraction ratio (<0.3) is more sensitive to changes in liver function (ie, intrinsic clearance or function hepatocytes). Conversely, hepatic clearance of drugs with high extraction ratio (>0.7) primarily depends on liver blood flow and is less affected by changes in liver function. Protein binding can be an important determinant of a drug's hepatic extraction ratio; however, changes to plasma protein binding are only relevant for drugs with high extraction ratios.

### References

1. Benet LZ, Hoener BA. Changes in plasma protein binding have little clinical relevance. *Clin Pharmacol Ther.* 2002;71(3):115-121.
2. Smith B, Yogaratnam D, Levasseur-Franklin KE, et al. Introduction to drug pharmacokinetics in the critically ill patient. *Chest.* 2012;141(5):1327-1336.

### 6. Correct Answer: B

**Rationale:**

First-pass metabolism is when a drug is metabolized between its site of administration and the site of sampling for measurement of drug concentration. One major therapeutic implication of extensive first-pass metabolism is that much larger oral doses are required to achieve equivalent plasma concentrations when compared with intravenous doses of the same drug. Therefore, drugs with significant first-pass metabolism require significant dose reduction when converting from oral to intravenous therapy.

### Reference

1. Pond SM, Tozer TN. First-pass elimination. Basic concepts and clinical consequences. *Clin Pharmacokinet.* 1984;9(1):1-25.

### 7. Correct Answer: A

**Rationale:**

Midazolam undergoes extensive hepatic metabolism via CYP3A4. Data suggest that therapeutic hypothermia decreases metabolic clearance by affecting the CYP450 system. Reduction in clearance may be due to diminished enzyme affinity for the drug, reduced speed of chemical reactions involved in metabolism, or both. Atracurium undergoes ester hydrolysis and Hofmann elimination (a nonbiologic process independent of renal, hepatic, or enzymatic function). Although Hofmann elimination may also be slowed during therapeutic hypothermia, both hydromorphone and midazolam are not metabolized via this process.

References

1. Tortorici MA, Kochanek PM, Poloyac SM, et al. Effects of hypothermia on drug disposition, metabolism, and response: a focus of hypothermia-mediated alterations on the cytochrome P450 enzyme system. *Crit Care Med*. 2007;35(9):2196-2204.
2. Van den Broek MPH, Groenendaal F, Egberts AC, et al. Effects of hypothermia on pharmacokinetics and pharmacodynamics: a systematic review of preclinical and clinical studies. *Clin Pharmacokinet*. 2010;49(5):277-294.

### 8. Correct Answer: B

**Rationale:**

Phenytoin is known to exhibit variably decreased absorption in the presence of enteral feeding solutions. The exact mechanism underlying this interaction is not fully established; however, majority of studies suggest that there is a physical incompatibility between phenytoin and certain components in the enteral feeding formulas. This interaction results in complexation of phenytoin particles and thus decreases bioavailability. Other studies suggest that binding to tube lumen or pH-related interactions may contribute to decreased bioavailability. In the above question, answer A is incorrect because phenytoin is not renally eliminated; therefore levels should not be affected by acute kidney injury. Answer C is incorrect because liver dysfunction might, if anything, increase phenytoin levels, which may result in phenytoin toxicity. However, this is unlikely to cause seizures. Lastly, phenytoin is highly protein bound. In states of hypoalbuminemia, the available (free) concentration of the drug may increase, resulting in phenytoin toxicity, but this is also unlikely to cause seizures.

References

1. Maka DA, Murphy LK. Drug-nutrient interactions: a review. *AACN Clin Issues*. 2000;11(4):580-589.
2. Yeung SCA, Ensom MH. Phenytoin and enteral feedings: does evidence support an interaction? *Ann Pharmacother*. 2000;34(7-8):896-905.

### 9. Correct Answer: A

**Rationale:**

The extent to which a drug is dialyzable is primarily dependent on physiochemical characteristics of the drug. These largely include molecular size, protein binding, volume of distribution, water solubility, and plasma clearance. The movement of drugs is largely determined by the size of the molecule in relation to the pore size of the dialysis membrane. As a general rule, smaller molecular weight substances will pass through the membrane more easily than larger size molecules. Another important factor in removal is the amount of unbound or free drug, across the membrane. Drugs with high protein binding (>80%) will have small plasma concentrations of unbound drug available for removal. Finally, a drug with a large volume of distribution is distributed widely through the tissue with low amounts of drug available in the plasma for removal. With these properties considered, answer A is the most appropriate.

Reference

1. Choi G, Gomersall CD, Tian Q, et al. Principles of antibacterial dosing in continuous renal replacement therapy. *Crit Care Med*. 2009;37:2268-2282.

### 10. Correct Answer: C

**Rationale:**

Urine alkalization will increase the reabsorption of basic drugs by making the drug nonionized and can enhance the elimination of acidic drugs by making the drug ionized. Data suggest that raising the urine pH 7.5 to 8 through the use of sodium bicarbonate enhances elimination of salicylates. An elevated pH is not a contraindication to use. In cases of salicylate toxicity, patients presenting in the early phase after ingestion generally have respiratory alkalosis due to direct stimulation of the respiratory center. As the absorption of the drug continues, an anion gap metabolic acidosis ensues. In this scenario sodium bicarbonate therapy is not used to prevent the development of a metabolic acidosis, but rather is used as a treatment to deprotonate the molecule, which both decreases concentration in the central nervous system and enhances excretion through renal tubular excretion.

References

1. Proudfoot AT, Krenzelok EP, Brent J, et al. Does urine alkalization increase salicylate elimination? If so, why? *Toxicol Rev*. 2003;22(3):129-136.
2. El-Sheikh AA, Masereeuw R, Russel FG. Mechanisms of renal anionic drug transport. *Eur J Pharmacol*. 2008;585(2-3):245-255.
3. Gabow PA, Anderson RJ, Potts DE, et al. Acid-base disturbances in the salicylate-intoxicated adult. *Arch Intern Med*. 1978;138(10):1481.

# 106

# ADVERSE EFFECTS OF DRUGS

Anoop Chhina and Avneep Aggarwal

1. A 55-year-old woman undergoes elective ventral hernia repair. Past medical history is significant for hypertension and asthma. She had uneventful induction of anesthesia. Five minutes after cefazolin was started for perioperative prophylaxis, the patient becomes hypotensive and progressively hypoxic with high peak airway pressures. Diphenhydramine, steroids, a H2-blocker, bronchodilators, and epinephrine are administered, with clinical improvement. A decision is made to postpone surgery, and she is transferred to the intensive care unit (ICU) for further management. Which of the following laboratory levels can help determine whether the episode was related to anaphylaxis as compared to asthma exacerbation?

   A. Pseudocholinesterase
   B. Tryptase
   C. Lipase
   D. Amylase

2. A 33-year-old woman is admitted to ICU s/p motor vehicle accident with traumatic brain injury, and CT scan of the head showed subdural hematoma without midline shift and bilateral frontal contusions. On day 2 of admission, she starts having seizures. She is given 1000 mg phenytoin and started on a maintenance dose. She remains in the ICU due to waxing and waning mental status. On day 5 as you are examining the patient, red-purple macules and papules are noticed on chest and abdomen, as well as on the bilateral upper and lower extremities. Similar lesions are also seen in mouth and genital area. Which of the following will help to differentiate Stevens-Johnson syndrome (SJS) from toxic epidermal necrolysis (TEN)?

   A. Presence of Nikolsky sign in SJS as compared to TEN
   B. Involvement of more than two mucosal surfaces in TEN as compared to two or less in SJS
   C. They are spectrum of same disease process; SJS is defined as affecting less than 10% body surface area (BSA), and TEN affects more than 30% BSA
   D. SJS occurs within 1 week of triggering factor, while TEN occurs more than 4 weeks after triggering agent

3. A 48-year-old woman with a history of poorly controlled hypertension, coronary artery disease, and chronic renal failure is admitted to ICU after presenting to emergency room (ER) with hypertensive emergency. Her blood pressure was controlled with sodium nitroprusside. After 32 hours of treatment, the patient develops agitation, confusion, and metabolic acidosis. Which of the following is used for the prevention/treatment of this adverse effect of nitroprusside?

   A. Thiocyanate
   B. Cyanocobalamin
   C. Thiosulfate
   D. Methylene blue

4. A 28-year-old woman presents to the emergency department with sudden onset of generalized fatigue, fever, chills, and blurry vision. She was recently diagnosed with urinary tract infection and started on Bactrim 2 days ago. On physical examination, her skin is mildly jaundiced. She has multiple purpura over her extremities. Laboratory tests reveal: Hemoglobin 8.0 g/dL, platelet count 57/mm³, and creatinine of 2.8 mg/dL. Of note, renal function was normal 4 days ago. On peripheral smear, multiple schistocytes are present (~2%). She is admitted to ICU due to metabolic disarray and for additional workup. She reports no history of illicit drug use, recent diarrhea, or no other significant past medical history. Vitals are heart rate 90 beats/min, blood pressure 130/74 mm Hg, temperature 38.7°C, and respiratory rate 18 breaths/min. Serum lactate dehydrogenase (LDH) is elevated. Serum ADAMTS13 level was send from emergency department, showed a mild reduction. Based on these findings what is most probable diagnosis?

   **A.** Immune thrombocytopenic purpura
   **B.** Thrombotic thrombocytopenic purpura
   **C.** Drug-induced thrombotic microangiopathy (DITMA)
   **D.** Disseminated intravascular coagulation

5. A 58-year-old woman is admitted to hospital with fever, productive cough, and shortness of breath. Chest x-ray is consistent with right lower lobe consolidation. She was treated as an outpatient for community-acquired pneumonia with oral ciprofloxacin, without improvement in symptoms. Medical history is significant for hypertension, gastroesophageal reflux disease (GERD), bipolar disorder, and depression. Her medications include carvedilol, omeprazole, aripiprazole, and amitriptyline. An ECG at time of admission shows normal sinus rhythm with prolonged QT interval.

   Which of the following medications should be discontinued FIRST based on patient's ECG findings?

   **A.** Aripiprazole
   **B.** Carvedilol
   **C.** Omeprazole
   **D.** Amitriptyline

6. A 48-year-old woman was recently admitted for pyelonephritis and discharged home on trimethoprim-sulfamethoxazole based on urinary culture results. She returns to the ER 5 days later with fever, nausea, and vomiting. Right-sided hydronephrosis was seen on renal ultrasound and the patient was admitted to ICU for presumed urosepsis and postureteric stent placement. On examination, widespread morbilliform itchy rash was noted all over the body. On physical examination, the patient is found to be febrile. Her mucous membranes are normal. She has 3 cm lymph nodes in the anterior cervical and axillary regions and a liver edge palpable 4 cm below the costal margin.

   Some facial swelling is also noted, but there was no difficulty in breathing. Medical history is otherwise unremarkable, and she was taking no other medications at home.

   Which of the following is the most appropriate next step in diagnosis of this patient?

   **A.** Skin biopsy
   **B.** No further testing
   **C.** Lymph node biopsy
   **D.** Complete blood count and liver chemistry

7. A 24-year-old man with no past medical history was scheduled for elective inguinal hernia repair under general anesthesia. Intraoperatively he becomes increasingly tachycardic and hyperthermic, and blood gas demonstrates severe metabolic acidosis. He is treated for malignant hyperthermia (MH) in the OR with good response and post procedure, is transferred to the ICU for close monitoring. Which of the following anesthetic agents used is most likely to trigger MH?

   **A.** Propofol
   **B.** Rocuronium
   **C.** Midazolam
   **D.** Succinylcholine

8. A 78-year-old woman with past medical history of hypertension, coronary artery disease, and stage III chronic kidney disease is admitted to ICU with symptoms of lethargy, altered mental status, hypotension, and bradycardia. On further history obtained from patient's daughter, she has been experiencing constipation and was taking over-the-counter laxatives. Over the past week, she had increased the magnesium-based laxative uptake to several times a day. On physical examination, her blood pressure is 90/62 mm of Hg, heart rate is 48 beats/min, and respiratory rate is 8 breaths/min. Her temperature is 37.4°C, and ECG shows sinus bradycardia. Her chemistries reveal a creatinine that has worsen from baseline, and her serum magnesium is 8.4 mg/dL. What is the next best step in immediate management of this patient?

A. Hold more laxative use, no treatment required
B. Urgent hemodialysis
C. Calcium chloride
D. Potassium chloride

# Chapter 106 ▪ Answers

**1.** Correct Answer: B

**Rationale:**
Mast cells have preformed mediators, including tryptase, which can be used to measure systemic mast cell activation. Concentrations of α-tryptase correlate with mast cell number, whereas β-tryptase concentrations are associated with acute mast cell activation. Total serum tryptase can be used to confirm a diagnosis of anaphylaxis, although samples need to be collected within 4 hours of a suspected anaphylactic reaction. β-tryptase levels are thought to peak 30 to 60 minutes after a reaction, with a half-life of 2 hours. Normal total tryptase ranges from 1 to 10 ng/mL. If baseline tryptase is >20 ng/mL in a patient without acute symptoms of anaphylaxis, indolent systemic mastocytosis should be suspected and further evaluation sought. Histamine elevation is short-lived after an anaphylactic episode; however, metabolites, such as *N*-methyl histamine and prostaglandins, can be measured in the urine for 24 hours after an anaphylactic event and may be useful for diagnosis. Other potentially useful biomarkers are being studied, including platelet-activating factor, bradykinin, chymase, and others. Amylase, lipase, and pseudocholinesterase are not mast cell mediators, so not related to the diagnosis of anaphylaxis.

## Reference
1. Makhija M. *Patterson's Allergic Diseases*. Lippincott Williams & Wilkins; 2018:868-869.

**2.** Correct Answer: C

**Rationale:**
This patient's presentation is consistent with SJS and TEN. SJS and TEN are severe acute inflammatory exfoliative skin reactions with unclear etiology usually triggered by medications or, less frequently, by upper respiratory infections. SJS and TEN are believed to be variants of same condition; Nikolsky sign is almost always present in both. Both TEN and SJS occur 1 to 3 weeks after exposure to inciting agent. The difference between the two is related to the percentage of BSA affected: SJS affects less than 10% and TEN affects greater than 30%, while a range of 10% to 30% is referred to as SJS/TEN overlap.

Pharmacologic triggers can be divided into drugs administered for shorter durations (eg, antibiotics such as trimethoprim/sulfamethoxazole, sulfonamides, cephalosporins, quinolones, and aminopenicillins) and medications administered chronically (eg, carbamazepine, oxicam nonsteroidal anti-inflammatory drugs, phenytoin, phenobarbital, allopurinol, and valproic acid).

Treatment consists of immediate discontinuation of the triggering agent and early transfer to a burn unit, which significantly reduces morbidity and mortality. Recent trials of immunosuppressive therapy, steroids, and immunoglobulins have not shown improvement in outcome. Application of silver nitrate may lead to cross-reactivity with antibiotics and is not recommended. Diagnosis is usually clinical and biopsy of affected areas is not required.

## References
1. Milliszewski MA, Kirchhof MG, Sikora S, Papp A, Dutz JP. Stevens-Johnson syndrome and toxic epidermal necrolysis: an analysis of triggers in implications for improving prevention. *Am J Med*. 2016;129(11):1221-1225.
2. Gerull R, Nelle M, Schaible T. Toxic epidermal necrolysis and Stevens-Johnson syndrome: a review. *Crit Care Med*. 2011;39(6):1521-1532.

**3.** Correct Answer: C

**Rationale:**

The signs and symptoms of the patient are consistent with cyanide toxicity from nitroprusside. Nitroprusside causes toxicity through release of cyanide and accumulation of thiocyanate. Most common symptoms of cyanide toxicity are changes in mental status, including convulsions, encephalopathy, coma, and even unexplained cardiac arrest. Metabolic acidosis can be present, though this may be a late event. Cyanide reacts in high affinity with metals such as ferric iron ($Fe^{3+}$) and cobalt and also binds to numerous critical enzyme systems in the body. Cyanide inhibits oxidative phosphorylation and thereby causes central nervous system and cardiovascular dysfunction due to cellular hypoxia. It does this by primarily binding to and inactivating the enzyme cytochrome oxidase (cytochrome a3).

Risk of cyanide toxicity can be decreased by utilizing nitroprusside at recommended doses for short period of time. Thiosulfate is a specific antidote for cyanide toxicity associated with nitroprusside infusion. Sodium thiosulfate removes cyanide from the blood through the action of the enzyme rhodanese. It has also been recommended that thiosulfate infusions be used for patients receiving high doses of nitroprusside. Cyanocobalamin is not effective as an antidote and is not capable of preventing cyanide toxicity. Hydroxocobalamin, a precursor of vitamin B12, may also be used to treat cyanide toxicity. It contains a cobalt moiety that binds intracellular cyanide forming cyanocobalamin.

Nitroprusside can cause a dose-dependent conversion of hemoglobin to methemoglobin. Methylene blue is used for treating methemoglobinemia, and not cyanide toxicity.

**References**
1. Hall AH, Dart R, Bogdan D. Sodium thiosulfate or hydroxocobalamin for the empiric treatment of cyanide poisoning? *Ann Emerg Med.* 2007;49(6):806-813.
2. Curry SC. Sodium nitroprusside. In: Brent H, et al. *Critical Care Toxicology.* Philadelphia, PA: Mosby; 2005:843-850.

**4.** Correct Answer: C

**Rationale:**

Thrombotic microangiopathy is characterized by platelet microthrombi in small vessels leading to thrombocytopenia and microangiopathic hemolytic anemia. Microthrombi may also lead to systemic effects like acute kidney injury, neurologic abnormalities, and cardiac ischemia. In this patient, the presence of schistocytes (>1%) with hemolytic anemia (anemia, jaundice, elevated LDH) is suggestive of microangiopathic hemolytic anemia. This, in addition to thrombocytopenia and the systemic symptoms, supports a diagnosis of thrombotic microangiopathy.

Schistocytes are not typical of disseminated intravascular coagulation and even, if present, are usually <0.5%. A higher percentage of schistocytes (>1%) suggests thrombotic microangiopathy.

Important causes of thrombotic microangiopathy include thrombotic thrombocytopenic purpura, hemolytic uremic syndrome, complement-mediated thrombotic microangiopathy, and DITMA. Thrombotic thrombocytopenic purpura is associated with a lesser degree of renal involvement (or no renal involvement), and the levels of ADAMTS13 (when available) are very low (<10%). Hemolytic uremic syndrome is usually accompanied by marked abdominal signs and symptoms (diarrhea, abdominal pain, nausea). Immune thrombocytopenic purpura is caused by immune-mediated destruction of platelets and not associated with microangiopathic hemolytic anemia.

This patient most likely has DITMA. DITMA is caused by either immune-mediated or toxin-mediated mechanisms. Various drugs have been implicated. Drugs known to cause immune-mediated DITMA include quinine, trimethoprim-sulfamethoxazole (Bactrim), and quetiapine. Common culprits in toxin-mediated DITMA are cancer chemotherapeutic agents, immunosuppressants (calcineurin inhibitors), and recreational drugs of abuse. The diagnosis of DITMA is made clinically, based on the findings of thrombotic microangiopathy with the appropriate history of exposure to a culprit drug. Immune-mediated DITMA is not dose dependent and occurs within 2 weeks of drug exposure, with a longer duration of exposure making the diagnosis less likely. ADAMTS13 activity is normal or only mildly decreased. ADAMTS13 activity <10% strongly supports a diagnosis of thrombotic thrombocytopenic purpura.

Management of DITMA involves discontinuation of culprit drug and supportive care. DITMA (caused by either immune- or toxin-mediated mechanisms) requires the presence of the drug to cause cellular damage. Thus, once the drug is cleared from the circulation, no further organ injury occurs.

**References**
1. George JN, Nester CM. Syndromes of thrombotic microangiopathy. *N Engl J Med.* 2014;371:654.
2. Hall JB, Schmidt GA, Wood LH, eds. *Principles of Critical Care.* 3rd ed. New York, NY: McGraw-Hill; 2005.
3. Hunt BJ. Bleeding and coagulopathies in critical care. *N Engl J Med.* 2014;370:847-859.

**5.** Correct Answer: D

**Rationale:**

Amitriptyline should be discontinued as the ECG demonstrates QT prolongation. Many medications prolong QT interval, including amitriptyline and ciprofloxacin; QT prolongation may be markedly increased in patients taking more than one medication with this effect. Other drugs that have been implicated include antiarrhythmic agents, antibiotics (including macrolides and fluoroquinolones), antipsychotics, and antidepressants. A corrected QT (QTc) interval greater than 500 ms is associated with increased risk of torsades de pointes (TdP). In cases of prolonged QT interval, all QT prolonging agents should be discontinued.

Beta-blockers (carvedilol) do not prolong QTc. An exception is sotalol, also a class III antiarrhythmic, which causes QT prolongation. Although rare, proton pump inhibitors (omeprazole) can cause prolonged QTc after chronic use (occurs due to hypomagnesemia). Aripiprazole is a quinolinone antipsychotic which unlike atypical antipsychotics may cause a decrease in QTc interval.

### References

1. Isbister GK, Page CB. Drug induced QT prolongation: the measurement and assessment of the QT interval in clinical practice. *Br J Clin Pharmacol*. 2013;76(1):48-57.
2. Roden DM. Drug induced prolongation of the QT interval. *N Engl J Med*. 2004;350:1013.

---

**6.** Correct Answer: D

**Rationale:**

She has a widespread morbilliform eruption with fever, facial edema, and lymphadenopathy that started 5 days after taking trimethoprim-sulfamethoxazole. This is typical of a systemic drug hypersensitivity syndrome known as drug reaction with eosinophilia and systemic symptoms (DRESS) syndrome. Diagnosis can be challenging in the presence of concurrent sepsis. DRESS is a rare life-threatening drug-induced hypersensitivity reaction. Clinical features typically includes skin eruption, hematologic abnormalities (atypical lymphocytosis and eosinophilia), lymphadenopathy, and internal organ involvement (including liver, kidneys, and lungs) that occurs 5 to 10 days after starting the offending medication. Lymph node biopsy and skin biopsy are not helpful in its diagnosis. Since it can be associated with multiorgan system involvement, additional laboratory testing including complete metabolic panel is indicated.

### Reference

1. Cacoub P, Musette P, Descamps V, et al. The DRESS syndrome: a literature review. *Am J Med*. 2011;124(7):588-597.

---

**7.** Correct Answer: D

**Rationale:**

MH is a rare, genetic, life-threatening condition that is a result of unregulated release of calcium from the sarcoplasmic reticulum. The incidence of MH episodes during anesthesia is between 1:10,000 and 1:250,000 anesthetics. It can be triggered by all volatile anesthetics and by succinylcholine. Halothane is most potent trigger for MH compared to the other volatile anesthetics. Classic signs of MH include hyperthermia, tachycardia, tachypnea, increased carbon dioxide production, increased oxygen consumption, acidosis, hyperkalemia, muscle rigidity, and rhabdomyolysis, all related to a hypermetabolic response. The syndrome is likely to be fatal if untreated. An increase in end-tidal carbon dioxide despite increased minute ventilation provides an early diagnostic clue. Dantrolene sodium is a specific antagonist and should be available wherever general anesthesia is administered. Increased understanding of the clinical manifestation and pathophysiology of MH has led to a decrease in mortality from 80% thirty years ago to less than 5% in 2006.

### References

1. Larach MG, Brandom BW, Allen GC, Gronert GA, Lehman EB. Malignant hyperthermia deaths related to inadequate temperature monitoring, 2007-2012: a report from the North American malignant hyperthermia registry of the malignant hyperthermia association of the United States. *Anesth Analg*. 2014;119(6):1359-1366.
2. Stoelting RK, Hillier SC. *Pharmacology and Physiology in Anesthetic Practice*, 4th ed. Philadelphia, PA: Lippincott Williams and Wilkins; 2006.
3. Halliday NJ. Malignant hyperthermia. *J Craniofac Surg*. 2003;14(5):800-802.
4. Roseberg H, Pollock N, Schiemann A, Bulger T, Stowell K. Malignant hyperthermia: a review. *Orphanet J Rare Dis*. 2015;10:93.

---

**8.** Correct Answer: C

**Rationale:**

Massive oral ingestion of magnesium can occasionally exceed renal excretory capacity, particularly if there is underlying renal insufficiency. Severe hypermagnesemia with life-threatening symptoms has been described with accidental poisoning with Epsom salts (almost 100% magnesium sulfate) in children, in laxative abusers, and during the treatment of a variety of drug overdoses using magnesium as a cathartic. In most such cases, initial treatment consists of cessation of magnesium-containing medications and administration of intravenous isotonic fluids (eg, normal saline) and a loop diuretic (eg, furosemide). Higher diuretic doses may be required in these patients since they have reduced glomerular filtration rate (GFR). Dialysis may be required in patients with severe or symptomatic hypermagnesemia who have end-stage renal disease (GFR less than 15 mL/min/1.73 m²) or who have moderate to severe acute kidney injury. Since preparation for hemodialysis often takes 1 hour or longer, patients with symptomatic hypermagnesemia should be immediately treated with intravenous calcium to reverse the neuromuscular and cardiac effects of hypermagnesemia. The usual dose is 100 to 200 mg of elemental calcium over 5 to 10 minutes.

### References

1. Schelling JR. Fatal hypermagnesemia. *Clin Nephrol*. 2000;53:61.
2. Weng YM, Chen SY, Chen HC, et al. Hypermagnesemia in a constipated female. *J Emerg Med*. 2013;44:e57.

# 107

# TOXINS AND POISONING

Paul S. Jansson and Jarone Lee

1. A 24-year-old male caterer is admitted to the ICU approximately 24 hours after ingesting what he described as a "sweet-tasting" liquid from the canned fuel used to heat the food. Fomepizole therapy was started promptly in the emergency department and toxic alcohol levels are sent to the lab and pending. On arrival to the ICU, he complains of being "in a snowstorm." What is the etiology for his visual changes?

   A. Focal (partial) seizure in the occipital lobe
   B. Direct damage to the retina and optic nerve
   C. Basal ganglia hemorrhage
   D. Vitamin $B_{12}$ (cobalamin) deficiency–induced neuron demyelination
   E. Substance-induced delirium

2. A 32-year-old male auto mechanic is transferred to your ICU from a small local hospital for consideration of dialysis. Two days prior, the patient ingested an entire jug of antifreeze at work on a dare. He was admitted to the local hospital for supportive care but developed progressive oliguric renal failure. On arrival to your hospital, a small amount of dark urine is present in the Foley catheter, which is sent to the lab for analysis. The lab calls you to tell you that there are crystals present in the urine. What is the likely composition of these crystals?

   A. Uric acid
   B. Calcium pyrophosphate
   C. Magnesium ammonium phosphate (struvite)
   D. Calcium oxalate
   E. Cysteine

3. A 28-year-old male is admitted from the emergency department after he was found unconscious at a party. The patient was given two doses of intranasal naloxone empirically with minimal improvement in his mental status. After he began to vomit, he was intubated for airway protection and placed on an infusion of propofol for sedation. His friends told the ED physicians that he ingested several tablets of crushed oxycodone, a "large number" of shots of liquor, and some of his friend's newly distilled moonshine. His ethanol level in the ED was 453 mg/dL and a toxicology screen was positive for oxycodone. On arrival to the unit, your intern suggests treating empirically with fomepizole given the moonshine ingestion. You reply that fomepizole therapy can be deferred at present because of the presence of:

   A. Oxycodone
   B. Propofol
   C. Ethanol
   D. Naloxone
   E. Moonshine

4. A 36-year-old female is admitted to the ICU for altered mental status after ingestion of an unknown substance in a suicide attempt. Laboratory studies in the emergency department were as follows:

   - Sodium 140 mEq/L
   - Potassium 4.0 mEq/L
   - Chloride 100 mEq/L
   - Bicarbonate 24 mEq/L
   - Blood urea nitrogen (BUN) 10 mg/dL
   - Glucose 100 mg/dL
   - Ethanol level 100 mg/dL
   - Measured serum osmolality 340 mOsm/kg

   Which of the following calculated values most strongly supports the diagnosis of a toxic alcohol ingestion?

   A. Osmolal gap >25 mOsm
   B. Osmolal gap <10 mOsm
   C. Anion gap >20 mEq
   D. Anion gap <10 mEq

5. A 41-year-old male was admitted from the emergency department for altered mental status after drinking a bottle of an unknown liquid. A venous blood gas and measures of the serum electrolytes, renal function, and anion gap were all normal and ethanol level was 100 mg/dL. On arrival to the floor, repeat labs demonstrate a measured serum osmolality that is 40 mOsm above the calculated value. The patient is found to be hypotensive and has a pH of 7.05 and an anion gap of 30 mEq. The next osmolal gap is nearly normal. Which of the following alcohols is NOT likely to be the ingested agent?

   A. Methanol
   B. Ethylene glycol
   C. Ethanol
   D. Propylene glycol
   E. Isopropyl alcohol

6. A 48-year-old male is well known to your hospital for his severe alcohol use disorder. In the emergency department a breathalyzer showed an ethanol level of 250 mg/dL, and he was noted to be more somnolent than usual. He then had an episode of emesis streaked with bright red blood. He was intubated for airway protection and admitted to the ICU. In the ICU, an elevated osmolal gap is noted and he is started empirically on fomepizole. The next day, an arterial blood gas is drawn with a pH of 7.38, but the patient does not awaken to participate in a spontaneous awakening trial/spontaneous breathing trial (SAT/SBT). What is the likely substance responsible for his continued altered mental status?

   A. Isopropyl alcohol
   B. Methanol
   C. Propylene glycol
   D. Ethylene glycol
   E. Ethanol

7. A 53-year-old female is well known to your hospital for her near-daily visits for acute alcohol intoxication. After a curious 3-day absence from the emergency department, she is brought in by local paramedics after being found, confused, in a local park. Her heart rate on arrival is 163 bpm and her blood pressure is 210/105. She is noted to be tremulous and diaphoretic and tells the ED that she quit alcohol "cold turkey" 3 days prior. Despite repeated doses of parenteral lorazepam, she continues to be in moderate-to-severe alcohol withdrawal and a continuous infusion of lorazepam is initiated. Assuming that the infusion is titrated to avoid oversedation, what acid-base disturbance would you expect to see with a prolonged infusion of lorazepam?

   A. Respiratory acidosis
   B. Respiratory alkalosis
   C. Metabolic acidosis
   D. Metabolic alkalosis
   E. Primary respiratory alkalosis with secondary metabolic acidosis

8. A 19-year-old male was brought to the emergency department of your hospital by his fraternity brothers after he "chugged" two full bottles of whiskey as part of a pledging ritual. EMS transported the patient to the emergency department where he was intubated for unresponsiveness. Point-of-care glucose was normal, as were serum electrolytes. An ethanol level is measured at 450 mg/dL. He is admitted to the ICU for further management. What is the appropriate next step in management?

   **A.** Immediate gastric lavage via placement of large-bore stomach (Ewald) tube
   **B.** Administration of activated charcoal
   **C.** Administer large volume crystalloid volume resuscitation for hemodilution
   **D.** Continue supportive care
   **E.** Consult nephrology for emergent dialysis

9. A 23-year-old female is admitted to the ICU after ingesting a bottle of medication in a suicide attempt. In the emergency department, the patient complained of abdominal pain and ringing in her ears, and would tell the physicians only that she bought the bottle of "pain medication" from a neighborhood convenience store earlier in the day. On arrival to the ICU, she is tachypneic and lethargic. What acid-base disturbance would you expect on blood gas analysis?

   **A.** Primary metabolic acidosis
   **B.** Primary respiratory alkalosis
   **C.** Mixed metabolic acidosis and respiratory alkalosis
   **D.** Primary metabolic acidosis with compensatory respiratory alkalosis
   **E.** Primary respiratory acidosis with compensatory metabolic acidosis

10. An 18-year-old male is admitted to your ICU after ingesting two "handfuls" of generic pain medications. In the emergency department, acetaminophen was not detected and a salicylate level was 20 mg/dL (therapeutic reference range 10-30 mg/dL). Upon arrival to the ICU, the patient complains of mild nausea and is mildly tachypneic. Lab testing in the ICU is notable for a pH of 7.50 and a repeat salicylate level of 35 mg/dL. What should be your next step in clinical management?

   **A.** Draw a repeat salicylate level in 2 hours
   **B.** Administer intravenous sodium bicarbonate
   **C.** Administer *N*-acetyl-cysteine (Acetadote)
   **D.** Endotracheally intubate the patient for anticipated respiratory failure
   **E.** Discharge the patient

# Chapter 107 ▪ Answers

**1.** Correct Answer: B

**Rationale:**
The patient likely ingested methanol, given the description of a "sweet-tasting" liquid from canned fuel. Methanol is present in many commercial and industrial products including windshield washer fluid, race car fuel, model airplane fuel, and as a byproduct of illicit distillation.

Although fomepizole was started promptly in the emergency department, the patient has likely already metabolized methanol to its toxic byproducts given that the ingestion occurred over 24 hours ago. Methanol is metabolized by alcohol dehydrogenase into formaldehyde and then again by aldehyde dehydrogenase into formic acid. Both formaldehyde and formic acid are toxic to the body.

**Metabolism of Methanol**

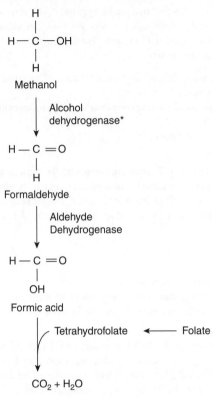

(Figure from Sivilotti MLA. Methanol and ethylene glycol poisoning. In: Grayzel J, ed. *UpToDate*. Waltham, Mass: UpToDate; 2018. www.uptodate.com. Accessed April 2, 2019.)

Formic acid (present in solution as formate) has direct cytotoxic action as a result of its inhibition of intramitochondrial oxygen transport, causing intracellular depletions of ATP. Formate is particularly toxic to the basal ganglia (causing hemorrhage and a Parkinsonian-type movement disorder) and to the retina and optic nerve (causing visual loss, classically described as "being in a snowstorm").

Although ethanol withdrawal can cause seizures, they are usually generalized. Methanol can cause hemorrhage or ischemia in the basal ganglia, but this typically manifests as a Parkinsonian movement disorder. Vitamin $B_{12}$ (cobalamin) deficiency is often seen in individuals with severe alcohol use disorder, but manifests as a megaloblastic anemia and a length-dependent neuronal dysfunction. Finally, the toxic alcohols can cause altered mental status, but visual changes are more likely due to retinal damage and not hallucinations or delirium.

References
1. Kruse JA. Methanol and ethylene glycol intoxication. *Crit Care Clin*. 2012;28:661-711.
2. McMartin K. Antidotes for poisoning by alcohols that form toxic metabolites. *Br J Clin Pharmacol*. 2016;81(2):505-515.
3. Kruse JA. Ethanol, methanol, and ethylene glycol. In: Vincent J-L, ed. *Textbook of Critical Care*. 7th ed. New York City: Elsevier; 2017:1270-1281.

**2.** Correct Answer: D

**Rationale:**
The patient likely ingested ethylene glycol, which lowers the boiling point of water and is a common ingredient in antifreeze. Its sweet taste contributes to a relatively high number of pediatric and pet animal overdoses. Like methanol, ethylene glycol is relatively nontoxic but is metabolized into substances that can directly harm the body.

The primary toxic metabolite of ethylene glycol is oxalic acid. Oxalic acid can bind directly to calcium in the blood and then precipitate out of solution as calcium oxalate. The most common site of precipitation is within the kidney, where it can cause renal tubular necrosis and renal failure. Calcium oxalate can also precipitate in the lungs, causing pulmonary edema, and in the heart, causing myocardial depression. In addition, precipitation of calcium out of the blood can cause hypocalcemia.

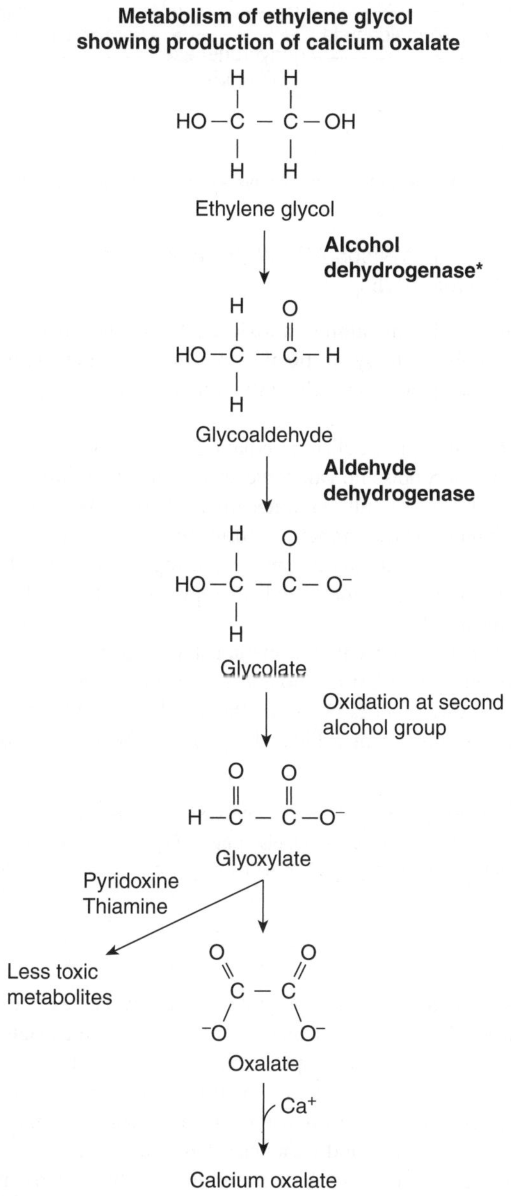

**Metabolism of ethylene glycol
showing production of calcium oxalate**

(Figure from Sivilotti MLA. Methanol and ethylene glycol poisoning. In: Grayzel J, ed. *UpToDate.* Waltham, Mass: UpToDate; 2018. www.uptodate.com. Accessed April 2, 2019.)

Uric acid and calcium pyrophosphate are common causes of gout and pseudogout, respectively, but are not typically seen with ethylene glycol overdose. Although magnesium ammonium phosphate (struvite) and cysteine are seen in some forms of kidney stones, they are not characteristic of ethylene glycol overdose.

References

1. Kruse JA. Methanol and ethylene glycol intoxication. *Crit Care Clin.* 2012;28:661-711.
2. McMartin K. Antidotes for poisoning by alcohols that form toxic metabolites. *Br J Clin Pharmacol.* 2016;81(2):505-515.
3. Kruse JA. Ethanol, methanol, and ethylene glycol. In: Vincent J-L, ed. *Textbook of Critical Care.* 7th ed. New York City: Elsevier; 2017:1270-1281.

**3.** Correct Answer: C

**Rationale:**
Fomepizole (4-methyl-1*H*-pyrazole) is a competitive inhibitor of alcohol dehydrogenase (ADH). For methanol and ethylene glycol, toxic effects of the alcohols occur not from the parent alcohol but from the metabolized intermediates (formic acid/formate in methanol and oxalic acid in ethylene glycol). These intermediates are typically produced from metabolism of the parent compound by ADH and then aldehyde dehydrogenase (ALDH). Further metabolism converts the toxic compounds into nontoxic breakdown products.

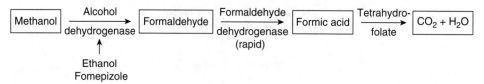

Metabolism of methanol. Fomepizole and ethanol both serve as competitive inhibitors of methanol at alcohol dehydrogenase.

(Figure from Suchard JR. Methanol. In: Wolfson AB, ed. *Harwood-Nuss' Clinical Practice of Emergency Medicine*. Philadelphia, PA: Wolters Kluwer; 2015.)

The purpose of fomepizole in the ingestion of a toxic alcohol is to decrease the production of toxic metabolites while allowing for later metabolic pathways to break down the toxic metabolites before they reach toxic concentrations. By inhibiting ADH, fomepizole slows the initial metabolism of the parent compound, allowing for downstream metabolism.

Like the toxic alcohols, the initial metabolism of ethanol is via ADH. In fact, ethanol has a 10- to 20-fold higher affinity for ADH than the toxic alcohols and can serve as a competitive inhibitor to the toxic alcohols at ADH. At ethanol levels above 100 mg/dL, ethanol fully saturates the ADH receptor, producing the same therapeutic effect as fomepizole. Interestingly, ethanol was traditionally used in the treatment of toxic alcohol ingestion before the creation of fomepizole; however, it is difficult to dose and sclerosing to the veins. Therefore, in the presence of ethanol co-ingestion with one of the toxic alcohols, fomepizole therapy can safely be delayed until the ethanol is metabolized to a level of approximately 100 mg/dL.

Oxycodone is likely contributing to his altered mental status and thus not a reason to defer therapy. Naloxone can serve as a reversal agent for opioids but has no effect on alcohol ingestion. Although propofol can be useful in the treatment of alcohol withdrawal, it does not affect the metabolism of the toxic alcohols and should not replace fomepizole as treatment. Finally, moonshine is likely the source of the patient's toxic alcohol—methanol—ingestion.

### References

1. McMartin K. Antidotes for poisoning by alcohols that form toxic metabolites. *Br J Clin Pharmacol*. 2016;81(2):505-515.
2. Brent J. Fomepizole for ethylene glycol and methanol poisoning. *N Engl J Med*. 2009;360(21):2216-2223.
3. Mycyk MB, Leikin JB. Antidote review: fomepizole for methanol poisoning. *Am J Ther*. 2003;10(1):68-70.

---

**4. Correct Answer: A**

**Rationale:**

Serum concentration levels of the toxic alcohols are not routinely available at most hospitals in time to guide management; they are more commonly used as confirmatory test. Therefore, the diagnosis of a toxic alcohol management depends on the clinical history, a high index of suspicion, and classic laboratory findings.

The toxic alcohols are rapidly absorbed from the gastrointestinal tract to the bloodstream as osmotically active substances. Therefore, measurement of the serum osmolality at or near the time of ingestion can reveal the presence of an osmotically active substance in the blood via an elevated osmolal gap.

The osmolal gap calculates the difference in the concentration of the known osmotically active agents in the blood and the actual concentration of osmotically active agents in the blood (Osmol gap = Measured osmolality – Calculated serum osmolality). A significant difference between the measured serum osmolality and the calculated serum osmolality implies that there is an "unmeasured osmol," which is likely a toxic alcohol. Although there is some individual variation in the osmolal gap, normal value is <10 and a gap of >25 increases specificity for a toxic ingestion in the proper clinical context.

The calculated osmolality is based on the concentration of the major osmotically active agents in blood: sodium, blood urea nitrogen (BUN), glucose, and ethanol and is calculated as follows:

$$Calculated\ osmolality = 2 \times Na^{+} + \frac{BUN}{2.8} + \frac{Glucose}{18} + \frac{Ethanol}{4.6}$$

In this case, the calculated osmolality would be as follows:

$$Calculated\ osmolality = 2 \times [140] + \frac{[10]}{2.8} + \frac{[100]}{18} + \frac{[100]}{4.6}$$

$$Calculated\ osmolality = 280 + 3.8 + 5.6 + 21.7$$

$$Calculated\ osmolality = 311.1$$

The osmolal gap is then calculated as:

$$Osmolal\ gap = Measured\ osmolality - Calculated\ osmolality$$

$$Osmolal\ gap = 340 - 311.1$$

$$Osmolal\ gap = 28.9$$

In the context of altered mental status, known ingestion of an unknown substance, and an osmolal gap of >25, a presumptive diagnosis of toxic alcohol ingestion can be made and treatment should be initiated while awaiting levels of the toxic alcohol from the lab. Although an elevated anion gap can be present after metabolism of some of the toxic alcohols (eg, methanol, ethylene glycol, and propylene glycol), the anion gap is normal in this patient, likely because of the recent ingestion.

### References

1. Kraut JA. Diagnosis of toxic alcohols: limitations of present methods. *Clin Toxicol.* 2015;53(7):589-595.
2. Kraut JA, Kurtz I. Toxic alcohol ingestions: clinical features, diagnosis, and management. *Clin J Am Soc Nephrol.* 2008;3(1):208-225.
3. Liamis G, Fillippatos TD, Liontos A, Elisaf MS. Serum osmolal gap in clinical practice: usefulness and limitations. *Postgrad Med.* 2017;129(4):456-459.
4. Nelson ME. Toxic alcohols. In: Walls RM, ed. *Rosen's Emergency Medicine – Concepts and Clinical Practice.* 9th ed. Philadelphia: Saunders; 2018:1829-1837.

**5.** Correct Answer: E

**Rationale:**

On arrival to the hospital, the patient has an elevated osmolal gap but a normal pH. All of the toxic alcohols are rapidly absorbed from the gastrointestinal tract and present in the blood as osmotically active compounds, which explains the initially elevated osmolol gap. (For more explanation of the osmolal gap, please see question 4.) A high osmolal gap in the setting of an ingested liquid is highly suspicious for ingestion of a toxic alcohol. If there is a delay in treatment because of a lack of fomepizole, the patient is able to metabolize the parent compound, which decreases the measured serum osmolality, explaining the near normalization of the osmolal gap. However, all of the toxic alcohols except for isopropyl alcohol (methanol, ethylene glycol, and propylene glycol) are metabolized into organic acids (formic acid, oxalic acid, and lactic acid, respectively) and produce a metabolic acidosis. In addition, because of its interference with mitochondrial respiration, methanol can produce a profound metabolic acidosis both by direct production of formic acid and by shifting cellular metabolism to an anaerobic process. Isopropyl alcohol is metabolized to acetone, which is a ketone, and is the only toxic alcohol that does not produce a metabolic acidosis.

Isopropyl alcohol (isopropanol) is metabolized by alcohol dehydrogenase (ADH) to acetone, a ketone.

(Figure from Sivilotti MLA. Isopropyl alcohol poisoning. In: Grayzel J, ed. *UpToDate.* Waltham, Mass: UpToDate; 2018. www.uptodate.com. Accessed April 2, 2019.)

The characteristic laboratory findings of methanol, ethylene glycol, and propylene glycol ingestion are described through the "mountain diagram." Initially, an elevated osmolal gap predominates whereas the anion gap is normal. Later in the ingestion, an elevated anion gap predominates whereas the osmolal gap is normal.

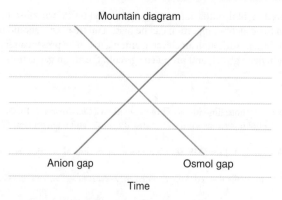

Mountain diagram

Anion gap          Osmol gap

Time

In metabolism of methanol, ethylene glycol and propylene glycol, the anion gap increases over time while the osmol gap decreases. Isopropyl alcohol (isopropanol) is metabolized by alcohol dehydrogenase (ADH) to acetone, a ketone.

### References

1. Kraut JA, Kurtz I. Toxic alcohol ingestions: clinical features, diagnosis, and management. *Clin J Am Soc Nephrol.* 2008;3(1):208-225.
2. Slaughter RJ, Mason RW, Beasley DM, Vale JA, Schep LJ. Isopropanol poisoning. *Clin Toxicol.* 2014;52(5):470-478.
3. Nelson ME. Toxic alcohols. In: Walls RM, ed. *Rosen's Emergency Medicine – Concepts and Clinical Practice.* 9th ed. Philadelphia: Saunders; 2018:1829-1837.

---

**6.** Correct Answer: A

**Rationale:**

Isopropyl alcohol is a common ingredient in some rubbing alcohols and nail polish removers. When ingested, it is a potent central nervous system (CNS) depressant, approximately two to four times more potent than the same dose of ethanol. In addition to its increased potency, the duration of action is approximately two to four times as long as ethanol.

Unlike the other toxic alcohols, where various metabolites are responsible for the toxic effects, isopropyl alcohol itself is responsible for the CNS depression. Therefore, inhibition of its metabolism via ethanol or fomepizole serves only to prolong the duration of action and is not indicated.

In this case, both the co-ingestion of ethanol and the iatrogenic administration of fomepizole have combined to maintain the toxic concentration of isopropyl alcohol in the blood and consequently the CNS depression and resultant altered mental status.

Isopropyl alcohol may be ingested in place of ethanol in an attempt to become inebriated and transdermal toxicity has been reported by "sponge bathing" in children. It is a potent gastrointestinal irritant when ingested enterically and may produce hemorrhagic gastritis. It is metabolized into acetone and can produce a characteristic "fruity" odor to the breath. Because acetone is a ketone, not an organic acid, metabolism of isopropyl alcohol does not produce the characteristic metabolic acidosis seen with other toxic alcohols.

Although ethanol may be contributing to the patient's altered mental status, isopropyl alcohol is a more potent CNS depressant and is likely the substance responsible for his altered mental status. Methanol, ethylene glycol, and propylene glycol can all produce an elevated anion gap but do not produce the same hemorrhagic gastritis or altered mental status as isopropyl alcohol.

### References

1. Kraut JA, Kurtz I. Toxic alcohol ingestions: clinical features, diagnosis, and management. *Clin J Am Soc Nephrol.* 2008;3(1):208-225.
2. Slaughter RJ, Mason RW, Beasley DM, Vale JA, Schep LJ. Isopropanol poisoning. *Clin Toxicol.* 2014;52(5):470-478.
3. Nelson ME. Toxic alcohols. In: Walls RM, ed. *Rosen's Emergency Medicine – Concepts and Clinical Practice.* 9th ed. Philadelphia: Saunders; 2018:1829-1837.

---

**7.** Correct Answer: C

**Rationale:**

Intravenous lorazepam is most commonly mixed in a solution of propylene glycol. Propylene glycol is metabolized by alcohol dehydrogenase (ADH) to lactaldehyde and then by aldehyde dehydrogenase (ALDH) into lactic acid. As an organic acid, lactic acid produces a metabolic acidosis.

Commonly used ICU medications that are mixed in propylene glycol include lorazepam (Ativan), diazepam (Valium), phenytoin (Dilantin), and phenobarbital. Prolonged or high-dose infusions of this medication can produce a lactic (metabolic) acidosis and resulting organ dysfunction including hypotension and dysrhythmias. Most propylene glycol overdoses are therefore iatrogenic and should be in the differential of any new lactic acidosis seen in the ICU. The treatment is supportive and involves discontinuing the offending medication.

Propylene Glycol is metabolized directly into lactic acid by alcohol dehydrogenase (ADH).

(Figure from Suchard JR. Isopropanol, acetone and other glycols. In: Wolfson AB, ed. *Harwood-Nuss' Clinical Practice of Emergency Medicine.* Philadelphia, PA: Wolters Kluwer; 2015.)

### References

1. Zosel A, Egelhoff E, Heard K. Severe lactic acidosis from iatrogenic propylene glycol overdose. *Pharmacother.* 2010;30(2):219.
2. Neale BW, Mesler EL, Young M, Rebuck JA, Weise WJ. Propylene glycol-induced lactic acidosis in a patient with normal renal function: a proposed mechanism and monitoring recommendations. *Ann Pharmacother.* 2005;39(10):1732-1736.
3. Horinek EL, Kiser TH, Fish DN, MacLaren R. Propylene glycol accumulation in critically ill patients receiving continuous intravenous lorazepam infusions. *Ann Pharmacother.* 2009;43(12):1964-1971.

### 8. Correct Answer: D

**Rationale:**

Ethanol is one of the most commonly used and abused intoxicants in the world. Most of the morbidity and mortality in the acute phase of ethanol ingestion is from accidental injury such as trauma. Ingestion of large volumes of alcohol or co-ingestion with other medications such as benzodiazepines or opioids can cause respiratory suppression and death. For most ethanol intoxication, clinical observation and ruling out other causes of altered mental status such as hypoglycemia is the mainstay of treatment. However, some patients may require tracheal intubation for airway protection and admission to the ICU.

Ethanol is absorbed quickly from the gastrointestinal tract into the bloodstream, typically within the first hour after ingestion. Therefore, gastric lavage is rarely indicated, even for acute intoxication, as it requires intubation and serves only to increase the risk of aspiration. Although activated charcoal can be used for certain poisonings immediately after ingestion, its use is contraindicated in patients with altered mental status. Furthermore, activated charcoal does not bind ethanol.

Many patients with alcohol intoxication will present with some aspect of hypovolemia due to increased diuresis from ethanol. However, administration of intravenous fluids does not aid in the metabolism of ethanol and large-volume crystalloid administration is not indicated in the management of acute alcohol ingestions. Additionally, large-volume crystalloid administration could lead to profound metabolic acidosis and electrolyte disturbances.

Alcohol dehydrogenase becomes quickly saturated at even low concentrations of ethanol, therefore elimination follows zero-order kinetics and a constant amount of alcohol is eliminated over time (typically 15-20 mg/dL per hour). People with alcohol abuse disorders typically metabolize alcohol at a higher rate (approximately 25-35 mg/dL per hour). Although hemodialysis can remove ethanol, it is typically reserved only for extreme cases causing severe hemodynamic instability.

### References

1. Darracq MA, Ly BT. Ethanol. In: Wolfson AB, ed. *Harwood-Nuss' Clinical Practice of Emergency Medicine.* 6th ed. Philadelphia: Lippincott Williams & Wilkins; 2015:1331-1336.
2. Finnell JT. Alcohol-related disease. In: Walls RM, ed. *Rosen's Emergency Medicine – Concepts and Clinical Practice.* 9th ed. Philadelphia: Saunders; 2018:1838-1851.
3. Cederbaum AI. Alcohol metabolism. *Clin Liver Dis.* 2012;16(4):667-685.

### 9. Correct Answer: C

**Rationale:**

The patient likely ingested salicylates, probably from aspirin (acetylsalicylic acid). Of the other common over-the-counter pain relievers, acetaminophen (Tylenol) manifests its toxicity with delayed liver damage. Common nonsteroidal anti-inflammatory medications (NSAIDs) such as ibuprofen (Motrin, Advil) or naproxen (Aleve) are typically well-tolerated, except in very large overdoses (above 100 mg/kg). Opioid pain medications, while not available over-the-counter in the United States, typically present with respiratory suppression.

Salicylate toxicity is most often seen in the context of aspirin overdoses but is also present in other common household products such as Pepto-Bismol (bismuth subsalicylate), topical salicylate creams (Aspercreme, Bengay), and oil of wintergreen, which can be particularly concentrated.

Initially, salicylates directly stimulate the medullary respiratory center, producing tachypnea and a metabolic alkalosis. As the salicylate is metabolized, it interferes with aerobic metabolism by uncoupling oxidative phosphorylation in the mitochondria, producing a metabolic acidosis.

In addition to the classic metabolic disturbances, salicylates initially provoke gastrointestinal distress with nausea, vomiting, and diarrhea, as well as tachypnea. As the poisoning progresses, tinnitus (ringing in the ears) occurs because of both central and peripheral effects. Late signs of salicylate toxicity include altered mental status, cerebral and pulmonary edema, hyperthermia, seizures, and ultimately death from cardiovascular collapse.

### References

1. O'Malley GF. Emergency department management of the salicylate-poisoned patient. *Emerg Med Clin North Am.* 2007;25(2):333-346.
2. Pearlman BL, Gambhir R. Salicylate intoxication: a clinical review. *Postgrad Med.* 2009;121(4):162-168.
3. Hatten BW. Aspirin and nonsteroidal agents. In: Walls RM, ed. *Rosen's Emergency Medicine: Concepts and Clinical Practice.* 9th ed. Philadelphia: Saunders; 2018:1858-1862.

---

**10.** Correct Answer: B

**Rationale:**

As evidenced by the rising salicylate level, the patient ingested aspirin (acetylsalicylic acid). Interestingly, aspirin tablets can aggregate in the stomach in overdose, forming a bezoar and delaying absorption. Given the rising salicylate level, empiric treatment for salicylate overdose should be initiated.

The mainstay of treatment for salicylate poisoning is administration of sodium bicarbonate. Because salicylic acid is a weak acid, alkalinization of the urine shifts the form of salicylic acid to the deprotonated form, "trapping" the ion in the urine and increasing excretion. Raising the serum pH limits tissue distribution by the same mechanism, "trapping" the ionic form in the bloodstream and out of sensitive areas such as the central nervous system. Given the rising salicylate level, high index of suspicion, and development of tachypnea, empiric sodium bicarbonate should be administered. Note that an elevated pH should not be seen as a contraindication to initiation of sodium bicarbonate therapy. In severe overdoses, hemodialysis may be indicated.

Although the initial stage of salicylate toxicity manifests as a respiratory alkalosis due to direct stimulation of the respiratory centers of the medulla, a profound metabolic acidosis develops later in the ingestion as a result of decoupling of oxidative phosphorylation. The minute ventilation required for respiratory compensation can be very high; therefore, endotracheal intubation should be reserved only for severe cases and should be performed quickly because of the risk for worsening acidosis from inadequate ventilation and resulting cardiovascular collapse.

Monitoring of the salicylate level can help guide therapy; it should be measured every 2 hours in an acute overdose until it drops below the toxic threshold. As the salicylate level is increasing, discharging the patient is premature.

### References

1. O'Malley GF. Emergency department management of the salicylate-poisoned patient. *Emerg Med Clin North Am.* 2007;25(2):333-346.
2. Pearlman BL, Gambhir R. Salicylate intoxication: a clinical review. *Postgrad Med.* 2009;121(4):162-168.
3. Hatten BW. Aspirin and nonsteroidal agents. In: Walls RM, ed. *Rosen's Emergency Medicine: Concepts and Clinical Practice.* 9th ed. Philadelphia: Saunders; 2018:1858-1862.
4. Dissanayake VL, Aks SE. Salicylates. In: Wolfson AB, ed. *Harwood-Nuss' Clinical Practice of Emergency Medicine.* 6th ed. Philadelphia: Lippincott Williams & Wilkins; 2015:1353-1357.

# 108

# DRUG OVERDOSES

DaMarcus Baymon and Jarone Lee

1. A 22-year-old previously healthy male was brought to the emergency department with nausea, vomiting, and a decline in mental status. T: 37°C, HR: 100, BP: 135/90, RR: 20, SpO$_2$: 92% on room air. Physical examination revealed pain in the RUQ upon palpation with slight jaundice. While in the emergency department, his mental status continued to decline precipitously. AST = 5116, ALT = 4300, PT-INR = 2.1, total bilirubin = 2.1. The patient was transferred to the ICU. What medication could be started empirically?

   A. Methylprednisolone
   B. N-acetylcysteine
   C. Hepatitis B immunoglobulin
   D. Heparin
   E. Azathioprine

2. An 84-year-old female with a history of hypertension and dementia presents to the emergency department with a fever, rigors, and chills. Vital signs: T: 38.9°C, HR: 110, BP: 70/50, RR: 20, SpO$_2$: 99%. After receiving 2.5 L of crystalloid solution in addition to broad-spectrum antibiotic therapy (cefepime, metronidazole, and vancomycin), she remains hypotensive and is started on Levophed. After several days in the ICU, the patient is noticeably more confused. She had a brief generalized seizure that was treated with Ativan. MRI and LP were negative. EEG showed triphasic waves with diffuse slowing. What medication may have caused the patient's mental status changes in the context of a negative neurological workup?

   A. Flagyl
   B. Vancomycin
   C. Cefepime
   D. Levophed
   E. Ativan

3. A 23-year-old male with hypermobile joints and vision loss was admitted to the ICU after a CT scan was concerning for an aortic dissection. He was placed on IV medications to control his HR and blood pressure. Over the next 24 hours he became lethargic, tachypneic, and short of breath. T: 37.1°C, HR: 62, BP: 115/70, RR: 30, SpO$_2$: 99% on room air. VBG: 7.10/28/90. Lactate: 6.

| 135 | 100 | 10 | |
|---|---|---|---|
| | | | 100 |
| 4 | 12 | 1.0 | |

What medication is causing this patient's metabolic derangement?

   A. Esmolol
   B. Nitroglycerin
   C. Labetalol
   D. Nitroprusside
   E. Nicardipine

4. A 47-year-old apple farmer presented to the emergency department after she was found down. In the trauma bay, her vital signs were: T: 36°C, HR: 35, BP: 105/70, RR: 35, SpO$_2$: 80% on room air. Physical examination was remarkable for wet and clammy skin with diminished pulses, bilateral wheezing, and copious secretions. She was intubated with rocuronium and etomidate. EMT and nursing began to feel ill with diaphoresis. Which pharmacological agent(s) will improve this patient's symptoms based on her underlying clinical syndrome?

   A. Repeat 0.5 mg of atropine
   B. Physostigmine
   C. Continuous epinephrine infusion
   D. Transcutaneous pacemaker
   E. 4 mg of atropine + pralidoxime chloride (2-PAM)

5. A 24-year-old previously healthy female graduate student has suffered from multiple witnessed seizures in the ED and is intubated for airway protection. Per report, EMS said they found multiple unidentified pill bottles next to her bed. Upon transfer to the ICU she is noted to have another seizure that occurred after she went into a pulseless wide complex tachycardia. ECG was obtained and revealed: PR 150, QRS 175, QTc 500 with right axis deviation, wide S in leads I and aVL, and deep terminal R in lead aVR. On examination, the patient has dilated pupils and a palpable mass in the suprapubic region. What is the most appropriate next step in treating this patient?

   A. Ammonium chloride
   B. Lidocaine
   C. Sodium bicarbonate
   D. Physostigmine
   E. Intralipid Infusion

# Chapter 108 ▪ Answers

1. Correct Answer: B

**Rationale:**
Based on the initial presentation of this patient, high clinical concern for acute hepatic failure exists. History is limited to the mental status of this patient, but the differential for acute hepatic failure includes acetaminophen toxicity, ischemic liver, hepatic thrombosis/veno-occlusive disease, autoimmune hepatitis, infectious hepatitis, drug toxicity, HELLP syndrome (hemolysis, elevated liver enzymes, and low platelets) if pregnant. Based on age and likelihood, N-acetylcysteine would be the most reasonable medication to start. Acetaminophen toxicity is the most common cause of acute hepatic failure in the United States. Acetaminophen ingestions greater than 10 g or 150 mg/kg are most commonly associated with acute hepatic failure. There are four stages of acute acetaminophen toxicity, which occur over 30 minutes to 4 weeks. The stages progress from nausea, vomiting, confusion to severe transaminitis with AST predominance, mild bilirubinemia, hypoglycemia, prolonged PT/INR with associated stupor. Patients are most vulnerable during stage III acute acetaminophen toxicity with associated stupor, coagulopathy, and metabolic derangement. If the patient can make it to stage IV/recovery phase, then full recovery without long-term sequelae is likely. Acute kidney injury can also be associated with acetaminophen toxicity, usually in the form of acute tubular necrosis. However, if the patient becomes oliguric, hepatorenal syndrome (HRS) must be considered and the patient should be transferred to a facility where liver transplantation is possible.

   Acetaminophen level should be checked at 4 hours and plotted on the Rumack nomogram. If the acetaminophen level exists beyond the treatment line, treat with N-acetylcysteine. N-acetylcysteine replenishes reduced glutathione and detoxifying NAPQI products created by the CYP2E1 enzyme that lead to oxidative damage to the liver. IV NAC should be started at 150 mg/kg or PO NAC at 140 mg/kg based on a 72-hour protocol. When administering NAC, monitor for a non-IgE–mediated anaphylactoid reaction.

   Methylprednisolone and azathioprine are used to treat autoimmune hepatitis, which is less likely in the patient's gender and age group. Hepatitis B immunoglobulin treats acute hepatitis B exposure. Heparin treats veno-occlusive disease and Budd-Chiari syndrome seen in patients with hypercoagulable history.

References
1. Wendon J, Bernal W. Acute liver failure. *N Engl J Med*. 2013;369:2525-2534.
2. Buckley NA, Dawson AH, Isbister GK. Treatments for paracetamol poisoning. *Br Med J*. 2016;353:i2579.
3. Hodgman MJ, Garrad AR. A review of acetaminophen poisoning. *Crit Care Clin*. 2012;28:499-516.

4. Mazer M, Perrone J. Acetaminophen-induced nephrotoxicity: pathophysiology, clinical manifestations, and management. *J Med Toxicol.* 2008;4(1):2.

5. Chiew AL, Gluud C, Brok J, Buckley NA. Interventions for paracetamol (acetaminophen) overdose. *Cochrane Database Syst Rev.* 2018;2:CD003328.

6. Andrade KQ, Moura FA, dos Santos JM, et al. Oxidative stress and inflammation in hepatic diseases: therapeutic possibilities of N-acetylcysteine. *Int J Mol Sci.* 2015;16(12):30269-30308.

## 2. Correct Answer: C

**Rationale:**

Cefepime, along with other cephalosporins, is a well-known neurotoxic antibiotic causing symptoms ranging from tardive dyskinesia, nonconvulsive status epilepticus, encephalopathy, confusion, and lethargy. Patients with impaired renal function are at increased risk for cefepime neurotoxicity. Cephalosporins have increased CNS penetration, leading to an imbalance of GABAergic and glutamatergic neurotransmission. Aminoglycosides may cause ototoxicity, peripheral neuropathy, and neuromuscular blockade. Carbapenems may cause seizures, myoclonus, and headache, whereas penicillins may cause tremors and tardive seizures. Fluoroquinolones are also known neurotoxic agents that may lead to encephalopathy and seizures. Antibiotic-related neurotoxicity is associated with increased mortality; therefore early diagnosis is key. Metronidazole may cause encephalopathy in patients, but patients usually have cerebellar signs and exhibit MRI abnormalities. The neurotoxic effects of metronidazole occur over weeks.

Vancomycin may cause red-man syndrome, acute renal failure, ototoxicity, and neutropenia. Vancomycin is not classically associated with neurotoxicity. Levophed is known to cause tachyarrhythmias. Ativan may cause sedation and delirium; however, a single dose should not cause persistent symptoms.

References:

1. Grill MF, Maganti RK. Neurotoxic effects associated with antibiotic use: management considerations. *Br J Clin Pharmacol.* 2011;72(3):381-393.

2. Bhattacharyya S, Darby RR, Raibagkar P, Castro LN, Berkowitz AL. Antibiotic-associated encephalopathy. *Neurology.* 2016;86(10):963-971.

3. Tamma PD, Avdic E, Li DX, Dzintars K, Cosgrove SE. Association of adverse events with antibiotic use in hospitalized patients. *JAMA Intern Med.* 2017;177(9):1308.

4. Bruniera FR, Ferreira FM, Saviolli LRM, et al. The use of vancomycin with its therapeutic and adverse effects: a review. *Eur Rev Med Pharmacol Sci.* 2015;19(4):694-700.

## 3. Correct Answer: D

**Rationale:**

This patient has an anion gap metabolic acidosis with a high lactate and normal renal function and glucose; tachypnea and shortness of breath is the respiratory compensation component. Nitroprusside is an antihypertensive that is known to cause cyanide toxicity when metabolized. Cyanide inhibits the function of cytochrome c leading to increased lactic acid production secondary to a decrease in aerobic metabolism. The degree of lactic acidosis correlates with the degree of toxicity. During nitroprusside administration, cyanide is converted to thiocyanate and exerted in the urine. The metabolism to thiocyanate occurs in the mitochondria. Renal insufficiency is an independent risk factor for developing cyanide toxicity during nitroprusside use.

Early cyanide toxicity presents with tachydysrhythmias, respiratory distress but can progress to flash pulmonary edema, seizures, and cardiopulmonary arrest. The skin may be bright red and the patient's breath may have a bitter almond scent. Nitroprusside can also prevent hypoxia-mediated vasoconstriction, leading to sustained V/Q mismatch, especially in those with congestive heart failure. Thrombocytopenia may occur as well.

Treatment includes thiosulfate, amyl-nitrite, and hydroxocobalamin. Thiosulfate produces a more renally excretable thiocyanate, which prevents cyanide and thiocyante buildup. Amyl-nitrite produces methemoglobin, to which cyanide will have a higher affinity for. Hydroxocobalamin can be used in the treatment and prophylaxis of cyanide toxicity by creating cyanocobalamin, which is excreted in the urine.

Nicardipine, esmolol, and labetalol toxicity is associated with hypotension and bradycardia. Nitroglycerin can be associated with severe hypotension when used in patients with recent myocardial infarctions who have taken sildenafil.

References

1. Hottinger DG, Beebe DS, Kozhimannil T, et al. Sodium nitroprusside in 2014: a clinical concepts review. *J Anaesthesiol Clin Pharmacol.* 2014;30(4):462-471.

2. Reade MC, Davies SR, Morley PT, Dennett J, Jacobs IC. Review article: management of cyanide poisoning. *Emerg Med Australas.* 2012;24(3):225-238.

3. Thompson JP, Marrs TC. Hydroxocobalamin in cyanide poisoning. *Clin Toxicol.* 2012;50(10):875-885.

4. Ghatak T, Samanta S. Methanol toxicity following esmolol infusion in a post-operative case of pheochromocytoma resection. *Saudi J Anesth.* 2013;7(4):484.

**4.** Correct Answer: E

**Rationale:**

Based on the constellation of signs of symptoms, this patient has suspected organophosphate poisoning from farming her land. Organophosphate poisoning presents with a cholinergic toxidrome of diarrhea, urination, miosis, bradycardia, bronchorrhea, bronchoconstriction, emesis, lacrimation, salivation (DUMBBBELSS) from action at muscarinic receptors via phosphorylation of serine side group, leading to inactivation of acetylcholinesterase enzyme. The inhibition has varying degrees of reversibility depending on the type of organophosphate that leads to a cholinergic syndrome. Patients can become quite hypotensive secondary to the extreme bradycardia and the degree of bronchoconstriction can lead to severe hypoxia. Bronchoconstriction, bronchorrhea, and bradycardia are important contributors to the mortality from organophosphate poisoning. However, if the nicotinic receptors are overstimulated in the sympathetic pathway, then patients may present with tachycardia, diaphoresis, and hypertension. If nicotinic receptors at the neuromuscular junction are affected, then patient may present with muscle paralysis and fasciculations.

Treatment of organophosphate poisoning includes atropine (a cholinergic antagonist), pralidoxime (2-PAM), prompt airway management, which may include intubation for securing the airway, and diazepam to treat seizures. Gastric lavage may be considered if the patient ingested an organophosphate within 1 hour of presentation to the emergency department. Pralidoxime (2-PAM) aids in the regeneration of acetylcholinerase by breaking the covalent bond that leads to the inactivity of acetylcholinerase. Atropine is titrated to heart rate and respiratory secretions. An infusion of pralidoxime should be continued until the patient is extubated or at least 12 hours have elapsed without the need for administration of atropine. Diazepam is the preferred agent in the management of seizures in patients with organophosphate poisoning. Patients should be monitored for a delayed cholinergic syndrome, which may have a delayed presentation up to weeks after the original exposure secondary to fat solubility of organophosphates.

It can be appropriate to repeat 0.5 mg of atropine, initate transcutaneous pacing, or consider an epinephrine infusion in the context of hypotension and bradycardia; however, high-dose atropine and 2-PAM would be the most appropriate next step in treatment. Physostigmine would worsen this patient's condition because acetylcholinerase would be further inhibited. This would lead to further elevated levels of acetylcholine at the synapse.

### References

1. Eddleston M. Novel clinical toxicology and pharmacology of organophosphorus insecticide self-poisoning. *Annu Rev Pharmacol Toxicol.* 2019;59(1):341-360.
2. Meddleston M, Buckley NA, Eyer P, Dawson AH. Management of acute organophosphorus pesticide poisoning. *Lancet.* 2008;371(9612):597-607.
3. Neumar RW, Otto CW, Link MS, et al. Part 8: adult advanced cardiovascular life support: 2010 American Heart Association Guidelines for cardiopulmonary resuscitation and emergency cardiovascular care. *Circulation.* 2010;122(18_suppl_3).

**5.** Correct Answer: C

**Rationale:**

Based on the clinical scenario, symptoms, and ECG findings, this patient likely overdosed on tricyclic antidepressants (TCAs). Examples of TCAs are nortriptyline, amitriptyline, doxepin, clomipramine, and imipramine. TCAs are weakly basic compounds that inhibit sodium channels, alpha-1-receptors, cholinergic receptors, histamine receptors, and serotonin and/or norepinephrine reuptake. Patients who overdose usually present with sinus tachycardia, hypotension, delirium, seizures, respiratory depression, dry mouth, urinary retention, and hyperthermia. Ventricular arrhythmias and bradycardia are also possible. Gastric lavage can be trialed if the ingestion occurred within 1 hour of arrival to a treating facility. First-line treatment of hypotension caused by TCA overdose is IV fluids; however, secondary to the cardiac effects of TCAs, sodium bicarbonate would be an appropriate next choice for this patient. Sodium bicarbonate is indicated when the pH <7.1, QRS >100, R/S ratio in aVR >0.7 hypotension, and/or arrhythmia events occur. Other ECG findings include QTc >415 to 430, wide/deep S in leads I and aVL, and acute right axis deviation. QRS >100 is predictive of seizure, whereas QRS >160 is predictive of ventricular arrhythmias. Although there are classic ECG findings as described above, sinus tachycardia is the most common ECG finding. If sodium bicarbonate is given, one must target a sodium concentration of 150 to 155 and pH of 7.5 to 7.55 and closely monitor for hypokalemia. Additionally, hyperventilation can aid in alkalizing the serum pH. Sodium bicarbonate displaces the TCA molecule from the cardiac myocytes as well as leading to decreased free TCA molecules in serum by increasing protein binding capacity. Large volumes of sodium bicarbonate or continuous infusions are necessary at times to reverse the cardiotoxicity. Magnesium sulfate can be helpful in refractory arrhythmias with associated long QTc. Benzodiazepines are used to treat seizures in TCA overdose as compared with phenytoin, which should be avoided secondary to its proarrhythmic effects in setting of TCA overdose.

Ammonium chloride acidifies the serum leading to more deleterious effects from TCAs owing to proarrhythmic nature in an acidic environment. Lidocaine is considered an adjunctive treatment of arrhythmias if the patient remains hemodynamically unstable despite initial treatment with bicarbonate. In theory, physostigmine would be appropriate for anticholinergic syndrome, but multiple studies have recommended to exclude its use in TCA overdose. In patients with suspected local anesthetic toxicity and continued circulatory collapse despite fluids, intralipid infusion should be considered, as the infusion will scavenge fat-soluble agents and slow the vasodilation.

References

1. Verbee FC. Tricyclic antidepressant poisoning: cardiovascular and neurological toxicity. *Neth J Crit Care*. 2016;24(2):16-19.
2. Body R, Bartram T, Azam F, Mackway-Jones K. Guidelines in Emergency Medicine Network (GEMNet): guideline for the management of tricyclic antidepressant overdose. *Emerg Med J*. 2011;28(4):347-368.
3. Ward C, Sair M. Oral poisoning: an update. *Continuing Education in Anesthesia Critical Care & Pain*. 2010;10(1):6-11.
4. Goldstein JN, Dudzinski DM, Erickson TB, Linder G. Case 12-2018: A 30-year-old woman with cardiac arrest. *N Engl J Med*. 2018;378(16):1538-1549.

# 109

# METABOLISM AND DRUG INTERACTIONS

Jeremy T. Rainey and Avneep Aggarwal

1. Which of the following correctly pairs the pharmacodynamics with the antibacterial agents?

   A. Oxacillin (time dependent), moxifloxacin (concentration dependent)
   B. Vancomycin (concentration dependent), cefazolin (time dependent)
   C. Daptomycin (time dependent), amikacin (concentration dependent)
   D. Levofloxacin (time dependent), meropenem (time dependent)

2. A 49-year-old male with a past medical history significant for hypertension and end-stage renal disease on hemodialysis is admitted to the ICU in septic shock from pneumonia. He is intubated and mechanically ventilated, and requires vasopressor support. Blood cultures grew multidrug–resistant *Acinetobacter baumannii*. You begin appropriate treatment. Over the course of several hours you begin to notice increasing vasopressor requirements and increasing peak airway pressures. Which of the following antimicrobial choices could adequately explain this scenario?

   A. IV polymyxin B without renal adjustment
   B. Meropenem allergy
   C. Inhaled colistin hypersensitivity
   D. IV tobramycin-induced bronchospasm

3. A 54-year-old man with a past medical history of cirrhosis is in the ICU 4 days after suffering severe burns to >40% of his body while at work. His respiratory status has been rapidly declining, and he is currently requiring BiPAP; however his P:F ratio is now <200 and his last chest radiograph supports your concern for acute respiratory distress syndrome. You make the decision to intubate and suspect that he will need continuous neuromuscular blockade. Which of the following neuromuscular blocking drugs will be most appropriate in this patient for intubation and continuous blockade?

   A. Succinylcholine (intubation), vecuronium (continuous)
   B. Rocuronium (intubation), rocuronium (continuous)
   C. Succinylcholine (intubation), atracurium (continuous)
   D. Rocuronium (intubation), cisatracurium (continuous)

4. A 48-year-old, male, liver transplant recipient is readmitted 4 months postsurgery because altered mental status. On examination, he is confused and agitated; the rest of the examination is unremarkable. A review of his medications indicates that he in on lisinopril, prednisone, and tacrolimus. Laboratory tests show Na 136, K 6.1, $HCO_3$ 17, Cl 108, blood urea nitrogen 42, creatinine 4.4. The results of his complete blood count and the rest of the chemistry profile are normal. CT scan of the brain is normal. What is the most likely cause of this patient's current presentation?

   A. Normal pressure hydrocephalus
   B. Meningitis
   C. Acute graft rejection
   D. Tacrolimus toxicity

5. A 19-year-old female with a past medical history of sensorineural deafness and mitochondrial encephalomyopathy lactic acidosis and strokelike episodes (MELAS) presented to the emergency room with slurred speech, tremor, and unsteady gait. Her physical examination revealed nystagmus, dysarthria, gait and limb ataxia. While in the ER, she had a generalized tonic-clonic seizure for which she was intubated. Phenytoin was also administered and an MRI was obtained that showed bilateral occipitotemporal lesions. She was transferred to the ICU. Phenytoin is discontinued and sodium valproate started. Laboratory results are unremarkable except for elevated lactate levels. EEG confirms seizure activity. Which of the following is most appropriate next step in management?

    **A.** Fluid resuscitation with ringer lactate @ 30 mL/kg
    **B.** Sodium valproate should be discontinued
    **C.** tPA should be administered emergently
    **D.** Empiric broad-spectrum antibiotics should be initiated

6. A 46-year-old male with a past medical history of COPD and uncontrolled diabetes is intubated and sedated in the ICU requiring inotropic and vasopressor support for septic shock due to pneumonia. Several days into his admission he develops bradycardia that is refractory to treatment, necessitating the placement of a transvenous catheter. Urinalysis is positive for myoglobin and his CK levels approach 50 000 U/L. You obtain a blood gas that reveals a pH of 7.13, $PaCO_2$ 39, $PaO_2$ 88, $HCO_3$ 13 with a base excess of $-8$. Propofol infusion syndrome (PRIS) is suspected. Which of the following is NOT a known triggering factor for this condition?

    **A.** Excessive carbohydrate intake
    **B.** Hydrocortisone therapy
    **C.** Epinephrine infusion
    **D.** Septic shock

7. A 62-year-old Cantonese woman with no significant past medical history is admitted to the ICU with intense nausea, vomiting, and diarrhea 24 hours after ingestion of an unknown mushroom. Laboratory studies are negative for Epstein-Barr, all forms of hepatitis, and antinuclear antibody. ALT and AST are elevated. On day 3 of admission, she goes into acute hepatic failure. Mushroom poisoning is suspected. Which of the following drugs is amatoxin uptake inhibitor?

    **A.** Thioctic acid
    **B.** Erythromycin
    **C.** Silibinin
    **D.** Methylprednisolone

8. Which of the following statements is most appropriate when considering the risk of arrhythmias between typical and atypical antipsychotics?

    **A.** Greater risk is seen with atypical antipsychotics compared with typical antipsychotics
    **B.** Greater risk is seen with typical antipsychotics compared with atypical antipsychotics
    **C.** Typical antipsychotics have a greater QTc increase than atypical antipsychotics
    **D.** There is no difference in the risk between the two

# Chapter 109 ▪ Answers

**1.** Correct Answer: A

**Rationale:**
The pharmacodynamics of the antimicrobial agents guide dosing regimen. There are two pharmacodynamic profiles that most antibacterial agents can be classified into (time-dependent and concentration-dependent), which must be considered for optimal efficacy of those agents.

    Time-dependent agents depend on duration above the minimum inhibitory concentration for optimal bactericidal activity. Here, the frequency of dosing is an important aspect of their antimicrobial effect because a higher frequency of administration will increase the duration of exposure to the drug. Examples of drugs in this category are beta-lactams, macrolides, linezolid, and vancomycin (see Table 109.1).

**TABLE 109.1 Time-Dependent Agents**

| Beta-lactams | Beta-lactamase sensitive | Penicillins |
|---|---|---|
| | Beta-lactamase resistant | Oxacillin, nafcillin, dicloxacillin |
| | Amoxicillin, ticarcillin, piperacillin | |
| | Cephalosporins | Cefazolin, cephalexin, cefuroxime, cefoxitin, ceftriaxone, cefepime |
| | Carbapenems | |
| | Monobactams | Aztreonam |
| | Beta-lactamase inhibitors | Tazobactam, avibactam, clavulanic acid |
| Vancomycin | | |
| Macrolides | Azithromycin, clarithromycin, erythromycin | |
| Oxazolidinones | Linezolid | |
| Tetracyclines | Doxycycline, tigecycline | |

On the other hand, antimicrobial effect of concentration-dependent agents depends on the concentration of free drug above the minimum inhibitory concentration. With these agents, increasing the amount or concentration of the drug relative to the minimum inhibitory concentration (or the area under the curve relative to the minimum inhibitory concentration) optimizes antimicrobial efficiency. And decreasing dosing frequency prevents accumulation of the drug and thereby reduces its side effects. Examples of drugs in this category are fluoroquinolones, aminoglycosides, daptomycin (see Table 109.2).

**TABLE 109.2 Concentration-Dependent Agents**

| Aminoglycosides | Amikacin, tobramycin, gentamicin, streptomycin |
|---|---|
| Fluroquinolones | Ciprofloxacin, levofloxacin, moxifloxacin |
| Daptomycin | |
| Polymyxins | Colistin, polymyxin B |
| Metronidazole | |

### References

1. Levison ME, Levison JH. Pharmacokinetics and pharmacodynamics of antibacterial agents. *Infect Dis Clin North Am.* 2009;23(4):791, vii. doi:10.1016/j.idc.2009.06.008.
2. Konaklieva MI. Molecular targets of β-lactam-based antimicrobials: beyond the usual suspects. *Antibiotics.* 2014;3(2):128-142. doi:10.3390/antibiotics3020128.
3. Douros A, Grabowski K, Stahlmann R. Safety issues and drug–drug interactions with commonly used quinolones. *Expert Opin Drug Metab Toxicol.* 2015;11(1):25-39. doi:10.1517/17425255.2014.970166.
4. Connors KP, Kuti JL, Nicolau DP. Optimizing antibiotic pharmacodynamics for clinical practice. *Pharmaceut Anal Acta.* 2013;4:214. doi:10.4172/2153-2435.1000214.

**2.** Correct Answer: C

**Rationale:**

The most likely culprit here is colistin. Colistin is a concentration-dependent bactericidal antibiotic that has both hydrophilic and lipophilic portions, which bind to the anionic lipopolysaccharides on the outer cell membrane of gram-negative bacteria leading to increased permeability of the cellular wall, causing leakage of cell contents, eventually resulting in cellular demise. Colistin has a narrow range of activity, primarily being utilized in the treatment of infections with *Pseudomonas aeruginosa* and *A.* baumannii. Colistin does NOT have activity against gram-positive bacteria such as *Burkholderia cepacia, Serratia marcescens, Moraxella catarrhalis, Proteus* spp., *Providencia* spp., and *Morganella morganii.*

Colistin is renally cleared and dose adjustments for IV forms in patients with kidney disease must be considered to avoid, or at least minimize, the potential nephrotoxic effects. Neurotoxicity is also of concern with the IV formulation of colistin. When administered in the aerosol form, up to approximately 10% of patients may develop hypersensitivity reactions, especially pulmonary symptoms such as bronchospasm, which in some cases can be quite severe. Pretreatment with bronchodilators can help assuage the occurrence or severity of this effect.

Polymyxin B is associated with lower rates of nephrotoxicity than colistin and does not need to be dose-adjusted for renal function. Inhaled tobramycin may cause bronchospasm, but IV formulations are less likely to.

### References

1. Domínguez-Ortega J, Manteiga E, Abad-Schilling C, et al. Induced tolerance to nebulized colistin after severe reaction to the drug. *J Investig Allergol Clin Immunol.* 2007;17(1):59-61.
2. Cunningham S, Prasad A, Collyer L, et al Bronchoconstriction following nebulised colistin in cystic fibrosis. *Arch Dis Child.* 2001;84:432-433.
3. Choi HK, Kim YK, Kim HY, Uh Y. Inhaled colistin for treatment of pneumonia due to colistin-only-susceptible acinetobacter baumannii. *Yonsei Med J.* 2014;55(1):118-125. doi:10.3349/ymj.2014.55.1.118.
4. Gupta S, Govil D, Kakar PN, et al. Colistin and polymyxin B: A re-emergence. *Indian J Crit Care Med.* 2009;13(2):49-53.

**3.** Correct Answer: D

**Rationale:**

When considering neuromuscular blocking agents in the critically ill, the physician must take into account the pathophysiology of the patient, the urgency with which he or she must secure a patient's airway, whether or not there is a need for continuous administration of a neuromuscular blocking agent, and the effects that agent will have on the patient.

Although succinylcholine is a very popular agent in the facilitation of intubation because of its rapid onset and short duration, its use in the critically ill population is limited for numerous reasons, primarily. Upregulation of extrajunctional nicotinic Ach receptors in this population can lead to a potentially adverse, if not fatal, hyperkalemia. Other contraindications for the use of succinylcholine include patients with or without a family history of malignant hyperthermia, muscular dystrophy, burns >48 hours (risk can be elevated for up to 1 year after the burn), spinal cord injury >24 hours, strokes >72 hours, and patients at risk for exaggerated hyperkalemia (rhabdomyolysis, hyperkalemic patients with ECG changes).

Non-depolarizing agents tend to have better safety profiles in the critically ill population. They do not cause fasciculations because of the competitive antagonism of the end plate. Rocuronium is the most commonly used alternative to succinylcholine for intubation in the critically ill because of its fairly rapid onset (approximately 60 seconds), intermediate duration, and low active metabolite production after metabolism. Rocuronium is excreted mainly through the biliary tract with minimal renal excretion. Thus, rocuronium infusion is not preferred in patients with cirrhosis. Vecuronium has a much longer onset time and has more renal excretion making it a poorer choice in the critically ill.

Cisatracurium and atracurium are other non-depolarizing agents that do not undergo hepatic metabolism, nor do they have hepatic or renal clearance. Atracurium is metabolized through nonspecific plasma esterases and Hoffman elimination. Atracurium can also lead to histamine release, causing flushing, tachycardia, and hypotension, which may make it less suitable in the critically ill. Cisatracurium is metabolized exclusively via Hoffman elimination and is approximately four times as potent as atracurium. Cisatracurium has no active metabolites and does not lead to histamine release and has a faster onset than atracurium, making it a better choice than atracurium in the critically ill.

### References

1. Bittner EA. Clinical use of neuromuscular blocking agents in critically ill patients. In: Post T, ed. *UpToDate.* Waltham, Mass: UpToDate; 2018. www.uptodate.com. Accessed October 3, 2018.
2. Van Miert MM, Eastwood NB, Boyd AH, Parker CJR, Hunter JM. The pharmacokinetics and pharmacodynamics of rocuronium in patients with hepatic cirrhosis. *Br J Clin Pharmacol.* 1997;44(2):139-144. doi:10.1046/j.1365-2125.1997.00653.x.
3. Fan E, Brodie D, Slutsky AS. Acute respiratory distress syndromeadvances in diagnosis and treatment. *JAMA.* 2018;319(7):698-710. doi:10.1001/jama.2017.21907.
4. Omera M, Hammad YM, Helmy AM. Rocuronium versus cisatracurium: onset of action, intubating conditions, efficacy and safety. *Alexandria J Anaesth Intens Care.* 2005;8:27-33.

**4.** Correct Answer: D

**Rationale:**

Tacrolimus is a calcineurin inhibitor that suppresses the immune system by preventing IL-2 production by T cells and is metabolized via CYP3A4. The adverse effects of the calcineurin inhibitors are primarily nephrotoxicity ranging from minimal to irreversible damage. In addition, tacrolimus may cause neurotoxicity, which can be severe enough to warrant immediate cessation of the medication. The need for frequent and specific monitoring of drug concentrations remains essential because the therapeutic dosing and pharmacokinetics of tacrolimus can demonstrate wide variability among recipients.

Antifungals, such as fluconazole, and multiple classes of antibiotics, such as macrolides, are known inhibitors of of the CYP3A4 system and can lead to increased and toxic blood levels of tacrolimus if not carefully monitored.

Normal-pressure hydrocephalus (NPH) is characterized by pathologically enlarged ventricular size with normal opening pressures on lumbar puncture. It classically presents with cognitive impairment, gait disturbance, and urinary incontinence. Secondary NPH can occur as a consequence of chronic meningitis or ongoing meningitis.

Calcineurin inhibitor toxicity should be part of the differential diagnosis in patients presenting with new renal and neurological toxicity, especially when multiple CYP inhibitors are being used in conjunction with one another.

### References

1. Paterson DL, Singh N. Interactions between tacrolimus and antimicrobial agents. *Clin Infect Dis.* 1997;25(6):1430-1440. doi:10.1086/516138.
2. Vanhove T, Bouwsma H, Hilbrands L, et al. Determinants of the magnitude of interaction between tacrolimus and voriconazole/posaconazole in solid organ recipients. *Am J Transplant.* 2017;17:2372-2380. doi:10.1111/ajt.14232.
3. Luo X, Zhu L, Cai N, Zheng L, Cheng Z. Prediction of tacrolimus metabolism and dosage requirements based on CYP3A4 phenotype and CYP3A5*3 genotype in Chinese renal transplant recipients. *Acta Pharmacol Sin.* 2016;37(4):555-560. doi:10.1038/aps.2015.163.

**5.** Correct Answer: B

**Rationale:**

The syndrome of MELAS is one of a complex group of heterogeneous multisystem disorders affecting the nervous system, which is maternally inherited and caused by mutations of mitochondrial DNA. Approximately 80% of MELAS cases are associated with an m.3243A>G mutation. Typical presenting symptoms include recurrent stroke-like episodes resulting in hemiparesis, hemianopia, cortical blindness, generalized seizure activity, recurrent migraine headaches, short stature, hearing loss, muscle weakness, and cardiomyopathy. MELAS usually presents in patients <40 years of age (though there have been described cases of onset after 40) with encephalopathy, lactic acidemia, and the presence of red fibers from skeletal muscle biopsy. MRI findings will reveal lesions that do not follow vascular territories with diffusion patterns that may be enhanced or mixed. Signal changes will not be static and may show faster resolution than what would be expected in true strokes.

Medications that affect mitochondrial function should be strictly avoided in patients with suspected MELAS. The underlying mechanism to the toxicity of valproic acid in these patients is its interference with and depression of mitochondrial beta oxidation of fatty acids and inhibition of oxidative phosphorylation, which can exacerbate underlying mitochondrial cytopathy.

Although elevated lactate and seizures can occur in sepsis, it is less likely based on her history and imaging. So antibiotics and fluid resuscitation will not be the first next step. Also, tPA is not indicated as MRI findings are not suggestive of acute ischemic stroke.

### References

1. Lin CM, Thajeb P. Valproic acid aggravates epilepsy due to MELAS in a patient with an A3243G mutation of mitochondrial DNA. *Metab Brain Dis.* 2007;1:105-109.
2. Chaudhry N, Patidar Y, Puri V. Mitochondrial myopathy, encephalopathy, lactic acidosis, and stroke-like episodes unveiled by valproate. *J Pediatr Neurosci.* 2013;8(2):135-137. doi:10.4103/1817-1745.117847.
3. Hsu YC, Yang FC, Perng CL, Tso AC, Wong LJ, Hsu CH. Adult-onset of mitochondrial myopathy, encephalopathy, lactic acidosis, and stroke-like episodes (MELAS) syndrome presenting as acute meningoencephalitis: a case report. *J Emerg Med.* 2012;43:e163-e166.
4. Finsterer J, Mahjoub SZ. Presentation of adult mitochondrial epilepsy. *Seizure.* 2013;22:119-123.

**6.** Correct Answer: A

**Rationale:**

PRIS is characterized by acute bradycardia (which may be refractory to treatment and that may progress to asystole, hypertriglyceridemia, hepatomegaly, metabolic acidosis, rhabdomyolysis, and myoglobinuria and is associated with propofol infusions >48 hours. Usually, doses at or exceeding 4 mg/kg/h are causative; however, there are case reports with smaller doses. Steroid use, vasopressors, low carbohydrate intake, poor tissue perfusion, sepsis, and cerebral injury have been shown to be associated PRIS; all of which may be seen in critical illness. The onset of PRIS is typically rapid and seen within 4 days of initiation. The mechanism of PRIS is poorly understood but may be related to direct mitochondrial respiratory chain inhibition or impaired mitochondrial fatty acid metabolism and blockage of beta-adrenoreceptors and cardiac calcium channels.

The best treatment is prevention and first-line therapy is immediate discontinuation of the infusion of propofol. Renal replacement therapy may become necessary because of metabolic acidosis, hyperkalemia, and rhabdomyolysis. Bradyarrhythmias can be managed with transthoracic or transvenous pacing and shock managed with the support of vasopressors and inotropes. Extracorporeal membrane oxygenation should be considered in cases of refractory PRIS. Ensuring adequate carbohydrate intake may also help to prevent PRIS development.

### References

1. Kam PC, Cardone D. Propofol infusion syndrome. *Anaesthesia.* 2007;62(7):690-701. doi: 10.1111/j.1365-2044.2007.05055.x.
2. Fodale V, La Monaca E. Propofol infusion syndrome: an overview of a perplexing disease. *Drug Saf.* 2008;31(4):293-303. doi:10.2165/00002018-200831040-00003.
3. Mirrakhimov AE, Voore P, Halytskyy O, et al. Propofol infusion syndrome in adults: a clinical update. *Crit Care Res Pract.* 2015;2015:260385.
4. Laquay N, Prieur S, Greff B, Meyer P, Orliaguet G. Propofol infusion syndrome. *Ann Fr Anesth Reanim.* 2010;29(5):377-386. doi:10.1016/j.annfar.2010.02.030.

**7.** Correct Answer: C

**Rationale:**

Patients ingesting mushrooms, such as *Amanita phalloides*, typically do so incidentally when foraging for mushrooms and mistake its identity for an edible mushroom. Patients usually suffer intoxication from the amatoxin of the mushroom (most commonly alpha-amanitin, which is heat stable and insoluble in water) and endure four clinical stages. The first stage is usually observed during the first 6 to 12 hours after mushroom ingestion and is known as the latent stage, where patients usually will not experience any symptoms. Severe muscarinic symptoms might be evident during the second stage, typically with severe gastritis, nausea, vomiting, abdominal pain, and severe diarrhea, which may be bloody or contain mucus. This second stage usually lasts between 12 to 24 hours. The third stage has been classified as a pseudo-remission period where the patient may begin to feel better, but unfortunately patients will rapidly progress to the fourth stage, which is characterized by acute liver failure with massive hepatocyte death. If not treated early, patients may go on to suffer multiorgan failure and death, which can be seen as early as 5 to 8 days after ingestion of the mushroom.

Silibinin, which is a water-soluble silymarin (a flavonolignan from milk thistle), inhibits the amatoxin uptake and penetration into hepatocytes and improves cellular survival in human hepatocytes exposed to alpha-amanitin. Silibinin is most effective when given within 24 to 48 hours of ingestion and is administered as an initial intravenous loading dose of 5 mg/kg followed by continuous infusion of 20 to 50 mg/kg/d for 6 to 8 days. Increased mortality or need for transplantation is seen when silibinin is administered >48 hours after ingestion. Other therapies that have been tried and abandoned include antibiotics, thioctic acids, steroids, hormones, and other antioxidants.

### References

1. Santi L, Maggioli C, Mastroroberto M, Tufoni M, Napoli L, Caraceni P. Acute liver failure caused by amanita phalloides poisoning. *Int J Hepatol.* 2012;2012:487480. doi:10.1155/2012/487480.
2. Cheung CW, Gibbons N, Johnson DW, Nicol DL. Silibinin-a promising new treatment for cancer. *Anti Cancer Agents Med Chem.* 2010;10:186-195. doi: 10.2174/1871520611009030186.
3. Loguercio C, Festi D. Silybin and the liver: From basic research to clinical practice. *World J Gastroenterol.* 2011;17(18):2288-2301. doi:10.3748/wjg.v17.i18.2288.
4. Li Y, Mu M, Yuan L, Zeng B, Lin S. Challenges in the early diagnosis of patients with acute liver failure induced by amatoxin poisoning: two case reports. *Medicine.* 2018;97(27):e11288. doi:10.1097/MD.0000000000011288.

**8.** Correct Answer: D

**Rationale:**

Typical antipsychotics exert their action by postsynaptic blockade of D2 dopamine receptors in the brain with extensive metabolism via the cytochrome P450 system, which makes this class quite dependent on adequate hepatic clearance to reduce systemic accumulation or drug-drug interactions. This class carries an increased risk for extrapyramidal side effects and tardive dyskinesia.

Atypical antipsychotics also have postsynaptic blockade of brain dopamine D2 receptors but they tend to have more serotonin 5HT-2 affinity than their dopamine affinity. This primarily separates them from typical antipsychotics. This serotonin receptor affinity is also what is suggested as the mechanism behind the lower incidence of extrapyramidal side effects seen in this class. This class is metabolized through the cytochrome P450 system, but there is individual drug variability that alters the risk for accumulation and drug-drug interactions (which is beyond the specific scope of this question).

Although there are clear differences in the extent of QTc prolongation between the two classes (haloperidol averages approximately 4.7 ms, quetiapine averages 14.5 ms), there does not seem to be a difference in the risk of arrhythmias, including Torsades de Pointes (TdP) between them. Patients taking either of these classes are approximately at a twofold increased risk of arrhythmias and TdP compared with patients not receiving these medications. Within the two classes, thioridazine (typical) and ziprasidone (atypical) have the highest risk of QTc prolongation and risk of TdP. Haloperidol does have a clinically significant risk; however, this is usually seen with doses of >35 mg/d. Of additional importance, QTc prolongation and TdP tend to occur when additional risk factors are present. These include age >65, preexisting cardiovascular disease, conduction disorders, brady or tachyarrythmias, female sex, electrolyte disturbances (hypokalemia, hypomagnesemia), supratherapeutic or toxic levels of accumulation, or concomitant administration of other drugs that interfere with cardiac conduction or drug metabolism.

### References

1. Huffman JC, Stern TA. QTc prolongation and the use of antipsychotics: a case discussion. *Primary Care Companion J Clin Psychiatry.* 2003;5(6):278-281.
2. Barr J, Fraser GL, Puntillo K, et al; American College of Critical Care Medicine. Clinical practice guidelines for the management of pain, agitation, and delirium in adult patients in the intensive care unit. *Crit Care Med.* 2013;41:263-306.
3. Ray WA, Chung CP, Murray KT, Hall K, Stein CM. Atypical antipsychotic drugs and the risk of sudden cardiac death. *N Engl J Med.* 2009;360(3):225-235. doi:10.1056/NEJMoa0806994.
4. Vieweg WVR. New generation antipsychotic drugs and qtc interval prolongation. *Primary Care Companion J Clin Psychiatry.* 2003;5(5):205-215.

# 110

# TOXICOLOGY AND DRUGS OF ADDICTION

Alexandra Plichta and Sheri M. Berg

1. The Rumack-Matthew nomogram is a risk stratification tool that should be employed when an overdose of which of the following medications is confirmed.

   A. Warfarin
   B. Salicylic acid
   C. Acetaminophen
   D. Digoxin

2. Which of the following, if present upon initial presentation in a patient with acute digoxin overdose, portends a poor prognosis?

   A. Visual disturbance
   B. An ECG showing a high-degree atrio-ventricular block
   C. Serum digoxin levels greater than 1 ng/mL
   D. A serum potassium concentration greater than 5.5 mEq

3. A patient is brought in to the emergency department after being found down by her mother. She admits to the attending physician that she ingested a large dose of her prescribed amitriptyline approximately seven hours prior. Which of the following pieces of information would be MOST helpful in risk stratification of likelihood of having a major cardiac or neurologic event due to her medication overdose?

   A. Ingested dose
   B. Peak serum amitriptyline concentration
   C. Serum potassium level
   D. QRS duration

4. A 29-year-old female is transferred to the intensive care unit (ICU) with a temperature of 104.5°F. Her only medical history includes herpes labialis and migraines, for which she regularly takes sumatriptan combined with ondansetron or metoclopramide for the associated severe nausea. She was initially admitted to the hospital for a cholecystectomy, which was complicated by vancomycin-resistant enterococcus (VRE) bacteremia, and she was treated with linezolid. She was started on appropriate empiric therapy and became acutely altered, tremulous, and febrile. Blood cultures were obtained and showed no growth. Which of the following would be the BEST initial therapy for this patient?

   A. Cyproheptadine
   B. Change antibiotic regimen
   C. Dantrolene
   D. Acetaminophen

5. A 58-year-old female is admitted to the ICU for a suspected infection. She is started on moxifloxacin and fluconazole. She is intubated and sedated and subsequently treated for gastroparesis with erythromycin. Which ECG finding is MOST likely associated with this patient's medication regimen?

    A. Prolonged QRS
    B. Widened QT interval
    C. Prolonged PR
    D. Presence of Osborn wave

6. A 55-year-old male who has a history of alcohol abuse disorder is brought to the emergency department after experiencing a generalized tonic-clonic seizure in prison. He was incarcerated 24 hours prior to presentation. After 24 hours on intravenous midazolam therapy, he continues to have delirium tremens. Which of the following strategies is the LEAST appropriate?

    A. Add gabapentin to current regimen
    B. Add phenobarbital to current regimen
    C. Continue administering midazolam until Clinical Institute Withdrawal Assessment from Alcohol—Revised (CIWA-Ar) score is less than 8 or until 50 mg midazolam is given
    D. Perform endotracheal intubation and start a propofol infusion

7. A 56-year-old male is admitted to the ICU overnight after admitting to snorting large quantities of cocaine. He is diaphoretic and agitated, with vital signs as follows: BP 223/150; rectal temperature 103.3°F. He endorses substernal chest pain, and his ECG shows ST segments that are depressed compared to his admission from one month ago. Which of the following is the LEAST appropriate treatment for this patient?

    A. Lorazepam
    B. Phentolamine
    C. Nitroglycerin
    D. Labetalol

8. A 20-year-old male is brought in by ambulance from a college campus with an altered mental status and appears to be floridly hallucinating. His blood pressure is 190/110 mm Hg and heart rate 129 beats per minute. A standard urine toxicology panel is negative. Which of the following is the MOST likely etiology?

    A. "Ecstasy" intoxication
    B. Amphetamine intoxication
    C. Synthetic cathinone intoxication
    D. New-onset schizophrenia presentation

# Chapter 110 ▪ Answers

1. Correct Answer: C

**Rationale:**

The Rumack-Matthew Nomogram helps to determine the risk of hepatotoxicity from acetaminophen (APAP) ingestion. It plots serum APAP concentration on a logarithmic scale against time (elapsed since acute ingestion). Note that the nomogram starts at 4 hours post-ingestion.

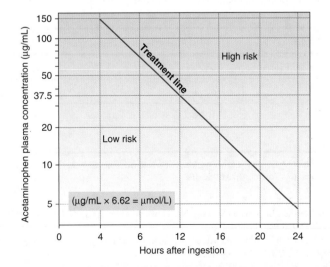

The nomogram was designed after observing two distinct populations of patients who had overdosed on acetaminophen:

- untreated patients that went on to develop transaminitis (AST or ALT >1,000 IU/L)
- untreated patients who maintained normal transaminase levels

A line divides these two populations. Those who fall above the line are high-risk and should be treated with N-acetylcysteine (NAC); those below are low-risk and do not need NAC therapy.

### References

1. Rumack BH, Peterson RC, Koch GG, Amara IA. Acetaminophen overdose. 662 cases with evaluation of oral acetylcysteine treatment. *Arch Intern Med*. 1981;141:380.
2. Rumack BH. Acetaminophen hepatotoxicity: the first 35 years. *J Toxicol Clin Toxicol*. 2002;40:3-20.
3. Hendrickson Robert G. Acetaminophen. In: Nelson LS, Lewin NA, Howland M, et al, eds. *Goldfrank's Toxicologic Emergencies*. 9th ed. New York: McGraw-Hill; 2011:483-499:chap 34. Print.
4. Pharmaceutical drug overdoses. In: Marino PL. *Marino's The ICU Book*. 4th ed. Philadelphia: Wolters Kluwer Health/Lippincott Williams & Wilkins; 2014:963-980:chap 54. Print.

---

**2.** Correct Answer: D

**Rationale:**

Hyperkalemia is a frequent finding in those with digoxin overdose. Serum potassium levels better predict mortality than either initial ECG changes or serum digoxin levels. However, successful treatment of the hyperkalemia does not change outcomes. The serum potassium level serves merely to prognosticate.

This phenomenon was discovered in a 1973 study of patients with acute digoxin poisoning before digoxin-specific antibody fragment was available. The raw data can be seen in figure and table that follow.

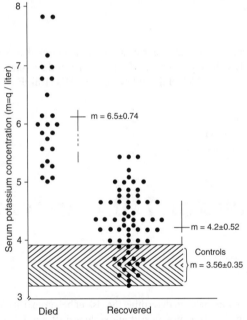

From Bismuth C, Gaultier M, Conso F, Efthymiou ML. Hyperkalemia in acute digitalis poisoning: prognostic significance and therapeutic implications. *Clin Toxicol*. 1973;6:153-162.

| SERUM K⁺ LEVEL (MEQ/L) | MORTALITY RATE | N |
|---|---|---|
| <5.0 | 0% | 58 |
| 5.0-5.5 | 40% | 15 |
| > 5.5 | 100% | 18 |
| | | 91 |

Data from Bismuth C, Gaultier M, Conso F, Efthymiou ML. Hyperkalemia in acute digitalis poisoning: prognostic significance and therapeutic implications. *Clin Toxicol*. 1973;6:153-162.

### References

1. Hack JB. Cardioactive steroids. In: Nelson LS, Lewin NA, Howland M, et al, eds. *Goldfrank's Toxicologic Emergencies*. 9th ed. New York: McGraw-Hill; 2011:936-945:chap 64. Print.
2. Bismuth C, Gaultier M, Conso F, Efthymiou ML. Hyperkalemia in acute digitalis poisoning: prognostic significance and therapeutic implications. *Clin Toxicol*. 1973;6:153-162.

3. Manini AF, Nelson LS, Hoffman RS. Prognostic utility of serum potassium in chronic digoxin toxicity: a case-control study. *Am J Cardiovasc Drugs*. 2011;11(3):173-178.

4. Kelly RA, Smith TW. Recognition and management of digitalis toxicity. *Am J Cardiol*. 1992;69:108-109.

## 3. Correct Answer: D

**Rationale:**

The mechanism by which tricyclic antidepressants (TCAs) such as amitriptyline exhibit their toxicity is by blockade of sodium ($Na^+$) channels. In the central nervous system, $Na^+$ channel blockade ultimately manifests as seizures. In the heart, $Na^+$ channel blockade leads to widening of the QRS and ventricular arrhythmias.

The 1985 study by Boehnert stratified patients into high- and low-risk categories based on the duration of their QRS.

In clinical toxicology, a QRS duration of 100 milliseconds after TCA poisoning is considered the upper limit of normal. As one can see from the original data, the negative predictive value of this is very high, while the positive predictive value is rather low (34% incidence of seizure, 14% incidence of ventricular arrhythmia in those with QRS >100 ms in above study). Also note that no ventricular arrhythmias occurred until the QRS duration was >160 ms.

$Na^+$ channel toxicity can be identified on an ECG by recognizing "R-axis deviation" of the terminal 40 milliseconds frontal plane QRS axis, which includes the presence of both

- S wave in lead I or aVL
- R wave in aVR

However, this finding is not specific to TCA overdose and can also be seen with pathophysiology leading to a large right ventricle or acute right ventricular strain.

### References

1. Boehnert MT, Lovejoy FH, Value of the QRS duration versus the serum drug level in predicting seizures and ventricular arrhythmias after an acute overdose of tricyclic antidepressants. *N Engl J Med*. 1985;313(8):474-479.

2. Clancy C. Electrophysiologic and electrocardiographic principles. In: Nelson LS, Lewin NA, Howland M, et al, eds. *Goldfrank's Toxicologic Emergencies*. 9th ed. New York: McGraw-Hill; 2011:314-329:chap 22. Print.

3. Liebelt EL, Francis PD, Woolf AD. ECG lead aVR versus QRS interval in predicting seizures and arrhythmias in acute tricyclic antidepressant toxicity. *Ann Emerg Med*. 1995;26(2):195-201.

## 4. Correct Answer: A

**Rationale:**

A change of antibiotic regimen is likely unnecessary, as the question stem suggests control of infection with clearance of blood cultures. Linezolid was the antimicrobial initiated to appropriately treat VRE bacteremia. When combined with agents this patient may be taking to treat her migraines and nausea (triptans, ondansetron, and metoclopramide), linezolid may precipitate serotonin syndrome (SS). Of the answer choices listed, cyproheptadine, a nonspecific serotonin antagonist, would be the most appropriate therapy.

### Drugs implicated in SS

| ANTIDEPRESSANTS | OTHER MEDICATIONS |
| --- | --- |
| - SSRIs:<br>  a. Sertraline (Zoloft)<br>  b. Paroxetine (Paxil)<br>  c. Fluoxetine (Prozac)<br>  d. Fluvoxamine (Luvox)<br>  e. Citalopram (Celexa)<br>  f. Escitalopram (Lexapro)<br>- SNRIs:<br>  a. Duloxetine (Cymbalta)<br>  b. Venlafaxine (Effexor)<br>  c. Desvenlafaxine (Pristiq)<br>- MAOIs<br>  a. Phenelzine (Nardil)<br>  b. Isocarboxazid (Marplan)<br>  c. Tranylcypromine (Parnate)<br>- TCAs<br>  a. Imipramine (Tofranil)<br>  b. Clomipramine (Anafranil)<br>  c. Doxepin<br>  d. Selegiline<br>- Mirtazapine (Remeron) | - Buspirone (Buspar)<br>- Valproate (Depakote)<br>- Analgesics:<br>  - Meperidine (Demerol)<br>  - Fentanyl (Sublimaze)<br>  - Tramadol (Ultram)<br>- Methylene blue, an MAOI<br>- Ondansatron (Zofran)<br>- Metoclopramide (Reglan)<br>- Triptans—sumatriptan (Imitrex)<br>- Ergot derivatives (ergotamine, methylergonovine)<br>- Linezolid (Zyvox), an MAOI<br>- Ritonavir (Norvir)<br>- Dextromethorphan<br>- MDMA (ecstasy, molly)<br>- St. John's wort |

MAOI, monoamine oxidase inhibitors; MDMA, 3,4-methyl enedioxy methamphetamine (ecstasy); SNRI, serotonin and norepinephrine reuptake inhibitors; SSRI, selective serotonin reuptake inhibitors; TCA, tricyclic antidepressants.

| | SEROTONIN SYNDROME (SS) | NEUROLEPTIC MALIGNANT SYNDROME |
|---|---|---|
| Symptoms | • Fever<br>• Altered mental status<br>• Autonomic hyperactivity<br>• Akathisia<br>• Tremor<br>• Hyperreflexia, clonus | • Fever<br>• Altered mental status<br>• Autonomic instability<br>• Rigidity |
| Causes | (See above list) | • Neuroleptics<br>• Metoclopromide (Reglan)<br>• Cessation of DA agonist (amantadine, bromocriptine, levodopa) |
| Treatment | • Stop culprit meds<br>• Supportive care<br>• Benzodiazepines<br>• If severe, consider paralysis<br>• Cyproheptadine | • Stop (or restart) culprit meds<br>• Supportive care<br>• Dantrolene (2-3 mg/kg/d up to 10 mg/kg/d) |

While the high temperature in the question stem may lead the reader to suspect refractory infection, severity of fevers in hospitalized patients has not been found to correlate with the likelihood of infection. The table that follows provides a framework for thinking about infectious and noninfectious causes of fever in the ICU.

## NONINFECTIOUS CAUSES OF FEVER IN ICU PATIENTS

- Alcohol/drug withdrawal
- Postoperative fever (48 h post-op)
- Blood transfusion reaction fevers[b]
- Drug fevers[b] (neuroleptic malignant syndrome[b])
- Neoplastic fevers
- Cerebral infarction/hemorrhage
- Subarachnoid hemorrhage
- Adrenal insufficiency (crisis)
- Myocardial infarction[a]
- Acute pancreatitis[a]
- Acalculous cholecystitis[a]
- Ischemic bowel
- Cirrhosis
- Gastrointestinal (GI) bleed[a]
- Aspiration pneumonitis
- Acute respiratory distress syndrome[a]
- Fat embolus
- Pulmonary embolism[a]/deep vein thrombosis
- Thrombophlebitis[a]
- Hematoma[a]
- Transplant rejection

[a]Indicates pathologies excluded by temperatures >102°F—per Cunha.
[b]Nnoninfectious disease with temperatures >102°F in ICU patients.
Adapted from Marik PE. Fever in the ICU. *Chest.* 2000;117(3):855-869 and Cunha BA. Fever in the critical care unit. *Crit Care Clin.* 1998;14(1):1-14.

### References

1. Boyer EW, Shannon M. The serotonin syndrome. *N Engl J Med.* 2005;352(11):1112-1120.
2. Graudins A, Stearman A, Chan B. Treatment of the serotonin syndrome with cyproheptadine. *J Emerg Med.* 1998;16(4):615.
3. Marik PE. Fever in the ICU. *Chest.* 2000;117(3):855-869.
4. Cunha BA. Fever in the critical care unit. *Crit Care Clin.* 1998;14(1):1-14.

**5.** Correct Answer: B

**Rationale:**

A number of medications have a known risk of prolonging QTc, which is defined as a QTc greater than 450 ms in males and greater than 460 ms in females. However, note that while some medications are known to prolong QTc, they are not necessarily associated with torsades de pointes (TdP) (amiodarone). Others have a known risk of TdP (erythromycin, haloperidol, ondansetron).

In this question, the patient was on amiodarone (a class III antiarrhythmic) and was started on moxifloxacin (a fluoroquinolone) and fluconazole, increasing her risk of developing a prolonged QTc. All three medications behave similarly to antipsychotics and produce this electrocardiographic finding by blocking potassium ($K^+$) channels.

| | ANTIPSYCHOTICS | TRICYCLIC ANTIDEPRESSANTS |
|---|---|---|
| **Channel blockade** | $K^+$ channels | $Na^+$ channel |
| **ECG finding** | Prolonged QTc | • Widened QRS<br>• R-axis deviation (terminal 40 ms)—see below |
| **Possible results** | Torsades de pointes | Ventricular arrhythmia |
| **Other implicated medications** | • Class IA antiarrhythmics<br>• Class III antiarrhythmics<br>• -azole antifungals<br>• Antimicrobials: macrolides, fluoroquinolones<br>• Protease inhibitors<br>• Methadone<br>• Citalopram (Celexa, SSRI)<br>• Diphenhydramine (Benadryl) | • Class IA antiarrhythmics<br>• Class IC antiarrhythmics<br>• Phenothiazines<br>• Amantadine<br>• Diphenhydramine (Benadryl)<br>• Carbamazepine (Tegretol)<br>• Cocaine |
| **Similar to** | Hypocalcemia | Hyperkalemia |
| **Therapy** | Defibrillate<br>Overdrive pace<br>Magnesium infusion (prevention) | $NaHCO_3$ |

Xenobiotics that cause $Na^+$ channel blockade prolong QTc by slowing cellular depolarization during phase 0. Thus QT duration increases because QRS duration increases while the ST segment duration remains essentially unchanged.

Xenobiotics that cause $K^+$ channel blockade prolong QTc by prolonging phases 2 and 3 (the plateau and repolarization phases). The ST segment is prolonged.

### References

1. Beach SR, Celano CM, Noseworthy PA, et al. QTc prolongation, torsades de pointes, and psychotropic medications. *Psychosomatics*. 2013;54(1):1-13.
2. Rautaharju PM, Surawicz B, Gettes LS, et al. AHA/ACCF/HRS recommendations for the standardization and interpretation of the electrocardiogram: part IV: the ST segment, T and U waves, and the QT interval: a scientific statement from the American Heart Association Electrocardiography and Arrhythmias Committee, Council on Clinical Cardiology; the American College of Cardiology Foundation; and the Heart Rhythm Society: endorsed by the International Society for Computerized Electrocardiography. *Circulation*. 2009;119:e241-e250.
3. Holstege CP, Eldridge DL, Rowden AK. ECG manifestations: the poisoned patient. *Emerg Med Clin N Am*. 2006;24(1):159-177.
4. Woosley RL, Heise CW, Romero KA. www.Crediblemeds.org. QTdrugs List, Accessed March 2019, AZCERT, Inc. 1822 Innovation Park Dr., Oro Valley, AZ 85755.

**6.** Correct Answer: A

**Rationale:**

The severity of the alcohol withdrawal is frequently stratified using the Clinical Institute Withdrawal Assessment for Alcohol—Revised (CIWA-Ar) scale. While patients with mild withdrawal symptoms (CIWA score 0-15) may be appropriate for ambulatory therapy with medications including chlordiazepoxide, oxazepam, and gabapentin, patients with moderate to severe withdrawal symptoms (CIWA-Ar score >16) are usually more appropriately treated as inpatients, with some warranting admission to the ICU. Any patient with seizures or delirium tremens (DT) should be started on intravenous benzodiazepines. The choice of agents and schedule of administration may be institution-dependent. Some patients' symptoms may persist through frequent and high doses of benzodiazepines (BZDs). It would be appropriate to add a second agent such as phenobarbital or propofol. Given propofol's propensity to depress ventilatory drive, especially when coadministered with BZDs, it would be most important to admit the patient to an ICU and secure the airway with an endotracheal tube prior to its initiation.

### References

1. Sullivan JT, Sykora K, Schneiderman J, et al. Assessment of alcohol withdrawal: the revised clinical institute withdrawal assessment for alcohol scale (CIWA-Ar). *Br J Addict*. 1989;84(11):1353.
2. Myrick H, Malcolm R, Randal PK, et al. A double-blind trial of gabapentin versus lorazepam in the treatment of alcohol withdrawal. *Alcohol Clin Exp Res*. 2009;33(9):1582-1588.

3. Victor M, Brausch C. The role of abstinence in the genesis of alcoholic epilepsy. *Epilepsia*. 1967;8(1):1-20.

4. Gold JA, Rimal B, Nolan A, Nelson LS. A strategy of escalating doses of benzodiazepines and phenobarbital administration reduces the need or mechanical ventilation in delirium tremens. *Crit Care Med*. 2007;35:724-730.

5. Gold JA, Nelson LS. Ethanol withdrawal. In: Nelson LS, Lewin NA, Howland M, et al, eds. *Goldfrank's Toxicologic Emergencies*. 9th ed. New York: McGraw-Hill; 2011:1134-1142:chap 78. Print.

## 7. Correct Answer: D

### Rationale:

This patient is displaying signs and symptoms of cocaine toxicity, including cocaine-related myocardial infarction. Of the choices listed, treatment with β-blockers is the least well-supported. First-line treatments may include sympatholysis with use of benzodiazepines such as lorazepam, α-adrenergic blockade with phentolamine, and vasodilation with nitroglycerin. The theoretical fear of use of β-blockers in cocaine overdose is the "unopposed alpha effect" whereby selective β-blockade leaves the patient with decreased cardiac chronotropy and inotropy (decreased cardiac output), while working against an increased afterload; a combination that could precipitate cardiovascular collapse. Even nonspecific β-blockers (with both anti-α and anti-β activity) such as labetalol are thought to have this effect. Though a number of more recent studies have described the safe use of β-blockers in this setting, it is still not a recommended practice.

### References

1. McCord J, Jneid H, Hollander JE, et al. Management of cocaine-associated chest pain and myocardial infarction: a scientific statement from the American Heart Association Acute Cardiac Care Committee of the Council on Clinical Cardiology. *Circulation*. 2008;117(14):1897-1907.

2. Richards JR, Garber D, Laurin EG, et al. Treatment of cocaine cardiovascular toxicity: a systematic review. *Clin Toxicol*. 2016;54(5):345-364.

3. Hoffman RS. Cocaine and beta-blockers: should the controversy continue? *Ann Emerg Med*. 2008;51(2):127.

## 8. Correct Answer: C

### Rationale:

Synthetic cathinones (aka "bath salts") are phenylethylamine derivatives, sharing the same core structure as amphetamines (methamphetamine, MDMA), as well as endogenous monoamines (epinephrine, norepinephrine, and dopamine). The effects of these drugs of abuse can be understood to some degree by comparing their ability to block reuptake of bioamines to different degrees:

**Differential effect on receptors: NET, DAT and SERT**

|  | SELECTIVITY OF NET VERSUS DAT | SELECTIVITY OF DAT > SERT |
|---|---|---|
| **Amphetamine** | threefold NET > DAT | 70-fold DAT > SERT |
| **Methamphetamine** | twofold NET > DAT | 30-fold DAT > SERT |
| **MDMA** | fivefold NET > DAT | 7-fold SERT > DAT |
| **Methcathinone** | 1:1 NET = DAT | 120-fold DAT > SERT |

MDMA, 3,4-methylenedioxymethamphetamine.

|  | CLINICAL EFFECT | PSYCHOSIS | CAN LEAD TO A LIFE-THREATENING HYPERTHERMIA? | ASSOCIATED WITH RENAL FAILURE? | ASSOCIATED WITH HYPONATREMIA? | ASSOCIATED WITH HYPOGLYCEMIA? |
|---|---|---|---|---|---|---|
| **Methamphetamine** | Hyperarousal, compulsivity, occasional paranoia | Common effect | Yes | Yes | No | No |
| **MDMA** | "Easily controlled altered state of consciousness with emotional and sensual overtones" | Occasional | Yes | Yes | Yes | No |
| **Methcathinone** | Stimulant and hallucinogenic effects. Increased energy, empathy, openness, and libido. | Most common effect | Yes | Yes | Yes | Yes |

Methamphetamine, MDMA, and bath salts act as sympathomimetics, which results clinically in hyperalertness, hypertension, tachycardia, mydriasis, and diaphoresis. Acute psychosis is the most common effect of bath salt ingestion, and can be present in the absence of the sympathomimetic symptoms.

Both MDMA and methamphetamine are highly likely to appear on a standard urine toxicology screen, whereas the heterogenous group of compounds within the singular group known as "bath salts" frequently evades detection on a standard assay. While new-onset schizophrenia may also present with similar clinical features, it would unlikely (by itself) present with perturbations in vital signs seen in this patient.

Bath salt intoxication can be treated with benzodiazepines, antipsychotics, and supportive care, with particular attention paid to renal function.

## References

1. Banks ML, Worst TJ, Rusyniak DE, et al. Synthetic cathinones ("bath salts"). *J Emerg Med.* 2014;46(5):632-642.
2. Kramer J, Fischman VS, Littlefield DC. Amphetamine abuse: pattern and effects of high doses taken intravenously. *JAMA.* 1967;201(5):305-309.
3. Winder GS, Stern N, Hosanagar A. Are "Bath Salts" the next generation of stimulant abuse? *J Subst Abuse Treat.* 2013;44(1):42-45.

# 111

# PSYCHOACTIVE MEDICATIONS

Archit Sharma and Anureet K Walia

1. A 55-year-old male with a past history of alcohol use disorder with a previous history of withdrawal seizures, hypertension, and cirrhosis presents to the emergency room requesting inpatient detoxification. The patient has been drinking 12 beers daily for the past 2 weeks. His initial lab work demonstrates a glomerular filtration rate >60, AST of 210 U/L, ALT of 152 U/L. Which of the following agents would be the best choice to use for this patient's alcohol detoxification?

   A. Chlordiazepoxide
   B. Diazepam
   C. Clorazepate
   D. Clonazepam
   E. Lorazepam

2. A 19-year-old male presents to the emergency department with agitation, altered mental status, and muscle rigidity. According to his girlfriend, his physician started him on a medication 2 weeks ago for schizophrenia and depression. During the clinical examination, he appears diaphoretic and has no clonus. His vital signs include a blood pressure of 185/90 mm Hg, temperature of 38.7°C, and pulse of 105 bpm. His lab data are significant for leukocytosis and elevated liver transaminases. Which of the following medications is most likely causing the patient's severe adverse reaction?

   A. Olanzapine 30 mg once daily
   B. Lithium 150 mg twice daily
   C. Bupropion 100 mg twice daily
   D. Clomipramine 25 mg once daily
   E. Chlordiazepoxide 5 mg three times daily

3. An 85-year-old patient is brought into the emergency room, after he was found comatose at home by his son. The patient has a known history of bipolar disorder and epileptiform seizures and is on medication for that. Vital examination reveals a BP of 112/56 mm Hg, a pulse rate of 96 bpm, a respiratory rate of 24 breaths/min, and a temperature of 36.7°C. His serum sodium is 115 mmol per liter. Which of the following medications is the most likely cause of his sodium imbalance?

   A. Lithium
   B. Olanzapine
   C. Carbamazepine
   D. Quetiapine
   E. Topiramate

4. A patient presents to the ED with confusion, myoclonus, diarrhea, hypotension, altered mental status, tachycardia, and a normal creatine phosphokinase (CPK). His family is able to confirm that he was recently started on a new medication by his psychiatrist for treatment of bipolar disorder, although they do not know the name of the medication or what kind of medication it was. Which one of the following is the most likely diagnosis and why?

   A. Neuroleptic malignant syndrome (NMS), because the patient is confused
   B. NMS, because rigidity is more commonly a part of serotonin syndrome
   C. Serotonin syndrome, because it commonly presents with hypertension
   D. NMS, because it usually presents with normal CPK
   E. Serotonin syndrome, because it more commonly presents with myoclonus and GI symptoms

5. A 37-year-old male with a past medical history of alcoholic cirrhosis presents to the ICU postoperatively, after having an open reduction and internal fixation of his femur fracture. He is currently intubated because of rib fractures, splinting, and concern for pulmonary contusions. He is currently sedated with dexmedetomidine and fentanyl infusions but is becoming more agitated and restless. The nurse requests a breakthrough dose of a benzodiazepine to keep him sedated. Which one of the following would be the best choice of medication in someone with impaired liver function?

   A. Diazepam
   B. Oxazepam
   C. Clonazepam
   D. Prazepam
   E. Estazolam

# Chapter 111 ▪ Answers

1. Correct Answer: E

**Rationale:**

In patients requiring alcohol detoxification who have evidence of liver disease or impairment, as evidenced in this patient by his elevated liver transaminases, lorazepam is the best option. Lorazepam does not have any active metabolites and is cleared from the patient's system more rapidly than other benzodiazepines, making it a preferable choice in patients with liver dysfunction. The other options are benzodiazepines, which can protect against alcohol withdrawal symptoms but would have a prolonged effect in patients with liver dysfunction. They require normal functioning of liver for their primary metabolism (diazepam undergoes oxidation and clonazepam undergoes nitroreduction).

References
1. Sachdeva A, Chandra M, Deshpande SN. A comparative study of fixed tapering dose regimen versus symptom-triggered regimen of lorazepam for alcohol detoxification. *Alcohol Alcohol.* 2014;49(3):287-291.
2. McKeon A, Frye MA, Delanty N. The alcohol withdrawal syndrome. *J Neurol Neurosurg Psychiatry.* 2008;79(8):854-862.
3. Kumar CN, Andrade C, Murthy P. A randomized, double-blind comparison of lorazepam and chlordiazepoxide in patients with uncomplicated alcohol withdrawal. *J Stud Alcohol Drugs.* 2009;70(3):467-474.

2. Correct Answer: A

**Rationale:**

This patient is likely experiencing neuroleptic malignant syndrome (NMS), a life-threatening reaction to an antipsychotic medication such as olanzapine. Characteristic symptoms include fever, altered mental status, muscle rigidity, and autonomic dysfunction. He presented with the classic symptoms of fever, altered mental status (mutism, agitation), muscle rigidity, and autonomic dysfunction (altered blood pressure, heart rate). Treatment involves stopping the medication and if clinically indicated, dantrolene, IV hydration, and benzodiazepines as needed. None of the other choices are antipsychotics, and hence do not cause NMS.

References
1. Strawn JR, Keck PE Jr, Caroff SN. Neuroleptic malignant syndrome. *Am J Psychiatry.* 2007;164(6):870-876.
2. Trollor JN, Chen X, Sachdev PS. Neuroleptic malignant syndrome associated with atypical antipsychotic drugs. *CNS Drugs.* 2009;23(6):477-492.
3. Picard LS, Lindsay S, Strawn JR, Kaneria RM, Patel NC, Keck PE Jr. Atypical neuroleptic malignant syndrome: diagnostic controversies and considerations. *Pharmacotherapy.* 2008;28(4):530-535.

**3.** Correct Answer: C

**Rationale:**

Certain medications are known to cause syndrome of inappropriate antidiuretic hormone (SIADH) secretion, leading to hyponatremia. Carbamazepine acts like a vasopressin-agonist and has antidiuretic effects. Altered sensitivity to serum osmolality by the hypothalamic osmoreceptors appears likely, but an increased sensitivity of the renal tubules to circulating ADH cannot be excluded. As such it can cause hyponatremia, especially in the elderly. Another medication that causes the same side effect is oxcarbazepine. Treatment includes discontinuing offending drug and fluid restriction, in addition to monitoring and correction of electrolyte balance. The other choices listed here are not known to cause SIADH.

References

1. Berghuis B, de Haan GJ, van den Broek MP, et al. Epidemiology, pathophysiology and putative genetic basis of carbamazepine-and oxcarbazepine-induced hyponatremia. *Eur J Neurol.* 2016;23(9):1393-1399.
2. Van Amelsvoort TH, Bakshi R, Devaux CB, Schwabe S. Hyponatremia associated with carbamazepine and oxcarbazepine therapy: a review. *Epilepsia.* 1994;35(1):181-188.
3. Prakash S, Bhatia PS, Raheja SG, Pawar M. Carbamazepine-induced hyponatremia. *Br J Anesth.* 2016;117(eLetters suppl).

**4.** Correct Answer: E

**Rationale:**

Both NMS and serotonin syndrome may present with mental status changes, autonomic instability, diaphoresis, and mutism. Both can have elevated CPK, but high CPK is more common in NMS because of the muscular rigidity. The key differentiating features between the two are that serotonin syndrome presents with myoclonus, hyperreflexia and GI symptoms, whereas NMS presents with muscle rigidity. Hence, this patient is most likely to have serotonin syndrome.

References

1. Perry PJ, Wilborn CA. Serotonin syndrome vs neuroleptic malignant syndrome: a contrast of causes, diagnoses, and management. *Ann Clin Psychiatry.* 2012;24(2):155-162.
2. Dosi R, Ambaliya A, Joshi H, Patell R. Case report: serotonin syndrome versus neuroleptic malignant syndrome: a challenging clinical quandary. *BMJ Case Rep.* 2014;2014
3. Sokoro AA, Zivot J, Ariano RE. Neuroleptic malignant syndrome versus serotonin syndrome: the search for a diagnostic tool. *Ann Pharmacother.* 2011;45(9):e50.

**5.** Correct Answer: B

**Rationale:**

Oxazepam is generally considered safer than many other benzodiazepines in patients with impaired liver function, primarily because it is metabolized by glucuronidation and does not require hepatic oxidation. Hence, oxazepam is less likely to accumulate and cause adverse reactions in the elderly or people with liver disease. Other options for patients with liver dysfunction are temazepam and lorazepam. They have short half-lives and do not have any active metabolites. Other benzodiazepines are less desirable in patients with hepatic dysfunction because they require the liver for their primary metabolism (diazepam undergoes oxidation and clonazepam undergoes nitroreduction) or have longer half-lives (prazepam and estazolam).

References

1. Shull HJ, Wilkinson GR, Johnson R, Schenker S. Normal disposition of oxazepam in acute viral hepatitis and cirrhosis. *Ann Intern Med.* 1976;84(4):420-425.
2. Klotz U, Avant GR, Hoyumpa A, Schenker S, Wilkinson GR. The effects of age and liver disease on the disposition and elimination of diazepam in adult man. *J Clin Invest.* 1975;55(2):347-359.
3. Greenblatt DJ, Divoll M, Harmatz JS, Shader RI. Oxazepam kinetics: effects of age and sex. *J Pharmacol Exp Ther.* 1980;215(1):86-91.

# RESEARCH, ADMINISTRATION, AND ETHICS

# 112

# RESEARCH AND BIOSTATISTICS

Edward A. Bittner

1. A study involving 100 patients assessed the efficacy of a high-flow nasal cannula (HFNC) administration in preventing intubation after chest trauma. Among 40 patients who received HFNC, 35 did not require intubation. Among the 60 patients who did not receive HFNC, 55 did not require intubation. The statistical test MOST appropriate to determine if HFNC use is associated with a reduction in the need for intubation is

   A. Chi-square test
   B. Analysis of variance
   C. Log-rank test
   D. A relative risk

2. An intensivist performs a study which examines the impact of a chlorhexidine bathing protocol on the incidence of new methicillin-resistant *Staphylococcus aureus* (MRSA) infections in the ICU. Based on her sample size calculation, 300 patients are needed for randomization to the two study groups (chlorhexidine vs. standard care), to detect a clinically meaningful difference with power of 0.8. However, due to cost constraints, only 200 patients are ultimately enrolled in the study. Statistical testing of the data reveals a lower incidence of MRSA infection in the chlorhexidine group compared with the standard care group ($P < .001$). Which of the following statements regarding interpretation of the findings is MOST correct?

   A. The chlorhexidine protocol is effective
   B. The chlorhexidine protocol is not effective
   C. A type 1 error is likely
   D. A type 2 error is likely

3. Statistical analysis of 20 patients with acute respiratory distress syndrome shows a mean cardiac output (CO) of 5 L/min with a standard deviation of 1 L/min. The distribution of CO in the population is normal. Which of the following statements is MOST accurate regarding interpretation of these data?

   A. Approximately 50% of the sample population would be expected to have a CO between 4 and 6 L/min
   B. Approximately 95% of the sample population would be expected to have a CO between 3 and 7 L/min
   C. Of the sample patients, 10 have a cardiac output greater than 5 L/min
   D. The mean and the median CO are the same in the sample of 20 patients

4. An investigator wants to compare a new noninvasive cardiac output measurement technology to cardiac output obtained from a pulmonary artery catheter using the thermodilution technique. Which of the following statistical methods is MOST appropriate for comparing the two techniques?

   A. Cohen's kappa statistic
   B. Correlation analysis
   C. Bland-Altman analysis
   D. Kaplan-Meier plot

**5.** A study is being designed to compare the efficacy of two analgesic regimens on pain scores of patients in the ICU. Which factor is MOST likely to increase the number of patients required to detect a difference between the two analgesic regimens?

    **A.** Low variability of individual responses to analgesic treatment
    **B.** Lack of randomization of patients to treatment regimens
    **C.** Little difference in the effectiveness of the two regimens
    **D.** Use of blinded rather than nonblinded observers

**6.** An investigator wants to evaluate the impact of a new anti-inflammatory agent on survival from septic shock. He randomizes 300 patients that develop septic shock to either receive the anti-inflammatory agent together with standard care or to receive standard care alone. He follows the two groups until ICU discharge. Which of the following is the most appropriate test to compare survival in the two groups?

    **A.** Log-rank test
    **B.** T-test
    **C.** Chi-square test
    **D.** Wilcoxon Rank Sum test

**7.** Which of the following Pearson correlation coefficients represents the strongest linear relationship between two variables?

    **A.** 0.85
    **B.** −0.80
    **C.** 1.25
    **D.** −0.95

**8.** An investigator wishes to perform analysis of retrospective cohort data to examine the impact of goal-directed fluid management (independent variable) on the need for renal replacement therapy (dependent variable) in patients suffering from major thermal injury. Potential confounding variables which the investigator wishes to control for in the analysis are age, baseline creatinine level, and sequential organ failure assessment score. Which method of regression analysis is MOST appropriate for this analysis?

    **A.** Simple linear
    **B.** Cox
    **C.** Multivariable linear
    **D.** Logistic

**9.** Receiver operator characteristic (ROC) curves comparing the performance of two biomarkers for early detection of sepsis are displayed in the figure that follows.

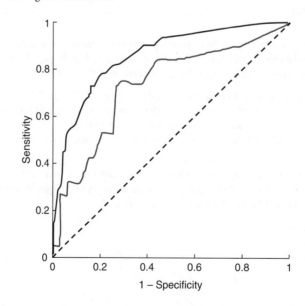

Based on the figure which of the following statements regarding the performance of the new biomarker is MOST likely true?

A. The existing biomarker (red) is a better predictor of sepsis than the new biomarker (blue).
B. There appears to be no difference in the performance of the two biomarkers for early detection of sepsis
C. The difference in the areas under the ROC curves for the two biomarkers can be used to compare their performance
D. The new biomarker (blue) appears to be a better predictor of septic shock than the existing biomarker (red) but not for sepsis

10. A clinical trial is performed to evaluate the impact of a new drug therapy for prevention of contrast-induced nephropathy (CIN) in patients with stage 2 or 3 chronic kidney disease (CKD). Three hundred patients are randomized to receive either the new drug therapy in combination with standard care versus standard care alone. After analyzing the trial data, the number needed to treat (NNT) is calculated to be 5. Which of the following statements regarding interpretation of the NNT in this study is most correct?

A. The relative risk reduction in CIN associated with receiving the new therapy is 0.1.
B. For every 5 patients receiving the new therapy, CIN will be prevented in one additional patient as compared with standard therapy alone.
C. The new therapy is five times more effective in preventing CIN than standard therapy.
D. The new therapy is more effective than an alternative prevention of CIN in patients with stage 4 CKD with an NNT of 15.

# Chapter 112 ▪ Answers

**1.** Correct Answer: A

**Rationale:**
The chi-square test measures the association between two categorical variables. In the question above, the categorical variables are HFNC and intubation and each patient can be classified as "YES" or "NO" based on these variables.

Analysis of variance is used to examine the differences in mean values of more than two groups. The log-rank test is used in analysis of time-to-end-point data to test for differences in hazard rates. Relative risk is a ratio of the probability of an event occurring in the exposed group versus the probability of the event occurring in the nonexposed group.

References
1. Bewick V, Cheek L, Ball J. Statistics review 8: qualitative data – tests of association. *Crit Care.* 2004;8:46-53.
2. Fisher MJ, Marshall AP, Mitchell M. Testing differences in proportions. *Aust Crit Care.* 2011;24:133-138.

**2.** Correct Answer: A

**Rationale:**
The power of a study is the likelihood that it will distinguish an effect of a certain size from chance. The study in the question was at risk for being underpowered given that the calculated sample size was not achieved. Nonetheless a difference was detected between groups, which suggests that the power was adequate for the effect measured.

In statistical hypothesis testing, a type I error is the rejection of a true null hypothesis (also known as a "false-positive" finding or conclusion), while a type II error is the failure to reject a false null hypothesis (also known as a "false-negative" finding or conclusion). Although a type 1 error is possible, it is unlikely given that p-value is <0.001.

References
1. Whitley E, Ball J. Statistics review 4: sample size calculations. *Crit Care.* 2002;6:335-341.
2. Scales DC, Rubenfeld GD. Estimating sample size in critical care clinical trials. *J Crit Care.* 2005;20:6-11.

**3.** Correct Answer: B

**Rationale:**
Quantitative clinical data follow a wide variety of distributions. By far the most common of these is symmetrical and unimodal, with a single peak in the middle and equal tails on either side. This distinctive bell-shaped distribution is known as "Normal." An important feature of the Normal distribution is that it is entirely defined by two quantities: its mean and its standard deviation (SD). The mean determines where the peak occurs, and the SD determines the

amount of variation or dispersion of data values. For normally distributed data, the standard deviation provides information on the proportion of observations above or below certain values. For example, 68% of data values fall within one standard deviation of the mean, approximately 95% are within two standard deviations, and about 99.7% lie within three standard deviations. For the question, approximately 68% of the sample population would be expected to have a CO between 4 and 6 L/min (mean ± 1 standard deviation) while approximately 95% of the sample population would be expected to have a CO between 3 and 7 L/min

Ten of the ARDS patients have could have a cardiac output greater than 5 L/min, but this is not necessary. For example, 2 patients could have a CO of 5.0, 9 with output < 5.0, and 9 with output > 5.0 L/min, resulting in a mean CO of 5.

The median and the mode are the same within the population from which the sample is drawn. However, these measures may differ in a sample drawn from the population due to the effects of random sampling.

### References

1. Whitley E, Ball J. Statistics review 2: samples and populations. *Crit Care.* 2002;6:143-148.
2. Moran JL, Solomon PJ. Statistics in review part I: graphics, data summary and linear models. *Crit Care Resusc.* 2007;9:81-90.

**4.** Correct Answer: C

**Rationale:**

Bland-Altman analysis is used to compare a measurement technique against a reference value, especially when the reference value may not be a true gold standard. Bland and Altman suggest that when a new technology has bias and precision comparable with the previous technology, then it may be accepted in the clinical setting. The Bland-Altman graph plots the difference between two techniques against their averages.

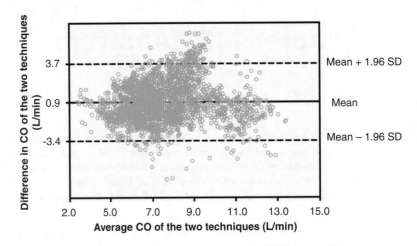

The resulting scatter diagram allows the clinician to determine the following:

- Bias—average difference, (ideal bias = 0)
- Precision—1 standard deviation that describes range for 68% of comparison points
- Limits of agreement—2 standard deviations that describe the range for 95% of comparison points

Correlation analysis (eg, the Pearson correlation coefficient) can be misleading in method agreement studies, since correlation measures linear association rather than agreement. Two methods of measurement can correlate well yet disagree greatly, as would occur if one method read consistently higher than the other. Furthermore, correlation typically depends on the range of measures being assessed, with wider ranges being assessed often resulting in higher correlations but not as a result of better agreement between the methods of measurement being assessed.

Cohen's kappa statistic uses Cohen's kappa coefficient (κ) to measure inter-rater agreement of qualitative (categorical) items. The Kaplan-Meier plots are used for estimating the survival function from lifetime data. The Mann-Whitney U-test is used to determine whether two independent samples of observations are drawn from the same or identical distributions.

### References

1. Odor PM, Bampoe S, Cecconi M. Cardiac output monitoring: validation studies-how results should be presented. *Curr Anesthesiol Rep.* 2017;7:410-415.
2. Cecconi M, Rhodes A, Poloniecki J, Della Rocca G, Grounds RM. Bench-to-bedside review: the importance of the precision of the reference technique in method comparison studies-with specific reference to the measurement of cardiac output. *Crit Care.* 2009;13:201.

**5.** Correct Answer: C

**Rationale:**

When designing a clinical trial to compare two or more groups, a key consideration is to know how many subjects must be enrolled to have adequate power to detect a difference between groups if such a difference exists. Even the most rigorously executed trial may fail to answer its research question if the sample size is too small. On the other hand, a trial with an inappropriately large sample will be more difficult to carry out, and it will not be cost effective.

Factors that influence the sample size include the following:

- Expected effect size (average difference between groups in the outcome of interest)
- Standard deviation in the population
- Acceptable level of significance
- Power of the study
- Underlying event rate in the population

A small difference in the effectiveness of treatment regimens (ie, effect size) will increase the sample size required to detect the difference as compared to detection of a larger effect size.

Randomization of treatment regimens is a means of controlling for confounders but does not affect sample size needed. Use of blinded rather than nonblinded observers can reduce the bias in a study but does not affect the sample size required.

References

1. Whitley E, Ball J. Statistics review 4: sample size calculations. *Crit Care.* 2002;6:335-341.
2. Rosner B. *Fundamentals of Biostatistics.* 8th ed. Boston: Brooks/Cole, Cengage Learning; 2016.

**6.** Correct Answer: A

**Rationale:**

Studies are often designed to compare the survival of two (or more) groups of patients. While the proportions of patients surviving at any specific time could be calculated, the weakness of this approach is that it does not provide a comparison of the total survival experience of the two groups, but rather gives a comparison at an arbitrary time point. The log-rank test is a popular method of comparing the survival of groups which takes the whole follow-up period into account. It accomplishes this by comparing estimates of the hazard functions of the two groups at each observed event time. The null hypothesis is that there is no difference between the groups in the probability of death at any time point. The log-rank test has the considerable advantage that it does not require knowledge about the shape of the survival curve or the distribution of survival times.

References

1. Bewick V, Cheek L, Ball J. Statistics review 12: survival analysis. *Crit Care.* 2004;8:389-394.
2. Bland JM, Altman DG. The logrank test. *BMJ.* 2004;328(7447):1073.

**7.** Correct Answer: D

**Rationale:**

Correlation is a measure of a monotonic association between two variables in which a change in the magnitude of one variable is associated with a change in the magnitude of another variable, either in the same or in the opposite direction. Most often, the term "correlation" is used in the context of such a linear relationship between two continuous, random variables, known as a Pearson product-moment correlation. To quantify the strength of the relationship, the correlation coefficient "r" from sample data is calculated. The value of "r" always lies between –1 and +1. A value of the correlation coefficient close to +1 indicates a strong positive linear relationship (ie, one variable increases with the other). A value close to –1 indicates a strong negative linear relationship (ie, one variable decreases as the other increases). A value close to 0 indicates no linear relationship; however, there could be a nonlinear relationship between the variables.

References

1. Bewick V, Cheek L, Ball J. Statistics review 7: correlation and regression. *Crit Care.* 2003;7:451-459.
2. Schober P, Boer C, Schwarte LA. Correlation coefficients: appropriate use and interpretation. *Anesth Analg.* 2018;126:1763-1768.

**8.** Correct Answer: D

**Rationale:**

A common question in the analysis of study data is whether a there is a statistical relationship between a dependent variable (Y) and independent variables ($X_1$, $X_2$, ...). A common method to answer this question is to employ regression analysis in order to model the relationship between the variables. The type of the regression model depends on the distribution of the dependent variable Y; if it is continuous and approximately normal, linear regression is used to model the relationship between Y and $X_1$. *Simple* linear regression is used when there is a single independent variable (X) and multiple linear regression when there are two or more independent variables ($X_1$, $X_2$, ...). If the dependent variable

Y is dichotomous (eg, YES/NO), then logistic regression is used; if modeling time-to-event (survival-type) data, Cox regression is used.

For analysis of the cohort study data in which the outcome (dependent) variable (eg, need for renal replacement therapy), is dichotomous, logistic regression is the regression model most appropriate to use.

### References

1. Bewick V, Cheek L, Ball J. Statistics review 7: correlation and regression. *Crit Care*. 2003;7:451-459.
2. Bewick V, Cheek L, Ball J. Statistics review 12: survival analysis. *Crit Care*. 2004;8:389-394.
3. Bewick V, Cheek L, Ball J. Statistics review 14: logistic regression. *Crit Care*. 2005;9:112-118.
4. Bender R. Introduction to the use of regression models in epidemiology. *Methods Mol Biol*. 2009;471:179-195.

---

**9.** Correct Answer: C

**Rationale:**

ROC curve analysis is used to assess the diagnostic accuracy of a test. It can also be used to compare the performance of more than one test for the same outcome. With ROC analysis, the sensitivity is plotted against 1-specificity for every cutoff point of the diagnostic test. Generally, a tradeoff is made between sensitivity and specificity, and a decision must be made regarding their relative performance. A perfect test (biomarker) would have sensitivity and specificity both equal to 1. The better the test the closer the ROC curve is to this ideal. The global performance of a diagnostic test can be quantified by calculating the area under the ROC curve (AUC). A greater AUC indicates better test performance. The ideal test would have an AUC of 1 whereas a random guess would have an AUC of 0.5.

In the figure, the position of the ROC curve for the new biomarker (blue) above and toward the left corner of the graph relative to the ROC curve for the existing biomarker (red) suggests that it may be a better in predicting early sepsis. A formal statistical test would be needed to determine whether the difference in AUCs of the two ROC curves is significant.

In the question, the performance of the two biomarkers was assessed for the early diagnosis of sepsis and not septic shock.

### References

1. Bewick V, Cheek L, Ball J. Statistics review 13: receiver operating characteristic curves. *Crit Care*. 2004;8:508-512.
2. Søreide K, Kørner H, Søreide JA. Diagnostic accuracy and receiver-operating characteristics curve analysis in surgical research and decision making. *Ann Surg*. 2011;253:27-34.

---

**10.** Correct Answer: B

**Rationale:**

The number needed to treat (NNT) estimates the number of patients who would need to be treated in order to obtain one more success than that obtained with a control treatment. The smaller the NNT, the more successful the intervention. The NNT is always in reference to a comparison group (in which patients receive placebo, no treatment, or some other treatment), a particular treatment outcome, and a defined period of treatment.

The NNT is calculated as the reciprocal of the absolute risk reduction (ARR) for a given treatment: NNT = 1/ARR.

While calculation of NNT is useful for describing the impact of a clinical treatment, it has some important limitations. First, an NNT is estimated from data obtained in a clinical trial, and therefore, the true value of the NNT may be higher or lower than the point estimate. A confidence interval for the NNT is useful in this regard because it can provide an indication of the range in which the true value of the NNT falls.

Second, it is inappropriate to compare NNTs across disease conditions, particularly when the outcomes of interest differ. Only if we have NNTs for different interventions for the same condition (and severity) and with the same outcome is it appropriate to directly compare NNTs.

Third, the NNT for a specified intervention in an individual patient depends not only on the nature of the treatment but also on the patient's risk at baseline. The concept of NNT assumes that a given intervention produces the same relative risk reduction whether the patient's risk at baseline is low, intermediate, or high. Since that risk may not be the same for all patients, an NNT that is provided by the literature may have to be adjusted for a given patient.

For the question, option B is the correct answer based on the definition of NNT. Option A is incorrect since the *relative* risk reduction cannot be calculated based on the data provided. The *absolute* risk reduction based on the NNT of 5 is 0.2 (1/5). Option C is an incorrect interpretation of the NNT while option D incorrect since it compares the NNTs of patient groups with different risks of CIN at baseline (stage 2-3 CKD vs. stage 4)

### References

1. Bewick V, Cheek L, Ball J. Statistics review 11: assessing risk. *Crit Care*. 2004;8:287-291.
2. Cook RJ, Sackett DL. The number needed to treat: a clinically useful measure of treatment effect. *BMJ*. 1995;310:452-454.

# 113

# ADMINISTRATION

Jason K. Bowman and Jarone Lee

1. A 75-year-old male is admitted to the ICU with combined heart failure exacerbation and multifocal pneumonia. He is currently on BiPAP and his only lines are two small peripheral IVs. You anticipate that he many require numerous procedures in the ICU within the first 24 to 48 hours. You consider talking to the patient and his family to obtain anticipatory consent for numerous specific common ICU procedures (intubation, bronchoscopy, arterial line, central venous access, etc), or just seeking a blanket consent for "all routine ICU interventions." What generally accepted aspects of informed consent may be violated by either of these methods of obtaining consent?

    A. Assessment of decision-making capacity
    B. Description of the proposed intervention(s)
    C. Discussion of risks and benefits of the proposed intervention(s) and alternatives
    D. Assessment of patient / proxy understanding and shared decision-making
    E. Ensuring voluntariness of consent

2. You are the director of an ICU in an academic center and are considering hiring NP and/or PA providers to work alongside residents under the supervision of the ICU attendings and fellows. Based on existing medical literature, ALL of the following appear to be true about the effect of integrating advanced practice providers in this manner EXCEPT for:

    A. Improved patient clinical outcomes
    B. Increased hospital costs for patients
    C. Decreased length of ICU admissions
    D. Similar or improved efficacy at invasive procedures
    E. Improved resident adherence to duty hours and conference attendance

3. Use of the Awakening and Breathing Coordination, Delirium Monitoring/ Management, and Early Exercise/ Mobility ("ABCDE") Bundle has been shown to have which of the following effects on ICU patients?

    A. Increased need for sedative medications
    B. Decreased risk of delirium
    C. More frequent need for reintubation
    D. Increased risk of patient self-extubation
    E. Shorter time to discharge

4. On morning rounds in the ICU, you wish to assess a patient for delirium. You would like to use the Confusion Assessment Method for ICU (CAM-ICU) scale. Which of the following is most important to assess in the patient, before using the CAM-ICU tool on them?

    A. Heart rate and blood pressure
    B. Fluid status
    C. If the patient has a history of psychiatric disease
    D. The patient's level of consciousness
    E. If the patient has risk factors for delirium in their history

5. During a busy shift as an ICU attending, you receive several requests for admission to your ICU from your hospital's emergency department and inpatient medical floor, as well as from another smaller hospital nearby that does not have an ICU. However, your unit currently only has one bed available. Effective and ethical ICU triage involves all of the following EXCEPT for:

    A. Assessing for specific patient need(s) that can only be addressed in an ICU
    B. Considering the patient's diagnosis, medical/surgical condition(s), and prognosis
    C. Balancing the ethical principle of distributive justice with obligation to individual patients
    D. Preferential use of standardized triage tools over case-by-case decisions from experienced clinicians
    E. Multidisciplinary discussion between ICU, emergency medicine, hospitalist medicine, surgery, and other allied health providers

6. You are leading a project to try and develop machine learning and decision tools in your ICU. Your team wishes to start by studying a topic for which machine learning has already been shown to demonstrate promising potential. All of the following topics fit this description EXCEPT:

    A. Sepsis detection
    B. Predicting complications in postsurgical ICU patients
    C. Deciding need for admission in patients diagnosed with pneumonia
    D. Predicting ICU readmission
    E. Predicting the need for prolonged mechanical ventilation

7. A 56-year-old female is admitted to the ICU for influenza and acute hypoxemic respiratory failure. On further review of her chart you note she also has advanced HIV complicated by AIDS and disseminated candidiasis. However, she has consistently declined antiretroviral therapy, but is still sexually active with her husband per prior notes, and previously reported intermittent use of protection. She arrives to the unit on BiPAP but you are able to briefly talk with her to try and assess her wishes and goals. The patient informs you that her husband is her healthcare proxy but tells you that he does not know about her HIV status, asks you to not disclose this to him, and further tells you that you cannot share this information without her consent because of HIPAA. A short time later her respiratory status further declines; she is successfully intubated, placed on a mechanical ventilator, and sedated. How should you proceed in subsequent conversations with her husband?

    A. Do not under any circumstances disclose the patient's HIV status to him because it's immoral to do so
    B. Tell him about her HIV status to allow him to better understand her medical condition and make informed decisions about her care
    C. Tell him about her HIV status so that he can obtain HIV testing himself
    D. Do not tell him because doing so is forbidden by HIPAA
    E. Both B and C

8. What is an example of a core aspect of critical care medicine that is not currently addressed by the US Department of Health and Human Services' contracted National Quality Forum (NQF), in the existing quality measures they have put forth?

    A. ICU length of stay
    B. In-hospital mortality rate
    C. Rate of catheter-associated bloodstream infections
    D. Delirium
    E. Sepsis management bundle

9. You have been tasked with researching and implementing tools to help better predict outcomes for patients in the ICU—both to improve clinical care and assist biomedical research. What are three of the major ICU predictive scoring systems in use today?

    A. APACHE (Acute Physiology and Chronic Health Evaluation), BISAP, and SAPS (simplified acute physiology score)
    B. $MPM_0$ (mortality probability model), SAPS, and TRISS
    C. APACHE, $MPM_0$, and SAPS
    D. BISAP, $MPM_0$, and TRISS
    E. APACHE, SAPS, and TRISS

10. Which of the following realms appears to often be the largest source of nosocomial actual/potential patient harm in the ICU?

   A. Medication error
   B. Problems with lines/drains/catheters
   C. Equipment failure
   D. Obstruction or leakage of artificial airway
   E. In appropriate silencing of an alarm

# Chapter 113 ▪ Answers

**1.** Correct Answer: C

**Rationale:**
Ethically obtained consent comprises numerous components, including (1) assessment of decision-making capacity, (2) discussion of pertinent information, (3) assessing comprehension, (4) ensuring voluntariness, (5) joint deliberation, (6) obtaining consent, and (7) documentation. Furthermore, discussion of pertinent information should include description of the proposed intervention (including listing the providers who will be participating), potential benefits and risks of the intervention, reasonable alternatives, and potential benefits and risks of those alternatives. The manner in which information is provided should be similar to how other clinicians would do so ("professional standard"), give details that a typical well-reasoning individual would want to know ("reasonable person standard"), and also answer the specific questions the patient/proxy has ("subjective standard").

   Obtaining consent for ICU patients presents numerous additional challenges. The patient is often unable to provide consent, proxies are not always present or available, a single ICU patient often needs numerous different procedures, and when an intervention is required it is often time-sensitive and needs to be done urgently or emergently. One method ICUs have adapted to try and address this challenge is to use "bundled consents" where a patient/proxy consents upfront to several commonly needed ICU procedures (intubation, central line, arterial line, etc). Another method is to use "blanket consents," which typically cover almost everything an ICU provider may need to do. These methods have been shown to result in markedly higher rates of consent obtained for procedures (increased from 53%-90% in one study) and improved family satisfaction.

   However, some argue that bundled or blanket consents may not allow for truly informed consent because the provider is not explaining the specific benefits and risks of an intervention (or alternatives to it) as they relate to the patient at a specific point in time in their ICU course. One potential way around this during conversations with a patient/proxy would be to describe for each intervention the common clinical scenario(s) in which it might be considered, such as intubation for respiratory failure, and the benefits / risks / alternatives that would likely exist in that situation.

References
1. Davis N, Pohlman A, Gehlbach B, et al. Improving the process of informed consent in the critically ill. *JAMA*. 2003;289(15):1963-1968.
2. Dhillon A, Tardini F, Bittner E, et al. Benefit of using a "bundled" consent for intensive care unit procedures as part of an early family meeting. *J Crit Care*. 2014;29(6):919-922.

**2.** Correct Answer: B

**Rationale:**
Use of NP and/or PA providers in the ICU is becoming increasingly common in the United States. Acute care/critical training for NPs has existed since 1995, and over 5000 have been certified to date. In contrast, PA providers all complete a broad, nonspecialized training and limited data exist on the number employed in an ICU setting. Collectively, only 4% to 6% of all NP/PA providers are acute care trained. Despite this, over 150 studies have examined the role of NP and/or PA providers in acute and critical care settings, and more than 30 have specifically examined their impact on patient care management.

   There is no evidence that using NP/PA providers results in increased costs for patients or the hospital. To the contrary, it appears that integrating them into multidisciplinary provider teams along with physicians and nurses leads to decreased hospital costs as well as cost savings to the patient. Numerous studies have compared NP/PA provider clinical outcomes to those of resident physicians in caring for acute care / critically ill patients, and shown similar outcomes or improved outcomes. One suggested reason for this is that resident physicians spend a relatively short portion of their residency working in the ICU, whereas in surveys it appears that the average NP/PA ICU provider reports having worked in that setting for several years or more. Furthermore, integration of NP/PA providers helps to provide clinical coverage and allow residents and fellows to attend didactics, conferences, fulfill other requirements outside of the ICU, and meet duty hours.

The increased ICU experience of many NP/PA providers compared to resident physicians rotating in the unit may also explain why integration of the former appears to have numerous other positive impacts on patient outcomes. However, many of the studies that have examined this topic had small sample sizes and short duration, and further study is needed.

## References

1. Kleinpell R, Ely W, Grabenkort R. Nurse practitioners and physician assistants in the intensive care unit: an evidence-based review. *Crit Care Med*. 2008;36(10):2888-2897.
2. Gershengorn H, Johnson M, Factor P. The use of nonphysician providers in adult intensive care units. *Am J Respir Crit Care Med*. 2012;185(6):600-605.
3. Kleinpell R, Ward N, Lynn K, et al. Provider to patient ratios for nurse practitioners and physician assistants in critical care units. *Am J Crit Care*. 2015;24(3):e16-e21.

## 3. Correct Answer: B

### Rationale:

Medical care bundles typically consistent of a small collection of evidence-based practices that, when performed consistently and collectively, have been shown to improve patient outcomes. Examples of these that are frequently used in ICUs include bundles intended to decrease urinary catheter-associated UTIs and ones aimed at reducing central line associated blood stream infections.

The ABCDE bundle was first described by Vasilevskis et al in 2010 and incorporates numerous evidence-based interventions with the collective stated goal of (1) improving collaboration among ICU team members, (2) standardizing care processes, and (3) breaking the cycle of oversedation and prolonged ventilation, which appear to cause delirium and weakness.

In subsequent studies, the ABCDE bundle has been shown to be beneficial in both mechanically ventilated and nonventilated ICU patients. Risk of delirium in particular appears to be markedly lower, with an adjusted odds ratio of 0.55 (risk reduced by almost half) for patients receiving ABCDE bundle care. Some of the other demonstrated benefits include reduced need for sedation medications, increased rate of out-of-bed ambulation, reduced ventilator days, and decreased hospital mortality. Use of the ABCDE bundle does not appear to result in more frequent need for reintubation or increased risk of patient self-extubation. It also does not appear to reduce time to discharge.

## References

1. Vasilevskis E, Speroff T, Pun B, et al. Reducing iatrogenic risks: ICU-Acquired delirium and weakness—crossing the quality chasm. *Chest*. 2010;138(5):1224-1233.
2. Balas C, Vasilevskis E, Olsen M, et al. Effectiveness and safety of the awakening and breathing coordination, delirium monitoring/management, and early exercise/mobility bundle. *Crit Care Med*. 2014;42(5):1024-1036.
3. Morandi A, Piva S, Ely E, et al. Worldwide survey of the "assessing pain, both spontaneous awakening and breathing trials, choice of drugs, delirium monitoring/management, early exercise/mobility, and family empowerment" (ABCDEF) bundle. *Crit Care Med*. 2017;45(11):e1111-e1122.
4. Marra A, Ely E, Pandharipande P, et al. The ABCDEF bundle in critical care. *Crit Care Clin*. 2017;33(2):225-243.
5. Bounds M, Kram S, Speroni K, et al. Effect of ABCDE bundle implementation on prevalence of delirium in intensive care unit patients. *Am J Crit Care*. 2016;25(6):535-544.
6. Ren X, Li JH, Peng C, et al. Effects of ABCDE bundle on hemodynamics in patients on mechanical ventilation. *Med Sci Monit*. 2017;23:4650-4656.

## 4. Correct Answer: D

### Rational:

Delirium is a commonly diagnosed condition in the ICU, with reported incidences in various studies ranging from 45% up to as high as 87%. Delirium is defined in The Diagnostic and Statistical Manual of Mental Disorders, Fifth Edition (DSM-5) in part as "a disturbance in attention (ie, reduced ability to direct, focus, sustain, and shift attention) and awareness (reduced orientation to the environment)." This typically develops over a short period of time (usually hours to a few days), represents a change from baseline attention and awareness, and tends to fluctuate in severity during the course of a day. Delirium can be further subclassified into hyperactive, hypoactive, or mixed type—with the latter two being the most commonly diagnosed in ICU patients.

Despite the fact that ICU delirium is quite common, the complex pathophysiology with regard to how it actually develops is not well understood. Some broad categories that are thought to potentially contribute to delirium include neurotransmitter imbalance, inflammation, impaired oxidative metabolism, and availability of large neutral amino acids. Numerous risk factors have been reported, which includes advanced age, infection, hypotension, metabolic disturbance, respiratory illness, immobilization, and critical illness. ICU patients who develop delirium appear to be at markedly higher risk for both morbidity and mortality. One recent systemic review and meta-analysis showed that ICU patients with delirium had a "significantly higher risk of mortality" (odds ratio 2.2), as well as longer durations of mechanical intubation, ICU stay, and overall hospital stay. Given this, guidelines recommend daily assessment for delirium in ICU patients.

The CAM-ICU is one of five currently validated screening tools to screen for delirium in adults. This and another tool, called the Intensive Care Delirium Screening Checklist (ICDSC), are the two best studied and most widely accepted. However, before using either method, clinicians must first assess the patient's level of sedation. Perhaps the most common way to do this is the Richmond Agitation–Sedation Scale. If patients have a score greater than −3, then they can be assessed using the CAM-ICU tool. The information listed in the other question answers above is also important to assess in your patients but is not specifically needed to screen for delirium with CAM-ICU.

### References

1. Kupfer D, Regier D, Narrow W, et al. *Diagnostic and Statistical Manual of Mental Disorders*. 5th ed. Washington, DC: American Psychiatric Publishing; 2013.
2. Salluh J, Wang H, Schneider E, et al. Outcome of delirium in critically ill patients: systematic review and meta-analysis. *Br Med J*. 2015;350(8011):h2538.
3. Girard T, Pandharipande P, Ely E. Delirium in the intensive care unit. *Crit Care*. 2008;12:s3.
4. Arumugam S, El-Menyar A, Al-Hassani A, et al. Delirium in the intensive care unit. *J Emerg Trauma Shock*. 2017;10(1):37-46.
5. Hayhurst C, Pandharipande P, Hughes C. Intensive care unit delirium: a review of diagnosis, prevention, and treatment. *Anesthesiology*. 2016;125(6):1229-1241.
6. Khan B, Guzman O, Campbell N, Comparison and agreement between the richmond agitation-sedation scale and the riker sedation-agitation scale in evaluating patients' eligibility for delirium assessment in the ICU. *Chest*. 2012;142(1):48-54.

---

**5.** Correct Answer: D

**Rationale:**

Critical care resources are often simultaneously vital, limited, and expensive. When this is combined with the inherent medical complexity of critically ill patients, it can make effectively and ethically triaging potential ICU admissions challenging. ICU care has been demonstrated to reduce mortality in patients who are critically ill, in particular within the first 3 days, suggesting that there is a "window of critical opportunity" and further emphasizing the importance of timeliness in ICU admissions.

Numerous critical care organizations have released guidelines intended to help aid clinicians in approaching the difficult task of ICU triage. Examples of these include the 2016 Society of Critical Care Medicine's "ICU Admission, Discharge, and Triage Guidelines," the 1997 American Thoracic Society's Bioethics Taskforce publication "Fair Allocation of Intensive Care Unit Resources," and the 2016 World Federation of Societies of Intensive and Critical Care Medicine report entitled "Triage Decisions in ICU Admission." Triage decisions should adhere to numerous fundamental principles including:

1. ICU care, when medically appropriate, is an essential component of a basic package of healthcare services that should be available to all
2. The duty of healthcare providers is to benefit an individual patient; when doing so unfairly they compromise the availability of resources needed by others
3. Providers should advocate for patients
4. Members of the provider team should collaborate
5. Care must be restricted in an equitable system
6. Decisions to give care should be based on expected benefit
7. Mechanisms for alternatives should be planned
8. Explicit policies should be written
9. Prior public notification is necessary

The actual process of ICU triage should consider in part the following:

1. Likelihood of benefit to the patient if admitted to the ICU
2. Impact of ICU treatment in improving the patient's quality of life
3. Duration of potential benefit
4. Urgency of the patient's condition (ie how close the patient is to death)
5. Amount of resources required for successful treatment

Three general models for triage have been proposed in previous critical care guidelines. These include the (1) prioritization model, where patients are categorized into four levels of priority based on likelihood of benefit from ICU admission, the (2) diagnosis model, where a list of specific diseases and conditions is used to decide which patients should be admitted to the ICU, and the (3) parameter model, where specific vital signs, laboratory findings, imaging or EKG results, or physical examination findings are used to guide decisions.

At present, there is a dearth of validated tools to assist in triage decisions. Although such tools will likely appear in coming years, no policy or tool can replace the clinical judgment of experienced clinicians such as those on a critical care multiprofessional team.

### References

1. Nates JL, Nunnally MS, Kleinpell RS, et al. ICU admission, discharge, and triage guidelines: a framework to enhance clinical operations, development of institutional policies, and further research. *Crit Care Med*. 2016;44(8):1553-1602.
2. Blanch L, Abillama FF, Amin P, et al. Triage decisions for ICU admission: report from the task force of the world federation of societies of intensive and critical care medicine. *J Crit Care*. 2016;36(C):301-305.
3. Klein D, Olivier A, Milner B, et al. Fair allocation of intensive care unit resources. American Thoracic Society. *Am J Respir Crit Care Med*. 1997;156(4 Pt 1):1282-1301.

**6.** Correct Answer: C

**Rationale:**

Machine learning is a rapidly expanding scientific field that focuses on both how computers learn from data as well as with the development of algorithms to help make this learning possible and more efficient. Given the incredible amount of patient data generated by a modern ICU each day, there is growing interest in using machine learning to analyze these massive datasets to provide more timely and effective care. However, critical care medicine presents numerous challenges to effectively implementing machine learning, including in part (1) compartmentalization of data across multiple systems, (2) data corruption, and (3) the incredible complexity inherent in most ICU patients.

After years of mostly hypothetical discussion on the value of machine learning in improving critical care medicine, within the past year or two numerous studies have been published reporting promising potential in specific topics. Some of these include sepsis detection (machine learning model detected sepsis in ICU patients 4-12 hours before clinical detection), predicting complications in postsurgical ICU patients (serious bleeding, kidney failure, mortality), predicting ICU readmission (which is associated with markedly worse outcomes), and predicting the need for prolonged mechanical ventilation (and need for tracheostomy).

However, great care must also be taken when designing, creating, testing, and implementing machine learning–based decision support systems (ML-DSS), as they can have unforeseen consequences and generate unexpected results. For example, studies examining computer-aided detection of radiology and EKG findings showed decreased sensitivity and accuracy when using them compared to non–computer-aided detection. Similarly, in a study of over 14 000 pneumonia patients that was presented in 2015, the researchers reported that their ML-DSS analyzed the provided data and decided that the patients at lowest risk of complication, and thus the safest to discharge on outpatient management, were those with asthma (C). In particular, machine learning systems struggle when dealing with intrinsic uncertainties and clinical scenarios where there is not a clear "right" answer but expert variation in practice style ("the art of medicine")—both of which are common in critical care medicine. Finally, because ML-DSS use algorithms that are typically inscrutable to clinicians (and with machine-learning / neural networks, that can be inscrutable even to the engineers who designed the system), there is concern that with cases less extreme than the pneumonia/asthma one mentioned above, incorrect results generated by the computer may not be detected by clinicians and could lead to patient harm. To help prevent these types of negative outcomes, ML-DSS products should offer explanations to clinicians of their results/recommendations, and clinicians must become familiar with the ML-DSS products they use—including possible limitations and sources of error.

Although the few existing machine learning generated ICU models (listed above) are still novel, initial comparisons of each of them with existing previously validated detection/prediction tools appear to suggest that they perform significantly better. Machine learning generated tools such as these, particularly once validated (preferably with prospective studies), have the potential to be integrated into ICU electronic health records to better facilitate early and excellent provider interventions. However, care must be taken in designing and implementing these ML-DSS tools to avoid potential harm to patients.

### References

1. Nemati S, Holder A, Razmi F, et al. An interpretable machine learning model for accurate prediction of sepsis in the ICU. *Crit Care Med*. 2018;46(4):547-553.
2. Meyer A, Zverinski D, Pfahringer B, et al. Machine learning for real-time prediction of complications in critical care: a retrospective study. *Lancet Respir Med*. 2018;6(12):905-914.
3. Rojas J, Carey K, Edelson D, et al. Predicting intensive care unit readmission with machine learning using electronic health record data. *Ann Am Thorac Soc*. 2018;15(7):846-853.
4. Desautels T, Das R, Calvert J, et al. Prediction of early unplanned intensive care unit readmission in a UK tertiary care hospital: a cross-sectional machine learning approach. *BMJ Open*. 2017;7(9):e017199.
5. Parreco J, Hidalgo A, Parks J, Kozol R, Rattan R. Using artificial intelligence to predict prolonged mechanical ventilation and tracheostomy placement. *J Surg Res*. 2018;228:179-187.
6. Sanchez-Pinto L, Luo Y, Churpek M. Big data and data science in critical care. *Chest*. 2018;154(5):1239-1248.
7. Johnson A, Ghassemi M, Nemati S, et al. Machine learning and decision support in critical care. *Proc IEEE Inst Electr Electron Eng*. 2016;104(2):444-466.
8. Pollard T, Celi L. Enabling machine learning in critical care. *ICU Manage Pract*. 2017;17(3):198-199.
9. Cabitza F, Rasoini R, Gensini GF. Unintended consequences of machine learning in medicine. *JAMA*. 2017;318(6):517-518.
10. Shortliffe E, Sepúlveda M. Clinical decision support in the era of artificial intelligence. *JAMA*. 2018;320(21):2199-2200.

**7.** Correct Answer: E

**Rationale:**

The Health Insurance Portability and Accountability Act (HIPAA) was passed in August 1996 and was intended to both make health care delivery more efficient and increase the percentage of Americans covered by health insurance. Several years later, in 1999 the US Department of Health and Human Services (HHS) proposed an additional HIPAA Privacy Rule, and the final iteration was issued in 2002. The HIPAA Privacy Rule controls how personally identifiable patient information can be stored, accessed, and used. In general, a patient's personally identifiable information cannot be stored, accessed, or used without their explicit permission. However, the HIPAA Privacy Rule was carefully designed to still allow healthcare researchers to access such data for research purposes—provided that they follow certain requirements and protocols.

This hypothetical case presents several challenging legal and ethical issues. First, providers are ethically obliged to provide proxies with all relevant information about the patient's medical condition and potentially contributory medical history to empower the proxy to make the best-informed decision possible on behalf of the patient. Because the patient's critical illness is likely due at least in part to her untreated AIDS, this is important information that would likely help her husband better understand her overall condition and prognosis. In general, disclosure is justified when: (1) the patient is at significant risk of unnecessary suffering; (2) the fully informed action of others (such as the medical proxy) is needed to prevent this suffering; (3) the action of others has a high probability of preventing suffering; and (4) the benefit that the patient can be expected to gain outweighs any harms, costs, or burdens that others are likely to incur by the proxy being fully informed.

Furthermore, the patient's AIDS and intermittently unprotected sex with her husband places him at serious risk for harm, and the ICU clinician has a duty to inform him so that he can get testing and/or treatment if desired by him.

HIPAA does not forbid sharing of patient information for either of these purposes. Furthermore, there is legal precedent (including the Tarasoff case of 1976) that healthcare professionals are not only protected but have a duty to act in cases such as this, even if doing so breaches confidentiality with the patient, in cases where not doing so would result in an imminent threat to the patient or to an identifiable third party. In this case, not fully informing the husband/proxy poses an imminent threat to the patient (not fully informed medical decision-making by the proxy) and to the proxy.

Finally, in challenging situations such as this one, remember that most hospitals have an ethics committee and legal representative, both of whom are typically available on-call and can help you do right by your patients and their families and provide the most clinically excellent, ethically, and legally defensible care possible.

### References

1. Nass S, Levit L, Gostin L, et al. Beyond the HIPAA privacy rule: enhancing privacy, improving health through research. In: *Institute of Medicine (US) Committee on Health Research and the Privacy of Health Information: The HIPAA Privacy Rule*. Washington, DC: National Academies Press (US); 2009. Available at https://www.ncbi.nlm.nih.gov/books/NBK9576/.
2. Vernillo A, Wolpe P, Halpern S. Re-examining ethical obligations in the intensive care unit: hiv disclosure to surrogates. *Crit Care*. 2007;11(2):125.

---

**8.** Correct Answer: D

**Rationale:**

In 2009, the US Department of Health and Human Services tasked the nonprofit organization National Quality Form (NQF) with developing quality and efficiency metrics for use within the US healthcare system. Over 600 of these metrics have been created to date, though only a small percentage of these are unambiguously attributable and/or relevant to ICU medicine. Some of these include ICU length of stay, in-hospital mortality rate, rate of catheter-associated bloodstream infections, and sepsis management bundle—but not avoidance of delirium.

The subsequent passage of the US Affordable Care Act in 2010 brought with it increased focus on incentivizing efficient and coordinated care, and subsequent federal legislative developments, such as the passage of the Medicare Access and CHIP Reauthorization Act of 2015, further prioritized value-based repayment models. As of this year (2018), it is estimated that 90% of all Medicare payments will be performance based and in the near future up to 10% of physicians' annual salary adjustments will be tied to performance.

Critical care medicine is a particularly important target for these national initiatives as ICU costs are high. The estimated total annual cost of ICU beds in the United States increased from $56.6 billion in 2000, to $81.7 billion in 2005, to approximately $108 billion in 2010. The number of ICU beds increased nationally during the same periods of time, but at a much lower rate—and roughly 75% of these new beds were created in only a small percentage (25%) of regions. However, it's important to also note that costs vary widely between different ICUs, also vary by day of ICU admission (the first day or two of an ICU stay typically costs more than the subsequent days), and are only one component of value in healthcare for the critically ill.

Given the lack of standardized metrics for evaluating quality and efficiency in ICU patients, some national critical care organizations are advocating to develop and test these metrics themselves instead of being constrained to those developed by a nonmedical third party (such as NQF). Others suggest that individual ICUs should be allowed to choose their own metrics—perhaps from a list of approved options.

Although the best pathway forward into value-based critical care delivery remains unclear and fiercely debated, what is certain is that it will profoundly impact the way future generations of ICU clinicians provide (and are reimbursed for) their expert subspecialty care.

### References

1. Nguyen A, Hyder J, Wanta B, et al. Measuring intensive care unit performance after sustainable growth rate reform: an example with the national quality forum metrics. *J Crit Care*. 2016;36:81-84.
2. Murphy D, Ogbu O, Coopersmith C. ICU director data: using data to assess value, inform local change, and relate to the external world. *Chest*. 2015;147(4):1168-1178.
3. Rubenfield G. *Do We Need More Public Reporting? Critical Care Canada Forum*. Presented November 5, 2011. Available at https://criticalcarecanada.com/presentations/2011/do_we_need_more_public_reporting.pdf

4. Chrusch C, Martin C. Quality improvement in critical care: selection and development of quality indicators. *Can Respir J.* 2016;2016:11.
5. Churpek M, Hall J. Measuring and rewarding quality in the ICU: the yardstick is not as straight as we wish. *Am J Respir Crit Care Med.* 2012;185(1):3-4.
6. Pastores S, Halpern N. Insights into intensive care unit bed expansion in the United States. National and Regional Analyses. *Am J Respir Crit Care Med.* 2015;191(4):365-366.
7. Halpern N, Pastores S. Critical care medicine beds, use, occupancy, and costs in the United States: a methodological review. *Crit Care Med.* 2015;43(11):2452-2459.

---

**9.** Correct Answer: C

**Rationale:**

The concept of using scoring systems based on physiologic data to try and predict ICU patient outcomes was first introduced over three decades ago. Since then, the three most commonly used ICU scoring systems have been the APACHE, $MPM_0$, and SAPS. Each of these has been updated numerous times over the years and offers various benefits and insights, their use is widely supported, and some European countries have made their use mandatory. They have each been validated in numerous regions of the world and in distinct different groups of ICU patients as well as specific subgroups such as critically ill cancer patients, cardiovascular, surgical, acute kidney injury requiring renal replacement therapy, and patients in need of extracorporeal membrane oxygen. Of note though, only the APACHE provides both mortality and length of stay predictions. Despite these benefits, in the United States only 10% to 15% of ICUs report using scoring systems such as these.

Ideally, a scoring system would have the following characteristics (1) scores calculated on the basis of easily/routinely recordable variables, (2) well calibrated and validated, (3) a high level of discrimination, (4) applicable to all patient populations in ICU, (5) can be used in different countries, health systems, or patient cohorts, and (6) the ability to predict mortality, functional status, or quality of life after ICU discharge. Scoring systems are typically described in terms of their "discrimination" and "calibration." Discrimination in this case refers to the ability of the scoring system to acutely predict the patients at highest risk for mortality. Discrimination is often described using a "receiver operating characteristic (ROC) curve," with ROC of 0.5 being no better than chance, and values >0.7, 0.8, and 0.9 being considered acceptable, excellent, and outstanding, respectively. Calibration measures how well actual outcomes match their predicted incidence across different groups and is often calculated with the Hosmer-Lemeshow C statistic. Ideally, a scoring system would perform equally well across all risk strata.

One metric generated by scoring systems and commonly used to evaluate ICU performance is the "standardized mortality ratio (SMR)," which is the ratio of the observed or actual patient mortality and the predicted general mortality for that hospital/unit/team over the same period of time. However, SMRs are significantly affected by outcomes in high-risk patient populations, as well as differences in patient population. For example, facilities that frequently transfer their sickest patients out to a quaternary facility may have a falsely low SMR, even if their ICU performance is not in fact as high. Simply reporting SMR does not account for differences in the patient population and does not convey details such as presenting acuity or patient comorbidities.

In summary, scoring systems such as the APACHE, $MPM_0$, and SAPS have the potential to help ICU clinicians better understand and predict patient outcomes to guide both clinical care and research. However, it is important to understand how a given scoring system works, when using it, and realize its potential weakness and limitations.

References

1. Breslow MJ, Badawi O. Severity scoring in the critically ill: part 1–interpretation and accuracy of outcome prediction scoring systems. *Chest.* 2012;141(1):245-252.
2. Breslow MJ, Badawi O. Severity scoring in the critically ill: part 2: maximizing value from outcome prediction scoring systems. *Chest.* 2012;141(2):518-527.
3. Vincent JL, Moreno R. Clinical review: scoring systems in the critically ill. *Crit Care.* 2010;14(2):207.
4. Kuzniewicz M, Vasilevskis E, Lane R, et al. Variation in ICU risk-adjusted mortality: impact of methods of assessment and potential confounders: impact of methods of assessment and potential confounders. *Chest.* 2008;133(6):1319-1327.
5. Salluh J, Soares M. ICU severity of illness scores: APACHE, SAPS and MPM. *Curr Opin Crit Care.* 2014;20(5):557-565.
6. Singh J, Gupta G, Garg R, et al. Evaluation of trauma and prediction of outcome using TRISS method. *J Emerg Trauma Shock.* 2011;4(4):446-449.
7. Wu B, Johannes R, Sun X, et al. The early prediction of mortality in acute pancreatitis: a large population-based study. *Gut.* 2008;57(12):1698-1703.

---

**10.** Correct Answer: A

**Rationale:**

Patients are at particularly high risk of inadvertent nosocomial harm while in the ICU. This is likely due to numerous factors including, in part, the complex medical condition(s) they are suffering from, the number of interventions performed on them daily by ICU staff (estimated to be over 140 interventions per day for each patient), and the busy and challenging environment of the ICU.

Sentinel events, which could or do harm the patient, are frequently underreported. The data that do exist, while thought to be an underestimate, suggest the rate of these is between 40 and 80 per 100 patient days in the ICU.

The largest study to date that has examined these events is the "Sentinel Events Evaluation (SEE) study," which studied patients in 205 ICUs around the world. In it, the following were shown to place the patient at higher risk for experiencing a sentinel event: (1) any organ failure, (2) a higher intensity in level of care, and (3) and time of exposure.

Given the relative frequency of potential harmful events in ICU patients, a great deal of research has gone into how to best improve timely and accurate reporting of these mistakes as well as how to avoid them. Nurses appear to typically be the most frequent reporters of potentially harmful events that occurred in the ICU, and reporting rates appear to improve when the method of reporting is simplified. (One study showed a three- to fourfold improvement in response rates by switching from a digital reporting system back to a simplified paper card system.) Numerous factors have been suggested as potentially decreasing the rate of potentially harmful events. Some of these include improved nurse to patient ratio, increased number of physicians, full-time ICU specialists, and others. However, some of the best evidence for beneficial effect appears to be around multidisciplinary ICU rounds and digital prescribing.

## References

1. Moreno R, Rhodes P, Donchin A. Patient safety in intensive care medicine: the declaration of Vienna. *Intensive Care Med.* 2009;35(10):1667-1672.
2. Valentin A, Capuzzo M, Guidet B, et al. Patient safety in intensive care: results from the multinational sentinel events evaluation (SEE) study. *Intensive Care Med.* 2006;32:1591-1598.
3. Rothschild J, Landrigan C, Cronin J, et al. The critical care safety study: the incidence and nature of adverse events and serious medical errors in intensive care. *Crit Care Med.* 2005;33(8):1694-1700.
4. Rothen H, Stricker U, Einfalt K, et al. Variability in outcome and resource use in intensive care units. *Intensive Care Med.* 2007;33(8):1329-1336.
5. Ilan R, Squires M, Panopoulos C, et al. Increasing patient safety event reporting in 2 intensive care units: a prospective interventional study. *J Crit Care.* 2011;26(4):431.e11-431.e18.

# 114

# TEACHING

Ryan J. Horvath

1. Several residents approach you, an intensivist, to mentor them through a Quality improvement (QI) project. You advise them that the three components of quality of care are structure, process, and outcome. Which of the following is an accepted model for approaching QI that you can suggest the residents use?

    A. Quality-adjusted life years (QALY)
    B. Structure-Process-Outcome cycle (SPO cycle)
    C. Plan-Do-Study-Act cycle (PDSA cycle)
    D. I-PASS
    E. Situation-Background-Assessment-Recommendation (SBAR)

2. During rounds in the intensive care unit (ICU), you begin discussing closed versus open ICU structure and processes that improve delivery of critical care with a group of residents and fellows. Which of the following has been associated with lower patient mortality across ICUs with divergent hospital structure (teaching hospital vs private practice), care team structure (solo intensivist vs mixed care team), and patient mix (surgical vs medical ICU)?

    A. Use of daily goals forms
    B. Dedicated ICU nursing managers and medical directors
    C. Avoidance of protocols (ie ventilator management, antibiotic usage, venous thromboembolism preventions, hypoglycemia management)
    D. Staffing models that rely heavily on residents, nurse practitioners, physician assistants, or other care extenders
    E. Multidisciplinary rounds at least twice daily

3. Recently, resident evaluations of their ICU rotations have revealed significant dissatisfaction with the traditional didactic teaching sessions. The director of the ICU asks you to develop a "flipped classroom" educational series for your ICU. Which of the following would be considered a model of a "flipped classroom"?

    A. Moving the location of teaching sessions out of the ICU and into an area away from clinical care and more conducive to learning.
    B. Instead of having attendings lecture to residents, allow residents to drive their own learning by asking questions of their staff during didactic sessions.
    C. Provide answers to problem sets or clinical questions to residents before teaching sessions to focus their learning.
    D. Completely abolish didactic classroom learning and initiate online-only learning modules.
    E. Have students first complete independent, self-directed education outside of the classroom and then do learning activities inside the classroom that builds upon prior work.

# Chapter 114 ▪ Answers

**1.** Correct Answer: C

**Rationale:**

Governmental agencies with healthcare oversight and hospital administration have placed increased focus on the delivery of quality health care in recent years. The Institute of Medicine defines quality care by six metrics: care that is safe, timely, effective, efficient, equitable, and patient centered. Quality care is not only a method by which hospitals and healthcare systems are judged but increasingly plays a role in their financial reimbursement. This incentivizes healthcare professionals to improve the quality of care that they deliver to patients.

The Institute for Healthcare Improvement recommends the PDSA cycle (answer C) model as an effective means of quality improvement. The first step in this model is to study the identified problem and come up with a Plan tailored to the environment and healthcare setting. The next steps are to implement a change or intervention (Do) and evaluate the results (Study). This information should be included in the improvement effort (Act), which can be further refined and improved in subsequent PDSA cycles.

QALY (answer A) is an outcome measure for clinical trials, I-PASS (answer D) and SBAR (answer E) are handoff tools commonly used in the ICU, and Structure-Process-Outcome (answer B) are the components of quality care, but not an accepted model for approaching QI.

## References

1. Curtis JR, Cook DJ, Wall RJ, et al. Intensive care unit quality improvement: a "how-to" guide for the interdisciplinary team. *Crit Care Med*. 2006;34:211-218.
2. Hahn J, Cummings BM. Quality Improvement and Standardization of Practice. In: Wiener-Kronish JP, ed. *Critical Care handbook of the Massachusetts General Hospital*. 6th ed. Philadelphia: Wolters Kluwer; 2016:575-588.

**2.** Correct Answer: A

**Rationale:**

There has been significant interest in the characteristics that improve outcomes in the ICUs. Across the Unites States, there is significant variation on the delivery of critical care including:

- ICU type: Medical ICU, surgical ICU, cardiac ICU, neuro ICU, burn ICU, etc.
- Structure: Open ICUs where the admitting physician remains the patient's primary caregiver after transfer to the ICU, and intensivists are available for consult purposes versus closed ICUs where there is a dedicated ICU care team including an intensivist who assumes primary responsibility for patients on transfer to the ICU.
- Hospital location: Large city versus rural.
- ICU team structure: Private practice solo practitioner intensivist, mixed structures with nurse practitioners and physician assistants, teaching hospitals with academic practice and resident teams, etc.
- Intensivist coverage: 24-hour in-house intensivist coverage, night home call intensivist coverage, etc.

Many studies exist that show incremental improvement in patient outcomes (usually low-level outcomes such as ventilator-free days or total ICU stay and not higher level outcomes such as overall morbidity and mortality) in individual or groups of ICUs before and after an intervention. However, with such variation in the structure and delivery critical care across the United States, it has been a challenge to extrapolate these finding more broadly.

In 2014, the United States Critical Illness and Injury Trails Group Critical Illness Outcomes Study (USCI-ITG-CIOS) studies the structure, process, and mortality across 69 divergent ICUs across the United States. Factors associated with lower mortality included use of a daily plan of care review (answer A) and lower bed-to-nurse ratios. 24-hour intensivist coverage and closed ICU status were not found to be associated with improved mortality.

## References

1. Checkly W, Martin GS, Brown SM, et al. Structure, process and annual intensive care unit mortality across 69 centers: United States Critical Illness and Injury Trials Group Critical Illness Outcomes Study (USCIITG-CIOS). *Crit Care Med*. 2014;42(2):344-356.
2. Frankel SK, Moss M. The effect of organizational structure and processes of care on ICU mortality as revealed by the USCI-ITG-critical illness outcomes study. *Crit Care Med*. 2014;42(2):463-464.

**3.** Correct Answer: E

**Rationale:**

Teaching in the ICU can be challenging for many reasons including: a wide range in learners from med students through residents and fellows; a wide range of past experiences from learners; varying acuity and volume of patients in the ICU; the fast-paced atmosphere that often allows little time without interruption. Additionally, learners are increasingly requesting more learner-centric opportunities as compared to more traditional didactic lectures. The "flipped classroom" model involves having students perform independent self-directed learning activities before education sessions, usually involving online modules, videos, etc. Educational sessions are then used to focus on reinforcing what was learned before the sessions. In this way, the method by which information is presented to learners is reversed or "flipped" compared to traditional educational sessions.

## References

1. Peets AD, McLaughlin K, Lockyer J, et al. So much to teach, so little time: a prospective cohort study evaluating a tool to select content for a critical care curriculum. *Crit Care.* 2008;12(5):R127.
2. Tainter CR, Wong NL, Cudemas-Desada GA, et al. The "Flipped Classroom" model for teaching in the intensive care unit: rationale, practical considerations, and an example of successful implementation. *J Intensive Care.* 2017;32(3):187-196.

# 115

## PSYCHOSOCIAL ISSUE AMONG PROVIDERS

Jennifer Cottral and William J. Benedetto

1. Classic symptoms of burnout syndrome (BOS) as defined by the Maslach Burnout Inventory (MBI) include all of the following EXCEPT:

   A. Exhaustion
   B. Moral distress
   C. Depersonalization
   D. Reduced personal accomplishment

2. What is the most commonly misused substance among physicians with substance use disorders?

   A. Alcohol
   B. Opioids
   C. Benzodiazepines
   D. Controlled stimulants

## Chapter 115 ▪ Answers

1. Correct Answer: B

   **Rationale:**
   BOS is a pattern of nonspecific signs and symptoms that result from work-related stressors, often seen in individuals with no history of psychological or psychiatric disorders. BOS was first described in healthcare workers in the 1970s, and by the 1980s, evaluation criteria became available through the design of a standard measurement instrument called the Maslach Burnout Inventory (MBI). The MBI quantifies the presence and severity of the three classic symptoms of BOS that include exhaustion, depersonalization, and reduced personal accomplishment. Exhaustion is physical and/or emotional fatigue related to devoting disproportionate time and effort to a task that is not perceived by the person to be beneficial. Depersonalization is feeling disconnected from one's work and colleagues and can manifest as negative, callous, and cynical behaviors. Reduced personal accomplishment is negatively evaluating one's job performance and the worth of one's work. Moral distress occurs when an individual knows the ethical action to take but feels constrained from taking this action. Moral distress can overlap with or contribute to BOS but is not a defined symptom of BOS as classically described by the MBI.

   References
   1. Moss M, Good VS, Gozal D, et al. An official critical care societies collaborative statement: burnout syndrome in critical care healthcare professionals: a call for action. *Crit Care Med*. 2016;44(7):1414-1421.
   2. Weber A. Burnout syndrome: a disease of modern societies? *Occup Med (Lond)*. 2000;50(7):512-517.
   3. Fourie C. Who is experiencing what kind of moral distress? Distinctions for moving from a narrow to a broad definition of moral distress. *AMA J Ethics*. 2017;19(6):578-584.

**2.** Correct Answer: A

**Rationale:**

An often-quoted prevalence of substance use disorders among physicians is 10% to 12%, which is based on a paper published over 25 years ago. More recent volunteer survey data among attending and trainee physicians suggest that the prevalence of substance use disorders among physicians is much higher, though predominantly represented by alcohol use disorder. Indeed, over the course of over 3 decades of research, alcohol has been the most frequently misused substance among physicians surveyed. This is also true for those physicians treated for substance use disorders, followed by opioids. Physicians have an ethical and (depending on the state) legal responsibility to report impaired colleagues. However, many are reluctant to report a colleague, even when the suspect is impaired or incompetent. This is due to belief that someone else was taking care of the problem, that nothing would happen as a result of the report, or due to fear of retaliation.

References

1.  Berge KH, Seppala MD, Schipper AM. Chemical dependency and the physician. *Mayo Clin Proc.* 2009;84(7):625-631.
2.  McLellan AT, Skipper GS, Campbell M, DuPont RL. Five year out- comes in a cohort study of physicians treated for substance use disorders in the United States. *BMJ.* 2008;337:a2038.
3.  Oreskovich MR, Shanafelt T, Dyrbye LN, et al. The prevalence of substance use disorders in American physicians. *Am J Addict.* 2015;24(1):30-38.
4.  Baldisseri MR. Impaired healthcare professional. *Crit Care Med.* 2007;35:S106-S116.
5.  Taub S, Morin K, Goldrich MS, Ray P, Benjamin R; Council on Ethical and Judicial Affairs of the American Medical Association. Physician health and wellness. *Occup Med.* 2006;56:77-82.
6.  DesRoches CM, Rao SR, Fromson JA, et al. Physicians' perceptions, preparedness for reporting, and experiences related to impaired and incompetent colleagues. *JAMA.* 2010;304:187-193.

# 116

# ETHICAL CONSIDERATIONS

Theresa Barnes, William J. Trudo, and Avneep Aggarwal

1. A 62-year-old man with new onset shortness of breath is admitted to the ICU with a large right-sided pleural effusion, requiring noninvasive positive pressure ventilation because of increased work of breathing. CT imaging is suggestive of lung cancer with metastasis to the liver. Prior to disclosing results of imaging to the patient, the patient's daughter asks to speak with you privately. She states that her father does not wish to know anything regarding his condition. What is the MOST appropriate next step?

   A. Determine why the daughter believes that her father does not want to know information regarding his diagnosis
   B. Ask the patient about his preferences for knowing results of imaging, likely diagnosis, and plans of care
   C. Further assess if the patient has capacity to make decisions
   D. Involve the ethics committee to determine if the patient is competent to make decisions

2. Which of the following is true regarding the concept of respect for autonomy?

   A. A patient may be coerced into a treatment by using a credible threat
   B. A patient may be persuaded into a treatment by using a legitimate argument
   C. Physicians are obligated to "do whatever the patient wants"
   D. If a patient refuses a treatment, there is no way a physician can be liable for injuries occurred owing to lack of treatment

3. A 78-year-old woman is admitted for choledocholithiasis, diagnosed by magnetic resonance cholangiopancreatography (MRCP), with mildly elevated liver function tests and serum bilirubin of 1.5 mg/dL. Serum amylase and lipase are normal and temperature is 37.1°C. Which of the following is LEAST appropriate to discuss while consenting the patient for endoscopic retrograde cholangiopancreatography (ERCP)?

   A. The diagnosis of choledocholithiasis and need for additional procedures after ERCP
   B. Propose and explain ERCP and alternative treatment options
   C. The contact information of family members not present
   D. The risks of refusing treatment

4. A 55-year-old male presents with a left middle cerebral artery stroke. Shortly after arriving at the hospital, his mental status declines, and he is intubated. His wife is his durable power of attorney for healthcare decisions. She notes that he did not want to end up, "connected to machines to keep him alive," and his living will states: "I do not want aggressive measures to extend my life." The neurointerventional team feels that his prognosis is likely good with an endovascular revascularization procedure, but the wife is hesitant to consent to this procedure. What is the most appropriate next step?

   A. Explore the patient's wishes with regard to medical care with his wife
   B. Proceed with the procedure without his wife's consent because it is likely lifesaving, and any delay may make his outcome worse
   C. Consult the hospital ethics committee
   D. Consult other members of the family and seek their consent for the procedure

**5.** Which of the following is the correct order for highest to lowest priority of surrogate decision makers for an incompetent adult patient?

   **A.** Individual appointed by patient, spouse, adult child, parent, adult sibling
   **B.** Individual appointed by patient, spouse, parent, adult child, adult sibling
   **C.** Individual appointed by patient, spouse, adult sibling, adult child, parent
   **D.** Individual appointed by patient, spouse, parent, adult sibling, adult child

# Chapter 116 ▪ Answers

**1.** Correct Answer: B

**Rationale:**

Patient autonomy involves the right to determine which treatment will and will not be accepted. The exertion of autonomy requires that the patient be free to make their own decision with adequate knowledge and freedom from controlling influences about their medical care. If a patient chooses to make a family member a healthcare proxy, the patient must do so independently, with the understanding that further medical information may be withheld from them. In this particular situation, a discussion with the patient would need to occur first (Answer B).

Family and group dynamics have a strong impact on decision making in many healthcare contexts. However, as the patient has not defined his daughter as a healthcare proxy, and there is no reason to question his decision-making capacity (no history of dementia, psychosis, intoxication, altered mental status, etc), it would be inappropriate at this time to relinquish the patient's right to know his medical details (Answer A and C).

With the information provided, there is no indication that the patient lacks decisional capacity. Legal determination of competency would need to be assessed if incapacity were established and the family was unable to come to a joint decision regarding care (Answer D).

References

1. Entwistle VA, Carter SM, Cribb A, McCaffery K. Supporting patient autonomy: the importance of clinician-patient relationships. *J Gen Intern Med.* 2010;25(7):741-745.
2. Jonsen AR, Siegler M, Winslade WJ. *Clinical Ethics: A Practical Approach to Ethical Decisions in Clinical Medicine.* 8th ed. New York: McGraw-Hill; 2015.

**2.** Correct Answer: B

**Rationale:**

A key point of informed consent of patients is the concept of respect for autonomy. In order to fulfill this principle, patients must be fully informed regarding risks, benefits, and alternative treatment options. Presenting information about different treatment options can include a component of persuasion, the act of influencing a decision with legitimate arguments (Answer B). For example, you might explain to a patient that the placement of a central venous catheter will ensure the safe delivery of vasoactive medications compared with a peripheral intravenous line. However, coercion with threats is not an appropriate method of communication when presenting treatment plans (Answer A). It would be inappropriate to say, "If you don't let us put in the central line, and we continue to use the peripheral IV for these medications, you'll lose your arm." In this case, the (somewhat) credible threat is coercion.

A physician cannot "do whatever the patient wants," if the patient does not have a proper understanding of all medical options (Answer C). Furthermore, if a patient refuses a treatment, the patient must have adequate understanding of the complications that could be associated with their refusal. If the patient is not truly making an informed refusal, then the physician may be liable for injury resulting from a lack of information held by the patient.

Reference

1. Waisel DB, Truog RD. Informed consent. *Anesthesiology.* 1997;87(4):968-978.

**3.** Correct Answer: C

**Rationale:**

There is a legal and ethical responsibility of a physician to provide sufficient information about medical procedures to a patient, allowing him or her to process the information and then choose an appropriate decision.

   Informed consent should include:

1. Reasoning behind and purpose of procedure, with potential need for further procedures
2. Explanation of procedure

3. Alternative options
4. Risks and benefits of procedure
5. Risks of refusing treatment

Unless the patient is determined by the medical provider to lack decisional capacity (intoxicated, delirious, demented, comatose, or is unable to remember/understand what is being said) or has been legally determined to lack competency, family members or a healthcare proxy do not need to be contacted or available during consent for the procedure (Answer C).

### References

1. Entwistle VA, Carter SM, Cribb A, McCaffery K. Supporting patient autonomy: the importance of clinician-patient relationships. *J Gen Intern Med.* 2010;25(7):741-745.
2. Mandava A, Pace C, Campbell B, Emanuel E, Grady C. The quality of informed consent: mapping the landscape. A review of empirical data from developing and developed countries. *J Med Ethics.* 2012;38(6):356-365.
3. White SM. Ethical and legal aspects of anesthesia for the elderly. *Anesthesia.* 2014;69(suppl 1):45-53.
4. Jonsen AR, Siegler M, Winslade WJ. *Clinical Ethics: A Practical Approach to Ethical Decisions in Clinical Medicine.* 8th ed. New York: McGraw-Hill; 2015.

**4.** Correct Answer: A

**Rationale:**

This patient lacks capacity to decide medical treatments secondary to his impaired mental status. Because his living will is somewhat vague regarding his wishes, the principle of substituted judgment should be followed. This principle calls for a surrogate decision maker to choose options for the patient based on their understanding of the patient's beliefs and values. The patient's wife, who is his durable power of attorney, is serving as the patient's legal surrogate decision maker in this case, and she has the final say with regard to medical treatments. It is appropriate to discuss the treatment with her and seek informed consent, and if she does not agree, explore her reasoning further (Answer A). She has the sole legal power to refuse any further medical treatments for her husband even if his prognosis is not necessarily terminal (Answer B). If other family members oppose this decision, they cannot overrule her choice (Answer D). If there is a lack of consensus among family members regarding treatment decisions, a hospital ethics committee consultation may be appropriate (Answer C).

### References

1. Bernat JL. *Clinical ethics and the law.* In: *Ethical issues in neurology.* 3rd ed. Philadelphia: Lippincott Williams & Wilkins; 2008:81-110.
2. Adelman EE, Zahuranec DB. Surrogate decision making in neurocritical care. *Continuum (Minneap Minn).* 2012;18(3):655-658.

**5.** Correct Answer: A

**Rationale:**

If an adult patient is deemed incapacitated, the hierarchy followed for surrogate decision makers is as follows:
1. Individual appointed by patient
2. Spouse
3. Adult child
4. Parent
5. Adult sibling

If the patient has an advance directive, then the surrogate decision maker should use this document to help guide their medical choices for the patient. The surrogate should also employ the substituted judgment principle, making choices that the incompetent individual would choose if they were competent.

### References

1. American Bar Association Commission on Law and Aging. *Default Surrogate Consent Statutes.* 2018. Available at https://www.americanbar.org/content/dam/aba/administrative/law_aging/2014_default_surrogate_consent_statutes.authcheckdam.pdf.
2. Buchanan AE, Brock DW. *Deciding for Others: The Ethics Of Surrogate Decision Making.* Cambridge: Cambridge University Press; 1989.

# 117

# PATIENT CONFIDENTIALITY, HEALTHCARE POLICY

Ryan J. Horvath

1. Which of the following is LEAST likely to reduce central line–associated bloodstream infections (CLABSI) in critically ill patients?

   A. Use of full body drapes when inserting central venous catheters (CVCs)
   B. Performing hand hygiene before placement or manipulation of CVCs
   C. Limiting number of people in the room during placement of the CVC to only those needed for placement and immediate patient care
   D. Routinely culturing the tip of CVCs on removal
   E. Avoidance of femoral vein CVCs if subclavian or internal jugular sites are available

2. Which of the following is MOST likely to reduce catheter-associated urinary tract infection (CAUTI) in the intensive care unit (ICU)?

   A. Routine use of urinary catheters for all postoperative patients
   B. Intermediate catheterization for patients with bladder emptying dysfunction
   C. Bladder irrigation with antimicrobial agents
   D. Maintain collecting systems above the level of the bladder
   E. Leave catheters unsecured to allow free movement of the collecting system

3. Under the *Standards for Privacy of Individually Identifiable Health Information* established under the Health Insurance Portability and Accountability Act of 1996 (HIPAA), which of the following is NOT a permitted disclosure of protected health information under "Public Interest and Benefit Activities"?

   A. Disclosure of the results of beta-HCG blood tests to the parents of a 15-year-old female recently admitted to the ICU
   B. Disclosure of an incident of abuse or neglect to government authorities
   C. Disclosure of protected information to the medical examiner in the case of a death in the ICU
   D. Disclosure of a diagnosis of measles to state authorities and the Centers for Disease Control
   E. Disclosure of protected information to the United Network for Organ Sharing (UNOS)

4. Regarding infection control in the ICU, which of the following are standard precautions shown to be most effective in decreasing the transmission of hospital-acquired infections?

   A. Positive pressure ICU rooms for all patients on "respiratory precautions"
   B. Limiting patient visitors to those patients on "contact precautions"
   C. Use of an alcohol-based hand cleanser or washing with soap and water between patient contacts
   D. Requiring ICU staff to wear dedicated clothing only for use in the ICU, and banning white coats as they are notorious fomites
   E. Use of sterile gloves and gowns as personal protective equipment during all patient interactions

5. The HIPAA Privacy Rule permits healthcare providers to disclose protected healthcare information concerning a patient with major depression, who has capacity and requests that his or her family not be contacted in which of the following situations?

   **A.** When the family member is the healthcare proxy
   **B.** When the healthcare provider perceives a serious patient safety concern
   **C.** When the family member is the spouse or next of kin
   **D.** When the healthcare provider does not agree with the patient's healthcare decisions
   **E.** When the healthcare provider believes that the patient's medical decisions are being influenced by their mental illness

# Chapter 117 ▪ Answers

**1.** Correct Answer: D

**Rationale:**
Many patients in the ICU will require CVCs for reasons including delivery of vital medication (ie vasopressors), nutrition (ie parenteral nutrition), and monitoring (ie central venous pressure monitoring). Morbidity from CVCs include adverse events from placement (ie hematoma, inadvertent arterial puncture, pneumothorax), thrombus, and CLABSI. CLABSI can arise from intraluminal or extraluminal contamination at any time from placement through routine use. The cost of CLABSI has been estimated to be as high as $45 000 for an individual patient and over $1 billion in annual healthcare costs nationwide.

CVC bundles have been developed to encourage methods that have been shown to reduce CLABSI. These methods include CVC training and education, centralizing CVC equipment into a central line cart; proper hand hygiene throughout placement and access of CVCs; proper personal protective equipment including hat and mask for everyone in the room and hat, mask, sterile gown, and gloves for practitioners placing CVCs; full body drapes; chlorhexidine-based antiseptic cleaning before placement, use of antimicrobial impregnated CVCs dressing sponges, changing dressing when they become loose or soiled, etc. Routine culture of the tip of CVC catheters (answer D) is not recommended as the tip can be easily contaminated by skin flora during removal.

References
1. Hahn J, Cummings BM. Quality improvement and standardization of practice. In: Wiener-Kronish JP, ed. *Critical Care handbook of the Massachusetts General Hospital*. 6th ed. Philadelphia: Wolters Kluwer; 2016:575-588.
2. O'Grady NP, Alexander M, Burns LA, et al. *Guidelines for the Prevention of Intravascular Catheter-Related Infections*. Centers for Disease Control; 2011. https://www.cdc.gov/infectioncontrol/guidelines/bsi/.

**2.** Correct Answer: B

**Rationale:**
Urinary catheters are commonplace in the ICU; however, infections related to their use can cause morbidity ranging from simple urinary tract infections to urosepsis. CAUTI-related costs are estimated to be only about $750 per patient; however, their high incidence leads to nearly $300 million in cost every year nationwide.

Similar to CVC bundles, catheter bundles have been developed to encourage methods shown to reduce CAUTI. These methods include only using catheters when absolutely indicated (including acute retention or obstruction, accurate monitoring of urine production in critical illness, with epidural use, peroneal wounds or certain surgeries); removing catheters as soon as reasonably possible, use of aseptic technique when placing or changing catheters or collection systems; maintaining collecting systems below the level of the bladder to avoid flow from the collecting system back into the bladder; securing catheters to prevent movement in the urethra; and using antimicrobial-coated catheters in high-risk populations. Bladder irrigation with antimicrobials is not recommended.

References
1. Gould CV, Umscheid CA, Agarwal RK, et al. *Guideline for Prevention of Catheter-Associated Urinary Tract Infections 2009*. Healthcare Infection Control Practices Advisory Committee, Centers for Disease Control. https://www.cdc.gov/infectioncontrol/guidelines/cauti/.
2. Hahn J, Cummings BM. Quality improvement and standardization of practice. In: Wiener-Kronish JP, ed. *Critical Care handbook of the Massachusetts General Hospital*. 6th ed. Philadelphia: Wolters Kluwer; 2016:575-588.

**3.** Correct Answer: A

**Rationale:**

The HIPAA was a revolutionary piece of legislation that, in addition to wide-ranging changes to health insurance regulation in the United States, established the *Standards for Privacy of Individually Identifiable Health Information.* This "Privacy Rule" established standards for the disclosure of protected health information to "covered entities" (including health plans, healthcare providers, and healthcare clearinghouses). One of the permitted uses and disclosures comes under "Public Interest and Benefit Activities."

These activities include: when required by law; public health activities (answer D); victims of abuse, neglect, or domestic violence (answer B); health oversight activities (answer C); judicial and administrative proceedings; law enforcement purposes; decedents; cadaveric organ, eye, or tissue donations (answer E); research; serious threat to health or safety; essential government functions; and workers' compensations. A juvenile's right to privacy concerning reproduction and especially pregnancy testing has been well established and thus disclosure of this protected information is not covered by HIPAA.

Reference

1. The United States Department of Health and Human Services, Office for Civil Rights. Summary of the HIPAA Privacy Rule. Revised 05/03.

**4.** Correct Answer: C

**Rationale:**

Hospital-acquired infections have come under increased scrutiny because of their cost both in patient morbidity and mortality and in healthcare dollars. It is recognized that the major method of transmission of most hospital-acquired infections is from healthcare workers transmitting microorganisms between patients through lack of proper hand hygiene, personal protective equipment, or through fomites on their person (objects that are likely to carry infection from one patient to another including stethoscopes, white coats, ties, etc). Therefore, limiting patient visitors (answer B) to individual rooms is unlikely to directly reduce transmission of disease between patients in the ICU where most rooms are single occupancy. No strategy has proven more effective and cost-efficient as proper hand hygiene (answer C) in reducing the spread of hospital-acquired infections.

In a positive pressure ICU room, the air pressure is higher in the room than the surrounding workspace, and although it can help to keep contagions from entering the room (as used in operating rooms), it can promote the spread of respiratory contagions (answer A). Therefore, patients with particularly virulent respiratory pathogens, such as tuberculosis (TB), are placed in negative pressure rooms. Use of sterile personal protective equipment versus regular personal protective equipment (answer E) and dedicated hospital clothing for the ICU (answer D) would certainly be an effective way of limiting fomites; however, these are costlier to implement and not as effective as good hand hygiene.

References

1. Hahn J, Cummings BM. Quality improvement and standardization of practice. In: Wiener-Kronish JP, ed. *Critical Care handbook of the Massachusetts General Hospital.* 6th ed. Philadelphia: Wolters Kluwer; 2016:575-588.
2. Siegel JD, Rhinehart E, Jackson M, et al. 2007 guideline for isolation precautions: preventing transmission of infectious agent in health care settings. *Am J Infect Control.* 2007;35(10 suppl 2):S65-S164. Last Updated February 15, 2017. Centers for Disease Control.

**5.** Correct Answer: B

**Rationale:**

The HIPAA allows for the disclosure of protected healthcare information concerning a patient with mental illness in a few very specific situations. If the patient is deemed competent, they retain agency to make their own healthcare decisions. Healthcare providers disagreeing with the patient's decisions (answer D) or believing that their mental illness is affecting their medical decision-making (answer E) is not sufficient to allow disclosure against the patient's wishes. Healthcare proxy status (answer A) or being a spouse or next of kin (answer C) does not supersede the patient's request for no information to be shared as long as they are not incapacitated. HIPAA provides allowances for disclosure of protected healthcare information concerning a patient with mental illness if the healthcare provider perceives a "serious and imminent threat to the health or safety of the patient or others and the family members are in a position to lessen the threat."

References

1. U.S. Department of Health and Human Services Office for Civil Rights. *HIPAA Privacy Rule and Sharing Information.* https://www.hhs.gov/sites/default/files/hipaa-privacy-rule-and-sharing-info-related-to-mental-health.pdf.
2. The United States Department of Health and Human Services, Office for Civil Rights. Summary of the HIPAA Privacy Rule. Revised 05/03.

# 118

# PALLIATIVE CARE AND END OF LIFE

Jennifer Cottral and William J. Benedetto

1. A 61-year-old male is admitted to the intensive care unit (ICU) intubated after an out-of-hospital cardiac arrest due to myocardial infarction complicated by anoxic brain injury. He has a history of severe chronic obstructive pulmonary disease (COPD) with home oxygen, poorly controlled insulin-dependent type II diabetes, chronic kidney disease, and severe peripheral vascular disease status post left above-the-knee amputation. The patient was assessed to be too high-risk for percutaneous coronary interventions, and two cardiac surgeons have deemed the patient a poor surgical candidate. Over the past 24 hours, the patient has remained on multiple high-dose vasopressors, has become anuric, his creatinine has tripled, and his potassium is 7.0 mEq/dL. The patient has not filled out an advance directive or assigned a healthcare proxy, and his next of kin includes his three children. After multiple family meetings, the patient's children continue to request renal replacement therapy despite concerns from the ICU team about its medical appropriateness. Which of the following is NOT a recommended step to conflict resolution based on the most recent multispecialty consensus statement regarding potentially inappropriate medical care in the ICU?

    A. Obtain a second medical opinion
    B. Provide review by an interdisciplinary hospital committee
    C. Offer legal counsel to surrogates
    D. Offer surrogates the opportunity for transfer to an alternate institution
    E. Enlist expert consultation to aid in achieving a negotiated agreement

2. The available evidence suggests that the impact of ICU-based palliative care includes all the following EXCEPT:

    A. Decrease ICU and hospital length of stay
    B. Decrease healthcare cost
    C. Improve communication with patient
    D. Increase in-hospital mortality

3. All the following have been shown to significantly reduce the rate of catheter-related bloodstream infections (CR-BSIs) occurring in the ICU EXCEPT:

    A. Handwashing
    B. Use of full-barrier precautions
    C. Cleaning the skin with chlorhexidine
    D. Avoiding the femoral site for cannulation
    E. Performing a time-out before line insertion

4. What is the 1-year mortality risk in a critically ill 67-year-old patient with platelets of $100 \times 10^9$/L requiring hemodialysis and mechanical ventilation on hospital day 21?

    A. 10% to 20%
    B. 30% to 40%
    C. 40% to 50%
    D. 60% to 70%
    E. >70%

5. Symptoms of postintensive care syndrome (PICS) include all of the following except:

   A. Cognitive dysfunction
   B. Psychiatric disturbances
   C. Metabolic syndrome
   D. Musculoskeletal weakness

6. A 64-year-old male with no known prior medical history was admitted 5 days ago with a large subarachnoid hemorrhage from a suspected ruptured cerebral aneurysm. His current vitals are blood pressure (BP) 105/70 mm Hg, heart rate 84 beats per minute, respiratory rate 16/min on volume control ventilation, and temperature 98.8°F. Laboratory data are all within normal limits. He has not received any central nervous system depressants or paralytics but makes no respiratory effort after 8 minutes of apnea. He is noted to have an intermittent bilateral finger tremor, though not in response to stimuli such as pain. All brainstem reflexes are absent. Does this patient meet the criteria for brain death based on the most recent recommendations by the Society of Critical Care Medicine?

   A. Yes
   B. No

7. All of the following conditions in a suspected organ donor are contraindications to organ donation EXCEPT:

   A. Bacteremia on appropriate antibiotics
   B. Grade II central nervous system tumor
   C. Hepatitis C virus (HCV) seropositive
   D. Human immunodeficiency virus (HIV) seronegative but meets the high-risk behavioral criteria for HIV infection
   E. All of the above
   F. None the above

8. In patients who are being considered for organ donation after cardiac death (DCD), all of the following are considered part of the United Network for Organ Sharing (UNOS) criteria for prediction of death within 60 minutes of withdrawal of life-sustaining treatment (LST), EXCEPT:

   A. Apnea
   B. Respiratory rate <8 or >30 breaths/min
   C. ≥3 vasopressors to maintain a mean arterial pressure (MAP) >65 mm Hg
   D. $Fio_2$ ≥0.5 and $Sao_2$ ≤92%
   E. Norepinephrine or phenylephrine ≥0.2 µg/kg/min

9. True or false: Withholding LST is permissible, but once started, it must be continued.

   A. True
   B. False

10. Match the following terms with their definitions:

| | TERMS | | DEFINITIONS |
|---|---|---|---|
| a | Living will | 1 | Medical orders addressing a range of topics likely to be relevant to the care of a patient near the end of life; other healthcare professionals (including emergency personnel) are required to follow them |
| b | Advance care planning | 2 | The process of clarifying goals, values, and preferences, usually through written documents and medical orders, about the type(s) of medical care a patient does or does not want under certain medical conditions |
| c | Medical orders for life-sustaining treatment | 3 | A type of advanced directive that specifies the type(s) of medical care a patient does or does not want under certain medical conditions, in the case that at a future time, the patient is not able to express those preferences |

| | TERMS | | DEFINITIONS |
|---|---|---|---|
| d | Do-not-resuscitate orders, do not hospitalize, do not intubate orders | 4 | Medical orders addressing the limitations of specific treatments near the end of life that are written within a healthcare facility but do not transfer to other care settings and are not necessarily followed by outside healthcare professionals |
| e | Durable power of attorney for health care | 5 | A type of an advanced directive that identifies the healthcare agent who will make medical decisions on behalf of a patient if the patient is incapable of making medical decisions |

**A.** a3, b5, c4, d2, e1
**B.** a5, b2, c3, d2, e1
**C.** a5, b5, c1, d4, e3
**D.** a3, b2, c1, d4, e5

# Chapter 118 ▪ Answers

**1.** Correct Answer: C

**Rationale:**

In 2015, a multispecialty group released a consensus statement regarding how ICU clinicians can and should respond to requests for potentially inappropriate treatment in the ICU with the goal to prevent intractable disagreements about the use of such treatments. This group recommended the use of the term "potentially inappropriate" rather than "futile" care to describe scenarios where a treatment may provide the effect desired by surrogates, but clinicians believe that certain ethical considerations justify not providing the treatment in question. If such a scenario arises and the surrogate(s) continue to request potentially inappropriate treatment despite intensive communication and negotiation with the ICU care team, the following approach recommended:

1. Enlist expert consultation to continue negotiation during the dispute resolution process
2. Give notice of the process to surrogates
3. Obtain a second medical opinion
4. Obtain review by an interdisciplinary hospital committee
5. Offer surrogates the opportunity to transfer the patient to an alternate institution
6. Inform surrogates of the opportunity to pursue extramural appeal
7. Implement the decision of the resolution process

Although surrogates should be informed of their right to seek extramural appeal (usually through seeking judicial review), clinicians and hospitals are not required to offer and/or provide legal counsel to surrogates.

Reference

1. Bosslet G, Pope T, Rubenfeld G, et al. An official ATS/AACN/ACCP/ESICM/SCCM policy statement: responding to requests for potentially inappropriate treatments in intensive care units. *Am J Respir Crit Care Med.* 2015;191(11):1318-1330.

**2.** Correct Answer: D

**Rationale:**

Palliative care in the ICU involves interprofessional support for both patients and families, attending to the spiritual, physical, and emotional domains of critical illness. Palliative care is often provided concomitantly with life-prolonging care and unlike hospice care, is not based on prognosis. Efforts to define outcomes and quantify the impact of ICU-based palliative care interventions are ongoing. Various meta-analyses and systematic review of the effect of ICU-based palliative care on a variety of outcomes suggest that palliative care interventions largely decrease hospital and ICU length of stay and a reduction in healthcare cost. While some studies suggest a reduction in in-hospital mortality, others show no effect. But there is no evidence to suggest that mortality increases with palliative care interventions (answer D). In addition, the results suggested that ICU-based palliative care led to improvement in the quality, quantity, and content of communication, decrease in symptoms of distress and anxiety among family members, decrease in procedures, decrease in the time between admission and comfort measures only, withdrawal of LSTs, and do-not-resuscitate orders.

## References

1. Aslakson RA, Curtis JR, Nelson JE. The changing role of palliative care in the ICU. *Crit Care Med.* 2014;42:2418-2428.
2. Aslakson RA, Bridges JF. Assessing the impact of palliative care in the intensive care unit through the lens of patient-centered outcomes research. *Curr Opin Crit Care.* 2013;19:504-510.
3. Mularski RA. Defining and measuring quality palliative and end-of-life care in the intensive care unit. *Crit Care Med.* 2006;34(11 suppl):S309-S316.
4. Mularski RA, Curtis JR, Billings JA, et al. Proposed quality measures for palliative care in the critically ill: A consensus from the Robert Wood Johnson Foundation Critical Care Workgroup. *Crit Care Med.* 2006;34:S404-S411.
5. Aslakson R, Cheng J, Vollenweider D, Galusca D, Smith TJ, Pronovost PJ. Evidence-based palliative care in the intensive care unit: a systematic review of interventions. *J Palliat Med.* 2014;17:219-235.

**3.** Correct Answer: E

**Rationale:**

CR-BSIs are a costly and often preventable source of morbidity and mortality in the ICU. The average cost per CR-BSI in the adult surgical ICU is estimated to be between $54 000 and $75 000. Many CR-BSIs are preventable, and studies have shown that implementing a variety of prevention strategies can significantly decrease the incidence of CR-BSIs. In a 2006 landmark paper, Provonost et al. demonstrated a nearly 50% decrease in CR-BSIs over 18 months with the implementation of five evidence-based procedures and identified as having the greatest effect on the rate of CR-BSIs and the fewest implementation barriers. These five procedures include the following: handwashing, using full-barrier precautions during the insertion of central venous catheters, cleaning the skin with chlorhexidine, avoiding the femoral site if possible, and removing unnecessary catheters. The preprocedure "time-out" is an important step in preventing error but does not impact CR-BSI rate.

## References

1. Hollenbeak CS. The cost of catheter-related bloodstream infections: implications for the value of prevention. *J Infus Nurs.* 2011;34:309-313.
2. Mermel LA. Prevention of intravascular catheter-related infections [Erratum in *Ann Intern Med.* 2000;133:5]. *Ann Intern Med.* 2000;132:391-402.
3. Blot K, Bergs J, Vogelaers D, Blot S, Vandijck D. Prevention of central line associated bloodstream infections through quality improvement interventions: a systematic review and meta-analysis. *Clin Infect Dis.* 2014;18(1):96-105.

**4.** Correct Answer: E

**Rationale:**

The ProVent score (Prognosis for Prolonged Ventilation Score) is a tool that aims to quantify risk of 1-year mortality among critically ill patients requiring prolonged mechanical ventilation. It is comprised of four easily measured variables recorded at day 21 of ventilation (see tables below). The ProVent score was originally derived from a prognostic model for 1-year mortality in medical, surgical, and trauma patients at a single academic hospital who required mechanical ventilation for at least 21 days. It was first described in 2008 by Carson et al. and over the past decade, has been validated at centers across the United States and overseas. The patient described above has a ProVent score of 4 (age >65 years, thrombocytopenia, hemodialysis).

**ProVent Model with Categorized Risk Variables**

| CATEGORICAL VARIABLE | NO. (%) | ODDS RATIO (95% CONFIDENCE INTERVAL) | BETA VALUE | POINTS |
|---|---|---|---|---|
| Age ≥65 y | 80 (31%) | 7.6 (3.8-15.5) | 2.03 | 2 |
| Age 50-64 y | 88 (34%) | 2.0 (1.0-3.9) | 0.67 | 1 |
| Platelets ≤150 × 10$^9$/L | 65 (25%) | 1.9 (0.9-3.9) | 0.65 | 1 |
| Vasopressors | 35 (13%) | 4.4 (1.6-12.6) | 1.49 | 1 |
| Hemodialysis | 34 (13%) | 2.4 (1.0-6.0) | 0.89 | 1 |

**ProVent score and observed 1-year mortality**

| PROVENTSCORE | NO. | OBSERVED MORTALITY PERCENT (95% CONFIDENCE INTERVAL) |
|---|---|---|
| 0 | 72 | 20 (10-29) |
| 1 | 60 | 36 (24-48) |
| 2 | 78 | 56 (45-68) |
| 3 | 36 | 81 (67-94) |
| 4 or 5 | 14 | 100 (77-100) |

References

1. Carson SS, Kahn JM, Hough CL, et al. A multicenter mortality prediction model for patients receiving prolonged mechanical ventilation. *Crit Care Med*. 2012;40(4):1171-1176.
2. Carson SS, Garrett J, Hanson LC, et al. A prognostic model for one-year mortality in patients requiring prolonged mechanical ventilation. *Crit Care Med*. 2008;36(7):2061-2069.
3. Leroy G, Devos P, Lambiotte F, Thévenin D, Leroy O. One-year mortality in patients requiring prolonged mechanical ventilation: multicenter evaluation of the ProVent score. *Crit Care*. 2014;18(4):R155. doi:10.1186/cc13994.
4. Jaiswal S, Sadacharam K, Shrestha RR, et al. External validation ofprognostic model of one-year mortality in patients requiring prolonged mechanical ventilation. *J Nepal Health Res Counc*. 2012;10:47-51.

**5.** Correct Answer: C

**Rationale:**

PICS was first described in 2012 after a Society of Critical Care Medicine conference created to improve long-term outcomes after critical illness for patients and their families. PICS is characterized by new or worsening problems in cognitive, psychiatric, or physical health that occur after a critical illness and persist after acute care hospitalization. Common symptoms are generalized weakness, fatigue, decreased mobility, sexual dysfunction, sleep disturbances, and cognitive impairment. Reported cognitive dysfunction includes memory disturbance or loss, slow mental processing, and poor concentration. Psychiatric disturbances include anxiety, depression, and posttraumatic stress disorder. Metabolic syndrome has not been associated with PICS. Many studies have attempted to identify risk factors for and the prevention of PICS, though are still in the early stages of discovery.

References

1. Needham DM, Davidson J, Cohen H, et al. Improving long-term outcomes after discharge from intensive care unit: report from a stakeholders' conference. *Crit Care Med*. 2012;40:502-509.
2. Casaer MP, Van den Berghe G. Nutrition in the acute phase of critical illness. *N Engl J Med*. 2014;370:1227.

**6.** Correct Answer: A

**Rationale:**

In 2015, the Society of Critical Care Medicine, the American College of Chest Physicians, and the Association of Organ Procurement Organizations released a joint consensus statement on the management of the potential organ donor in the ICU. Included in these guidelines is the mandate that clinicians should incorporate the most recent recommendations provided by the Quality Standards Subcommittee of the American Academy of Neurology (AAN). Within these AAN recommendations is the assertion that complex motor activity (such as finger tremor in the patient described in the question stem) can sometimes occur in patients who meet the criteria for brain death and as such, its presence does not exclude the diagnosis of brain death.

References

1. Kotloff RM, Blosser S, Fulda GJ, et al. Management of the potential organ donor in the ICU: Society of Critical Care Medicine / American College of Chest Physicians/ Association of Organ Procurement Organizations Consensus Statement. *Crit Care Med*. 2015;43:1291-1325.
2. Wijdicks EFM, Varelas PN, Gronseth GS, et al.: Evidence-based guideline update: determining brain death in adults. Report of the Quality Standards Subcommittee of the American Academy of Neurology. *Neurology*. 2010;74:1911-1918.

**7.** Correct Answer: F

**Rationale:**

Based on the most recent multiorganizational guidelines regarding management of the potential organ donor in the ICU, all of the aforementioned conditions are NOT considered contraindications for organ donation consideration.

Organs from bacteremic donors have been successfully donated with few transmitted infections when the donor received pathogen-specific antibiotics for a minimum of 48 hours before procurement. As such, the most recent guidelines recommend that bacteremic organ donors receive pathogen-specific antibiotic therapy for at least 48 hours, even if this delays organ procurement. Patients with histologically low-grade central nervous system tumors (grades I–II) and no history of craniotomy, brain irradiation, or ventricular shunts have a low risk of tumor transmission. Organs from a HCV-seropositive donor can be used in HCV-positive recipients. Based on behavioral criteria that define donors at increased risk of having acquired HIV infection, the estimated risk of undetected viremia among seronegative donors is sufficiently low to not disqualify from organ donation consideration. For adults, the risk of undetected viremia among seronegative donors at increased risk of having acquired HIV infection is the following (per 10 000 donors): IV drug users (12.1), men who have had sex with other men (10.2), commercial sex workers (6.6), inmates of correctional facilities (2.3), persons exposed to HIV-infected blood in the past 12 months (1.5), for persons who have had sex with a high-risk individual in the past 12 months (0.7), and hemophiliacs (0.09).

**Reference**

1. Kotloff RM, Blosser S, Fulda GJ, et al. Management of the potential organ donor in the ICU: Society of Critical Care Medicine / American College of Chest Physicians / Association of Organ Procurement Organizations Consensus Statement. *Crit Care Med.* 2015;43:1291-1325.

**8.** Correct Answer: C

**Rationale:**

A widely adopted protocol for donation after circulatory determination of death (DCDD) involves transferring a patient being considered for DCD to an operating room where circulatory function is monitored and LST is withdrawn. The patient is observed until circulatory function ceases or until 60 minutes pass. If cessation of circulatory function does not occur within 60 minutes, the patient is returned to the ICU and organ procurement is aborted. Although the majority of deaths are determined using cardiac (rather than brain) death criteria, a disproportionately low number of donated organs are procured via DCD. One hypothesized reason is the difficulty in predicting death within 60 minutes of withdrawal of LST. Accurately predicting the timing of cardiac death also has emotional, logistical, and financial consequences on all those involved including the donor family, recipient, and transplant teams. One of the widely used tools to predict cardiac death within 60 minutes of withdrawal of LST is the UNOS Consensus Committee Criteria (see below). These criteria were prospectively validated in a single-center study and demonstrated that among patients with 0, 1, 2, and 3 UNOS DCD criteria, 29%, 52%, 65%, and 82% died within 60 minutes of withdrawal of LST, respectively.

**UNOS Consensus Committee Criteria for Prediction of Death Within 60 Minutes of Withdrawal of LST**

- Apnea
- Respiratory rate <8 or >30 breaths/min
- Dopamine ≥15 µg/kg/min
- Left or right ventricular assist device
- Venoarterial or venovenous extracorporeal membrane oxygenation
- Positive end-expiratory pressure ≥10 and $Sao_2$ ≤92%
- $Fio_2$ ≥0.5 and $Sao_2$ ≤92%
- Norepinephrine or phenylephrine ≥0.2 µg/kg/min
- Pacemaker unassisted heart rate <30
- IABP 1:1 or dobutamine or dopamine ≥10 µg/kg/min and CI ≤ 2.2 L/min/m²
- IABP 1:1 and CI ≤1.5 L/min/m²

CI, cardiac index; $Fio_2$, fraction of inspired oxygen; IABP, intra-aortic balloon pump; $Sao_2$, arterial oxygen saturation.

**References**

1. Kotloff RM, Blosser S, Fulda GJ, et al. Management of the potential organ donor in the ICU: Society of Critical Care Medicine / American College of Chest Physicians / Association of Organ Procurement Organizations Consensus Statement. *Crit Care Med.* 2015;43:1291-1325.
2. DeVita MA, Brooks MM, Zawistowski C, et al. Donors after cardiac death: Validation of identification criteria (DVIC) study for predictors of rapid death. *Am J Transplant.* 2008;8:432-441.

**9.** Correct Answer: B

**Rationale:**

There are a number of misunderstood medicolegal principles relevant to care of the critically ill. One of these principles involves whether there is a distinction between decisions to withhold or withdraw treatments. For example, it has been demonstrated that healthcare professionals disagree on whether there is an ethical difference between forgoing a life support measure and stopping it once it has been started. However, the American College of Critical Care Medicine (ACCM) recommends that clinicians should make no distinction between decisions to withhold or to withdraw treatment. In their consensus statement, the ACCM emphasizes the importance of preventing barriers for clinicians to initiate treatments where the value of a specific intervention within the context of a patient's clinical course (for example, hemodialysis) can only be determined after a trial of therapy.

References

1. Meisel A. Legal myths about terminating life support. *Arch Intern Med.* 1991;151:1497-1502.
2. Solomon MZ, O'Donnell L, Jennings B, et al. Decisions near the end of life: professional views on life-sustaining treatments. *Am J Public Health.* 1993;83:14-23.
3. Truog RD, Campbell ML, Curtis JR, et al. Recommendations for end-of-life care in the intensive care unit: a consensus statement by the American College of Critical Care Medicine. *Crit Care Med.* 2008;36:953-963.

**10.** Correct Answer: D

Reference

1. Institute of Medicine. *Dying in America: Improving Quality and Honoring Individual Preferences Near the End of Life.* Washington, DC: National Academies Press; 2014.

# 119

# ORGAN DONATION

Nandini C. Palaniappa and Kevin C. Thornton

1. A patient in the ICU has been declared brain dead after a traumatic brain injury and the family has agreed to organ donation in accordance with the patient's prior wishes. He is found to have a sodium of 148 mEq/L with urine output of 200 mL/h over the past 4 hours. Urine osmolality is150 mOsm/L. What is the most appropriate therapy?

   A. Desmopressin 0.5 to 2 μg IV
   B. Continue maintenance fluids at current rate of 100 mL/h
   C. Bolus 2 L of normal saline
   D. Continue to monitor urine output until organ harvesting

2. The ICU team caring for a patient who was admitted 4 days ago with traumatic brain injury believes the patient has a norecoverable neurologic injury and is planning on performing a brain death examination later in the day. Who is the most appropriate person to speak to the family regarding potential organ donation?

   A. Transplant team
   B. ICU attending physician
   C. Organ procurement organization in-house coordinator
   D. Bedside nurse

3. Which of the following is NOT a general guideline for hemodynamic management of organ donors?

   A. Mean arterial pressure greater than 60 mm Hg
   B. Urine output of 1 mL/kg/h
   C. Intravascular volume replacement with crystalloids
   D. Intravascular volume replacement with hydroxyethyl starch (HES)

4. Which is a generally accepted threshold of donor organ suitability for lung transplantation?

   A. P/F >200 on 5 cm $H_2O$ PEEP
   B. P/F >300 on 10 cm $H_2O$ PEEP
   C. P/F >300 on 5 cm $H_2O$ PEEP
   D. P/F >400 on 7 cm $H_2O$ PEEP

# Chapter 119 ▪ Answers

---

**1.** Correct Answer: A

**Rationale:**

The hypothalamic-pituitary axis (HPA) is particularly vulnerable to ischemia. Vasopressin, which is produced in the hypothalamus, transported to the posterior pituitary, then released by the posterior pituitary, is decreased in up to 80% of patients with brain death, leading to central diabetes insipidus (DI). Arginine vasopressin (AVP) deficiency can lead to diuresis and is characterized by dilute urine and hypertonic plasma. Urine osmolality is often less than 200 mOsm/L in central DI, and one can confirm the diagnosis with fluid restriction and failure of urine osmolality to increase more than 30 mOsm/L in the first few hours.

Treatment of central DI consists of desmopressin administration. Desmopressin is a vasopressin analogue with greater affinity for the V2 receptor (present in the distal collecting duct) than the V1 receptor on vascular smooth muscle. Dosing can vary, but can be between 0.5 µg and 2 µg IV. Additional dosing is required approximately every 6 hours and should be titrated based on urine output, urine osmolality, and serum sodium.

**Reference**

1. Kotloff RM, Blosser S, Fulda GJ, et al; Society of Critical Care Medicine/American College of Chest Physicians/Association of Organ Procurement Organizations Donor Management Task Force. Management of the potential organ donor in the ICU. *Crit Care Med.* 2015;43(6):1291-1325.

---

**2.** Correct Answer: C

**Rationale:**

Initial discussions with families regarding organ donation are an essential part of the organ donation process. Ideally, the person who speaks to family members for authorization (or consent) for organ donation is someone who is familiar with the process and has experience in guiding and supporting family members through the organ donation process. As such, some centers have organ procurement organization coordinators who are ideally suited for this task.

Although the ICU attending and bedside nurse may have developed a relationship with the family, conversations to consent for organ donation may be viewed as a conflict of interest. The same principle applies to transplant team members who wish to approach families of patients who may become organ donors. In the situation that a transplant team member is caring for or has cared for the patient, for instance, as the trauma critical care attending, that attending should transfer care to another physician in order to participate in the organ procurement.

**References**

1. Kotloff RM, Blosser S, Fulda GJ, et al; Society of Critical Care Medicine/American College of Chest Physicians/Association of Organ Procurement Organizations Donor Management Task Force. Management of the potential organ donor in the ICU. *Crit Care Med.* 2015;43(6):1291-1325.
2. Gries CJ, White DB, Truog RD, et al. An Official American Thoracic Society/International Society for Heart and Lung Transplantation/Society of Critical Care Medicine/Association of Organ and Procurement Organizations/United Network of organ sharing statement: ethical and policy considerations in organ donation after circulatory determination of death. *Am J Respir Crit Care Med.* 2013;188(1):103-109.

---

**3.** Correct Answer: D

**Rationale:**

The primary hemodynamic goal of organ donors is to maximize organ perfusion for organ preservation by maintaining normovolemia, an adequate blood pressure, and adequate cardiac output. Specific goals include mean arterial pressure of 60 to 70 mm Hg, urine output of 1 to 3 mL/kg/h, minimization of pressor dosage, left ventricular ejection fraction of at least 45%, initial volume replacement with crystalloids or colloids, and avoidance of HES for colloidal resuscitation. The use of HES can lead to acute kidney injury and has been shown to be associated with delayed graft function and graft failure.

**References**

1. Cittanova ML, Leblanc I, Legendre C, Mouquet C, Riou B, Coriat P. Effect of hydroxyethylstarch in brain-dead kidney donors on renal function in kidney-transplant recipients. *Lancet.* 1996;348(9042):1620-1622.
2. Kotloff RM, Blosser S, Fulda GJ, et al; Society of Critical Care Medicine/American College of Chest Physicians/Association of Organ Procurement Organizations Donor Management Task Force. Management of the potential organ donor in the ICU. *Crit Care Med.* 2015;43(6):1291-1325.
3. Wood KE, Becker BN, McCartney JG, D'Alessandro AM, Coursin DB. Care of the potential organ donor. *N Engl J Med.* 2004;351(26):2730-2739.

**4.** Correct Answer: C

**Rationale:**

Generally, a P/F ratio greater than 300 mm Hg in the donor is considered acceptable for lung donation. In donors who fail to meet this requirement, donor management protocols that include diuresis, therapeutic bronchoscopy, chest physiotherapy, and lung recruitment can improve oxygenation. Of note, bronchoscopy should be performed in all potential lung donors, both to assess for occult aspiration and infection and to perform therapeutic airway clearance.

Additional ideal lung donor criteria include:

- Age <55 years
- Smoking history <20 pack-years
- Clear chest x-ray
- $PaO_2$ >300 mm Hg with $FiO_2$ 100% and PEEP of 5 cm $H_2O$
- Absence of chest trauma
- No evidence of aspiration or sepsis
- No prior cardiothoracic surgery
- No organisms seen on donor sputum Gram stain
- No purulent secretions or gastric contents on bronchoscopy
- No history of significant chronic lung disease

With regard to ventilation strategies, potential donors should undergo lung-protective ventilation with tidal volumes of 6 to 8 mL/kg ideal body weight.

### References

1. Kotloff RM, Blosser S, Fulda GJ, et al; Society of Critical Care Medicine/American College of Chest Physicians/Association of Organ Procurement Organizations Donor Management Task Force. Management of the potential organ donor in the ICU. *Criti Care Med.* 2015;43(6):1291-1325.
2. Mascia L, Pasero D, Slutsky AS, et al. Effect of a lung protective strategy for organ donors on eligibility and availability of lungs for transplantation. *JAMA.* 2010;304(23):2620.
3. Wood KE, Becker BN, McCartney JG, D'Alessandro AM, Coursin DB. Care of the potential organ donor. *N Engl J Med.* 2004;351(26):2730-2739.

# MISCELLANEOUS

# 120

# PROCEDURES

Jennifer Cottral and William J. Benedetto

1. A 67-year-old female is on two vasopressors for septic shock and needs invasive arterial hemodynamic monitoring. Right radial artery cannulation is attempted twice without success, followed by successful cannulation of the right brachial artery by landmark technique. Several days later, the patient complains of right thumb tingling and is noted to be unable to abduct her right thumb. Iatrogenic nerve injury related to arterial cannulation is suspected. Which respective artery and nerve is most commonly associated with this pattern of injury in arterial cannulation for invasive hemodynamic monitoring?

   A. Radial artery, radial nerve
   B. Radial artery, median nerve
   C. Brachial artery, radial nerve
   D. Brachial artery, median nerve

2. A 67-year-old female with hypertension and osteoporosis is brought to the emergency department after a mechanical fall on her left side. She appears dyspneic, pale, and diaphoretic, and primary survey reveals extensive ecchymoses forming around her lower left chest. Her initial vitals include heart rate 115 beats/min (normal sinus rhythm), blood pressure 85/55 mm Hg, respiratory rate 30 breaths/min, SPO$_2$ 91%. You suspect a tension pneumothorax and plan to perform an emergent needle decompression. According to the most recent Advanced Trauma Life Support guidelines, the correct placement of a large bore needle for emergent decompression of a suspected tension pneumothorax is:

   A. Second intercostal space, midclavicular
   B. Third intercostal space, midaxillary
   C. Fourth intercostal space, midclavicular
   D. Fifth intercostal space, midaxillary
   E. Sixth intercostal space, midaxillary

3. A 27-year-old male pedestrian struck at high speed by a motor vehicle has just arrived in the emergency department. First-responders in the field report that they were unable to obtain intravenous (IV) access, with initial vitals including heart rate 120 beats/min (normal sinus rhythm), blood pressure 110/80 mm Hg, respiratory rate 20 breaths/min. The patient's vitals in the ED are HR 125 beats/min (normal sinus rhythm), blood pressure 90/65 mm Hg, respiratory rate 25 breaths/min. The patient appears confused and has a positive FAST examination, and primary survey is notable for compound fractures of both femurs. Out of concern for decompensated hypovolemic shock, you decide to secure intraosseous (IO) access for volume resuscitation. Which of the following IO sites will allow for volume to be infused at the fastest rate?

   A. Sternum
   B. Proximal humerus
   C. Proximal tibia
   D. Distal tibia

4. A 68-year-old female with a history of juvenile rheumatoid arthritis and severe COPD is admitted to the ICU for impending respiratory failure in the setting of a COPD exacerbation. Vitals are blood pressure 150/90 mm Hg, heart rate 97 beats/min, SPO$_2$ 89% with oxygen delivered via a non-rebreather face mask, respiratory rate 32 breaths/min. After induction for intubation, the patient is noted to have significantly limited neck range of motion and mouth opening. Attempts at direct laryngoscopy by two providers failed, and inadequate tidal volumes are achieved via bag and mask ventilation. Vitals are now blood pressure 160/100 mm Hg, heart rate 110 beats/min, and SPO$_2$ 81%. According to the most recent practice guidelines for management of the difficult airway, what is the most appropriate next step in the management of this patient?

A. Wake the patient up and consider awake intubation
B. Attempt intubation with video-assisted laryngoscopy
C. Percutaneous needle cricothyrotomy
D. Insertion of a supraglottic airway

5. A 59-year-old man with hypertension and a 40-pack-year smoking history presents to the emergency department with acute onset tearing chest pain that radiates to his back. Initial vitals include a blood pressure of 140/90 mm Hg, heart rate 73 beats/min (normal sinus rhythm), and SPO$_2$ 97% on room air. An acute type A aortic dissection is suspected. En route to his CT chest angiogram, the patient becomes less responsive and is noted to have blood pressure 80/60 mm Hg, heart rate 120 beats/min in sinus tachycardia. A quick bedside transthoracic echo reveals:

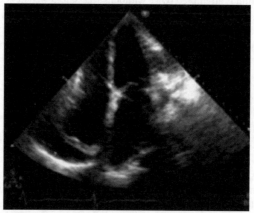

(Figure from Adler Y, Charron P, Imazio M, et al. 2015 ESC guidelines for the diagnosis and management of pericardial diseases: the task force for the diagnosis and management of pericardial diseases of the European Society of Cardiology (ESC). *Eur Heart J.* 2015;36:2921.)

The next best step in the management of this patient is:

A. Immediate-acting vasodilator to prevent extension of dissection flap
B. Immediate and blind subxiphoid pericardiocentesis
C. Echo-guided controlled pericardial drainage
D. Emergent surgery for repair of type A aortic dissection

6. A 64-year-old female with hypertension, hyperlipidemia, morbid obesity, and steroid-dependent ulcerative colitis was admitted to the ICU 11 days ago for respiratory failure due to community-acquired pneumonia. Repeated attempts at weaning from mechanical ventilation were unsuccessful, and she underwent a challenging percutaneous tracheostomy placement 7 days ago where the tracheostomy was placed below the fourth tracheal ring. Over the past few hours the patient has required frequent tracheal suctioning for small amounts of frank blood. Upon examination of the patient's stoma site, you notice pulsating bright red blood emerge from the tracheal tube. After a prompt bronchoscopy, the next best step in the management of this patient is:

A. Orotracheal intubation
B. Overinflate the tracheostomy cuff
C. Immediate bedside surgical exploration
D. Digital compression via stoma

7. A 21-year-old male is admitted to the ICU for respiratory distress due suspected Ludwig angina. The patient's respiratory status rapidly deteriorates and three attempts at endotracheal intubation by different providers failed because of suspected complete airway obstruction. Vitals are blood pressure 150/90 mm Hg, heart rate 120 beats/min (normal sinus rhythm), SPO$_2$ 65%. An emergent surgical airway is called for and a needle cricothyrotomy is performed, with difficulty, with a 14 g angiocatheter. The angiocatheter is connected via a Y-connector to an oxygen delivery system at 100 psi and the patient is manually ventilated at 25 breaths per minute. Vitals are now blood pressure 80/40 mm Hg, heart rate 130 beats/min (normal sinus rhythm), SPO$_2$ 89%, and the patient's rhythm quickly deteriorates to ventricular fibrillation. All of the following likely contributed to this patient's hemodynamic collapse EXCEPT:

   A. Small cannula internal diameter
   B. Complete airway obstruction
   C. Esophageal perforation
   D. High oxygen flow rate
   E. low inspiratory to expiratory ratio

8. A 73-year-old female who is admitted to the hospital after a traumatic fall needs central access for vasopressor support. The following images correspond (in no particular order) to the views that facilitate internal jugular vein, subclavian vein, and femoral vein cannulation.

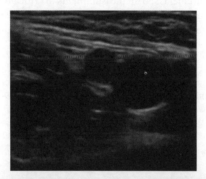

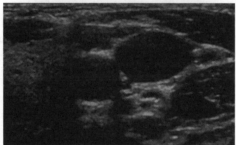

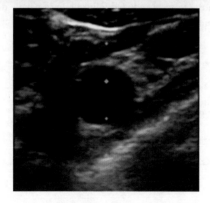

Arrange the above ultrasound images in the following order of veins imaged: subclavian, internal jugular, and femoral.

   A. 1, 2, 3
   B. 1, 3, 2
   C. 2, 1, 3
   D. 2, 3, 1
   E. 3, 2, 1
   F. 3, 1, 2

# Chapter 120 ▪ Answers

**1.** Correct Answer: D

**Rationale:**

Invasive arterial blood pressure monitoring is essential to the management of hemodynamically unstable patients and in patients who require tight blood pressure management. Although noninvasive blood pressure (NIBP) monitoring has advantages as many of the complications associated with arterial lines (eg, bleeding, infection, thrombosis) are avoided, the overall incidence of arterial line–related adverse events is low. Common sites of arterial cannulation in adults include the following arteries: radial, femoral, axillary, and less commonly, brachial, ulnar, dorsalis pedis. Brachial artery cannulation carries a theoretical risk of median nerve injury because this nerve runs close to the brachial artery in the antecubital fossa. Median nerve injury can present as numbness and paresthesia in the median nerve distribution, as well as the inability to abduct or oppose the thumb. However, in a recent retrospective observational study of over 20 000 patients undergoing brachial arterial line placement, not a single reported nerve injury plausibly related to brachial artery cannulation was discovered.

NIBP measurements in critically ill patients carry their own risk, as a recent study demonstrated that, compared with arterial blood pressure measurements, NIBP measurements in critically ill patients overestimated systolic blood pressures during hypotensive events. In this study, NIBP measurements were also found to be less sensitive in assessing patients' risk of developing acute kidney injury when traditional hypotension thresholds (systolic blood pressure ≤90 mm Hg) were used.

### References

1. Scheer B, Perel A, Pfeiffer UJ. Clinical review: complications and risk factors of peripheral arterial catheters used for haemodynamic monitoring in anesthesia and intensive care medicine. *Crit Care*. 2002;6:199-204.
2. Singh A. Brachial arterial pressure monitoring during cardiac surgery rarely causes complications. *Anesthesiology*. 2017;126(6):1065-1076.
3. Lehman LW. Methods of blood pressure measurement in the ICU. *Crit Care Med*. 2013;41(1):34-40.

**2.** Correct Answer: D

**Rationale:**

The most recent Advanced Trauma Life Support (ATLS) guidelines from 2018 recommend that a large, over-the-needle catheter be placed at the fifth interspace, slightly anterior to the midaxillary line for needle decompression of a tension pneumothorax. These guidelines reflect recent evidence that challenges the traditional ATLS recommendation that needle decompression occur at the second intercostal space, midclavicular line. In an observational study of over-the-needle catheter placement into the anterior chest wall by paramedics, confirmatory imaging revealed that in 44% of patients the catheter was placed too medial, thus risking inadvertent cardiac and/or mediastinal injury. Additionally, a recent systematic review and meta-analysis demonstrated that chest wall thickness was correlated with needle decompression failure rate, and that the anterior chest had the largest mean chest wall thickness and correspondingly highest mean failure rate. This same study demonstrated that the anterior axial line of the fourth and fifth intercostal space correlated with the lowest predicted failure rate of needle decompression in multiple populations. The 10th edition of the ATLS guidelines recommends needle decompression occurs slightly anterior to midaxillary line at the fifth intercostal space.

|  | SECOND ICS-MCL | FOURTH/FIFTH ICS-MAL | FOURTH/FIFTH ICS-AAL |
|---|---|---|---|
| Mean chest wall thickness (P = 0.08) | 42.79 mm (95% CI, 38.78-46.81 | 39.85 mm (95% CI, 28.70-51.00) | 34.33 mm (95% CI, 28.20-40.47) |
| Mean failure rate (P = 0.01) | 38% (95% CI, 24-54) | 31% (95% CI, 10-64) | 13% (95% CI, 8-22) |

AAL, anterior axillary; ICS, intercostal space; MAL, midaxillary; MCL, midclavicular.

### References

1. American College of Surgeons Committee on Trauma. *Advanced Trauma Life Support (ATLS)*. 10th ed. Chicago, IL: American College of Surgeons; 2018.
2. Netto FA, Shulman H, Rizoli SB, Tremblay LN, Brenneman F, Tein H. Are needle decompressions for tension pneumothraces being performed appropriately for appropriate indications? *Am J Emerg Med*. 2008;26:597-602.
3. Laan DV, Vu TD, Thiels CA, et al. Chest wall thickness and decompression failure: a systematic review and metaanalysis comparing anatomic locations in needle thoracostomy. *Injury*. 2016;47(4):797-804.

**3.** Correct Answer: A

**Rationale:**

IO access is a quick and safe method for obtaining parenteral access in patients with difficult venous access. Several studies have shown that when peripheral intravenous (IV) access is difficult to obtain, the procedure for placement of an IO line is both shorter and has a higher success rate on first attempt compared with insertion of a central venous catheter or an ultrasound-guided peripheral venous catheter. Crystalloid, colloid, and all resuscitation drugs can be given by the IO route, but peak flow rates vary by site of IO placement and are greatly enhanced by use of a pressure bag inflated to 300 mm Hg. Although studies vary in the maximal flow rates obtained at each IO placement site, the highest IO flow rates (both with and without use of a pressure bag) are consistently achieved at the sternum, followed by the proximal humerus and proximal tibia. Whether flow rates are faster at the proximal humerus versus the proximal tibia remains a question because some studies show faster rates at the IO humeral site, whereas others show faster rates at the IO proximal tibia (though notably, not to a level of statistical significance). One study comparing flow rates in the same patient at both the humeral and tibial site showed no significant difference in flow rates between tibial and humeral sites, with or without pressure bag infusion. Flow rates have been demonstrated to be more than twice as fast in the proximal tibia compared with the distal tibia both with and without the use of pressure bags.

| IO ACCESS SITE | FLOW RATES IN mL/min[a] | | | |
| | PUGA ET AL, 2016 | HAMMER ET AL, 2015 | PASLEY ET AL, 2015 | ONG ET AL, 2009 |
| --- | --- | --- | --- | --- |
| Sternum | (150.0)[h] | 53.2 (112)[h] | 93.7 | – |
| Proximal humerus | (104.9)[b] | 15.9 (60)[b] | 57.1 | 84.4 (153.2)[c] |
| Proximal tibia | – | 26.9 (69)[b] | 30.7 | 73 (165.3)[c] |

[a]When available, values are provided without (and with) the use of a pressure bag.
[b]300 mm Hg of pressure applied.
[c]Unspecified amount of pressure applied.

References

1. Petitpas F, Guenezan J, Vendeuvre T, Scepi M, Oriot D, Mimoz O. Use of intra-osseous access in adults: a systematic review. *Crit Care*. 2016;20(1):102.
2. Puga T, Montez D, Philbeck T, Davlantes C. Adequacy of intraosseous vascular access insertion sites for high-volume fluid infusion. *Crit Care Med*. 2016;44(12):143.
3. Hammer N, Möbius R, Gries A, Hossfeld B, Bechmann I, Bernhard M. Comparison of the fluid resuscitation rate with and without external pressure using two intraosseous infusion systems for adult emergencies, the CITRIN (Comparison of InTRaosseous infusion systems in emergency medicINe)-study. *PLoS One*. 2015;10(12):e0143726.
4. Pasley J, Miller CH, DuBose JJ, et al. Intraosseous infusion rates under high pressure: a cadaveric comparison of anatomic sites. *J Trauma Acute Care Surg*. 2015;78(2):295-299.
5. Ong M, Chan Y, Oh J, Ngo A. An observational, prospective study comparing tibial and humeral intraosseous access using the EZ-IO. *Am J Emerg Med*. 2009;27(1):8-15.
6. Tan BK, Chong S, Koh ZX, Ong ME. EZ-IO in the ED: an observa- tional, prospective study comparing flow rates with proximal and distal tibia intraosseous access in adults. *Am J Emerg Med*. 2012;30(8):1602-1606.

**4.** Correct Answer: D

**Rationale:**

Guidelines for airway management developed for the operating room setting are often extrapolated to the ICU environment, although an ICU patient might be physiologically very different. Intubations in the ICU often occur in patients who are hemodynamically unstable and hypoxemic, often with metabolic and coagulation derangements. Tracheal intubation is one of the highest risk procedures performed in the ICU, and airway-related events in ICU are associated with significant morbidity and mortality. For example, a recent British audit project revealed that 61% of airway-related events in ICU were associated with death or permanent neurological damage compared with 14% in operating room. In light of these findings, guidelines for the management of tracheal intubation in critically ill adults were recently published and specifically address issues often seen in the ICU such as suboptimal preoxygenation conditions and hemodynamic instability. Both American Society of Anesthesiologists and British Difficult Airway Society guidelines recommend placement of a supraglottic airway if both laryngoscopy and facemask ventilation have failed.

### References

1. Lapinsky SE. Endotracheal intubation in the ICU. *Crit Care*. 2015;19(1):258.
2. Perbet S, Jong AD, Delmas J, et al. Incidence of and risk factors for severe cardiovascular collapse after endotracheal intubation in the ICU: a multicenter observational study. *Crit Care*. 2015;19:257.
3. Griesdale DE, Bosma TL, Kurth T, Isac G, Chittock DR. Complications of endotracheal intubation in the critically ill. *Intensive Care Med*. 2008;34(10):1835-1842.
4. Ahmed A, Azim A. Difficult tracheal intubation in critically ill. *J Intensive Care*. 2018;6:49. https://doi.org/10.1186/s40560-018-0318-4.
5. Higgs A, McGrath BA, Goddard C, et al. Guidelines for the management of tracheal intubation in critically ill adults. *Br J Anesthesia*. 2018;120:323-352.
6. Apfelbaum JL, Hagberg CA, Caplan RA, et al. Practice guidelines for management of the difficult airway. *Anesthesiology*. 2013;118:251-270.

**5.** Correct Answer: C

**Rationale:**

This patient is experiencing cardiac tamponade associated with aortic rupture, which is a life-threatening complication of an acute type A aortic dissection (AADA). Although pericardial fluid collection is a common complication of AADA, only a subset of patients will experience cardiac tamponade (estimated incidence between 8% and 31%). Patients with cardiac tamponade as a result of AADA have been shown to have a twofold risk of in-hospital death compared with AADA patients without tamponade. Although prompt surgical repair of this patient's presumed aortic dissection is necessary, he is currently hemodynamically unstable and may die prior surgical correction if no action is taken to drain the hemopericardium. The most recent guidelines recommend that in the setting of aortic dissection with hemopericardium, controlled pericardial drainage of small volumes should be considered to stabilize the patient temporarily with a goal to maintain blood pressure around 90 mm Hg (class IIa). Historically, pericardiocentesis was contraindicated in tamponade associated with AADA out of concern that complete drainage of the hemopericardium would cause a large increase in systolic blood pressure, thus leading to intensified bleeding and extension of the aortic dissection. However, recent studies have shown that controlled pericardial drainage in hypotensive patients with AADA-related tamponade is a safe and effective way to restore perfusion without inducing hypertension. Controlled pericardial drainage involves echo-guided placement of an 8 Fr pigtail catheter into the pericardial space, followed by aspiration of the hemopericardium in increments of a few milliliters while watching for the desired hemodynamic response. Given the availability of echocardiography, blind procedures including pericardiocentesis must not be done in order to avoid the risk of injury to nearby structures (myocardium, liver, lung, etc). Although vasodilators are useful in patients with AADA without tamponade, recent guidelines recommend against the use of vasodilators and diuretics in the presence of cardiac tamponade.

### References

1. Tsukube T, Okita Y. Cardiac tamponade due to aortic dissection: clinical pictureand treatment with focus on pericardiocentesis. *E-Journal of Cardiology Practice*. 2017;15(18). Retrieved from https://www.escardio.org/Journals/E-Journal-of-Cardiology-Practice/Volume-15/Cardiac-tamponade-due-to-aortic-dissection-clinical-picture-and-treatment-with-focus-on-pericardiocentesis.
2. Yehuda A, Charron P, Imazio M, et al. ESC Guidelines for the diagnosis and management of pericardial diseases: the task force for the diagnosis and management of pericardial diseases of the European Society of Cardiology (ESC). *Eur Heart J*. 2015;36(42):2921–2964.
3. Cruz I, Stuart B, Caldeira D, Morgado G, et al. Controlled pericardiocentesis in patients with cardiac tamponade complicating aortic dissection: experience of a center without cardiothoracic surgery. *Eur Heart J Acute Cardiovasc Care*. 2015;4(2):124-128.
4. Hayashi T, Tsukube T, Yamashita T, et al. Impact of controlled pericardial drainage on critical cardiac tamponade with acute type-A aortic dissection. *Circulation*. 2012;126(11 suppl 1):S97-S101.

**6.** Correct Answer: B

**Rationale:**

The patient likely has a fistula communicating between the trachea and the innominate artery (tracheoinnominate fistula, or TIF). TIF is a life-threatening complication of tracheostomy placement usually occurring within the first 3 weeks after placement in 0.1% to 1% of patients undergoing the procedure (either surgically or percutaneously). Mortality from TIF approaches 100% without prompt diagnosis, emergency management, and definitive surgical intervention. Although the differential diagnosis of tracheostomy bleeding is broad, there should be strong suspicion of a TIF if the bleed is brisk and pulsating. The innominate artery typically crosses the trachea at the level of the ninth tracheal ring but can be as high as the sixth tracheal ring (see the figure that follows).

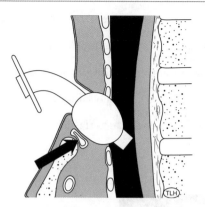
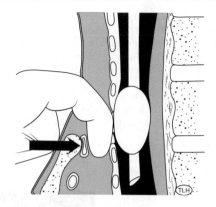

Partial withdrawal of tracheostomy tube
with the tracheostomy cuff hyperinflated
to tamponade the innominate artery

Utley maneuver. Digital pressure of
innominate artery against sternum to
tamponade the innominate artery

Manual innominate artery occlusion of the innominate artery tracheostomy. Black arrow = innominate artery. (Graphic adapted from Thorp A, Hurt TL, Kim TY, et al. Tracheoinnominate artery fistula: a rare and often fatal complication of indwelling tracheostomy tubes. *Pediatr Emerg Care*. 2005;21:763-766.)

Many risk factors for TIF have been described, including pressure necrosis from high cuff pressure, repetitive contact of the tracheal tube tip with the tracheal mucosa, exposures that render the endotracheal mucosa friable (such as chronic steroids or nascent radiation), and a tracheostomy placed too low (below the third tracheal ring). A protocolized approach to immediate management of a suspected TIF as a bridge to emergent surgical intervention has been described. Depending on the briskness of the bleed, a bronchoscopy can be performed to explore the etiology of the hemoptysis. In the presence of active, suspected arterial bleed, the tracheostomy cuff should be overinflated. If the bleeding is not controlled by this maneuver, the patient should be orotracheally intubated while digital compression is applied to the innominate artery through the tracheostomy opening. The patient should then be emergently transported to the operative room for definitive surgical management.

## References

1. Grant CA, Dempsey G, Harrison J, Jones T. Tracheo-innominate artery fistula after percutaneous tracheostomy: three case reports and a clinical review. *Br J Anaesth*. 2006;96:127-131.
2. Gasparri MG, Nicolosi AC, Almassi GH. A novel approach to the management of tracheoinnominate artery fistula. *Ann Thorac Surg*. 2004;77:1424-1426.
3. Bradley PJ. Bleeding around a tracheostomy wound: what to consider and what to do? *J Laryngol Otol*. 2009;123:952-956.
4. Ridley RW, Zwischenberger JB. Tracheo-innominate fistula: surgical management of an iatrogenic disaster. *J Laryngol Otol*. 2006;120:676-680.
5. Epstein SK. Late complications of tracheostomy. *Respir Care*. 2005;50:542-549.

**7.** Correct Answer: C

**Rationale:**
Needle (cannula) cricothyrotomy is an airway rescue procedure recommended in several airway guidelines to be used during a "Can't Intubate Can't Oxygenate" (CICO) emergency. It involves the passing an over-the-needle catheter through the cricothyroid membrane in a patient with respiratory failure in whom less invasive techniques are either not likely to be successful or have failed. The needle cricothyrotomy is meant to provide temporary oxygenation and ventilation via percutaneous transtracheal ventilation until a definitive airway can be secured urgently rather than emergently. After entering the cricothyroid membrane with a large bore needle, a catheter is advanced over the needle and connected to an oxygen source (with pressure not to exceed 50-60 psi) with manual intermittent insufflation achieving an inspiration-to-expiration (I:E) ratio of approximately 1 to 4 (eg, 12 breaths per minute). Expiration through the transtracheal catheter is insufficient to prevent hypercarbia and lung hyperinflation from air trapping, so a partially patent airway is at least necessary for passive exhalation in order to avoid severe barotrauma, airway rupture, and death. Several reports in both animal models and human studies have described factors associated with hemodynamic collapse during transtracheal ventilation, including cannula internal diameters less than 2.5 to 2.8 mm (the average 14 g angiocath internal diameter is less than 2.5 mm), complete airway obstruction, and I:E ratios less than 1:4 or 1:9.

## References

1. Apfelbaum JL, Hagberg CA, Caplan RA, et al. Practice guidelines for management of the difficult airway. *Anesthesiology*. 2013;118:251-270.
2. Frerk C, Mitchell V, McNarry A, et al. Difficult airway society 2015 guidelines for management of the unanticipated difficult intubation in adults. *Br Aournal Anaesth*. 2015;115:827-848.

3. American College of Surgeons Committee on Trauma. *Advanced Trauma Life Support (ATLS)*. 10th ed. Chicago, IL: American College of Surgeons; 2018.
4. Patel RG: Percutaneous transtracheal jet ventilation: a safe, quick, and temporary way to provide oxygenation and ventilation when conventional methods are unsuccessful. *Chest*. 1999;116:1689-1694.
5. Neff CC, Pfister RC, Sonnenberg E. Percutaneous transtracheal ventilation: experimental and practical aspects. *J Trauma*. 1983;23:84-90.
6. Stothert JC, Stout MJ, Lewis LM, et al. High-pressure percutaneous transtracheal ventilation: the use of large gauge intravenous type catheters in the totally obstructed airway. *Am J Emerg Med*. 1990;8(3):184-189.
7. Ahn W, Bahk JH, Lim YJ. The "gauge" system for the medical use. *Anesth Analg*. 2002;95:1125.

---

**8.** Correct Answer: E

**Rationale:**

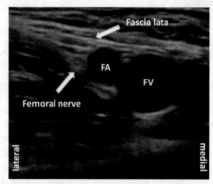

FA = femoral artery, FV = femoral vein. (Figure from Forouzan A, Masoumi K, Motamed H, et al. Nerve stimulator versus ultrasound guided femoral nerve block; a randomized clinical trial. *Emerg (Tehran)*. 2017;5(1):e54.)

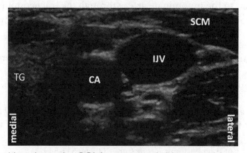

CA = carotid artery, IJV = internal jugular vein, SCM = sternocleidomastoid muscle, TG = thyroid gland. (Figure from Rezayat T, Stowell JR, Kendall JL, Turner E, Fox JC, Barjaktarevic I. Ultrasound-guided cannulation: time to bring subclavian central lines back. *West J Emerg Med*. 2016;17:216-221.)

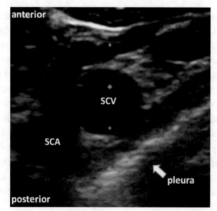

SCA = subclavian artery, SCV = subclavian vein (Figure from Rezayat T, Stowell JR, Kendall JL, Turner E, Fox JC, Barjaktarevic I. Ultrasound-guided cannulation: time to bring subclavian central lines back. *West J Emerg Med*. 2016;17:216-221.)

# 121

# PREGNANCY

Brett Elo and Mariya Geube

1. A 34-year-old G2P1 female with no prior cesarean sections is transferred to the intensive care unit following an urgent cesarean section for failure to progress despite augmentation with oxytocin. The case was complicated by uterine atony causing postpartum hemorrhage (PPH). The estimated blood loss was 2.5 L. The OB massive transfusion protocol was activated, and blood loss was replaced with 4 units of packed red blood cells, 2 units of fresh frozen plasma, 1-six pack of platelets, and tranexamic acid (TXA). On arrival, the patient is hemodynamically unstable on a phenylephrine infusion. Which of the following laboratory values should be immediately corrected?

   A. PTT of 46 s
   B. INR of 1.6
   C. Platelet count of $103 \times 10^9$/L
   D. Fibrinogen level of 163 mg/dL
   E. All of the above

2. A 27-year-old G1P0 healthy female delivers a healthy newborn under labor epidural anesthesia. Shortly after delivery of the placenta, the patient complains of shortness of breath and dizziness, followed by convulsions and cardiovascular collapse. The patient is intubated, resuscitated with fluids and pressors, and brought to the intensive care unit. The obstetrical team suspects amniotic fluid embolism. What initial findings are expected on bedside transesophageal echocardiographic examination (TEE)?

   A. Normal left and right ventricular function
   B. Severe left ventricular hypokinesis
   C. Large thrombus burden at the bifurcation of the right and left pulmonary artery
   D. Acute right ventricular dilation and severe dysfunction
   E. Right ventricular systolic pressure of 75 mm Hg

3. A 35-year-old G5P4 African American female at 40 weeks of gestation undergoes an urgent cesarean section for poor fetal heart rate tracings after being admitted for labor induction. Postoperatively, the patient becomes progressively short of breath, tachycardic, and hypotensive. A rapid response team is called in the recovery area for hypoxia, and the patient is placed on a non-rebreather to maintain $SpO_2$ >92%. A bedside transthoracic echocardiography is performed and the left ventricle appears to be severely hypokinetic and dilated. The patient is admitted to the intensive care unit for further management. Which of the following statements is true regarding peripartum cardiomyopathy (PPCM)?

   A. Approximately 50% of patients with PPCM regain normal left ventricular function by 6 months
   C. Beta blockers, diuretics, and ACE inhibitors are contraindicated in the postpartum period
   D. The risk of PPCM in subsequent pregnancies is very low
   E. The majority of patients do not recover normal LV function and require heart transplantation

**4.** A 27-year-old female with a past medical history of severe pulmonary hypertension secondary to a ventricular septal defect becomes pregnant despite warnings from expert obstetricians. At 27 weeks, the patient presents to the emergency room with shortness of breath and is admitted to an intensive care unit for hemodynamic monitoring. Several hours after admission, she becomes comatose, apneic, and pulseless. Which of the following is NOT true regarding the treatment of cardiac arrest in pregnancy?

**A.** If possible, IV access should be obtained in the upper extremity
**B.** Uterine displacement must be achieved by placing the patient 15 to 30° left lateral decubital position
**C.** After 10 minutes of unsuccessful resuscitation efforts, a cesarean section should be performed in the operating room
**D.** Chest compressions should be performed 1 to 2 cm higher on the sternum in pregnant patients
**E.** Defibrillation energy doses should remain the same as in nonpregnant patients

**5.** A 30-year-old G4P3 female presents at 35 weeks' gestation with changes in vision and headaches. At triage, her blood pressure is elevated at 149/91 mm Hg and her urine analysis is positive for protein. Initial blood work is within normal limits. Decision is made to treat with steroids to improve fetal lung maturity. Two days later, the patient complains of severe right upper quadrant pain with nausea and vomiting. A repeat metabolic panel reveals elevated aspartate aminotransferase, alanine aminotransferase, and lactate dehydrogenase. Platelet count and hemoglobin are downtrending. One day after an uneventful cesarean section, the patient again complains of severe right upper quadrant pain and becomes hypotensive and lethargic. The critical care team responds to a code, and STAT labs show a hemoglobin level of 5.2 g/dL, with a bedside ultrasound showing free fluid in the abdominal cavity. Which of the following is the most likely diagnosis?

**A.** Uterine hemorrhage
**B.** Splenic rupture
**C.** GI bleeding
**D.** Ruptured liver hematoma
**E.** Intravascular hemolysis

# Chapter 121 ■ Answers

**1.** Correct Answer: D

**Rationale:**
Postpartum hemorrhage continues to present a great challenge to obstetricians and anesthesiologists and represents a major cause of maternal mortality (between 3.5% and 12%). In the last decade, the incidence of postpartum hemorrhage has shown an uptrend, mainly because of an accompanying increase in maternal morbidity. Patient's risk factors include uterine atony and placenta accreta, percreta, and increta. The four T's classify etiologies into:
- Tone—atony
- Tissue—retained products of conception or abnormal placental attachment (accreta, percreta, increta)
- Trauma—rupture, laceration
- Thrombin—preexisting or acquired coagulation abnormalities

Along with replacing blood loss with packed red blood cells, fresh frozen plasma, and platelets in a 1:1:1 ratio, fibrinogen levels in obstetrical patients are of utmost importance in evaluating/predicting the severity of postpartum hemorrhage. Normal fibrinogen levels at the end of pregnancy are higher (373-619 mg/dL) than in nonpregnant patients (233-496 mg/dL). Decrease in fibrinogen level below 200 mg/dL has been found to be a strong predictor for severe postpartum hemorrhage. Replacement of fibrinogen with either cryoprecipitate or fibrinogen concentrate has been shown to reduce the need for transfusion of blood products by up to 33%.

References
1. Landau R, Ciliberto CG, Vuilleumier PH. Management of obstetric hemorrhage. In: Santos AC, Epstein JN, Chaudhuri K. eds. *Obstetric Anesthesia*. 1st ed. New York, NY: McGraw-Hill; 2015.
2. Butwick AJ. Postpartum hemorrhage and low fibrinogen levels: the past, present and future. *Int J Obstet Anesth*. 2013;22:87-91.
3. Bell SF, Rayment R, Collins PW, Collis RE. The use of fibrinogen concentrate to correct hypofibrinogenaemia rapidly during obstetric haemorrhage. *Int J Obstet Anesth*. 2010;19:218-223.
4. Ahmed S, Harrity C, Johnson S, et al. The efficacy of fibrinogen concentrate compared with cryoprecipitate in major obstetric haemorrhage—an observational study. *Transfus Med*. 2012;22:344-349.
5. Wikkelsoe AJ, Afshari A, Stensballe J, et al. The FIB-PPH trial: fibrinogen concentrate as initial treatment for postpartum haemorrhage: study protocol for a randomised controlled trial. *Trials*. 2012;13:110.

**2.** Correct Answer: D

**Rationale:**

Diagnosis of amniotic fluid embolism (AFE) remains a diagnosis of exclusion and can easily be mistaken for many other syndromes including eclampsia, high neuraxial block, local anesthetic toxicity, pulmonary embolism, hemorrhage, oxytocin reaction, and anaphylaxis, among others. The condition is characterized by initial cardiovascular collapse, which may or may not include seizures, followed by disseminated intravascular coagulation and clinical bleeding, leading ultimately to end organ damage.

Contrary to historical belief, the term "embolism" is a misnomer, and the phenomenon is now thought to be an immunological reaction resulting from cytokine activation and inflammation, rather than an "embolic phenomenon," which causes obstructive shock. Nonetheless, there are echocardiographic findings that aid in the diagnosis of AFE. Initially, TEE may reveal severe right ventricular dilation and systolic dysfunction, secondary to pulmonary vasoconstriction and right ventricular pressure overload. In short-axis view at the midpapillary level, there is a D-shaped left ventricle in systole and diastole, with the interventricular septum deviated to the left, because of the increased right ventricular pressure. Because the changes in the geometry of the right ventricle occur abruptly, there is no time for the right ventricle to adapt to the new loading conditions and systolic failure is imminent. With the decrease in the right ventricular ejection, the left ventricular preload and stroke volume decreases as well. In case of acute increase in the right ventricular afterload, the right ventricular systolic pressure is expected to be low, because of the inability of the acutely overloaded right ventricle to eject against high pulmonary artery resistance. High right ventricular systolic pressure is typically observed with chronic pulmonary arterial hypertension and hypertrophy of the right ventricle, which occurs over long period of time. As a late sign of amniotic fluid embolism, due to myocardial ischemia, TEE may show worsening left ventricular systolic function.

## Reference

1. James CF, Feinglass NG, Menke DM, et al. Massive amniotic fluid embolism: diagnosis aided by emergency transesophageal echocardiography. *Int J Obstet Anesth.* 2004;13:279-283.

**3.** Correct Answer: A

**Rationale:**

PPCM occurs in approximately 1:3200 deliveries in the United States. The condition is defined as new onset systolic heart failure presenting in the last month of pregnancy up to 5 months postpartum in a female with no history of cardiac disease. African American women, advanced maternal age, and multiparity are all risk factors for postpartum cardiomyopathy.

The diagnosis of PPCM can be delayed as symptoms such as mild shortness of breath, tachycardia, and lower extremity edema can be typical in pregnancy. The diagnosis is typically made by echocardiography revealing an LVEF of <45%, with or without LV dilation in a woman with no prior history of cardiac disease.

Management includes heart failure medications, such as beta blockers, diuretics, digoxin, with the addition of angiotensin converting enzyme inhibitors for afterload reduction in the postpartum period. Temporary inotropic support may be necessary in most severe cases. Anticoagulation may be necessary as patients with a depressed ejection fraction are at risk for thromboembolic events. In severe cases, an intra-aortic balloon pump or left ventricular assist device may be necessary until symptoms improve or until heart transplantation, which is required in up to 6% to 11% of patients with PPCM.

In the United States, approximately 50% of patients with recover from PPCM within 6 months. Those with a left ventricular ejection fraction of <35% at the time of diagnosis have a much higher morbidity and mortality, with less chance of recovery.

## References

1. Landau R, Ciliberto CG, Vuilleumier PH. Management of obstetric hemorrhage. In: Santos AC, Epstein JN, Chaudhuri K. eds. *Obstetric Anesthesia.* 1st ed. New York, NY: McGraw-Hill; 2015.
2. Elkayam U. Clinical characteristic of PPCM in the US: diagnosis, prognosis and management. *J Am Coll Cardiol.* 2011;58(7):659-670.
3. Sliwa K, Hilfiker-Kleiner D, Petrie MC, et al; Heart Failure Association of the European Society of Cardiology Working Group on Peripartum Cardiomyopathy. Current state of knowledge and etiology, diagnostic, management and therapy of peripartum cardiomyopathy: a position statement from the Heart Failure Association of the European Society of Cardiology Working Group on peripartum cardiomyopathy. *Eur J Heart Fail.* 2010;12:767-778.
4. Desplantie O, Tremblay-Gravel M, Avram R, et al. The medical treatment of new-onset cardiomyopathy: a systematic review of prospective studies. *Can J Cardiol.* 2015;31(12):1421-1426.

**4.** Correct Answer: C

**Rationale:**

Although cardiac arrest in pregnant patients is a rare event, it is important to understand the key differences between resuscitation in pregnant versus nonpregnant patients. The modifications to standard resuscitation are based on anatomical and physiological changes in pregnancy.

The "4-minute rule" describes better fetal outcome at greater than 24 to 25 weeks' gestation when delivery occurs within 5 minutes of mother's arrests. An emergent perimortem cesarean section is recommended at 4 minutes after cardiac arrest if there is no response to resuscitation efforts, with goals for delivery of the fetus at 5 minutes. The location of cesarean section has been debated, but studies have shown that moving the patient to the operating room may delay care and result in worse outcomes. Therefore, it is reasonable and may be recommended to perform the emergency cesarean section at the bedside.

Pregnant patients with a fundal height at, or above, the umbilicus experience decreased venous return in supine position secondary to inferior vena cava compression. It is important to place intravenous access in the upper extremity to ensure proper drug and fluid delivery during resuscitation. If IV access cannot be obtained, the humerus can be used for intraosseous access in emergency.

For appropriate cardiac output from chest compressions, it is imperative to either place the patient in left lateral decubitus position or provide manual displacement of the uterus to the left in order to release the aortocaval compression.

The pregnant patient in cardiopulmonary arrest is at high aspiration risk and immediate attempts should be made to secure the airway to prevent hypoxemia and pulmonary aspiration.

Because the gravid uterus displaced the abdominal contents and diaphragm, chest compressions should be adjusted 1 to 2 cm cephalad in a pregnant patient.

There is no difference in transthoracic impedance between pregnant and nonpregnant patients. Therefore, for a pregnant patient who requires an electrical shock for a fatal arrhythmia, no modification to standard adult doses of defibrillation is recommended.

### References

1. Landau R, Ciliberto CG, Vuilleumier PH. Management of obstetric hemorrhage. In: Santos AC, Epstein JN, Chaudhuri K. eds. *Obstetric Anesthesia.* 1st ed. New York, NY: McGraw Hill; 2015.
2. Jeejeebhoy FM, Zelop CM, Lipman S, et al; American Heart Association Emergency Cardiovascular Care Committee, Council on Cardiopulmonary, Critical Care; Perioperative and Resuscitation; Council on Cardiovascular Diseases in the Young, and Council on Clinical Cardiology. Cardiac arrest in pregnancy: a scientific statement from the American Heart Association. *Circulation.* 2015;132:1737-1773.
3. Robbins KS, Martin SR, Wilson WC. Intensive care considerations for the critically ill parturient. In: Resnick R, Creasy RK, Iams JD, Lockwood CJ, Moore T, Greene MF, eds. *Creasy and Resnick's Maternal-Fetal Medicine.* 7th ed. Philadelphia, PA: Elsevier Saunders; 2014:1182-1214.
4. Mhyre JM, Tsen LC, Einav S, Kuklina EV, Leffert LR, Bateman BT. Cardiac arrest during hospitalization for delivery in the United States, 1998 -2011. *Anesthesiology.* 2014;120:810-818.

**5.** Correct Answer: D

**Rationale:**

HELLP syndrome stands for hemolysis, elevated liver enzymes, and low platelet count. It is usually, but not always, associated with severe preeclampsia. HELLP syndrome can cause a variety of complications that increase maternal morbidity and mortality, including placental abruption, stroke, disseminated intravascular coagulation, acute renal failure, acute respiratory distress syndrome, and as in this case, liver hemorrhage.

Pathognomonic for HELLP syndrome is microangiopathic hemolytic anemia. Schistocytes are seen on peripheral smear. Elevated bilirubin (1.2 mg/dL) and lactate dehydrogenase (>600 U/L) are common, along with elevated aspartate aminotransferase (<70 U/L), ALT (>50 U/L), and decreased platelet count. The diagnosis of HELLP syndrome can be difficult as many other clinical conditions can present with similar symptoms, including idiopathic thrombocytopenic purpura, hemolytic uremic syndrome, and acute fatty liver of pregnancy.

Severe right upper quadrant pain can be an ominous sign for development of subcapsular liver hematoma. A ruptured subcapsular liver hematoma is considered surgical emergency. The diagnosis is made by ultrasound, computed tomography, or magnetic resonance imaging. Management of liver hematoma may vary from vessel embolization by interventional radiology, to abdominal exploration and even liver transplantation in severe cases.

### Reference

1. Bateman B, Polley LS. Hypertensive disorders. In: Chestnut DH, Polley LS, Wong CA, Tsen LC, eds. *Chestnut's Obstetric Anesthesia: Principles and Practice.* 5th ed. Philadelphia, PA: Saunders; 2014:825-859.

# 122

# DERMATOLOGICAL DISORDERS

Howard Zee and Abraham Sonny

1. An 18-year-old female is brought to the emergency department with a new-onset rash. Her mother states that over the past few days, she has had a fever of 102°F, as well as appeared lethargic. She had initially presented to an urgent care center where a rapid strep test was found to be negative, and she was started on antibiotics. Her past medical history is remarkable for seizure disorder and trigeminal neuralgia, and she reports that her medications were recently switched by her neurologist. You notice a macular rash involving her lips, eyes, and most of her chest and back. When palpating the rash, you notice the skin sloughs off with little pressure.

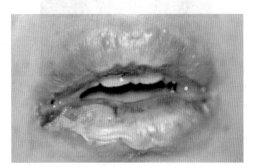

From Fleisher GR, Ludwig S, Baskin MN. *Atlas of Pediatric Emergency Medicine*. Philadelphia, PA: Lippincott Williams & Wilkins; 2004.

Which of the following agents is LEAST likely to be the cause of her current disease?

A. Phenytoin
B. Carbamazepine
C. Sulfamethoxazole-trimethoprim
D. Ibuprofen
E. Valproic acid

2. A 63-year-old man was transferred from the floor to the intensive care unit (ICU) overnight due to hypotension refractory to fluid administration. He was initially admitted to the hospital after an injury during his most recent fishing trip off of the Florida coast. His past medical history was significant for diet-controlled type 2 diabetes mellitus and hypertension. Vital signs reveal a heart rate of 110 beats/minute, blood pressure of 75/40 mm Hg, and temperature of 102°F. He appears somnolent and his right arm appears to be warm, edematous, and covered in bullae. There appears to be 2-cm laceration over the ipsilateral shoulder. Lab values are as follows: hemoglobin 9 g/dL, white blood cell count 24,000/μL, sodium 132 mEq/L, creatinine 2.7 mg/dL, glucose 200 mg/dL, and C-reactive protein 20 mg/dL. Initial blood culture results identified a single gram-negative organism. Given his presentation, you have a high suspicion for which of the following causative organisms:

A. *Escherichia coli*
B. *Vibrio vulnificus*
C. *Aeromonas hydrophila*
D. *Salmonella enterica*
E. *Enterococcus faecalis*

3. A 27-year-old male with a past medical history of rheumatoid arthritis is admitted to the ICU after a fall. The patient was found down on a forest hiking trail. During the fall he suffered head trauma. You are evaluating the patient on his second hospital day. On physical examination, you notice a rash that involves his face, neck, and arms, but spares the trunk. The rash is maculopapular with streaking patterns, occasional black, spots and occasional bullae (in the figure that follows).

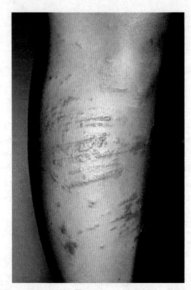

From Arndt KA, Hsu JTS. *Manual of Dermatologic Therapeutics (Lippincott Manual Series)*. 8th ed. Philadelphia, PA: Wolters Kluwer Health; 2014.

During this hospitalization, he was started on levetiracetam for seizure prophylaxis as well as cefazolin due to a concern for infection. What would be the best next step in management?

A. Stop the levetiracetam
B. Stop the cefazolin
C. Continue medications and provide supportive measures
D. Biopsy the rash
E. Draw an antinuclear antibody (ANA)

4. A 44-year-old male admitted to the hospital with a 3-day history of fevers, cough, pruritus, and rash. The patient notes he was in his usual state of health until the night before his admission. His past medical history is significant for hypertension, hyperlipidemia, and gout. He was seen by his primary care physician 2 weeks ago, and he was started on allopurinol and hydrochlorothiazide. On physical examination, you note a morbilliform rash that appears to cover his thorax and upper extremities as well as tender lymphadenopathy. His metabolic panel shows serum sodium 141 mEq/L, potassium 4.6 mEq/L, chloride 110 mEq/L, bicarbonate 23 mg/dL, urea 30 mg/dL, creatinine 2.0 mg/dL, and glucose 210 mg/dL. Liver function tests showed aspartate aminotransferase 500 U/L and alanine aminotransferase 450 U/L. Additional lab tests reveal a white blood cell count of 20,000 cells/μL, hemoglobin 12 g/dL, platelets 100,000/μL, and an absolute eosinophil count of 1600 cells/μL (normal <350). A dermatology consult was placed for evaluation and biopsy, but the results were still pending.

Which of the following criteria would help establish the appropriate diagnosis?

A. Hemoglobin, white blood cell count, creatinine, bilirubin
B. Fever, lymphadenopathy, body surface area (BSA) involved, number of organs involved
C. Biopsy findings, hemoglobin, albumin
D. Creatinine, bilirubin, INR
E. AST, ALT, albumin, platelet count

5. A 35-year-old female presented with chest pain, dyspnea, and cough. She reported a history of recurrent polyarthralgias but has never been evaluated for autoimmune disorders. On physical examination, she has a maculopapular erythematous rash localized to her arms, cheeks, and bridge of her nose. She said she has tried to avoid the sun as she tends to develop severe sunburns. Her laboratory results were significant for a hemoglobin 9.5 g/dL, white blood cell count 17,000/μL, and creatinine 1.3 mg/dL. Urinalysis reveals significant proteinuria. Dermatology was consulted, and a biopsy was taken for analysis. Histology revealed vacuolar dermatitis with lymphocytic infiltrate. Direct immunofluorescence of the sample demonstrated immunoreactants depositing at the dermal-epidermal junction. Other laboratory results include positive ANA, positive anti-Sm antibody, and negative antihistone antibody. Which of the following is the MOST likely diagnosis?

A. Drug-induced lupus
B. Psoriatic arthritis
C. Cellulitis
D. Systemic lupus erythematosus (SLE)
E. Amyloidosis

# Chapter 122 ■ Answers

1. Correct Answer: D

**Rationale:**

| CLASSIFICATION | % BODY SURFACE AREA (BSA) INVOLVED |
| --- | --- |
| SJS | <10 |
| SJS/TEN overlap | 10-30 |
| TEN | >30 |

This patient's presentation is consistent with toxic epidermal necrolysis (TEN). The new rash after initiation of a new antibiotic and antiepileptic medication involving almost half of her total BSA further supports this. She also demonstrates mucosal involvement as well as a positive Nikolsky sign, which are discussed below. Stevens-Johnson syndrome (SJS) is a life-threatening dermatological disorder that exists on a spectrum of disease, including TEN. The classification of the disease is determined by how much of the total body surface area is involved.

The most common cause is a drug reaction, but it can also be triggered by infection. Although oxicam NSAIDs have been implicated with SJS, ibuprofen (**answer D**) has not. Other drugs identified as having a strong association with SJS/TEN include sulfonamides (**answer C**), quinolones, cephalosporin antibiotics, allopurinol, nevirapine, etoricoxib, and antiepileptic drugs, for example, phenytoin (**answer A**), phenobarbital, carbamazepine (**answer B**), valproic acid (**answer E**), and lamotrigine. It is important to remember that many antiepileptic drugs are also used to treat other neurological disorders such as trigeminal neuralgia. *Mycoplasma pneumonia* and human immunodeficiency virus infection have also been associated with SJS/TEN. Malignancy and certain HLA-haplotypes are also implicated as risk factors. Although the mechanism is not completely understood, it appears that cytotoxic T-cells and natural killer cells release granulysin, a cytotoxic mediator that plays a key role in the keratinocyte apoptosis.

24 to 72 hours prior to cutaneous involvement, patients classically present with fever and other flu-like symptoms. Affected skin will demonstrate epidermal detachment and necrosis. The lesions are typically erythematous macules with centers that can be purpuric or necrotic but may be also bullous. Mucous membranes in more than one anatomical distribution are typically involved (eg, oral, ocular, genital, or anal). A classical physical examination finding of detachment of the entire epidermal layer with pressure is referred to as the Nikolsky sign, which is seen in this patient. In order to definitively diagnose SJS or TEN, a skin biopsy is required demonstrating full-thickness epidermal necrosis.

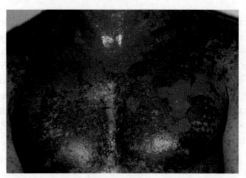

TEN from nevirapine. From Goodheart HP. *Goodheart's Photoguide of Common Skin Disorders*. 2nd ed. Philadelphia, PA: Lippincott Williams & Wilkins; 2003.

While patients are often on a multitude of medications in the ICU, the first step should be identification of and stopping suspected medication. Supportive management is the cornerstone of treatment for these patients, as many authors advocate transferring to a burn intensive care unit for severe disease. The optimal strategy for wound care has not been established. However, fluid resuscitation of 2 mL/kg/% BSA involved in the first 24 hours and targeting patient room temperature to 30 to 32°C are recommended. Depending on respiratory involvement, mechanical ventilation may be necessary. Other adjuncts including steroids and intravenous immunoglobulin have been described, but their benefit has not been proven. A dermatological consult, as well as early ophthalmological consult is crucial. Depending on the extent of the disease, a urologic or gynecologic consult may also be appropriate.

### References

1. Gerull R, Nelle M, Schaible T. Toxic epidermal necrolysis and Stevens-Johnson syndrome: a review. *Crit Care Med*. 2011;39(6):1521-1532.
2. Zimmermann S, Sekula P, Venhoff M, et al. Systemic immunomodulating therapies for Stevens-Johnson syndrome and toxic epidermal necrolysis. *JAMA Dermatol*. 2017;153(6):514.
3. Schneider J, Cohen P. Stevens-Johnson syndrome and toxic epidermal necrolysis: a concise review with a comprehensive summary of therapeutic interventions emphasizing supportive measures. *Adv Ther*. 2017;34(6):1235-1244.
4. Borchers A, Lee J, Naguwa S, Cheema G, Gershwin M. Stevens–Johnson syndrome and toxic epidermal necrolysis. *Autoimmun Rev*. 2008;7(8):598-605.

---

**2.** Correct Answer: B

**Rationale:**

Skin and soft tissue infections (SSTI) are a collection of infectious disease processes of variable etiology and severity. SSTI includes superficial infections such as impetigo and cellulitis, as well as systemic and invasive processes such as toxic shock syndrome and necrotizing soft tissue infections (NSTI).

This patient presents with septic shock, which appears to be secondary to an NSTI. Necrotizing fasciitis (NF), a type of NSTI, involves the fascial layer and can progress rapidly if not recognized and treated surgically in a timely fashion. It is not always easy to distinguish NF from less invasive or superficial infections such as cellulitis. Risk factors for developing NF include immunosuppression, malignancy, blunt or penetrating trauma, and recent surgery. Extremities are the most commonly involved site of infection. However, the groin, head, and neck can also be at risk. This patient's physical examination findings of upper extremity erythema, edema, and bullae are consistent with an NSTI. The diagnosis of NF can only be established in the operating room after surgical exploration, as it requires direct visualization of the tissue planes.

Although the most common responsible organisms for SSTIs are gram-positive bacteria, for example, *Staphylococcus aureus* and *Streptococcus pyogenes*, certain pathologies can be caused by gram-negative organisms or anaerobes. *V. vulnificus* (**answer B**) is a gram-negative bacillus of warm saltwater environments. Given this patient's history of fishing off of the Florida coast, the history of penetrating trauma, and the bullous appearance of his NSTI and the single gram-negative organism culture, the suspicion for *V. vulnificus* is high. *A. hydrophila* (**answer C**) can also cause NF, but is typically associated with freshwater or brackish water environments, and would be less likely in this patient. *E. coli* (**answer A**) and *S. enterica* (**answer D**), while also possible, are also less likely given his history. *E. faecalis* (**answer E**) is a gram-positive coccus and is unlikely given the gram stain results.

Computed tomography is thought to be the best imaging modality for NF. Imaging findings include soft tissue edema and presence of gas in the tissue planes, although formal diagnosis still requires surgical exploration. Another clinical tool is the Laboratory Risk Indicator for Necrotizing Fasciitis (LRINEC) score. *See table that follows.*

| LABORATORY TEST | RESULT | SCORE |
|---|---|---|
| C-reactive protein | <15 mg/dL | 0 |
| | ≥15 mg/dL | 4 |
| White Blood Cell Count (×10,000/μL) | <15 | 0 |
| | 15-25 | 1 |
| | >25 | 2 |
| Hemoglobin (g/dL) | >13.5 | 0 |
| | 11-13.5 | 1 |
| | <11 | 2 |
| Sodium (mEq/L) | ≥135 | 0 |
| | <135 | 2 |
| Creatinine (mg/dL) | ≤1.6 | 0 |
| | >1.6 | 2 |
| Glucose (mg/dL) | ≥180 | 0 |
| | <180 | 1 |

The purpose of LRINEC score is to try to differentiate patients into high-risk (score ≥8), moderate-risk (score ≥6-7), and low-risk (score <6) categories using routine laboratory tests in order to identify patients that would benefit from early operative intervention. However, several recent studies have emphasized that a low LRINEC score alone is not sufficient to rule out NF. Additionally, it is important to initiate standard care for septic shock, including blood cultures, broad-spectrum antibiotics, and supportive therapy.

### References

1. Burnham JP, Kirby JP, Kollef MH. Diagnosis and management of skin and soft tissue infections in the intensive care unit: a review. *Intensive Care Med*. 2016;42(12):1899-1911.
2. Bonne SL, Kadri SS. Evaluation and management of necrotizing soft tissue infections. *Infect Dis Clin North Am*. 2017;31(3): 497-511.
3. Breyre A, Frazee BW. Skin and soft tissue infections in the emergency department. *Emerg Med Clin North Am*. 2018;36(4): 723-750.
4. Wong C-H, Khin L-W, Heng K-S, Tan K-C, Low C-O. The LRINEC (laboratory risk indicator for necrotizing fasciitis) score: a tool for distinguishing necrotizing fasciitis from other soft tissue infections. *Crit Care Med*. 2004;32(7):1535-1541.
5. Fernando SM, Tran A, Cheng W, et al. Necrotizing soft tissue infection: diagnostic accuracy of physical examination, imaging, and LRINEC score. *Ann Surg*. 2019;269(1):58-65.

**3.** Correct Answer: C

**Rationale:**
On his physical examination, the rash appears to be distributed in a pattern consistent with exposed skin surfaces, specifically those not typically covered by clothing. As he was found unconscious in the forest, the suspicion for allergic contact dermatitis should be high. His new exposure to an antiepileptic (**answer A**) and an antibiotic (**answer B**) should also raise suspicion of a drug rash. Contact dermatitis appears within minutes to hours of contact with the allergen, whereas drug rashes appear hours to days after initiation. The characteristics of the rash, including appearance and distribution (sparing of the trunk) make an allergic contact dermatitis more likely than a drug reaction. Although an ANA (**answer E**) may be positive in this patient due to his history of rheumatoid arthritis, this test would not be helpful in making the diagnosis. Typical biopsy results show spongiotic dermatitis with collections of Langerhans cells and eosinophils. However, contact dermatitis is typically made as a clinical diagnosis and does not require biopsy.

This patient's clinical picture is consistent with a specific type of allergic contact dermatitis commonly caused by plants of the Anacardiaceae family and the genus *Toxicodendron*, including poison ivy. Poison ivy dermatitis is caused the plant oil urushiol. Roughly half of all adults will have a clinical reaction when exposed to poison ivy, and it is thought to be due to sensitization earlier in life. Allergic contact dermatitis, as a category, is caused by a type IV delayed-type hypersensitivity reaction. The differential diagnosis includes other forms of allergic contact dermatitis, drug reactions, cellulitis, and arthropod reactions.

The rash appears erythematous but may include macula, papula, or bullae. Rarely, the resin, if not removed, produces a black appearance due to oxidation. It typically appears in a linear or streak-like appearance in exposed areas, as only damaged plants will cause exposure to urushiol. As previously mentioned, this is a clinical diagnosis, and thus biopsy may not be beneficial. The gold standard for diagnosing allergic contact dermatitis is patch testing, which involves applying patches with the specific allergen in question to the patients back. However, this is meant to be done as an outpatient test and may not be helpful in the acute setting when there is still active inflammation.

Unfortunately, there is no one specific therapy except preventing further exposure. For patients admitted to the hospital, it is important that on presentation all clothing that may have been exposed should be removed and washed or discarded. Oral systemic steroids may help with recovery when the rash is severe or widespread.

### References

1. Kostner L, Anzengruber F, Guillod C, Recher M, Schmid-Grendelmeier P, Navarini AA. Allergic contact dermatitis. *Immunol Allergy Clin North Am.* 2017;37(1):141-152. doi:10.1016/j.iac.2016.08.014.
2. Mowad CM, Anderson B, Scheinman P, Pootongkam S, Nedorost S, Brod B. Allergic contact dermatitis. *J Am Acad Dermatol.* 2016;74(6):1029-1040. doi:10.1016/j.jaad.2015.02.1139.
3. Rosa G, Fernandez AP, Vij A, et al. Langerhans cell collections, but not eosinophils, are clues to a diagnosis of allergic contact dermatitis in appropriate skin biopsies. *J Cutan Pathol.* 2016;43(6):498-504. doi:10.1111/cup.12707.
4. Prok L, McGovern T. Poison ivy (Toxicodendron) dermatitis. In: Post TW, ed. *UpToDate.* Waltham, MA: UpToDate Inc. https://www.uptodate.com. Accessed on March 10, 2019.

## 4. Correct Answer: B

### Rationale:

Given the patient's symptoms, physical examination, and laboratory findings, this patient has a probable diagnosis of drug reaction with eosinophilia and systemic symptoms (DRESS). DRESS is also referred to as drug-induced hypersensitivity syndrome.

Although the pathogenesis of DRESS is not entirely understood, an inappropriate immune response, viral reactivation, and genetic mutation may contribute. Immunologically, it appears to involve proliferation of T-cells in response to the causative medication and eosinophilia from cytokine release. Certain genetic mutations that alter enzyme function may lead to the production of metabolites that may stimulate the immune response. Herpes group (eg, human herpes virus-6 and Epstein-Barr virus) viral reactivation often occurs simultaneously which further stimulates the immune response, but it is unclear if the infection is causative or reactive. Allopurinol, antiepileptics (eg, lamotrigine, carbamazepine, phenobarbital), antibiotics, and antiretrovirals have all been implicated.

Patients typically present with fever, rash, lymphadenopathy as well as multiple organ system involvement. Symptoms typically appear 2 to 8 weeks after initiation of the causative drug, and this delay in onset of symptoms is characteristic for DRESS. On examination, patients often demonstrate an erythematous morbilliform rash that involves the upper thorax, face, and upper extremities, but can spread to the lower extremities. The rash may appear maculopapular and be accompanied by significant edema, especially facial swelling. The liver and kidney are the most frequently involved visceral organs and may demonstrate varying degrees of hepatitis and renal impairment. Lung involvement may cause acute respiratory distress syndrome and cardiac involvement often presents with myocarditis.

There can be leukocytosis, significant eosinophilia, and thrombocytopenia. Should a skin biopsy be performed, lymphocytic infiltrate and eosinophils in the superficial dermal layers is characteristic.

### Scoring system for DRESS

| ITEM | | PRESENT | ABSENT | |
|---|---|---|---|---|
| Fever ≥38.5°C (101.3°F) | | 0 | −1 | |
| Enlarged lymph nodes (>1 cm size, at least two sites) | | 1 | 0 | |
| Eosinophilia: ≥700% or ≥10% (leukopenia) | ≥1500% or ≥20% (leukopenia) | 1 | 2 | 0 |
| Atypical lymphocytes | | 1 | 0 | |
| Rash ≥50% of body surface area | | 1 | 0 | |
| Rash suggestive (≥2 of facial edema, purpura, infiltration, desquamation) | | 1 | 0 | |
| Skin biopsy suggesting alternative diagnosis | | −1 | 0 | |
| Organ involvement: 1 | ≥2 | 1 | 2 | 0 |
| Disease duration >15 days | | 0 | −2 | |
| Investigation for alternative cause (blood cultures, ANA, serology for hepatitis viruses, mycoplasma, chlamydia) ≥3 done and negative | | 1 | 0 | |

Total score <2: excluded; 2-3: possible; 4-5: probable; ≥6: definite

The RegiSCAR scoring system (see table above) is useful for diagnosing DRESS, but clinicians should be aware that certain criteria are more useful retrospectively than at the time of presentation (e.g., disease duration >15 days, evaluation for other potential causes). Each of the incorrect answers (**answers A, C, D, and E**) includes some criteria that are useful and some criteria that are nondiagnostic. This patient presented with fever, tender lymphadenopathy, involvement of the entire upper body and face, and evidence of kidney and liver involvement (**answer B**). He additionally had an absolute eosinophil count ≥1500. His score is 6, which would be diagnostic.

### References

1. Husain Z, Reddy BY, Schwartz RA. DRESS syndrome. *J Am Acad Dermatol.* 2013;68(5). doi:10.1016/j.jaad.2013.01.033.
2. Mockenhaupt M. Drug reaction with eosinophilia and systemic symptoms (DRESS). In: Post TW, ed. *UpToDate.* Waltham, MA: UpToDate Inc. https://www.uptodate.com. Accessed on March 10, 2019.
3. Kardaun S, Sekula P, Valeyrie-Allanore L, et al. Drug reaction with eosinophilia and systemic symptoms (DRESS): an original multisystem adverse drug reaction. Results from the prospective RegiSCAR study. *Br J Dermatol.* 2013;169(5):1071-1080. doi:10.1111/bjd.12501.

**5.** Correct Answer: D

**Rationale:**

The likely diagnosis in this patient is SLE, which is part of a spectrum of autoimmune diseases (**answer D**). Although not fully understood, SLE appears to be the result of a complex interplay between genetic predisposition, hormonal abnormalities, and a multitude of immune abnormalities. The pathogenesis is believed to be due to creation of autoantibodies, inappropriate complement activation, and amplification of this autoimmune response. Diagnosing SLE can be challenging given its protean manifestations. Clinicians often utilize the existing classification criteria to help with the diagnosis. The 2012 Systemic Lupus International Collaborating Clinics (SLICC) criteria require four positive features (out the 17) with at least one clinical and one immunological criteria to diagnose SLE.

### SLICC CRITERIA

| CLINICAL CRITERIA | IMMUNOLOGICAL CRITERIA |
| --- | --- |
| Acute cutaneous lupus | ANA |
| Chronic cutaneous lupus | Anti-dsDNA |
| Nonscarring alopecia | Anti-Sm |
| Oral or nasal ulcers | Antiphospholipid |
| Arthralgia | Low complement |
| Serositis | Direct Coomb's test |
| Renal involvement | |
| Neurological involvement | |
| Hemolytic anemia | |
| Leukopenia or lymphopenia | |
| Thrombocytopenia | |

This patient demonstrates many of the classical symptoms including fatigue, fever, and arthralgias. Although the classic finding is a facial butterfly rash, often referred to as a malar rash, patients can develop rashes in other sun-exposed areas due to their photosensitivity. Histological findings on skin biopsy do not confirm diagnosis of SLE, but provide supporting evidence when the other clinical features are indeterminate. Biopsy typically shows vacuolar changes at the dermal-epidermal junction with lymphocytic infiltrate. The diagnosis can be further supported by direct immunofluorescence showing immunoreactants at the dermal-epidermal junction.

Drug-induced lupus can present with similar features as SLE and usually occurs after chronic drug exposure, typically months after exposure. Drug-induced lupus is classically associated with positive antihistone antibody and/or ss-DNA antibodies, and thus our patient is less likely to have drug-induced lupus (**answer A**). Psoriatic arthritis (**answer B**) can cause significant polyarthralgias, but the skin findings are typically plaque-like lesions. If biopsied, epidermal hyperplasia and parakeratosis can be seen on histology. Parakeratosis refers to the retention of nuclei in the stratum cornei. Psoriatic disease does not typically cause kidney disease even with visceral involvement. While an infection is possible, the distribution of the rash and the multiorgan involvement make cellulitis less likely (**answer C**). However, if biopsied, cellulitic lesions would show neutrophilic infiltration with subepidermal edema without formation of abscesses. In amyloidosis (**answer E**), amyloid can deposit in the skin to cause thickening or subcutaneous nodules, but this is not consistent with this patient's presentation. Biopsy of these skin lesions would show amyloid deposits in the papillary dermis.

## References

1. Aberle T, Bourn RL, Chen H, et al. Use of SLICC criteria in a large, diverse lupus registry enables SLE classification of a subset of ACR-designated subjects with incomplete lupus. *Lupus Sci Med.* 2017;4(1). doi:10.1136/lupus-2016-000176.

2. Merola J. Overview of cutaneous lupus erythematosus. In: Post TW, ed. *UpToDate.* Waltham, MA: UpToDate Inc. https://www.uptodate.com. Accessed on March 10, 2019.

3. Crowson AN, Magro C. The cutaneous pathology of lupus erythematosus: a review. *J Cutan Pathol.* 2001;28(1):1-23. doi:10.1034/j.1600-0560.2001.280101.x.

4. Wallace D. Diagnosis and differential diagnosis of systemic lupus erythematosus in adults. Post TW, ed. *UpToDate.* Waltham, MA: UpToDate Inc. https://www.uptodate.com. Accessed on March 10, 2019.

# 123

# THERMOREGULATORY DISORDERS

Sonia John and Abraham Sonny

1. A 35-year-old male is brought to the emergency department and is found to be diaphoretic, clammy, and agitated. He has altered mental status, slurred speech, and a core temperature 40°C. He was playing basketball outdoors prior. After further workup, the diagnosis of exertional heat stroke is made. Which among the following does NOT have a role in treatment?

   A. Antipyretics
   B. Cooling blankets
   C. Immersion in ice water
   D. Evaporative cooling

2. A 22-year-old female with no significant past medical or surgical history is admitted to the intensive care unit (ICU) with worsening respiratory failure. She was being treated on the floor for pneumonia and is receiving noninvasive ventilation. On admission to ICU, she is found to be tachypneic with increasing work of breathing, and her mentation is altered. On airway examination, both thyromental distance and mouth opening are more than 3 fingerbreadth and her Mallampati score is 2. You decide to institute invasive mechanical ventilation. Once equipment and personnel are ready, propofol and succinylcholine are administered to facilitate endotracheal intubation. After 90 seconds, direct laryngoscopy is attempted, but you have difficulty opening her mouth and note marked masseter muscle rigidity.

   Which among the following conditions is known to be associated with this presentation?

   A. Neuroleptic malignant syndrome (NMS)
   B. Malignant hyperthermia (MH)
   C. Hypokalemic periodic paralysis
   D. Temporomandibular joint dysfunction

3. A 48-year-old gentleman with no significant past medical history underwent uncomplicated Whipple procedure for pancreatic cancer. On postoperative day 1, laboratory data are notable for a white blood cell count of 19 000/μL. His abdominal wound appears mildly erythematous and appropriately tender, with no drainage. Auscultation reveals some crackles at the bases bilaterally. His heart rate is 100 beats/min, respiratory rate 20/min, pulse oximetry 97% on room air, and temperature of 38.4°C. Which of the following is the most likely cause of fever in this patient?

   A. Surgical site infection
   B. Acute deep venous thrombosis
   C. Postoperative inflammatory response
   D. Urinary tract infection
   E. Atelectasis

4.  A 24-year-old male with past medical history significant for gastroesophageal reflux disease (GERD), orthostatic hypotension, history of smoking and alcohol use, and newly diagnosed bipolar disorder was admitted to the ICU from emergency department. He presents with tachycardia, muscle rigidity, labile blood pressure, fever, lactate of 8 mmol/L, and creatine phosphokinase of 74 000 IU/L in the setting of being found down at a fraternity party. Blood alcohol levels were consistent with intoxication. Urine toxicology screen was negative. Nonspecific electrocardiogram (EKG) changes were noted. What drug or medication is most likely to be responsible for his presentation?

    A.  Olanzapine
    B.  Pantoprazole
    C.  Alcohol intoxication
    D.  Sertraline

# Chapter 123 ▪ Answers

1.  Correct Answer: A

    **Rationale:**
    Heat stroke can be divided into two types: classic (nonexertional) heat stroke and exertional heat stroke. Heat stroke is generally defined as a core body temperature in excess of 40°C (104°F). Generally classic (nonexertional) heat stroke affects older individuals with underlying chronic medical conditions (cardiovascular disease, neurologic, or psychiatric disorders), obesity, anhidrosis, physical disability, extremes of age, the use of recreational drugs such as alcohol or cocaine, and certain prescription drugs (beta-blockers, diuretics, or anticholinergic agents), which impair thermoregulation and interference with access to hydration or attempts at cooling. Exertional heat stroke generally occurs in younger individuals and typically present after long periods in the outdoors with high temperatures. Patients should be treated promptly with cooling measures. Presenting symptoms include tachycardia (arrhythmias), hypotension, flushing, oliguria, pulmonary crackles, and neurologic abnormalities. Metabolic acidosis and respiratory alkalosis are the most common abnormalities. If left untreated, can result in acute respiratory distress syndrome, disseminated intravascular coagulation, acute kidney injury, hepatic injury, hypoglycemia, rhabdomyolysis, and seizures.

    Initial treatment involves ensuring airway, breathing, circulation, and rapid cooling. Continuous core temperature monitoring should be performed with a rectal/esophageal probe, and cooling measures should ensue to a target temperature of 38°C to 39°C (100.4°F-102.2°F) in order to reduce the risk of iatrogenic hypothermia. Adequate cooling measures involve evaporative and convective cooling. This can be performed with the patient stripped of blankets and clothing and sprayed with a mist of lukewarm water while fans blow air over the moist skin. Intravenous benzodiazepines such as lorazepam may also improve body cooling. Immersing the patient in ice water is an efficient, noninvasive method of rapid cooling, but it may be harmful in the elderly and may complicate monitoring and intravenous access. Water ice therapy can also be used, which is composed of a patient sitting supine on a porous stretcher positioned on top of a tub of ice water. Cold thoracic and peritoneal lavage result in rapid cooling, however is invasive. Other adjuncts include cooled oxygen, cooling blankets, and cool ambient air. There are no definitive studies that support any particular approach to cooling in classic heat stroke. Pharmacologic therapy such as dantrolene has no role in the treatment of heat stroke. Acetaminophen and aspirin also have no role in management of heat stroke as the underlying mechanism does not involve a change in the hypothalamic set point, and these medications may exacerbate complications such as hepatic injury or disseminated intravascular coagulation. Furthermore, salicylates can contribute to hyperthermia by uncoupling oxidative phosphorylation.

    Reference
    1.  Mechem CC. Severe nonexertional hyperthermia (classic heat stroke) in adults. *UpToDate*. https://www.uptodate.com/contents/severe-nonexertional-hyperthermia-classic-heat-stroke-in-adults?search=heat%20stroke&source=search_result&selectedTitle=1~62&usage_type=default&display_rank=1. Accessed October 18, 2018.

2.  Correct Answer: B

    **Rationale:**
    Masseter muscle spasm has been implicated as an early indicator of susceptibility to MH. However, the proportion of patients with masseter spasm who go on to develop MH is unknown. Medications associated with MH include inhaled anesthetics (ether, halothane, enflurane, isoflurane, desflurane, sevoflurane) and succinylcholine. The onset could be explosive if succinylcholine is used. The classical manifestation of fulminant MH is muscle rigidity, unexplained sinus tachycardia, ventricular arrhythmias, increase in $PaCO_2$ despite adequate ventilation (if intubated),

unexplained respiratory and metabolic acidosis, increase in core body temperature >38.8°C, masseter muscle spasm, cardiac arrest, disseminated intravascular coagulation, and myoglobinuria. Prompt diagnosis is essential and should include arterial/venous blood sampling for measurement of creatine phosphokinase, acid-base status, and electrolytes, particularly potassium. If development of MH is suspected, dantrolene should be reconstituted in sterile water and administered as 2.5 mg/kg IV every 5 to 10 minutes, up to a cumulative dose of 10 mg/kg. Management is largely supportive, and metabolic derangements may be treated symptomatically. In this patient, treatment consists of delivering 100% oxygen via bag and mask ventilation, hyperventilation, and administering an intubating dose of a nondepolarizing neuromuscular blocker to attempt direct laryngoscopy.

This patient has not received any medications that would be likely to induce NMS, making it an unlikely diagnosis. Hypokalemic periodic paralysis is a rare, autosomal dominant channelopathy characterized by muscle weakness and paralysis with associated reduction in serum potassium. The times at which it presents are usually after strenuous exercise, sleep, high carbohydrate meals, or meals with high loads of sodium content, and large fluctuations in temperature. Since the patient had normal mouth opening before administration of succinylcholine, temporomandibular joint dysfunction is unlikely.

### Reference

1. Zhou J. *Malignant Hyperthermia and Muscle Related Disorders Miller's Anesthesia.* Elsevier Inc; 2015:1287-1314.e8;chap 43. https://phstwlp2.partners.org:2093/#!/content/book/3-s2.0-B9780702052835000436?scrollTo=%23hl0000456.

---

**3.** Correct Answer: C

**Rationale:**

Fever is the most common morbidity in the postoperative period. Roughly 20% of postoperative fevers are related to infection and around 80% are related to noninfectious causes. Therefore, it is important to differentiate a potentially infectious cause from a noninfectious cause.

Early postoperative fever (as in this patient) is usually caused by the inflammatory stimulus of surgery and resolves spontaneously. It is a manifestation of cytokine release caused by tissue trauma (due to surgery). Endogenous pyrogens include cytokines interleukins 1 and 6, tumor necrosis factor alpha, interferon beta and gamma, and prostaglandin E2, which attaches to the prostaglandin receptors in the hypothalamus to produce the new temperature set point. Fever-associated cytokines released from tissue trauma do not necessarily signal infection. Typically, the magnitude of tissue trauma is correlated with the degree of fever response. Since, atelectasis and fever occur frequently after surgery, atelectasis is often described as a reason for unexplained postoperative fever. However, their concurrence has been shown to be coincidental rather than causal. Though this patient might have atelectasis, it is not the cause of postoperative fever.

Other important differentials for postoperative fever include surgical site infection, acute deep venous thrombosis, urinary tract infection, nosocomial pneumonia, and drug fever. Patients at high risk of developing infection include those undergoing bowel operation, preoperative infection, immunodeficiency, indwelling vascular access, mechanical heart valves, or intensive care admission and those with persistent fevers over 101°F for more than 48 hours. However, if no infection was present preoperatively, infectious causes are less likely in the first 1 to 2 postoperative days. Drugs that are considered culpable for inducing fevers include allopurinol, carbamazepine, lamotrigine, phenytoin, sulfasalazine, vancomycin, minocycline, dapsone, and sulfamethoxazole. The risk of drug-induced fever is higher in elderly and HIV-infected patients.

### Reference

1. Clark L. *Perioperative Management of Complications: Fever, Respiratory, Cardiovascular, Thromboembolic, Urinary Tract, Gastrointestinal, Wound, and Operative Site Complications; Neurologic Injury; Psychological Sequelae Comprehensive Gynecology 25.* Elsevier Inc; 2017:583-620.e14. https://phstwlp2.partners.org:2093/#!/content/book/3-s2.0-B9780323322874000259?scrollTo=%23hl0001742.

---

**4.** Correct Answer: A

**Rationale:**

NMS occurs in roughly 0.2% of those using neuroleptics. Presentation is precipitated in the setting of dehydration/malnutrition and in newly diagnosed individuals with medication adjustments. It commonly presents with high fever (>40°C), diffuse muscle rigidity, and rhabdomyolysis. It requires two or more of the following features for definitive diagnosis: autonomic instability (tachycardia, labile blood pressures), mental status changes, leukocytosis, and elevated creatine phosphokinase. It can also manifest with bradykinesia, chorea, dystonia, dysphagia, dysarthria, or aphonia, seizures, and tremor. The severity of rhabdomyolysis can be correlated with creatine phosphokinase levels, presence of myoglobin, myoglobinuria, metabolic acidosis, and azotemia. If untreated, NMS has a mortality rate as high as 10%. Treatment includes bromocriptine and dantrolene along with supportive care.

This patient's presentation is most consistent with NMS, likely triggered by recent initiation of olanzapine and dehydration in the setting of acute alcohol intoxication. Other differential diagnosis to consider (in appropriate clinical context) would be infection of the central nervous system, drug-induced Parkinsonism, drug overdose (psychostimulants, antidepressants, lithium, anticholinergics), alcohol or drug withdrawal, side effects of nonpsychotropic dopamine-depleting drugs (reserpine, metoclopramide, prochlorperazine, promethazine), cholinergic rebound, serotonin syndrome, thyrotoxicosis, and malignant hyperthermia. The following table shows differentiating features between NMS, serotonin syndrome, and malignant hyperthermia.

|  | Neuroleptic Malignant Syndrome | Serotonin Syndrome | Malignant Hyperthermia |
|---|---|---|---|
| Inciting factors | Dopamine blockers | Serotonergic agents | Inhalational anestheticsSuccinylcholine |
| Timing | Gradual onset | Abrupt onset | Abrupt onset (rarely hours later) |
| Vital signs | Hypertension, tachycardia, tachypnea, hyperthermia | Hypertension, tachycardia, tachypnea, hyperthermia | Hypertension, tachycardia, hypercarbia, tachypnea, hyperthermia |
| Course | Rapidly resolving | Prolonged | Prolonged without definitive treatment |
| Neurologic symptoms | Lead pipe rigidity, decreased reflexes, normal pupils | Increased muscular tone, tremors, choreoathetoid movements, hyperreflexia, clonus, mydriasis | Increased muscle rigidity, masseter muscle spasm (often may not be generalized) |
| Bowel sounds | Normal to decreased | Hyperactive | Normal to decreased |

### Reference

1. Manu P. *Medical Consultation in Psychiatry; Goldman-Cecil Medicine.* Vol 434. Elsevier Inc; 2016:2625-2629.e2. https://phstwlp2.partners.org:2093/#!/content/book/3-s2.0-B9781455750177004347?scrollTo=%23hl0000331.

Alexandra Plichta, Amanda S. Xi, John Hwabejire, Rachel Steinhorn, Edward Bittner, Sheri Berg, and Abraham Sonny

1. Which of the following patients with acute acetaminophen (APAP) overdose is the LEAST likely to benefit from N-acetylcysteine (NAC) therapy?

   A. A 35-year-old man with depression, found down at home with multiple empty medication bottles, including Tylenol
   B. A 28-year-old 50 kg woman with hypertension, who called EMS 4 hours taking 5 g of APAP
   C. A 28-year-old woman with chronic back pain, who has a serum APAP level of 170 µg/mL 4 hours after an acute ingestion
   D. A 35-year-old man with hemochromatosis, who misread the label and took an order of magnitude too much Tylenol. His serum level on presentation 4 hours after ingestion is 140 µg/mL

2. An 89-year-old female is admitted to the ICU with a past medical history of cardiac disease. According to EMS, there were multiple empty medication bottles at the scene. Upon review of the intake ECG, you notice atrial fibrillation with a ventricular rate of 51 and frequent premature ventricular contractions (PVCs). Over the course of the night, she becomes progressively more bradycardic and hypotensive. Of the choices provided, what would be the BEST next step in management?

   A. Place a double-lumen central venous catheter (CVC) and begin hemodialysis
   B. Administer a modified immunoglobulin
   C. Administer IV bicarbonate to increase urinary pH
   D. Administer calcium as a therapy for hyperkalemia

3. A 23-year-old male with a past medical history significant for schizophrenia is admitted to the ICU following an intentional overdose of olanzapine and quetiapine. Which of the following is NOT a symptom of overdose with antipsychotics?

   A. QT prolongation
   B. Stupor
   C. Bradycardia
   D. Hypotension

4. A 29-year-old female with a past medical history of treatment refractory depression, which has been somewhat controlled with amitriptyline and venlafaxine, is admitted to the ICU following a supposed drug overdose. Her mother reports that the vial of amitriptyline was empty. What is the molecular mechanism underlying the toxicity of tricyclic antidepressants (TCAs) in overdose?

   A. $Na^+$ channel antagonism
   B. $Ca^{2+}$ channel antagonism
   C. Profound sympatholysis
   D. Uncoupling of the $Na^+$-$K^+$ ATPase

**5.** A 58-year-old female is admitted to the intensive care unit for a suspected infection. She is started on moxifloxacin and fluconazole. She is intubated and sedated and subsequently treated for gastroparesis with erythromycin. Her rhythm degenerates into a polymorphic ventricular tachycardia (VT), and arterial wave pressure tracing appears substantially dampened despite flushing of the tubing. Which of the following is the next best step in management?

   **A.** Initiate overdrive pacing
   **B.** Start an infusion of magnesium sulfate
   **C.** Defibrillate
   **D.** Start an infusion intravenous lipid emulsion (ILE) therapy

**6.** A 64-year-old male with a history of alcoholism and countless admissions for withdrawal seizures is admitted to the ICU after he was found down on the street. Which of the following is FALSE regarding alcohol withdrawal syndromes?

   **A.** Hallucinations are usually present in both alcoholic hallucinosis and delirium tremens.
   **B.** Autonomic instability is usually present in both alcoholic hallucinosis and delirium tremens.
   **C.** Sensorium is usually normal in alcoholic hallucinosis.
   **D.** There are different mortality rates associated with the diagnoses of delirium tremens versus alcoholic hallucinosis.

**7.** A 27-year-old male is admitted to the ICU after he presented to the emergency department with chest pain after bingeing on cocaine. A CT scan demonstrated a type B aortic dissection. Which of the following is NOT a major molecular mechanism by which cocaine elicits its effects?

   **A.** Norepinephrine reuptake inhibition peripherally
   **B.** Increased glutamatergic neurotransmission centrally
   **C.** Downregulation of gamma-aminobutyric acid (GABA) neurotransmission centrally
   **D.** Sodium channel blockade of the myocardium

**8.** Which of the following opioid withdrawal syndromes is MOST likely to be fatal?

   **A.** A 35-year-old female who is addicted to heroin and is incarcerated without further access to opioids or opioid replacement therapy.
   **B.** A 66-year-old man with a prior coronary artery bypass who is addicted to heroin, found down on the street, and given 4 mg of naloxone IV.
   **C.** A 66-year-old female with a prior left anterior descending artery stent and with known fentanyl addiction, who is found down and intubated by EMS. She is given naloxone IV in escalating doses, starting with 0.04 mg.
   **D.** A 35-year-old female with no significant past medical or social history who is undergoing monitored anesthesia care with midazolam and fentanyl and is mistakenly given 40 mg of IV naloxone at the end of the case.

**9.** A 31-year-old female presents to the emergency department after she was found down by her boyfriend. He admits that they were using "many different drugs" the previous night. Which of the following physical examination findings will NOT help to differentiate a patient who ingested methamphetamine from one who ingested a week supply of oxybutynin?

   **A.** Skin temperature
   **B.** Pupil reactivity
   **C.** Moisture of mucous membranes
   **D.** Presence of perspiration

**10.** You are called to the intensive care unit to perform an anesthetic for an emergent bedside reexploration on a 60-year-old woman with a past medical history of atrial fibrillation (on a heparin infusion) and diabetes (on a regular insulin infusion) who is postoperative day #3 from an emergent small bowel resection. Two hours prior to your arrival, she had a cardiac arrest with return of spontaneous circulation (ROSC) for presumed hypovolemia from intraperitoneal hemorrhage.

A transthoracic echocardiogram from 3 days prior notes:

- Left ventricle (LV): Decreased LV systolic function, with LV ejection fraction 36%, and segmental wall motion abnormalities at the apex with basal sparing
- Right ventricle (RV): RV is dilated, RV systolic function is severely decreased, RV is diffusely hypokinetic

- No aortic valve pathology
- Mild mitral regurgitation
- Mild tricuspid regurgitation, estimated RV systolic pressure (RVSP) 30 mm Hg

Immediately after administering 50 mg of protamine, the patient's arterial line tracing shows a drop from a systolic blood pressure of 96 to 46 mm Hg with subsequent pulseless electrical activity (PEA). Which of the following is the MOST likely explanations for this observed reaction?

A. Direct systemic vasodilation
B. Direct mast cell degranulation
C. IgE-mediated mast cell degranulation
D. Constriction of pulmonary vasculature

11. A 35-year-old male with a history of intravenous drug abuse presents to the ICU postoperatively from an abscess drainage of the right upper extremity due to persistent pressor requirement in the postanesthesia care unit (PACU). He was a difficult peripheral IV cannulation preoperatively and required multiple attempts. A peripheral IV was eventually placed in the left upper extremity near the wrist. Upon arrival to the ICU, he complains of persistent left thumb and index finger burning on the posterior aspect. What structure is implicated in this injury?

A. Median nerve
B. Ulnar nerve
C. Radial nerve
D. Musculocutaneous nerve

12. A 45-year-old male with a history of multiple psychiatric illnesses presents to the ICU as a transfer from a medical floor after a rapid response is called on the floor due to concern for respiratory failure. During the last 24 hours, he is given a total of 60 mg of haloperidol for agitation. When he arrives on the unit, he is agitated and rigid. His heart rate is 130 beats/min; temperature is 40°C; blood pressure is 160/80 mm Hg. What is the next step in management?

A. Electroconvulsive therapy
B. Stop the causative agent
C. Administer dantrolene
D. Administer haloperidol

13. You are called to the bedside of a patient because the peripherally inserted central catheter (PICC) line (arrow) is no longer drawing back. A chest x-ray (CXR) is ordered and shows:

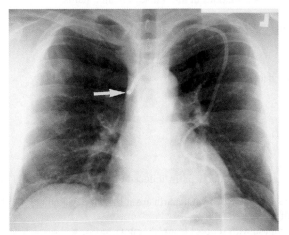

Image from Collins J, Stern EJ. *Chest radiology: The essentials.* 3rd ed. Philadelphia, PA: Wolters Kluwer; 2014:75.

Which of the following is NOT a typical complication of this finding?

A. Hemopericardium
B. Vascular perforation
C. Pleural effusion
D. Pneumothorax

**14.** A 45-year-old male with history of recurrent bilateral urinary calculi and infection is admitted to ICU with suspicion of urosepsis. On arrival to ICU, he is found to be in respiratory failure and hence is quickly intubated and placed on mechanical ventilation. He is ventilated with volume control ventilation (8 mL/kg ideal body weight) and has no inspiratory efforts. He is receiving moderate dose of norepinephrine infusion to maintain a mean arterial pressure (MAP) >65 mm Hg. His arterial pressure waveform follows.

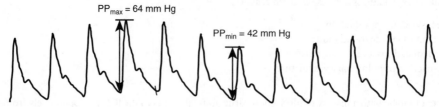

Adapted from Michard F. Changes in arterial pressure during mechanical ventilation. *Anesthesiology.* 2005;103(2):419-428.

What is the next best step in management?

**A.** 1 L lactated Ringer's
**B.** Add epinephrine
**C.** No further intervention
**D.** Obtain STAT echocardiogram

**15.** A rapid response is called on an 18-year-old female due to seizure. She was recently diagnosed with acute lymphocytic leukemia, and chemotherapy has just been started. She is intubated on the floor and transferred to the unit. A basic metabolic panel is likely to show:

**A.** Hypocalcemia
**B.** Hypophosphatemia
**C.** Hypokalemia
**D.** Hypouricemia

**16.** In assessing delirium using the Confusion Assessment Method for ICU Patients (CAM-ICU), which is NOT required to be present to diagnose delirium?

**A.** Acute onset of changes or fluctuations in the course of mental status
**B.** Inattention
**C.** Disorganized thinking
**D.** Combative behavior

**17.** Which coagulation factor decreases in pregnancy?

**A.** Protein C
**B.** Factor VII
**C.** Factor XII
**D.** Factor XIII

**18.** Which of the following statements about heparin-induced thrombocytopenia (HIT) is FALSE?

**A.** Patients of any age, receiving any type of heparin are at risk for developing HIT antibodies.
**B.** Bleeding is commonly seen with HIT.
**C.** Diagnosis of HIT is clinical with support from laboratory testing.
**D.** Testing for heparin-PF4 antibody is recommended in patients with suspected HIT.

**19.** In conjunction with the infectious disease department, your unit is trying to improve compliance with hand washing in the setting of contact isolation patients. The team plans an intervention and proposes to employ Plan-Do-Study-Act (PDSA) cycles. Which of the following is NOT part of a PDSA cycle?

**A.** Plan
**B.** Do
**C.** Study
**D.** Assess

20. An investigator wishes to study transthoracic echocardiograms performed by trainees. In the trial of 100 echocardiograms, 10 cases of endocarditis were correctly identified, 15 cases were incorrectly identified as endocarditis, 70 cases were correctly ruled out for endocarditis, and 5 cases of endocarditis were missed. What is the positive predictive value of this test?

    A. 40%
    B. 67%
    C. 82%
    D. 93%

21. Which of the following criteria is part of the 2016 definition of sepsis (Sepsis-3)?

    A. Systemic inflammatory response syndrome (SIRS)
    B. Hypotension unresponsive to fluids
    C. Confirmation of at least one positive blood culture
    D. Life-threatening organ dysfunction

22. A 26-year-old man is admitted to the ICU with septic shock from a perforated appendix. He is treated with abscess drainage, fluid resuscitation, broad-spectrum antimicrobials (vancomycin, cefepime, metronidazole), and norepinephrine for blood pressure support. Vitamin C, thiamine, and hydrocortisone are administered as adjuncts. While his shock improves, his blood glucose levels remain elevated by point-of-care (POC) testing while laboratory testing reveals normoglycemia. What is the most likely cause of the discrepancy between the POC and laboratory glucose levels?

    A. Hydrocortisone
    B. Cefepime
    C. Thiamine
    D. Vitamin C

23. Endogenous molecules released from damaged host cells that provoke inflammation in sepsis are referred to as:

    A. Damage-associated molecular patterns (DAMPs)
    B. Pathogen-associated molecular patterns (PAMPs)
    C. Inflammasomes
    D. Toll-like receptors (TLRs)

24. Development of acute kidney injury (AKI) in sepsis is most likely attributable to which of the following etiologies?

    A. Reduced renal blood flow
    B. Hypotension
    C. Acute tubular necrosis
    D. Microvascular dysfunction

25. A 70-year-old man has a PEA arrest immediately following intubation for respiratory failure. To facilitate the intubation etomidate and rocuronium had been administered. He received chest compressions and epinephrine and had ROSC after 10 minutes. To facilitate decision-making after ROSC, a neurologic examination is desired. Administration of which of the following medications would be most appropriate to facilitate this examination?

    A. Neostigmine
    B. Sugammadex
    C. Flumazenil
    D. Naloxone

26. A 27-year-old man presents to the emergency department with the "worst headache of his life," and imaging reveals a subarachnoid hemorrhage. Which of the following statements regarding ICU triage is MOST appropriate for this patient?

    A. Admit to a general ICU
    B. Triage to the ICU based on the patient's severity of illness score
    C. Transfer to the ICU within 6 hours of presentation
    D. Admit to an ICU with 24/7 inhouse intensivist staffing

27. A 49-year-old, 70 kg man is admitted to the ICU after large volume aspiration resulting from a small bowel obstruction. He is intubated and initial ventilator settings are tidal volume 420 mL, respiratory rate 27 breaths/min, positive end-expiratory pressure (PEEP) 5 cm $H_2O$, 100% $FiO_2$, and the arterial blood gas is pH 7.30/ $pCO_2$ 39 mm Hg/ $pO_2$ 57 mm Hg on those settings. He undergoes bronchoscopy with evidence of and successful evacuation of aspirated material from the airways. Chest radiograph reveals diffuse bilateral alveolar opacities. A recruitment maneuver is performed, and the PEEP is increased to 10 cm $H_2O$ with subsequent arterial blood gas of pH 7.32/ $pCO_2$ 40 mm Hg/ $pO_2$ 60 mm Hg.

    Which of the following is the next best step in diagnosis of the patient's hypoxemia?

    A. Pulmonary embolism—protocol CT scan
    B. Cardiac catheterization
    C. Echocardiogram with bubble study
    D. Bronchoalveolar lavage

28. Which of the following statements regarding the performance of a passive leg raise (PLR) test for assessment of fluid responsiveness is MOST correct?

    A. It should only be performed in a spontaneously breathing patient.
    B. It should start with the patient in the supine position.
    C. It should be assessed by a direct measurement of cardiac output.
    D. It should be assessed after waiting more than a minute for volumetric equilibration.

29. For the management of gastrointestinal dysmotility in critically ill patients, erythromycin differs from metoclopramide in which of the following ways?

    A. Erythromycin is more effective as a prokinetic agent than metoclopramide.
    B. Combination therapy with erythromycin and metoclopramide is not more effective than administration of either agent alone.
    C. Erythromycin is a motilin agonist while metoclopramide acts as an agonist of dopamine receptors.
    D. Tachyphylaxis to the prokinetic effects develops with erythromycin but not metoclopramide.

30. A 55-year-old woman with ideal body of 50kg has developed acute respiratory distress syndrome (ARDS) as a result of intra-abdominal sepsis. She is currently being mechanically ventilated with tidal volume 300 mL, respiratory rate 30 breaths/min, PEEP 8 cm $H_2O$, and 40% $FiO_2$. Her peak pressure is 37 cm $H_2O$ and plateau pressure is 34 cm $H_2O$. Her most recent arterial blood gas is pH 7.31, $PCO_2$ 44 mm Hg, and $PO_2$ 80 mm Hg. Which of the following values is the BEST estimate of the driving pressure during mechanical ventilation?

    A. 4 cm $H_2O$
    B. 14 cm $H_2O$
    C. 26 cm $H_2O$
    D. 29 cm $H_2O$

31. A 76-year-old male who has been in a rehabilitation facility for 3 months after sustaining a traumatic brain injury was brought to the emergency room with a 3-day history of nausea, vomiting, and unremitting abdominal pain. On examination, he was febrile with a maximum temperature of 102.5°F and hypotensive with a systolic BP of 82 mm Hg. His heart rate was 92 beats/min, in sinus rhythm. A midline laparotomy scar was evident. He has a history of hypertension, coronary heart disease, and atrial fibrillation and is currently on aspirin, simvastatin, and metoprolol and had a complete blood count (CBC) which showed a WBC of 13,000/mm³. Two large bore peripheral IV catheters were placed and 2 L of Ringer's lactate promptly administered, without any significant hemodynamic changes. A right internal jugular central venous line was promptly placed; he was pan-cultured, given a single dose of IV piperacillin-tazobactam and started on norepinephrine and vasopressin infusions. He was promptly admitted to the surgical intensive care unit (SICU) where a focused abdominal ultrasound showed a distended gallbladder with a 4 mm wall thickness, mild pericholecystic fluid, and gallbladder sludge. What is the next appropriate next step?

    A. Laparoscopic cholecystectomy
    B. Percutaneous cholecystostomy tube (PCT) placement
    C. Open cholecystectomy
    D. Endoscopic retrograde cholangiopancreatography (ERCP)
    E. Resuscitation with 5% albumin

**32.** A 52-year-old male with a history of chronic alcoholism and liver cirrhosis presented to the emergency room with a 3-day history of difficulty breathing, abdominal distension, and altered mental status. His liver function enzymes were all significantly elevated. Abdominal ultrasound showed massive ascites with splinting of the right hemidiaphragm. He underwent a large volume paracentesis and was admitted to the ICU. While in the ICU, bleeding from the paracentesis site which was initially controlled with digital pressure was noted. The patient soon became hypotensive and was started on vasopressors. A right IJ central line was placed. However, this required two attempts as the right common carotid artery was inadvertently punctured on the first attempt. Three hours later, he was noted to have an expanding hematoma at the right IJ puncture site with deviation of his trachea to the left, increasing dyspnea and a systolic BP of 90 mm Hg. International normalized ratio (INR) was 4.5, with increased bleeding from the paracentesis site. The next best step in the management of this patient is:

A. Emergent neck exploration
B. 1:1:1 transfusion of packed red blood cells (PRBCs), fresh frozen plasma (FFP), and platelets
C. Endotracheal intubation
D. CT angiogram of the neck
E. Exploratory laparotomy and control of abdominal bleeding

**33.** A 63-year-old female with no significant past medical history underwent exploratory laparotomy and extensive cytoreductive surgery with right hemicolectomy and ileotransverse anastomosis for mucinous adenocarcinoma of the appendix. She was admitted to the SICU for her immediate postoperative care with patient-controlled epidural anesthesia for pain control and extubated on postoperative day 1. Beginning from postoperative day 3 into postoperative day 4, she was noted to be having persistent tachycardia that was unresponsive to volume resuscitation and adequate pain control. She had mild right lower quadrant tenderness. ECG showed sinus tachycardia, and bedside echocardiography was unimpressive. Noninvasive duplex ultrasonography was negative for deep venous thrombosis. The next step in management of this patient should be:

A. CT abdomen and pelvis with oral and intravenous contrast
B. Abdominal ultrasound
C. Formal transthoracic ultrasound
D. Intravenous broad-spectrum antibiotics
E. Esophagogastroduodenoscopy and colonoscopy

**34.** A 65-year-old female presented to the emergency department with a 5-day history of nausea, vomiting, and left lower quadrant abdominal pain. She had abdominal tenderness and rebound tenderness on physical examination. CT scan of the abdomen and pelvis showed perforated diverticulitis. She received 2 L of Ringer's lactate and is taken emergently to the operating room for exploratory laparotomy. Intraoperatively, she was found to have a perforated sigmoid diverticulitis with spillage of bowel contents into the abdomen. She had sigmoid colectomy, anastomosis of the descending colon to the upper rectum, and thorough irrigation of the abdominal cavity with 3 L of warm normal saline mixed with antibiotics. The abdomen was then closed. She received 3 L of crystalloids and 2 units of packed red cells intraoperatively and was transferred to the ICU. She remains intubated on mechanical ventilation. Her resuscitation was continued with Ringer's lactate at 150 mL/h. About 12 hours after arrival in the SICU, she became oliguric with elevated peak airway pressures. Her nasogastric tube output was negligible, and bladder pressure was 31 mm Hg. The next critical step in this patient's care is what?

A. Increase in PEEP
B. Increase in the dosage of intravenous sedative
C. CT scan of the abdomen and pelvis with oral and intravenous contrast
D. Decompressive laparotomy
E. Administration of intravenous furosemide to improved urine output

**35.** A 73-year-old male had laparoscopic cholecystectomy for acute calculous cholecystitis 2 weeks ago followed by an uncompleted immediate postoperative course. He now presents to the emergency department with a 2-day history of upper abdominal pain, nausea, and vomiting. He is febrile to 101.5°F, and hypotensive with a systolic BP of 86 mm Hg. His abdomen is distended on physical examination with right upper quadrant tenderness and his WBC count was 14,000/mm³. A CT scan of the abdomen and pelvis showed a large amount of perihepatic, right paracolic, and left paracolic regions. He is given 3 L of intravenous crystalloids, started on broad-spectrum antibiotics, and admitted to the ICU. What is the next best step in the patient's management?

A. CT-guided drainage of intra-abdominal fluid collection
B. Endoscopic retrograde cholangiopancreatography
C. Magnetic resonance cholangiopancreatography
D. Exploratory laparotomy
E. Intravenous vitamin C, hydrocortisone, and thiamine

36. A 70-year-old male with a history of coronary artery disease successfully underwent an endovascular repair of a 7 cm abdominal aortic aneurysm and was admitted to the ICU for neurovascular monitoring. On postoperative day 2, he was started on clear liquid diet. About 6 hours later, he had increasing left upper quadrant pain and nausea with slight difficulty breathing. Physical examination revealed generalized abdominal distention and localized tenderness in the left upper quadrant. An abdominal x-ray showed a markedly dilated stomach with a nonobstructive bowel gas pattern. Which of the following interventions should be performed next?

    A. Aggressive bowel regimen
    B. Placement of a nasogastric tube
    C. High-flow nasal oxygen
    D. Noninvasive ventilation with bilevel positive airway pressure (BiPAP)
    E. Upper gastrointestinal endoscopy

37. A 23-year-old male was involved in a high-speed motor vehicle crash. He sustained multiple pelvic and lower extremity fractures. He is hemodynamically stable and is admitted to the ICU. His serum creatine phosphokinase is 29,500 U/L. Which of the following measures should be instituted to reduce the risk of AKI?

    A. Aggressive fluid resuscitation
    B. IV mannitol
    C. Alkalinization of the urine
    D. Hemodialysis
    E. Intravenous urogram

38. A 55-year-old female was having a right internal jugular central venous line placed under ultrasound guidance. She required multiple attempts before successful cannulation of the vein. Following the central line placement, her oxygen decreased from 97% to 86% on 2 L/min nasal cannula with hypotension. Bedside ultrasound of the chest revealed absence of lung sliding on the right. What is the next best step in the patient's management?

    A. Administration of vasopressors
    B. Fluid resuscitation
    C. Immediate chest CT scan
    D. Right tube thoracostomy
    E. Endotracheal intubation

39. During a bedside open tracheostomy on a 75-year-old female in the ICU, the respiratory therapist noted extreme difficulty in ventilating the patient after placement of the tracheostomy tube and removal of the endotracheal tube. The patient's peak airway pressures were elevated, along with hemodynamic instability and subcutaneous emphysema involving the head and neck. What is the most likely underlying pathophysiology?

    A. Bleeding from the injury to the anterior jugular veins
    B. Rupture of preexisting pulmonary bullae
    C. Abdominal compartment syndrome
    D. Massive hemothorax
    E. Tension pneumothorax

40. A 71-year-old female patient is admitted to the intensive care unit with hypotension and shortness of breath. She received 2 L crystalloids over 2 hours, however, continues to be hypotensive and requires moderate doses of phenylephrine to maintain MAP above 65 mm Hg. Also, she is receiving supplemental oxygen via high-flow nasal cannula ($FiO_2$ 50%, 50 L/min). Her past medical history is significant for congestive heart failure and chronic obstructive pulmonary disease (COPD). A bedside ultrasound is performed to assess fluid responsiveness. The following image is obtained:

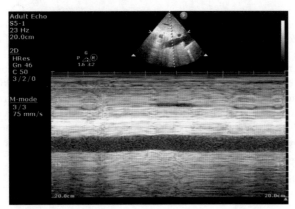

M mode through inferior vena cava in subcostal view.

Which among the following is true regarding volume responsiveness in this patient?

A. Patient is fluid responsive
B. Unable to interpret fluid responsiveness
C. Patient is fluid overloaded
D. Patient is fluid responsive to 5% albumin

41. A 54-year-old woman is admitted to the ICU for hypoxemic respiratory failure secondary to pneumonia. Her oxygen saturation is 90% on high-flow nasal cannula (FiO$_2$ 60%, 60 L/min). She is also in septic shock and needs a high-dose norepinephrine infusion to keep MAP above 65 mm Hg, despite adequate fluid resuscitation. You decide to place a central venous line for vasopressor infusion. During ultrasound-guided central line placement in the right internal jugular vein, the patient coughs; and blood pressure abruptly decreases from 110/54 to 90/45 mm Hg and her heart rate increases from 90 to 120 beats/min in sinus rhythm. A bedside transthoracic echocardiogram shows a hyperdynamic left ventricle and a mildly hypokinetic right ventricle. What is the next best step in management?

A. Discontinue PEEP
B. Aspirate the central line
C. Increase FiO$_2$ to 100%
D. Chest tube placement

42. A 59-year-old woman is placed on peripheral venoarterial extracorporeal membrane oxygenation (VA-ECMO) for pneumonia with septic shock complicated by stress cardiomyopathy with a decrease in left ventricular ejection fraction to 10%. On ECMO day 2, she develops frothy secretions from the endotracheal tube, and chest radiograph shows diffuse consolidations. Her arterial line waveform demonstrates decreased pulsatility, and inferior ST wave depressions are noted on ECG. What is the most likely transthoracic echocardiogram finding?

A. Left ventricle distension
B. Papillary muscle rupture
C. Right ventricle distension
D. Patent foramen ovale (PFO)

43. A 67-year-old man with a history of dilated cardiomyopathy with an ejection fraction of 20% is admitted with septic shock secondary to pyelonephritis. He is placed on VA-ECMO for shock unresponsive to fluid resuscitation and vasopressors. The heparin infusion rate required to maintain a therapeutic activated clotting time increases from 10,000 units/24 hours to 20,000 units/24 hours over his admission. On ECMO day 6, the patient begins to bleed from venous access sites, and a clot is noted in the ECMO oxygenator. Pre-ECMO labs were hemoglobin 9 g/dL and platelets 110,000/mm$^3$; labs now show hemoglobin 8 g/dL, platelets 55,000/mm$^3$, and coagulation studies remarkable only for an activated partial thromboplastin time (aPTT) of 70 seconds. What is the most likely diagnosis?

A. Heparin resistance
B. Disseminated intravascular coagulation
C. Supratherapeutic heparin dose
D. Heparin-induced thrombocytopenia

44. A 34-year-old woman with a history of hereditary hemorrhagic telangiectasia (HHT) is admitted to the ICU intubated and sedated following an exploratory laparotomy for a stab wound to the abdomen. Sedation is weaned on postoperative day 1; the patient's mental status is maintained at Richmond Agitation Sedation Scale (RASS) 0, and she passes a spontaneous breathing trial (SBT). During injection of hydromorphone in her central line, the luer-lock hub becomes disconnected and the line is left open to air. Moments later, blood pressure decreases to 85/45 mm Hg, heart rate rises to 110 beats/min in sinus tachycardia, and respiratory rate increases from 8 to 25 breaths/min. ST elevations are noted in leads II, III, and aVF on telemetry, and the patient suddenly exhibits a left facial droop. After hemodynamic stability is achieved, an emergent noncontrast head computed tomography shows no acute bleeding but did find an area of low attenuation in the left frontal lobe. In addition to ongoing hemodynamic support, what is the next best step in management?

    A. Cardiac catheterization with percutaneous coronary intervention
    B. Hyperbaric oxygen therapy (HBOT)
    C. Heparin infusion
    D. Tissue plasminogen activator initiation

45. A 78-year-old man with a history of COPD is admitted to the ICU intubated and sedated after colectomy with loop ileostomy creation for perforated diverticulitis. It is postoperative day 3, and despite broad-spectrum antibiotic therapy and fluid resuscitation, the patient continues to require a norepinephrine infusion to maintain MAP above 65 mm Hg. Blood glucose is 130 mg/dL. What is the best option for administering nutrition?

    A. With normoglycemia, initiate nutrition after day 7
    B. Total parenteral nutrition (TPN)
    C. Enteral tube feeds
    D. Dextrose infusion

46. A 67-year-old male with a history of severe COPD and morbid obesity remains intubated in the ICU POD 2 following an exploratory laparotomy and small bowel resection. Your respiratory therapist informs you that she has been having difficulty ventilating the patient despite changing from volume-control to pressure-control ventilation. You are then called stat to the room by his nurse, as his ECG demonstrates sinus bradycardia at 40 beats/min with associated hypotension (60/42 mm Hg). You are unable to palpate a carotid pulse. Your team initiates chest compressions and administers epinephrine. What is the most appropriate next step in managing this patient?

    A. Administer a bronchodilator
    B. Remove the endotracheal tube and reintubate
    C. Needle decompression in the second intercostal space
    D. Disconnect the patient from the ventilator circuit
    E. Obtain a chest x-ray

47. An 84-year-old female is admitted to your ICU following surgical repair of her complex right hip fracture. She has a history significant for moderate aortic stenosis, hypertension, and COPD on 2 L/min oxygen via nasal cannula at home. All of the following interventions are recommended to reduce the risk of ventilator-associated pneumonia (VAP), EXCEPT:

    A. Elevation of head of bed at least 30 degrees
    B. Early tracheostomy
    C. Daily SBTs
    D. Noninvasive positive-pressure ventilation (NIPPV)
    E. Minimize sedation

48. Your patient has been in the ICU for over 2 weeks and it is noted that her CVC has been in place since admission. You are concerned that it should be changed, as you are worried about a possible infection from the catheter. Which of the following statements regarding catheter-related bloodstream infections (CRBSIs) is true?

    A. CVCs should be replaced weekly.
    B. CRBSI is diagnosed when blood cultures drawn from the catheter are positive.
    C. Arterial lines carry a negligible risk of CRBSI.
    D. Skin preparation with chlorhexidine/alcohol is more effective than povidone iodine in preventing CRBSI.
    E. The most common pathogens in CRBSI are gram-negative rods.

**49.** A 67-year-old male is postoperative day 2 following a Whipple for pancreatic cancer. The surgeon requests that his Foley catheter be removed. Which of the following statements regarding catheter-associated urinary tract infection (CAUTI) is true?

A. External urinary catheters have similar rates of complications compared with indwelling catheters.
B. Asymptomatic catheter-associated bacteriuria should be treated to reduce the risk of developing systemic infection.
C. Intermittent catheterization does not reduce the risk of CAUTI.
D. Indwelling catheters should be replaced at regular intervals to reduce the risk of CAUTI.
E. Screening for bacteriuria is not effective in reducing CAUTI.

**50.** A 51-year-old female is admitted to the ICU following a pneumonectomy for cavitary tuberculosis. She reports that she may have received treatment "many years ago" but does not recall if she completed the full course of recommended therapy. All of the following statements regarding tuberculosis precautions are true EXCEPT:

A. The patient should be placed in a negative-pressure isolation room.
B. Empiric therapy for tuberculosis with a four-drug regimen should be initiated immediately.
C. Contact precautions are not necessary.
D. Airborne precautions can be discontinued if a tuberculin skin test is negative.
E. A bacterial filter should be placed on the ventilator circuit.

**51.** A 63-year-old female was admitted to the ICU following the development of septic shock, secondary to a presumed pneumonia. She has been treated with antibiotics for 1 week and has improved clinically. Your team is planning to extubate her this evening. When preparing to extubate this patient, all of the following criteria should be met EXCEPT?

A. Rapid shallow breathing index of less than 100
B. Minimal secretions
C. Presence of cuff leak
D. Successful SBT lasting 30 minutes using continuous positive airway pressure (CPAP) 5
E. Ability to follow commands

**52.** You care called to evaluate an 81-year-old male who has had an acute worsening of his already tenuous respiratory status. He has a remote history of a liver transplant, COPD, and recently diagnosed diffuse large B-cell lymphoma and is currently receiving a course of antibiotics for pneumonia. When speaking with his family, you discover he was admitted to the hospital 2 days ago via MedFlight from a community hospital in Georgia. You note that his oxygen saturation is 86% on high-flow nasal cannula and he is using accessory muscles to breathe. You obtain an arterial blood gas: pH 7.27, $PaO_2$ 56 mm Hg, $PaCO_2$ 49 mm Hg. His rhythm is atrial fibrillation with a heart rate of 115 beats/min and blood pressure of 80/55 mm Hg. You perform an urgent bedside echo:

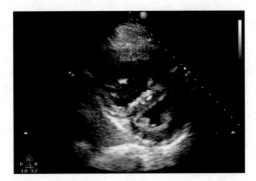

Given what the beside echo shows, what is the most likely cause of this patient's shock?

A. Distributive
B. Hypovolemic
C. Cardiogenic
D. Obstructive
E. Unable to determine at this time

**53.** A 53-year-old female is admitted to the ICU in severe respiratory distress and circulatory shock. Her medical history is significant only for widely metastatic breast cancer to which she is currently undergoing systemic chemotherapy. Her vasopressor therapy has been steadily rising over the past 2 hours and you elect to place a PA catheter. Based on the image that follows, which of the following data sets would be obtained?

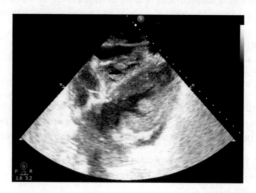

|   | HR | CVP | PA | CO | SVR |
|---|-----|-----|-------|-----|------|
| A | 120 | 1 | 10/5 | 4 | 1800 |
| B | 80 | 7 | 20/10 | 4 | 1300 |
| C | 50 | 25 | 45/30 | 3 | 1800 |
| D | 120 | 25 | 45/30 | 3 | 2000 |
| E | 150 | 2 | 12/8 | 6 | 500 |

**54.** A 56-year-old female with a history of tetraplegia following a bicycle accident over 10 years ago is admitted to the ICU following a ureteroscopy for multiple stone extraction. She has known recurrent UTIs and was recently in the ICU a few months ago for pyelonephritis complicated by urosepsis. The last urine culture obtained from that time was *E coli*, resistant to quinolones and cephalosporins. Her vital signs after a 2 L fluid bolus are temperature 38.8°C, heart rate 130 beats/min, blood pressure 75/50 mm Hg, and respiratory rate 25 breaths/min. She appears to be shivering and drowsy but does answer questions appropriately. What is the next step in your management of this patient?

**A.** Call her primary urology team and recommend repeat ureteroscopy
**B.** Start empiric vancomycin and cefepime and initiate vasopressor therapy
**C.** Start empiric meropenem and repeat the fluid bolus
**D.** Start empiric meropenem and initiate vasopressor therapy

**55.** A 31-year-old male is admitted to the ICU after he dived from a boat in shallow water and presumably hit his head on the bottom of the lake. He was pulled immediately from the water and reports that he "cannot feel" his arms or legs. Primary survey is notable for Glasgow Coma Scale (GCS) 15, absence of sensation below clavicles, and inability to move his arms and legs. His has weak cough and intermittent desaturations that resolve with deep nasal suctioning. Chest and abdominal CT scan are remarkable for a 5mm pneumothorax and grade 2 splenic laceration. MRI demonstrates a C6 subluxation injury with resulting spinal cord compression and edema at C4-C7 level. His blood pressure is 70/30 mm Hg, heart rate 50 beats/min, and $O_2$ saturation is 94%, with supplemental oxygen via facemask. What is the primary etiology of his hemodynamic instability and impending shock state?

**A.** Spinal shock
**B.** Neurogenic shock
**C.** Obstructive shock
**D.** Septic shock
**E.** Hypovolemic shock

**56.** A 66-year-old male has been in the ICU for 5 days following a mandibular resection and partial glossectomy. He has failed a speech and swallow examination and is unable to safely intake orally. Your team would like to start him on some form of nutrition and an enteral feeding tube is placed. Which of the following statements regarding nutrition in the ICU is true?

A. Gastric residual volumes should be frequently measured to monitor for feeding intolerance.
B. Initiation of enteral nutrition should be delayed until signs of return of bowel function.
C. Early enteral nutrition decreases mortality.
D. Protein has the lowest respiratory quotient.
E. A postpyloric tube should be placed for enteral feeding.

57. A 74-year-old female is in postoperative day 1 following a sigmoid resection for colon cancer. Her past medical history is significant for a right-sided stroke 5 years ago (she has some residual left upper extremity weakness), hypertension, and coronary artery disease (coronary stents placed 1 year ago). She takes a full-dose aspirin and clopidogrel at home, which were both held for her procedure. She now complains of chest pain and shortness of breath. Her ECG shows 2 mm ST elevations in V2-V4 leads. Her vital signs are heart rate 72 beats/min, blood pressure 92/55 mm Hg, and $SpO_2$ 95% on room air. Labs are remarkable for troponin 3.8 ng/mL and lactate 8 mmol/L. A cardiology consult is obtained, and an emergent cardiac catheterization is planned. What would be another appropriate initial treatment modality at this time?

    A. Dopamine
    B. 1L crystalloid bolus
    C. Dobutamine
    D. Norepinephrine
    E. No other intervention necessary besides immediate cardiac catheterization

58. A 79-year-old male with a history significant for dementia, hypertension, and diabetes mellitus was admitted from his skilled nursing facility for failure to thrive. He was not able to safely take per orally due to risk of aspiration. A nasogastric tube is placed and enteral feeding initiated on hospital day 2. Labs the following day are notable for phosphate 0.6 mg/dL, total calcium 5.5 mg/dL, magnesium 1.2 mg/dL, potassium 2.6 mEq/L, and albumin 1.4 g/dL. Of the following choices, which is the most appropriate regarding the next step in management of this patient?

    A. Increase enteral feeds
    B. Temporarily stop enteral feeding
    C. Switch to TPN
    D. Initiate workup for hyperparathyroidism
    E. Increase phosphate, magnesium, and potassium content in enteral feeds

59. You are called urgently for an intubation in the emergency department for a young woman who was found stumbling out of a subway terminal confused and with labored breathing. She has copious oral secretions and appears to have recently vomited. As you prepare to intubate, the patient has a seizure. You hear of other patients arriving from the same subway station with a similar presentation and suspect a terrorist attack with a biologic or chemical weapon. Which agent is most likely?

    A. Sarin
    B. Chlorine
    C. Phosgene
    D. Cyanide
    E. Anthrax

60. A 32-year-old female with a history of severe depression and multiple suicide attempts is brought to the emergency department by her mother after she admitted to ingesting 10 pills of lorazepam. She is somnolent but does wake up following sternal rub. She is hemodynamically stable and is maintaining oxygen saturations of 94% on room air. What is the next step in managing this patient?

    A. Administer 2 mg of flumazenil
    B. Intubate her for inability to protect her airway
    C. Continue to observe her with continuous telemetry monitoring
    D. Directly admit her to an inpatient psychiatry unit
    E. Obtain a stat head CT

61. A 34-year-old male was admitted to the intensive care unit 1 week ago after polytrauma sustained after a motor vehicle accident. Major injury burden includes multiple rib fractures, lung contusion, splenic laceration, and lower extremity long bone fractures. His ventilator settings are pressure support ventilation with a pressure support of 5 cm $H_2O$ over PEEP of 8 cm $H_2O$ and $FiO_2$ of 30%. His minute ventilation remains high at 13 L/min. His vital are BP 130/70 mm Hg, HR 82 beats/min, and respiratory rate 30 breaths/min. An arterial blood gas is drawn to evaluate further.

pH 7.29
Bicarbonate 14 mEq/L
pCO$_2$ 30 mm Hg
pO$_2$ 105 mm Hg

Additional lab results are:

Na 138 mEq/L
K 3.5 mEq/L
Cl 110 mEq/L
Albumin 3.8 mg/dL
Creatinine 2.8 mg/dL

Urine electrolytes:

Na 40 mEq/L
K 10 mEq/L
Cl 15 mEq/L

What is the next best step in management of this patient?

A. 1 L normal saline
B. Enteral bicarbonate replacement
C. Hemodialysis
D. Loop diuretics

62. A 48-year-old female presents to the intensive care unit with 2-day history of abdominal pain and vomiting. Her past medical history is significant for recurrent small bowel obstruction and multiple abdominal surgeries in the past. Vitals are blood pressure 80/40 mm Hg, heart rate 112 beats/min, and temperature 37°C. An arterial blood gas is drawn with the following results:

pH 7.31
Bicarbonate 19 mEq/L
pCO$_2$ 37 mm Hg
Na 138 mEq/L
K 4 mEq/L
Cl 98 mEq/L
Albumin 3.0 mg/dL

What type of acid-base abnormality is seen in this patient?

A. Anion gap and normal anion gap metabolic acidosis
B. Unable to determine with given information
C. Metabolic acidosis and metabolic alkalosis
D. Normal anion gap metabolic acidosis

63. A 65-year-old male with past medical history of congestive heart failure, diabetes, and COPD presents with shortness of breath. He reports progressive shortness of breath for the last 5 days. He is admitted to the intensive care unit for hypoxemia and is placed on noninvasive mechanical ventilation. On examination, the jugular venous pressure is elevated. His vitals are blood pressure 110/70 mm Hg, heart rate 102 beats/min, and respiratory rate 28 breaths/min.

Arterial blood gas shows
pH 7.26
Bicarbonate 14 mEq/L
pCO$_2$ 30 mm Hg
Laboratory data
Na 132 mEq/L
Chloride 98 mEq/L
K 4.5 mEq/L
Albumin 3 mg/dL
Blood glucose 105 mg/dL

What is the next best step in investigating the cause of this acid-base abnormality?

A. Urine anion gap
B. Serum lactic acid
C. Beta-hydroxy butyrate
D. Urine chloride
E. Serum osmolar gap

64. A 72-year-old patient is admitted to intensive care unit with altered mental status. Her past medical history is remarkable for recent hospitalization for periprosthetic hip infection, for which she underwent a prosthesis explant. She was discharged to rehabilitation center 1 week ago, on a 6-week course of cefepime for hip osteomyelitis.

To evaluate the cause of the altered mentation, a CT scan of the head and lumbar puncture is done, both with negative results. After ruling out other etiologies, she is suspected to have cefepime-induced neurotoxicity.

Which among the following is NOT useful in management of cefepime-induced neurotoxicity?

A. Hemodialysis
B. Antiepileptic medications
C. Discontinuation of cefepime
D. Corticosteroids

65. A 66-year-old female presents to intensive care unit with altered mental status. Her past medical history is significant for diabetes on metformin, chronic back pain recently started on gabapentin, chronic kidney disease, COPD, and recent-onset hypertension on hydrochlorothiazide and lisinopril. She has no history of fall, and her vital signs at admission are within normal limits. Her laboratory data are as follows:

Na 118 mEq/L
Cl 95 mEq/L
Creatinine 1.3 mg/dL
Glucose 85 mg/dL

What medication is the moist likely culprit for this patient's hyponatremia?

A. Metformin
B. Gabapentin
C. Lisinopril
D. Hydrochlorothiazide

66. An 82-year-old frail looking female presents to the emergency room with failure to thrive. She reports having diarrhea for last 2 days. She currently weighs 45 kg, with 10 kg weight loss in last 6 months. Vitals are blood pressure 82/40 mm Hg, heart rate 108 beats/min, and respiratory rate 24 breaths/min. Lungs are clear to auscultation. She is lethargic but oriented to time, place, and person.

Laboratory blood work shows the following:

Na 121 mEq/L
K 3.2 mEq/L
Cl 95 mEq/L
Creatinine 1.5 mg/dL
Hemoglobin 9 g/dL
Serum osmolality 270 mOsm/kg
Urine Na 5 mEq/L

What is the next best step in management of her hyponatremia?

A. Resuscitation with normal saline
B. Diuresis with loop diuretics
C. Water restriction
D. Start salt tablets

67. The previous patient receives 1 L normal saline with improvement in blood pressure. Repeat sodium in 4 hours shows sodium to be 118 mEq/L. Now, she appears more confused and is only oriented to self. You decide to start an infusion of hypertonic saline and check serum sodium levels every 2 hours.

What is the benefit of adding desmopressin to this patient's treatment regimen?

**A.** For rapid correction of hyponatremia
**B.** To treat occult diabetes insipidus
**C.** Prevent inadvertent overcorrection of hyponatremia
**D.** For evaluating cause of hyponatremia

68. A 45-year-old male with Crohn disease presents to the intensive care unit after urgent exploratory laparotomy, extensive lysis of adhesions, and small bowel resection for small bowel obstruction. Past medical history is significant for bipolar disorder on quetiapine. He was on lithium previously but was stopped 5 years ago. On postoperative day 1, he was noted to have a high urine output (300-400 mL/h). Blood and urine electrolytes were sent to investigate the etiology. His serum sodium was 155 mEq/L and serum osmolarity, 315 mOsm/Kg. His urine sodium was 5 mEq/L and urine osmolarity, 214 mOsm/Kg. His preoperative serum sodium was 143 mEq/L.

What is the next best step in management?

**A.** Decrease intravenous maintenance fluids by half
**B.** Restart lithium
**C.** Start 5% dextrose water intravenously
**D.** Start desmopressin

69. A 66-year-old male presents with perforated diverticulitis and undergoes urgent exploratory laparotomy and sigmoid resection. His past medical history is significant for hypertension, diabetes on insulin, COPD, and bipolar disorder on lithium. The operative course is complicated by intra-abdominal spillage of bowel contents and hypotension requiring vasopressors. Postoperatively, he is brought to the intensive care unit for close monitoring. On postoperative day 2, he develops acute mental status changes and slurred speech. Vital signs are with in normal limits. CT scan of the head was done which was unremarkable.

Laboratory data show:

Na 144 mEq/L
Cl 100 mEq/L
K 4.0 mEq/L
Creatinine 1.8 mg/dL
Urea 56 mg/dL
Hb 10 g/dL

What is the most likely cause for the neurological symptoms seen in this patient?

**A.** Abrupt reduction in lithium levels
**B.** Acute lithium toxicity
**C.** Chronic lithium toxicity
**D.** Unrelated to lithium

70. A 62-year-old male is admitted to intensive care unit with intra-abdominal sepsis. He developed septic cardiomyopathy 2 days later, with a left ventricular ejection fraction of 25%. So, a pulmonary artery catheter was placed to guide fluid management. The pulmonary artery catheter is wedged to determine the left ventricular end-diastolic pressure. Which point in the waveform correctly represents the wedge pressure?

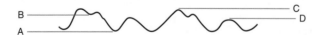

**A.** Point A
**B.** Point B
**C.** Point C
**D.** Point D

71. A 71-year-old male with is admitted to ICU with COPD exacerbation. At admission, his vitals are BP 110/72 mm Hg, heart rate 78 beats/min, normal sinus rhythm, temperature 38°C, respiratory rate 22 breaths/min, and oxygen saturation 93% on 5 L oxygen via nasal cannula. Next day, the patient complains of palpitations, and you find him to be tachycardic in 130 beats/min. His blood pressure is 100/68 mm Hg. The following rhythm is noticed.

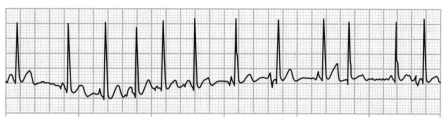

Adapted from Appendix 1: Atlas of electrocardiography. In: Barash PG, Cullen BF, Stoelting RK, et al. *Clinical Anesthesia*. Philadelphia, PA: Lippincott, Williams & Wilkins; 2013.

What is the next best step in management?

A. Cardioversion
B. Beta blockade
C. Digoxin
D. Anticoagulation
E. Echocardiogram

72. A 55-year-old male with chronic liver disease is admitted to ICU with decompensated cirrhosis. He is known to have portopulmonary hypertension and is on sildenafil. A pulmonary artery catheter is placed to guide therapy and the following measurements were obtained. Calculate the pulmonary vascular resistance (PVR) in dyne sec/cm$^5$.

| Cardiac output | 5.2 L/min |
| --- | --- |
| Mean arterial blood pressure | 91 mm Hg |
| Mean pulmonary arterial pressure | 28 mm Hg |
| Pulmonary capillary wedge pressure | 14 mm Hg |
| Central venous pressure | 12 mm Hg |

A. 215
B. 1215
C. 2.7
D. Cannot be calculated with the given information

73. A 47-year-old diabetic male presents to the intensive care unit in distributive shock. On examination, the likely source is soft-tissue infection of his leg. Which among the following is NOT a component of the 1-hour (Surviving Sepsis Campaign) sepsis bundle?

A. Obtaining blood cultures before antibiotics
B. Starting 30 mL/kg of crystalloid resuscitation
C. Serum procalcitonin before antibiotics
D. Serum lactate concentration

74. Which one among the following parameters is NOT used in calculating the qSOFA (quick Sequential Organ Failure Assessment) score described in Sepsis-3 recommendations?

A. Respiratory rate
B. Serum lactate
C. Blood pressure
D. Mental status

75. A 55-year-old female patient is admitted to the intensive care unit with a diagnosis of septic shock. She received 30 mL/kg of crystalloid resuscitation in the emergency department. Currently, she is receiving a moderate dose (14 μg/min) of norepinephrine infusion to maintain a MAP above 65 mm Hg. Based on Surviving Sepsis Guidelines, additional fluid resuscitation can be based on which among the following parameters?

A. Central venous pressure (CVP)
B. Central venous oxygen saturation
C. Response to PLR
D. Pulmonary capillary wedge pressure

**76.** A patient presents to the intensive care unit in atrial fibrillation with rapid ventricular rate and is short of breath. He is known to have paroxysmal atrial fibrillation which was first detected after he underwent mechanical mitral valve replacement for severe rheumatic mitral stenosis. He has been therapeutically anticoagulated with warfarin for the mechanical mitral valve.

In the past, he has underwent cardioversion three times for symptomatic atrial fibrillation. Now, he is started on amiodarone for rhythm control, since he is short of breath while in atrial fibrillation. What is the impact of coadministering amiodarone and warfarin?

A. Warfarin and amiodarone cannot be coadministered
B. Decrease warfarin dose
C. Increase warfarin dose
D. Amiodarone has no impact on warfarin dose

**77.** A 61-year-old male presents with altered mental status 6 days after craniotomy and resection of meningioma. CT head is unremarkable. A lumbar puncture is done which is suggestive of bacterial meningitis. He is empirically started on vancomycin and ceftriaxone for empiric coverage. His cerebrospinal fluid (CSF) culture grows *Serratia marcescens*; resistant to ampicillin and cefazolin, sensitive to ceftriaxone.

Which of the following is the next best step?

A. Stop vancomycin, continue ceftriaxone
B. Continue both vancomycin and ceftriaxone
C. Stop vancomycin and ceftriaxone, start meropenem
D. Stop vancomycin and ceftriaxone, start penicillin G

**78.** A 34-year-old male is admitted to the ICU after a motor vehicle crash and associated polytrauma. Major injuries include multiple rib fractures, lung contusions, and traumatic brain injury. He was intubated on arrival due to poor mental status. Five days into his ICU stay, he remains intubated and mechanically ventilated. He develops increased tan-colored respiratory secretions and increasing oxygen requirements and is febrile. He is empirically started on broad-spectrum antibiotics—vancomycin and cefepime. Preliminary results are available from respiratory culture, shows Stenotrophomonas. Antibiotic resistance patterns are not yet available.

Which among the following alterations in antimicrobial therapy is most appropriate?

A. Stop all antibiotics
B. Stop cefepime, and start meropenem
C. Add trimethoprim-sulfamethoxazole
D. Stop vancomycin and cefepime, and start penicillin G
E. No change to current regimen

**79.** A 55-year-old female has been admitted to the intensive care unit for hypoxemic respiratory failure presumably from exacerbation of COPD. She is being treated with steroids, broad-spectrum antibiotics, and diuresis. A urinary catheter is placed for monitoring urinary output after diuresis. Four days later, she continues to have leukocytosis, and hence, urine, blood, and respiratory cultures are sent to investigate leukocytosis. The urine analysis shows candida species.

What is the next best step, while urine culture data are pending?

A. Start fluconazole
B. Start micafungin
C. CT scan of the abdomen
D. Change the urinary catheter

**80.** A 55-year-old male patient is admitted to the intensive care unit with hypoxemic respiratory failure, AKI, altered mental status, and distributive shock. He is undergoing treatment for acute lymphocytic leukemia and received an infusion of chimeric antigen receptor modified T cells 3 days ago.

Which among the following therapies would be most beneficial?

A. Tocilizumab
B. Abciximab
C. Intravenous immunoglobulin
D. Plasma exchange

81. A 60-year-old patient was admitted in the intensive care unit with pneumonia, hypoxemic respiratory failure, and altered mental status. He was intubated and mechanically ventilated upon arrival to the intensive care unit. His past medical history is significant for hypertension and COPD. Five days later, despite improvement in lung function, his mental status does not. Thyroid function tests are sent to evaluate for causes of altered mental status.

Which among the following is expected to be elevated in critical illness?

A. Thyroid-stimulating hormone
B. Total T4
C. T3
D. rT3

82. A 68-year-old male patient undergoes transvenous extraction of a right ventricular pacemaker lead due to lead malfunction and implantation of a new lead. His past medical history is significant for coronary artery disease, sick sinus syndrome, and diabetes. He is found to have a new small pericardial effusion after the lead explant and so is admitted to the ICU for hemodynamic monitoring. Over the next 8 hours, he is progressively hypotensive, and you perform a bedside echo. Left ventricular function is hyperdynamic, and the following images are obtained.

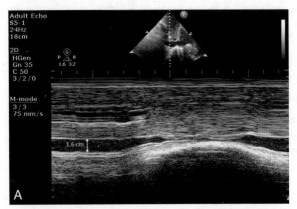

M mode through inferior vena cava in subcostal view

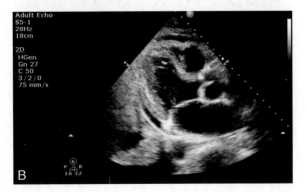

Parasternal long axis view

What is the next best step in management?

A. Urgent pericardiocentesis
B. Administer 1 L normal saline
C. No further intervention
D. Start inotropes

**83.** A 67-year-old male with no significant past medical history is admitted to the ICU following angiography and embolization of a lingual artery pseudoaneurysm after developing significant oropharyngeal hemorrhage following resection of a 1 cm oropharyngeal squamous cell carcinoma. The left common femoral artery was used as the access point. Six hours later, he developed coldness of his left foot with absence of the left popliteal, dorsalis pedis, and posterior tibial pulses. The most likely cause of this is:

    **A.** Low-flow state
    **B.** Embolus to the left common femoral artery
    **C.** Thrombosis of the left common femoral artery
    **D.** Left iliofemoral deep venous thrombosis
    **E.** Excessive compression with sequential compression devices

**84.** Which among the following statements accurately represent the latest 2016 Surviving Sepsis Guideline recommendations?

    **A.** Volume resuscitation needs to be guided by early goal-directed therapy.
    **B.** All available sites should be sampled for microbial culture before initiating antibiotic therapy.
    **C.** Antibiotics need to be administered within 1 hour of presumed sepsis.
    **D.** Resuscitation and metabolic stabilization for at least 24 hours is recommended before operative intervention for source control.

**85.** A 55-year-old male patient is transferred to your ICU (from an outside hospital) on high-dose inotropes for cardiogenic shock. Urgent transthoracic echocardiogram on arrival shows:

Left ventricular hypertrophy, small left ventricular cavity, left ventricular ejection fraction of 25% with wall motion abnormalities in left circumflex distribution, mild right ventricular dysfunction, mild mitral regurgitation, no aortic regurgitation or aortic stenosis.

An intra-aortic balloon pump (IABP) is inserted for left ventricular support as he is being prepared for cardiac catheterization. But the patient becomes severely hypoxemia and requires intubation.

In this patient, which among the following conditions will cause worsening of hypoxemia after insertion of an IABP?

    **A.** Hypertrophic obstructive cardiomyopathy
    **B.** Ventricular septal defect
    **C.** Papillary muscle rupture
    **D.** Left main coronary obstructive lesion

# Appendix Answers

**1.** Correct Answer: B

**Rationale:**
The number 150 can help a clinician to distinguish between groups of patients who may and may not need NAC therapy after APAP ingestion.

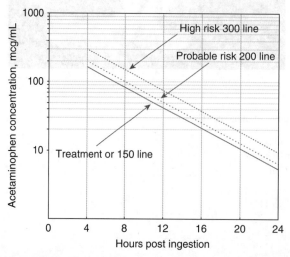

- A toxic dose is greater than 150 mg/kg.
- Start NAC therapy if APAP serum level is greater than 150 µg/mL 4 hours after ingestion (the first time point on the nomogram).
  - Most guidelines outside of the United States use the "200 line" instead of this "150 line." The 200 line was initially used in the United States but was lowered to 150 µg/mL to increase sensitivity.
  - Patients with certain comorbidities including chronic alcoholism and other liver disease may benefit from a "100-line," or a more sensitive threshold, before starting NAC.
- The NAC loading dose is 150 mg/kg IV (140 mg/kg PO).

### References

1. Heard KJ. Acetylcysteine for acetaminophen poisoning. *N Engl J Med.* 2008;359(3):285-292.
2. Waring WS, Robinson ODG, Stephen AFL, et al. Does the patient history predict hepatotoxicity after acute paracetamol overdose? *Q J Med.* 2008;101(2):121-125.
3. Vale JA, Proudfoot AT. Paracetamol (acetaminophen) poisoning. *Lancet.* 1996;346(8974):547-552.
4. Hodgman MJ, Garrard AR. A review of acetaminophen poisoning. *Crit Care Clin.* 2012;28(4):499-516.

**2.** Correct Answer: B

**Rationale:**

This clinical scenario is most consistent with an ingestion of digoxin leading to toxicity. Virtually any arrhythmia is possible in digoxin overdose, save rapid supraventricular tachycardias. Bidirectional VT is almost pathognomonic of digoxin toxicity, but is a rare finding. Most commonly, one will see rhythms with AV junctional blocks of varying degrees and ventricular ectopy. Slow or regularized atrial fibrillation (AFib) or flutter (AFlutter) is also highly suggestive of digoxin overdose.

**Cardiac Dysrhythmias Associated With Digoxin Toxicity**

| Myocardial Irritability Causing Dysrhythmias | Primary Conduction System Dysfunction Causing Dysrhythmia |
|---|---|
| • AFib and AFlutter w/ AV block<br>• Nonparoxysmal atrial tachydysrhythmias w/ AV block<br>• Premature ventricular contractions (PVCs)<br>• Nonsustained ventricular tachycardia (NSVT)<br>• Ventricular bigeminy<br>• Bidirectional VT<br>• VT<br>• VFib | • AV dissociation<br>• Exit blocks<br>• High-degree AV block<br>• His-Purkinje dysfunction<br>• Junctional tachycardia<br>• SA nodal arrest<br>• Sinus bradycardia |

Adapted from Cardiac dysrhythmias associated with cardioactive steroid poisoning. In: Hoffman RS, Howland MA, Lewin NA, Nelson LS, Goldfrank LR, eds. *Goldfrank's Toxicologic Emergencies.* 10th ed. McGraw-Hill Education; 2015.

Hemodialysis (HD) would be a poor choice of therapy, as digoxin cannot be dialyzed. It may be a more appropriate choice in certain instances of salicylate (acetylsalicylic acid [ASA]) or lithium toxicity, as those compounds are able to be hemodialyzed.

Administration of intravenous bicarbonate, a way to alkalinize the urine in order to promote trapping and excretion, is a first-line therapy for ASA overdose if the patient does not meet criteria for HD.

Hyperkalemia can be a common finding in digoxin overdose, though it serves only to prognosticate: its treatment will not lead to improvement in outcome. It has been classically thought, based on theoretical molecular mechanisms, that administering exogenous calcium can lead to "stone heart," or impaired diastolic function leading to a hypocontractile state. Despite the fact that recent literature does not support this belief, many believe IV calcium to be potentially dangerous in situations of digoxin overdose.

The best treatment would be administration of digoxin-specific antibody fragment derived from sheep, marketed as Digibind and DigiFab.

## INDICATIONS FOR USE OF DIGOXIN-SPECIFIC ANTIBODY FRAGMENTS

- Any digoxin-related life-threatening dysrhythmias (regardless of digoxin level)
- K+ >5 mEq/L (after acute digoxin poisoning)
- Chronic elevation of serum digoxin level associated with any of the following:
  - Dysrhythmias
  - Significant GI symptoms
  - Altered mental status
- Serum digoxin level >15 ng/mL at any time
- Serum digoxin level >10 ng/mL 6 hour post ingestion
- Acute ingestion of 10 mg of digoxin in an adult
- Acute ingestion of 4 mg of digoxin in a child
- Poisoning with a nondigoxin cardioactive steroid

Adapted from Indications for administration of digoxin-specific antibody fragments (DSFab). In: Hoffman RS, Howland MA, Lewin NA, Nelson LS, Goldfrank LR, eds. *Goldfrank's Toxicologic Emergencies*. 10th ed. McGraw-Hill Education; 2015.

### References

1. Hack JB. Chapter 64: Cardioactive steroids. In: Nelson LS, Lewin NA, Howland M, et al, eds. *Goldfrank's Toxicologic Emergencies*. 9th ed. New York: McGraw-Hill; 2011:936-945.
2. Howland M. Chapter A20: Digoxin-specific antibody fragments. In: Nelson LS, Lewin NA, Howland M, et al, eds. *Goldfrank's Toxicologic Emergencies*. 9th ed. New York: McGraw-Hill; 2011:946-951.
3. Levine M, Nikkanen H, Pallin DJ. The effects of intravenous calcium in patients with digoxin toxicity. *J Emerg Med*. 2011;40(1)41-46.
4. Kelly RA, Smith TW. Recognition and management of digitalis toxicity. *Am J Cardiol*. 1992;69(18):108G-118G.

---

**3.** Correct Answer: C

**Rationale:**

Antipsychotics include first-generation antipsychotics (typical antipsychotics, neuroleptics), as well as newer second-generation antipsychotics (atypical antipsychotics). Examples of each are included in the table below.

| FIRST-GENERATION ANTIPSYCHOTICS | SECOND-GENERATION ANTIPSYCHOTICS |
|---|---|
| - Haloperidol (Haldol)<br>- Fluphenazine (Prolixin)<br>- Pimozide (Orap)<br>- Perphenazine (Trilafon)<br>- Chlorpromazine (Thorazine) | - Clozapine (Clozaril)<br>- Risperidone (Risperdal)<br>- Olanzepine (Zyprexa)<br>- Quetiapine (Seroquel)<br>- Lurasidone (Latuda)<br>- Paliperidone (Invega) |

In addition to their primary (intended) effect as dopamine (D2) receptor antagonists, antipsychotics (atypicals > typicals) exhibit varying degrees of effects on other receptors. This is responsible for many of their adverse side effects. These include histamine ($H_1$), adrenergic ($\alpha_1$), and muscarinic ($M_1$) receptor antagonism, which can be thought of as the "HAM" effects.

| RECEPTOR | EFFECTS OF ANTIPSYCHOTIC MEDICATIONS (RECEPTOR BLOCKADE) |
|---|---|
| $H_1$ | Sedation |
| $\alpha_1$ | Orthostatic hypotension (dizziness) → reflex tachycardia |
| $M_1$ | Anticholinergic side effects (dry mouth, blurry vision, constipation, urinary retention) |

Of the choices listed, bradycardia is least likely, as the patient is more likely to experience orthostatic hypotension with a reflex tachycardia.

### References

1. Voicu VA, Rădulescu F, Gheorghe M. Pharmacodynamic and therapeutic effects of antipsychotics. Modulation and neurobiological resetting. *Ther Clin Pharmacol Toxicol*. 2008;12(1):11-25.
2. Miron IC, Baroană VC, Popescu F, Ionică F. Pharmacological mechanisms underlying the association of antipsychotics with metabolic disorders. *Curr Health Sci J*. 2013;40(1):12-17.

**4.** Correct Answer: A

**Rationale:**

Tricyclic antidepressants (TCAs) act as sodium (Na$^+$) channel blockers. As there are a large number of Na$^+$ channels in the heart and central nervous system (CNS), the toxicity of TCAs are readily seen in these organs/systems. Drugs that cause cardiac Na$^+$ channel blockade slow Na$^+$ influx into the cell and delay the depolarization phase (phase 0) of the ventricular myocyte action potential. This results in widening of the QRS complex. In severe cases, this may lead to a sinusoidal pattern on electrocardiogram, possible ventricular tachycardia with degeneration to ventricular fibrillation, and eventual asystole. A similar phenomenon can be seen with hyperkalemia, as well as overdose with:

- Class IA antiarrhythmics
- Class IC antiarrhythmics
- Phenothiazines
- Cocaine
- Quinine (an isomer of quinidine), hydroxychloroquine (Plaquenil)
- Carbamazepine (Tegretol)
- Diphenhydramine (Benadryl)
- Bupropion (Wellbutrin)

Sinus tachycardia is more commonly seen in TCA overdose, as many of these compounds have anticholinergic or sympathomimetic properties. Bradycardias are therefore rare but can be seen if Na$^+$ channel blockade is so significant that the cardiac pacemaker tissue is affected, resulting in pacemaker cells which are slow to depolarize. Noting bradycardias in a TCA-overdose patient is an ominous sign and should be treated immediately with administration of IV sodium bicarbonate.

References

1. Clancy C. Chaper 22: Electrophysiologic and electrocardiographic principles. In: Nelson LS, Lewin NA, Howland M, et al, eds. *Goldfrank's Toxicologic Emergencies*. 9th ed. New York: McGraw-Hill; 2011:314-329.
2. Holstege CP, Eldridge DL, Woden AK. ECG manifestations: the poisoned patient. *Emerg Med Clin N Am*. 2006;24(1):159-177.
3. Harrigan RA, Brady WJ. ECG abnormalities in tricyclic antidepressant ingestion. *Am J Emerg Med*. 1999;17(4):387-393.

**5.** Correct Answer: C

**Rationale:**

The triad of medications this patient is on increases the risk of a prolonged QT interval. Torsade de pointes (TdP) is a polymorphic VT that occurs in the setting of a prolonged QT and may be either nonsustained or sustained. It is usually a nonperfusing rhythm (as is suggested in our patient with hypotension), can rapidly degenerate into ventricular fibrillation, and therefore urgent treatment with defibrillation is warranted. Because TdP is a polymorphic ventricular tachycardia, synchronized cardioversion may not be possible, in which case defibrillation (unsynchronized cardioversion) may be performed.

Magnesium sulfate (MgSO$_4$) IV may be given in a conscious (hemodynamically stable) patient to treat self-limited TdP episode or prevent their recurrence. Magnesium boluses (1-2 g) are repeated or infusion is initiated until QTc duration drops below 500 ms. If patients are refractory to magnesium infusion, one may consider overdrive (transvenous, either atrial or ventricular) pacing at about 70 to 100 beats/min, as the pauses that trigger TdP are less likely to occur at faster heart rates.

While not the BEST therapy at this point, ILE warrants further discussion. Guy Weinberg at University of Illinois, Chicago has done substantial work involving ILE therapy, the gold standard treatment for local anesthetic systemic toxicity (LAST). However, recent reviews detail the successful use of ILE in humans with toxicity from bupropion-/lamotrigine-induced cardiac arrest, reversal of sertraline-/quetiapine-induced coma, and improvement of shock due to verapamil and beta-blocker overdose. In one case report, a 17-year-old female with bupropion and lamotrigine overdose had cardiovascular collapse which was refractory to standard advanced cardiac life support (ACLS) algorithm. She had ROSC 1 minute after intralipid administration.

References

1. Drew BJ, Ackerman MJ, Funk M, et al. Prevention of torsade de pointes in hospital settings: A scientific statement from the AHA and American College of Cardiology Foundation. *Circulation*. 2010;121(8):1047-1060.
2. Tzivoni D, Banai S, Benhorin J, et al. Treatment of torsade de pointes with magnesium sulfate. *Circulation*. 1988;77(2):392-397.
3. Yap YG, Camm AJ. Durg induced QT prolongation and torsades de pointes. *Heart*. 2003;89(11):1363-1372.
4. Ozcan MS, Weinberg G. Intravenous lipid emulsion for treatment of drug toxicity. *J Intensive Care Med*. 2014;29(2):59-70.
5. Weinberg GL. Lipid emulsion infusion: resuscitation for local anesthetic and other drug overdose. *Anesthesiology*. 2012;117(1):180-187.

6. Sirianni AJ, Osterhoudt KC, Calello DP, et al. Use of lipid emulsion in the resuscitation of a patient with prolonged cardiovascular collapse after overdose of bupropion and lamotrigine. *Ann Emerg Med.* 2008;51(4):412-415.

7. Cave G, Harvey M. Intravenous lipid emulsion as antidote beyond local anesthetic toxicity: a systematic review. *Acad Emerg Med.* 2009;16(9):815-824.

---

**6.** Correct Answer: B

**Rationale:**

Alcoholic hallucinosis (AH) and delirium tremens (DTs) share many features, yet it is critical to differentiate the two clinically, as they carry different mortality risks. Presence of hallucinations is the uniting feature of both syndromes. However, where vital signs and sensorium are usually normal in AH, they are both usually abnormal in DTs. These features are summarized in the table below.

| | HALLUCINATIONS | VSs | SENSORIUM |
|---|---|---|---|
| Alcoholic hallucinosis | YES—usually visual, sometimes auditory or tactile | Normal (usually) | Normal |
| Delirium tremens | YES | Abnormal (usually) <br>• inc HR <br>• inc BP <br>• inc temp | CLOUDED—disoriented |

**References**

1. Adams VM. The effect of alcohol on the nervous system. *Res Publ Assoc Nerv Ment Dis.* 1953;32:526-573.
2. Gold JA, Nelson LS. Chapter 78: Ethanol withdrawal. In: Nelson LS, Lewin NA, Howland M, et al, eds. *Goldfrank's Toxicologic Emergencies.* 9th ed. New York: McGraw-Hill; 2011:1134-1142.

---

**7.** Correct Answer: C

**Rationale:**

Cocaine is known to act on several different receptors to produce its clinical effects:

1. Biogenic amine (norepinephrine [NE], epinephrine [epi], dopamine [DA], and serotonin [5-HT]) reuptake inhibition, acting as an indirect sympathomimetic
   a. Increased levels of catecholamines (NE > epi) leads to increased stimulation of adrenergic receptors ($\alpha_1 \gg \alpha_2$, $\beta_1$, $\beta_2$), which leads to the cardiac and peripheral vasoconstriction frequently seen with cocaine intoxication.
   b. Increased levels of 5-HT in the CNS lead to the euphoria well-described with cocaine intoxication.
   c. Increased levels of DA in the CNS fuel the reward pathway that frequently leads to cocaine addiction.
2. Sodium ($Na^+$) channel blockade
   a. Cocaine was the first local anesthetic, discovered (and subsequently abused) by pioneering surgeon, William Stewart Halsted. Like other local anesthetics, cocaine decreases the cell membrane permeability to $Na^+$, thereby blocking conduction. In neurons, this blockade manifests as local anesthesia, while in the heart it manifests as a widened QRS complex on ECG, and as negative inotropy in cardiac myocytes.
3. Increased glutamate (Glu) concentration
   a. Increased concentrations of Glu (an excitatory neurotransmitter) in the CNS leads to the psychomotor agitation seen with cocaine intoxication.

Downregulation of GABA$_A$ receptors is a well-known change in chronic alcohol use as an adaptation to overstimulation of the receptor by ethanol. In chronic alcohol use, Glu receptors (excitatory) are upregulated in response to increased GABA$_A$ (inhibitory) neurotransmission.

**References**

1. Tella SR, Schindler CW, Goldberg SR. Cocaine: cardiovascular effects in relation to inhibition of peripheral neuronal monoamine uptake and central stimulation of the sympathoadrenal system. *J Pharmacol Exp Ther.* 1993;267(1):153.
2. Smith JA, Mo Q, Guo H, et al. Cocaine increases extraneuronal levels of aspartate and glutamate in the nucleus accumbens. *Brain Res.* 1995;683(2):264.
3. Most D, Ferguson L, Harris RA. Molecular basis of alcoholism. *Handb Clin Neurol.* 2014;125:89-111.

---

**8.** Correct Answer: B

**Rationale:**

While agonists of GABA receptors (ethanol, benzodiazepines, barbiturates) are classically known to be associated with a potentially fatal withdrawal syndrome, opioid withdrawal can also carry a significant mortality rate. Voluntary or involuntary abstinence from opioids (such as answer choice A) is known to result in an uncomfortable withdrawal syndrome, which includes the following signs and symptoms:

## SYMPTOMS OF OPIOID WITHDRAWAL

- Insomnia
- Yawning
- Mydriasis
- Lacrimation
- Rhinorrhea
- Vomiting
- Diarrhea
- Piloerection
- Diaphoresis
- Myalgias
- Mild tachycardia and hypertension

In an opioid-dependent patient, an opioid withdrawal that is precipitated by the administration of an opioid antagonist like naloxone differs from one that is brought about by abstinence. One review article purports that "in patients treated for severe pain with an opioid, high-dose naloxone and/or rapidly infused naloxone may cause catecholamine release and consequently pulmonary edema and cardiac arrhythmias." Fatal opioid withdrawal syndromes have been reported after ultrarapid opioid detoxification (UROD).

Experts in the field support the use of naloxone in these patient populations with the desired goal of return of adequate spontaneous ventilation rather than full arousal. Most patients should respond to 0.04 to 0.05 mg of naloxone IV, with "rapid escalation as warranted by the clinical situation." While a starting dose of 0.4 mg naloxone is appropriate in nonopioid-dependent patients, it should be avoided in opioid-dependent patients.

### References

1. Nelson LS, Olsen Dean. Chapter 38: Opioids. In: Nelson LS, Lewin NA, Howland M, et al, eds. *Goldfrank's Toxicologic Emergencies*. 9th ed. New York: McGraw-Hill; 2011:559-578.
2. Howland M, Nelson LS, Chapter A6: Opioid antagonists. In: Nelson LS, Lewin NA, Howland M, et al, eds. *Goldfrank's Toxicologic Emergencies*. 9th ed. New York: McGraw-Hill; 2011:579-585.
3. Bracken MB, Shepard MJ, Collins WF, et al. A randomized controlled trial of methylprednisolone or naloxone in the treatment of acute spinal cord injury. *N Engl J Med*. 1990;322(20):1405-1411.
4. Van Dorp EL, Yassen A, Dahan A. Naloxone treatment in opioid addiction: the risks and benefits. *Expert Opin Drug Safety*. 2007;6(2):125-132.
5. Kienbaum P, Thürauf N, Michel MC, Scherbaum N, Gastpar M, Peters J. Profound increase in epinephrine plasma concentration and cardiovascular stimulation following μ-opioid receptor blockade in opioid addicted patients during barbiturate anesthesia for acute detoxification. *Anesthesiology*. 1998;88(5):1154-1161.
6. Michaelis LL, Hickey PR, Clark TA, et al. Ventricular irritability associated with the use of naloxone hydrochloride. *Ann Thorac Surg*. 1984;18:608-624.
7. Hamilton RJ, Olmedo RE, Shah S, et al. Complications of ultrarapid opioid detoxification with subcutaneous naltrexone pellets. *Acad Emerg Med*. 2002;9:63-68.
8. Flacke JW, Flacke WE, Williams GD. Acute pulmonary edema following naloxone reversal of high-dose morphine anesthesia. *Anesthesiology*. 1977;47:376-378.
9. Prough DS, Roy R, Bumgarner J. Acute pulmonary edema in healthy teenagers following conservative doses of intravenous naloxone. *Anesthesiology*. 1984;60:485-486.
10. Schwartz JA, Koenigsberg MD. Naloxone-induced pulmonary edema. *Ann Emerg Med*. 1987;16:1294-1296.
11. Tanaka GY. Hypertensive reaction to naloxone. *JAMA*. 1974;228:25-26.

**9.** Correct Answer: A

**Rationale:**

This question asks you to differentiate between sympathomimetic (amphetamine) and anticholinergic (oxybutynin) toxidromes. Many similarities exist between the two toxidromes on physical examination, including presence of dilated pupils, tachycardia, warm skin to touch, and a flushed appearance. The provider must look to other examination findings to differentiate the two:

|  | ANTICHOLINERGIC | SYMPATHOMIMETIC |
| --- | --- | --- |
| Pupil reactivity | Unreactive | Reactive |
| Bowel sounds | Decreased | Normal |
| Bladder | Distended | Normal |
| Mucous membranes | Dry | Normal |
| Perspiration | Absent | Present |

Adapted from Vincent JL, Moore FM. *Textbook of Critical Care*. 7th ed. Philadelphia, PA: Elsevier; 2011.

One may remember the signs and symptoms of anticholinergic (muscarinic) toxicity with the popular mnemonic "blind as a bat, red as a beet, hot as a hare, dry as a bone, made as a hatter."

| MNEMONIC | MEANING | MUSCARINIC MECHANISM |
|---|---|---|
| Blind as a bat | Blurry vision | • Loss of ability to accommodate (adjust near and far vision by adjusting lens thickness via contraction of ciliary muscles)<br>• Ciliary muscles possess muscarinic receptors, and accommodation is thus blocked in an anticholinergic toxidrome and preserved in a sympathetic toxidrome |
| Red as a beet | Flushed skin (red appearance) | • Peripheral vasodilation is a compensatory mechanism to facilitate cooling, as cholinergic blockade prevents ability to dissipate heat via sweating (see below)<br>• Adrenergic stimulation results in both sweating and peripheral vasoconstriction |
| Hot as a hare | Warm skin/hyperpyrexia | • Occurs as the patient loses ability to sweat as a cooling mechanism (see below) |
| Dry as a bone | Dry mucous membranes | • Though sweat glands are part of the sympathetic nervous system, they are innervated by parasympathetic nerve fibers (both nicotinic and muscarinic neurotransmission)<br>• Anticholinergic overdose would inhibit sweating, while sympathomimetic overdose would preserve this function |
| Full as a flask | Full urinary bladder/urinary retention | • Muscarinic stimulation will increase detrusor muscle contraction and decrease urethral sphincter contraction (promoting urination)<br>• Oxybutinin's intended effect is to reduce urinary frequency in those with overactive bladder by antagonizing muscarinic receptors in the urinary bladder |
| Mad as a hatter | Altered mental status: agitation, delirium, psychosis ("Lilliputian hallucinations") | • By antagonism of CNS cholinergic receptors |

## References

1. Farmer B, Seger DL. Chapter 153: Poisoning: overview of approaches for evaluation and treatment. In: Vincent J, Abraham E, Moore FA, et al, eds. *Textbook of Critical Care*. 7th ed. Philadelphia: Elsevir; 2017:1070-1077.
2. Liebelt EL. Chapter 73: Cyclic antidepressants. In: Nelson LS, Lewin NA, Howland M, et al, eds. *Goldfrank's Toxicologic Emergencies*. 9th ed. New York: McGraw-Hill; 2011:1049-1059.

**10.** Correct Answer: D

**Rationale:**

This patient had preexisting right ventricular dysfunction as one may interpret from the echocardiogram. The patient's RVSP appears to be within normal limits, which can be due to a combination of factors including decompensated RV systolic function (an RV that is to weak to mount a significant forward flow) and volume loading (hypovolemia vs. euvolemia at the time of the examination).

Intravenous administration of protamine has several deleterious effects which can include

• Anaphylaxis
• Urticaria
• Bronchospasm
• Hypotension
• Transient increase in pulmonary artery pressure
• Cardiovascular collapse
• Death

The cellular and molecular mechanisms by which these events occur are not completely understood but are thought to include

- IgE-mediated reactions
- Potentiation of IgE-mediated histamine release
- Direct, nonimmunologic histamine release from mast cells
- Complement activation
- Inhibition of serum carboxypeptidase
- Elevation of thromboxane B2 and 6-keto-PGF1a levels causing pulmonary artery pressure increases

| REACTION TYPE | CLINICAL PRESENTATION | DESCRIPTION |
|---|---|---|
| Type I | Hypotensive | Likely secondary to histamine release |
| Type II | Allergic | |
| Type IIA | Anaphylactic | |
| Type IIB | Anaphylactoid, early | |
| Type IIC | Anaphylactoid, delayed | |
| Type III | Acute pulmonary hypertension | Diagnosed clinically when the following is seen after protamine administration<br>• Increased PAP<br>• RV failure<br>• Decreased systemic BP<br>Etiology unclear<br>• Immunological + nonimmunological factors contribute<br>Risk factors<br>• Preexisting pulmonary HTN<br>• Prior exposure to protamine or NPH insulin<br>• Vasectomy<br>• Allergy to vertebrate fish |

All of the answer choices and all three types of protamine reactions can cause hypotension; systemic hypotension in a patient with an already failing right ventricle can lead to RV ischemia and cardiac arrest; however the *most likely* explanation in this patient is a type III reaction, which worsens the patient's already-ailing right heart.

Risk factors for anaphylaxis to or other adverse reactions from protamine include patients with
- A prior history of protamine-containing insulin (NPH) or IV protamine use (significantly increased risk)
- A vasectomy, as they have IgE to protamine due to immunologic response to systemic absorption of sperm that occurs after vasectomy (probably at risk)
- A fish allergy due to cross-reactivity between salmon and protamine (no great evidence)

References
1. Pannu BS, Sanghavi DK, Guru PK, Reddy DR, Iyer VN. Fatal right ventricular failure and pulmonary hypertension after protamine administration during cardiac transplantation. *Indian J Crit Care Med*. 2016;20(3):185-187.
2. Gupta SK, Veith FJ, Ascer E, et al. Anaphylactoid reactions to protamine: An often lethal complication in insulin-dependent diabetic patients undergoing vascular surgery. *J Vasc Surg*. 1989;9(2):342-350.
3. Nicklas RA, Bernstein IL, Li JT, et al. Protamine. *J Allergy Clin Immunol*. 1998;101(6):S507-S509.

**11.** Correct Answer: C

**Rationale:**
The superficial branch of the radial nerve is often in close proximity to the cephalic vein of the wrist and can be damaged during blood draws or intravenous cannulation. This often presents as burning pain during the blood draw or peripheral intravenous line insertion. In this case, the patient likely had damage to the superficial branch of the radial nerve during his IV placement.

References
1. Horowitz SH. Peripheral nerve injury and causalgia secondary to routine venipuncture. *Neurology*. 1994;44(5):962-964.
2. Andrea A, Gonzales JR, Iwanaga J, Oskouian RJ, Tubbs RS. Median nerve palsies due to injections: a review. *Cureus*. 2017;9(5):e1287. Published 2017 May 29. doi:10.7759/cureus.1287.

**12.** Correct Answer: B

**Rationale:**

This patient presents with the classic tetrad of neuroleptic malignant syndrome (NMS), including fever, rigidity, mental status changes, and autonomic instability in the setting of haloperidol. NMS is associated with first-generation neuroleptic agents such as haloperidol and fluphenazine; however it is implicated in lower-potency and second-generation antipsychotic medications as well. The mainstay of treatment for NMS is stopping the causative agent—in this case, haloperidol. Additionally, patients with NMS should receive supportive care to avoid potentially life-threatening complications of the syndrome.

**Reference**

1. Tse L, Barr AM, Scarapicchia V, Vila-rodriguez F. Neuroleptic malignant syndrome: a review from a clinically oriented perspective. *Curr Neuropharmacol.* 2015;13(3):395-406.

**13.** Correct Answer: D

**Rationale:**

The PICC line migrates into the azygos vein. Due to its size (azygos vein is 6-7 mm in diameter while the superior vena cava is typically 1.5-2 cm in diameter) and opposing blood flow, cannulation of azygos vein leads to a higher risk of perforation. It has been reported that up to 19% of azygos vein cannulations led to perforation. Additional potential complications of azygos vein cannulation are often sequelae of perforation and include pleural effusion and hemopericardium. Pneumothorax is not a typical complication of azygos vein cannulation.

**References**

1. Talari G, Oyewole-eletu S, Talari P, Parasramka S. Migration of peripherally inserted central catheter likely into the azygos vein: a conservative management. *BMJ Case Rep.* 2016;2016.
2. Langston CT. The aberrant central venous catheter and its complications. *Radiology.* 1971;100:55-59.
3. Granata A, Figuera M, Castellino S, Logias F, Basile A. Azygos arch cannulation by central venous catheters for hemodialysis. *J Vasc Access.* 2006;7:43-45.

**14.** Correct Answer: A

**Rationale:**

Latest Surviving Sepsis Guidelines 2016 recommend using dynamic indices of volume responsiveness to guide fluid therapy in patients with sepsis. Dynamic parameters of fluid responsiveness are calculated based on measurement of change in stroke volume resulting from breathing-based changes in left ventricular preload. If stroke volume increases significantly from intrathoracic pressure-induced increase in preload, administration of an external fluid bolus will also have the same effect. Since stroke volume is difficult to measure, changes in pulse pressure obtained from an arterial line tracing is a commonly used surrogate.

It has been shown that variations in pulse pressure or stroke volume (called pulse pressure variation or stroke volume variation) of a magnitude greater than 15% are associated with positive response to fluid challenge (increase in blood pressure and cardiac output). Conversely, when variations are less than 10%, no hemodynamic benefit to volume resuscitation is seen. These measurements are best validated in patients without respiratory efforts (after neuromuscular blockade) and are on positive-pressure ventilation, as in our patient. Pulse pressure variation is calculated based on the equation:

$$\text{Pulse pressure variation (\%)} = \frac{PP\,max - PP\,min}{(PP\,max + PP\,min)/2} \times 100$$

The patient in the question has a pulse pressure variation of 41%, based on the figure. This favors administration of more intravenous fluids to treat hypotension.

**Reference**

1. Rhodes A, Evans LE, Alhazzani W, et al. Surviving sepsis campaign: International guidelines for management of sepsis and septic shock: 2016. *Crit Care Med.* 2017;45(3):486-552.

**15.** Correct Answer: A

**Rationale:**

Tumor lysis syndrome is a disease-related emergency in patients with hematologic cancers. Patients with non-Hodgkin lymphoma or acute leukemia are at the highest risk of developing this syndrome; however its incidence is increasing among other cancers. Tumor lysis syndrome occurs due to tumor cell content release into the bloodstream, which leads to hyperuricemia, hyperkalemia, hyperphosphatemia, and hypocalcemia. These electrolyte derangements can lead to renal failure, cardiac arrhythmias, seizures, and death from multiorgan failure.

Reference

1. Howard SC, Jones DP, Pui CH. The tumor lysis syndrome. *N Engl J Med.* 2011;364(19):1844-1854.

**16.** Correct Answer: D

**Rationale:**

Delirium is a common pathology encountered in the ICU setting. The Confusion Assessment Method for ICU Patients is a validated delirium assessment instrument that allows for rapid, valid, and reliable assessment of delirium, even in mechanically ventilated patients. Combative behavior is not one of the primary features assessed in CAM-ICU.

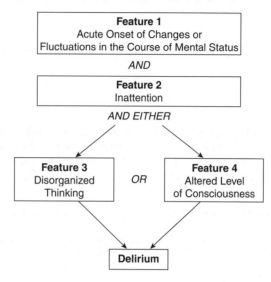

Reference

1. Ely EW, Inouye SK, Bernard GR, et al. Delirium in mechanically ventilated patients: validity and reliability of the Confusion Assessment Method for the Intensive Care Unit (CAM-ICU). *JAMA.* 2001;286(21):2703-2710. doi:10.1001/jama.286.21.2703.

**17.** Correct Answer: D

**Rationale:**

The process of hemostasis is complex and is further complicated in pregnancy due to physiologic changes. In a normal pregnancy, most coagulation factors increase; however it is notable that factor XIII and protein S actually decrease.

| HEMOSTATIC PARAMETER | CHANGE AT TERM PREGNANCY (% CHANGE) |
| --- | --- |
| Factors II and V | No change |
| Fibrinogen | Increases more than 100% |
| Factor VII | Up to 1000% increase |
| Factors VIII, IX, X, XII, and VWF | Increase more than 100% |
| Factor XI | Variable |
| Factor XIII | Up to 50% decrease |
| Protein C | No change |
| Protein S | Up to 50% decrease |
| D-dimer | Up to 400% increase |
| Platelet count | Up to 20% decrease |

From Katz D, Beilin Y. Disorders of coagulation in pregnancy. *Br J Anaesth.* 2015;115(suppl 2):ii75-ii88.

Reference

1. Katz D, Beilin Y. Disorders of coagulation in pregnancy. *Br J Anaesth.* 2015;115(suppl 2):ii75-ii88.

**18.** Correct Answer: B

**Rationale:**

Heparin-induced thrombocytopenia (HIT) is an immune-mediated drug reaction caused by antibodies that activate platelets in the setting of heparin administration. Although patients will become thrombocytopenic, bleeding is rare. Thromboembolic complications are more common in HIT and can occur in both arterial and venous vascular systems. The "4 Ts" are commonly used to determine the pretest probability of HIT and include thrombocytopenia, timing of platelet count fall, thrombosis, and other potential causes for thrombocytopenia. Although laboratory testing is important, HIT is a clinical diagnosis. As part of laboratory workup, heparin-PF4 antibody testing is recommended; however, since these results may not be immediately available, treatment should not be delayed pending laboratory confirmation.

Reference

1. Ahmed I, Majeed A, Powell R. Heparin induced thrombocytopenia: diagnosis and management update. *Postgrad Med J.* 2007;83(983):575-582.

**19.** Correct Answer: D

**Rationale:**

Walter Shewhart and Edward Deming's work on iterative processes later evolved into the four stages of the PDSA cycle. Application of PDSA cycles promotes small-scale interventions in order to provide quicker assessment and increased adaptability for change. In order to drive quality improvement in medicine, methods such as PDSA cycles have been introduced as a tool to use when crafting a quality improvement project.

References

1. Deming WE. *Out of the crisis, 1986.* Cambridge, MA: Massachusetts Institute of Technology Center for Advanced Engineering Study, 1991; xiii, 507.
2. Taylor MJ, Mcnicholas C, Nicolay C, Darzi A, Bell D, Reed JE. Systematic review of the application of the plan-do-study-act method to improve quality in healthcare. *BMJ Qual Saf.* 2014;23(4):290-298.

**20.** Correct Answer: A

**Rationale:**

In this question, the true positive (TP) is 10, false positive (FP) is 15, true negative (TN) is 70, and false negative (FN) is 5.

|  | ENDOCARDITIS | NOT ENDOCARDITIS | TOTAL |
| --- | --- | --- | --- |
| Positive on TTE | 10 | 15 | 25 |
| Negative on TTE | 5 | 70 | 75 |
| Total | 15 | 85 | 100 |

PPV = TP/(TP + FP)
PPV = 10/(10 + 15) = 0.4 or 40%

NPV = TN/(TN + FN)
NPV = 70/(70 + 5) = 0.93 or 93%

Sensitivity = TP/(TP + FN)
Sensitivity = 10/(10 + 5) = 0.67 or 67%

Specificity = TN/(TN + FP)
Specificity = 70/(70 + 15) = 0.82 or 82%

Reference

1. Preoperative assessment, premedication, & perioperative documentation. In: Butterworth JFIV, Mackey DC, Wasnick JD, eds. *Morgan & Mikhail's Clinical Anesthesiology.* 6th ed. New York, NY: McGraw-Hill; 2018. Available at: http://accessanesthesiology.mhmedical.com/content.aspx?bookid=2444&sectionid=193847252. Accessed June 02, 2019.

**21.** Correct Answer: D

**Rationale:**

The first consensus definition of sepsis was proposed at an international conference in 1992. Sepsis (Sepsis-1) was defined as the identification of two or more SIRS criteria, in addition to a known or suspected infection. SIRS criteria included four clinical signs that, when altered, were thought to induce an inflammatory response: temperature, heart rate, respiratory rate, and white blood cell count. The definition of sepsis was subsequently revised in 2001 (Sepsis-2) by expanding the criteria defining SIRS as well as defining organ dysfunction variables indicative of severe sepsis.

In 2016, a new consensus definition was published (Sepsis-3) which defined sepsis as "a life-threatening organ dysfunction caused by dysregulated host response to infection." In contrast to prior definitions, Sepsis-3 replaced "systemic inflammatory response" with "dysregulated host response," and "systemic inflammatory response syndrome" (SIRS) has been replaced with "sequential organ failure assessment" (SOFA). The reasons for changing the definition from Sepsis-1 to Sepsis-3 included an overwhelming focus on inflammation in prior definitions; a misleading continuum between sepsis, severe sepsis, and septic shock; SIRS criteria lacking adequate sensitivity and specificity.

### References
1. Singer M, Deutschman CS, Seymour CW, et al. The third international consensus definitions for sepsis and septic shock (sepsis-3). *JAMA*. 2016;315:801-810.
2. Nunnally ME, Patel A. Sepsis – What's new in 2019? *Curr Opin Anaesthesiol*. 2019;32:163-168.

---

**22.** Correct Answer: D

**Rationale:**

Significant discrepancies between POC and central laboratory-analyzed blood glucose values have been reported in patients receiving high-dose vitamin C (mean of 225 vs. 138 mg/dL, respectively). High doses of vitamin C may falsely elevate glucose level readings when measured with certain POC glucometers employing glucose dehydrogenase-pyrroloquinoline quinone amperometric methods. These discrepancies are often inconsistent over time and can range widely. A falsely elevated POC blood glucose measurement may result in overly aggressive insulin therapy, resulting in iatrogenic hypoglycemia, and has been reported to have contributed to patient mortality in at least one case.

### References
1. Flannery AH, Bastin MLT, Magee CA, Bensadoun ES. Vitamin C in sepsis: when it seems too sweet, it might (literally) be. *Chest*. 2017;152:450-451.
2. Moskowitz A, Andersen LW, Huang DT, et al. Ascorbic acid, corticosteroids, and thiamine in sepsis: a review of the biologic rationale and the present state of clinical evaluation. *Crit Care*. 2018;22:283.
3. Kahn SA, Lentz CW. Fictitious hyperglycemia: point-of-care glucose measurement is inaccurate during high-dose vitamin C infusion for burn shock resuscitation. *J Burn Care Res*. 2015;36:e67-e71.

---

**23.** Correct Answer: A

**Rationale:**

In sepsis, the host loses local-regional containment of an infection, and the body is systemically exposed to microbes, microbial components, and products of damaged tissue. The innate immune system, composed mainly of macrophages, monocytes, granulocytes, natural killer cells, and dendritic cells, has evolved to detect PAMPs including components of bacterial, fungal, and viral pathogens (e.g., endotoxin and 9-glucan) and DAMPs which are endogenous molecules released from damaged host cells, (e.g., ATP, mitochondrial DNA, and high mobility group box 1).

DAMPs and PAMPs activate the innate immune through pattern recognition receptors (PRRs) on the surface of immune cells (e.g., TLRs or in the cytosol (e.g., NOD-like receptors), initiating transcription of type I interferons and proinflammatory cytokines such as tumor necrosis factor (TNF)-α, interleukin (IL)-1, and IL-6. Some of these pattern recognition receptors (mostly nucleotide-binding oligomerization domain [NOD]-like receptors) can assemble into molecular complexes termed inflammasomes, which are important in the maturation and secretion of the very potent cytokines IL-1β and IL-18, that can trigger programmed cell death termed pyroptosis.

### References
1. Gotts JE, Matthay MA. Sepsis: pathophysiology and clinical management. *BMJ*. 2016;353:i1585.
2. Delano MJ, Ward PA. The immune system's role in sepsis progression, resolution, and long-term outcome. *Immunol Rev*. 2016;274:330-353.

---

**24.** Correct Answer: D

**Rationale:**

Acute kidney injury (AKI) is common in severe sepsis and substantially increases morbidity and mortality. Although in the past septic AKI has been attributed to reduced renal perfusion and widespread tubular necrosis, recent studies have challenged this notion, by showing, for example, that AKI occurs in the setting of normal or increased renal blood flow; and that it is characterized not by acute tubular necrosis or apoptosis, but rather by heterogeneous areas of colocalized sluggish peritubular blood flow and tubular epithelial cell oxidative stress. Evidence has also shown that microvascular dysfunction, inflammation, and the metabolic response to inflammatory injury are fundamental pathophysiologic mechanisms that may explain the development of sepsis-induced AKI.

### References
1. Gómez H, Kellum JA. Sepsis-induced acute kidney injury. *Curr Opin Crit Care*. 2016;22:546-553.
2. Prowle JR, Bellomo R. Sepsis-associated acute kidney injury: macrohemodynamic and microhemodynamic alterations in the renal circulation. *Semin Nephrol*. 2015;35:64-74.

**25.** Correct Answer: B

**Rationale:**

Sugammadex is the first selective antagonist to reverse neuromuscular blockade induced by rocuronium and vecuronium. Importantly, sugammadex has the capacity to rapidly and predictably reverse even deep neuromuscular blockade. Administration of sugammadex to the patient in this question will reverse the rocuronium received during intubation thereby facilitating neurologic examination.

Acetylcholinesterase inhibitors, such as neostigmine, have traditionally been used for reversal of nondepolarizing neuromuscular blocking agents. However, these drugs have significant limitations, such as indirect mechanisms of reversal, limited and unpredictable efficacy, and undesirable autonomic responses.

Flumazenil is a benzodiazepine antagonist, and naloxone is an opioid antagonist. Since the patient did not receive either benzodiazepines or opioids, the administration of these antagonists would not be indicated for this patient.

References

1. Ezri T, Boaz M, Sherman A, Armaly M, Berlovitz Y. Sugammadex: an update. *J Crit Care Med*. 2016;2:16-21.
2. Karalapillai D, Kaufman M, Weinberg L. Sugammadex. *Crit Care Resusc*. 2013;15:57-62.
3. Pani N, Dongare PA, Mishra RK. Reversal agents in anesthesia and critical care. *Indian J Anaesth*. 2015;59:664-669.

**26.** Correct Answer: C

**Rationale:**

In 2016, the Society of Critical Care Medicine published ICU Admission, Discharge, and Triage (ADT) Guidelines to provide a comprehensive framework to guide practitioners in making informed decisions in ADT process. The ADT guidelines contain recommendations classified as "strong" (grade 1) or "weak" (grade 2) based on certainty of the evidence, assessment of the balance of risks and benefits, relevant values and preferences, and burdens and costs of interventions. Guideline recommendations relevant to the patient in this question include:

- The admission of neurocritically ill patients to a neuro-ICU is suggested, especially for patients with a diagnosis of intracerebral hemorrhage or head injury (grade 2C). Evidence suggests that neurocritically ill patients show improved outcomes when compared with the treatment in a general ICU, especially for intracerebral hemorrhage and head injury.
- Scoring systems are not recommended for use in isolation to determine ICU admission or discharge because they are not accurate in predicting individual mortality (grade 2C).
- Minimizing the transfer time of critically ill patients from the emergency department to the ICU (<6 hour in nontrauma patients) has been associated with improved outcomes in several studies and is recommended (grade 2D).
- A 24-hour/7-day intensivist model is not recommended if the ICU has a high-intensity staffing model (grade 1A). Around-the-clock on-site intensivist coverage is not recommended since it may not be feasible for all ICUs because of the shortage of available intensivists, the financial constraints required, and the lack of evidence supporting the approach.

Reference

1. Nates JL, Nunnally M, Kleinpell R, et al. ICU admission, discharge, and triage guidelines: a framework to enhance clinical operations, development of institutional policies, and further research. *Crit Care Med*. 2016;44:1553-1602.

**27.** Correct Answer: C

**Rationale:**

In patients with the ARDS an acute increase in right ventricular afterload secondary to increased PVR may result in acute cor pulmonale (ACP) and/or right-to-left shunting through a PFO. The prevalence of ACP and PFO has recently been reported to be 22% to 25% and 16% to 19%, respectively, in ARDS. Shunt of blood through a PFO may worsen ARDS-induced hypoxemia, thereby limiting the beneficial effects of recruitment maneuvers such as PEEP trials. Echocardiography is valuable for the diagnosis of ACP and PFO in mechanically ventilated patients with ARDS.

Aspirated material is frequently liquid in nature and disperses rapidly. Hence routine bronchoscopy with lavage is not indicated. However, in the event that the aspirate is predominantly particulate in nature with clear radiographic evidence of lobar collapse or major atelectasis, a therapeutic bronchoscopy may be helpful. While pulmonary embolism may cause severe hypoxemia, it is unlikely given the clinical vignette provided in the question.

References

1. Mekontso Dessap A, Boissier F, Leon R, et al. Prevalence and prognosis of shunting across patent foramen ovale during acute respiratory distress syndrome. *Crit Care Med*. 2010;38:1786-1792.
2. Legras A, Caille A, Begot E, et al. Acute respiratory distress syndrome (ARDS)-associated acute cor pulmonale and patent foramen ovale: a multicenter noninvasive hemodynamic study. *Crit Care*. 2015;19:174.
3. Raghavendran K, Nemzek J, Napolitano LM, Knight PR. Aspiration-induced lung injury. *Crit Care Med*. 2011;39:818-826.

**28.** Correct Answer: C

**Rationale:**

The PLR is a test that predicts whether a patient is "fluid responsive," that is, whether cardiac output will increase by 10% to 15% with volume expansion. By transferring a volume of venous blood (approximately 300 ml) from the lower body to the right heart, the PLR mimics a fluid challenge. However, no fluid is infused, and the hemodynamic effects rapidly dissipate, thereby avoiding the risks of fluid overload. PLR has the advantage of remaining reliable under conditions in which measures of fluid responsiveness based on the respiratory variations of stroke volume cannot be used, such as when patients are spontaneous breathing, are having arrhythmias, have low lung compliance, or are receiving low tidal volume ventilation.

The method of performing a PLR is important because it fundamentally affects its hemodynamic effects and therefore the reliability of the test. The PLR should start from the semirecumbent and not the supine position. Adding trunk lowering to leg raising mobilizes venous blood from the large splanchnic compartment, thus magnifying the increasing effects of leg elevation on cardiac preload and increasing the test's sensitivity.

The effects of the PLR should be assessed by a direct measurement of cardiac output and not by the measurement of blood pressure. Although the arterial pulse pressure is positively correlated with stroke volume, it also depends on arterial compliance and pulse wave amplification which could be altered during PLR, impeding the use of pulse pressure as a surrogate of stroke volume to assess PLR effects.

Finally the measurement of cardiac output during PLR must be able to detect short-term changes since the PLR effects may vanish after 1 minute. Techniques which provide cardiac output measurements in "real time," such as arterial pulse contour analysis, echocardiography, esophageal Doppler, or pulse contour analysis of arterial pressure, can be used.

References

1. Maizel J, Airapetian N, Lorne E, et al. Diagnosis of central hypovolemia by using passive leg raising. *Intensive Care Med.* 2007;33:1133-1138.
2. Monnet X, Teboul JL. Passive leg raising: five rules, not a drop of fluid! *Crit Care.* 2015;19:18.

**29.** Correct Answer: A

**Rationale:**

Gastrointestinal dysmotility is a common feature of critical illness, with a number of potentially significant consequences including malnutrition secondary to reduced feed tolerance, pulmonary aspiration, VAP, bacterial overgrowth, and possible translocation causing sepsis. Prokinetic pharmacotherapy is a mainstay for the management of disordered upper gastrointestinal dysmotility.

Erythromycin and, to a lesser extent, metoclopramide accelerate gastric emptying in the critically ill and improve the success of nasogastric feeding. Erythromycin, a macrolide antibiotic, promotes upper gastrointestinal motility as a motilin receptor agonist. It acts on enteric neurons and smooth muscle cells of the gastric antrum and proximal small bowel and is commonly used in critically ill patients. Metoclopramide, a dopamine receptor antagonist, promotes gastric emptying by acting as an antagonist to the inhibitory actions of dopamine on the motility of the gut, increasing lower esophageal sphincter tone and sensitizing the gastrointestinal system to acetylcholine. Tachyphylaxis to the prokinetic effects develops with both erythromycin and metoclopramide. Erythromycin and metoclopramide appear more potent when they are used in combination, and tachyphylaxis is reduced.

References

1. Chapman MJ, Nguyen NQ, Deane AM. Gastrointestinal dysmotility: clinical consequences and management of the critically ill patient. *Gastroenterol Clin North Am.* 2011;40:725-739.
2. Fraser RJ, Bryant L. Current and future therapeutic prokinetic therapy to improve enteral feed intolerance in the ICU patient. *Nutr Clin Pract.* 2010;25:26-31.
3. Nguyen NQ, Chapman MJ, Fraser RJ, et al. Erythromycin is more effective than metoclopramide in the treatment of feed intolerance in critical illness. *Crit Care Med.* 2007;35:483-489.
4. Nguyen NQ, Chapman M, Fraser RJ. Prokinetic therapy for feed intolerance in critical illness: one drug or two? *Crit Care Med.* 2007;35:2561-2567.

**30.** Correct Answer: C

**Rationale:**

In patients without spontaneous breathing efforts (i.e., sedated and/or paralyzed on controlled mechanical ventilation), the driving pressure of the respiratory system is defined as the difference between plateau pressure and positive end-expiratory pressure (Pplat − PEEP). For this patient, the driving pressure is calculated as Pplat − PEEP = 34 cm $H_2O$ − 8 cm $H_2O$ = 26 cm $H_2O$

Evidence from both a post hoc analysis of previous randomized controlled trials and a subsequent meta-analysis suggests that driving pressure is a strong predictor of mortality in patients with ARDS. Importantly, the meta-analysis suggested targeting driving pressure below 13 to 15 cm $H_2O$ although it remains unclear how to best reduce the driving pressure as part of a ventilatory strategy at the bedside.

In the presence of spontaneous breathing efforts, the negative change in pleural pressure generated by spontaneous breathing becomes additive to the distending pressure; therefore, driving pressure may be underestimated without considering these efforts. In these circumstances, the plateau pressure should be measured using a brief inspiratory hold to calculate actual driving pressure.

## References

1. Aoyama H, Yamada Y, Fan E. The future of driving pressure: a primary goal for mechanical ventilation? *J Intensive Care.* 2018;6:64.
2. Amato MBP, Meade MO, Slutsky AS, et al. Driving pressure and survival in the acute respiratory distress syndrome. *N Engl J Med.* 2015;372:747-755.
3. Aoyama H, Pettenuzzo T, Aoyama K, Pinto R, Englesakis M, Fan E. Association of driving pressure with mortality among ventilated patients with acute respiratory distress syndrome. *Crit Care Med.* 2017;46:1.

---

**31.** Correct Answer: B

**Rationale:**

The clinical, laboratory, and imaging findings in this patient are consistent with septic shock secondary to acute cholecystitis. The patient was initially resuscitated with IV fluids without any improvement in his hemodynamics and started on vasopressors as a result. He has been started on broad-spectrum antibiotics. To ensure source control, the acute cholecystitis needs to be addressed. The three options available to this patient include PCT placement, laparoscopic cholecystectomy, and open cholecystectomy. Because of his hemodynamic instability and significant comorbidities, this patient is a very high-risk surgical candidate. Therefore, PCT placement would be the best of the three options here. PCT involves image-guided placement of a drainage tube into the gallbladder, commonly using the Seldinger technique. This ensures initial aspiration of bile followed by continuous drainage. As a result, the gallbladder is decompressed, and the infection is controlled. The technical success rate is reported to be between 95% and 100%. One unique advantage of PCT is that it can be done at the bedside. This is important in critically ill ICU patients who are too unstable to travel to the operating room or tolerate the additional stress of a surgical procedure. It is also relatively quick to perform and rapidly achieves source control. Performing a laparoscopic cholecystectomy in this patient would be fraught with difficult as the patient is unlikely to tolerate the pneumoperitoneum required for safe laparoscopy due to his hemodynamic instability. An open cholecystectomy would be an option if resources for performance of PCT placement are unavailable, but it is not the first option. There is no indication for ERCP in this patient. Resuscitation with albumin does not address the source of infection in this patient.

## References

1. Gulaya K, Desai S, Sato K. Percutaneous cholecystostomy: evidence-based current clinical practice. *Semin Intervent Radiol.* 2016;33(4):291-296.
2. Bakkaloglu H, Yanar H, Guloglu R, et al. Ultrasound guided percutaneous cholecystostomy in high-risk patients for surgical intervention. *World J Gastroenterol.* 2006;12(44):7179-7182.

---

**32.** Correct Answer: C

**Rationale:**

This critically ill patient has multiple acute issues going on simultaneously: he has a potentially compromised airway due to mechanical compression of the trachea by a rapidly expanding hematoma; hemodynamic instability from the expanding hematoma and bleeding from a prior paracentesis site; coagulopathy; altered mental status most likely due to hepatic encephalopathy; and severe liver disease. The order in which these clinical issues are addressed matters. Among these issues, airway compromise is imminently life-threatening; therefore, securing the patient's airway should be the first priority. Thus, endotracheal intubation would be the next best step in management. Once this is done, the patient's hypotension and coagulopathy should be rapidly corrected by transfusion with the appropriate blood products. Unlike the trauma patient who requires immediate operative exploration with an expanding neck hematoma, this patient may not need to have a surgical exploration. After securing the airway and correction of the coagulopathy, the bleeding should stop spontaneously. Once hemodynamically stable for travel, a CT angiogram of the neck can then be obtained to define the extent of the hematoma and determine if there is still active hemorrhage. Exploratory laparotomy is not indicated at this time in this patient. Bleeding from the paracentesis site should stop with correction of the coagulopathy. If not, the patient should be considered for angiographic embolization for hemorrhage control.

## References

1. Baron RM. Point: should coagulopathy be repaired prior to central venous line insertion? Yes. *Chest.* 2012;141(5):1139-1142.
2. Goldhaber SZ. Counterpoint: should coagulopathy be repaired prior to central venous line insertion? No. *Chest.* 2012;141(5):1142-1144.

**33.** Correct Answer: A

**Rationale:**

This patient is in postoperative day 4 after extensive cytoreductive surgery with right hemicolectomy and ileotransverse anastomosis. Persistent tachycardia despite adequate pain control that is unresponsive to fluid resuscitation is most likely from anastomotic leak. ECG and bedside echocardiography in this patient revealed no cardiovascular cause of the patient's tachycardia. With a negative duplex ultrasonography for deep venous thrombosis, the chance of a pulmonary embolism is very low. For a surgical patient with tachycardia, a cause that is related to the actual surgery should always be entertained in the differential diagnosis. The consequences of delayed diagnosis of an anastomotic leak are severe, as rapid intra-abdominal sepsis, septic shock, and multiple organ dysfunction syndrome can occur. The investigation of choice to rule out an anastomotic leak is a CT scan of the abdomen and pelvis with oral and intravenous contrast. The classic radiologic findings associated with anastomotic leak include extraluminal air, extraluminal fluid, and extravasation of contrast into the peritoneal cavity. Once the diagnosis is made, a rapid decision should be made regarding whether the patient should be taken back to the operating room for reexploration of the abdomen or whether percutaneous drain placement would be employed in management.

References

1. Lynn ET, Chen J, Wilck EJ, El-Sabrout K, Lo CC, Divino CM. Radiographic findings of anastomotic leaks. *Am Surg.* 2013;79(2):194-197.
2. Gesser B, Eriksson O, Angenete E. Diagnosis, treatment, and consequences of anastomotic leakage in colorectal surgery. *Int J Colorectal Dis.* 2017;32(4):549-556.

**34.** Correct Answer: D

**Rationale:**

This patient presented with a recent exploratory laparotomy for intra-abdominal sepsis and resuscitation with a fairly large volume of intravenous fluid; has the appropriate clinical context and typical signs of abdominal compartment syndrome: oliguria, elevated peak airway pressure, and elevated bladder pressure. Abdominal compartment syndrome is a life-threatening condition that is characterized by rapid development of multiple organ failure. Early recognition and rapid institution of appropriate therapy is key to halt systemic organ failure. When it is suspected, measurement of bladder pressure as a surrogate for intra-abdominal pressure is performed, and if elevated, along with the appropriate signs, decompressive laparotomy is indicated. If untreated, the mortality from abdominal compartment syndrome is uniformly 100%. Decompressive laparotomy releases the intra-abdominal pressure and reverses the mechanical complications of this condition. The abdomen is usually temporarily closed. Since excess fluid resuscitation is a risk factor, it is important to be cautious with further resuscitation. CT scan of the abdomen and pelvis is not indicated, since this is a clinical diagnosis. The oliguria in this condition is not responsive to administration of furosemide. Increase in PEEP and administration of sedatives, may become necessary, but is not the next critical step.

References

1. De Backer D. Abdominal compartment syndrome. *Crit Care.* 1999;3(6):R103-R104.
2. Hecker A, Hecker B, Hecker M, Riedel JG, Weigand MA, Padberg W. Acute abdominal compartment syndrome: current diagnostic and therapeutic options. *Langenbecks Arch Surg.* 2016;401(1):15-24.

**35.** Correct Answer: A

**Rationale:**

This patient is likely experiencing a biliary leak as a complication of laparoscopic cholecystectomy. Most commonly, the biliary leak could be either from the cystic duct stump or an intraoperative injury to the common bile duct. The presence of fever, hypotension, abdominal distension, right upper quadrant tenderness, leukocytosis, and a large amount of free intraperitoneal fluid is indicative of sepsis secondary to biliary peritonitis. The patient is being appropriately resuscitated, has been started on intravenous antibiotics, and has been admitted to the ICU for hemodynamic monitoring. To achieve source control, a CT-guided drainage of the intra-abdominal fluid collection should be performed. Exploratory laparotomy is usually not the first option; it is indicated if source control is not achieved with percutaneous drainage. While magnetic resonance cholangiopancreatography and ERCP can help in delineating the biliary anatomy, source control with drainage takes priority. ERCP may eventually be needed for stent placement in case of cystic stump or common bile duct leak. Use of intravenous vitamin C, hydrocortisone, and thiamine would be of minimal or no benefit if adequate source control is not achieved.

References

1. Lee CM, Stewart L, Way LW. Postcholecystectomy abdominal bile collections. *Arch Surg.* 2000;135(5):538-542.
2. Ahmad F, Saunders RN, Lloyd DM, Robertson GSM. An algorithm for the management of bile leak following laparoscopic cholecystectomy. *Ann R Coll Surg Engl.* 2007;89(1):51-56.

**36.** Correct Answer: B

**Rationale:**

The presence of increasing left upper quadrant pain, nausea, and generalized abdominal distension after commencement of clear liquid diet is suggestive of postoperative ileus. This is confirmed by the abdominal x-ray finding of distended stomach and nonobstructive bowel gas pattern. The slight difficulty in breathing is most likely due to splinting of the diaphragm by the abdominal distension. Placement of a nasogastric tube would offer this patient immediate symptomatic relief. The patient should then be kept NPO till there is evidence of return of bowel function. Electrolyte derangements should be corrected. While the patient may benefit from an aggressive bowel regimen at some point, it is not the next step in the setting of a markedly distended stomach. There is no indication for an upper gastrointestinal endoscopy. High-flow nasal oxygen and noninvasive ventilation with BiPAP are unlikely to provide benefit in this patient.

References

1. Luckey A. Mechanisms and treatment of postoperative ileus. *Arch Surg.* 2003;138(2):206-214.
2. Resnick J, Greenwald DA, Brandt LJ. Delayed gastric emptying and postoperative ileus after nongastric abdominal surgery: part I. *Am J Gastroenterol.* 1997;92(5):751-762.

**37.** Correct Answer: A

**Rationale:**

A markedly elevated serum creatine kinase in a blunt trauma patient is highly suggestive of rhabdomyolysis. In this condition, damage to skeletal muscle is marked by the release into the plasma of muscle constituents such as creatine kinase, potassium, and myoglobin. AKI is one of the feared complications of rhabdomyolysis from any cause, with any incidence of 4% to 33%. The pathogenesis is thought to be due to acute tubular necrosis from release of free radicals rather than simple mechanical damage of renal tubules by myoglobin. Aggressive fluid resuscitation is the primary means of preventing acute tubular necrosis in this situation. Evidence for urine alkalinization is equivocal and thus not favored. So long as urine output is adequate, generally in the range of 100 to 200 mL/h, administration of IV mannitol or hemodialysis is not necessary. There is no role for intravenous urogram in this condition

References

1. Madrazo Delgado M, Uña Orejón R, Redondo Calvo FJ, Criado Jiménez A. Ischemic rhabdomyolysis and acute renal failure. *Rev Esp Anestesiol Reanim.* 2007;54(7):425-435.
2. Pezzi M, Giglio AM, Scozzafava A, Serafino G, Maglio P, Verre M. Early intensive treatment to prevent kidney failure in post-traumatic rhabdomyolysis: case report. *SAGE Open Med Case Rep.* 2019;7:2050313X19839529.

**38.** Correct Answer: D

**Rationale:**

The absence of lung sliding following multiple attempts for central line placement in a patient is consistent with a diagnosis of pneumothorax. In this patient, with absence of lung sliding, decrease in oxygen saturation, and hemodynamic instability, the most likely diagnosis is tension pneumothorax. Once this assessment is made, the clinician should proceed with immediate tube thoracostomy (chest tube placement). Needle decompression with a long angiocath needle may be used as a temporizing measure, but it is not a substitute for chest tube placement. The diagnosis of tension pneumothorax is largely clinical and does not require a CT scan of the chest. Administration of vasopressors and fluid resuscitation will not correct the mechanical obstruction from the tension pneumothorax, neither would endotracheal intubation.

References

1. Kim KH. Tension pneumothorax after attempting insertion of a central venous catheter. *Acute Crit Care.* 2018;33(4):280-281.
2. Day MW. Tension pneumothorax from central line placement. *Nursing.* 2006;36(11):80.

**39.** Correct Answer: E

**Rationale:**

The combination of extreme difficulty with bagging the patient, elevated peak airway pressure, subcutaneous emphysema, and hemodynamic instability is consistent with tension pneumothorax. This could result from perforation of the posterior tracheal wall or from placement of the tracheostomy tube in a false passage and subsequent positive-pressure ventilation into the false passage. Given that there is a direct communication between the pleural cavity and the neck spaces, it is easy to understand why this can happen. Immediate recognition is key. If the tracheostomy tube is in a false passage, the patient should be endotracheally reintubated if possible and ventilated from above while a needle decompression followed by chest tube placement should be performed. Once the airway is secure and the pneumothorax adequately drained with a chest tube, the neck should be reexplored and the tracheostomy tube appropriately placed. In this challenging situation, bronchoscopy should be performed to confirm appropriate placement of the tracheostomy tube before removal of the endotracheal tube. Perforation of the posterior tracheal wall may require surgical repair.

References

1. Gupta P, Modrykamien A. Fatal case of tension pneumothorax and subcutaneous emphysema after open surgical tracheostomy. *J Intensive Care Med.* 2014;29(5):298-301.
2. Matsumura S, Kishimoto N, Iseki T, Momota Y. Tension pneumothorax after percutaneous tracheostomy. *Anesth Prog.* 2017;64(2):85-87.

---

**40.** Correct Answer: B

**Rationale:**

The association between volume responsiveness and inferior vena cava (IVC) ultrasound (diameter and collapsibility) is well studied. Various studies and meta-analyses have shown that IVC collapsibility is not associated with volume responsiveness in a spontaneously breathing patient. This is especially true for patients in respiratory distress. Increased work of breathing creates large swings in intrathoracic pressure creating a collapsible IVC, irrespective of volume status. On the other hand, lack of collapsibility cannot be used to rule out volume responsiveness. Hence, IVC collapsibility cannot be used to measure volume responsiveness in this patient (option B).

Respiratory variation of IVC performs better as a diagnostic tool in mechanically ventilated patients, where IVC collapsibility with respiration is moderately predictive of volume responsiveness. But, a lack of IVC collapsibility cannot be used to rule out volume responsiveness, even in mechanically ventilated patients. IVC collapsibility does not give information on the type of fluid likely to be successful in eliciting a response to volume challenge.

Reference

1. Long E, Oakley E, Duke T, et al. Does respiratory variation in inferior vena cava diameter predict fluid responsiveness: a systematic review and meta-analysis. *Shock.* 2017;47(5):550-559.

---

**41.** Correct Answer: C

**Rationale:**

Venous air embolism (VAE) occurs with entrainment of air into the vasculature due to a multitude of causes, most of them iatrogenic. Any condition that creates a negative pressure gradient favoring entry of air from the environment into the bloodstream represents a risk, including not just the prototypical surgical sources but also angiography, trauma, endoscopy, and central line placement. The incidence varies widely based on etiology, with the frequency of VAE associated with central line placement ranging anywhere from 1 in 47 to 1 in 3000 in different case series. Despite optimal positioning and techniques, interventional radiology studies demonstrate a VAE incidence of 0.13%. The morbidity and mortality of VAE depend on both the rate of air infusion and the volume entrained. The adult human lethal volume has been described as approximately 200 to 300 mL at a rate of 100 mL/s, which can be accomplished with a 14 gauge needle and a 5 cm $H_2O$ pressure differential. A low CVP (especially in a spontaneously breathing patient) can increase the risk of VAE by creating a more favorable pressure gradient for air entrainment. Large VAEs (3-5 mL/kg) can create a right ventricular air lock with resultant partial to complete RV outflow obstruction, right heart failure leading to hypotension and outright cardiovascular collapse. Smaller or slower emboli lead to obstruction at the level of the pulmonary vasculature, producing vasoconstriction and vascular inflammation and a resultant V/Q mismatch. The pulmonary hypertension produced causes RV strain.

The symptoms of VAE are nonspecific and rely primarily on patient history and a high clinical suspicion. An awake patient may cough and endorse dyspnea or a sense of impending doom. Other pulmonary findings include a decrease in end-tidal carbon dioxide, $SpO_2$, and $PaO_2$, with an increase in $PaCO_2$. Tachyarrhythmias are the most common ECG finding, and myocardial ischemia may develop in the setting of hypotension. Pulmonary artery and CVPs often increase due to right heart strain. Transesophageal ultrasound remains the most sensitive tool to confirm diagnosis, capable of detecting as little as 0.02 mL/kg of air, but is invasive and requires a skilled operator to employ.

Treatment of VAE focuses on prevention of further air entrainment and support of end-organ perfusion. During central line placement, the patient should be placed in Trendelenburg position and hydrated beforehand to maximize CVP relative to atmosphere. With spontaneous negative-pressure ventilation in an awake patient, avoid vein puncture during inspiration, which maximizes thoracic negative pressure. Supportive measures include institution of high-flow oxygen with an $FiO_2$ 100%, which will both support tissue oxygenation and aid in nitrogen elimination, directly reducing embolus volume, vasopressors to support perfusion, inotropy for acute right ventricular strain, and intravascular volume to increase venous return. Rapid initiation of ACLS may become necessary with cardiopulmonary collapse, especially in the case of right ventricular air lock.

References

1. Gordy S, Rowell S. Vascular air embolism. *Int J Crit Illn Inj Sci.* 2013;3(1):73-76.
2. Mirski M, Lele A, Fitzsimmons L, Toung T. Diagnosis and treatment of vascular air embolism. 2007;106:164-177.

**42.** Correct Answer: A

**Rationale:**

Mechanical circulatory support with VA-ECMO (via peripheral cannulation) relies on retrograde aortic flow to perfuse organs, and one key limitation of this strategy is the significant increase in left ventricle (LV) afterload. This leads to LV distension, which in turn can cause pulmonary edema and increased myocardial wall stress due to persistently elevated LV end-diastolic pressure. The impairment in myocardial recovery can in turn delay ECMO weaning. Frequent echocardiograms and daily chest radiographs, in addition to close hemodynamic monitoring, can assist in identifying this phenomenon. Decreased pulsation in the arterial waveform suggests that the LV is not ejecting against the high afterload produced by ECMO flows.

Indications for LV decompression include no observed LV ejection (a closed aortic valve), refractory pulmonary edema or hemorrhage, distended left atrium and LV with elevated pressures, LV thrombus due to stasis, or significant aortic regurgitation. Treatment strategies to unload and decompress the left ventricle include pharmacologic, interventional, and surgical. Pharmacologic support with inotropy to support LV function is often the first step. Interventional approaches include transseptal left atrial decompression with balloon atrial septostomy or atrial vent insertion, pulmonary artery vents, IABP placement, or Impella placement. Direct decompression of the left ventricle is typically accomplished surgically in the operating room. The timing of LV decompression is still debated, but literature in pediatric and adult populations suggests that early decompression is associated with better LV recovery and improved likelihood of weaning from ECMO.

### References

1. Ong CS, Hibino N. Left heart decompression in patients supported with extracorporeal membrane oxygenation for cardiac disease. *Postepy Kardiol Interwencyjnej.* 2017;13(1):1-2.
2. Makdisi G, Wang IW. Extra corporeal membrane oxygenation (ECMO) review of a lifesaving technology. *J Thorac Dis.* 2015;7(7):E166-E176.

**43.** Correct Answer: D

**Rationale:**

Both bleeding and thrombosis are common complications of ECMO, and adequate anticoagulation is a key therapy for prevention of circuit thrombosis. While no standardized targets have been established, a goal aPTT of 60 to 80 seconds or activated clotting time of 160 to 180 seconds are often used. The combination of bleeding and thrombosis suggests HIT or disseminated intravascular coagulation (DIC). HIT remains a clinical diagnosis supported by confirmatory laboratory testing, and in the event of high clinical suspicion, initiation of treatment should not be delayed pending confirmation with a positive heparin-PF4 antibody screen. The "4 Ts" of HIT (see table) is a common diagnostic standard that includes the degree of thrombocytopenia, timing of onset, thrombosis, and ruling out of other causes. Treatment consists of discontinuing heparin infusion and starting infusion of an alternate anticoagulant that will not cross-react with HIT antibodies, typically the direct thrombin inhibitors bivalirudin or argatroban. Platelet levels should return to normal and thrombotic events stop after discontinuation of heparin.

DIC can be triggered by sepsis or by ECMO circuit thrombosis itself and is associated with generalized coagulation test abnormalities, including elevated aPTT, PTT, INR, and low fibrinogen, with a characteristic thromboelastogram profile. Treating the underlying cause with aggressive antibiotic therapy for infection or exchange of the ECMO circuit in the case of thrombosis is critical. Antifibrinolytic therapy such as tranexamic acid may be a helpful adjunct in cases that involve severe fibrinolysis.

Heparin resistance on ECMO is typically due to acquired antithrombin III deficiency and may result in thrombosis without bleeding. It is defined as the need for an excessive amount of heparin (commonly defined as >35,000 units/24 hours) to maintain an aPTT or ACT in the therapeutic range. Antithrombin III and antifactor Xa levels can verify the diagnosis and assess whether the current heparin dose is therapeutic. A subtherapeutic aPTT combined with a low ATIII and an anti-Xa level in the therapeutic range would suggest that heparin resistance is present but that the current heparin dose is appropriate.

| THE 4TS OF HIT | | | |
| --- | --- | --- | --- |
| VARIABLE | SCORE | | |
| | 20 | 1 | 0 |
| Thrombocytopenia | >50% fall, or nadir 20-100,000/mm³ | 30%-50% fall, or nadir 10-19,000/mm³ | <30% fall, or nadir <10,000/mm³ |
| Timing of onset after heparin initiation | 5-10 days, or <1 day if recent prior heparin exposure | Day >10, or <1 day if heparin exposure 30-100 days prior | <4 days without history of recent heparin exposure |

THE 4TS OF HIT

| VARIABLE | SCORE | | |
|---|---|---|---|
| | 20 | 1 | 0 |
| Thrombosis | New thrombosis | Progressive, recurrent, or suspected thrombosis | None |
| Other causes | None | Possible | Definite |

The 4T scoring system is widely used to estimate the probability of HIT, with pretest probability based on sum of points: 0-3 = low, 4-5 = medium, and 6-8 = high probability. A score of <4 points has a high negative predictive value, while intermediate scores have a lower positive predictive value and should be followed up with confirmatory lab testing.

### References

1. Sidebotham D. Troubleshooting adult ECMO. *J Extra Corpor Technol.* 2011;43(1):27-32.
2. Ahmed I, Majeed A, Powell R. Heparin induced thrombocytopenia: diagnosis and management update. *Postgrad Med J.* 2007;83(983):575-582.

---

**44.** Correct Answer: B

**Rationale:**

A venous air embolism (VAE) always has the potential to become an arterial embolism if a connection between the two systems exists and a right-to-left pressure gradient favors paradoxical air embolism (PAE). The symptoms of PAE depend on which arterial bed the air is entrained into and are prototypically cerebral or cardiac. In contrast to the nonspecific altered mental status secondary to global hypoperfusion seen in VAE, cerebral PAE results in focal ischemia with hemiparesis or hemianopsia. Similarly, entrainment of paradoxical air in the coronary arteries causes ST segment depression or elevation, depending on the degree of occlusion. Irritation of the left ventricle can also produce malignant arrhythmias.

The most common source of paradoxical embolism is a PFO, which is present in 30% of the population. PEEP in a ventilated patient can increase the CVP and hypothetically favor increased right-to-left shunting in patients with a PFO. Other conditions result in an increased in shunt fraction across the pulmonary vasculature, including severe COPD, cirrhosis, and pulmonary arteriovenous malformations.

Hereditary hemorrhagic telangiectasia (HHT) is an autosomal dominant vascular disorder with a prevalence between 1:5000 and 1:8000. It is characterized by the combination of epistaxis, gastrointestinal bleeding, and iron-deficiency anemia, along with mucocutaneous telangiectasias on the lips and oral mucosa. These patients are also at increased risk of arteriovenous malformations in the pulmonary (50% incidence), hepatic (30%), and cerebral (10%) circulation, which can place them at risk of severe systemic complications. Pulmonary AVMs in particular can be associated with paradoxical thrombotic, gas, or septic emboli resulting in ischemic stroke or brain abscesses.

VAE and PAE are treated primarily by prevention of further air entrainment and support of tissue perfusion with supplemental oxygen, vasopressors, fluid resuscitation, and ACLS algorithm in the case of cardiovascular collapse. HBOT is one additional modality that both accelerates nitrogen reabsorption with high oxygen tension and directly decreases the embolism size with increased pressure in accordance with Boyle's law. HBOT has been shown to improve neurologic deficits following arterial air embolism, and early initiation of therapy demonstrates greater benefits. Limitations to HBOT include both the availability of a hyperbaric chamber and the difficulties in managing a critically ill patient during hyperbaric therapy.

### References

1. Gordy S, Rowell S. Vascular air embolism. *Int J Crit Illn Inj Sci.* 2013;3(1):73-76.
2. McDonald J, Bayrak-Toydemir P, Pyeritz R. Hereditary hemorrhagic telangiectasia: An overview of diagnosis, management, and pathogenesis. *Genetics in Medicine.* 2011;13(7):607-616.
3. Blanc P, Boussuges A, Henriette K, Sainty J, Deleflie M. Iatrogenic cerebral air embolism: importance of an early hyperbaric oxygenation. *Intensive Care Medicine.* 2002;28(5):559-563.

---

**45.** Correct Answer: C

**Rationale:**

The acute phase of sepsis is characterized by an inflammatory catabolic state that breaks down glycogen, lipid, and muscle to mobilize the body's calorie stores. The rapid loss of lean body mass often results in an ICU-acquired weakness that can impair return to baseline function even after successful discharge from the hospital. Underfeeding in the ICU course can lead to increased mortality and long-term quality of life impairment. Nutritional support guidelines recommend initiation of enteral nutrition in mechanically ventilated patients within 24 to 48 hours of ICU admission. The Surviving Sepsis 2016 Guidelines likewise suggest early initiation of enteral feeding rather than a complete fast, intravenous glucose only, or early parenteral nutrition. One other key advantage is the preservation of gut function and integrity. Lack of enteral nutrition is associated with villous atrophy, reduced mucosal thickness, and increased intestinal permeability. Animal studies show higher translocation of bacteria due to the decrease in gut integrity, although conclusive evidence of translocation in humans remains to be documented. These changes reverse with the addition of enteral nutrition, and the maintenance of trophic or hypocaloric enteral feeding is recommended even in cases where the patient cannot tolerate full enteral feeding and requires intravenous supplementation.

When to initiate TPN remains a matter of debate, although most guidelines recommend waiting 7 days to start TPN except in cases of significant pre-ICU malnourishment. The addition of TPN to inadequate enteral nutrition after 8 days was found to result in a shorter duration of mechanical ventilation, lower rate of infection, fewer days on renal replacement therapy, and lower risk of cholestasis as compared to TPN initiation within the first 48 hours of ICU admission. Indications for TPN rather than enteral feeding include small bowel obstruction, complete pseudo-obstruction, active gastrointestinal bleeding, high-output enteric fistulas, and short gut syndrome with insufficient residual function to absorb adequate enteral nutrition.

### References

1. Wischmeyer PE. Nutrition therapy in sepsis. *Crit Care Clin*. 2018;34(1):107-125.
2. Casaer MP, Mesotten D, Hermans G, et al. Early versus late parenteral nutrition in critically ill adults. *N Engl J Med*. 2011;365:506-517.

---

**46.** Correct Answer: D

**Rationale:**

Intrinsic PEEP, also known as auto-PEEP or air trapping, is a serious complication of mechanical ventilation and can lead to significant hemodynamic instability. Patients with obstructive airway disease with reduced expiratory flow (e.g., asthma, COPD) are at especially high risk for auto-PEEP with mechanical ventilation. Auto-PEEP reduces cardiac preload and can culminate in obstructive shock and cardiac arrest similar to a tension pneumothorax. Cardiac arrest following intubation and mechanical ventilation, particularly in patients with obstructive lung disease, should raise suspicion for auto-PEEP. Disconnecting from the Ambu bag or ventilator should be the first intervention in cases of suspected auto-PEEP.

Bronchodilators can help patients with COPD; however, it is not an appropriate plan of action in this hemodynamically unstable patient. He is not demonstrating other signs of possible tension pneumothorax (unilateral absence of breath sounds, distended neck veins). Obtaining a CXR may be helpful if mainstem intubation, pulmonary edema, or pneumothorax are suspected; however in this case, it would not be the most appropriate next step in management.

### References

1. Barash PG, Cullen BF, Stoelting RK, et al, eds. Chapter 57: Critical care medicine. In: *Clinical Anesthesia*. 8th ed. Philadelphia: Lippincott, Williams & Wilkins; 2017.
2. Laghi F., Goyal A. Auto-PEEP in respiratory failure. *Minerva Anestesiologica* 2012;78(2):201-221.

---

**47.** Correct Answer: B

**Rationale:**

Ventilator-associated pneumonia (VAP) is diagnosed in 5% to 15% of patients on mechanical ventilation and carries significant morbidity and mortality. VAP increases the duration of mechanical ventilation and ICU length of stay and has a mortality of about 10%.

The most effective way to prevent VAP is to minimize duration of mechanical ventilation. Recent evidence-based recommendations for VAP prevention include the following:

- Use noninvasive positive-pressure ventilation (NIPPV) if possible
- Decrease duration of mechanical ventilation by minimizing sedation and performing daily SBTs
- Elevate head of bed 30 to 45 degrees
- Oral hygiene with chlorhexidine
- Use endotracheal tubes with subglottic secretion drainage ports if patients are likely to be intubated for more than 2 to 3 days

Interventions that are *not* recommended for VAP prevention include early tracheostomy, stress ulcer prophylaxis, and monitoring gastric residual volumes. Monitoring for regurgitation or vomiting is sufficient for detection for feeding intolerance and risk of aspiration.

### References

1. Klompas M, Branson R, Eichenwald EC, et al. Strategies to prevent ventilator-associated pneumonia in acute care hospitals: 2014 update. *Infect Control Hosp Epidemiol*. 2014;35(8):915-936.
2. Maselli DJ, Restrepo Marcos I. Strategies in the prevention of ventilator-associated pneumonia. *Ther Adv Respir Dis*. 2011;5:131-141.

**48.** Correct Answer: D

**Rationale:**

Catheter-related bloodstream infections (CRBSIs) carry significant morbidity and cost. Diagnosis requires a positive blood culture from the catheter *and* a matching positive blood culture obtained from another site. The catheter must have been in place for at least 48 hours prior to positive blood cultures, and other sources of bacteremia should be ruled out. A positive blood culture from the catheter with negative blood culture from another site is suggestive of line colonization or contaminant. The most common pathogens are coagulase-negative staphylococci, *Staphylococcus aureus*, enterococci, and *Candida*; gram-negative rods are responsible for only about 20% of infections. A recent meta-analysis showed that arterial lines do in fact carry a risk of CRBSI with an incidence of 3.4/1000 arterial catheters.

Key recommendations in recent Centers for Disease Control and Prevention (CDC) guidelines for CRBSI prevention include:

- Do not replace CVCs unless clinically indicated; routine replacement of CVCs does not reduce the risk of CRBSI
- Maximal sterile barrier precautions are required for CVC insertion and guidewire exchange and include sterile gown and gloves, mask, cap, and full body drape
- Avoid femoral line placement in obese adult patients
- Avoid subclavian placement in patients with end-stage renal disease due to risk of causing subclavian vein stenosis
- Chlorhexidine with alcohol for skin disinfection is more effective compared with povidone iodine or alcohol
- Replace dressings on CVC at minimum of every 7 days unless loose or soiled
- Placement of peripheral arterial lines requires a cap, mask, sterile gloves, small sterile drape, and chlorhexidine for skin preparation. Femoral and axillary arterial lines require maximal sterile barrier precautions described above for CVCs

References

1. Barash PG, et al. *Critical Care Medicine. Clinical Anesthesia.* 8th ed. Philadelphia: Wolters Kluwer; 2013:1635-1660.
2. O'Horo JC, Maki DG, Krupp AE, Safdar N. Arterial catheters as a source of bloodstream infection: a systematic review and meta-analysis. *Crit Care Med.* 2014;42(6):1334-1339.
3. O'Grady NP. *Guidelines for the Prevention of Intravascular Catheter-Related Infections*; 2011. Available at: https://www.cdc.gov/ infectioncontrol/guidelines/ bsi/background/prevention-strategies.html.

**49.** Correct Answer: E

**Rationale:**

Catheter-associated urinary tract infection is the most preventable healthcare-acquired infection. The most effective method to prevent CAUTI is to remove indwelling catheters as soon as they are no longer indicated. Each day a urinary catheter is in place carries up to 10% risk of developing bacteriuria. There are several alternatives to an indwelling urinary catheter. Intermittent straight catheterization reduces the risk of CAUTI compared with indwelling catheters and is recommended in patients with urinary retention. External catheters ("condom catheters") have a reduced rate of complications compared with indwelling catheters and are recommended in male patients with incontinence. Routine catheter exchange in the absence of infection does not reduce the risk of CAUTI and is not recommended.

Symptomatic CAUTI should be treated with antibiotics. Asymptomatic catheter-associated bacteriuria should *not* be treated with antibiotics. Monitoring for asymptomatic bacteriuria is not recommended.

Acceptable indications for indwelling urinary catheters according to CDC guidelines:

- Acute urinary retention
- Close monitoring of urine output in critically ill patients
- Incontinence in setting of open sacral or perineal wounds (incontinence is otherwise not an indication for indwelling catheters)
- Comfort care at end of life

References

1. Tenke P, Köves B, Johansen TE. An update on prevention and treatment of catheter-associated urinary tract infections. *Curr Opin Infect Dis.* 2014;27(1):102-107.
2. O'Grady NP. *Guidelines for the Prevention of Intravascular Catheter-Related Infections*; 2011. Available at: https://www.cdc.gov/ infectioncontrol/guidelines/ bsi/background/prevention-strategies.html.

**50.** Correct Answer: D

**Rationale:**

*Mycobacterium tuberculosis* (MTB) outbreaks in healthcare facilities have been attributed to delayed diagnosis and inadequate precautions. MTB is transmitted through respiratory droplets. The risk of transmission is especially high for healthcare workers in close contact with respiratory secretions, including intubation, suctioning, and bronchoscopy. When MTB disease is suspected, airborne precautions should be instituted immediately, including admitting the patient to a negative-pressure room and requiring healthcare workers to wear fit-tested N95 respirators. Before each use of an N95 respirator, the user should confirm a tight mask seal by positive- and negative-pressure leak tests. In the positive-pressure leak test, the wearer exhales with hands around the corners of the mask; if airflow is detected, there is a leak around the mask. In the negative-pressure leak test, the wearer inhales deeply; the mask should move closer to the face, indicating a tight seal. A bacterial filter should be applied to the ventilator circuit.

Airborne precautions should only be discontinued when (1) the patient is found to have another condition that explains the symptoms or (2) there are three negative sputum acid-fast bacilli (AFB) smears obtained 8 to 24 hours apart. A tuberculin skin test is unreliable in patients with active MTB disease and/or human immunodeficiency virus (HIV) due to anergy and cannot be used to rule out MTB in these patients.

MTB is not acquired through surfaces; contact precautions are therefore not necessary. If the suspicion for MTB disease is high and the patient is critically ill, empiric therapy for TB disease should begin with a four-drug regimen to prevent development of resistance.

### Reference

1. Centers for Disease Control and Prevention. Guidelines for preventing the transmission of *Mycobacterium tuberculosis* in health-care settings, 2005. *MMWR*. 2005;54(RR-17).

---

### 51. Correct Answer: E

**Rationale:**

Key criteria for extubation in the ICU include resolution of the indication for intubation, adequate gas exchange, ability to protect the airway (including strong cough and minimal secretions), stable hemodynamics, and absence of airway obstruction. The ability to follow commands is not a requirement for extubation. Delirium, dementia, or other neurological disorders may impair a patient's ability to follow commands but are not indications for intubation so long as the patient is able to protect the airway.

The amount of pressure support, if any, to provide during a SBT and the duration of the trial are controversial. Disconnecting from the ventilator and breathing with a T-piece requires the most patient effort. However, studies comparing SBT with a T-piece versus low-pressure support ventilation showed no difference in the rate of reintubation. Recent guidelines for ventilator weaning now recommend inspiratory pressure support (5-8 cm $H_2O$) over T-piece or CPAP during SBT. A study comparing SBT lasting 30 minutes versus 2 hours showed no difference in rate of reintubation. However, these findings may not apply to patients at high risk of reintubation, and it has been suggested that high-risk patients should meet more stringent criteria for extubation (e.g., prolonged T-piece trial).

The rapid shallow breathing index, calculated by respiratory rate/tidal volume, is helpful in identifying patients likely to fail extubation. Rapid shallow breathing index greater than 100 is associated with extubation failure. The absence of a cuff leak implies airway obstruction, and extubation should not be attempted in the absence of leak. However, the presence of a cuff leak does not eliminate the possibility of significant airway obstruction after extubation.

### References

1. Esteban A, Alía I, Gordo F, et al. Extubation outcome after spontaneous breathing trials with T-tube or pressure support ventilation. The Spanish Lung Failure Collaborative Group. *Am J Respir Crit Care Med*. 1997;156(2 Pt 1):459-465.
2. Perren A, Domenighetti G, Mauri S, Genini F, Vizzardi N. Protocol-directed weaning from mechanical ventilation: clinical outcome in patients randomized for a 30-min or 120-min trial with pressure support ventilation. *Intensive Care Med*. 2002;28:1058-1063.
3. Thille AW, Richard JC, Brochard L. The decision to extubate in the intensive care unit. *Am J Respir Crit Care Med*. 2013;187(12):1294-1302.
4. Ouellette DR, Patel S, Girard TD, et al. Liberation from mechanical ventilation: an Official American College of Chest Physicians/American Thoracic Society Clinical Practice Guidelines. *Chest*. 2017;151(1):166-180.

---

### 52. Correct Answer: D

**Rationale:**

This patient has an enlarged right ventricle. His hypoxemic respiratory failure is likely secondary from a pulmonary embolism. Clues to this diagnosis include his recent air travel and newly diagnosed malignancy, all increasing his risk of deep venous thrombosis and pulmonary embolism. Focused bedside cardiac ultrasonography can be extremely valuable in the rapid evaluation of patients presenting with shock. This is a parasternal short axis view which can be obtained by placing the ultrasound probe in the left third to fifth intercostal spaces with the marker facing the left shoulder. Normally, the right ventricle should be smaller than the left ventricle, and the interventricular septum should bow into the right ventricle due to the higher filling pressures of the left ventricle. This image is notable for a dilated right ventricle and flattened interventricular septum resulting in a D-shaped left ventricle (see image that follows), findings highly concerning for pulmonary embolism in the setting of acute hemodynamic instability. Live images may show McConnell sign: akinesis of right ventricular midwall with preserved apical function. Pulmonary embolism is a type of obstructive shock. Other etiologies of obstructive shock include tension pneumothorax and cardiac tamponade.

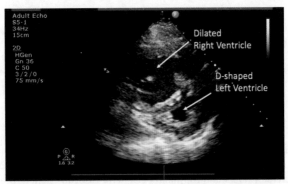

Distributive shock (e.g., due to sepsis or anaphylaxis) would show underfilled and hyperdynamic ventricles, not signs of right ventricle overload as seen here. Cardiogenic shock is a possibility given evidence of cardiac ischemia on ECG, however the absence of a dilated left ventricle makes this less likely.

### Reference

1. Chapter 11: Echocardiographic diagnosis and monitoring of right ventricular function. In: Levitov AB, Mayo PH, Slonim AD. *Critical Care Ultrasonography*. The McGraw-Hill Companies, Inc.; 2014.

---

**53.** Correct Answer: D

### Rationale:

This subcostal view shows a pericardial effusion with right ventricle collapse, which is highly concerning for tamponade in the presence of hemodynamic instability. A PA line would show elevated and theoretically "equal" CVP and PA pressures due to impaired ventricle filling and elevated systemic vascular resistance (SVR, a compensatory response to obstructive shock). HR would be elevated as a compensatory response to maintain cardiac output in the setting of reduced stroke volume. Physical examination findings might include muffled heart sounds, distended neck veins, and pulsus paradoxus (Beck triad).

Choice A is consistent with hypovolemic shock with low CVP, PA pressures, and compensatory elevated HR and SVR. While the ventricles appear underfilled on echocardiography, this is more likely due to restricted filling. It can also be difficult to assess ventricular filling on long-axis views; the parasternal short axis midpapillary view is most reliable for volume assessment. Choice B is normal values. Choice C is consistent with cardiogenic shock with an inappropriately low HR (perhaps in the setting of conduction block or beta blocker use). Choice E is consistent with distributive shock with low CVP, PA pressures, SVR, and compensatory elevated HR and cardiac output.

### Reference

1. Marino PL. The pulmonary artery catheter. *The ICU Book*. 4th ed. Philadelphia: Wolters Kluwer, 2014:135-150.

---

**54.** Correct Answer: D

### Rationale:

This patient's presentation is concerning for postoperative urosepsis, and therefore, empiric broad-spectrum antibiotic therapy should be initiated immediately. Given her last known urine culture was resistant to cephalosporins, cefepime is not the best choice of drugs, nor does she have a need for vancomycin; hence, meropenem would be the most appropriate antibiotic at this time. In addition, she has already received a fluid bolus and remains hypotensive and in shock; hence, initiating vasopressor therapy at this time is warranted. Norepinephrine is the first-line vasopressor in septic shock and should be titrated to a goal MAP 65. Vasopressin may be added to reduce the norepinephrine requirement and should be added in general, given the relative "vasopressin deficiency" that is seen in patients with septic shock. Patients undergoing surgical procedures to remove kidney stones are at risk for urosepsis secondary to manipulation of the urinary tract. Signs of sepsis frequently surface within 6 hours of the surgical procedure.

The latest Sepsis-3 guidelines offer the qSOFA criteria as a simple bedside screening tool for evaluating patients with possible sepsis. The qSOFA criteria are based on physical examination and vital signs: respiratory rate > 22 breaths/min, altered mental status, and systolic blood pressure < 100 mm Hg. A qSOFA score > 2 in a patient with suspected infection (as this patient has) should prompt further workup for sepsis and organ dysfunction including cultures, CBC, metabolic panel, and lactate. The cornerstone of sepsis treatment is timely initiation of broad-spectrum antibiotics (ideally within 1 hour).

Postoperative urosepsis following stone removal surgery can occur simply from manipulation of the urinary tract and does not necessarily indicate a retained stone. Returning to the OR for repeat ureteroscopy is not currently indicated for this patient at this time.

## References

1. Singer M, Deutschman CS, Seymour CW, et al. The third international consensus definitions for sepsis and septic shock (sepsis-3). *JAMA*. 2016;315(8):801-810.
2. Mariappan P, Tolley DA. Endoscopic stone surgery: minimizing the risk of post-operative sepsis. *Curr Opin Urol*. 2005;15(2).
3. Rhodes A et al. Surviving sepsis campaign: International guidelines for management of sepsis and septic shock: 2016. *Crit Care Med*. 2017;45(3).

## 55. Correct Answer: B

**Rationale:**

Given the nature of his injury and MRI findings, his hemodynamic instability is most likely due to neurogenic shock. Cervical spinal cord injury interrupts input to the sympathetic neurons in the spinal cord (located T1-L2) and leading to loss of cardioaccelerator fibers, inotropy, and peripheral vasoconstriction. Bradycardia and hypotension resolve over time as the spinal cord sympathetic nerves develop automaticity.

Neurogenic shock, which refers to the hemodynamic changes seen with a sympathectomy, is often confused with spinal shock. Spinal shock describes transient flaccid muscle weakness following spinal cord injury. Obstructive shock could be seen in tension pneumothorax, but a small pneumothorax is unlikely to cause the degree of hemodynamic instability seen here. Hypovolemic shock is also unlikely to explain his degree of hemodynamic instability. In pure hypovolemic shock, 30% to 40% of blood volume must be lost before hypotension results (class III shock), and a grade 2 splenic laceration would be unlikely to cause this degree of bleeding. Hypovolemic and obstructive shock would also be accompanied by compensatory tachycardia, not seen here. While trauma patients are certainly at risk for infection, septic shock would be unlikely to have developed this early.

### Reference

1. Ruiz IA, Squair JW, Phillips AA, et al. Incidence and natural progression of neurogenic shock after traumatic spinal cord injury. *J Neurotrauma*. 2018;35(3).

## 56. Correct Answer: C

**Rationale:**

Early enteral nutrition in the ICU has been shown to reduce the risk of infection and mortality. Enteral nutrition promotes gut integrity, which provides a barrier to infection. Enteral nutrition is strongly preferred to parenteral nutrition, which carries risk of infection, hypertriglyceridemia, and liver dysfunction. However, parenteral nutrition may be unavoidable in cases of severe malabsorption (e.g., short gut syndrome).

The most recent ASPEN guidelines advocate strongly for early enteral feeding in the ICU within 24 to 48 hours of admission and address concerns related to enteral feeding. Initiation of enteral nutrition should not be delayed until there are clear "signs of contractility" namely bowel sounds, flatus, or stool. A postpyloric tube is not required for all patients receiving enteral nutrition but should be considered in patients at high risk for aspiration or with signs of gastric feeding intolerance. Guidelines recommend against routinely checking gastric residual volumes as a way to assess feeding tolerance. The "head of the bed" should be elevated to 30 to 45 degrees to reduce aspiration risk, and prokinetic agents, such as erythromycin and metoclopramide, could be considered in patients with feeding intolerance.

### Reference

1. McClave SA et al. Guidelines for the provision and assessment of nutrition support therapy in the adult critically ill patient: Society of Critical Care Medicine (SCCM) and American Society for Parenteral and Enteral Nutrition (A.S.P.E.N.). *J Parenter Enteral Nutr*. 2016;40(2):159-211.

## 57. Correct Answer: C

**Rationale:**

This patient likely has cardiogenic shock due to an acute myocardial infarction (MI). She has evidence of organ hypoperfusion, with an elevated lactate and would benefit from an inotropic agent while undergoing revascularization. Dobutamine is a beta-1 and beta-2 agonist with inotropic and chronotropic effects and is the preferred agent in cardiogenic shock. Dobutamine can cause a mild decrease in SVR due to its beta-2 agonism, and patients should be monitored closely for development of hypotension. Norepinephrine has beta-1 effects as well but increases afterload and therefore can adversely affect cardiac output secondary to its intrinsic alpha-1 agonism. Norepinephrine is therefore not the preferred inotrope in cardiogenic shock but could be used in addition to dobutamine to counteract hypotension.

A fluid bolus is not likely to be beneficial in cardiogenic shock, as cardiac filling pressures are typically elevated. A fluid bolus may even be harmful by worsening of any pulmonary edema that could be present. Dopamine is associated with significant increased risks of dysrhythmias and should be avoided in cardiogenic shock.

### Reference

1. De Backer D, Biston P, Devriendt J, et al. Comparison of dopamine and norepinephrine in the treatment of shock. *N Engl J Med*. 2010;362:779-789.

**58.** Correct Answer: B

**Rationale:**

This patient has severe hypophosphatemia and other electrolyte disturbances coinciding with initiation of nutrition which is concerning for refeeding syndrome. His history of dementia and failure to thrive in combination with a low serum albumin suggest he is chronically malnourished and puts him at high risk for refeeding syndrome. When refeeding syndrome is suspected, the first step is to temporarily stop feeding while aggressively repleting electrolytes.

While exact criteria for refeeding syndrome have not been established, it can be broadly defined as severe electrolyte and fluid shifts following initiation of nutrition (most commonly hypophosphatemia, hypomagnesemia, and hypokalemia). Electrolyte depletion occurs due to sudden increased utilization. Clinical symptoms of refeeding syndrome include encephalopathy, heart failure, edema, arrhythmias, respiratory failure, and arrhythmias. Refeeding syndrome typically begins within the first 72 hours after initiating nutrition. Malnourished patients are at high risk for refeeding syndrome; risk factors include alcoholism, anorexia nervosa, low body mass index, and low prealbumin.

Enteral feeds should not be increased if refeeding syndrome is suspected. Electrolyte content can be adjusted when feeding is restarted, but electrolyte repletion should be intravenous initially. Feeds should be restarted at a lower rate or calorie content. Hypophosphatemia can be seen in hyperparathyroidism, but refeeding syndrome is more likely in this scenario. This patient's calcium level is also not consistent with hyperparathyroidism (his corrected calcium level for low albumin is 8.5 mg/dL, which is normal).

Reference

1. Friedli N, Stanga Z, Sobotka L, et al. Revisiting the refeeding syndrome: results of a systematic review. *Nutrition.* 2017;35:151-160.

**59.** Correct Answer: A

**Rationale:**

This patient's presentation is concerning for organophosphate exposure. Organophosphates are found in pesticides, although use has decreased in the United States per the Environmental Protection Agency. Organophosphates used as chemical weapons are called nerve agents and include tabun, sarin, and soman. Nerve agent exposure can occur via inhalation, skin exposure, or ingestion. Organophosphates inhibit acetylcholinesterase. Excessive stimulation of muscarinic receptors produces signs of parasympathetic stimulation: defecation, urination, miosis, bradycardia, bronchorrhea, bronchospasm, emesis, lacrimation, and salivation (mnemonic DUMBBBELS). It is important to remember that anticholinergic crisis can include signs of sympathetic stimulation due to activation of nicotinic receptors in the sympathetic ganglia. Stimulation of nicotinic receptors at the neuromuscular junction produces fasciculations and weakness progressing to paralysis (similar to succinylcholine). The signs of nicotinic stimulation can be remembered by the mnemonic "Monday-Tuesday-Wednesday-Thursday-Friday" (mydriasis-tachycardia-weakness-hypertension-fasciculations). CNS symptoms of organophosphate toxicity include headache, agitation, confusion, seizures, and coma. Death is usually caused by respiratory insufficiency (aspiration, bronchospasm, CNS depression, or weakness) or seizures.

Chlorine and phosgene gases cause respiratory failure resembling ARDS and is managed supportively. Cyanide can be aerosolized as used as a chemical weapon; its hallmark is severe lactic acidosis caused by inhibition of cytochrome oxidase. *B. anthracis* is a gram-positive spore-producing bacillus (anthrax) that can be used as a biologic weapon. Inhalation of Anthrax spores is highly lethal and produces a flulike syndrome progressing to dyspnea, hemoptysis, and chest pain with widened mediastinum on CXR.

Reference

1. King AM, Aaron CK. Organophosphate and carbamate poisoning. *Emerg Med Clin N Am.* 2015;33:133-151.

**60.** Correct Answer: C

**Rationale:**

Luckily for this patient, benzodiazepines are rarely the sole cause of a fatal drug overdose and do not cause severe respiratory depression or hemodynamic instability unless ingested with other sedatives, such as opiates or alcohol. Overdoses of benzodiazepines are typically treated with supportive care and watchful waiting. Flumazenil is a benzodiazepine receptor antagonist; however it is rarely used for overdoses when the patient is stable, for fear that it will precipitate withdrawal, namely seizures. She will likely benefit from admission to an inpatient psychiatry ward; however, she should be monitored in the emergency department or on a floor that has telemetry capabilities, until her mental status improves. She does arouse and is maintaining adequate oxygen saturations, so intubation is not indicated at this time. A head CT scan is not indicated at this time, given the lack of a trauma history and lack of focal deficits; her altered mental status can be explained by the overdose of lorazepam.

Reference

1. An H, Godwin J. Flumazenil in benzodiazepine overdose. *CMAJ.* 2016;188(17-18):E537.

**61.** Correct Answer: B

**Rationale:**

This patient's high minute ventilation is likely driven by respiratory compensation to his metabolic acidosis. Thus, further evaluation to identify the etiology of his metabolic acidosis is essential.

Based on blood gas analysis, he has partially compensated metabolic acidosis. The anion gap is $Na - Cl - HCO_3 = 138 - 110 - 14 = 14$. Hence, this patient has normal anion gap metabolic acidosis. Two main etiologies for normal anion gap metabolic acidosis are renal and gastrointestinal loss of bicarbonate. This can be further evaluated by measuring urine anion gap. A positive value of urine anion gap suggests renal bicarbonate wasting. On the other hand, a negative value of urine anion gap suggests gastrointestinal loss of bicarbonate. This patient's urine anion gap is positive (urine $Na + K - Cl = 40 + 10 - 15 = 35$). The likely cause for his metabolic acidosis is renal bicarbonate losses, likely from AKI. It is typically seen in patients recovering from AKI and typically resolves in a few weeks. Meanwhile, this acidosis is managed by providing bicarbonate replacement.

The acidosis is not severe enough to necessitate hemodialysis, and no other indications for hemodialysis exist. Hypoperfusion and hypovolemia cause lactic acidosis, which results in anion gap metabolic acidosis. The absence of anion gap metabolic acidosis in this patient makes hypovolemia less likely, and thus additional fluid bolus is not needed. There is no indication for loop diuretics in this patient.

References

1. Rastegar M, Nagami GT. Non-anion gap metabolic acidosis: a clinical approach to evaluation. *Am J Kidney Dis.* 2017;69(2):296-301.
2. Adeva-Andany MM, Fernández-Fernández C, Mouriño-Bayolo D, Castro-Quintela E, Domínguez-Montero A. Sodium bicarbonate therapy in patients with metabolic acidosis. *ScientificWorldJournal.* 2014;2014:627673.

**62.** Correct Answer: C

**Rationale:**

This patient has metabolic acidosis based on the pH of 7.31 and a decreased serum bicarbonate. The anion gap here is $Na - Cl - HCO_3 = 138 - 98 - 19 = 21$. The anion gap corrected for serum albumin is = anion gap + $2.5 \times (4 - \text{serum albumin}) = 21 + 2.5 (4 - 3) = 23.5$. Thus, this patient has anion gap metabolic acidosis. To identify any coexisting acid-base abnormality, we need to calculate delta ratio = (anion gap − 12)/ (24 − bicarbonate). Here, the delta ratio is $(23.5 - 12)/(24 - 19) = 2.3$.

In the presence of anion gap metabolic acidosis, a delta ratio of >2 suggests concomitant metabolic alkalosis. A delta ratio of 1:2 suggests pure anion gap metabolic acidosis and a delta ratio of <1 suggests concomitant normal anion gap metabolic acidosis. Hence, our patient has both anion gap metabolic acidosis and metabolic alkalosis (option C). In this patient, the anion gap acidosis is likely from hypovolemia causing lactic acidosis, and the metabolic alkalosis is from loss of gastric acid from vomiting.

Reference

1. Reddy P, Mooradian AD. Clinical utility of anion gap in deciphering acid-base disorders. *Int J Clin Pract.* 2009;63(10):1516-1525.

**63.** Correct Answer: B

**Rationale:**

Based on the arterial pH, this patient has uncompensated metabolic acidosis. Investigating etiology of metabolic acidosis requires calculation of anion gap = $Na - Cl - HCO_3 = 132 - 98 - 14 = 20$. Anion gap corrected for albumin is = anion gap + $2.5 \times (4 - \text{serum albumin}) = 20 + 2.5 (4 - 3) = 22.5$. Thus, the patient has anion gap metabolic acidosis. To identify any coexisting acid-base abnormality, we need to calculate delta ratio = (anion gap − 12)/ (24 − bicarbonate). Here, the delta ratio is $(22.5 - 12)/(24 - 14) = 1$. A delta ratio of 1 suggests pure anion gap metabolic acidosis.

Since the patient does not have normal anion gap metabolic acidosis, urine anion gap is not useful. Urine chloride is used to identify different etiologies of metabolic alkalosis and so not useful for this patient. The initial step in identifying cause of anion gap metabolic acidosis is to investigate presence of usual culprits, specifically lactate and ketones. Based on this patient's history, he likely has congestive heart failure exacerbation and related tissue hypoperfusion. Hence, lactic acidosis is the most likely culprit. Since blood glucose is normal, ketoacidosis is unlikely. If no common causes of anion gap metabolic acidosis are identified, serum osmolar gap is measured to help identify uncommon causes.

Reference

1. Kraut JA, Madias NE. Metabolic acidosis: pathophysiology, diagnosis and management. *Nat Rev Nephrol.* 2010;6(5):274-285.

**64.** Correct Answer: D

**Rationale:**

Cefepime is a widely used antibiotic with neurotoxicity attributed to its ability to cross the blood-brain barrier. Symptoms include depressed consciousness, encephalopathy, aphasia, myoclonus, seizures, and coma. Known risk factors are renal dysfunction, excessive dosing, preexisting brain injury, and elevated serum cefepime concentrations. Symptoms typically occur 3 to 4 days after starting therapy and are easy to overlook, since they are similar to metabolic encephalopathy seen among many critically ill patients. Since approximately 85% of cefepime is excreted unchanged by the kidneys, renal dysfunction can dramatically increase the half-life. Hence, epileptiform activity with abnormal EEG findings is most commonly noted in patients with renal dysfunction. Symptoms improve with drug removal (discontinuation or hemodialysis), or treatment interventions (antiepileptic administration).

Reference

1. Payne LE, Gagnon DJ, Riker RR, et al. Cefepime-induced neurotoxicity: a systematic review. *Crit Care*. 2017;21(1):276.

**65.** Correct Answer: D

**Rationale:**

Diuretics cause diuresis and natriuresis. However, thiazide diuretics result in more sodium loss than water loss resulting in hyponatremia. On the other hand, loop diuretics cause more water loss than sodium loss, usually causing hypernatremia. Hence, the likely culprit for this patient's hyponatremia is the recently started hydrochlorothiazide. Diuretic use is one of the most common causes of drug-induced hyponatremia. Metformin and gabapentin are not associated with hyponatremia. Angiotensin-converting enzyme inhibitors (lisinopril) have been associated with hyponatremia due to increase in antidiuretic hormone secretion, however, is very rare.

Reference

1. Liamis G, Milionis H, Elisaf M. A review of drug-induced hyponatremia. *Am J Kidney Dis*. 2008;52(1):144-153.

**66.** Correct Answer: A

**Rationale:**

Based on the laboratory data (low sodium and low serum osmolality), the patient has hypotonic hyponatremia. Hypotonic hyponatremia is further classified into hypovolemia, euvolemic, and hypervolemic presentations. This patient's clinical presentation is consistent with hypovolemia (low blood pressure, no pulmonary edema on auscultation, low urine sodium, and history of diarrhea). Thus, this patient likely has hypovolemic hypotonic hyponatremia from sodium and water loss via gastrointestinal tract and poor oral intake. The recommended treatment strategy is volume resuscitation with normal saline. The recommended rate of correction is 6 to 12 mEq/L in 24 hours. Sodium should be frequently monitored to prevent inadvertent overcorrection. If hyponatremia persists after achieving euvolemia, salt tablets may be started. Water restriction and loop diuretics have no role in management of hypotonic hypovolemic hyponatremia.

Reference

1. Braun MM, Barstow CH, Pyzocha NJ. Diagnosis and management of sodium disorders: hyponatremia and hypernatremia. *Am Fam Physician*. 2015;91(5):299-307.

**67.** Correct Answer: C

**Rationale:**

It is recommended to start hypertonic saline in patients with severe symptomatic hyponatremia, as in this patient. Since this patient was in a state of hypovolemia, the antidiuretic hormone secretion would be at its maximum. Increasing serum sodium or volume resuscitation would lead to rapid reduction in secretion of antidiuretic hormone, leading to unwanted free water diuresis. This in turn results in a rise of serum sodium to a level higher than what is expected with the amount of hypertonic saline administered. Overcorrection of sodium increases the risk of osmotic demyelination (previously called central pontine myelinolysis). Studies have shown that adding desmopressin to the regimen (for the first 2 days) allows a more controlled rise of serum sodium by preventing free water diuresis.

References

1. Braun MM, Barstow CH, Pyzocha NJ. Diagnosis and management of sodium disorders: hyponatremia and hypernatremia. *Am Fam Physician*. 2015;91(5):299-307.
2. MacMillan TE, Tang T, Cavalcanti RB. Desmopressin to prevent rapid sodium correction in severe hyponatremia: a ystematic review. *Am J Med*. 2015;128(12):1362.e15-1362.e24.

**68.** Correct Answer: C

**Rationale:**

Polyuria, hypernatremia, and a urine osmolarity lower than serum osmolarity suggest diabetes insipidus. Chronic lithium ingestion leads to decreased renal concentrating capacity, which may evolve into nephrogenic diabetes insipidus if the patient continues to take lithium. The decreased urinary concentrating capacity is fairly common, occurring in up to 40% of patients taking lithium, though overt diabetes insipidus is less common. In most patients, stopping lithium leads to resolution of diabetes insipidus; however it can be irreversible after long-term therapy. Hence, based on his history of lithium intake in the past, he likely has nephrogenic diabetes insipidus which has persisted despite stopping lithium.

It was not apparent preoperatively since we would have been drinking water to compensate for free water loss in urine. However, postoperatively after major bowel surgery, he would be nil per oral and so is not able to maintain the compensatory polydipsia. The best strategy in this patient would be to replace free water losses intravenously, until the patient is able to take adequate water orally (option C). Desmopressin is useful in central diabetes insipidus, but not in nephrogenic diabetes insipidus, as in this case. Restarting lithium or decreasing maintenance fluids has no role in management.

References

1. Moug SJ, McKee RF, O'Reilly DS, Noble S, Boulton-Jones M. The perioperative challenge of nephrogenic diabetes insipidus: a multidisciplinary approach. *Surgeon.* 2005;3(2):89-94.
2. Irefin SA, Sonny A, Harinstein L, Popovich MJ. Postoperative adverse effects after recent or remote lithium therapy. *J Clin Anesth.* 2014;26(3):231-234.

**69.** Correct Answer: B

**Rationale:**

Lithium is freely filtered through the glomeruli but about 80% is reabsorbed via the proximal tubule. Lithium is widely distributed in the body and is transported similar to sodium by kidneys. Hence, states in which there is a negative sodium balance (e.g., dehydration, congestive heart failure, cirrhosis) lead to marked reduction in fractional excretion of lithium resulting in elevated serum levels. Due to tissue saturation with lithium, chronic lithium patients may manifest toxicity even with small elevations in serum lithium level when compared with acute toxicity.

Manifestations of lithium toxicity are predominantly neurological. They range from drowsiness, slurred speech and psychomotor slowing to seizure, coma, and death in severe cases. Withholding lithium therapy is usually sufficient. But, if symptoms worsen or become life-threatening, despite stopping lithium, hemodialysis needs to be strongly considered.

This patient's BUN to creatinine ratio (BUN:Cr > 20:1) suggests a prerenal physiology (dehydration). This promotes renal reabsorption of lithium predisposing the patient to acute lithium toxicity.

References

1. Grandjean EM, Aubry JM. Lithium: updated human knowledge using an evidence-based approach: part III: clinical safety. *CNS Drugs.* 2009;23(5):397-418.
2. Timmer RT, Sands JM. Lithium intoxication. *J Am Soc Nephrol.* 1999;10:666-674.

**70.** Correct Answer: B

**Rationale:**

The pulmonary capillary wedge pressure is used as a surrogate to estimate the left ventricular end-diastolic pressure. Thus, the portion of the waveform corresponding to the end of diastole (at the very end of ventricular filling and at the end of the atrial kick) will provide the best estimate of left ventricular end-diastolic pressure. The portions of the cardiac cycle associated the venous waveform (central venous or pulmonary venous) are explained below:

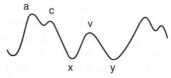

| a-wave | Atrial contraction |
| --- | --- |
| c-wave | Bulging of the atrioventricular valve from ventricular systole |
| v-wave | Filling of the atria during systole (atrioventricular valves closed) |
| x-descent | Atrial relaxation |
| y-descent | Early ventricular filling during ventricular diastole |

The location on the left atrial pressure wave that best reflects end-diastolic pressure is the point just prior to the c-wave. Point B (option B) corresponds to the point in the waveform just prior to c-wave, and hence is the correct answer.

Another important challenge in determining the wedge pressure occurs in patients with large intrathoracic pressure swings, such as in positive-pressure ventilation or labored spontaneous breathing. In such instances, measurement of wedge pressure at the end expiratory best estimates the left ventricular end-diastolic pressure.

### References

1. Barash PG, Cullen BF, Stoelting RK, et al. Chapter 25: Commonly used monitoring techniques. *Clinical Anesthesia*. Philadelphia: Lippincott, Williams & Wilkins; 2013.
2. Miller RD. Chapter 45: Cardiovascular monitoring. *Miller's Anesthesia*. W B Saunders Company; 2015.

### 71. Correct Answer: B

**Rationale:**

The ECG strip demonstrates an irregular narrow complex tachycardia. The most common differential is atrial fibrillation. However, presence of P waves before the QRS complex rules out atrial fibrillation. This rhythm strip shows multisite or multifocal atrial tachycardia. Multifocal atrial tachycardia is a form of supraventricular tachycardia (heart rate > 100 beats/min) where the atrial contraction occurs from the impulse generated by different clusters of cells outside of the sinoatrial node. Thus, different morphologies of P waves are present in multifocal atrial tachycardia. The arrhythmia is called a multifocal atrial rhythm or wandering atrial pacemaker if the rate is between 60 and 100 beats/min.

It is seen in older patients and is typically associated with exacerbations of COPD or other lung disease. It usually arises in the context of an underlying medical condition, and treatment of the underlying cause typically results in its resolution. If the tachycardia is symptomatic and sustained (as in our patient), beta blockade or calcium channel blockers are effective. Multifocal atrial tachycardia may be associated with or precede atrial fibrillation. There is no role for DC cardioversion or for antiarrhythmic agents in multifocal atrial tachycardia. This rhythm is typically not representative of an ischemic etiology and further cardiac workup is not necessary.

### Reference

1. Barash PG, Cullen BF, Stoelting RK, et al. *Clinical Anesthesia: Appendix 1: Atlas of Electrocardiography*. Philadelphia: Lippincott, Williams & Wilkins; 2013.

### 72. Correct Answer: A

**Rationale:**

Discussion: PVR is calculated as follows:

$$PVR\left(dyne\text{-}sec/cm^5\right) = \frac{\left(MPAP\ in\ mm\ Hg - PCWP\ in\ mm\ Hg\right)X\ 80}{Cardiac\ output\ in\ \frac{L}{min}}$$

MPAP: mean pulmonary arterial pressure, PCWP: pulmonary capillary wedge pressure, 80 is the conversion factor to equalize measurement units and obtain PVR in its most commonly reported unit, dyne-sec/ cm$^5$. The normal range of PVR is 20 to 120 dyne-s/cm$^5$. In this patient, PVR = (28 − 14) × 80/5.2 = 215 dynes-s/cm$^5$.

### Reference

1. Hensley FA, Martin DE, Gravlee GP. Chapter 1: Cardiovascular physiology: a primer. *A Practical Approach to Cardiac Anesthesia*. Philadelphia: Lippincott, Williams & Wilkins; 2012.

### 73. Correct Answer: C

**Rationale:**

Surviving Sepsis Campaign bundle was published in 2018, which calls for recognizing sepsis as a medical emergency, similar to acute myocardial infarction or stroke, where early diagnosis and appropriate immediate management improves outcomes. The elements of the bundle intended to be initiated in the first hour are (1) measure lactate, (2) blood cultures before antibiotics, (3) broad-spectrum antibiotics, (4) initial resuscitation (30 mL/kg crystalloids) for hypotension or lactate >4 mmol/L, and (5) vasopressors to maintain MAP > 65 mm Hg. Serum procalcitonin is not a required aspect of the bundle.

### Reference

1. Levy MM, Evans LE, Rhodes A. The surviving sepsis campaign bundle: 2018 update. *Crit Care Med*. 2018;46(6):997-1000.

**74.** Correct Answer: B

**Rationale:**

The definitions of sepsis, septic shock, and organ dysfunction have largely remained unchanged for more than 2 decades prompting the development of the Sepsis-3 guidelines. Sepsis is a syndrome defined as life-threatening organ dysfunction caused by a dysregulated host response to infection. SIRS criteria are no longer recommended to diagnose sepsis, since SIRS may simply reflect an appropriate host response which is frequently adaptive. A new screening criteria, qSOFA was therefore coined comprising of three components: altered mentation, systolic BP < 100 mm Hg, and respiratory rate > 22 breaths/min. In patients with a suspicion of infection, qSOFA score >2 identifies patients who are likely to have a prolonged ICU stay or in-hospital mortality, from sepsis. This simple scoring system will allow early identification and triage of patients with (or at risk for) sepsis, enabling early intervention. Lactate is a component of qSOFA assessment.

References

1. Singer M, Deutschman CS, Seymour CW, et al. The third international consensus definitions for sepsis and septic shock (sepsis-3). *JAMA*. 2016;315(8):801-810.
2. Seymour CW, Liu VX, Iwashyna TJ, et al. Assessment of clinical criteria for sepsis: for the third international consensus definitions for sepsis and septic shock (sepsis-3). *JAMA*. 2016;315(8):762-774.

**75.** Correct Answer: C

**Rationale:**

Early effective fluid resuscitation is crucial for stabilization of sepsis-induced tissue hypoperfusion or septic shock. Early goal-directed therapy, based on the protocol published by Rivers et al., uses a series of "goals" that included CVP and central venous oxygen saturation (option A and B). This approach has now been challenged following the failure to show a mortality reduction in three subsequent large multicenter randomized controlled trials. The same holds true for other static measurements of right or left heart pressures or volumes (option D). Dynamic measures of assessing whether a patient requires additional fluid have been shown to be superior in predicting those patients who will respond to a fluid challenge by increasing stroke volume. After initial resuscitation (30 mL/kg crystalloids over 3 hours), further volume resuscitation in septic shock should be guided by dynamic indices of volume responsiveness. Dynamic indices of volume responsiveness include PLR (option C), fluid challenges against stroke volume measurements, or the variations in systolic pressure, pulse pressure, or stroke volume to changes in intrathoracic pressure induced by mechanical ventilation.

Reference

1. Rhodes A, Evans LE, Alhazzani W, et al. Surviving sepsis campaign: international guidelines for management of sepsis and septic shock: 2016. *Crit Care Med*. 2017;45(3):486-552.

**76.** Correct Answer: B

**Rationale:**

Warfarin anticoagulation is challenging because of its narrow therapeutic range and the wide variation in inter-individual response and consequent requirement to vary dosage. Warfarin is metabolized to inactive form predominantly by hepatic microsomal enzymes (cytochrome P450). Polymorphisms in the CYP2C9 gene affect the rate at which patients metabolize S-warfarin, the most active enantiomer of the drug. Amiodarone can interact with warfarin metabolism by inhibiting CYP2C9. It leads to increased anticoagulant effects of warfarin and thus warrants close monitoring and reduction in warfarin dose (option B). Some studies report effects within 1 week of coadministration, while other report effects many weeks later dependent on the final maintenance dose of amiodarone.

Reference

1. Santos PC, Soares RA, Strunz CM, et al. Simultaneous use of amiodarone influences warfarin maintenance dose but is not associated with adverse events. *J Manag Care Spec Pharm*. 2014;20(4):376-381.

**77.** Correct Answer: C

**Rationale:**

Serratia species can cause a wide spectrum of human infections that can involve the urinary tract, bloodstream, skin and soft tissue, bone, respiratory tract, CNS, and eye. Serratia is associated with nosocomial infections and hospital-associated outbreaks and should prompt evaluation for a potential common source outbreak. Serratia species are intrinsically resistant to ampicillin, amoxicillin, ampicillin-sulbactam, amoxicillin-clavulanate, narrow-spectrum cephalosporins, cephamycins, cefuroxime, macrolides, tetracyclines, nitrofurantoin, and colistin.

*S. marcescens* and several other *Serratia* species encode an inducible, chromosomal AmpC beta-lactamase. AmpC gene–mediated resistance is seen in *Serratia*, *Pseudomonas*, *Acinetobacter*, *Citrobacter*, and *Enterobacter*

(SPACE organisms). It mediates resistance to several beta-lactam antibiotics, such as penicillins and first-generation cephalosporins (e.g., cefazolin), but resistance to later-generation cephalosporins may not be detected on initial antibiotic susceptibility tests. However, treatment with third-generation cephalosporins usually leads to selection of mutants which are resistant to higher-generation cephalosporins leading to treatment failures. This is especially important in CNS infections, where the risk of emergence of AmpC-mediated resistance during therapy is high due to need for prolonged antibiotic therapy.

Hence in this patient, though resistance patterns show susceptibility to ceftriaxone, the potential for inducible resistance is high. So, escalating to meropenem is the best option. Vancomycin can be stopped since no gram-positive organisms were isolated.

### Reference

1. Meini S, Tascini C, Cei M, et al. AmpC β-lactamase-producing Enterobacterales: what a clinician should know. *Infection.* 2019;47(3):363-375.

## 78. Correct Answer: C

**Rationale:**

This patient likely has ventilator-associated pneumonia. Stenotrophomonas maltophilia is a multidrug-resistant gram-negative bacillus that is an opportunistic pathogen, particularly among hospitalized patients. Due to widespread multidrug-resistance, antibiotic options are limited and clinical data are limited regarding optimal therapy. High levels of resistance are seen to penicillin, cephalosporins, and carbapenems. More than 95% of the isolates are still susceptible to trimethoprim-sulfamethoxazole and thus is recommended as first-line therapy. Alternatives include fluroquinolones, minocycline, and tigecycline. Vancomycin and cefepime needs to be continued until respiratory culture data are finalized, since multiple pathogens can be present in ventilator-associated pneumonia.

### Reference

1. Brooke JS. Stenotrophomonas maltophilia: an emerging global opportunistic pathogen. *Clin Microbiol Rev.* 2012;25(1):2-41.

## 79. Correct Answer: D

**Rationale:**

In many instances, a report from the clinical laboratory indicating candiduria represents colonization or procurement contamination of the specimen and not invasive candidiasis. Even if infection of the urinary tract by Candida species can be confirmed, antifungal therapy is not always warranted. When candiduria is found, changing or removing the catheter can be anticipated to clear the candiduria in 20% to 40% of individuals (option D). Elimination of predisposing factors, such as discontinuing antibiotics that are no longer necessary and removal of indwelling bladder catheters, is recommended whenever feasible. If candiduria fails to resolve despite these measures, a more deep-seated infection should be suspected, and imaging of the kidneys and collecting system is indicated. Treatment with antifungal agents is not recommended unless the patient belongs to a group at high risk for dissemination, that is, neutropenic patients, very low-birth-weight infants, and patients who will undergo urologic manipulation.

### Reference

1. Pappas PG, Kauffman CA, Andes DR, et al. Clinical Practice Guideline for the Management of Candidiasis: 2016 Update by the Infectious Diseases Society of America. *Clin Infect Dis.* 2016;62(4):e1-e50.

## 80. Correct Answer: A

**Rationale:**

Chimeric antigen receptor therapy targeting CD19 is an effective treatment for refractory B-cell malignancies, especially acute lymphoblastic leukemia. As immune-based therapies for cancer become potent, more effective, and more widely available, optimal management of their unique toxicities becomes increasingly important. Cytokine release syndrome (CRS) is a potentially life-threatening toxicity that has been observed following administration of natural and bispecific antibodies and, more recently, following adoptive T-cell therapies for cancer. CRS is characterized by fever, hypotension, and respiratory insufficiency associated with elevated serum cytokines, including interleukin-6 (IL-6).

Tocilizumab is anti–IL-6 receptor monoclonal antibody approved for treatment of rheumatoid arthritis, juvenile idiopathic arthritis, and polyarticular juvenile rheumatoid arthritis. Retrospective data have shown that immunosuppression using tocilizumab with or without corticosteroids is effective against CRS and has been approved (by FDA) as the first-line therapy against severe life-threatening CRS (option A).

Abciximab is a glycoprotein IIb/IIIa receptor antagonist used as an antiplatelet agent. Intravenous immunoglobulin and plasma exchange has no current role in treatment of CRS.

### References

1. Lee DW, Gardner R, Porter DL, et al. Current concepts in the diagnosis and management of cytokine release syndrome. *Blood.* 2014;124(2):188-195.
2. Le RQ, Li L, Yuan W, et al. FDA approval summary: tocilizumab for treatment of chimeric antigen receptor t cell-induced severe or life-threatening cytokine release syndrome. *Oncologist.* 2018;23(8):943-947.

---

**81.** Correct Answer: D

**Rationale:**

Thyroid function should not be assessed in seriously ill patients unless there is a strong suspicion of thyroid dysfunction. However, when measured, most with critical illness have low serum concentrations of both thyroxine (T4) and triiodothyronine (T3). Serum thyroid-stimulating hormone (TSH) concentration also may be low in patients who may have acquired transient central hypothyroidism. It is possible that the changes in thyroid function during severe illness are protective in that they prevent excessive tissue catabolism.

Thyroid hormone metabolism pathways are depicted below, which will help understand thyroid dysfunction of critical illness.

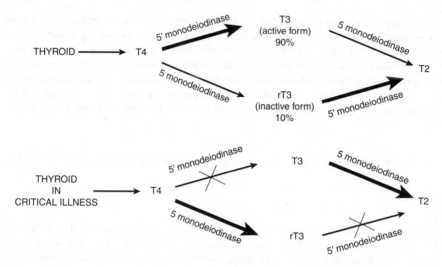

T3 is the active form of thyroid hormone. T4 is converted to T3 by 5' monodeiodinase and rT3 by 5 monodeiodinase. normally. Majority of T4 (90%) is converted to T3, the active form of the hormone. But in critical illness, cytokines and cortisol inhibit 5' monodeiodinase, leading to low T3 levels. On the other hand, rT3 is the product of 5-monodeiodination of T4, and 5 monodeiodinase is induced in (nonthyroid) critical illness, especially in the setting of hypoxia or ischemia. This leads to high levels of rT3 and lower levels of T3. Also, total T4 is low in critical illness due to reduction in binding proteins (thyroxine-binding globulin, transthyretin, and albumin).

### Reference

1. Van den Berghe G. Non-thyroidal illness in the ICU: a syndrome with different faces. *Thyroid.* 2014;24(10):1456-1465.

---

**82.** Correct Answer: B

**Rationale:**

Transvenous lead extractions are associated with a consistent rate of significant procedure-related complications. Some of them are life-threatening and occur from damage to structures adherent to the pacemaker lead. These complications include vascular laceration, pericardial effusion, cardiac tamponade, cardiac arrest, and tricuspid regurgitation, among others.

A small, nonexpanding, hemodynamically insignificant pericardial effusion can be managed expectantly with close observation in the intensive care unit. Hemodynamically significant effusion with tamponade physiology requires immediate percutaneous pericardial drainage or sternotomy.

Echocardiographic monitoring is instrumental in diagnosing cardiac tamponade in these patients. Important echocardiographic features of tamponade are right atrial collapse during systole and right ventricular collapse during diastole. The parasternal long-axis view of this patient shows a circumferential pericardial effusion. However, the image is in diastole (since aortic valve is closed), but WITHOUT right ventricular collapse.

Another important feature of cardiac tamponade is jugular venous distension or elevated CVP. American Society of Echocardiography uses the following criteria to estimate right atrial pressure (CVP) in spontaneously breathing patients based on IVC diameter and collapsibility.

| IVC DIAMETER | IVC COLLAPSIBILITY | ESTIMATED RIGHT ATRIAL PRESSURE |
| --- | --- | --- |
| <2.1 cm | >50% | 3 mm Hg |
| <2.1 cm | <50% | 8 mm Hg |
| >2.1 cm | >50% | 8 mm Hg |
| >2.1 cm | <50% | 15 mm Hg |

The IVC of this patient is 1.6 cm and 100% collapsible, making his estimated CVP ~ 3 mm Hg. A low CVP and absence of right ventricular diastolic collapse rule out tamponade, and hence, pericardiocentesis is not required. This is likely a stable, small pericardial effusion with no hemodynamic effects from the effusion. Inotropes are not necessary since left ventricular function is not depressed. A hyperdynamic left ventricle and low CVP likely suggest hypovolemia, and thus a bolus of intravenous fluid (or volume challenge) would be most appropriate, while other causes of hypovolemia is investigated.

### References

1. Sonny A, Wakefield BJ, Sale S, et al. Transvenous lead extraction: A Clinical Commentary for Anesthesiologists. *J Cardiothorac Vasc Anesth.* 2018;32(3):1101-1111.
2. Lang RM, Badano LP, Mor-Avi V, et al. Recommendations for cardiac chamber quantification by echocardiography in adults: an update from the American Society of Echocardiography and the European Association of Cardiovascular Imaging. *J Am Soc Echocardiogr.* 2015;28(1):1-39.

---

**83.** Correct Answer: C

**Rationale:**

This patient developed acute limb ischemia secondary to thrombosis of the left common femoral artery. This was the access site used for the angiography and embolization. Typically, the access site is compressed for about 30 minutes after the conclusion of the procedure to ensure hemostasis. In a patient with a hypercoagulable disorder, this necessary compression may predispose to clot formation, therefore the treating team should be on the look out for this. Serial peripheral vascular examination is the quickest way of diagnosing this condition. This patient has no significant cardiac history; therefore, an embolus to the left common femoral artery is unlikely. A low-flow state would cause generalized hypoperfusion to both extremities. Deep venous thrombosis or the use of sequential compression devices do not typically result in acute limb ischemia.

### References

1. Wongwanit C, Hahtapornsawan S, Chinsakchai K, et al. Catheter-directed thrombolysis for acute limb ischemia caused by native artery occlusion: an experience of a university hospital. *J Med Assoc Thai.* 2013;96(6):661-668.
2. Acar RD, Sahin M, Kirma C. One of the most urgent vascular circumstances: Acute limb ischemia. *SAGE Open Med.* 2013;1:2050312113516110.

---

**84.** Correct Answer: C

**Rationale:**

The 2016 Surviving Sepsis Guidelines incorporate latest evidence-based recommendation in diagnosis and treatment of sepsis. Early goal-directed therapy based on CVP or central venous oxygen saturation is no longer recommended (option A). After initial resuscitation (30 mL/kg crystalloids over 3 hours), further volume resuscitation should be guided by dynamic indices of volume responsiveness. Intravenous antimicrobial therapy should be initiated as soon as possible, within 1 hours of recognition of sepsis (option C). Each hour delay in administration of effective antimicrobial therapy is associated with a measurable increase in mortality in various studies. Routine microbiologic cultures should be obtained before initiation of antimicrobial therapy from all sites considered to be potential sources of infection. "Pan culture" of all sites that could potentially be cultured should be discouraged, because this practice can lead to inappropriate antimicrobial use (option B). Infectious foci suspected to cause septic shock should be controlled as soon as possible following successful initial resuscitation. Without adequate source control, some more severe presentations will not improve despite rapid resuscitation and appropriate antimicrobials. Hence, prolonged efforts at medical stabilization prior to source control for severely ill patients, particularly those with septic shock, are generally not warranted (option D).

### Reference

1. Rhodes A, Evans LE, Alhazzani W, et al. Surviving sepsis campaign: International guidelines for management of sepsis and septic shock: 2016. *Crit Care Med.* 2017;45(3):486-552.

**85.** Correct Answer: A

**Rationale:**

Intra-aortic balloon pump (IABP) counterpulsation is used for mechanical hemodynamic support. It is inserted into the proximal descending aorta, where it inflates during diastole and deflates during systole. Inflation during diastole augments systemic diastolic pressure, thereby improving coronary perfusion. On the other hand, deflation during systole, decreases left ventricular afterload. This in turn increases cardiac output; and reduces left ventricular wall stress and myocardial oxygen demand.

Ventricular septal defect typically causes left-to-right shunting, increases pulmonary blood flow, and causes pulmonary edema. Insertion of IABP will reduce left ventricular afterload, decreases left-to-right shunting, and hence reduces pulmonary edema in this scenario. Papillary muscle rupture leads to severe mitral regurgitation and also causes pulmonary edema. However, afterload reduction achieved by IABP will decrease the regurgitant volume and thereby decrease pulmonary edema. IABP would increase coronary perfusion in a patient with a left main coronary lesion. This would result in improved myocardial oxygen delivery, improved left ventricular ejection fraction, and thereby reduced pulmonary edema.

But, patients with hypertrophic obstructive cardiomyopathy are at risk for systolic anterior motion of the mitral valve and worsening of mitral regurgitation with afterload reduction. Hence, IABP insertion would lead to worsening of pulmonary edema in patients with left ventricular outflow tract obstruction from hypertrophic obstructive cardiomyopathy. From among the list of options presented, only hypertrophic obstructive cardiomyopathy (option A) will result in worsening of pulmonary edema with IABP.

References

1. Santa-Cruz RA, Cohen MG, Ohman EM. Aortic counterpulsation: a review of the hemodynamic effects and indications for use. *Catheter Cardiovasc Interv.* 2006;67(1):68.
2. Takamura T, Dohi K, Satomi A, et al. Intra-aortic balloon pump induced dynamic left ventricular outflow tract obstruction and cardiogenic shock after very late stent thrombosis in the left anterior descending coronary artery. *J Cardiol Cases.* 2012;6(5):e1 37-e140.

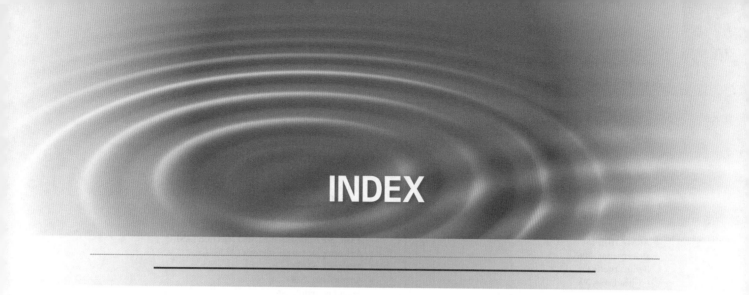

# INDEX

Note: Page numbers followed by "t" indicates tables.